Oxidative Stress, Disease and Cancer

Oxidative Stress, Disease and Cancer

Edited by Keshav K. Singh

Roswell Park Cancer Institute,
New York, USA

ICP

Imperial College Press

Published by

Imperial College Press
57 Shelton Street
Covent Garden
London WC2H 9HE

Distributed by

World Scientific Publishing Co. Pte. Ltd.
5 Toh Tuck Link, Singapore 596224
USA office: 27 Warren Street, Suite 401-402, Hackensack, NJ 07601
UK office: 57 Shelton Street, Covent Garden, London WC2H 9HE

Library of Congress Cataloging-in-Publication Data
Oxidative stress, disease, and cancer / editor, Keshav Singh.
p. ; cm.
Includes bibliographical references and index.
ISBN 1-86094-609-7 (alk. paper)
1. Oxidative stress--Pathophysiology. 2. Diseases--Etiology. 3. Cancer--Etiology.
I. Singh, Keshav K.
[DNLM: 1. Oxidative Stress--physiology. 2. Disease--etiology. 3. Neoplasms--etiology.
QZ 180 O977 2005]
RB170.O962 2005
616.3'907--dc22

2005054505

British Library Cataloguing-in-Publication Data
A catalogue record for this book is available from the British Library.

Typeset by Stallion Press
Email: enquiries@stallionpress.com

Printed in Singapore by Mainland Press

The book is dedicated to the memory of
my brother and sister:

Krishna K. Singh (1948–2004)
Uma Singh (1955–2002)

Contents

Contributors

Ashok Agarwal
The Cleveland Clinic Foundation
Glickman Urological Institute
9500 Euclid Avenue
Cleveland, OH 44195, USA

Christine Ambrosone
Department of Epidemiology
Roswell Park Cancer Institute
Elm & Carlton Streets
Buffalo, NY 14263, USA

J Anastassopoulou
National Technical University of Athens
Chemical Engineering Department, Radiation Chemistry and Biospectroscopy
9 Iroon Polytechnioy,
Zografou 15780, Greece

Svetlana Arbuzova
Interregional Medico-Genetic Center
Central Hospital, Clinic Number 1
57 Artem Street, 83000 Donetsk, Ukraine

Roberta Assaloni
Department of Pathology and Medicine
University of Udine
P. le S. Maria della Misericordia
33100 Udine, Italy

Chris Benz
The Buck Institute for Age Research
8001 Redwood Blvd.
Novato, CA 94945, USA

Hari K Bhat
Department of Environmental Health Sciences
Columbia University
Mailman School of Public Health
60 Haven Avenue, B1
New York, NY 10032, USA

Jeffrey Blumberg
Friedman School of Nutrition Science and Policy
Jean Mayer USDA Human Nutrition Research Center on Aging
Tufts University
Boston, MA 02111, USA

Jennifer S. Carew
Department of Molecular Pathology
The University of Texas, MD Anderson Cancer Center
Houston, TX 77030, USA

Antonio Ceriello
Chair, Internal Medicine
Department of Pathology and Medicine
University of Udine
P. le S. Maria della Misericordia
33100 Udine, Italy

Chung-Yen Chen
Friedman School of Nutrition Science and Policy
Jean Mayer USDA Human Nutrition Research Center on Aging
Tufts University
Boston, MA 02111, USA

Yin-Chiu Chen
Department of Biochemistry
National Yang-Ming University
School of Life Science
Taipei 112, Taiwan

Marcus S. Cooke
Department of Cancer Studies and Molecular Medicine
University of Leicester
P.O. Box 65, RKCSB, Leicester Royal Infirmary
University Hospitals of Leicester NHS Trust
Leicester, LE2 7LX, UK

Howard Cuckle
Reproductive Epidemiology, Leeds Screening Center
University of Leeds
Gemini Park, Sheepscar Way
Leeds, LS7 3JB, UK

Roberto Da Ros
Department of Pathology and Medicine
University of Udine
P. le S. Maria della Misericordia
33100 Udine, Italy

Ian W. Dawes
Ramaciotti Centre for Gene Function Analysis
School of Biotechnology and Biomolecular Sciences
University of New South Wales
Sydney 2052, Australia

T. Paul A. Devasagayam
Radiation Biology and Health Sciences Division
Bhabha Atomic Research Centre
Mumbai, 400-085, India

Marco d'Ischia
Department Organic Chemistry and Biochemistry
University of Naples Federico II
Via Cinthia 4, I-80126 Naples, Italy

Wulf Droge
Division of Immunochemistry
The German Cancer Research Center
DKFZ, Im Neuenheimer Feld 280
69120 Heidelberg, Germany

Emily M. Dunner
Eskitis Centre for Cell and Molecular Therapeutics and School of Biomolecular and Biomedical Sciences
Griffith University
Nathan 4111, Queensland, Australia

Thomas Dziubla
Department of Pharmacology
University of Pennsylvania
School of Medicine
Philadelphia, PA 19104, USA

Anne Eckert
Neurobiology Research Laboratory
Psychiatric University
Clinic Basel
Wilhelm Klein-Strasse 27
CH-4025 Basel, Switzerland

Lena Ekstrom
Department of Laboratory
Medicine
Division of Clinical Pharmacology
Karolinska Institutet
Huddinge University Hospital
SE-14186, Stockholm, Sweden

Mark Evans
Department of Cancer Studies and
Molecular Medicine
University of Leicester
P.O. Box 65, RKCSB, Leicester
Royal Infirmary
University Hospitals of Leicester
NHS Trust
Leicester, LE2 7LX, UK

Kurt Fagerstedt
Helsinki University
Department of Biological and
Environmental Sciences
Division of Plant Biology, Viikki
Biocenter, P.O. Box 56
FIN-00014 Helsinki, Finland

Prabhat C. Goswami
Department of Radiation Oncology
University of Iowa
B180 Medical Laboratories
Iowa City, IA 52242, USA

Peng Huang
Department of Molecular Pathology
The University of Texas,
MD Anderson Cancer Center
Houston, TX 77030, USA

Michael F. Hughes
US Environmental Protection Agency
Office of Research and Development,
MD-74
National Health and Environmental
Research Laboratory
Research Triangle Park, NC 27711,
USA

Hiroko P. Indo
Department of Oncology
Kagoshima University Graduate School
of Medical and Dental Sciences
Sakuragaoka, Kagoshima 890-8544,
Japan

Sofian Johar
Cardiovascular Division
King's and St. Thomas' School of
Medicine
King's College London
New Medical School Bldg., 1st Floor
Bessemer Road, SE5 9PJ, UK

Santosh K. Katiyar
Departments of Dermatology,
Environmental
Health Sciences, Center for Aging
Clinical Nutrition Research Center and
Comprehensive Cancer Center
University of Alabama at Birmingham
1670 University Blvd.
Birmingham, AL 35294, USA

Hirotoshi Kato
National Institute of Radiological
Sciences
Chiba 260-8555, Japan

Seiji Kawano
Department of Clinical Pathology and Immunology
Faculty of Medical Sciences
Graduate School of Medicine
Kobe University
7-5-1, Kusunokicho, Chuo-ku
Kobe 650-0017 Hyogo, Japan

Uta Keil
Department of Pharmacology, Biocenter
University of Frankfurt
Marie-Curie-Str. 9, D-60439
Frankfurt am Main, Germany

KT Kitchin
US Environmental Protection Agency
Office of Research and Development, MD-74
National Health and Environmental Research Laboratory
Research Triangle Park, NC 27711, USA

Michael Koval
Emory University School of Medicine
Division of Pulmonary, Allergy and Critical Care Medicine
Whitehead Biomedical Research Building
615 Michael Street, Suite 205M
Atlanta, GA 30322, USA

Shunichi Kumagai
Department of Clinical Pathology and Immunology
Faculty of Medical Sciences
Graduate School of Medicine
Kobe University
7-5-1, Kusunokicho, Chuo-ku
Kobe 650-0017 Hyogo, Japan

Cheng-Feng Lee
Department of Biochemistry
National Yang-Ming University School of Life Science
Taipei 112, Taiwan

Jee-Yoong Leong
Cardiac Surgical Research Unit
Alfred Hospital & Baker Institute
PO Box 315, Prahran
3181 Victoria, Australia

Yiwei Li
Department of Pathology
Karmanos Cancer Institute
Wayne State University School of Medicine
715 Hudson Webber Cancer Research Center
110 East Warren Drive
Detroit, MI 48201, USA

Jie Liao
Ernest Mario School of Pharmacy
Department of Chemical Biology
Rutgers, The State University of New Jersey
Piscataway, NJ 08854-8020, USA

Chun-Yi Liu
Department of Biochemistry
National Yang-Ming University School of Life Science
Taipei 112, Taiwan

Ching-You Lu
Department of Biochemistry
National Yang-Ming University School of Life Science
Taipei 112, Taiwan

Louise Lyrenas
Division of Biochemical Toxicology
Institute of Environmental Medicine
Karolinska Institutet
Box 210, SE-17177 Stockholm, Sweden

Yi-Shing Ma
Department of Biochemistry
National Yang-Ming University
School of Life Science
Taipei 112, Taiwan

Philip MacCarthy
Cardiovascular Division
King's and St. Thomas' School of Medicine
King's College London
New Medical School Bldg., 1st Floor
Bessemer Road, SE5 9PJ, UK

C. Madeddu
Universita de Cagliari Policlinico Universitario
Cattedra e Divisione di Oncologia Medica
Presidio di Monserrato, SS 554. bivio Sestu
09042 Monserrato (Cagliari), Italy

Hideyuki J. Majima
Department of Oncology
Kagoshima University Graduate School of Medical and Dental Sciences
Sakuragaoka, Kagoshima 890-8544, Japan

P. Manini
Department Organic Chemistry and Biochemistry
University of Naples Federico II
Via Cinthia 4, I-80126 Naples, Italy

Giovanna Mantovani
Universita de Cagliari Policlinico Universitario
Cattedra e Divisione di Oncologia Medica
Presidio di Monserrato, SS 554. bivio Sestu
09042 Monserrato (Cagliari), Italy

Silvana Marasco
Cardiac Surgical Research Unit
Alfred Hospital & Baker Institute
PO Box 315, Prahran
3181 Victoria, Australia

Rosario Maselli
Department of Experimental and Clinical Medicine
Section of Respiratory Diseases
University "Magna Graecia" of Catanzaro
Via Tommaso Campanella 115
88100 Catanzaro, Italy

Simon Melov
The Buck Institute for Age Research
8001 Redwood Blvd.
Novato, CA 94945, USA

Ralf Morgenstern
Institute of Environmental Medicine
Karolinska Institute
Division of Biochemical Toxicology
Box 210, SE-17177 Stockholm, Sweden

Shigeatsu Motoori
First Department of Medicine
Chiba University School of Medicine
Chiba 260-0856, Japan

Florian L. Muller
Department of Cellular and Structural Biology
University of Texas Health Science Center
San Antonio, TX 78229-3900, USA

Silvia Muro
Department of Pharmacology
University of Pennsylvania School of Medicine
Philadelphia, PA 19104, USA

Vladimir R. Muzykantov
Department of Pharmacology
University of Pennsylvania School of Medicine
Philadelphia, PA 19104, USA

Yoshimichi Nakatsu
Department of Medical Biophysics and Radiation Biology
Faculty of Medical Sciences
Kyushu University
Fukuoka 812-8582, Japan

A. Napolitano
Department Organic Chemistry and Biochemistry
University of Naples Federico II
Via Cinthia 4, I-80126 Naples, Italy

Toshihiko Ozawa
National Institute of Radiological Sciences
Chiba 260-8555, Japan

Giovanni Pagano
Italian National Cancer Institute
G. Pascale Foundation
I-80131 Naples, Italy

Girolamo Pelaia
Department of Experimental and Clinical Medicine
Section of Respiratory Diseases
University "Magna Graecia" of Catanzaro
Via Tommaso Campanella 115
88100 Catanzaro, Italy

Salvatore Pepe
Cardiac Surgical Research Unit
Alfred Hospital & Baker Institute
PO Box 315, Prahran
3181 Victoria, Australia

Kevin Pong
Neuroscience Discovery Research,
Wyeth Research, CN-8000,
Princeton, NJ 08543, USA

Lene Juel Rasmussen
Department of Life Sciences and Chemistry
Roskilde University
DK-4000 Roskilde, Denmark

Franklin L Rosenfeldt
Cardiac Surgical Research Unit
Alfred Hospital & Baker Institute
PO Box 315, Prahran
3181 Victoria, Australia

Jun Saegusa
Department of Dermatology
University of California, Davis
Research III/UCDMC
One Shields Avenue, Davis, CA 95616, USA

Enrique Samper
The Buck Institute for Age Research
8001 Redwood Blvd.
Novato, CA 94945, USA

Fazlul H. Sarker
Department of Pathology
Karmanos Cancer Institute
Wayne State University School of Medicine
715 Hudson Webber Cancer Research Center
110 East Warren Drive
Detroit, MI 48201, USA

Katrin Schüssel
Department of Pharmacology, Biocenter
University of Frankfurt
Marie-Curie-Str. 9, D-60439
Frankfurt am Main
Germany

Mutsuo Sekiguchi
Department of Biology and Frontier Research Center
Fukuoka Dental College
Fukuoka 814-0193, Japan

Darren N. Seril
Ernest Mario School of Pharmacy
Department of Chemical Biology
Rutgers, The State University of New Jersey
Piscataway, NJ 08854-8020, USA

Ajay M. Shah
Cardiovascular Division
King's and St. Thomas' School of Medicine
King's College London
New Medical School Bldg., 1st Floor
Bessemer Road, SE5 9PJ, UK

Keshav K. Singh
Department of Cancer Genetics
Roswell Park Cancer Institute
Elm & Carlton Streets
Buffalo, NY 14263, USA

Anatoly Starkoc
Neurology and Neuroscience
Weill Medical College
Cornell University
A501, 445 E 69th Street,
New York, NY 10021, USA

Shigeaki Suenaga
Department of Oncology
Kagoshima University Graduate School of Medical and Dental Sciences
Sakuragaoka, Kagoshima 890-8544, Japan

Theo Theophanides
National Technical University of Athens
Radiation Chemistry and Biospectroscopy
9 Iroon Polytechnioy
Zografou 15780, Greece

J. C. Tilak
Radiation Biology and Health Sciences Division
Bhabha Atomic Research Centre
Mumbai, 400-085, India

Kazuo Tomita
Department of Oncology
Kagoshima University Graduate School of Medical and Dental Sciences
Sakuragaoka, Kagoshima 890-8544, Japan

Shinya Toyokuni
Department of Pathology and Biology of Diseases
Graduate School of Medicine
Kyoto University
Yoshida-Konoe-cho, Sakyo-ku
Kyoto 606-8501, Japan

Holly van Remmen
Department of Cellular and Structural Biology
University of Texas Health Science Center
San Antonio, TX 78229-3900, USA

Kendall B. Wallace
Department of Biochemistry and Molecular Biology
University of Minnesota School of Medicine
1035 University Drive, Duluth, MN 55812, USA

Dianne J. Watters
Eskitis Centre for Cell and Molecular Therapeutics and
School of Biomolecular and Biomedical Sciences
Griffith University
Nathan 4111, Queensland, Australia

Chia-Yu Wei
Department of Biochemistry
National Yang-Ming University
School of Life Science
Taipei 112, Taiwan

Yau-Huei Wei
Department of Biochemistry
National Yang-Ming University
School of Life Science
Taipei 112, Taiwan

Shi-Bei Wu
Department of Biochemistry
National Yang-Ming University School of Life Science
Taipei 112, Taiwan

Chung S. Yang
Ernest Mario School of Pharmacy
Department of Chemical Biology
Rutgers, The State University of New Jersey
Piscataway, NJ 08854-8020, USA

Guan-Yu Yang
Ernest Mario School of Pharmacy
Department of Chemical Biology
Rutgers, The State University of New Jersey
Piscataway, NJ 08854-8020, USA

Hsiu-Chuan Yen
School of Medical Technology
Chang Gung University
Kwei-Shan, TaoYuan 333, Taiwan

Yan Zhou
Department of Molecular Pathology
The University of Texas, MD Anderson Cancer Center
Houston, TX 77030, USA

Elena Zotova
Division of Biochemical Toxicology
Institute of Environmental Medicine
Karolinska Institutet
Box 210, SE-17177 Stockholm, Sweden

Preface

The ability of cells to reduce oxygen to produce energy is fundamental to aerobic life. Unfortunately, production of energy by reduction of dioxygen leads to the generation of reactive oxygen species that cause oxidative stress. It is now well established that oxidative stress causes extensive damage to cellular components, which can lead to a number of diseases, including cancer. The purpose of the book is to provide a comprehensive review of the most up-to-date knowledge of the sources and molecular mechanisms of oxidative stress and its role in disease and cancer. The book also focuses on the novel agents and methods that can be employed to prevent oxidative stress and associated diseases.

Over 35 of the leading experts in the oxidative stress field have contributed to this book. Their expertise ranges from basic to translational to therapeutic aspects of oxidative stress-associated diseases. I am greatly indebted to the contributing authors for their enthusiasm cooperation and the responsibility they took in writing chapters in their area of expertise and bringing this book to fruition. I thank my colleagues John Cowell, Barbara Henderson, Thomas Shows, John Subjeck, Christine Ambrosone, Ivan Still, and Andrei Bakin for stimulating discussion on oxidative stress. I am also grateful to Donna Ovak for secretarial help and to members of my laboratory. Finally, I thank my wife, Kylie, and children, Vijay and Anita, for their patience and support while putting together this monograph.

This book is organized into three broad sections. In the first section, the authors review the most recent data on the basic mechanism of oxidative stress. In the second section, oxidative stress leading to several diseases and cancer are discussed. In the third section of the book, current strategies employed in the prevention and treatment of oxidative stress-related diseases are discussed.

Keshav K. Singh
Spring 2006

1 Yin and Yang of Mitochondrial ROS

Anatoly Starkov and Kendall B. Wallace

1. Introduction

For many, it is a firm paradigm that mitochondria are the major source of reactive oxygen species (ROS) in mammalian cells; dissenters consider these complicated organelles the major target of oxidative stress, whereas conformists argue that mitochondria are both the source and target of intracellular ROS, subject to conditions. All these views are possibly correct because the reality is that there is not enough data yet to support any scientifically based conclusion on the role of mitochondria in the intracellular ROS metabolism. Being able to produce ROS at least *in vitro*, mammalian mitochondria also possess powerful, multi-leveled high-capacity ROS defense systems that are not well studied. It is not yet understood what function — ROS production or ROS scavenging — prevails in mitochondria *in vivo*. This review attempts to introduce major elements of both ROS producing and detoxifying systems mitochondria encompassing the state of the art *circa* 2004. Summarized are the major findings regarding the mitochondrial sites of ROS production, the regulation of ROS production, and the ROS defense systems relevant primarily to the mammalian mitochondria.

2. Multiplicity of ROS-Producing Sources in Mitochondria

Although about 50% of all the land in Holland lies below sea level, the assiduous and diligent Hollanders created numerous dikes and channels and other things to hold the sea back so that the land can be put to good use. A familiar fable tells the story that long ago, in a city named Haarlem, there lived a boy named Peter who was just eight years old, but he was very smart and swift-minded. One rainy day as he walked home after a visit to the countryside all by himself, he suddenly heard a sound of water springing from a small hole in the dike. Peter examined that situation and quickly calculated that the pressure of the water would make the hole huge pretty soon causing the dike to burst in a wall of water bringing flood and disaster to the town below! He immediately saw a solution; Peter got onto the dike and stuck his finger in the hole. It was cold and dark and he started feeling quite miserable. He knew no help would come to his rescue soon but decided rather to die holding the water back than betray his beautiful country. There he was, an eight-year-old boy lying on his tummy on a cold damp dike holding the flood with his finger all through the night. When dawn broke, a cleric walked by and saw Peter, and inquired about what was going on. Peter's answer was simple: "I am holding the water back," he said, "Please get help!" And help he got, the compassionate cleric climbed up to his side and put his palm over the boy's small hand to prevent his tired finger from falling out of the hole in the dike. Haarlem was saved and the boy has been revered as Holland's national hero ever since.

Hydraulic analogy with a dike and a hole illustrates the essence of mitochondrial ROS production. A source of ROS is like a hole in the dike; it brings more damage the longer it is left unpatched, and eventually destroys the "city of Mitochondrion." The major difference however is the number of fingers required to prevent a disaster.

Thermodynamically, numerous mitochondrial enzymes and enzyme complexes are capable of one-electron reduction of oxygen.[1] ROS production by at least nine of the mammalian mitochondrial enzymes has so far been reported by various laboratories; it is highly likely that additional ROS sources will be discovered as many more researchers started exploring the field in the last four years than during the last four decades. Although all nine ROS-producing enzymes are more or less ubiquitously present in mammalian mitochondria, their capacity in producing ROS varies greatly and there is always a tissue specificity factor as everything is expressed to different levels in different tissues. Owing to the metabolic heterogeneity of tissues and our limited knowledge of life's mechanics, it is not surprising that singling out a ROS-producing source as the major one *in vivo* might be difficult if not impossible, scientifically speaking.

The nine known sources of ROS in mitochondria (marked by stars) are shown on Fig. 1 in the context of location within a mitochondrion. ROS production by Complex I (C-I) and Complex III (bc1) will be discussed in separate sections, as well as numerous ROS-detoxifying systems presented on Fig. 1. This section introduces the remaining seven ROS-producing enzymes.

(1) *Mitochondrial cytochrome b5 reductase* is located in the outer mitochondrial membrane. The enzyme is widely distributed in mammalian tissues.[2] It oxidizes cytoplasmic NAD(P)H and reduces cytochrome b5, another protein of the outer membrane. Cytochrome b5 reductase may be involved in regeneration of ascorbate because it catalyzes the reduction of ascorbyl free radical back to ascorbate in mammalian liver[2] and in yeast mitochondria.[3] It may play some important role in human brain cells; it is elevated in schizophrenics thus implying having a role in aetiology of the disease.[4,5] There is a single report that mitochondrial cytochrome b5 reductase using NADH as an electron donor may produce superoxide with a very high rate ~300 nmol superoxide per min per mg protein.[5] Few other details or other studies on this subject are currently available.

(2) *Monoamine oxidases (MAO-A and MAO-B, EC 1.4.3.4)* are also located in the outer mitochondrial membrane and ubiquitously expressed in various mammalian tissues. These enzymes catalyze the oxidation of biogenic amines accompanied by the release of H_2O_2. MAOs of brain mitochondria play a central role in the turnover of monoamine neurotransmitters; numerous detailed and extensive reviews covering almost every aspect of these enzymes can be found elsewhere. The amount of H_2O_2 that MAOs can generate may substantially exceed the amount produced by any other mitochondrial source of ROS. Tyramine oxidation by rat brain mitochondria produced H_2O_2 with a rate $\sim$50 times higher than that exerted by Complex III inhibited with antimycin A.[6] The latter ROS-producing system has long been considered as one of the most "productive" sources of ROS in mitochondria (discussed later). Mitochondrial MAO enzymes may also be a major source of H_2O_2 in tissues in ischemia,[7,8] aging,[9] and upon oxidation of exogenous biogenic amines.[10] An increase in MAO activity and

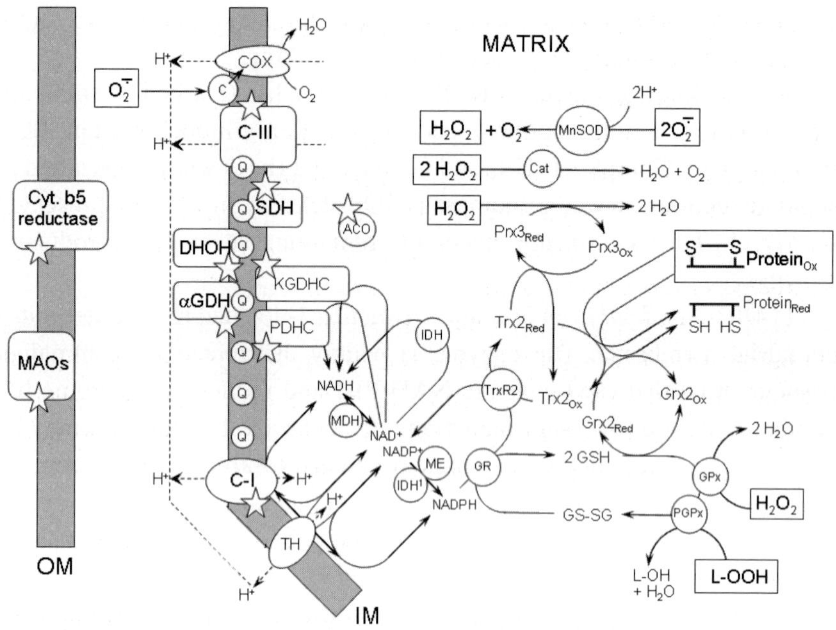

Fig. 1. *Known sources of ROS and ROS-detoxifying systems in mitochondria.* Selected ROS-producing enzymes and ROS-detoxifying systems are shown in a context of their location within mitochondria. See text for further detail. *Abbreviations:* COX, cytochrome c oxidase; C, cytochrome c, C-III, Complex III; MnSOD, mitochondrial manganese superoxide dismutase; Cat, catalase; SDH, succinate dehydrogenase; ACO, aconitase; $Prx3_{red}$, peroxiredoxin reduced; $Prx3_{ox}$, peroxiredoxin oxidized; Q, coenzyme Q; DHOH, dihydroorotate dehydrogenase; KGDHC, a-ketoglutarate dehydrogenase complex; αGDH, α-glycerophosphate dehydrogenase; PDHC, pyruvate dehydrogenase complex; IDH, isocitric dehydrogenase, NAD^+-dependent; $Trx2_{red}$, thioredoxin-2 reduced; $Trx2_{ox}$, thioredoxin-2 oxidized; $Grx2_{red}$, glutaredoxin-2 reduced; $Grx2_{ox}$, glutaredoxin-2 oxidized; TrxR2, thioredoxin-2 reductase; MDH, malate dehydrogenase; IDH^1, isocitric dehydrogenase, $NADP^+$-dependent; ME, malic enzyme $NADP^+$-dependent; GR, glutathione reductase; GSH, reduced glutathione; GS-SG, oxidized glutathione dipeptide; GPx, glutathione peroxidase; PGPx, phospholipid hydroperoxide glutathione peroxidase; C-I, Complex I; TH, transhydrogenase; Cyt. B5 reductase, cytochrome b5 reductase; MAOs, mono amine oxidases A and B; ME, malic enzyme; OM, outer mitochondrial membrane; IM, inner mitochondrial membrane. Other symbols: ROS species that are detoxified by the corresponding systems are shown enclosed in a square frame; stars indicate sources of ROS.

MAO-catalyzed H_2O_2 production may be responsible for the mitochondrial damage in Parkinson's disease.[11]

(3) *Dihydroorotate dehydrogenase (DHOH, EC1.3.3.1 or EC1.3.99.11)* is located at the outer surface of inner mitochondrial membrane. It catalyzes the conversion of dihydroorotate to the pyrimidine base, orotate, which is a step in the *de novo* synthesis of uridine monophosphate. The latter is involved in the formation of DNA and RNA. The DHOH is ubiquitously distributed in mammalian tissues.[12] In the absence of its natural electron acceptor, coenzyme Q of inner mitochondrial membrane, reduced DHOH can produce H_2O_2 *in vitro*.[12] The DHOH has frequently been considered as a mitochondrial source of superoxide.[13,14] However, in a more recent study the same authors concluded that superoxide production during dihydroorotate oxidation was from Complex III rather than from DHOH[15] and explained this and other discrepancies by the lower quality of mitochondrial preparation in the earlier study. Therefore, the capacity of DHOH to produce superoxide requires further clarification.

(4) *Mitochondrial dehydrogenase of α-glycerophosphate* (Glycerol-3-Phosphate Dehydrogenase, mGPDH, EC 1.1.99.5) is also located at the outer surface of inner mitochondrial membrane. It is a FAD-linked enzyme catalyzing the oxidation of glycerol-3-phosphate to dihydroxyacetone phosphate and utilizing mitochondrial coenzyme Q as electron acceptor. The mGPDH is involved in lipid metabolism and in the so-called glycerol phosphate shuttle capable of regenerating cytosolic NAD^+ from the NADH formed in glycolysis. Homozygous mice with disrupted mGPDH survive but have decreased viability and lower body weight than their wild type littermates.[16] The enzyme expression is upregulated in hyperthyroid animals.[17,18] It is ubiquitously but unevenly expressed in various mouse tissues with brown fat, muscle, and brain possessing the highest activity of mGPDH.[19] The activity of mGPDH is also high in flying muscles in insects.[20] Mitochondria from mouse tissues[21] and from *Drosophila* fly[22] produce H_2O_2 upon oxidation of sn-glycerol-3-phosphate, a substrate of mGPDH. The mechanism of mGPDH-mediated ROS production was studied in *Drosophila* mitochondria, it appeared that most of H_2O_2 was produced by the enzyme *per se* whereas about 30% was produced at Complex I site because of reverse electron transfer from mGPDH to that site[22] as discussed later in this chapter.

(5) *Succinate dehydrogenase complex* (SDH, succinate:ubiquinone oxidoreductase, Complex II, EC1.3.5.1) is a flavoprotein located at the inner surface of inner mitochondrial membrane. The enzyme oxidizes succinate to fumarate using coenzyme Q as an electron acceptor. Although oxidation of succinate by good-quality mitochondria from most mammalian tissues can produce ROS with a high rate, the source of ROS is Complex I, not SDH. The mechanism involves reverse electron transfer from SDH-reduced coenzyme Q to Compelx I. Nevertheless, isolated SHD reconstructed in liposomes can produce ROS by itself.[23] Authors concluded that reduced FAD of SDH generates ROS in the absence of its electron acceptor.[23] There is also a report implying that SDH can generate ROS in submitochondrial particles.[24] However the conclusion was based solely on the inhibition of ROS production by carboxin, a specific inhibitor of SDH. The same inhibitor also suppressed antimycin-induced ROS production and ROS production supported by NADH oxidation. The former is thought to originate from Complex III (discussed later) that is not inhibited by carboxin whereas the effect of carboxin on NADH-supported ROS production may not be readily explained either. Therefore, it is unclear whether SDH produces ROS *in situ*, in mitochondria.

(6) *Mitochondrial aconitase* (m-aconitase, EC4.2.1.3) is an enzyme localized to the matrix space of mitochondria; it participates in tricarboxylic acid cycle catalyzing a conversion of citrate to isocitrate. The enzyme contains an iron-sulfur cluster that can be oxidized by superoxide, inactivating m-aconitase.[25] Recently, it was found that isolated aconitase oxidized by either superoxide or hydrogen peroxide produces hydroxyl radical.[26] The authors proposed that similar continuous hydroxyl radical production may occur upon superoxide-driven redox-cycling of aconitase in mitochondria.[26]

(7) *Ketoglutarate dehydrogenase complex* (KGDHC, 2-oxoglutarate dehydrogenase) is an integral mitochondrial enzyme tightly bound to the inner mitochondrial membrane on the matrix side.[27] In the tricarboxylic acid cycle, it catalyzes the oxidation of α-ketoglutarate to succinyl-CoA using NAD^+ as electron acceptor. Structurally, KGDHC is composed of multiple copies of three enzymes: α-ketoglutarate dehydrogenase (E1k subunit, EC 1.2.4.2), dihydrolipoamide succinyltransferase (E2k subunit, EC 2.3.1.12), and lipoamide dehydrogenase (E3 subunit, EC 1.6.4.3). The E3

component of KGDHC is a flavin-containing enzyme; it is identical to the E3 component of another integral mitochondrial enzyme located in the matrix, *pyruvate dehydrogenase* (PDHC). The E3 component is also known as *dihydrolipoamide dehydrogenase* (Dld) which is ubiquitously present in mammalian mitochondria. Two recent studies demonstrated that both PDHC and KGDHC can generate superoxide and hydrogen peroxide; ROS production was shown with isolated purified enzymes from bovine heart[28,29] and in isolated brain mitochondria.[28] The source of ROS in KGDHC and PDHC appears to be the *dihydrolipoamide dehydrogenase* component.[28] Earlier, isolated *dihydrolipoamide dehydrogenase* was shown to produce ROS.[30] In mitochondria and with isolated enzyme, ROS production from KGDHC and PDHC was stimulated by a decrease in availability of its natural electron acceptor, NAD^+.[28,29]

To summarize, we would like to emphasize that although these seven sources were shown to produce ROS, in experiments with isolated enzymes or in mammalian mitochondria, their contribution to ROS production has not yet been estimated in mitochondria under physiological conditions. That does not mean of course that it can not be done; genetic engineering and biophysical approaches are ripe and quite suitable for such studies.

3. ROS Production at Complex I of Mitochondrial Respiratory Chain

Mitochondrial Complex I, "Rotenone-Sensitive Mitochondrial NADH-Ubiquinone Oxidoreductase", provides a major entry point into respiratory chain for electrons derived from the oxidation of various substrates in the mitochondrial tricarboxylic acid cycle. It is a very important enzyme catalyzing the oxidation of NADH in the mitochondrial matrix by coenzyme Q dissolved in the inner mitochondrial membrane. It utilizes the energy of NADH oxidation to generate protonmotive force that is used to synthesize ATP or other work that mitochondria perform. Many scientists insist that in addition to that, Complex I routinely generates significant amounts of ROS.

Several research groups have demonstrated that Complex I preparations can generate ROS[1,31,32] when reduced with NADH, although there is no consensus about the specific site of ROS production in Complex I.[32–34] The published studies differ widely in approaches, sources of mitochondria and techniques employed for Complex I isolation so the lack of consistency in results is not surprising.

A few studies attempted localizing the ROS producing site or sites within Complex I by using inhibitors of electron transfer. One of the earliest studies[35] demonstrated that isolated Complex I supplemented with NADH can generate superoxide. ROS generation apparently required a reduced ubiquinone molecule because it was inhibited by rotenone which blocks electron transfer from electron-carrying components of Complex I to ubiquinone.[35] The same authors also demonstrated an enhancement of ROS production in Complex I by added quinones,[35] which was later confirmed by others.[36] An inhibition of ROS production in NADH-reduced Complex I by rotenone is a unique observation; in other studies cited in this chapter rotenone either enhanced ROS production by NADH-reduced Complex I or had no effect.

Studies with both isolated Complex I and submitochondrial particles demonstrated that ROS producing site is located between a rotenone-sensitive site and a flavin[37–40] and that there may be not one but two superoxide producing sites in that region.[41] Others suggested that the ROS producing site in Complex I is exactly the flavin[34,42] or a complex of bound half-reduced NAD* with the flavin of the enzyme.[43] The sum of presently available data favors the idea that ROS is most likely produced by one of the electron-transferring iron-sulfur centers that are localized in Complex I between the flavin and the rotenone–sensitive site,[39,40] not by a flavin *per se*. That may of course change as our knowledge of electron transfer mechanics in Complex I becomes more detailed.

At the intact mitochondria level, two major experimental paradigms are employed in studies on ROS production attributed to Complex I. The first, both historically and by the frequency of use, is ROS production resulting from so-called reverse electron transfer in the mitochondrial respiratory chain. Discovered in experiments with submitochondrial particles,[37] it was the first reaction of ROS production in mitochondria studied in detail. Reverse electron transfer (RET) is a term describing a set of redox reactions in the mitochondrial respiratory chain that allows electrons to flow from coenzyme Q to NAD^+ instead of oxygen. It is not yet clear whether or not it is a physiologically relevant phenomenon. RET requires a combination of several factors to occur simultaneously. In submitochondrial particles, it requires the presence of succinate to reduce coenzyme Q, the electron flow should be inhibited downstream, either at the level of Complex III or at cytochrome c oxidase and an additional source of energy such as hydrolyzable ATP should be present to "push" the electrons from coenzyme Q against the redox potential difference toward reduction of NAD^+. And of course, submitochondrial particles should be of very good quality having no significant impairments to their respiratory chain components or the lipid membrane. If all these conditions are met, a succinate and ATP-dependent reduction of added NAD^+ can be observed that is associated with a massive production of H_2O_2.[1,37] Both the NAD^+ reduction and the production of H_2O_2 can be prevented by Complex I inhibitors acting at the rotenone-binding site, thereby indicating that the site of ROS production is located somewhere in the Complex I upstream of that site. Neither NAD^+ *per se* nor the electron flow to NAD^+ is required for ROS production; however more ROS is produced in the presence of NAD^+.[43]

In mitochondria, RET does not require ATP and an inhibition of electron flow toward oxygen. It requires only the presence of a $FADH_2$-linked substrate to reduce coenzyme Q directly, and the presence of high membrane potential. These conditions are usually met by incubating mitochondria under resting state conditions (so-called "State 4" respiration) in the presence of succinate or α-glycerophosphate.[22,33,44] In mitochondria, RET supports very high rates of ROS production. Rodent heart and brain mitochondria oxidizing succinate in State 4 conditions can produce H_2O_2 with rates ranging from 0.5 to 3 nmols H_2O_2 per minute per mg of mitochondrial protein.[44–47] That amounts to 5–20% of their total oxygen consumption rate under State 4 conditions. RET-induced ROS production is regulated by the amplitude of mitochondrial electrical membrane potential[44–47] so that a 10% decrease in the membrane potential inhibits ROS production by 90%. It is therefore inhibited by any energy-dissipating process, whether it is ATP synthesis, Ca^{2+} uptake, or a chemical-induced uncoupling. RET-supported ROS production is also apparently suppressed by acidification of the mitochondrial matrix.[48] This may be viewed as additional indirect evidence that it originates from Complex I; it is known that ROS production by Complex I in submitochondrial particles is higher at more alkaline pH.[38,49] And of course, RET-supported ROS production in intact mitochondria is inhibited by rotenone because it blocks the flow of electrons from coenzyme Q to Complex I.

The second experimental paradigm in research on ROS production by Complex I starts where the first ends. It has long been known that rotenone induces ROS production by mitochondria oxidizing NAD-linked substrates such as pyruvate or glutamate plus malate. Rotenone-induced ROS production is not regulated by the membrane potential, but it depends on pH[38,49] and also on the degree of reduction of matrix pyridine nucleotides.[33] Rotenone-induced ROS production rates are generally about 5–10% of those induced by succinate-supported RET. It is not known if the same or different sites are involved in RET and rotenone-induced ROS production.

Regarding the physiological relevance of these two experimental paradigms, both may be equally meaningful. The essence of RET-paradigm is high membrane potential that is needed to overcome a redox potential difference between coenzyme Q and a site in Complex I that produces ROS. This condition could occur *in vivo* when mitochondria are in a "resting" non-phosphorylating state, or their phosphorylation is inhibited by a toxic compound. The essence of rotenone-induced ROS production is an over-reduction of intrinsic Complex I electron carriers and mitochondrial pyridine nucleotides. This may also occur *in vivo* due to a xenobiotic or a pathology preventing electron transfer from either Complex I to coenzyme Q or at any point downstream the respiratory chain. For example, a release of cytochrome c from mitochondria due to apoptotic stimuli would result in an enhanced ROS production from Complex I.[33] Switching of mitochondria into State 4 non-phosphorylating conditions also enhances ROS production by mitochondria oxidizing NAD-linked substrates, but to a 10–20 times lesser degree than in the case of RET. This is because in the absence of Complex I inhibitors, ROS production supported by NAD-linked substrates is also stimulated by high membrane potential. However, the dependence of ROS production rate on the amplitude of membrane potential is not so steep as in the case of RET.[47]

It should be understood that there is no evidence directly supporting the hypothesis that mitochondrial Complex I (or in fact any other mitochondrial ROS producing site) is producing ROS *in vivo*. All the evidence on ROS production by Complex I was obtained *in vitro* with isolated mitochondria and *extrapolated* to various *in vivo* situations.

Complex I of the mitochondrial electron transport chain has been viewed as a major site of mitochondrial ROS production.[32,39,50,51] There are three principal types of experiments that contributed to this concept: (*a*) experiments demonstrating that isolated Complex I preparations or submitochondrial particles generate ROS in the presence of NADH, (*b*) experiments with rotenone–inhibited mitochondria oxidizing NAD-dependent substrates, and (*c*) experiments with isolated mitochondria under conditions favoring RET from succinate to Complex I. The latter reaction generates large amounts of ROS.[1,31] However, the possibility of RET under physiological conditions is not yet established. The interpretation of *b*) and *c*) -type experiments with intact mitochondria suffers from inherent uncertainty because the source of ROS could actually be something that is in a redox equilibrium with intramitochondrial NAD(P)H. This difficulty also applies to experiments demonstrating the dependence of mitochondrial ROS production on the amplitude of the membrane potential[44–47] or intramitochondrial NAD(P)H/NAD(P)$^+$ ratio.[33,47] Logistically, such experiments do not allow one *to quantify* the contribution of Complex I to mitochondrial ROS production. The same argument applies to *a*) -type experiments involving submitochondrial particles by their virtue of being mitochondrial fragments devoid of most of normal mitochondrial content and lacking normal mitochondrial enzyme interactions.

Therefore, whether or not Complex I is a significant source of ROS in intact mitochondria *in vivo* is a complicated issue. There is even evidence that argues against the concept that Complex I in mitochondria, or in submitochondrial particles, can generate ROS at all, even in the presence of its inhibitors. The absence of a correlation between the inhibition of Complex I activity by rotenone and other inhibitors and the production of ROS by submitochondrial particles was interpreted as an indication of the presence of a superoxide–producing rotenone-binding site other than Complex I.[52] The finding that H_2O_2 production is frequently reported as being almost absent in the presence of succinate and rotenone,[34,50] is intriguing because intramitochondrial NAD(P)H/NAD(P)$^+$ ratio under such conditions is high. It is puzzling that Complex I does not generate ROS with at least the same efficiency under these circumstances, as observed with NAD-linked substrates with rotenone.[50] Stimulatory effects of ADP[50] and Ca^{2+} [53–57] on mitochondrial ROS production are also intriguing because both Ca^{2+} uptake/retention, and ADP-induced oxidative phosphorylation dissipate energy and would be expected to decrease the level of reduction of Complex I and hence, the ROS production. Even more intriguing is the fact that the stimulatory effect of the Complex I inhibitor rotenone on ROS production is in fact, species and tissue–dependent, as ROS stimulation by rotenone varies from ~300% in guinea pig to 0% in horse heart submitochondrial particles[39] and in whole intact rat heart mitochondria,[58] to inhibition of ROS production in mouse kidney mitochondria.[21] Therefore, whether or not Complex I is a major site of ROS production continues to be a complicated issue indeed.

4. Q-Cycle and the Mechanism of ROS Production at Complex III

Historically, the first mitochondrial site producing ROS was identified at the Complex III (bc1 complex, ubiquinone:cytochrome c reductase) of the mitochondrial respiratory chain.[59] The primary ROS produced at this site is superoxide,[49,60–63] which quickly dismutates forming H_2O_2.[64]

4.1. *The Q-cycle model of the coenzyme Q oxidation*

The scheme on Fig. 2A illustrates the mechanism of Complex III–catalyzed coenzyme Q (CoQ) oxidation known as the "Q-cycle." The reaction starts from the oxidation of the CoQ quinol (**QH_2**) in a bifurcated electron transfer reaction at the **Q_o-site** of the complex. The first electron is transferred to a high reduction potential chain consisting of the iron sulfur protein (**ISP**, or Rieske protein), cytochrome c1 (**Cyt.c1**) and cytochrome c (**Cyt.c**) and cytochrome c oxidase (not shown). This reaction leaves a semiquinone (**Q_o^{*-}**), which is very unstable. This semiquinone donates the second electron to the low reduction potential chain consisting of two cytochromes b, **cyt b_l** and **cyt b_h**, which serve as a pathway routing the electrons to the **Q_i-site**. There, these electrons reduce another CoQ molecule. To provide two electrons required for the complete reduction of CoQ quinone at the Q_i-site, the Q_o-site oxidizes two QH_2 molecules in two successive turnovers. The first electron at the Q_i-site generates a stable semiquinone (**Q_i^{*-}**) that is reduced to a quinol by the second electron.[65–67]

Recently, the structures of bc1 complexes isolated from bovine, chicken, and rabbit mitochondria were determined by x-ray crystallography,[66,68,69] and the structural changes induced by the major inhibitors of the bc1 complex were also determined. The data support the Q-cycle model. A novel finding of great importance is that the extramembrane domain of the ISP is mobile and undergoes a large scale movement to shuttle the electron from the quinol at the Q_o-site to the cytochrome c1.[66,68,69]

4.2. *The site and source of electrons for the superoxide formation*

An unstable semiquinone formed in the Q_o center is believed to be the one-electron donor responsible for the superoxide formation.[35,62,63,70–72] This semiquinone has; however, never been detected.[1,31,73] The effects of specific Complex III inhibitors played therefore the most important role for identification of both the site and the source of superoxide production.

Figure 2A shows the sites of action of three most frequently used inhibitors of Complex III. Myxothiazol prevents the binding of QH_2 at the Q_o-site, stigmatellin prevents the transfer of first electron to ISP, and antimycin A interrupts the transfer of the second electron to the Q_i-site.

The hypothesis that semiquinone in Q_o center is the donor of electrons for the reduction of oxygen to superoxide is based primarily on the following experimental observations:

(1) The quinone of inner mitochondrial membrane is obligatory required for the antimycin A-induced superoxide production in bc1 complex.[62,70]

(2) The specific inhibitors of the bc1 complex affect the production of superoxide in a remarkable agreement with their effect on the formation of the putative semiquinone at the center Q_o. According to the classical Q-cycle hypothesis, inhibitors acting at the quinone-reducing center (Q_i), e.g. antimycin A, should stimulate superoxide formation by inhibiting semiquinone oxidation, as illustrated by the Fig. 2B. The inhibitor prevents the transfer of the second electron to the Q_i-site, thus "switching off" the low potential chain. This results in the accumulation of unstable semiquinone at Q_o-site and increases the probability of its side reaction with oxygen. However, the inhibitors of the Q_o site, such as myxothiazol or stigmatellin, should inhibit superoxide production by preventing semiquinone formation.[1,31,65,67] Myxothiazol inhibits semiquinone formation at center Q_o by displacing quinol at its binding site, whereas stigmatellin specifically blocks the first electron transfer reaction from quinol to ISP[1,31,65,67] thereby preventing the semiquinone formation.

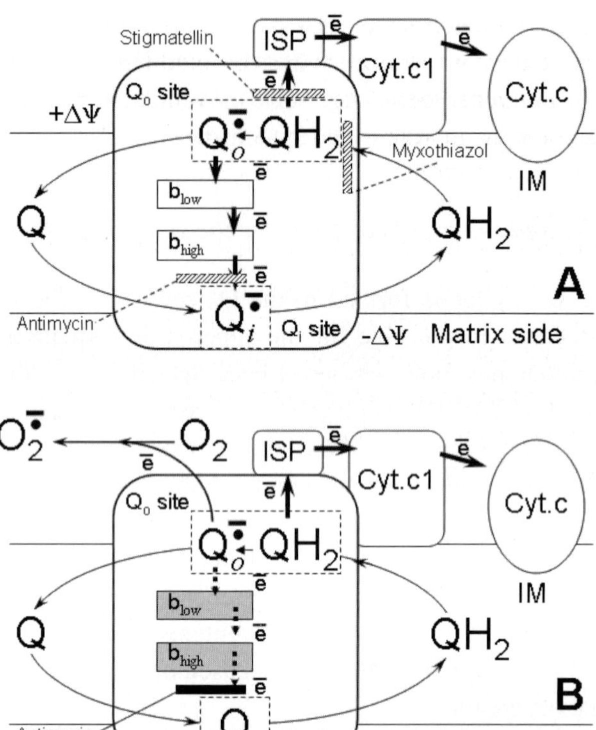

Fig. 2. The Q-cycle model of the coenzyme Q oxidation. The scheme A indicates the sites of action of most frequently used inhibitors of bc1 complex.The scheme B illustrates the mechanism of bc1–catalyzed coenzyme Q (CoQ) oxidation known as the "Q-cycle". The reaction starts from the oxidation of the CoQ quinol (**QH_2**) in a bifurcated electron transfer reaction at the **Q_o-site** of the complex. The first electron is transferred to a high reduction potential chain consisting of the iron sulfur protein (**ISP**, Rieske protein), cytochrome c1 (**Cyt.c1**) and cytochrome c (**Cyt.c**) and further to cytochrome c oxidase (not shown). The remaining semiquinone ($\mathbf{Q_o^{*-}}$) is unstable. It donates the second electron to the low reduction potential chain consisting of two cytochromes b, **cyt b_l** and **cyt b_h**, which serve as a pathway conducting electrons to the **Q_i-site**. There, these electrons reduce another CoQ molecule. To provide two electrons required for the complete reduction of CoQ quinone at the Q_i-site, the Q_o-site oxidizes two QH_2 molecules in two successive turnovers. The first electron at the Q_i-site generates a stable semiquinone ($\mathbf{Q_i^{*-}}$) that is reduced to a quinol by the second electron.[65–67]

Therefore, antimycin A should stimulate the superoxide production as it was demonstrated,[1,31] whereas myxothiazol should both prevent and inhibit the effect of antimycin. Indeed, myxothiazol was reported to inhibit superoxide production in mammalian mitochondria.[44,62,71,72,74,75] Stigmatellin was also shown to both prevent and suppress the antimycin A–induced ROS production.[76,77]

(3) Another observation strongly supporting both the Q-cycle hypothesis and that of superoxide production by the semiquinone in the center Q_o was made by Turrens *et al.* These authors demonstrated that succinate-supported antimycin-induced H_2O_2 production by the mitochondrial particles can be strongly inhibited by removing of cytochrome c from the particles, and restored by replenishing the cytochrome c. This observation can best be explained within the framework of the Q-cycle hypothesis, according to which the removal of the cytochrome c should prevent the oxidation of c1 and ISP and therefore the transfer of the first electron from the QH_2 (Fig. 2A) and thereby the formation of semiquinone at the center Q_o. At the same time, this observation rules out both the ISP and the quinol as sources of ROS because they remain fully reduced in the absence of cytochrome c.[72] Another observation made in the same study was that myxothiazol suppressed ROS production. It effectively excluded cytochromes b as reductants donating electrons for superoxide formation because both cyt. b_l and cyt.b_h remained fully reduced. Authors concluded that "by exclusion of other possibilities" ubisemiquinone at the center Q_o was the only reduced electron carrier in complex III capable of producing superoxide.[72]

(4) More evidence that superoxide is most likely produced by the oxidation of semiquinone at the center Q_o was obtained in the studies of Dr. Konstantinov and colleagues. Using an EPR superoxide probe Tiron (1,2-dihydroxybenzo-3,5-disulfonate) they directly demonstrated superoxide production by inside-out submitochondrial particles reduced by succinate.[63] These particles produced superoxide when inhibited by antimycin A (or a similarly acting inhibitor) but not when inhibited with cyanide alone or with antimycin + cyanide, exactly as it would be expected if the superoxide was produced by the semiquinone at the center Q_o.[63] Further studies by Konstantinov's group demonstrated that the effects of center

Q_o inhibitors mucidin, 2,3-dimercaptopropanol, and myxothiazol on the superoxide production were also exactly as expected, that is inhibitory.[71,78]

4.3. *The unexplained features of the superoxide production mechanism at the Complex III*

Earlier studies uncovered several puzzling features characterizing antimycin-inducible superoxide production at bc1-complex. While being relevant to the molecular mechanism of the superoxide production, all of them have yet to receive an explicit explanation.

Redox–dependence. The superoxide production[a] by antimycin–inhibited submitochondrial particles exerts a bell-shaped dependence on the redox poise of the respiratory chain,[71,77] rather than a sigmoidal dependence that would be expected for an unstable Q_o-site allocated semiquinone.[71] Such a redox behavior characterizes a stable semiquinone formed at equilibrium via a reversible dismutation of a quinone and a quinol, that is incompatible with an unstable semiquinone species at center Q_o as a source of superoxide.[71] The mechanism of this phenomenon was reported[71] has been, and continues to be, under investigation in 1983.

Another peculiar recent observation is that myxothiazol[b] can also induce ROS production by Complex III, albeit with a different redox-dependence and much lower rate of production than that in the presence of antimycin A.[77] This observation was confirmed and expanded in experiments with isolated yeast bc1 complex[79,80] and with isolated bovine and yeast bc1-complex.[81] Muller *et al.* proposed a reasonable explanation for a shape of the redox-dependence of myxothiazol-induced ROS production and hypothesized that another semiquinone at Q_o-center can be a source of electrons for the myxothiazol-induced superoxide formation.[80]

"*Wrong*" *sidedness of superoxide production.* Earlier studies demonstrated that antimycin-induced superoxide production can be detected with submitochondrial particles (SMPs) but not with intact mitochondria.[63,76]

---

[a]Measured as H_2O_2 production.

[b]This does not contradict a statement that myxothiazol suppresses antimycin-stimulated ROS production. Myxothiazol per se induces ROS production whereas it both prevents and inhibits the ROS production induced by antimycin.

Given the complexity and high capacity of various mitochondrial ROS-destroying systems, failure of detecting superoxide production by the intact mitochondria is not overly surprising. It may be explained by the presence of SOD[76,82] in the mitochondrial matrix; experimental artifacts such as a direct reaction of a superoxide probe Tyron with cytochrome c[63,83] might also mask superoxide production. It is the release of superoxide by the inside-out SMPs that has to be somehow explained. The problem is that superoxide–generating Q_o-site is located closer to the inner surface of the SMPs whereas a superoxide-detecting probe (a spin-trapping chemical or cytochrome c) is always outside of the particles. This disposition implies that either the probe or the superoxide molecules should be membrane-permeable. However, the study[63] employed a negatively charged spin-trapping chemical Tyron which is unlikely to penetrate the SMP membrane;[63] the negatively charged superoxide ion is also not expected to penetrate the membrane easily.[c] Several studies demonstrated that mitochondria do release detectable Complex III-generated superoxide into the external space.[82,89,90] However, these studies provide no explanation how the superoxide produced at the Q_o-site can be released toward the matrix side of the mitochondrial membrane; neither have they allowed dismissing earlier observations with SMPs as erroneous.

The effect of uncouplers. Protonophorous uncouplers of oxidative phosphorylation such as FCCP stimulate the antimycin-induced H_2O_2 production by mitochondria.[70,91,92] Other energy-dissipating agents including Ca^{2+} and ionophores valinomycin and gramicidin also stimulate the H_2O_2 production by isolated mitochondria.[92] It was suggested[70,92] that uncouplers stimulate the H_2O_2 production by dissipating the small electrical potential across the mitochondrial membrane that still can be generated even in the presence of antimycin.[93] However, the mechanism of the membrane potential effect on the superoxide production by a semiquinone at Q_o-center is not apparent. Under the experimental conditions of Cadenas

[c]The ability of superoxide molecule to penetrate lipid membranes is circumstantial. Some studies demonstrated that superoxide can easily penetrate the plasma membrane of erythrocytes or even liposomes by means of an anion channel,[84–86] whereas other studies found that the penetration of superoxide though the membranes of thylakoids and phospholid liposomes is too slow or otherwise insignificant to be of any importance.[86–88] To the best of our knowledge, the permeability of mitochondrial membranes to superoxide was not reported.

and Boveris,[92] uncoupling of mitochondria could stimulate the antimycin-induced H_2O_2 production by multiple mechanisms, e.g. by affecting the intramitochondrial succinate to fumarate ratio thereby shifting the redox poise of the respiratory chain (discussed above), or by increasing the permeability of mitochondrial membrane to protons thereby promoting the semiquinone reaction with oxygen.[94] What makes the stimulatory effect of uncouplers interesting is that it apparently rules out a semiquinone at the center Q_o of bc1 complex as the major site of ROS production by metabolically competent mitochondria. It is firmly established that high membrane potential stimulates whereas uncouplers strongly inhibit ROS production by coupled functional mitochondria (discussed elsewhere in this manuscript).

The pH dependence of ROS production. The maximum of the pH dependence of the superoxide and hydrogen peroxide production by antimycin-inhibited mitochondria[70] or sonicated mitochondrial fragments[60] is distinctly shifted toward alkaline conditions ($pH>7.5$). Whereas this fact has never received an explanation, it might be of interest in regards to the role of this mechanism of ROS production under some pathological conditions. Obviously, any metabolic conditions acidifying a tissue milieu, such as lactic acidosis, would suppress this mechanism of ROS production by mitochondria.

The quinone concentration dependence of ROS production. ROS generation by antimycin-inhibited mitochondrial particles was shown to depend linearly on the amount of enzyme-reducible ubiquinone in the mitochondrial membrane.[62,70] These experiments were performed with mitochondrial membranes that were extracted with acetone to remove most of endogenous ubiquinone. The extraction rendered the membrane particles practically incapable of both the electron transport from succinate to cytochrome c and the ROS production. Re-incorporation of various amounts of ubiquinone restored both activities. Surprisingly, the activity of succinate dehydrogenase (employed to reduce the re-incorporated quinone) and the rate of electron transport through the bc1 complex (measured as succinate-cytochrome c reductase activity, in the absence of antimycin) were saturated at much lower amounts of re-incorporated ubiquinone than ROS production.[62] The latter increased linearly with an increase in amount of succinate-reducible ubiquinone.[62] It is also of interest that re-incorporation of less lipophylic ubiquinone-3 resulted in generation significantly less ROS than re-incorporation of more lipophylic ubiquinone-10.[70]

4.4. *The mechanism of superoxide production at Complex III*

Despite the recent advances in understanding of the structure of the bc1 complex, a mechanism of superoxide production is not yet known. There is little doubt that semiquinone at center Q_o is the most likely species responsible for the reduction of oxygen to superoxide (or even the only capable one);[1,31,95] there are however, uncertainties about how it does it. This is primarily due to the fact that unstable semiquinone at the center Q_o has yet to be demonstrated.[1,31,73]

The published data allow for multiple models of Q_o-site quinone occupancy, which significantly complicates the interpretation of the experimental data on the superoxide production at the site.[79,80] Not a least important fact is that relatively little research efforts were invested in solving the mechanism of superoxide production *per se;* most data was obtained in attempts to prove the validity of Q-cycle scheme of electron transfer in Complex III.

Any molecular mechanism explaining how the superoxide is produced by the Q_o-site originated semiquinone would have to account both for the known structural features of bc1 complex and for the unusual characteristics of the process as described above. An interesting recent idea is that the superoxide may be produced by a semiquinone that escaped from the Q_o-site.[79] However, we do not think that such an escape is possible in the absence of some severe conformational distortions of the bc1-complex resulting from binding of antimycin-like inhibitor or perhaps, a mutation affecting the Q_o-site.

5. Mitochondrial ROS Detoxifying Systems

Decades–long fascination of researchers with the phenomenology of mitochondrial ROS production has shadowed the fact that mammalian mitochondria possess a complicated multi-leveled ROS defense network of enzymes and non-enzymatic antioxidants. The complexity of this network has just begun to be appreciated, and several new elements have been discovered recently. A systematic study of mitochondrial ROS defenses is yet to be performed, and a tissue-specific expression of many ROS-detoxifying enzymes is an additional complication to the understanding of its functioning. The enormity of the subject precludes us from providing a comprehensive review of mitochondrial ROS defenses. This chapter describes selected, primarily enzymatic subsystems (Fig. 3) that most likely represent mainstream mitochondrial ROS detoxifying pathways. It should however be kept in mind that the latter are yet to be established and that not all enzymes are present in mitochondria from every tissue.

5.1. *Membrane lipid peroxide removal systems*

The "perimeter" layer of ROS defenses is formed by the systems protecting lipids of mitochondrial membranes from peroxidation. These are chiefly α-tocopherol (α-TPH) and phospholipid hydroperoxide glutathione peroxidase (where present). The α-TPH is a ubiquitous lipid soluble directly operating non-enzymatic antioxidant dissolved in mitochondrial membranes. It can reduce lipid radicals "on contact" and requires regeneration for continuous operation. It can be regenerated by reduced coenzyme Q within mitochondrial membranes or by water–soluble ascorbic acid at the water/membrane interface. A physiological role, redox chemistry, tissue-specific distribution in mitochondria and other aspects of α-TPH have repeatedly and comprehensively been reviewed elsewhere and will not be addressed here (see Packer[96] for a recent review and Lass[97] for distribution and content in rodents mitochondria).

5.2. *Phospholipids hydroperoxide glutathione peroxidase*

Phospholipids hydroperoxide glutathione peroxidase (PHGPx, GPx4, EC 1.11.1.12) is a mitochondrial selenoenzyme that belongs to the glutathione peroxidase family and utilizes glutathione. It catalyzes the reduction of phospholipid hydroperoxides to corresponding alcohols (Diagram 1), but it can also react with H_2O_2, cholesterol peroxides,[98,99] and even with thymine peroxide.[100]

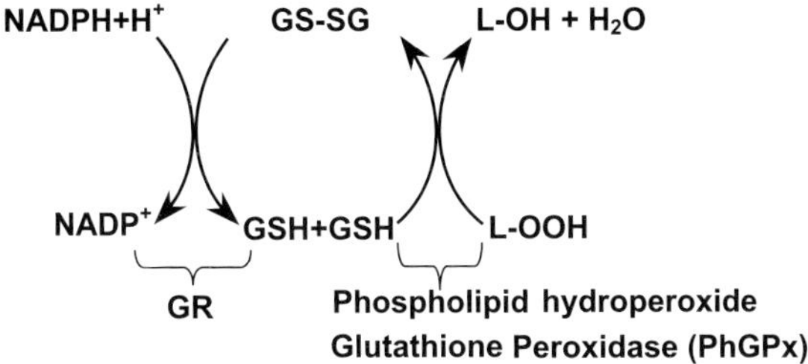

Diagram 1. Lipoperoxide Reduction Catalyzed by GPx4.

It is the only enzyme known to reduce peroxidized phospholipids within membranes and it is thought to play an important role in cellular ROS defense system.[101] Homozygous knockout mice completely lacking GPx4 die *ab utero*, but heterozygous mice are viable and fertile.[102] Mouse embryonic fibroblasts derived from GPx4 heterozygous animals were highly sensitive to paraquat, H_2O_2, tert-butylhydroperoxide, and gamma-irradiation.[102] Overexpression of mitochondrial GPx4 in cells increased their resistance to several mitochondrial toxins inducing oxidative stress[103] and suppressed apoptotic changes including cytochrome c release from mitochondria, tentatively by inhibiting the peroxidation of a mitochondrial lipid cardiolipin.[104]

GPx4 is synthesized in two isoforms, a short form and a long form (L-form) containing a leader sequence that is required for transport to mitochondria.[103] Detailed information on tissue distribution of mitochondrial (L-form) GPx4 is not available, except that it is absent in mouse liver,[105] and that L-form RNA transcript is present only in testis among murine tissues.[106] In rat tissues, it is also highest in testis but some traces of L-form RNA transcript could also be detected in kidney, intestine, and cortex.[107] Such narrow tissue specificity raises some doubts whether GPx4 is of any importance in mitochondria from tissues other than testis. In brain and testis mitochondria, GPx4 activity was localized in the inner mitochondrial membrane.[108,109] It is however possible that the activity was due to other enzymes or a contamination with non-mitochondrial GPx4.

6. Superoxide Removal Systems

6.1. *MnSOD*

The second layer of ROS defenses is formed by enzymes dealing with primary ROS generated in mitochondria, superoxide radical and H_2O_2. The former is a substrate for mitochondrial manganese-containing superoxide dismutase (MnSOD, a.k.a. SOD2, EC 1.15.1.1). This enzyme is located exclusively inside the mitochondrial matrix; its only known function is to facilitate a dismutation of superoxide radical to H_2O_2 (Diagram 2), thereby protecting mitochondrial iron-sulfur cluster containing enzymes from the superoxide attack.[110]

$$2O_2^{\cdot -} \xrightarrow[\text{MnSOD}]{2H^+} O_2 + H_2O_2$$

Diagram 2. Superoxide Removal by MnSOD.

This fascinating enzyme is apparently very important because homozygous MnSOD knockout mice do not survive longer than a few days after birth.[111,112] However, heterozygous mutant mice possessing only 50% of MnSOD activity and protein in their mitochondria are viable and fertile and do not develop any apparent abnormalities.[111,112] A 50% deficiency in MnSOD did not result in an increased sensitivity to oxidative stress-promoting hyperoxia[113] even when animals were exposed to lethal levels of oxygen.[114] The MnSOD deficient mice live as long and age at the same rate as wild type mice despite having more accumulated DNA damage and cancer occurrence later in life.[115] However, heart mitochondria isolated from these apparently healthy animals exerted signs of severe oxidative damage manifested as significant inhibition of mitochondrial Complex I and respiration with NAD-linked substrates, inhibition of aconitase, and increased sensitivity to Ca^{2+}-induced damage to mitochondrial integrity.[116] Mitochondria isolated from hearts of MnSOD–deficient mice exerted ~2.4% (~4 mV) higher membrane potential than mitochondria from wild type mice, that led authors to propose differences in the endogenous proton leak through inner mitochondrial membrane.[116] Similar damage was found in liver mitochondria isolated from MnSOD deficient mice.[117]

A sum of these and other data indicates that MnSOD is an important part of mitochondrial ROS defense system. It does not require any co-factors so the efficiency of this system in superoxide removal is determined by the amount of MnSOD enzyme present in mitochondria. The MnSOD activity is unevenly distributed among different tissues; in mice, the activity in liver and kidneys is highest followed by brain and heart, muscle, and spleen, with lungs exerting the lowest MnSOD activity, almost 20 times lower than that in liver.[118]

Whereas heterozygous MnSOD deficient mice are apparently healthy, an overexpression of MnSOD to 6–10 times above the normal level resulted in developmental abnormalities and decreased fertility of mice.[119] It is not clear what caused these abnormalities.

6.2. *Cytochrome c*

In addition to MnSOD, mitochondria possess another system capable of efficient superoxide removal. The intermembrane space of mitochondria contains ~0.7 mM cytochrome c[120] that can be alternatively reduced by either the respiratory chain or superoxide.[121] This ability of cytochrome c to react with superoxide is well known and widely used to measure the superoxide production. The reduced cytochrome c is regenerated (oxidized) by its natural electron acceptor, cytochrome c oxidase (Diagram 3).

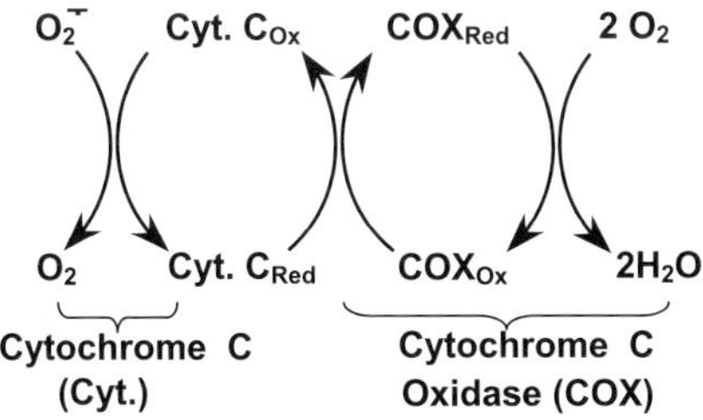

Diagram 3. Superoxide Removal by Cytochrome c.

The antioxidant properties of cytochrome c were demonstrated *in vitro* in experiments with isolated mitochondria,[122] but the physiological role and *in vivo* efficiency of this superoxide-scavenging system remains to be explored. It deserves to be examined in detail also because if operational *in vivo*, it would be the only known ROS-defense system that generates useful metabolic energy while detoxifying superoxide without producing toxic products. All other ROS–defense systems (except catalase) either consume energy for their regeneration or produce toxic products, such as H_2O_2. In contrast, oxidation of cytochrome c by cytochrome c oxidase generates protonmotive force that mitochondria can use to produce ATP, as was demonstrated in experiments with heart mitochondria exposed to the exogenously generated superoxide.[123]

7. Hydrogen Peroxide Removal Systems

7.1. *Catalase*

The product of MnSOD reaction is H_2O_2 which *per se* can be quite toxic to cells and mitochondria and has to be detoxified by other enzymes. One such enzyme is catalase (EC 1.11.1.6.), which converts H_2O_2 into O_2 and H_2O (Diagram 4).

$$2H_2O_2 \xrightarrow[\text{Catalase}]{} O_2 + H_2O$$

Diagram 4. Hydrogen Peroxide Removal by Catalase.

In murine tissues, catalase activity is highest in liver followed by kidneys, lungs, heart and brain.[124] It is thought that catalase is present only in heart mitochondria, where it comprises up to 0.025% of all protein.[125] The presence of catalase was also demonstrated in rat brain cortex mitochondria, where its content is developmentally regulated.[126]

The role of catalase in mitochondrial ROS-defense network is not well understood. Even in heart mitochondria, the contribution of catalase to H_2O_2 removal is thought to be insignificant compared to that of glutathione peroxidase, another H_2O_2–detoxifying enzyme.[127] The role of catalase in ROS-defenses in brain mitochondria is not known.

Recently, knockout mice lacking catalase activity were generated.[124] These mice develop normally and do not show any apparent pathology. However, their brain mitochondria appeared to suffer more damage than mitochondria isolated from brains of wild type mice subjected to a physical impact brain injury. These experiments suggest that catalase may be dispensable under normal circumstances. In pathology, the role of catalase in ROS defense may be dependent on the type of tissue and the model of oxidant-mediated tissue injury.[124]

7.2. *Glutathione*

A staple of mitochondrial H_2O_2 defense network is a small tripeptide compound called glutathione. Glutathione (GSH, L-g-glutamyl-L-cysteinylglycine) is composed of cysteine, glutamic acid and glycine; its active group is the thiol (–SH) of cysteine. Various aspects of GSH metabolism, biochemistry, functions, and analysis have recently been extensively reviewed.[128,129] Mitochondria contain ~10–12% of total GSH amount in a cell, but due to their relatively small matrix volume the concentration of GSH in mitochondrial matrix is somewhat higher than that in cytosol.[130] Mitochondria lack enzymes needed for GSH biosynthesis; intramitochondrial pool of GSH is replenished by rapid net uptake of GSH from cytosol.[131–133] There are several systems capable of transporting GSH into mitochondria, including specialized low and high affinity GSH-transporters[132] and dicaboxylate and 2-oxoglutarate carriers.[133] On "average", the concentration of glutathione within mitochondria is in the range from 2 to 14 mM[130,131,134]; about ~90% of gluthatione is in its reduced form, GSH.[130,134,135] Actual concentrations of total (reduced + oxidized) glutathione in mitochondria vary depending on the metabolic state, age, and tissue.[134] However, since published estimates for steady-state levels of H_2O_2 in the matrix of mitochondria are in the low micromolar range,[136] it is likely that even a significant decrease in GSH levels may not have an impact on H_2O_2 detoxification by GSH–dependent enzymes. The question is then to what threshold level GSH can be depleted without impairing mitochondrial H_2O_2 scavenging capacity. For rat heart mitochondria, the threshold level of GSH depletion was determined experimentally to be ~50%.[137] An increase in mitochondrial H_2O_2 emission was observed only after ~50% depletion of GSH. After that threshold was reached, GSH loss corresponded to a linear increase in H_2O_2 production by mitochondria.[137]

7.3. *Glutathione-S-transferase*

Mitochondria utilize GSH in two major ways, as a recyclable electron donor and as a consumable in conjugation reactions.[128] The latter are catalyzed by glutathione-S-transferases (GST, EC 2.5.1.18), several isoforms of which are present in mitochondria.[138] These enzymes protect mitochondria from various toxins including products of lipid peroxidation such as 4-hydroxynonenal by adding a GSH molecule to a toxin; GSH is consumed and has to be replenished by the uptake from cytosol.[131–133] A sufficiently large intramitochondrial pool of GSH ensures an efficient operation of a GST-based detoxifying system.

7.4. *Glutathione reductase*

Reduced glutathione can either scavenge superoxide and hydroxyl radical non-enzymatically or by serving as an electron-donating substrate to several enzymes involved in ROS-detoxifying.[128] In either case, GSH is oxidized to GSSG that cannot be exported to cytosol[139] and has to be reduced back to GSH in the mitochondrial matrix. The reduction is catalyzed by a specific enzyme glutathione reductase (GR, GSSG reductase, GSR, EC1.8.1.7, formerly EC1.6.4.2) which is present in the matrix of mitochondria.[108,140–142] This enzyme utilizes intramitochondrial NADPH as a source of electrons for the reduction of GSSG to GSH (Diagram 5).

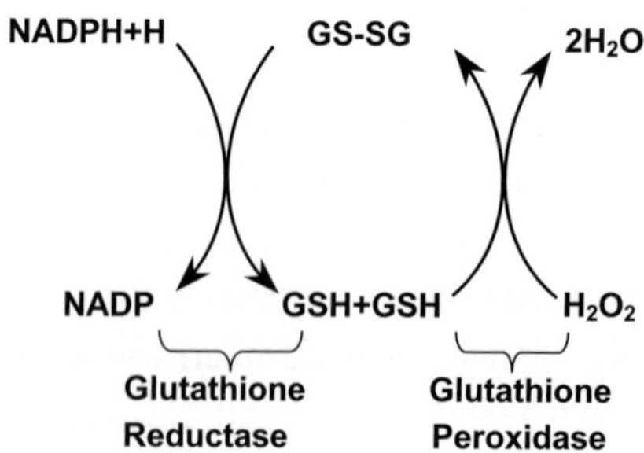

Diagram 5. Glutathione Reduction by GR.

In turn, mitochondrial NADPH can be regenerated by two major pathways, which are the substrate-dependent reduction by dehydrogenases of mitochondrial matrix and protonmotive force-dependent hydride ion transfer reaction utilizing intramitochondrial NADH to reduce $NADP^+$. The former pathway is catalyzed primarily by $NADP^+$-dependent isocitrate dehydrogenase (mNADP-IDH, IDPm, ICD1, EC 1.1.1.42) and by malic enzyme (NADP-ME, EC 1.1.1.40)[135]; the latter is catalyzed by a protein of inner mitochondrial membrane, nicotinamide nucleotide transhydrogenase (TH, E.C.1.6.1.2).[143]

7.5. *A quintessence of the GSH-dependent mitochondrial ROS-defense network*

The dual nature of NADPH regeneration pathways (Fig. 3) is a quintessence of the GSH-dependent mitochondrial ROS-defense network. It establishes the link between the mitochondrial ability to defend themselves against both endogenously and exogenously generated ROS, their bioenergetics prowess and oxidative capacity. In mitochondria, ROS detoxifying dissipates energy derived from a flow of carbon either directly, by oxidizing malate and isocitrate, or indirectly, by consuming protonmotive force generated by

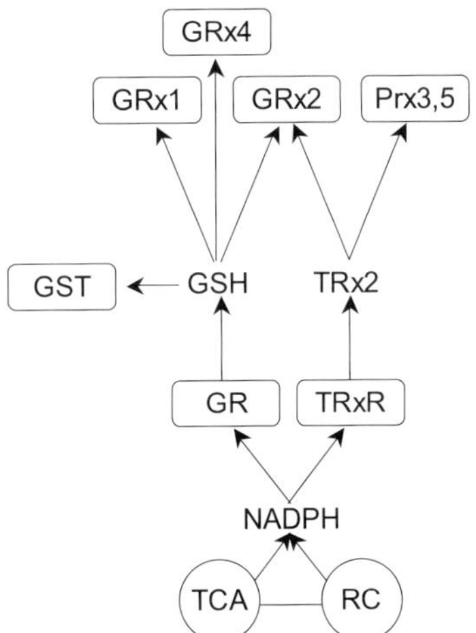

Fig. 3. *Hierarchy of ROS-detoxifying systems in relation to the source of energy — Abbreviations*: TCA, tricarboxylic acids cycle; RC, mitochondrial respiratory chain; GR, glutathione reductase; TrxR, thioredoxin reductase; GSH, reduced glutathione; Trx2 thioredoxin-2; GST, glutathione-S-transferase; GPx1 glutathione peroxidase-1; GPx4, phospholipid hydroperoxide glutathione peroxidase; Grx2 glutaredoxin-2; Prx3,5 peroxiredoxins 3 and 5.

oxidation of any substrate (including malate and isocitrate). In either case, energy is spent to detoxify ROS instead of being used for other functions such as ATP synthesis. In either case, energy is used to regenerate NADPH that is used to regenerate GSH that serves as an electron donor for various ROS-detoxifying systems. However, the enzymes involved in NADPH reduction are differentially expressed in various tissues thereby defining which pathway of GSH-regeneration in mitochondria would dominate in a specific mammalian tissue. It is conceivable that tissue specificity of GSH-regenerating pathways results in tissue-specific mitochondrial resistance to ROS or ROS-related toxin challenges.

Without knowing which pathway contributes more to NADPH reduction, it might be impossible to predict how mitochondrial ROS defenses would be affected by a toxin in different tissues. For example, a protonophorous uncoupler like 2,4-dinitrophenol (DNP) dissipates the protonmotive force thereby rendering TH–catalyzed $NADP^+$ reduction inoperable. It may be anticipated that DNP would have more impact on mitochondrial GSH reduction level and ROS-defenses in mouse heart mitochondria than in brain mitochondria that express only 14% of TH than that in heart mitochondria.[144] However, mouse brain mitochondria possess 3 to 7 times higher activity of malic enzyme (depending on mouse strain)[145] whereas their NADP isocitrate dehydrogenase activity is about 20 times lower than that of heart mitochondria.[146] Both the accumulation of malate and isocitrate in mitochondria and their oxidation rate are individually controlled by the protonmotive force that is affected by the uncoupler. Hence, the effect of DNP on mitochondrial NADPH, GSH and ROS defenses may be quite different depending on the comparative efficiency of all three $NADP^+$ reduction pathways under specific experimental conditions for a specific tissue. Unfortunately, in real life such extended information is rarely available. Therefore, an effect of a toxin on mitochondrial ROS defenses has to be evaluated experimentally rather than assumed. On the bright side, the multiplicity of NADP reduction pathways ensures the robustness, flexibility and efficiency of mitochondrial GSH-linked ROS defense network.

7.6. *Hypothetical antioxidant function of NAD(P)H*

It should be noted that some authors hypothesize that NAD(P)H *per se* can serve as a directly operating non-enzymatic antioxidant.[147] Their reasoning is that mammalian mitochondria contain high concentrations of NADH and NADPH (~3–5 mM of each),[148] and that both NADH and NADPH readily react with oxygen-centered radicals such as trioxocarbonate and nitrogen dioxide, thereby scavenging them and preventing them from causing damage to mitochondrial proteins and DNA. Although such reactions usually result in formation of superoxide radical and further H_2O_2, and NAD(P)* radical can further propagate ROS formation reactions, authors hypothesize that mitochondrial MnSOD and glutathione peroxidase are sufficient to prevent ROS build up.[147] However, this original hypothesis should yet somehow account for a well-established fact that mitochondrial ROS production is strongly stimulated at high levels of NAD(P)H reduction.

7.7. *Glutathione peroxidase*

Classical glutathione peroxidase (GPx1, cGPx, EC 1.11.1.9.) is likely the best studied mitochondrial enzyme that utilizes GSH for the reduction of H_2O_2 to H_2O (Diagram 5). This selenoenzyme is ubiquitously expressed in mammalian tissues[149] and can be detected in various cellular compartments and in mitochondrial matrix[108,140,150,151] and intermembrane space;[108] the same gene encodes both the mitochondrial and extramitochondrial GPx1.[152] The enzyme is not specific toward its substrate and can react with both the H_2O_2 and organic hydroperoxides such as cumene hydroperoxide and tert-butyl hydroperoxide. The latter two compounds are frequently used to detect the enzyme activity in tissue samples *in vitro*.[153] The glutathione peroxidase activity is high in liver, kidney and heart mitochondria and somewhat lower in brain and skeletal muscle mitochondria; however the detailed information on the expression and activity of GPx1 in mitochondria from different mammalian tissues is not available.[105]

Some authors suggest that glutathione peroxidase is the most important enzyme in H_2O_2 removal even in heart mitochondria where catalase is present.[127] Overexpression of Grx1 protected cells against various oxidants.[154,155] Because of that, GPx1 was long thought to be an important part of cellular and mitochondrial ROS-defense network and a potential pharmacological target. These beliefs were shaken when it was discovered that homozygous knockout mice possessing no GPx1 activity are healthy, fertile, develop normally and do not show any signs of tissue damage and oxidative stress.[156–159] That would imply that GPx1 is dispensable.

However, other studies revealed that GPx1 knockout mice are significantly more sensitive than wild type mice to a number of toxins known to induce severe oxidative stress, including paraquat, N-methyl-4-phenyl-1,2,3,6-tetrahydropyridine, and 3-nitropropionic acid.[160–162] Another study with knockout mice found mild growth retardation, slightly elevated H_2O_2 production and uncoupling in liver but not in heart mitochondria, and a remarkable absence of accumulation of lipid peroxides or any other signs of oxidative damage in heart and liver mitochondria from homozygous GPx1 knockout mice.[105] The sum of data obtained with GPx1 knockout mice favor the idea that it is more involved in protection of tissues and mitochondria against acute oxidative stress induced by xenobiotics rather than being a major defense against low-level endogenous mitochondrial ROS production.

7.8. *Peroxiredoxins and other oxins*

Peroxiredoxins, or thioredoxin-dependent peroxide reductases, are recently discovered peroxidases that reduce H_2O_2 and lipid hydroperoxides[163,164] (Diagram 6).

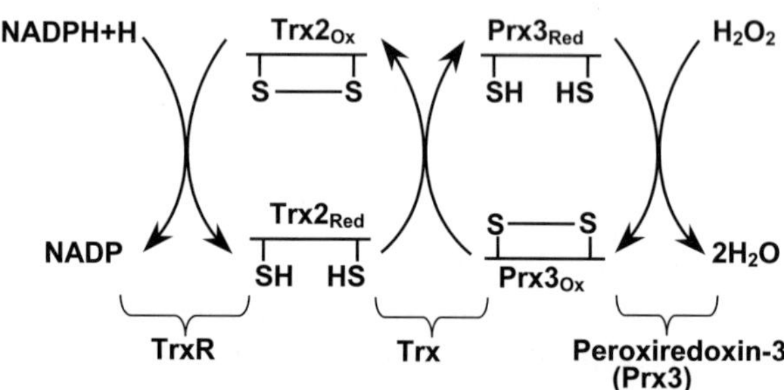

Diagram 6. Reaction Catalyzed by Prx.

Two isoforms of peroxiredoxins (Prx or Prdx) were found in mammalian mitochondria, Prx3 and Prx5. Prx3 (SP-22) is ubiquitously present in mitochondria from various rat tissue, with the highest amount found in heart and adrenal tissue, followed by liver and brain.[165] Similar Prx3 gene expression was found in bovine tissues except that it was highest in adrenal gland.[166] Prx3 gene expression can be induced by oxidative stress; Prx3 apparently functions as an antioxidant in heart mitochondria[167] and in neuronal mitochondria[168] protecting them *in vivo* against oxidative damage. However, the capacity and efficiency of Prx3 in H_2O_2 removal compared to those of other mitochondrial systems are not yet known.

Prx5 is the newest member of peroxiredoxins family discovered in mitochondria. Prx5 gene is also ubiquitously expressed in bovine tissues, with the highest level found in testis.[166] Overexpression of human Prx5 in mitochondria of hamster ovary cells protected them from H_2O_2-induced oxidative damage thereby suggesting a role for this protein in mitochondrial ROS defense network.[169]

A regeneration of both Prx3 and Prx5 to their active form is performed by mitochondrial disulfide oxidoreductase thioredoxin (Trx2) that is a part of so-called mitochondrial thioredoxin system. The backbone of the latter is composed of Trx2 that is a substrate for thioredoxin reductase (TrxR2) that in turn utilizes intramitochondrial NADPH as a hydrogen donor for the Trx2 reduction (Diagram 7).

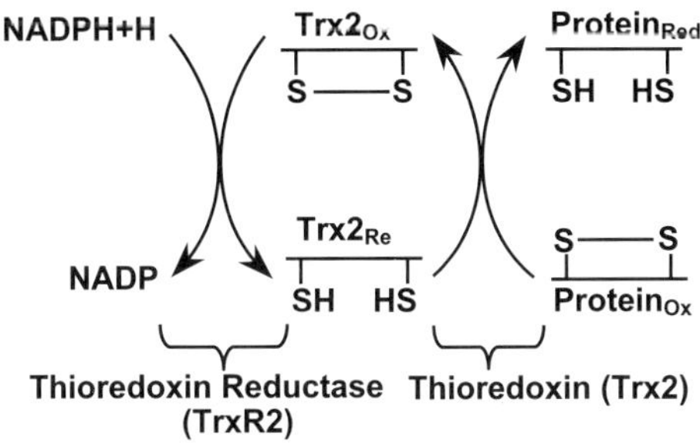

Diagram 7. Thioredoxin system.

Therefore, efficient operation of Prx3 and Prx5 is dependent upon an efficient regeneration of mitochondrial NADPH, similar to the GSH-linked systems described above. Glutaredoxin (Grx2) is also a member of this family of proteins and it can catalyze Trx-disulfide oxidoreduction reactions (Diagram 8).

However, it is different in that it can reduce both protein disulfides in dithiol reactions and catalyze monothiol reductions of mixed disulfides with GSH.[170] Thioredoxins reduce efficiently only protein disulfides.

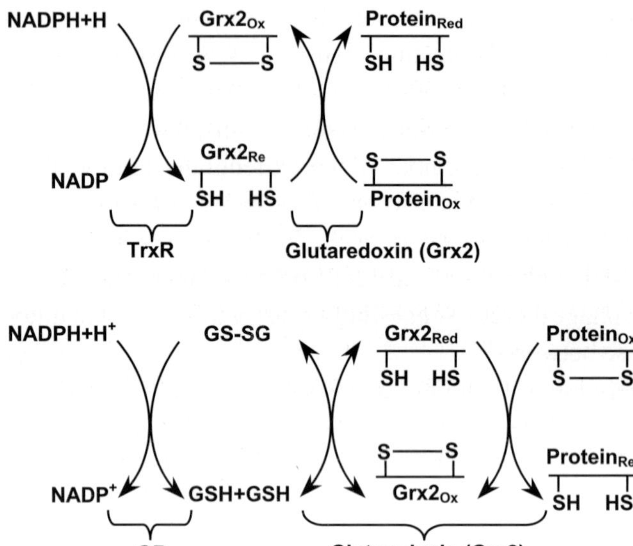

Diagram 8. Glutaredoxin system.

Thioredoxin and thioredoxin reductase (TrxR, EC1.8.1.9., formerly EC1.6.4.5.) and glutaredoxin are ubiquitous proteins present in many if not all tissues and performing a multitude of functions aside of their role in cellular antioxidant defenses. A wealth of information on tissue distribution, genetics, functions, reaction mechanism, and other aspects of these proteins is available.[171,172] However, not much is known about specific mitochondrial isoforms of these proteins, Trx2, TrxR2, and Grx2, and even less is known about their specific role in mitochondrial ROS defenses. In murine tissues, different levels of mRNA transcripts for Trx2, Grx2, and TrxR2 were detected in spleen, lung, liver, kidney, brain, heart, and testis. The levels of Trx2, TrxR2 and Grx2 mRNAs were different from each other and did not follow any apparent pattern of coordinated transcription.[173] The mitochondrial thioredoxin system seems to be essential for mammalian development because a disruption of Trx2 gene in the mouse resulted in massive apoptosis during early embryogenesis and embryonic lethality.[174] However, overexpression of Trx2 or TrxR2, or both, does not necessarily improve cell survival or resistance to ROS-promoting factors, indicating that perhaps an unidentified variable controls the effect of these proteins.[175]

Summarizing this section, we should note that the role of these disulfide reductases in mitochondrial ROS defenses remains to be explored. A wealth of information that is available regarding the antioxidant, cell signaling, and other important functions performed by non-mitochondrial isoforms of these proteins leaves no doubt that they can play a significant role in mitochondrial ROS defenses; that does not mean they do play that role. Instrumental might and wonders of modern day genetic engineering have proven that at least some of these proteins are obligatory for cell survival. That does not yet explain how their primary antioxidant functions provide for that cell survival, if the said functions have anything to do at all with that. There are plenty of examples when proteins perform several functions, with those that we do not know about being much more important than the one we can measure. Therefore, there are plenty of mitochondrial ROS-defense systems but their functioning as a fully integrated system remains to be explored. More experimental work is needed to reveal the roles and capacities of individual mitochondrial ROS-detoxifying systems in protection of mitochondria and cells from ROS.

8. Mitochondrial ROS Production in Pathologies

A compelling body of evidence indicates that oxidative stress is intimately involved in pathways leading to cell death and tissue damage. The role of endogenous ROS in etiology of various diseases and protective strategies have been extensively reviewed elsewhere[176] and will not be covered here. Instead, we shall focus on the mitochondrially produced ROS and two least recognized aspects of the problem. The first aspect is a surprising shortage of studies where an increase in *mitochondrial* (as opposed to "source is not known") ROS production associated with a disease was actually demonstrated rather than hypothesized. The second aspect that has just begun emerging in recent studies is an apparent controversy between the high energy requirements for ROS production by most known mitochondrial sites and a generally poor state of mitochondrial energy production observed in a pathology-affected tissue. The questions then arise — what are the mitochondrial sites that boost their ROS production in pathologies, and how does it happen. Regarding the highly popular emphasis placed on the role of mitochondrially produced ROS in *almost every* human disease including the most common one, ageing, the absence of answers on these questions comes as a bit of a surprise. In this chapter we review the state of the art in this field in light of the knowledge of mechanistic aspects of mitochondrial ROS production as described in previous sections.

8.1. *Types of mechanisms enhancing mitochondrial ROS production*

A multitude of mitochondrial sites that produce ROS suggest that there are many potential routes that could result in an increased ROS production by mitochondria in a pathology-affected tissue. However, all these routes could be arbitrarily divided into three major groups, one consisting of mechanisms ("active-type") contributing to an increase in ROS production *per se* by mitochondria, the other uniting all the mechanisms ("passive-type") contributing to a decrease in mitochondrial ROS scavenging capabilities, and the third representing a special case when the two occur simultaneously. Although the "observable" outcome would always be an increase in an apparent mitochondrial ROS production, there are essential nuances.

The active-type mechanisms consume energy for ROS production, thus diverting a flow of reducing equivalents produced by oxidation of substrates to energy dissipation. ROS production by these mechanisms does double damage to a cell, by using huge catabolic capacity of mitochondria to generate harmful ROS while simultaneously decreasing the availability of energy needed for repairing ROS-induced damage and for ROS detoxifying. Obviously, such mechanisms would result ultimately in cell death unless compensated by an increase in activity/content of catalytic energy-independent ROS-detoxifying elements, such as catalase, MnSOD, cytosolic SOD, and in content of lipid and water-soluble antioxidants. The active-type mechanisms may for example include:

(i) a toxic intervention: a toxin-induced inhibition of Complexes I or III in mitochondrial respiratory chain or other redox-active enzymes preventing them from reacting with their physiological electron acceptors so that these complexes and enzymes would become over-reduced and prone to react with oxygen;

(ii) a mutational damage: a mutation-induced damage to the same complexes or other redox-active enzymes such that part of normal flow of electrons in these enzymes become diverted to superoxide production;

(iii) a peroxidative attack: anything inducing a chain-propagating peroxidation of mitochondrial lipids, such as iron loading of mitochondria;

(iv) a metabolic deregulation; anything elevating mitochondrial membrane potential above the normal level for that metabolic state, such as an ATPase mutation;

(v) an assembly failure: an improper assembly of mitochondrial redox-active multicomponent enzymes such as PDHC or KGDHC or respiratory chain complexes that would result in overall diversion of a normal electron flow toward ROS formation. Of course, any combinations of these mechanisms are possible, too.

The passive-type mechanism could perhaps be less damaging or even not lethal at all, thereby being responsible for a sustained elevation in mitochondrial ROS production and chronic oxidative stress. The passive-type mechanisms could play a major role in slow-developing diseases such as various neurodegenerative conditions. These mechanisms could be difficult to detect in experiments with isolated mitochondria where a mitochondrial ROS production is measured; they should however be detectable by examining mitochondrial ROS-scavenging capacity[142] or by directly assessing the content and activity of mitochondrial antioxidant systems.

The third type of the mechanism that is fairly relevant to various pathologies is a combination of both an active-type and a passive-type ROS producing mechanism. It is best represented by an increase in mitochondrial ROS production caused by mitochondrial permeability transition. It will be discussed in more detail later in this chapter.

8.2. *Complex I as a site of enhanced ROS production*

Unless induced by a toxin or a mutation-inflicted damage to Complex I, a poor state of mitochondrial bioenergetics is generally incompatible with an enhanced ROS production from Complex I of mitochondrial respiratory chain. The ROS production from this site requires high membrane potential that is hardly expected if the bioenergetics of mitochondria is suppressed. This argument is also valid for the lipoamide dehydrogenase, malate dehydrogenase, and other putative mitochondrial ROS-producing dehydrogenases that draw upon matrix pyridine nucleotides as their electron acceptors. The ROS production from these sites requires high NADH to NAD^+ ratio that is not to be expected if the bioenergetics is poor. These are maladies of an excess, so to speak.

One may argue that it is not correct to limit a mutation-inflicted damage just to Complex I *per se*, as from the previous sections it follows that interruption or suppression of electron flow at any site between Complex I and oxygen should stimulate ROS production. It is correct, however in that case ROS would be produced by all sites upstream of the site of inhibition, not by Complex I alone. However, it is conceivable that an inherited or acquired mutation in Complex I could result in a diversion of a normal electron flow within the complex toward an increased production of ROS. When such a mutation is found, it will be very interesting to examine what particular subunit of Complex I is involved in this elevated ROS production.

A deficiency in Complex I could be associated with an enhanced intracellular ROS production[177–180]; however it is unlikely that it was of mitochondrial origin. It was also demonstrated that a deficiency in NADH:cytochrome c reductase activity (that may reflect Complex I deficiency or some damage to Complex I) somehow resulted in an elevated superoxide production by isolated mitochondrial fragments oxidizing NADH[177] *in vitro*. Although there was no obvious correlation between the rate of ROS production and a degree of deficiency in NADH:cytochrome c reductase,[177,179] these and other data do not contradict the hypothesis that a damage or a deficiency in Complex I *in vivo* might indeed result in an elevated mitochondrial ROS production. Future experiments with mitochondria harboring a mutation in Complex I associated with Leber's hereditary optic neuropathy may provide additional data in support of this hypothesis.[181]

8.3. *Complex III as a site of enhanced ROS production*

Enhanced ROS production by the mitochondrial Complex III would perhaps not require high membrane potential or a high NAD(P)H/NAD(P)+ ratio in the mitochondrial matrix. However, the mitochondrial Complex III-derived ROS production in the absence of antimycin or a similar inhibitor is yet to be demonstrated. In fact, the sum of available *in vitro* data on the mechanism of ROS production at this site and the absence of confirmatory *in vivo* data clearly indicate that while it could have produced ROS *in vivo*, it obviously does not, unless severely damaged by antimycin A, myxotiazol, or other inhibitor. Nevertheless, it is conceivable that many man-made environmental, agricultural, and habitual toxins might be able to cause an antimycin-like inhibition of Complex III and stimulate mitochondrial ROS production in an affected tissue; these toxicities just await to be demonstrated.

A deficiency in Complex III activity originating from a mutation in mtDNA in a patient with Parkinsonism resulted in an increased intracellular ROS production in transmitochondrial cybrids.[182] Future experiments should establish whether that increase was due to mitochondrially produced ROS or due to a decrease in mitochondrial ROS scavenging capacity resulting from impaired bioenergetics associated with diminished Complex III activity.[182]

8.4. *ATPase mutation may enhance ROS production*

A mutation in this or that mitochondrial enzyme that enhances mitochondrial ROS production has yet to be demonstrated. However, a mitochondrial mutation that results in an elevated steady state level of cytosolic ROS has been recently demonstrated. A T8993G point mutation in mtDNA targets one of the subunit (MTATP6) of mitochondrial ATPase and impairs oxidative phosphorylation in two mitochondrial disorders.[183] Experiments with transmitochondrial cybrid cells harboring this mutation revealed higher cytosolic ROS, impaired mitochondrial ATP synthesis, and elevated mitochondrial membrane potential.[183] Although mitochondrial ROS production *per se* was not measured, it is not unlikely that a mutation inhibiting an energy-dissipating process (oxidative phosphorylation) would increase the membrane potential thereby stimulating mitochondrial ROS production.

8.5. *Ischemia reperfusion enhances mitochondrial ROS production*

There exists an acute shortage in relevant published experimental data regarding the mitochondrial ROS production in diseases and pathologies. Although a deficiency in this or that mitochondrial enzyme would frequently result in impaired bioenergetics, it does not necessarily mean an enhanced mitochondrial ROS production. Similarly, an increase in cytosolic steady-state ROS levels does not necessarily mean that it originates from mitochondria, even if it appears to respond on mitochondrial inhibitors. In almost all studies of oxidative stress associated with pathology the mitochondrial ROS production *per se* has not actually been examined.

A notable exception is an elevated mitochondrial ROS production associated with ischemia and reperfusion-induced tissue damage. Ischemia-reperfusion associated ROS production has been studied most extensively in heart tissue where it is manifested by three phenomena: an elevated ROS production during the ischemia phase, a "burst" in ROS production upon the onset of reperfusion that fades in a few minutes, and an elevated ROS production observed in reperfused tissue.[184] It is well established that mitochondria isolated from either ischemic or reperfused heart tissue exert an enhanced ROS production compared to mitochondria isolated from control tissue.[185–188] A significant decrease in Complex III activity was also observed, that perhaps contributed to a conclusion that Complex III is responsible for the enhanced ROS production.[187] However, it would be more likely that ROS was actually generated by Complex I and/or dehydrogenases in mitochondrial matrix. This is because mitochondrial ROS production was measured in the presence of Complex I inhibitor rotenone and succinate as oxidative substrate; these conditions are known to stimulate ROS production by Complex I and matrix dehydrogenases. Other studies[186,188] report a significant decrease in NAD-linked respiration and/or Complex I activity and increased ROS production by mitochondria isolated from ischemic or reperfused heart tissue. The measurements were performed under conditions favoring increased ROS production by Complex I and/or matrix dehydrogenases (State 4 respiration supported by NAD-linked substrates).[186,188]

It is not known what causes a decrease in Complex I activity and an increase in ROS production from this site in mitochondria during ischemia and reperfusion. An accumulation of long chain unsaturated fatty acids such as arachidonic acid may be the factor responsible for both phenomena.[186] Another likely mechanism could be the opening of mitochondrial permeability transition pore during the reperfusion phase (reviewed later in this chapter), because most of the results obtained with ischemic mitochondria were also obtained with control mitochondria that were allowed to accumulate Ca^{2+}.[186]

Apparently, *in situ* tissue conditions and/or factors affecting mitochondria are not obligatory for stimulating mitochondrial ROS production by reperfusion. Isolated liver mitochondria subjected to anoxia *in vitro* exerted an elevated superoxide production upon reperfusion.[189] Authors suggested that it was caused by the oxidation of ubisemiquinone that could have accumulated during the anoxic phase[189]; it is however clear that something else could be equally responsible for such a burst as everything redox-capable in mitochondria becomes over-reduced during the anoxia phase.

It should be noted that ischemia-induced increase in mitochondrial ROS production may be a tissue-specific phenomenon. A study[190] failed to detect an increase in ROS production by mitochondria isolated from rat brain subjected to a post-decapitative ischemia; no decline in mitochondrial Complex I or III activities was noted either.[190] However, their experimental model was different from those where an increase in mitochondrial ROS production was observed in that the ischemia was not followed by a reperfusion.[190]

8.6. *Mitochondrial Ca^{2+} accumulation per se unlikely enhances ROS production*

There are numerous reports implying that a massive mitochondrial accumulation of Ca^{2+}, another prominent phenomenon associated with ischemia and reperfusion,[191,192] somehow promotes ROS production.[53,54,57,193,194]

The Ca^{2+} uptake *per se* should suppress ROS production because it dissipates the $\Delta\Psi$ and decreases the level of NAD(P)H reduction in mitochondria. It also induces collateral energy expenditures caused by Ca^{2+} recycling and re-phosphorylating of ATP hydrolyzed during the phase of active transport. This reasoning was proved experimentally; ROS production by mitochondria oxidizing NAD-linked substrates was severely suppressed both during the active Ca^{2+} uptake and for a prolonged period after the accumulation has been completed.[195]

It is also unlikely that Ca^{2+} accumulation could stimulate ROS production by affecting dehydrogenases in mitochondrial matrix. Although Ca^{2+} in the low micromolar range stimulates the activity of several dehydrogenases including pyruvate dehydrogenase complex, isocitrate dehydrogenase, and α-ketoglutarate dehydrogenase complex,[196,197] a massive Ca^{2+} accumulation actually inhibits the activity of the very same dehydrogenases[198,199] as well as the overall NAD-linked respiratory activity and phosphorylation in mitochondria.[200,201] Upon reperfusion, Ca^{2+} is accumulated in mitochondria well above normal, physiological matrix concentration.[191,192] Therefore, it is unlikely that Ca^{2+} effect on matrix dehydrogenases is responsible for Ca^{2+}-associated stimulation of ROS production observed upon reperfusion of ischemic tissues.

8.7. *Ca^{2+}-induced mitochondrial permeability transition may be responsible for an increase in ROS production*

The most dramatic pathological event associated with over-accumulation of Ca^{2+} by mitochondria is the opening of a large pore in the inner mitochondrial membrane. This is a unique mitochondrial phenomenon that was extensively studied for over 20 years yet is far from being well-understood. Mitochondrial permeability transition pore (PTP) is thought to be a large channel in the inner mitochondrial membrane which is normally closed and can be opened by Ca^{2+} overloading and other factors including oxidative stress. Structural changes such as partial release of the cytochrome c typically accompanies the PTP,[202–206] as well as loss of mitochondrial matrix pyridine nucleotides[207] and other solutes such as glutathione.[208] The various characteristics of PTP and its importance and involvement in etiology of various diseases and in cell death are extensively reviewed elsewhere.[202,205]

Several reports demonstrate that opening of PTP correlates with an increase in ROS production by isolated mitochondria[56,209] and in cells.[210] It is conceivable that PTP-induced changes in mitochondrial structure and content are the major reason for increased ROS production observed in ischemia-reperfusion models. It is also most likely the main mechanism for an increase in mitochondrial ROS production in other pathologies that are associated with abnormal Ca^{2+} regulation, such as glutamate neurotoxicity.[210] Another prominent example of a condition where PTP opening is responsible for an increase in mitochondrial ROS production is so-called "ROS-induced ROS release". This is an interesting phenomenon described by Dr. Zorov *et al.*[211] that consist of an increase in mitochondrial ROS production induced by an exposure of mitochondria to increasing levels of exogenously generated ROS. In the experiments of Dr. Zorov and colleagues, ROS were generated incrementally and spatially in the mitochondria–rich regions *in situ* in intact myoblasts by a laser irradiation of a photoactive ROS-producing chemical. Several mitochondrial parameters including their membrane potential, ROS production, and PTP opening were monitored simultaneously using a confocal microscopy technique. It appeared that photodynamically ROS triggered the PTP opening in mitochondria that resulted in depolarization of the membrane potential and secondary increase in mitochondrial ROS production.[211] This study is of primary importance as it is the first direct demonstration of *in situ* ROS production by mitochondria that had undergone PTP opening.

According to the classification presented earlier in this chapter, PTP-induced ROS production represents a combination of both the active and the passive-type mechanisms. A PTP opening in mitochondrial inner membrane should induce a genuine increase in ROS production from several mitochondrial sites, primarily from Complex I and substrate dehydrogenases of mitochondrial matrix. This is illustrated in Fig. 4. Small solutes with the molecular weight less than 1,500 Da are released from mitochondrial matrix upon the onset of PTP. This includes matrix pyridine nucleotides,[207] that are released downward the gradient of their concentration, as mitochondrial concentrations of NAD and NADP are ~10 times higher than their concentrations in a cell cytosol.[148] However, the substrates of mitochondrial dehydrogenases are still available, and this results in over-reduction of substrate dehydrogenases in the mitochondrial matrix due to the lack of their natural electron acceptor (pyridine nucleotides). This would stimulate ROS production by the NAD-linked enzymes such as dihydrolipoamide dehydrogenase and malate dehydrogenase, as described in a previous section of this manuscript. Complex I is also expected to increase its ROS production because a PTP opening induces partial loss of cytochrome c from mitochondria thereby inhibiting the respiratory chain and inducing Complex I over-reduction.

All the active mitochondrial antioxidant systems become dysfunctional shortly after the PTP occurs. This is because in the absence of proton gradient and sufficient supply of NADH and NADPH mitochondrial reduced glutathione cannot be regenerated and is eventually depleted, in addition to its direct release into cell cytosol downward the concentration gradient.[130] This results in an impaired ROS scavenging by mitochondria.

Normal state

Parameter	Status
Matrix [Ca^{2+}]	Normal
Protonmotive force (Δp)	High
Matrix $NADH/NAD^+$	High
Matrix $NADPH/NADP^+$	High
Matrix GSH/GSSG	High
GR, GPx, mxDH	High
ROS scavenging	High
ROS production	Moderate
ROS release	Low

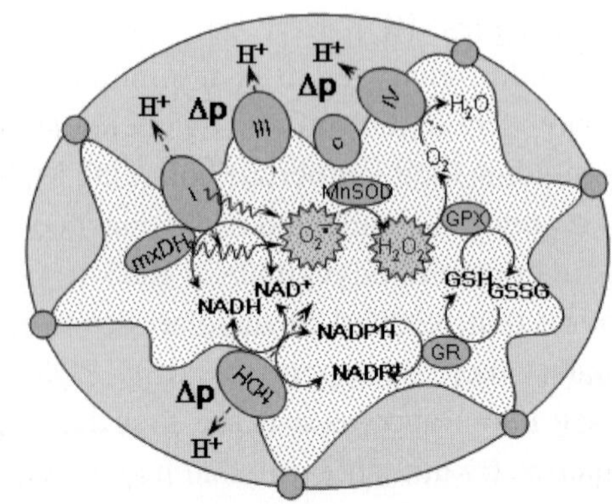

Massive Ca^{2+} accumulation

Parameter	Status
Matrix [Ca^{2+}]	High
Protonmotive force (Δp)	Low
Matrix $NADH/NAD^+$	Low
Matrix $NADPH/NADP^+$	Low
Matrix GSH/GSSG	High
GR, GPx, mxDH	Low
ROS scavenging	Low
ROS production	Low
ROS release	Low

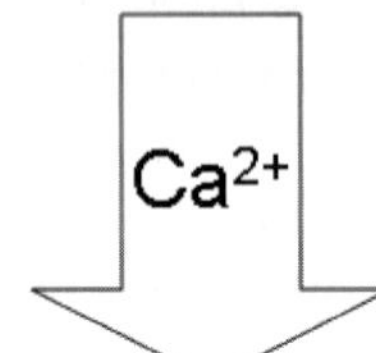

Permeability Transition

Parameter	Status
Matrix [Ca^{2+}]	Ext
Protonmotive force (Δp)	None
Matrix $NADH/NAD^+$	Ext
Matrix $NADPH/NADP^+$	Ext
Matrix GSH/GSSG	Ext
GR, GPx, mxDH	Low
ROS scavenging	Low
ROS production	High
ROS release	High

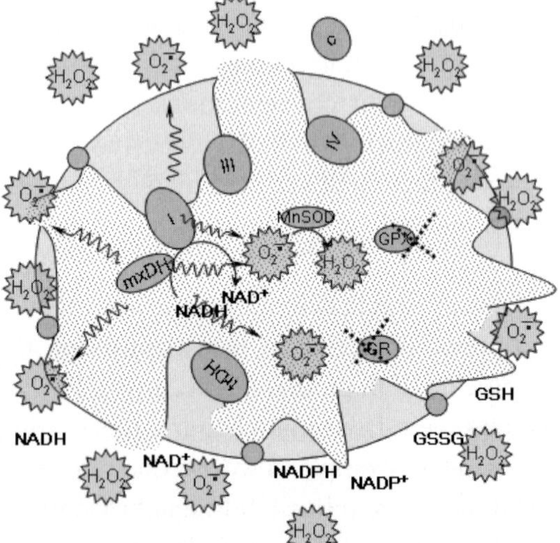

Fig. 4. Effect of massive Ca2+ accumulation and mitochondrial permeability transition on ROS production. See text for details.

9. Postscriptum

A huge wave in interest in mitochondrial free radicals production mechanisms is growing internationally. Hopefully, it will deliver advanced knowledge about the functioning and regulation of mitochondrial ROS generating and detoxifying systems and their role in the life and death of cells. Research on mitochondrial ROS production and detoxifying mechanisms has been a side-bar, rather than a mainstream subject of modern biology for far too long. The subject of mitochondrial free radicals has not yet fully embraced the power of post-genome era tools and conceptions and hypothesis-driven approaches. Nevertheless, even with the present patchwork state of knowledge, the emerging complexity and degree of interactions in mitochondrial ROS-related systems is impressive. With carefully designed and conclusive advances in our understanding of these complex and integrated systems, the potential significance of mitochondrial ROS in regulating tissue bioenergetics and pathogenesis may deserve distinct recognition as critical control points in Maps of Biochemical Pathways.

References

1. Turrens JF. Mitochondrial formation of reactive oxygen species. *J. Physiol.* 552: 335–344 (2003).
2. Nishino H, Ito A. Subcellular distribution of OM cytochrome b-mediated NADH-semidehydroascorbate reductase activity in rat liver. *J. Biochem. (Tokyo)* 100: 1523–1531 (1986).
3. Lee JS, Huh WK, Lee BH, Baek YU, Hwang CS, Kim ST, Kim YR, Kang SO. Mitochondrial NADH-cytochrome b(5) reductase plays a crucial role in the reduction of D-erythroascorbyl free radical in *Saccharomyces cerevisiae*. *Biochim. Biophys. Acta* 1527: 31–38 (2001).
4. Whatley SA, Curti D, Marchbanks RM. Mitochondrial involvement in schizophrenia and other functional psychoses. *Neurochem. Res.* 21: 995–1004 (1996).
5. Whatley SA, Curti D, Das Gupta F, Ferrier IN, Jones S, Taylor C, Marchbanks RM. Superoxide, neuroleptics and the ubiquinone and cytochrome b5 reductases in brain and lymphocytes from normal and schizophrenic patients. *Mol. Psychiatry* 3: 227–237 (1998).

6. Hauptmann N, Grimsby J, Shih JC, Cadenas E. The metabolism of tyramine by monoamine oxidase A/B causes oxidative damage to mitochondrial DNA. *Arch. Biochem. Biophys.* 335: 295–304 (1996).
7. Simonson SG, Zhang J, Canada AT, Jr, Su YF, Benveniste H, Piantadosi CA. Hydrogen peroxide production by monoamine oxidase during ischemia-reperfusion in the rat brain. *J. Cereb. Blood Flow Metab.* 13: 125–134 (1993).
8. Kunduzova OR, Bianchi P, Parini A, Cambon C. Hydrogen peroxide production by monoamine oxidase during ischemia/reperfusion. *Eur. J. Pharmacol.* 448: 225–230 (2002).
9. Maurel A, Hernandez C, Kunduzova O, Bompart G, Cambon C, Parini A, Frances B. Age-dependent increase in hydrogen peroxide production by cardiac monoamine oxidase A in rats. *Am. J. Physiol. Heart Circ. Physiol.* 284: H1460–1467 (2003).
10. Carvalho F, Duarte JA, Neuparth MJ, Carmo H, Fernandes E, Remiao F, Bastos ML. Hydrogen peroxide production in mouse tissues after acute d-amphetamine administration. Influence of monoamine oxidase inhibition. *Arch. Toxicol.* 75: 465–469 (2001).
11. Kumar MJ, Nicholls DG, Andersen JK. Oxidative alpha-ketoglutarate ehydrogenase inhibition via subtle elevations in monoamine oxidase B levels results in loss of spare respiratory capacity: implications for Parkinson's disease. *J. Biol. Chem.* 278: 46432–46439 (2003).
12. Loffler M, Becker C, Wegerle E, Schuster G. Catalytic enzyme histochemistry and biochemical analysis of dihydroorotate dehydrogenase/oxidase and succinate dehydrogenase in mammalian tissues, cells and mitochondria. *Histochem. Cell. Biol.* 105: 119–128 (1996).
13. Forman JH, Kennedy J. Superoxide production and electron transport in mitochondrial oxidation of dihydroorotic acid. *J. Biol. Chem.* 250: 4322–4326 (1975).
14. Forman HJ, Kennedy J. Dihydroorotate-dependent superoxide production in rat brain and liver. A function of the primary dehydrogenase. *Arch. Biochem. Biophys.* 173: 219–224 (1976).
15. Dileepan KN, Kennedy J. Complete inhibition of dihydro-orotate oxidation and superoxide production by 1,1,1-trifluoro-3-thenoylacetone in rat liver mitochondria. *Biochem. J.* 225: 189–194 (1985).
16. Brown LJ, Koza RA, Everett C, Reitman ML, Marshall L, Fahien LA, Kozak LP, MacDonald MJ. Normal thyroid thermogenesis but reduced viability and adiposity in mice lacking the mitochondrial glycerol phosphate dehydrogenase. *J. Biol. Chem.* 277: 32892–32898 (2002).

17. Lee YP, Lardy HA. Influence of thyroid hormones on L-alpha-glycerophosphate dehydrogenases and other dehydrogenases in various organs of the rat. *J. Biol. Chem.* 240: 1427–1436 (1965).
18. Dummler K, Muller S, Seitz HJ. Regulation of adenine nucleotide translocase and glycerol 3-phosphate dehydrogenase expression by thyroid hormones in different rat tissues. *Biochem. J.* 317 (Pt 3): 913–918 (1996).
19. Koza RA, Kozak UC, Brown LJ, Leiter EH, MacDonald MJ, Kozak LP. Sequence and tissue-dependent RNA expression of mouse FAD-linked glycerol-3-phosphate dehydrogenase. *Arch. Biochem. Biophys.* 336: 97–104 (1996).
20. Estabrook RW, Sacktor B. Alpha-Glycerophosphate oxidase of flight muscle mitochondria. *J. Biol. Chem.* 233: 1014–1019 (1958).
21. Kwong LK, Sohal RS. Substrate and site specificity of hydrogen peroxide generation in mouse mitochondria. *Arch. Biochem. Biophys.* 350: 118–126 (1998).
22. Miwa S, St-Pierre J, Partridge L, Brand MD. Superoxide and hydrogen peroxide production by Drosophila mitochondria. *Free Radic. Biol. Med.* 35: 938–948 (2003).
23. Zhang L, Yu L, Yu CA. Generation of superoxide anion by succinate-cytochrome c reductase from bovine heart mitochondria. *J. Biol. Chem.* 273: 33972–33976 (1998a).
24. McLennan HR, Degli Esposti M. The contribution of mitochondrial respiratory complexes to the production of reactive oxygen species. *J. Bioenerg. Biomembr.* 32: 153–162 (2000).
25. Gardner PR. Aconitase: sensitive target and measure of superoxide. *Methods Enzymol.* 349: 9–23 (2002).
26. Vasquez-Vivar J, Kalyanaraman B, Kennedy MC. Mitochondrial aconitase is a source of hydroxyl radical. An electron spin resonance investigation. *J. Biol. Chem.* 275: 14064–14069 (2000).
27. Maas E, Bisswanger H. Localization of the alpha-oxoacid dehydrogenase multienzyme complexes within the mitochondrion. *FEBS Lett.* 277: 189–190 (1990).
28. Starkov AA, Fiskum G, Chinopoulos C, Lorenzo BJ, Browne SE, Patel MS, Beal MF. Mitochondrial alpha-ketoglutarate dehydrogenase complex generates reactive oxygen species. *J. Neurosci.* 24: 7779–7788 (2004).
29. Tretter L. Adam-Vizi V. Generation of reactive oxygen species in the reaction catalyzed by alpha-ketoglutarate dehydrogenase. *J. Neurosci.* 24: 7771–7778 (2004).

30. Bunik VI, Sievers C. Inactivation of the 2-oxo acid dehydrogenase complexes upon generation of intrinsic radical species. *Eur. J. Biochem.* 269: 5004–5015 (2002).
31. Turrens JF. Superoxide production by the mitochondrial respiratory chain. *Biosci. Rep.* 17: 3–8 (1997).
32. Lenaz G. The mitochondrial production of reactive oxygen species: mechanisms and implications in human pathology. *IUBMB Life* 52: 159–164 (2001).
33. Kushnareva Y, Murphy AN, Andreyev A. Complex I-mediated reactive oxygen species generation: modulation by cytochrome c and NAD(P)+ oxidation-reduction state. *Biochem. J.* 368: 545–553 (2002).
34. Liu Y, Fiskum G, Schubert D. Generation of reactive oxygen species by the mitochondrial electron transport chain. *J. Neurochem.* 80: 780–787 (2002).
35. Cadenas E, Boveris A, Ragan CI, Stoppani AO. Production of superoxide radicals and hydrogen peroxide by NADH-ubiquinone reductase and ubiquinol-cytochrome c reductase from beef-heart mitochondria. *Arch. Biochem. Biophys.* 180: 248–257 (1977).
36. Genova ML, Pich MM, Biondi A, Bernacchia A, Falasca A, Bovina C, Formiggini G, Parenti Castelli G, Lenaz G. Mitochondrial production of oxygen radical species and the role of coenzyme Q as an antioxidant. *Exp. Biol. Med.* (*Maywood*) 228: 506–513 (2003).
37. Hinkle PC, Butow RA, Racker E, Chance B. Partial resolution of the enzymes catalyzing oxidative phosphorylation. XV. Reverse electron transfer in the flavin-cytochrome beta region of the respiratory chain of beef heart submitochondrial particles. *J. Biol. Chem.* 242: 5169–5173 (1967).
38. Takeshige K, Minakami S. NADH- and NADPH-dependent formation of superoxide anions by bovine heart submitochondrial particles and NADH-ubiquinone reductase preparation. *Biochem. J.* 180: 129–135 (1979).
39. Herrero A, Barja G. Localization of the site of oxygen radical generation inside the complex I of heart and non-synaptic brain mammalian mitochondria. *J. Bioenerg. Biomembr.* 32: 609–615 (2000).
40. Genova ML, Ventura B, Giuliano G, Bovina C, Formiggini G, Parenti Castelli G, Lenaz G. The site of production of superoxide radical in mitochondrial Complex I is not a bound ubisemiquinone but presumably iron-sulfur cluster N2. *FEBS Lett.* 505: 364–368 (2001).
41. Kang D, Narabayashi H, Sata T, Takeshige K. Kinetics of superoxide formation by respiratory chain NADH- dehydrogenase of bovine heart mitochondria. *J. Biochem.* (*Tokyo*) 94: 1301–1306 (1983).

42. Kudin AP, Bimpong-Buta NY, Vielhaber S, Elger CE, Kunz WS. Characterization of superoxide-producing sites in isolated brain mitochondria. *J. Biol. Chem.* 279: 4127–4135 (2004).
43. Krishnamoorthy G, Hinkle PC. Studies on the electron transfer pathway, topography of iron-sulfur centers, and site of coupling in NADH-Q oxidoreductase. *J. Biol. Chem.* 263: 17566–17575 (1988).
44. Korshunov SS, Skulachev VP, Starkov AA. High protonic potential actuates a mechanism of production of reactive oxygen species in mitochondria. *FEBS Lett.* 416: 15–18 (1997).
45. Hansford RG, Hogue BA, Mildaziene V. Dependence of H2O2 formation by rat heart mitochondria on substrate availability and donor age. *J. Bioenerg. Biomembr.* 29: 89–95 (1997).
46. Votyakova TV, Reynolds IJ. DeltaPsi(m)-dependent and -independent production of reactive oxygen species by rat brain mitochondria. *J. Neurochem.* 79: 266–277 (2001).
47. Starkov AA, Fiskum G. Regulation of brain mitochondrial H2O2 production by membrane potential and NAD(P)H redox state. *J. Neurochem.* 86: 1101–1107 (2003).
48. Lambert AJ, Brand MD. Superoxide production by NADH: ubiquinone oxidoreductase (complex I) depends on the pH gradient across the mitochondrial inner membrane. *Biochem. J.* 382: 511–517 (2004).
49. Turrens JF, Boveris A. Generation of superoxide anion by the NADH dehydrogenase of bovine heart mitochondria. *Biochem. J.* 191: 421–427 (1980).
50. Barja G. Mitochondrial oxygen radical generation and leak: sites of production in states 4 and 3, organ specificity, and relation to aging and longevity. *J. Bioenerg. Biomembr.* 31: 347–366 (1999).
51. Sipos I, Tretter L, Adam-Vizi V. Quantitative relationship between inhibition of respiratory complexes and formation of reactive oxygen species in isolated nerve terminals. *J. Neurochem.* 84: 112–118 (2003).
52. Ramsay RR, Singer TP. Relation of superoxide generation and lipid peroxidation to the inhibition of NADH-Q oxidoreductase by rotenone, piericidin A, and MPP^+. *Biochem. Biophys. Res. Commun.* 189: 47–52 (1992).
53. Dykens JA. Isolated cerebral and cerebellar mitochondria produce free radicals when exposed to elevated CA^{2+} and Na^+: implications for neurodegeneration. *J. Neurochem.* 63: 584–591 (1994).
54. Kowaltowski AJ, Castilho RF, Vercesi AE. Ca^{2+}-induced mitochondrial membrane permeabilization: role of coenzyme Q redox state. *Am. J. Physiol.* 269: C141–C147 (1995).

55. Kowaltowski AJ, Castilho RF, Vercesi AE. Opening of the mitochondrial permeability transition pore by uncoupling or inorganic phosphate in the presence of Ca^{2+} is dependent on mitochondrial-generated reactive oxygen species. *FEBS Lett.* 378: 150–152 (1996).
56. Kowaltowski AJ, Naia-da-Silva ES, Castilho RF, Vercesi AE. Ca^{2+}-stimulated mitochondrial reactive oxygen species generation and permeability transition are inhibited by dibucaine or Mg^{2+}. *Arch. Biochem. Biophys.* 359: 77–81 (1998b).
57. Kowaltowski AJ, Netto LE, Vercesi AE. The thiol-specific antioxidant enzyme prevents mitochondrial permeability transition. Evidence for the participation of reactive oxygen species in this mechanism. *J. Biol. Chem.* 273: 12766–12769 (1998a).
58. Chen Q, Vazquez EJ, Moghaddas S, Hoppel CL, Lesnefsky EJ. Production of reactive oxygen species by mitochondria: central role of complex III. *J. Biol. Chem.* 278: 36027–36031 (2003).
59. Jensen PK. Antimycin-insensitive oxidation of succinate and reduced nicotinamide-adenine dinucleotide in electron-transport particles. I. pH dependency and hydrogen peroxide formation. *Biochim. Biophys. Acta* 122: 157–166 (1966).
60. Loschen G, Azzi A, Richter C, Flohe L. Superoxide radicals as precursors of mitochondrial hydrogen peroxide. *FEBS Lett.* 42: 68–72 (1974).
61. Dionisi O, Galeotti T, Terranova T, Azzi A. Superoxide radicals and hydrogen peroxide formation in mitochondria from normal and neoplastic tissues. *Biochim. Biophys. Acta* 403: 292–300 (1975).
62. Boveris A, Cadenas E, Stoppani AO. Role of ubiquinone in the mitochondrial generation of hydrogen peroxide. *Biochem. J.* 156: 435–444 (1976).
63. Grigolava IV, Ksenzenko M, Konstantinob AA, Tikhonov AN, Kerimov TM. Tiron as a spin-trap for superoxide radicals produced by the respiratory chain of submitochondrial particles. *Biokhimiia* 45: 75–82 (1980).
64. Sawyer DT, Valentine JS. How super is superoxide? *Acc. Chem. Res.* 14: 393–400 (1981).
65. Trumpower BL. The protonmotive Q cycle. Energy transduction by coupling of proton translocation to electron transfer by the cytochrome bc1 complex. *J. Biol. Chem.* 265: 11409–11412 (1990).
66. Zhang Z, Huang L, Shulmeister VM, Chi YI, Kim KK, Hung LW, Crofts AR, Berry EA, Kim SH. Electron transfer by domain movement in cytochrome bc1. *Nature* 392: 677–684 (1998b).
67. Crofts AR, Barquera B, Gennis RB, Kuras R, Guergova-Kuras M, Berry EA. Mechanism of ubiquinol oxidation by the bc(1) complex: different domains

of the quinol binding pocket and their role in the mechanism and binding of inhibitors. *Biochemistry* 38: 15807–15826 (1999).

68. Iwata S, Lee JW, Okada K, Lee JK, Iwata M, Rasmussen B, Link TA, Ramaswamy S, Jap BK. Complete structure of the 11-subunit bovine mitochondrial cytochrome bc1 complex. *Science* 281: 64–71 (1998).
69. Kim H, Xia D, Yu CA, Xia JZ, Kachurin AM, Zhang L, Yu L, Deisenhofer J. Inhibitor binding changes domain mobility in the iron-sulfur protein of the mitochondrial bc1 complex from bovine heart. *Proc. Natl. Acad. Sci. USA* 95: 8026–8033 (1998).
70. Boveris A, Chance B. The mitochondrial generation of hydrogen peroxide. General properties and effect of hyperbaric oxygen. *Biochem. J.* 134: 707–716 (1973).
71. Ksenzenko M, Konstantinov AA, Khomutov GB, Tikhonov AN, Ruuge EK. Effect of electron transfer inhibitors on superoxide generation in the cytochrome bc1 site of the mitochondrial respiratory chain. *FEBS Lett.* 155: 19–24 (1983).
72. Turrens JF, Alexandre A, Lehninger AL. Ubisemiquinone is the electron donor for superoxide formation by complex III of heart mitochondria. *Arch. Biochem. Biophys.* 237: 408–414 (1985).
73. Junemann S, Heathcote P, Rich PR. On the mechanism of quinol oxidation in the bc1 complex. *J. Biol. Chem.* 273: 21603–21607 (1998).
74. Konstantinov AA, Peskin AV, Popova E, Khomutov GB, Ruuge EK. Superoxide generation by the respiratory chain of tumor mitochondria. *Biochim. Biophys. Acta* 894: 1–10 (1987).
75. Zoccarato F, Cavallini L, Deana R, Alexandre A. Pathways of hydrogen peroxide generation in guinea pig cerebral cortex mitochondria. *Biochem. Biophys. Res. Commun.* 154: 727–734 (1988).
76. Raha S, McEachern GE, Myint AT, Robinson BH. Superoxides from mitochondrial complex III: the role of manganese superoxide dismutase. *Free Radic. Biol. Med.* 29: 170–180 (2000).
77. Starkov AA, Fiskum G. Myxothiazol induces H_2O_2 production from mitochondrial respiratory chain. *Biochem. Biophys. Res. Commun.* 281: 645–650 (2001).
78. Ksenzenko M, Konstantinov AA, Khomutov GB, Tikhonov AN, Ruuge EK. Relationships between the effects of redox potential, alphathenoyltrifluoroacetone and malonate on O_2 and H_2O_2 generation by submitochondrial particles in the presence of succinate and antimycin. *FEBS Lett.* 175: 105–108 (1984).

79. Muller F, Crofts AR, Kramer DM. Multiple Q-cycle bypass reactions at the Qo site of the cytochrome bc1 complex. *Biochemistry* 41: 7866–7874 (2002).
80. Muller FL, Roberts AG, Bowman MK, Kramer DM. Architecture of the Qo site of the cytochrome bc1 complex probed by superoxide production. *Biochemistry* 42: 6493–6499 (2003).
81. Sun J, Trumpower BL. Superoxide anion generation by the cytochrome bc1 complex. *Arch. Biochem. Biophys.* 419: 198–206 (2003).
82. Nohl H, Hegner D. Do mitochondria produce oxygen radicals *in vivo*? *Eur. J. Biochem.* 82: 563–567 (1978).
83. Miller RW, Rapp U. The oxidation of catechols by reduced flavins and dehydrogenases. An electron spin resonance study of the kinetics and initial products of oxidation. *J. Biol. Chem.* 248: 6084–6090 (1973).
84. Lynch RE, Fridovich I. Permeation of the erythrocyte stroma by superoxide radical. *J. Biol. Chem.* 253: 4697–4699 (1978).
85. Gus'kova RA, Ivanov, II, Kol'tover VK, Akhobadze VV, Rubin AB. Permeability of bilayer lipid membranes for superoxide ($O^{2-\bullet}$) radicals. *Biochim. Biophys. Acta* 778: 579–585 (1984).
86. Mao GD, Poznansky MJ. Electron spin resonance study on the permeability of superoxide radicals in lipid bilayers and biological membranes. *FEBS Lett.* 305: 233–236 (1992).
87. Takahashi MA, Asada K. Superoxide anion permeability of phospholipid membranes and chloroplast thylakoids. *Arch. Biochem. Biophys.* 226: 558–566 (1983).
88. Frimer AA, Strul G, Buch J, Gottlieb HE. Can superoxide organic chemistry be observed within the liposomal bilayer? *Free Radic. Biol. Med.* 20: 843–852 (1996).
89. Han D, Williams E, Cadenas E. Mitochondrial respiratory chain-dependent generation of superoxide anion and its release into the intermembrane space. *Biochem. J.* 353: 411–416 (2001).
90. St-Pierre J, Buckingham JA, Roebuck SJ, Brand MD. Topology of superoxide production from different sites in the mitochondrial electron transport chain. *J. Biol. Chem.* 277: 44784–44790 (2002).
91. Loschen G, Flohe L, Chance B. Respiratory chain linked H_2O_2 production in pigeon heart mitochondria. *FEBS Lett.* 18: 261–264 (1971).
92. Cadenas E, Boveris A. Enhancement of hydrogen peroxide formation by protophores and ionophores in antimycin-supplemented mitochondria. *Biochem. J.* 188: 31–37 (1980).

93. Klingenberg M, Rottenberg H. Relation between the gradient of the ATP/ADP ratio and the membrane potential across the mitochondrial membrane. *Eur. J. Biochem.* 73: 125–130 (1977).
94. Nohl H, Gille L, Schonheit K, Liu Y. Conditions allowing redox-cycling ubisemiquinone in mitochondria to establish a direct redox couple with molecular oxygen. *Free Radic. Biol. Med.* 20: 207–213 (1996).
95. Skulachev VP. Role of uncoupled and non-coupled oxidations in maintenance of safely low levels of oxygen and its one-electron reductants. *Q. Rev. Biophys.* 29: 169–202 (1996).
96. Packer L, Weber SU, Rimbach G. Molecular aspects of alpha-tocotrienol antioxidant action and cell signalling. *J. Nutr.* 131: 369S–373S (2001).
97. Lass A, Forster MJ, Sohal RS. Effects of coenzyme Q10 and alpha-tocopherol administration on their tissue levels in the mouse: elevation of mitochondrial alpha-tocopherol by coenzyme Q10. *Free Radic. Biol. Med.* 26: 1375–1382 (1999).
98. Thomas JP, Maiorino M, Ursini F, Girotti AW. Protective action of phospholipid hydroperoxide glutathione peroxidase against membrane-damaging lipid peroxidation. *In situ* reduction of phospholipid and cholesterol hydroperoxides. *J. Biol. Chem.* 265: 454–461 (1990).
99. Maiorino M, Thomas JP, Girotti AW, Ursini F. Reactivity of phospholipid hydroperoxide glutathione peroxidase with membrane and lipoprotein lipid hydroperoxides. *Free Radic. Res. Commun.* 12–13 (Pt 1): 131–135 (1991).
100. Bao Y, Jemth P, Mannervik B, Williamson G. Reduction of thymine hydroperoxide by phospholipid hydroperoxide glutathione peroxidase and glutathione transferases. *FEBS Lett.* 410: 210–212 (1997).
101. Imai H, Nakagawa Y. Biological significance of phospholipid hydroperoxide glutathione peroxidase (PHGPx, GPx4) in mammalian cells. *Free Radic. Biol. Med.* 34: 145–169 (2003).
102. Yant LJ, Ran Q, Rao L, Van Remmen H, Shibatani T, Belter JG, Motta L, Richardson A, Prolla TA. The selenoprotein GPX4 is essential for mouse development and protects from radiation and oxidative damage insults. *Free Radic. Biol. Med.* 34: 496–502 (2003).
103. Arai M, Imai H, Koumura T, Yoshida M, Emoto K, Umeda M, Chiba N, Nakagawa Y. Mitochondrial phospholipid hydroperoxide glutathione peroxidase plays a major role in preventing oxidative injury to cells. *J. Biol. Chem.* 274: 4924–4933 (1999).
104. Nomura K, Imai H, Koumura T, Kobayashi T, Nakagawa Y. Mitochondrial phospholipid hydroperoxide glutathione peroxidase inhibits the release of

cytochrome c from mitochondria by suppressing the peroxidation of cardiolipin in hypoglycaemia-induced apoptosis. *Biochem. J.* 351: 183–193 (2000).

105. Esposito LA, Kokoszka JE, Waymire KG, Cottrell B, MacGregor GR, Wallace DC. Mitochondrial oxidative stress in mice lacking the glutathione peroxidase-1 gene. *Free Radic. Biol. Med.* 28: 754–766 (2000).
106. Knopp EA, Arndt TL, Eng KL, Caldwell M, LeBoeuf RC, Deeb SS, O'Brien KD. Murine phospholipid hydroperoxide glutathione peroxidase: cDNA sequence, tissue expression, and mapping. *Mamm. Genome.* 10: 601–605 (1999).
107. Pushpa-Rekha TR, Burdsall AL, Oleksa LM, Chisolm GM, Driscoll DM. Rat phospholipid-hydroperoxide glutathione peroxidase. cDNA cloning and identification of multiple transcription and translation start sites. *J. Biol. Chem.* 270: 26993–26999 (1995).
108. Panfili E, Sandri G, Ernster L. Distribution of glutathione peroxidases and glutathione reductase in rat brain mitochondria. *FEBS Lett.* 290: 35–37 (1991).
109. Godeas C, Sandri G, Panfili E. Distribution of phospholipid hydroperoxide glutathione peroxidase (PHGPx) in rat testis mitochondria. *Biochim. Biophys. Acta* 1191: 147–150 (1994).
110. Gardner PR, Raineri I, Epstein LB, White CW. Superoxide radical and iron modulate aconitase activity in mammalian cells. *J. Biol. Chem.* 270: 13399–13405 (1995).
111. Li Y, Huang TT, Carlson EJ, Melov S, Ursell PC, Olson JL, Noble LJ, Yoshimura MP, Berger C, Chan PH *et al.* Dilated cardiomyopathy and neonatal lethality in mutant mice lacking manganese superoxide dismutase. *Nat. Genet.* 11: 376–381 (1995).
112. Lebovitz RM, Zhang H, Vogel H, Cartwright J, Jr, Dionne L, Lu N, Huang S, Matzuk MM. Neurodegeneration, myocardial injury, and perinatal death in mitochondrial superoxide dismutase-deficient mice. *Proc. Natl. Acad. Sci. USA* 93: 9782–9787 (1996).
113. Tsan MF, White JE, Caska B, Epstein CJ, Lee CY. Susceptibility of heterozygous MnSOD gene-knockout mice to oxygen toxicity. *Am. J. Respir. Cell. Mol. Biol.* 19: 114–120 (1998).
114. Jackson RM, Helton ES, Viera L, Ohman T. Survival, lung injury, and lung protein nitration in heterozygous MnSOD knockout mice in hyperoxia. *Exp. Lung. Res.* 25: 631–646 (1999).
115. Van Remmen H, Ikeno Y, Hamilton M, Pahlavani M, Wolf N, Thorpe SR, Alderson NL, Baynes JW, Epstein CJ, Huang TT, Nelson J, Strong R, Richardson A. Life-long reduction in MnSOD activity results in increased

DNA damage and higher incidence of cancer but does not accelerate aging. *Physiol. Genomics* 16: 29–37 (2003).
116. Van Remmen H, Williams MD, Guo Z, Estlack L, Yang H, Carlson EJ, Epstein CJ, Huang TT, Richardson A. Knockout mice heterozygous for Sod2 show alterations in cardiac mitochondrial function and apoptosis. *Am. J. Physiol. Heart. Circ. Physiol.* 281: H1422–1432 (2001).
117. Williams MD, Van Remmen H, Conrad CC, Huang TT, Epstein CJ, Richardson A. Increased oxidative damage is correlated to altered mitochondrial function in heterozygous manganese superoxide dismutase knockout mice. *J. Biol. Chem.* 273: 28510–28515 (1998).
118. Van Remmen H, Salvador C, Yang H, Huang TT, Epstein CJ, Richardson A. Characterization of the antioxidant status of the heterozygous manganese superoxide dismutase knockout mouse. *Arch. Biochem. Biophys.* 363: 91–97 (1999).
119. Raineri I, Carlson EJ, Gacayan R, Carra S, Oberley TD, Huang TT, Epstein CJ. Strain-dependent high-level expression of a transgene for manganese superoxide dismutase is associated with growth retardation and decreased fertility. *Free Radic. Biol. Med.* 31: 1018–1030 (2001).
120. Hackenbrock CR, Chazotte B, Gupte SS. The random collision model and a critical assessment of diffusion and collision in mitochondrial electron transport. *J. Bioenerg. Biomembr.* 18: 331–368 (1986).
121. McCord JM, Fridovich I. The utility of superoxide dismutase in studying free radical reactions. II. The mechanism of the mediation of cytochrome c reduction by a variety of electron carriers. *J. Biol. Chem.* 245: 1374–1377 (1970).
122. Korshunov SS, Krasnikov BF, Pereverzev MO, Skulachev VP. The antioxidant functions of cytochrome c. *FEBS Lett.* 462: 192–198 (1999).
123. Mailer K. Superoxide radical as electron donor for oxidative phosphorylation of ADP. *Biochem. Biophys. Res. Commun.* 170: 59–64 (1990).
124. Ho YS, Xiong Y, Ma W, Spector A, Ho DS. Mice lacking catalase develop normally but show differential sensitivity to oxidant tissue injury. *J. Biol. Chem.* 279: 32804–32812 (2004).
125. Radi R, Turrens JF, Chang LY, Bush KM, Crapo JD, Freeman BA. Detection of catalase in rat heart mitochondria. *J. Biol. Chem.* 266: 22028–22034 (1991).
126. Del Maestro R, McDonald W. Subcellular localization of superoxide dismutases, glutathione peroxidase and catalase in developing rat cerebral cortex. *Mech. Ageing. Dev.* 48: 15–31 (1989).

127. Antunes F, Han D, Cadenas E. Relative contributions of heart mitochondria glutathione peroxidase and catalase to H_2O_2 detoxification in *in vivo* conditions. *Free Radic. Biol. Med.* 33: 1260–1267 (2002).
128. Dringen R. Metabolism and functions of glutathione in brain. *Prog. Neurobiol.* 62: 649–671 (2000).
129. Pastore A, Federici G, Bertini E, Piemonte F. Analysis of glutathione: implication in redox and detoxification. *Clin. Chim. Acta* 333: 19–39 (2003).
130. Wahllander A, Soboll S, Sies H, Linke I, Muller M. Hepatic mitochondrial and cytosolic glutathione content and the subcellular distribution of GSH-S-transferases. *FEBS Lett.* 97: 138–140 (1979).
131. Griffith OW, Meister A. Origin and turnover of mitochondrial glutathione. *Proc. Natl. Acad. Sci. USA* 82: 4668–4672 (1985).
132. Martensson J, Lai JC, Meister A. High-affinity transport of glutathione is part of a multicomponent system essential for mitochondrial function. *Proc. Natl. Acad. Sci. USA* 87: 7185–7189 (1990).
133. Chen Z, Lash LH. Evidence for mitochondrial uptake of glutathione by dicarboxylate and 2-oxoglutarate carriers. *J. Pharmacol. Exp. Ther.* 285: 608–618 (1998).
134. Rebrin I, Kamzalov S, Sohal RS. Effects of age and caloric restriction on glutathione redox state in mice. *Free Radic. Biol. Med.* 35: 626–635 (2003).
135. Vogel R, Wiesinger H, Hamprecht B, Dringen R. The regeneration of reduced glutathione in rat forebrain mitochondria identifies metabolic pathways providing the NADPH required. *Neurosci. Lett.* 275: 97–100 (1999).
136. Boveris A, Cadenas E. *Cellular Sources and Steady-State Levels of Reactive Oxygen Species*. Marcel Dekker, New York, 1997.
137. Han D, Canali R, Rettori D, Kaplowitz N. Effect of glutathione depletion on sites and topology of superoxide and hydrogen peroxide production in mitochondria. *Mol. Pharmacol.* 64: 1136–1144 (2003).
138. Raza H, Robin MA, Fang JK, Avadhani NG. Multiple isoforms of mitochondrial glutathione S-transferases and their differential induction under oxidative stress. *Biochem. J.* 366: 45–55 (2002).
139. Olafsdottir K, Reed DJ. Retention of oxidized glutathione by isolated rat liver mitochondria during hydroperoxide treatment. *Biochim. Biophys. Acta* 964: 377–382 (1988).
140. Kozhemiakin LA, Bulavin DV, Udintsev AV, Smirnov VV. The subcellular distribution of the glutathione system enzymes in the brain tissue of the rat. *Tsitologiia* 35: 58–63 (1993).
141. Kelner MJ, Montoya MA. Structural organization of the human glutathione reductase gene: determination of correct cDNA sequence and identification

of a mitochondrial leader sequence. *Biochem. Biophys. Res. Commun.* 269: 366–368 (2000).

142. Zoccarato F, Cavallini L, Alexandre A. Respiration-dependent removal of exogenous H_2O_2 in brain mitochondria: inhibition by Ca^{2+}. *J. Biol. Chem.* 279: 4166–4174 (2004).
143. Hoek JB, Rydstrom J. Physiological roles of nicotinamide nucleotide transhydrogenase. *Biochem. J.* 254: 1–10 (1988).
144. Arkblad EL, Egorov M, Shakhparonov M, Romanova L, Polzikov M, Rydstrom J. Expression of proton-pumping nicotinamide nucleotide transhydrogenase in mouse, human brain and C elegans. *Comp. Biochem. Physiol. B Biochem. Mol. Biol.* 133: 13–21 (2002).
145. Bernstine EG. Genetic control of mitochondrial malic enzyme in mouse brain. *J. Biol. Chem.* 254: 83–87 (1979).
146. Stein AM, Stein JH, Kirkman SK. Diphosphopyridine nucleotide specific isocitric dehydrogenase of mammalian mitochondria. I. On the roles of pyridine nucleotide transhydrogenase and the isocitric dehydrogenases in the respiration of mitochondria of normal and neoplastic tissues. *Biochemistry* 6: 1370–1379 (1967).
147. Kirsch M, De Groot H. NAD(P)H, a directly operating antioxidant? *FASEB J.* 15: 1569–1574 (2001).
148. Tischler ME, Hecht P, Williamson JR. Effect of ammonia on mitochondrial and cytosolic NADH and NADPH systems in isolated rat liver cells. *FEBS Lett.* 76: 99–104 (1977).
149. Lenzen S, Drinkgern J, Tiedge M. Low antioxidant enzyme gene expression in pancreatic islets compared with various other mouse tissues. *Free Radic. Biol. Med.* 20: 463–466 (1996).
150. Utsunomiya H, Komatsu N, Yoshimura S, Tsutsumi Y, Watanabe K. Exact ultrastructural localization of glutathione peroxidase in normal rat hepatocytes: advantages of microwave fixation. *J. Histochem. Cytochem.* 39: 1167–1174 (1991).
151. Asayama K, Yokota S, Dobashi K, Hayashibe H, Kawaoi A, Nakazawa S. Purification and immunoelectron microscopic localization of cellular glutathione peroxidase in rat hepatocytes: quantitative analysis by postembedding method. *Histochemistry* 102: 213–219 (1994).
152. Esworthy RS, Ho YS, Chu FF. The Gpx1 gene encodes mitochondrial glutathione peroxidase in the mouse liver. *Arch. Biochem. Biophys.* 340: 59–63 (1997).
153. Chance B, Sies H, Boveris A. Hydroperoxide metabolism in mammalian organs. *Physiol. Rev.* 59: 527–605 (1979).

154. Mirault ME, Tremblay A, Beaudoin N, Tremblay M. Overexpression of seleno-glutathione peroxidase by gene transfer enhances the resistance of T47D human breast cells to clastogenic oxidants. *J. Biol. Chem.* 266: 20752–20760 (1991).
155. Sies H, Sharov VS, Klotz LO, Briviba K. Glutathione peroxidase protects against peroxynitrite-mediated oxidations. A new function for selenoproteins as peroxynitrite reductase. *J. Biol. Chem.* 272: 27812–27817 (1997).
156. Spector A, Yang Y, Ho YS, Magnenat JL, Wang RR, Ma W, Li WC. Variation in cellular glutathione peroxidase activity in lens epithelial cells, transgenics and knockouts does not significantly change the response to H_2O_2 stress. *Exp. Eye Res.* 62: 521–540 (1996).
157. Cheng WH, Ho YS, Ross DA, Valentine BA, Combs GF, Lei XG. Cellular glutathione peroxidase knockout mice express normal levels of selenium-dependent plasma and phospholipid hydroperoxide glutathione peroxidases in various tissues. *J. Nutr.* 127: 1445–1450 (1997).
158. Ho YS, Magnenat JL, Bronson RT, Cao J, Gargano M, Sugawara M, Funk CD. Mice deficient in cellular glutathione peroxidase develop normally and show no increased sensitivity to hyperoxia. *J. Biol. Chem.* 272: 16644–16651 (1997).
159. Cheng WH, Ho YS, Valentine BA, Ross DA, Combs GF, Jr, Lei XG. Cellular glutathione peroxidase is the mediator of body selenium to protect against paraquat lethality in transgenic mice. *J. Nutr.* 128: 1070–1076 (1998).
160. de Haan JB, Bladier C, Griffiths P, Kelner M, O'Shea RD, Cheung NS, Bronson RT, Silvestro MJ, Wild S, Zheng SS, Beart PM, Hertzog PJ, Kola I. Mice with a homozygous null mutation for the most abundant glutathione peroxidase, Gpx1, show increased susceptibility to the oxidative stress-inducing agents paraquat and hydrogen peroxide. *J. Biol. Chem.* 273: 22528–22536 (1998).
161. Klivenyi P, Andreassen OA, Ferrante RJ, Dedeoglu A, Mueller G, Lancelot E, Bogdanov M, Andersen JK, Jiang D, Beal MF. Mice deficient in cellular glutathione peroxidase show increased vulnerability to malonate, 3-nitropropionic acid, and 1-methyl-4-phenyl-1,2,5,6-tetrahydropyridine. *J. Neurosci.* 20: 1–7 (2000).
162. Zhang J, Graham DG, Montine TJ, Ho YS. Enhanced N-methyl-4-phenyl-1,2,3,6-tetrahydropyridine toxicity in mice deficient in CuZn-superoxide dismutase or glutathione peroxidase. *J. Neuropathol. Exp. Neurol.* 59: 53–61 (2000).
163. Fujii J, Ikeda Y. Advances in our understanding of peroxiredoxin, a multi-functional, mammalian redox protein. *Redox. Rep.* 7: 123–130 (2002).

164. Wood ZA, Schroder E, Robin Harris J, Poole LB. Structure, mechanism and regulation of peroxiredoxins. *Trends Biochem. Sci.* 28: 32–40 (2003).
165. Chae HZ, Kim HJ, Kang SW, Rhee SG. Characterization of three isoforms of mammalian peroxiredoxin that reduce peroxides in the presence of thioredoxin. *Diabetes Res. Clin. Pract.* 45: 101–112 (1999).
166. Leyens G, Donnay I, Knoops B. Cloning of bovine peroxiredoxins-gene expression in bovine tissues and amino acid sequence comparison with rat, mouse and primate peroxiredoxins. *Comp. Biochem. Physiol. B Biochem. Mol. Biol.* 136: 943–955 (2003).
167. Araki M, Nanri H, Ejima K, Murasato Y, Fujiwara T, Nakashima Y, Ikeda M. Antioxidant function of the mitochondrial protein SP-22 in the cardiovascular system. *J. Biol. Chem.* 274: 2271–2278 (1999).
168. Hattori F, Murayama N, Noshita T, Oikawa S. Mitochondrial peroxiredoxin-3 protects hippocampal neurons from excitotoxic injury *in vivo*. *J. Neurochem.* 86: 860–868 (2003).
169. Banmeyer I, Marchand C, Verhaeghe C, Vucic B, Rees JF, Knoops B. Overexpression of human peroxiredoxin 5 in subcellular compartments of Chinese hamster ovary cells: effects on cytotoxicity and DNA damage caused by peroxides. *Free Radic. Biol. Med.* 36: 65–77 (2004).
170. Johansson C, Lillig CH, Holmgren A. Human mitochondrial glutaredoxin reduces S-glutathionylated proteins with high affinity accepting electrons from either glutathione or thioredoxin reductase. *J. Biol. Chem.* 279: 7537–7543 (2004).
171. Fernandes AP, Holmgren A. Glutaredoxins: glutathione-dependent redox enzymes with functions far beyond a simple thioredoxin backup system. *Antioxid. Redox. Signal* 6: 63–74 (2004).
172. Gromer S, Urig S, Becker K. The thioredoxin system — from science to clinic. *Med. Res. Rev.* 24: 40–89 (2004).
173. Jurado J, Prieto-Alamo MJ, Madrid-Risquez J, Pueyo C. Absolute gene expression patterns of thioredoxin and glutaredoxin redox systems in mouse. *J. Biol. Chem.* 278: 45546–45554 (2003).
174. Nonn L, Williams RR, Erickson RP, Powis G. The absence of mitochondrial thioredoxin 2 causes massive apoptosis, exencephaly, and early embryonic lethality in homozygous mice. *Mol. Cell. Biol.* 23: 916–922 (2003).
175. Patenaude A, Murthy MR, Mirault ME. Mitochondrial thioredoxin system: effects of TrxR2 overexpression on redox balance, cell growth, and apoptosis. *J. Biol. Chem.* 279: 27302–27314 (2004).
176. Droge W. Free radicals in the physiological control of cell function. *Physiol. Rev.* 82: 47–95 (2002).

177. Pitkanen S, Robinson BH. Mitochondrial complex I deficiency leads to increased production of superoxide radicals and induction of superoxide dismutase. *J. Clin. Invest.* 98: 345–351 (1996).
178. Swerdlow RH, Parks JK, Miller SW, Tuttle JB, Trimmer PA, Sheehan JP, Bennett JP, Jr, Davis RE, Parker WD, Jr. Origin and functional consequences of the complex I defect in Parkinson's disease. *Ann. Neurol.* 40: 663–671 (1996).
179. Luo X, Pitkanen S, Kassovska-Bratinova S, Robinson BH, Lehotay DC. Excessive formation of hydroxyl radicals and aldehydic lipid peroxidation products in cultured skin fibroblasts from patients with complex I deficiency. *J. Clin. Invest.* 99: 2877–2882 (1997).
180. Barrientos A, Moraes CT. Titrating the effects of mitochondrial complex I impairment in the cell physiology. *J. Biol. Chem.* 274: 16188–16197 (1999).
181. Genova ML, Pich MM, Bernacchia A, Bianchi C, Biondi A, Bovina C, Falasca AI, Formiggini G, Castelli GP, Lenaz G. The mitochondrial production of reactive oxygen species in relation to aging and pathology. *Ann. NY Acad. Sci.* 1011: 86–100 (2004).
182. Rana M, de Coo I, Diaz F, Smeets H, Moraes CT. An out-of-frame cytochrome b gene deletion from a patient with Parkinsonism is associated with impaired complex III assembly and an increase in free radical production. *Ann. Neurol.* 48: 774–781 (2000).
183. Mattiazzi M, Vijayvergiya C, Gajewski CD, DeVivo DC, Lenaz G, Wiedmann M, Manfredi G. The mtDNA T8993G (NARP) mutation results in an impairment of oxidative phosphorylation that can be improved by antioxidants. *Hum. Mol. Genet.* 13: 869–879 (2004).
184. Becker LB. New concepts in reactive oxygen species and cardiovascular reperfusion physiology. *Cardiovasc. Res.* 61: 461–470 (2004).
185. Ledenev AN, Ruuge EK. Generation of superoxide radicals by ischemic heart mitochondria. *Bull. Eksp. Biol. Med.* 100: 303–305 (1985).
186. Turrens JF, Beconi M, Barilla J, Chavez UB, McCord JM. Mitochondrial generation of oxygen radicals during reoxygenation of ischemic tissues. *Free Radic. Res. Commun.* 12–13 (Pt 2): 681–689 (1991).
187. Petrosillo G, Ruggiero FM, Di Venosa N, Paradies G. Decreased complex III activity in mitochondria isolated from rat heart subjected to ischemia and reperfusion: role of reactive oxygen species and cardiolipin. *FASEB. J.* 17: 714–716 (2003).
188. Paradies G, Petrosillo G, Pistolese M, Di Venosa N, Federici A, Ruggiero FM. Decrease in mitochondrial complex I activity in ischemic/reperfused rat

heart: involvement of reactive oxygen species and cardiolipin. *Circ. Res.* 94: 53–59 (2004).

189. Du G, Mouithys-Mickalad A, Sluse FE. Generation of superoxide anion by mitochondria and impairment of their functions during anoxia and reoxygenation *in vitro*. *Free Radic. Biol. Med.* 25: 1066–1074 (1998).
190. Cino M, Del Maestro RF. Generation of hydrogen peroxide by brain mitochondria: the effect of reoxygenation following postdecapitative ischemia. *Arch. Biochem. Biophys.* 269: 623–638 (1989).
191. Dux E, Mies G, Hossmann KA, Siklos L. Calcium in the mitochondria following brief ischemia of gerbil brain. *Neurosci. Lett.* 78: 295–300 (1987).
192. Zaidan E, Sims NR. The calcium content of mitochondria from brain subregions following short-term forebrain ischemia and recirculation in the rat. *J. Neurochem.* 63: 1812–1819 (1994).
193. Fiskum G. Mitochondrial participation in ischemic and traumatic neural cell death. *J. Neurotrauma.* 17: 843–855 (2000).
194. Nicholls DG, Budd SL. Mitochondria and neuronal survival. *Physiol. Rev.* 80: 315–360 (2000).
195. Starkov AA, Polster BM, Fiskum G. Regulation of hydrogen peroxide production by brain mitochondria by calcium and Bax. *J. Neurochem.* 83: 220–228 (2002).
196. Hansford RG, Zorov D. Role of mitochondrial calcium transport in the control of substrate oxidation. *Mol. Cell. Biochem.* 184: 359–369 (1998).
197. Vandecasteele G, Szabadkai G, Rizzuto R. Mitochondrial calcium homeostasis: mechanisms and molecules. *IUBMB Life* 52: 213–219 (2001).
198. Lai JC, Cooper AJ. Brain alpha-ketoglutarate dehydrogenase complex: kinetic properties, regional distribution, and effects of inhibitors. *J. Neurochem.* 47: 1376–1386 (1986).
199. Lai JC, DiLorenzo JC, Sheu KF. Pyruvate dehydrogenase complex is inhibited in calcium-loaded cerebrocortical mitochondria. *Neurochem. Res.* 13: 1043–1048 (1988).
200. Villalobo A, Lehninger AL. Inhibition of oxidative phosphorylation in ascites tumor mitochondria and cells by intramitochondrial Ca^{2+}. *J. Biol. Chem.* 255: 2457–2464 (1980).
201. Roman I, Clark A, Swanson PD. The interaction of calcium transport and ADP phosphorylation in brain mitochondria. *Membr. Biochem.* 4: 1–9 (1981).
202. Zoratti M, Szabo I. The mitochondrial permeability transition. *Biochim. Biophys. Acta* 1241: 139–176 (1995).

203. Lemasters JJ, Nieminen AL, Qian T, Trost LC, Herman B. The mitochondrial permeability transition in toxic, hypoxic and reperfusion injury. *Mol. Cell. Biochem.* 174: 159–165 (1997).
204. Lemasters JJ, Nieminen AL, Qian T, Trost LC, Elmore SP, Nishimura Y, Crowe RA, Cascio WE, Bradham CA, Brenner DA, Herman B. The mitochondrial permeability transition in cell death: a common mechanism in necrosis, apoptosis and autophagy. *Biochim. Biophys. Acta* 1366: 177–196 (1998).
205. Bernardi P, Scorrano L, Colonna R, Petronilli V, Di Lisa F. Mitochondria and cell death. Mechanistic aspects and methodological issues. *Eur. J. Biochem.* 264: 687–701 (1999).
206. He L, Lemasters JJ. Regulated and unregulated mitochondrial permeability transition pores: a new paradigm of pore structure and function? *FEBS Lett.* 512: 1–7 (2002).
207. Di Lisa F, Menabo R, Canton M, Barile M, Bernardi P. Opening of the mitochondrial permeability transition pore causes depletion of mitochondrial and cytosolic NAD^+ and is a causative event in the death of myocytes in post-ischemic reperfusion of the heart. *J. Biol. Chem.* 276: 2571–2575 (2001).
208. Anderson MF, Sims NR. The effects of focal ischemia and reperfusion on the glutathione content of mitochondria from rat brain subregions. *J. Neurochem.* 81: 541–549 (2002).
209. Maciel EN, Vercesi AE, Castilho RF. Oxidative stress in Ca^{2+}-induced membrane permeability transition in brain mitochondria. *J. Neurochem.* 79: 1237–1245 (2001).
210. Perez Velazquez JL, Frantseva MV, Carlen PL. *In vitro* ischemia promotes glutamate-mediated free radical generation and intracellular calcium accumulation in hippocampal pyramidal neurons. *J. Neurosci.* 17: 9085–9094 (1997).
211. Zorov DB, Filburn CR, Klotz LO, Zweier JL, Sollott SJ. Reactive oxygen species (ROS)-induced ROS release: a new phenomenon accompanying induction of the mitochondrial permeability transition in cardiac myocytes. *J. Exp. Med.* 192: 1001–1014 (2000).

2 Intracellular Oxidative Stress Caused by Ionizing Radiation

Hideyuki J. Majima, Hiroko P. Indo, Kazuo Tomita, Shigeaki Suenaga, Shigeatsu Motoori, Hirotoshi Kato, Hsiu-Chuan Yen, and Toshihiko Ozawa

1. The Effects of Radiation on Mammalian Cells

The effects of radiation on cells and the consequences have been studied for more than 40 years. It has been concluded that a major target is DNA, and the mechanism of cell death is related to double strand breaks (dsb).[1] The process of cell death involves two mechanisms: direct action in which radiation is absorbed in a cell directly by DNA, and indirect effects in which radiation interacts with other atoms or molecules in the cell (particularly water) to produce free radicals that are able to diffuse far enough to reach and damage the critical targets, e.g. DNA, and may result in cell death (Fig. 1).[1,2]

Ito tried to quantify ionization processes and the number of $HO^{\bullet}$ radicals produced by 1 Gy ionizing irradiation by simulating the electron track using a Monte Carlo program (ETRACK).[2] The mammalian cell nucleus (3–10 μm diameter) contains as much as 3×10^9 nucleotide pairs (1.9×10^{12} Dalton, 3.1 pg) of DNA. The number of ionizing events and the subsequent reactive oxygen species (ROS) created in the cell nucleus are proportional to the absorbed dose. For example, taking into account a cell nucleus diameter of 5 μm (65 pg as water equivalent), which receives an absorbed dose of 1 Gy, there are $\sim 1.36 \times 10^4$ ionizing hits [assuming G(ion) value = 3.3] and $\sim 8.87 \times 10^3$ $HO^{\bullet}$ radicals ($G(HO^{\bullet})$ value = 2.95) after initial recombination within the spur in the cell nucleus. A single strand break (ssb)

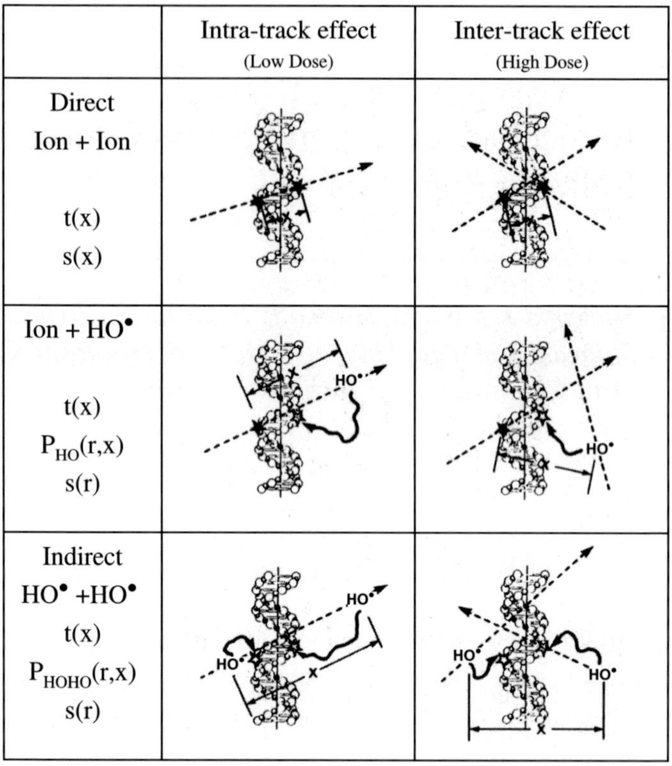

	Intra-track effect (Low Dose)	Inter-track effect (High Dose)
Direct Ion + Ion t(x) s(x)		
Ion + HO$^{\bullet}$ t(x) P_{HO}(r,x) s(r)		
Indirect HO$^{\bullet}$ +HO$^{\bullet}$ t(x) P_{HOHO}(r,x) s(r)		

Fig. 1. A model of the dsb breaks of DNA with electron tracks. Direct action through ionization hits and indirect action through HO$^{\bullet}$ radicals are considered. Also, the intratrack effect and the intertrack effect are treated separately.[2]

is assumed to take place through either ionization or HO$^{\bullet}$ radical hits on the molecules composing the backbone of the DNA strand (–O–P–O–C_5–C_4–C_3–). As a first approximation, the ssb probability is assumed to be proportional to the mass of the backbone of DNA. Under such simplified conditions, 360 ssbs (cell^{-1} Gy^{-1}) are created randomly by ionization hits, and 235 ssbs (cell^{-1} Gy^{-1}) by HO$^{\bullet}$ radicals, in the cell nucleus. These results are consistent with the experimental values of the ssb frequency (several hundreds of ssbs cell^{-1} Gy^{-1}).[3] A dsb takes place around an ssb when a second ssb occurs in close proximity. Figure 1 shows models of dsbs of DNA. They are categorized as intratrack effects, single-track effects, and intertrack effects. In each case, the strand break mechanisms are classified as direct action and indirect action. The dsb probabilities of an intratrack effect were calculated for both direct and indirect actions by Ito.[4] The direct action (ion + ion) dsb probability is calculated and found to vary between 0.74 (^{60}Co) and 1.50 (523 eV) as the percentage of the total ssb. As the DNA dsb target function, **S**(x), of finding the pair strand has the maximum probability at a distance between 1 and 2 nm, the dsb probability is higher for lower-energy electrons, whose hit distance is short. The direct action dsb depends on the track structure and cannot be influenced by chemical modifications. The probability of a dsb through indirect action is calculated to vary between 0.80 and 1.59 (ionization + $HO^\bullet$) and between 0.02 and 0.03 ($HO^\bullet + HO^\bullet$) as the percentage of the total ssb. Indirect dsbs occur more frequently than do direct dsbs because indirect action depends on the diffusion of the $HO^\bullet$ radical, which has a longer interaction distance, and the yield is strongly influenced by chemical modifiers such as radical scavengers or sensitizers around a DNA molecule. As indirect dsbs takes place more efficiently when the initial distance of hits is short, it also depends on the track structure. Thus, a lower-energy electron also has a higher yield of indirect dsbs. The number of indirect dsbs by produced $HO^\bullet + HO^\bullet$ is an order of magnitude smaller than that of dsbs produced by ion + $HO^\bullet$. The yield is linear with absorbed dose at low dose levels. The total dsb probability was calculated to be 1.56 and 1.69 times that of the total ssb value, for ^{60}Co and 280 kVp X-rays, respectively. The ratio for X-rays is comparable with the experimental value (irreparable strand break) of about 1% in mouse V79 cells.[3]

Free radical formation after irradiation has been studied by many researchers.[5] The formation of free radicals by ionizing radiation through indirect action would be as follows:[5]

$$
\begin{aligned}
H_2O &\xrightarrow{\text{irradiation}} H_2O^+ + e^- \\
e^- + H_2O &\longrightarrow H_2O^- \\
H_2O^+ &\longrightarrow H^+ + HO^\bullet \\
H_2O^- &\longrightarrow H^\bullet + HO^- \\
H^\bullet + H^\bullet &\longrightarrow H_2 \\
HO^\bullet + HO^\bullet &\longrightarrow H_2O_2 \\
H^\bullet + HO^\bullet &\longrightarrow H_2O \\
H_2O + H^\bullet &\longrightarrow H_2 + HO^\bullet \text{ (this equation might not be so important)} \\
H_2O_2 + HO^\bullet &\longrightarrow H_2O + HO_2^\bullet \text{ (hydroperoxyl radical)}
\end{aligned}
$$

And an organic substance (RH) will also react as

$$\mathrm{RH} + \mathrm{OH}^{\bullet} \longrightarrow \mathrm{R}^{\bullet} + \mathrm{H_2O}$$
$$\mathrm{RH} + \mathrm{H}^{\bullet} \longrightarrow \mathrm{R}^{\bullet} + \mathrm{H_2}$$
$$\mathrm{RH} \xrightarrow{\text{irradiation}} \mathrm{R}^{\bullet} + \mathrm{H}^{\bullet}.$$

Many free radicals readily react with oxygen, forming other reactive oxygen species (ROS). For example,

$$\begin{aligned}
\mathrm{O_2} + \mathrm{H}^{\bullet} &\longrightarrow \mathrm{HO_2^{\bullet}}\\
\mathrm{O_2} + \mathrm{e^-_{aq}} &\longrightarrow \mathrm{O_2^{\bullet -}}\\
\mathrm{O_2^{\bullet -}} + \mathrm{H^+} &\rightleftarrows \mathrm{HO_2^{\bullet}}\\
2\mathrm{HO_2^{\bullet}} &\longrightarrow \mathrm{H_2O_2} + \mathrm{O_2}\\
\mathrm{R}^{\bullet} + \mathrm{O_2} &\longrightarrow \mathrm{RO_2^{\bullet}}\\
\mathrm{RO_2^{\bullet}} + \mathrm{RH} &\longrightarrow \mathrm{RO_2H} + \mathrm{R}^{\bullet}.
\end{aligned}$$

As described above, ionizing radiation has been shown to generate ROS in a variety of cells.[6] Recent evidence suggests that ROS play an important role in cell death and signal transduction by ionizing radiation.[7] When water, the most abundant intracellular material, is exposed to ionizing radiation, decomposition reactions occur, which form a variety of free radicals and molecular products.[8] These products can peroxidize membrane lipids and attack proteins or DNA.[9] However, most ROS are hydroxyl radicals with a rate constant (k_{obs}) of $1.1 \times 10^{10}\,\mathrm{M^{-1}\,s^{-1}}$ for reaction with DNA; therefore the decay time is estimated to be nanoseconds.[5,10,11] Figure 2 shows a schematic of the timescale of radiation-induced events in mammalian cells.[11] It is believed that the initial cellular events caused by irradiation take place in microseconds and are followed by consequential DNA repair. However, recent studies have shown that other cytosol organelles, i.e. the cellular membrane, Golgi apparatus, endoplasmic reticulum, mitochondria, etc., are involved in the intracellular effects of radiation, in terms of transduction and translocation of cell death signals.[12,13]

Mechanisms of apoptosis[14] reveal two major pathways: (1) the FAS pathway and (2) the mitochondria pathway;[15,16] FAS is the death receptor pathway and the other is the mitochondrial pathway[15] (summarized in Fig. 3).

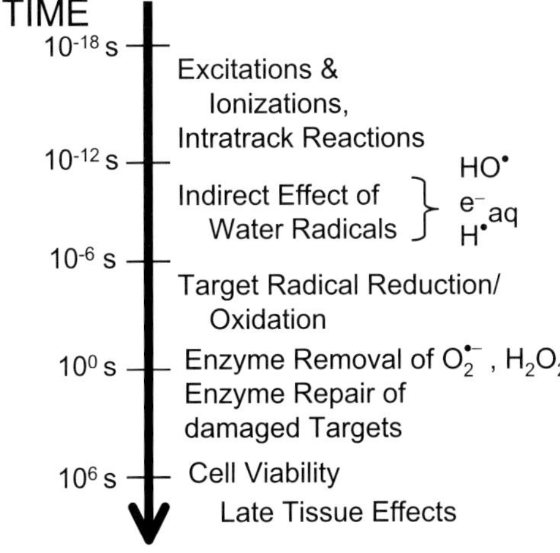

Fig. 2. A schematic of the timescale of radiation-induced events in mammalian cells.[11]

The death receptor pathway is triggered by members of the death receptor superfamily such as tumor necrosis factor receptor I (TNFR), TNF-related apoptosis inducing ligand receptor (TRAILR), and FAS/CD95. Binding of the FAS/CD95 ligand to FAS/CD95 induces receptor clustering and formation of a death-inducing signaling complex. This complex activates procaspase-8 to caspase-8 through FAS-associated death domain protein (FADD).[17] It has been shown that a cellular FADD like interleukin 1-converting enzyme inhibitory protein (c-FLIP) inhibits caspase-8 activation from procaspase-8.[18] Cell surface FAS-L is shed by matrix metalloproteases (MMPs)[19] and the activity is, in turn, tightly regulated by tissue inhibitor of metalloproteases (TIMs).[20] Ionizing radiation activates stress-activated protein kinase/jun amino terminal kinase (SAPK/JNK) pathways and leads to FAS expression.[21] Mitogen-activated protein kinase phosphatase 1 (MKP1, CL100) inhibits the activity of SAPK.[22]

The mitochondrial pathway is triggered in response to extracellular cues and internal insults such as DNA damage.[16] These diverse response pathways, including the activation of p53 and activation of bcl2-associated X protein (Bax), converge on mitochondria and result in cytochrome c

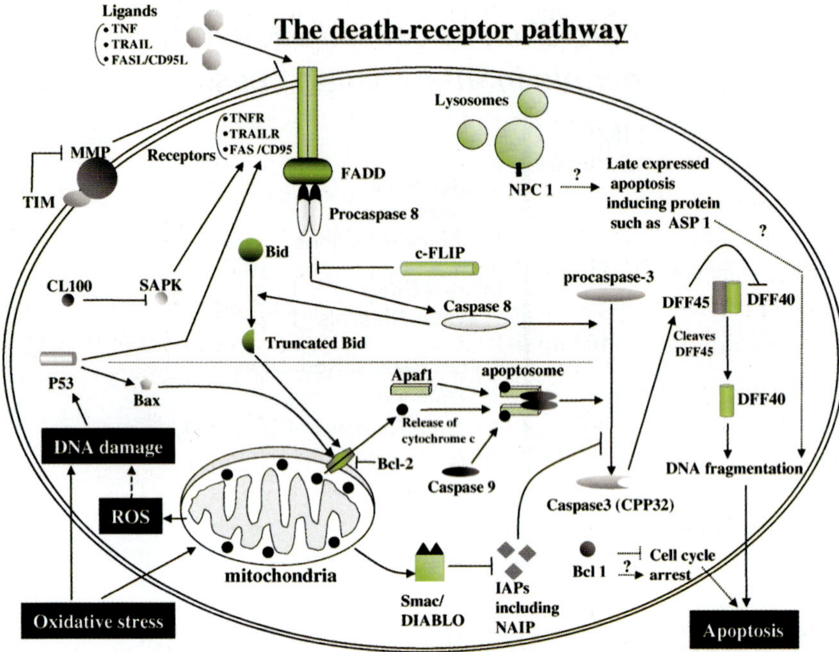

Fig. 3. Schematic diagram of two major apoptotic pathways: the death receptor pathway and the mitochondrial pathway. Binding ligands to death receptors triggers the death receptor pathway, and activation of the mitochondrial pathway is observed extensively in response to extracellular cues such as irradiation.

release from mitochondria.[15] Released cytochrome c binds to procaspase-9 and apoptotic protease activating factor 1 (Apaf-1) to form the apoptosome. Bcl2 is an apoptosis inhibitory protein that exists in mitochondria and inhibits cytochrome c release from the mitochondria.[23] Inhibitors of apoptosis proteins (IAPs) including neuronal apoptosis inhibitory protein (NAIP) are known to inhibit apoptosis and are antagonized by the second mitochondria-derived activator of caspase/direct inhibitor of apoptosis protein binding protein with the low PI (Smac/DIABLO) protein, which is released from mitochondria.[24–27] It has been reported that the BH3 interacting death domain agonist (Bid) provides the cross-talk and integration between the death receptor and mitochondrial pathways.[28]

After caspase-8 activation or apoptosome formation, the death receptor and mitochondrial pathways converge at the level of caspase-3 (cystein protease protein 32; CPP32) activation and progress apoptosis activating DNA fragmentation factor 40 (DFF40).[15,29] DNA fragmentation factor 45 (DFF45) is known to inhibit DFF40 and is cleaved by CPP32.[30] Expression of apoptosis-specific protein (ASP1) is a relatively late event in the apoptotic process, occurring downstream of caspase activity.[31] Niemann-Pick disease type C (NPC) is an inherited lipid storage disorder caused by mutations in the NPC 1 gene in humans.[32] The knockout mice of this gene die untimely during early postnatal development.[33] It has been reported that heterozygous mutation of this gene selectively blocks cholesterol trafficking to the endoplasmic reticulum (ER) and are protected from cholesterol-induced apoptosis.[34] Bcl 1 (cyclin D1) is the cell cycle regulator and is involved in apoptosis through its expression level.[35–37] Moreover, heat-shock proteins act at multiple steps in the pathway to modulate apoptosis (not shown in Fig. 3).[38,39]

2. Evidence of Intracellular Mitochondrial Generation of ROS Following Ionizing Irradiation and Subsequent Apoptosis

Mechanisms of apoptosis have been well studied, and two major pathways, i.e. the FAS and mitochondria pathways,[15,16] have been discovered as described above. However, it is not clear whether any ROS besides hydroxyl radicals generated by ionizing irradiation contribute to apoptosis. To answer this question, the authors performed a series of experiments to examine the relationships among intracellular ROS and nitric oxide (NO) generation, lipid peroxidation, and subsequent apoptosis.

A novel fluorescent probe, HPF, which detects intracellular ROS-generation, has been developed and has made it possible to detect selectively hydroxyl radicals and peroxynitrites.[40] Our studies showed clearly that intracellular ROS were generated during the irradiation and the extent of ROS increased as a function of time following irradiation, reaching a maximum at 2 hours after irradiation and declining thereafter (Fig. 4). These results indicate clearly that intracellular ROS increase after irradiation. Furthermore, our results clearly show that ROS are generated from

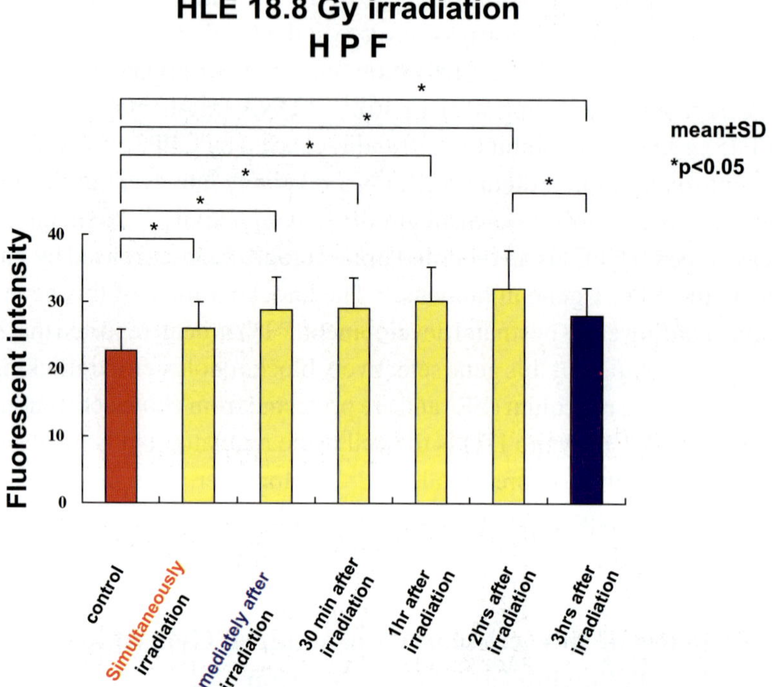

Fig. 4. The amount of intracellular ROS was detected using a novel fluorescent probe, HPF, which detects selectively hydroxyl radicals, using a confocal microscope. Intracellular ROS generated during the irradiation, and the amount of ROS, increased as a function of time following irradiation, reaching a maximum at 2 hours after irradiation and declining thereafter. It is noted that hydroxyl radicals produced by ionizing radiations should disappear in nanoseconds to microseconds (Fig. 2).[11] Surprisingly, the relative amounts of hydroxyl radicals detected at 2 h after irradiation were more easily and quantitatively detected compared with those detected during the irradiation.

mitochondria (Fig. 5). It is noted that hydroxyl radicals produced by ionizing radiation should disappear in nanoseconds to microseconds (Fig. 2).[11] Surprisingly, the relative amounts of hydroxyl radicals detected at 2 hours after irradiation were much more compared with those detected during the irradiation (Fig. 4).

ROS, such as superoxide, hydrogen peroxide, and hydroxyl radicals, are molecules that contain oxygen and have a higher reactivity than ground-state molecular oxygen. There was a suggestion that among these

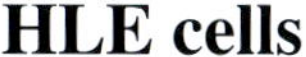

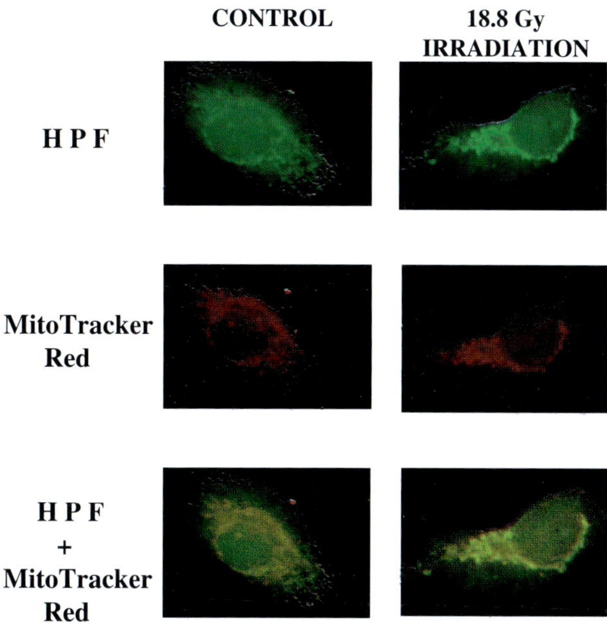

Fig. 5. Representative images of live cells examined for ROS detection using HPF in vector-transfected HLE cells (control cells) with or without X-irradiation. For the irradiated cells, ROS were examined 2 h after 18.8 Gy X-irradiation or at the peak times. To locate mitochondria, the same cells were stained with MitoTracker Red CMXRos. Merged double images of HPF and MitoTracker were obtained to identify ROS generation in mitochondria. Most of the ROS generation was localized in mitochondria, as shown by the yellow color (green plus red) in the double image of HPF fluorescence and Mitotracker. For irradiated cells, the HPF fluorescent image seemed increased.

free radicals, superoxide is a major factor in oxygen toxicity (superoxide theory of oxygen toxicity).[41,42] However, it has a limited reactivity with most biological molecules, raising questions about its toxicity *per se*.[43] To account for the toxicity of superoxide *in vivo*, the secondary generation of a more reactive hydroxyl radical is suggested to occur through a superoxide-assisted Fenton reaction. The production of a hydroxyl radical by this reaction needs the interaction of superoxide, hydroxyl peroxide, and a suitably chelated iron, all kept at low concentrations *in vivo* because of efficient defense systems. The rate constant for the reduction of Fe^{3+} by the superoxide has a wide range, from $<10^2$ to $10^9\ M^{-1}\ s^{-1}$.[44] It can be assumed that other cellular constituents, such as ascorbic acid, can reduce iron and are present in much higher concentrations than superoxide.[45] However, this study, using a novel fluorescent probe that specifically detected the hydroxyl radical and appeared to be generated from mitochondria (Fig. 4), suggests that hydroxyl radical production from superoxide is the superoxide-assisted Fenton reaction through the Haber–Weiss reaction. However, other reactions may play important roles in superoxide toxicity.

Among the reactions, the reaction between superoxide radicals and nitric oxide (NO) to form peroxynitrite has become the center of attention. Superoxide radicals can react with NO to form peroxynitrite with a high rate constant because NO contains an unpaired electron.[46] Peroxynitrite is a potent biological oxidant, which has recently been implicated in diverse forms of free radical-induced tissue injury.[47,48] The reaction of peroxynitrite with membrane lipid induces a phospholipid membrane peroxidation product without the need for iron.[49] A variety of aldehydes have been generated as final products when lipid hydroperoxides further react with iron ions or break down. Among them, 4-hydroxy-2-nonenal (HNE) is a highly toxic nine-carbon α,β-unsaturated aldehyde that can be generated by the peroxidation of ω-6-unsaturated fatty acids, such as arachidonic and linoleic acids.[50–52] In biological systems, HNE originates almost exclusively from phospholipid-bound arachidonic acid and may be the most reliable and sensitive marker of lipid peroxidation.[50] *In vitro* studies have revealed that at relatively high concentrations, HNE causes rapid cell death associated with the depletion of sulfhydryl groups, disturbances in calcium homeostasis, inhibition of key metabolic enzymes, and inhibition of protein and DNA synthesis.[50]

It is essential for aerobic organisms to possess enzymatic and non-enzymatic antioxidant defense systems that deal with ROS produced as a result of aerobic respiration. One important family of enzymes is that of superoxide dismutase (SOD) (EC 1.15.1.1).[53] This family of enzymes is a class of metalloproteins that catalyzes the dismutation of superoxide radicals into hydrogen peroxide and molecular oxygen.[41,42] Hydrogen peroxide is further degraded to water by other antioxidant enzymes, such as glutathione peroxidase (GPx) (EC 1.11.1.9) and catalase (EC 1.11.1.6). In mammalian cells, there are three types of superoxide dismutase: cytosolic CuZn superoxide dismutase (CuZnSOD), mitochondrial manganese superoxide dismutase (MnSOD),[54] and extracellular superoxide dismutase (ECSOD).[55]

Several studies have shown that mitochondria produce superoxide, mainly from complexes I and III of the electron transport system, which are located in the inner membrane of mitochondria.[56,57] Majima *et al.* reported the first evidence of MnSOD, which could protect against apoptosis.[58] Production of ROS from the electron transport chain may result in oxidative stress in cells and may result in apoptotic cell death.[58–60] It is noted that MnSOD is an essential enzyme, which scavenges superoxide in mitochondria.[54] The biological importance of MnSOD has been demonstrated in many reports, and the expression of MnSOD is essential for the survival of aerobic life and the development of cellular resistance to oxygen radical-mediated toxicity.[58,61] In addition, our results suggested that existence of MnSOD in mitochondria should be important in prevention of cell death caused by X-rays (Figs. 6–9).[61] Our previous study also showed that MnSOD without MTS could not prevent cellular injuries caused by hypoxia-reoxygenation insults, but authentic MnSOD could do so.[62] These results suggest that only when MnSOD is located in mitochondria, after proper post-translational import and processing,[63–66] is it efficient in protecting against cellular injuries by oxidative stress, and they also indicate that mitochondria are primary sites of oxidant-induced cellular oxidative injuries.

Recent studies suggest that the apoptosis of neuronal cells induced by oxidative stress can be mediated by HNE, the major alkenal formed from oxidative degradation of membrane lipids;[67] also, HNE can directly mediate apoptotic and differentiating effects in K562 cells.[68] Our study shows that the mitochondrial ROS, the levels of HNE, and the apoptotic index are correlated with each other (Fig. 10).[61] There is a possibility that mitochondrial ROS forms HNE and that this might help to release the cytochrome c from mitochondria and induce apoptosis. MnSOD might be able to prevent this course by reducing the production of mitochondrial ROS and HNE. Figures 11 and 12 show schematic diagrams of the proposed hypothesis on how mitochondrial ROS and lipid peroxidation products accelerate cell death, and its inhibition by

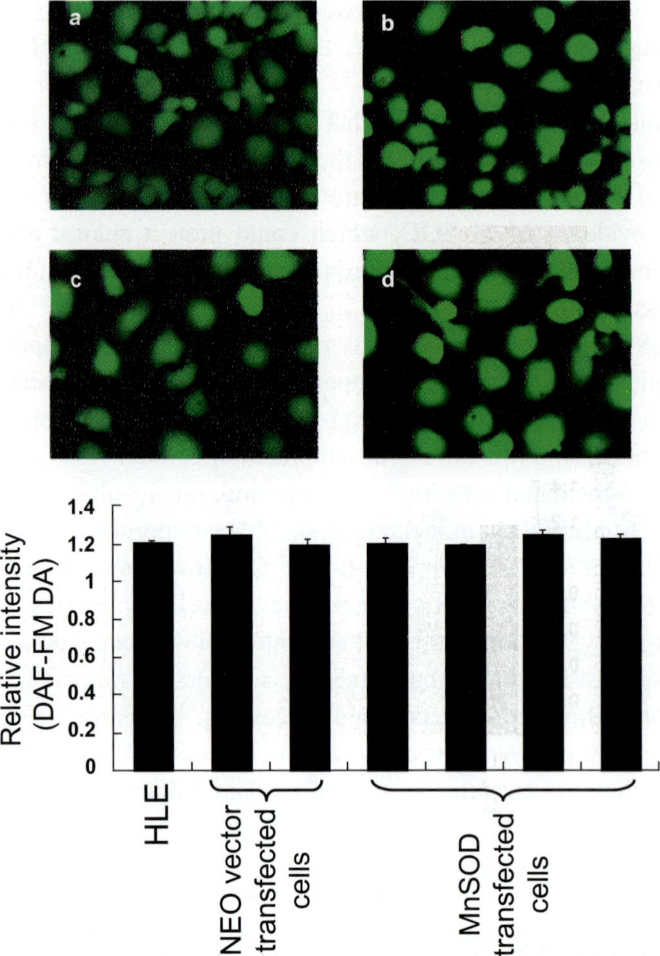

Fig. 6. Intracellular NO• generation. One hour after irradiation, the cell culture medium was replaced by a modified Hanks' balanced salt solution and loaded with DAF-FM DA by incubation for 30 min at 37°C in the presence of 10 μM dye. Bioimages of DAF-FM DA were acquired using a confocal laser microscope and a 3CCD camera: (a) non-irradiated HLE (parental cell); (b) HLE after 15 Gy irradiation; (c) non-irradiated MnSOD-clone-13 (MnSOD transfectants); (d) MnSOD-clone-13 after 15 Gy irradiation; (e) fluorescent intensity on 15 Gy irradiation divided by the intensity on sham (0 Gy) irradiation, i.e., the relative fluorescent intensity. Note that the intracellular NO was almost equally increased at 15 Gy in all cells used in the experiment ($p = 0.50$).[61]

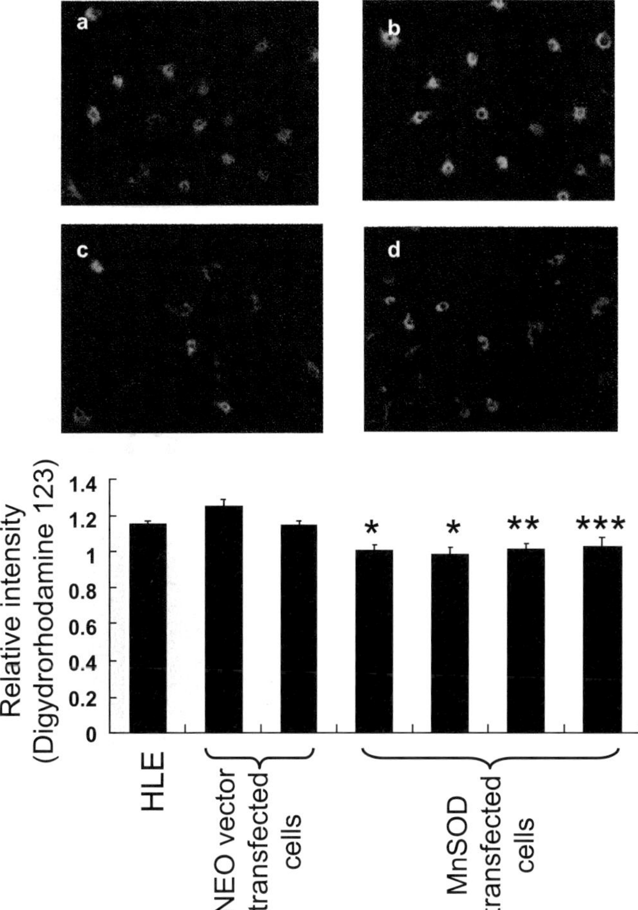

Fig. 7. Intracellular ROS generation. The cell culture medium was replaced by modified HBSS at pH 7.3 and irradiated. After irradiation, the cells were incubated for 60 min at 37°C and loaded with dihydrorhodamine 123 (DHR) by incubation for an additional 30 min at 37°C in the presence of $10\,\mu g\,ml^{-1}$ dye: (a) non-irradiated NEO-clone-1 (control plasmid transfected cell); (b) NEO-clone-1 after 15 Gy irradiation; (c) non-irradiated MnSOD-clone-7 (MnSOD transfectants); (d) MnSOD-clone-7 after 15 Gy irradiation; (e) fluorescent intensity on 15 Gy irradiation divided by the intensity on sham (0 Gy) irradiation, i.e., the relative fluorescent intensity. Note that the generation of mitochondrial ROS was suppressed in Mn-SOD transfected cells. $^*p < 0.05$ versus HLE, and/or NEO-clone-1, and/or NEO-clone-2.[61]

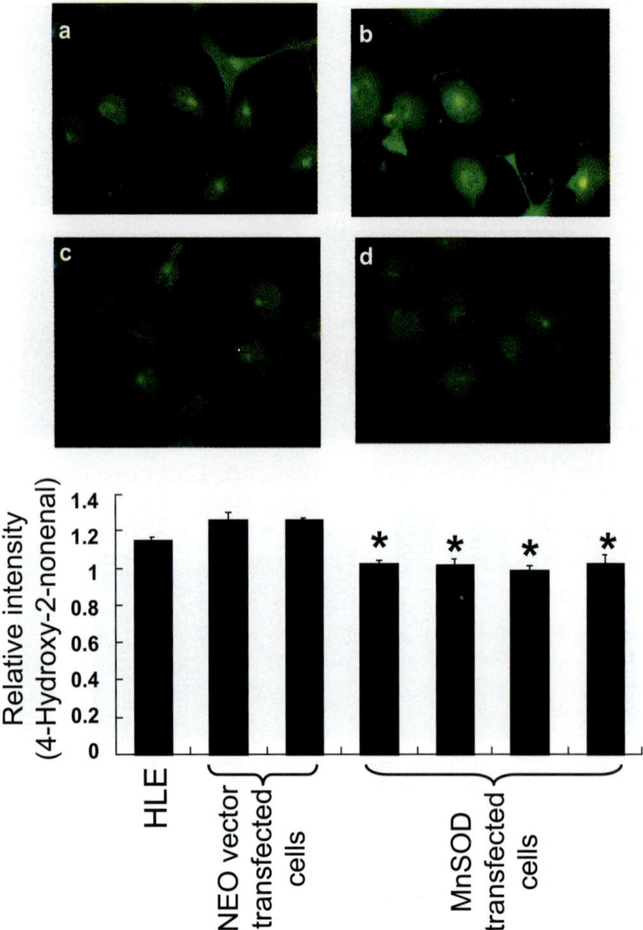

Fig. 8. Intracellular HNE generation. HNE is a highly toxic nine-carbon α,β-unsaturated aldehyde that can be generated by the peroxidation of ω6-unsaturated fatty acids; it may be the most reliable and sensitive marker of lipid peroxidation. Two hours after irradiation, the cells were fixed and membranes were permiabilized by incubation in 95% ethanol with 5% acetic acid. After washing, the cells were incubated in a blocking serum and in anti-HNE mouse monoclonal antibody: (a) immunofluorescent staining of non-irradiated NEO-clone-2 (control plasmid-transfected cell) by anti-HNE antibody; (b) NEO-clone-2 after 15 Gy irradiation; (c) non-irradiated MnSOD-clone-6 (MnSOD transfectant); (d) MnSOD-clone-6 after 15 Gy irradiation; (e) fluorescent intensity on 15 Gy irradiation divided by the intensity on sham (0 Gy) irradiation, i.e. the relative fluorescent intensity. Note that the generation of intracellular HNE production was suppressed in MnSOD transfected cells. $^*p < 0.05$ versus HLE, and/or NEO-clone-1, and/or NEO-clone-2.[61]

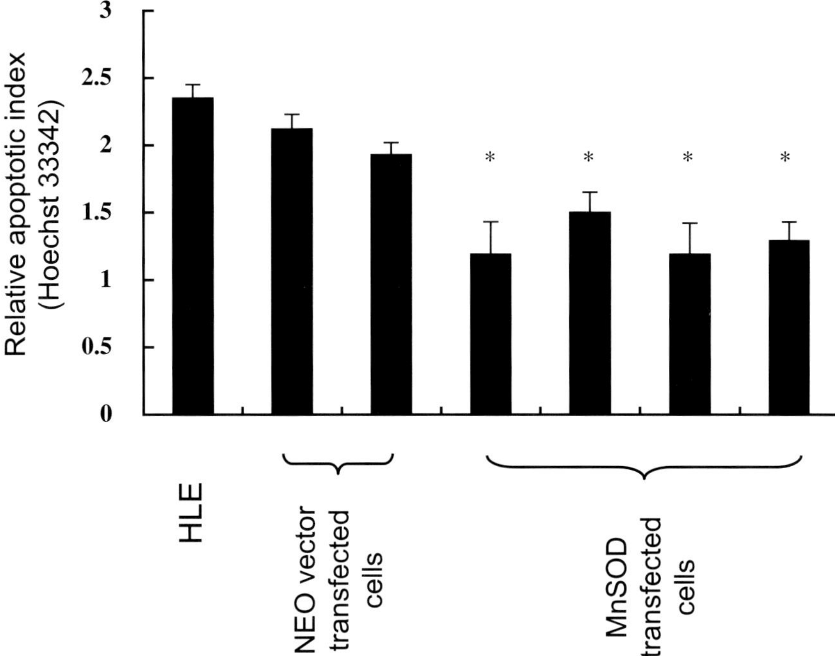

Fig. 9. Relative apoptotic index of the MnSOD-transfected clones, control plasmic transfections, and parental cells. Cells were fixed and assessed by microscopic examination of nuclear chromatin condensation and fragmentation using Hoechst 33342 staining. $^{*}p < 0.05$ versus HLE, and/or NEO-clone-1, and/or NEO-clone-2.[61]

MnSOD. These results suggest that MnSOD might play an important role in protecting cells against radiation-induced apoptosis by controlling the generation of mitochondrial ROS and intracellular lipid peroxidation (Fig. 12). Figure 13 shows a schematic of the timescale of classical radiation-induced events in mammalian cells[11] and one of our new observation of apoptosis caused by mitochondrial generation of ROS. It is noted that generation of ROS from mitochondria occurs after X-irradiation (Fig. 13). These results indicate that ROS generation from mitochondria is an important and early event conveying apoptotic signals[15] and also that mitochondria are the primary target for ionizing radiation-induced apoptosis.

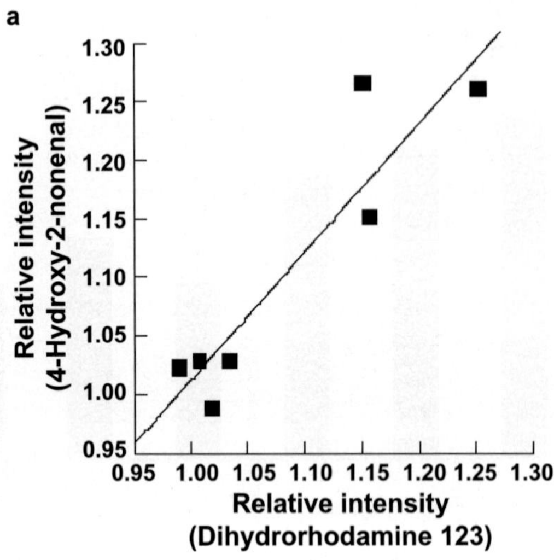

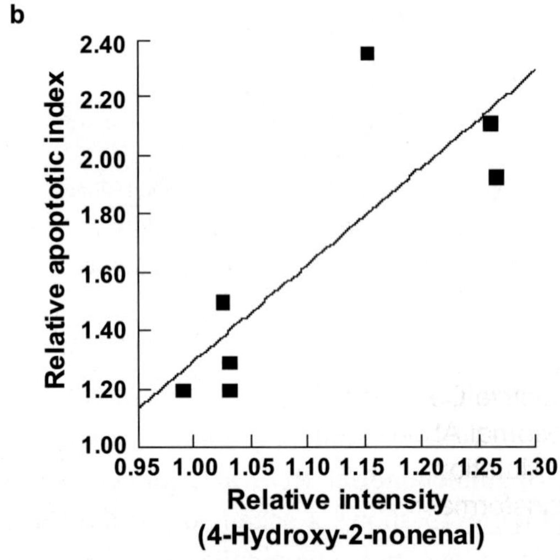

Fig. 10. Correlation between mitochondrial ROS, intracellular lipid peroxidation product, and cell death. (a) Linear-regression analysis showing the relationship between the relative DHR staining intensity (mitochondrial ROS) and the relative HNE staining intensity (intracellular lipid peroxidation products) after irradiation ($r = 0.922$, $p = 0.0013$); (b) relation between the relative HNE staining intensity and the relative apoptosis index ($r = 0.822$, $p = 0.020$). Intracellular lipid peroxidation products have a strong correlation with apoptotic cell death.[61]

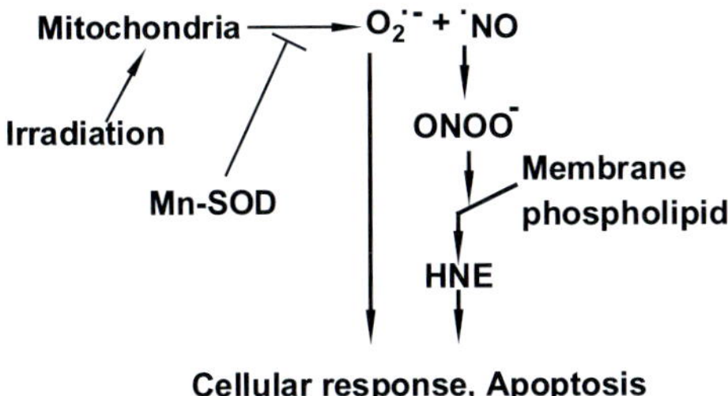

Fig. 11. A schematic diagram of a hypothesis on how ROS generation and lipid peroxidation products affect cell death, and its prevention by MnSOD after irradiation.[61]

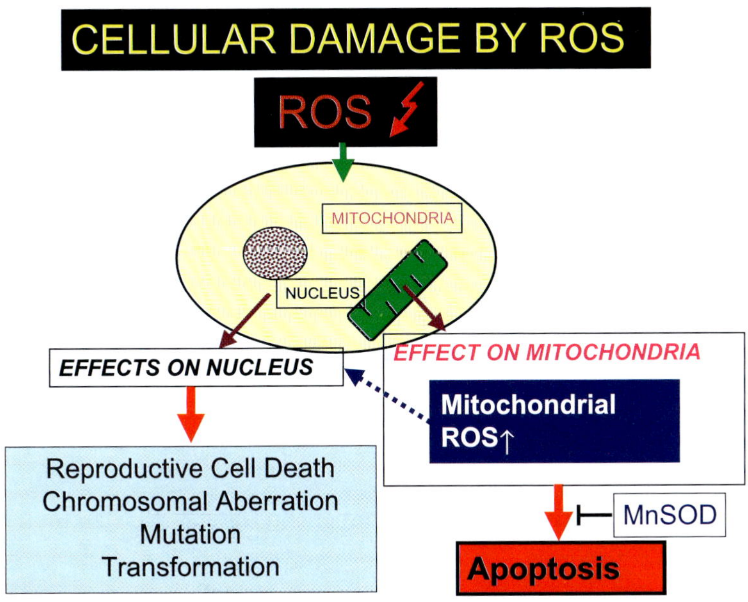

Fig. 12. A schematic diagram of effects of X-irradiation on nucleus that cause DNA strand breaks and subsequent reproductive cell death, chromosomal aberration, and mutation and transformation on mitochondria, which causes apoptosis and is prevented by MnSOD.

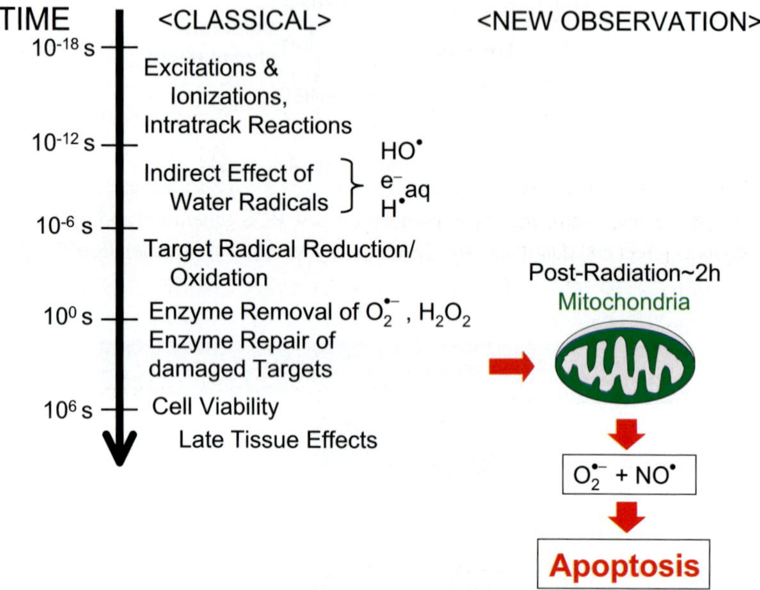

Fig. 13. A schematic of the timescale of radiation-induced events in mammalian cells (from Ref. 11) and one of our new observation of apoptosis caused by mitochondrial generation of ROS. It is noted that generation of ROS from mitochondria occurs after X-irradiation.

Acknowledgments

The authors thank Profs. Garry R. Buettner and Daret K. St Clair for helpful discussions.

References

1. Hall HJ (ed.) DNA strand breaks and chromosomal aberrations. In: *Radiobiology for the Radiologist*, 4th edn. J.B. Lippincott Company, Philadelphia, 1994, pp. 15–27.
2. Ito A. Electron track simulation for microdosometry. In: Jenkins TM, Melson WR, Rindi A (eds.) *Monte Carlo Transport of Electrons and Photons*. Plenum Publishers, New York, 1988, pp. 361–382.

3. Sakai K, Okada S. Radiation-induced DNA damage and cellular lethality in cultured mammalian cells. *Radiat. Res.* 98: 479–490 (1984).
4. Ito A. Calculation of double strand break probability of DNA for low LET radiations based on Track structure analysis. In: Okamoto K (ed.) *Nuclear and Atomic Data for Radiotherapy and Related Radiobiology*. TECDOC Series 413, IAEA Publication, Vienna, 1987.
5. Coggle JE (ed.) *Biological Effects of Radiation*. Taylor & Francis, London, 1983.
6. Riley PA. Free radicals in biology: oxidative stress and the effects of ionizing radiation. *Int. J. Radiat. Biol.* 65: 27–33 (1994).
7. Schmidt-Ullrich RK, Dent P, Grant S, Mikkelsen RB, Valerie K. Signal transduction and cellular radiation responses. *Radiat. Res.* 153: 245–257 (2000).
8. Wallace SS. Enzymatic processing of radiation-induced free radical damage in DNA. *Radiat. Res.* 150(5 Suppl): S60–S79 (1998).
9. Halliwell B, Gutteridge JMC (eds.) Oxidative stress: adaptation, damage, repair and death. In: *Free Radicals in Biology and Medicine*, 3rd edn. Oxford University Press, Oxford, 1999, pp. 246–350.
10. Buettner GR, Jurkiewicz BA. Catalytic metals, ascorbate and free radicals: combinations to avoid. *Radiat. Res.* 145: 532–541 (1996).
11. Chapman JD. Biophysical models of mammalian cell inactivation by radiation. In: Meyn RE, Withers HR (eds.) *Radiation Biology in Cancer Research.* Raven Press, New York, 1980, pp. 21–32.
12. Rudner J, Jendrossek V, Belka C. New insights in the role of Bcl-2, Bcl-2 and the endoplasmic reticulum. *Apoptosis* 7: 441–447 (2002).
13. Dent P, Yacoub A, Contessa J, Caron R, Amorino G, Valerie K, Hagan MP, Grant S, Schmidt-Ullrich R. Stress and radiation-induced activation of multiple intracellular signaling pathways. *Radiat. Res.* 159: 283–300 (2003).
14. Kerr JFR, Searle J. Apoptosis its nature and kinetic role. In: *Radiation Biology in Cancer Research*. Raven Press, New York, 1980, pp. 367–384.
15. Hengartner MO. The biochemistry of apoptosis. *Nature* 407: 770–776 (2000).
16. Rich T, Allen RL, Wyllie AH. Defying death after DNA damage. *Nature* 407: 777–783 (2000).
17. Muzio M, Stockwell BR, Stennicke HR, Salvesen GS, Dixit VM. An induced proximity model for caspase-8 activation. *J. Biol. Chem.* 273: 2926–2930 (1998).
18. Irmler M, Thome M, Hahne M, Schneider P, Hofmann K, Steiner V, Bodmer JL, Schroter M, Burns K, Mattmann C, Rimoldi D, French LE, Tschopp J. Inhibition of death receptor signals by cellular FLIP. *Nature* 388: 190–195 (1997).

19. Powell WC, Fingleton B, Wilson CL, Boothby M, Matrisian, LM. The metalloproteinase matrilysin proteolytically generates active soluble Fas ligand and potentiates epithelial cell apoptosis. *Curr. Biol.* 9: 1441–1447 (1999).
20. Brew K, Dinakarpandian D, Nagase H. Tissue inhibitors of metalloproteinases: evolution, structure and function. *Biochim. Biophys. Acta* 1477: 267–283 (2000).
21. Kuwabara M, Takahashi K, Inanami O. Induction of apoptosis through the activation of SAPK/JNK followed by the expression of death receptor Fas in X-irradiated cells. *J. Radiat. Res.* 44: 203–209 (2003).
22. Franklin CC, Srikanth S, Kraft AS. Conditional expression of mitogen-activated protein kinase phosphatase-1, MKP-1, is cytoprotective against UV-induced apoptosis. *Proc. Natl. Acad. Sci. USA* 95: 3014–3019 (1998).
23. Ruvolo PP, Deng X, May WS. Phosphorylation of Bcl2 and regulation of apoptosis. *Leukemia* 15: 515–521 (2001).
24. Liston P, Fong WG, Korneluk RG. The inhibitors of apoptosis: there is more to life than Bcl2. *Oncogene* 22: 8568–8580 (2003).
25. Robertson GS, Crocker SJ, Nicholson DW, Schulz JB. Neuroprotection by the inhibition of apoptosis. *Brain Pathol.* 10: 283–292 (2000).
26. Du C, Fang M, Li Y, Li L, Wang X. Smac, a mitochondrial protein that promotes cytochrome c-dependent caspase activation by eliminating IAP inhibition. *Cell* 102: 33–42 (2000).
27. Verhagen AM, Ekert PG, Pakusch M, Silke J, Connolly LM, Reid GE, Moritz RL, Simpson RJ, Vaux DL. Identification of DIABLO, a mammalian protein that promotes apoptosis by binding to and antagonizing IAP proteins. *Cell* 102: 43–53 (2000).
28. Barnhart BC, Alappat EC, Peter ME. The CD95 type I/type II model. *Semin. Immunol.* 15: 185–193 (2003).
29. Liu X, Li P, Widlak P, Zou H, Luo X, Garrard WT, Wang X. The 40-kDa subunit of DNA fragmentation factor induces DNA fragmentation and chromatin condensation during apoptosis. *Proc. Natl. Acad. Sci. USA* 95: 8461–8466 (1998).
30. Widlak, P. The DFF40/CAD endonuclease and its role in apoptosis. *Acta Biochim. Pol.* 47: 1037–1044 (2000).
31. Grand RJ, Milner AE, Mustoe T, Johnson GD, Owen D, Grant ML, Gregory CD. A novel protein expressed in mammalian cells undergoing apoptosis. *Exp. Cell Res.* 218: 439–451 (1995).
32. Carstea ED, Morris JA, Coleman KG, Loftus SK, Zhang D, Cummings C, Gu J, Rosenfeld MA, Pavan WJ, Krizman DB, Nagle J, Polymeropoulos MH, Sturley SL, Ioannou YA, Higgins ME, Comly M, Cooney A, Brown A,

Kaneski CR, Blanchette-Mackie EJ, Dwyer NK, Neufeld EB, Chang TY, Liscum L, Strauss JF III, Ohno K, Zeigler M, Carmi R, Sokol J, Markie D, O'Neill RR, van Diggelen OP, Elleder M, Patterson MC, Brady RO, Vanier MT, Pentchev PG, Tagle DA. Niemann-Pick C1 disease gene: homology to mediators of cholesterol homeostasis. *Science* 277: 228–231 (1997).

33. Erickson RP, Bernard O. Studies on neuronal death in the mouse model of Niemann-Pick C disease. *J. Neurosci. Res.* 68: 738–744 (2002).
34. Feng B, Yao PM, Li Y, Devlin CM, Zhang D, Harding HP, Sweeney M, Rong JX, Kuriakose G, Fisher EA, Marks AR, Ron D, Tabas I. The endoplasmic reticulum is the site of cholesterol-induced cytotoxicity in macrophages. *Nat. Cell Biol.* 9: 781–792 (2003).
35. Weitzman JB, Fiette L, Matsuo K, Yaniv M. JunD protects cells from p53-dependent senescence and apoptosis. *Mol. Cell* 6: 1109–1119 (2000).
36. Pidgeon GP, Kandouz M, Meram A, Honn KV. Mechanisms controlling cell cycle arrest and induction of apoptosis after 12-lipoxygenase inhibition in prostate cancer cells. *Cancer Res.* 62: 2721–2727 (2002).
37. Shi C, Yu L, Yang F, Yan J, Zeng H. A novel organoselenium compound induces cell cycle arrest and apoptosis in prostate cancer cell lines. *Biochem. Biophys. Res. Commun.* 309: 578–583 (2003).
38. Jaattela, M. Escaping cell death: survival proteins in cancer. *Exp. Cell Res.* 248: 30–43 (1999).
39. Xanthoudakis S, Nicholson DW. Heat-shock proteins as death determinants. *Nat. Cell Biol.* 2: E163–E165 (2000).
40. Setsukinai K, Urano Y, Kakinuma K, Majima HJ, Nagano T. Development of novel fluorescence probes that can reliably detect reactive oxygen species and distinguish specific species. *J. Biol. Chem.* 278: 3170–3175 (2003).
41. Halliwell B, Gutteridge JMC (eds.) Antioxidant defences. In: *Free Radicals in Biology and Medicine*, 3rd edn. Oxford University Press, Oxford, Oxford, 1999, pp. 105–245.
42. Fridovich I. Superoxide radical and superoxide dismutases. *Annu. Rev. Biochem.* 64: 97–112 (1995).
43. Sawyer DT, Valentine JS. How super is superoxide? *Acc. Chem. Res.* 14: 393–400 (1981).
44. Winterbourn CC. Comparison of superoxide with other reducing agents in the biological production of hydroxyl radicals. *Biochem. J.* 182: 625–628 (1979).
45. Babbs CF, Griffin DW. Scatchard analysis of methane sulfinic acid production from dimethyl sulfoxide: a method to quantify hydroxyl radical formation in physiologic systems. *Free Radic. Biol. Med.* 6: 493–503 (1989).

46. Blough NV, Zafiriou OC. Reaction of superoxide with nitric oxide to form peroxonitrite in alkaline aqueous solution. *Inorg. Chem.* 24: 3502–3504 (1985).
47. Beckman JS, Beckman TW, Chen J, Marshall PA, Freeman, BA. Apparent hydroxyl radical production by peroxynitrite: implications for endothelial injury from nitric oxide and superoxide. *Proc. Natl. Acad. Sci. USA* 87: 1620–1624 (1990).
48. Keller JN, Kindy MS, Holtsberg FW, St. Clair DK, Yen HC, Germeyer A, Steiner SM, Bruce-Keller AJ, Hutchins JB, Mattson MP. Mitochondrial manganese superoxide dismutase prevents neural apoptosis and reduces ischemic brain injury: suppression of peroxynitrite production, lipid peroxidation, and mitochondrial dysfunction. *J. Neurosci.* 18: 687–697 (1998).
49. Radi R, Beckman JS, Bush KM, Freeman BA. Peroxynitrite-induced membrane lipid peroxidation: the cytotoxic potential of superoxide and nitric oxide. *Arch. Biochem. Biophys.* 288: 481–487 (1991).
50. Esterbauer H, Schaur RJ, Zollner H. Chemistry and biochemistry of 4-hydroxynonenal, malonaldehyde and related aldehydes. *Free Radic. Biol. Med.* 11: 81–128 (1991).
51. Pryor WA, Porter NA. Suggested mechanisms for the production of 4-hydroxy-2-nonenal from the autoxidation of polyunsaturated fatty acids. *Free Radic. Biol. Med.* 8: 541–543 (1990).
52. Spitz DR, Malcolm RR, Roberts RJ. Cytotoxicity and metabolism of 4-hydroxy-2-nonenal and 2-nonenal in H_2O_2-resistant cell lines. Do aldehydic by-products of lipid peroxidation contribute to oxidative stress? *Biochem. J.* 267: 453–459 (1990).
53. McCord JM, Fridovich I. Superoxide dismutase. An enzymic function for erythrocuprein (hemocuprein). *J. Biol. Chem.* 244: 6049–6055 (1969).
54. Weisiger RA, Fridovich I. Mitochondrial superoxide dismutase: site of synthesis and intramitochondrial localization. *J. Biol. Chem.* 248: 4793–4796 (1973).
55. Fukai T, Siegfried MR, Ushio-Fukai M, Cheng Y, Kojda G, Harrison DG. Regulation of the vascular extracellular superoxide dismutase by nitric oxide and exercise training. *J. Clin. Invest.* 105: 1631–1639 (2000).
56. Boveris A, Cadenas E. Mitochondrial production of superoxide anions and its relationship to the antimycin insensitive respiration. *FEBS Lett.* 54: 311–314 (1975).
57. Takeshige K, Minakami S. NADH- and NADPH-dependent formation of superoxide anions by bovine heart submitochondrial particles and NADH-ubiquinone reductase preparation. *Biochem. J.* 180: 129–135 (1979).

58. Majima HJ, Oberley TD, Furukawa K, Mattson MP, Yen HC, Szweda LI, St. Clair DK. Prevention of mitochondrial injury by manganese superoxide dismutase reveals a primary mechanism for alkaline-induced cell death. *J. Biol. Chem.* 273: 8217–8224 (1998).
59. Mattson MP. Apoptosis in neurodegenerative disorders. *Nat. Rev. Mol. Cell Biol.* 1: 120–129 (2000).
60. Mattson MP, Duan W, Pedersen WA, Culmsee C. Neurodegenerative disorders and ischemic brain diseases. *Apoptosis* 6: 69–81 (2001).
61. Motoori S, Majima HJ, Ebara M, Kato H, Hirai F, Kakinuma S, Yamaguchi C, Ozawa T, Nagano T, Tsujii H, Saisho H. Overexpression of mitochondrial manganese superoxide dismutase protects against radiation-induced cell death in the human hepatocellular carcinoma cell line, HLE. *Cancer Res.* 61: 5382–5388 (2001).
62. Hirai F, Motoori S, Kakinuma S, Tomita K, Indo HP, Kato H, Yamaguchi T, Yen H-C, St. Clair DK, Nagano T, Ozawa T, Saisho H, Majima HJ. Mitochondrial signal lacking manganese superoxide dismutase failed to prevent cell death by reoxygenation following hypoxia in a human pancreatic cancer cell line, KP4. *Antioxid. Redox Signal.* 6: 523–535 (2004).
63. Doonan S, Marra E, Passarella S, Saccone C, Quagliariello E. Transport of proteins into mitochondria. *Int. Rev. Cytol.* 91: 141–186 (1984).
64. Martinus RD, Ryan MT, Naylor DJ, Herd SM, Hoogeraad NJ, Høj PB. Role of chaperones in the biogenesis and maintenance of the mitochondrion. *FASEB J.* 9: 371–378 (1995).
65. Mihara K, Omura T. Cytoplasmic chaperones in precursor targeting to mitochondria: the role of MSF and hsp70. *Trends Cell Biol.* 6: 104–108 (1996).
66. Lithgow T. Targeting of proteins to mitochondria. *FEBS Lett.* 476: 22–26 (2000).
67. Kruman I, Bruce-Keller AJ, Bredesen D, Waeg G, Mattson MP. Evidence that 4-hydroxynonenal mediates oxidative stress-induced neuronal apoptosis. *J. Neurosci.* 17: 5089–5100 (1997).
68. Cheng J-Z, Singhal SS, Saini M, Singhal J, Piper JT, Van Kuijk FJ, Zimniak P, Awasthi YC, Awasthi S. Effects of mGST A4 transfection on 4-hydroxynonenal mediated apoptosis and differentiation of K562 human erythroleukemia cells. *Arch. Biochem. Biophys.* 372: 29–36 (1999).

3 Oxidative Damage to Mitochondria

Jai C. Tilak and Thomas P.A. Devasagayam

1. Introduction — Significance of Mitochondria in Cell/Metabolism

1.1. *General description and significance*

Mitochondria are functionally important subcellular organelles. Oxidative damage to them can have serious consequences. There are a large number of studies on this topic in recent years. It is almost impossible to cover all of them. We attempt to include more recent ones that pertain to this subject matter. There are two closely related chapters namely on "Mitochondrial ROS Production" (Chapter 1) and "Oxidative Stress and Mitochondrial Diseases" (Chapter 21) whose subject matter may overlap some portions of this chapter.

The term *Mitochondria* was introduced at the turn of the century and is based on their appearance as threadlike granules in the light microscope. Mitochondria are among the most prominent structures in most cells. In the electron micrograph, each mitochondrion is observed to be made up of a double bilayer membrane. The outer bilayer is a simple membrane that encloses the entire organelle. The inner bilayer has a variable number of infoldings called cristae, which served to increase the surface area greatly. Mitochondria are the site of cellular respiration, and thus are the cell's center of energy production.[1]

Mitochondria are composed of four compartments, each with quite different compositions, activities and functions: a porous outer membrane, permeable to molecules smaller than about 6 kDa; and intermembrane space containing a number of specialized proteins, but which is continuous with the cytoplasm for small molecules; a convoluted and invaginated inner membrane containing the enzymes of oxidative phosphorylation and a series of metabolic carrier proteins; the mitochondrial matrix containing enzymes for many different metabolic pathways, including the citric acid cycle, fatty acid oxidation and the urea cycle. Mitochondria also contain their own DNA (mtDNA), which in mammals encodes 13 polypeptides, along with the 22 tRNA genes and two rRNA genes necessary for their translation. All 13 mitochondrially-encoded polypeptides are components of the respiratory chain or the F_0F_1 ATP synthase. Mitochondria arise from the binary fission of pre-existing mitochondria and although they are generally thought of as discrete organelles, within the cell they may continually fuse and separate to form reticular networks.[2]

Recent electron microscopic (EM) tomography is providing important new insights into the internal organization of mitochondria. The standard baffle model for cristae structure, called into question years ago, has now clearly been shown to be inaccurate. Depending on source and conformational state, cristae can vary from simple tubular structures merging with the inner boundary membrane through tubular structures 28 nm in diameter. The structural information provided by EM tomography has important implications for mitochondrial bioenergetics, biogenesis and the role of mitochondria in apoptosis.[3]

New live cell imaging techniques indicate that mitochondria exist in the living cell as a continuous interconnected mitochondrial reticulum, or "MR," closely associated with the endoplasmic reticulum (ER). Ca^{2+} ions released from ER in response to hormonal stimulation might thus be preferentially transferred into the mitochondrial matrix causing the local activation of ATP synthesis.[4]

The mitochondrion is known as the "power plant" of the cell. All processes involved in the growth of cells require energy. In most cases, free energy is supplied by the hydrolysis of one of the high-energy phosphoanhydride bonds in adenosine triphosphate (ATP). The energy released powers many otherwise energetically unfavorable events. ATP is needed in a multitude of pathways and is termed "universal currency" of chemical energy, found in all types of organisms.[5]

1.2. *History of study of mitochondria and its significance*

Biochemical research tends to move forward at an uneven pace that depends on new technologies, on the novel insights of investigators involved, and even on the vagaries of the funding sources available for research projects. Nowhere is this more evident than in the area of mitochondrial research.[6] What started out as a quest to define the principles of biological energy conservation has largely been replaced by attempts to understand the molecular basis of several human diseases. As a result, mitochondria are receiving increased attention from investigators with varied interests and backgrounds. Novel techniques are now being used to study both mitochondrial structure and functioning, and these methods are leading to a redefining of long-lived views about the basic biology of the organelle.

Work in the late 1940s and early 1950s by David Green, Albert Lehninger and others first demonstrated that mitochondria are the centers of energy metabolism within the cells. Since then isolated mitochondria have been studied extensively to understand the mechanism of energy conservation, especially the process of oxidative phosphorylation. This work has already resulted in several landmarks in biochemistry, beginning with the development of the concept of chemi-osmosis, which was rewarded with a Nobel Prize to Peter Mitchell. Studies on the ATP synthase have provided unexpected insight into the elegance of biological machinery. Strong evidence has been obtained that this large protein complex functions as a rotary motor, work that led to the awarding of the Nobel Prize in Chemistry to Paul Boyer and John Walker in 1997.

Rutter and Rizzuto[4] explain the key roles this organelle plays as a regulator of Ca^{2+} levels and a participant in Ca^{2+} signaling within the cell. A reticular morphology has important advantages in Ca^{2+} homeostasis, just as it has for energy metabolism by acting as an intracellular cable for membrane potential. This can, at any time, produce energy in one part of the cell, while using energy in another distant part. Another recent surprise regarding mitochondrial functioning comes with studies that place this organelle at the center of programmed cell death, or apoptosis. The evidence that the mitochondrion participates in apoptosis through regulated release of selected proteins is overwhelming. Cytochrome c is one of these proteins, which means that this small hemoprotein has a dual role: it functions in electron transfer and programmed cell death. The importance of apoptosis to medicine cannot be overstated. Perturbation of the equilibrium between cell proliferation and the equally physiologically relevant programmed cell death can explain many serious medical conditions. Cancer could be viewed as much as a reduced rate of cell death as it can as an increase in the rate of cell division. Neurological disorders, including Parkinson's and Alzheimer's disease are being rethought in terms of increased rates of programmed cell death in selected areas of the brain. The role of the mitochondrion in apoptosis is only one reason that clinicians now study this organelle, and for the emergence of what is now called mitochondrial medicine.

Researchers involved in mitochondrial medicine are faced with several issues related to the multiplicity of the mitochondrial genome. Most mutations are heteroplasmic — that is, they occur in some, but not all, copies of the mtDNA. Patients then present with variable symptoms, the severity of which depends on the proportion of mutated mtDNAs. Moreover these diseases are often tissue-specific. How mtDNA mutations are generated is also the focus of much attention. mtDNA is badly positioned in the cell because it is close to respiratory chain components and the unwanted by-products of electron transfer, namely the formation of free radicals. These free radicals including superoxides and hydroxyl radicals are potent mutagens.

1.3. *Oxidative phosphorylation*

Most human cells contain substantial numbers of mitochondria in their cytoplasm whose principal function is ATP synthesis by oxidative phosphorylation (OxPHOS). Mitochondria make ATP by passing electrons derived from the oxidation of food down the respiratory chain to react with oxygen, using the redox energy to translocate protons across the inner membrane. This establishes a proton electrochemical potential gradient (negative inside) and a pH gradient (basic inside), which drives ATP synthesis by the F_0F_1ATP synthase. The mitochondrial inner membrane also contains a number of metabolite carriers, which export ATP from the matrix and allow other metabolites to enter without dissipating the proton electrochemical potential gradient. Thus mitochondria supply most of our ATP and consume nearly all of the oxygen we breathe.[2]

During metabolism, glucose and fatty acids (the principal sources of energy in animal and most other non-photosynthetic cells) are metabolized to CO_2. The complete aerobic degradation of glucose to CO_2 and H_2O is coupled to the synthesis of as many as 32 molecules of ATP. In eukaryotic cells and in bacteria, the initial enzymatically catalyzed chemical reactions in the pathway of glucose degradation occur in cytosol. In eukaryotes, the final steps occur in mitochondria, together with generation of most of the ATP. Similarly, the final stages of metabolism of fatty acids can also occur in mitochondria.

Mitochondria use a process called chemi-osmosis, to generate ATP from ADP and Pi. The immediate energy sources that power this reaction are the proton concentration gradient and the membrane electric potential, collectively termed the proton-motive force. In mitochondria, energy from the metabolism of sugars, fatty acids, and other substances culminating in their oxidation by O_2, is used to pump protons across mitochondrial membrane, generating a proton-motive force.

Mitochondria have four enzyme complexes: Complex I — CoQ reductase complex; Complex II — succinate-CoQ reductase complex; Complex III — $CoQH_2$-cytochrome c reductase complex; and Complex IV — cytochrome c-cytochrome c oxidase complex. Reducing equivalents in the form of NADH and $FADH_2$ of the Krebs cycle enter the electron transport chain through complexes I and II, respectively. Electrons are then transferred through a series of redox couples with the final electron acceptor being O_2 leading to the formation of H_2O.[5]

The mitochondrion lies at the "heart" of cell life and cell death. That we must breathe oxygen to stay alive is simply the consequence of the demand of our mitochondria for oxygen. About 98% of inhaled oxygen is consumed by mitochondria. They provide the energy required for almost all cellular processes — to allow muscle to contract (for instance cardiac muscle and smooth muscle in the gut, the vasculature, and the lungs), to maintain ionic gradients in excitable cells, to allow the accumulation of secreted material into vesicles, and to permit the vesicle fusion and cycling necessary for the secretion of hormones and neurotransmitters.[7]

An emerging and important site of action for nitric oxide ($NO^\bullet$) within cells is the mitochondrial inner membrane, where $NO^\bullet$ binds to and inhibits members of the electron transport chain, complex III and cytochrome c oxidase.[8] In this study, we present evidence for a consumption of NO in the mitochondrial membrane in the absence of substrate, in a non-saturable process that is O_2 dependent. This consumption modulates inhibition of cytochrome c oxidase by $NO^•$. It is evident that the partition of NO into mitochondrial membranes has a major impact on the ability of $NO^•$ to control mitochondrial respiration.

1.4. *Other functions of mitochondria*

Quite apart from the provision of ATP, mitochondria play important roles in aspects of normal physiology. These include the transduction pathway that underlies the secretion of insulin in response to glucose by β-cells and possibly in the sensing of oxygen tension in the carotid body and pulmonary vasculature. Mitochondria also house key enzyme systems quite distinct from those required for intermediary metabolism — the rate-limiting enzymes in steroid biosynthesis, the synthesis of haem, and even carbonic anhydrase required for acid secretion in the stomach. By accumulating calcium when cytosolic calcium levels are high, mitochondria play subtle roles in coordinating the complexities of intracellular calcium signaling pathways that may be extremely important in the finer aspects of cell regulation. The physiological "uncoupling" plays a central role as a heat-generating mechanism in non-shivering thermogenesis in young mammals. Production of free radical species by mitochondria may play a key role as a signaling mechanism, for instance, in the regulation of ion-channel activities and also in initiating cyto-protective mechanisms in stressed cells.[7]

Mitochondria contribute to the maintenance of the intracellular Ca^{2+} homeostasis by taking up and releasing the cation via separate and specific pathways.[9] The molecular details of the release pathway are elusive but its stimulation by the cross-linking of some vicinal thiols and consequently NAD^+ hydrolysis are known. Thiol cross-linking and NAD^+ hydrolysis can be achieved by addition of peroxynitrite ($ONOO^-$). Intramitochondrially formed $ONOO^-$ stimulates the specific NAD^+-linked Ca^{2+} release from mitochondria. Findings that upon Ca^{2+} uptake mtNOS is stimulated, that $ONOO^-$ is formed, and that Ca^{2+} is subsequently released from intact mitochondria suggest the existence of a feedback loop, which prevents overloading of mitochondria with Ca^{2+}.

2. Source of ROS in Mitochondria

Mitochondria are important sources of ROS generation. Molecular oxygen is chemically inert, which allows the maintenance of biomolecules in the presence of oxygen which otherwise would readily oxidize. To circumvent spin inversion, single electrons are transferred to refill the two vacant positions of the orbital. This physicochemical principle is also obeyed in cell respiration being carried out in mitochondria where the reduction of oxygen to water occurs by the consecutive transfer of four single electrons leading to the formation of three ROS, namely superoxide ($O_2^{\bullet-}$), hydrogen peroxide (H_2O_2) and hydroxyl radical ($^{\bullet}OH$).[10]

By virtue of the redox reactions carried out during electron transport this process has attracted considerable attention as a potential source of oxygen derived radicals during normal physiological processes and as a result of disturbances in metabolic homeostasis. During normal cellular metabolism, free radicals are produced at the NADH-coenzyme Q reductase (complex I) and cytochrome c oxidase (complex III) components of the mitochondrial electron transport chain. Any event that diminishes electron transport distal to respiratory chain components capable of transferring an electron to O_2 would be expected to result in an increase in the rate of oxygen radical production.[5]

Being an important source of ROS generation mitochondria also form major targets of oxidative damage. Such damage can lead to reduced cellular functions resulting from loss of energy generation and in cell death. As the electrons traverse complex I, III and IV, protons are pumped out of the matrix through these complexes and into the intermembrane space to create an electrochemical gradient. These protons can then move back into the matrix by traversing a channel in the membrane component of the ATP synthase, driving the synthesis of ATP. Therefore, oxygen consumption is coupled to ADP phosphorylation through the mitochondrial membrane potential.[11] The mitochondrial respiratory chain is a powerful source of ROS (see figure below), primarily the $O_2^{\bullet-}$ and consequently H_2O_2, either as a product of superoxide dismutase (SOD) or by dis-proportionation. It is calculated that 1–4% of oxygen reacting with the respiratory chain is incompletely reduced to ROS.[12]

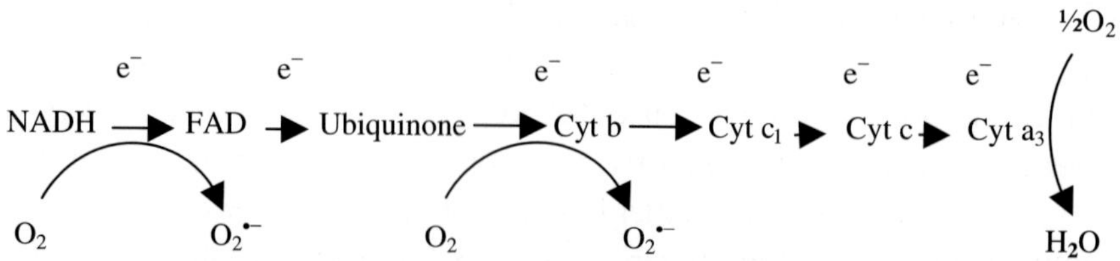

ROS production by mitochondria increases after a period of anoxia, during ischemia-reperfusion and defective oxidative phosphorylation (e.g. such as in ADP/ATP antiporter or ANT• deficient mice).[11,13] Highly energized mitochondria are also dangerous for the cell since the reduced state of respiratory chain electron carriers supports the formation of $O_2^{\bullet-}$ by one-electron transfer reactions. Consequently mild uncoupling of mitochondria reduces their ability to generate ROS.[14]

Superoxide is itself damaging and also reacts to form further reactive oxidants, by dismutation of H_2O_2, which can decompose to the •OH, and by reaction with nitric oxide to form $ONOO^-$. Although there are still considerable uncertainties about the extent of mitochondrial oxidative damage *in vivo*, its potential severity was illustrated by mice lacking Mn-SOD, which died shortly after birth while mice lacking Cu, Zn-SOD, the cytosolic form of the enzyme, survived.[2]

Increasing the degree of fatty acid unsaturation of heart mitochondria increases oxidative damage to their lipids and proteins, and can also increase their rates of mitochondrial oxygen radical generation in situations in which the degree of reduction of Complex III is higher than normal. These observations strengthen the notion that the relatively low double bond content of the membranes of long-lived animals could have evolved to protect them from oxidative damage.[15]

Recently, two independent research groups detected the presence of a calcium-dependent nitric oxide synthase (NOS) facing the matrix side of the inner mitochondrial membrane. Further studies showed that the product of this enzyme xNO was also able to block mitochondrial respiration. Therefore, the presence of an intra-mitochondrial NOS suggests that the resulting xNO may have a physiological role controlling respiration and electron flow under certain conditions. As a result of the inhibition of mitochondrial respiration, superoxide formation by complex I (NADH-deoxygenase) is likely to increase leading to an increased production of H_2O_2 and $ONOO^-$. One of the consequences of the resulting oxidative stress may be the opening of permeability transition pores, accompanied by the release of cytochrome c into the cytoplasm, triggering apoptosis.

The majority of superoxide that is produced on a daily basis in most organisms comes from the mitochondrial respiratory chain produced by a non-enzymatic mechanism.[16] Ubisemiquinone (UQ_{10}) species generated in the course of electron transport reactions in the respiratory chain donate electrons to oxygen and provide a constant source of superoxide:

$$UQ_{10}^{-} + O_2 = O_2^{-} + UQ_{10}$$

Superoxide itself can be toxic, especially through inactivation of proteins that contain iron-sulfur centers such as aconitase and succinate dehydrogenase and mitochondrial NADH-ubiquinone oxidoreductase. A second much more damaging species, the $^{\bullet}OH$, can arise. It is very reactive, with an estimated physiological half-life of the order of 10^{-9} seconds. It causes peroxidative damage to proteins, lipids and DNA and is formed by at least two mechanisms.

Superoxide can also react with nitric oxide to form the damaging oxidant $ONOO^{-}$, which is more reactive than either precursor. Nitric oxide diffuses easily into mitochondria and may also be produced there. Consequently, mitochondrial $O_2^{\bullet -}$ production initiates a range of damaging reactions through the production of $O_2^{\bullet -}$, H_2O_2, Fe^{2+}, $^{\bullet}OH$, and $ONOO^{-}$, which can damage lipids, proteins, and nucleic acids. Mitochondrial function is particularly susceptible to oxidative damage, leading to decreased mitochondrial ATP synthesis, cellular calcium dyshomeostasis, and induction of the mitochondrial permeability transition, all of which predispose cells to necrosis or apoptosis.[17]

The assumption that mitochondria are the major intracellular source of ROS was essentially based on *in vitro* experiments with isolated mitochondria.[10] The transfer of these data to the living cell may, however, be incorrect. One of the most critical electron transfer steps in the respiratory chain is the electron bifurcation from ubiquinol to the cytochrome bc_1 complex. This electron bifurcation requires the free mobility of the head domain of the Rieske iron-sulfur protein. Inhibition of electron bifurcation by antimycin A causes leakage of single electrons to oxygen, which results in the release of ROS.

ROS formation observed with isolated mitochondria does not allow conclusions to be drawn about *in vivo* conditions. Experimental evidence was provided which draws attention to the ubiquinol/cytochrome bc_1 redox couple as a potential ROS source. Any impediment of regular redox exchange at this site was found to result in the release of single electrons to dioxygen out of sequence. In agreement with this basic finding, Nohl *et al.*[10] believe that incorporation of oxidized fatty acids into the inner mitochondrial membrane of lipophilic xenobiotics will be a trigger of intracellular ROS from mitochondria.

Mitochondria contain antioxidant enzymes, including SOD (Mn form) glutathione peroxidase, phospholipid hydroperoxide glutathione peroxidase and lipid soluble antioxidants such as vitamin E and reduced Co Q.[18,19] Ubiquinol may exert its antioxidant function indirectly by reducing the α-tocopheroxyl radical back to vitamin E or directly as a quencher of oxygen or lipid peroxyl radicals.[20]

3. Historical Aspect of Oxidative Damage to Mitochondria

Ottolenghi[21] was among the first to observe oxidative damage in mitochondria. Non-enzymic oxidation of unsaturated lipids has been shown to occur in a number of tissue preparations including mitochondria. The non-enzymic formation of lipid peroxide in mitochondrial suspensions upon addition of ascorbic acid and iron salts and the quantitative relationships between these reactants were presented. Mitochondria suspensions do not form lipid peroxides upon incubation, but rapid peroxide formation takes place when relatively small amounts of ascorbic acid are added to the incubation mixture. This reaction occurs equally well in mitochondrial suspensions previously boiled under nitrogen for 20 minutes and is apparently non-enzymic. Peroxide formation and ascorbic acid oxidation progress at comparable rates and reach apparent end points at the same time. The rate of lipid peroxide formation in the mitochondrial-ascorbic acid system is increased by ferrous ions. The increase is proportional to the concentration of iron in the range of $0.5–2.0 \times 10^{-6}$ M by extrapolation, the amount of iron present in the mitochondria can be estimated as 1×10^{-6} M. The catalytic effect of ferric ions is approximately 1/30 that of ferrous. This is probably due to the inability of the ferric ion to penetrate to the site of reaction because both ferric and ferrous ions are equally catalytic when an aqueous suspension of lecithin is substituted for mitochondria. Additional evidence of the importance of metal ions in the mitochondrial-ascorbic acid reaction is the inhibitory action of ethylenediaminetetraacetic acid (EDTA). Total inhibition of lipid peroxide formation occurs at $5 \times 10^{-6} M$ EDTA. Peroxide formation also occurs when larger amounts of ferrous salts are added to the mitochondrial suspensions in the absence of ascorbic acid. The reaction proceeds at a fast rate, and the amount of peroxide formed is roughly proportional to the amount of iron added. When an excess of mitochondria is used, the concentration of ascorbic acid limits the total peroxide production. This suggests that the basic mechanism of these reactions is a co-oxidation of unsaturated lipid and ascorbic acid. The bivalent state of the metal is of definite importance in the mitochondrial system as shown by the failure of the ferric salts to cause a comparable increase in the rate of the reaction.

In exploring possible mechanisms for the ascorbate-induced lysis of mitochondria reported earlier, Hoffsten *et al.*[22] have studied the formation of "lipid peroxide" during swelling or lysis of mitochondria by several agents. The correlation between the appearance of "lipid peroxide" and the beginning of swelling are so close in the ascorbate studies that it is not possible to say with certainty whether "lipid peroxide" formation begins first and is the cause of lysis. The changes in double bonds in unsaturated fatty acids of the membranes might in themselves lead to permeability or structural changes. In addition, the lipid peroxides behave something like free radicals and can lead to oxidation of thiol, dithiol, or other group of the membrane. These studies were followed by Hunter *et al.*[23] They reported that the possibility that ascorbate- and reduced glutathione-induced swelling and lysis of mitochondria were dependent on some metal, such as iron, which was contaminating reagents, or even the non-heme iron in mitochondria led us to investigate the action of added iron. The ferrous iron was of special interest as a result of its role in several reactions catalyzed by ascorbate. Unlike swelling induced by many other substances such as phosphate and thyroxine, swelling with ascorbate, reduced glutathione, or Fe^{++} is not dependent on endogenous or added substrates. There is a close correlation between lipid peroxide formation and swelling or lysis induced by Fe^{++}, just has been observed with ascorbate and oxidized plus reduced glutathione. Whether or not such effects contribute to physiological control or pathological phenomena remains to be seen, but these studies with isolated mitochondria provide additional information about structure and permeability control in the mitochondrial membranes.

Fe^{++} ion induces a swelling and lysis of mitochondria, which is quite different from electron-transported swelling. Although cyanide and antimycin A partially inhibit Fe^{++}-induced swelling, the concentrations required are higher than those necessary for respiratory chain inhibition. Uncouplers of oxidative phosphorylation, such as DNP, have no effect. Lipid peroxide formation is very well correlated swelling and lysis. Accelerators and inhibitors of this type of swelling affect lipid peroxidation formation in an exactly parallel fashion. Formation of lipid peroxide, possibly in some lipoproteins associated with electron transport and energy transfer or phosphorylation, causes first permeability increase and swelling. Extensive lipid peroxidation leads to lysis and disintegration.

Wills[24] reported that lipid peroxides, as measured by the thiobarbituric acid method, are formed in homogenates of many different tissues after incubation. Separated mitochondria form lipid peroxides after incubation. Iron, either in an inorganic form or as a heme complex, is likely to form an important part of the catalytic system in lipid peroxidation in the mitochondrial fraction. Ascorbate stimulates peroxide formation in mitochondrial suspensions. Lipid peroxides may be important as a factor causing, or a stage in, general membrane damage and they have been implicated in damage to mitochondrial membrane. The above studies formed the basis for such several later studies on oxidative damage to mitochondria. This was followed by studies on oxidative damage in mitochondria during aging and chemical toxicities as well as prevention by antioxidants. In recent years oxidative damage in relation to disease and apoptosis is the major focus of study in mitochondrial research.

4. Significance of Mitochondrial Oxidative Damage in Relation to Membrane Damage and Disease Development

Damage by ROS/RNS to mitochondrial components includes lipid peroxidation (LP), protein oxidation and mitochondrial DNA (mtDNA) mutations.[11,16] LP might be particularly harmful in mitochondria, that contain cardiolipin as a major component of the inner mitochondrial membrane, and which is required for the activity of cytochrome oxidase. Protein oxidation, which occurs as a result of oxidative stress, has been described to affect respiratory chain enzymes.[13,25,26]

Susceptibility of four major rat tissues to oxidative damage in terms of lipid peroxidation induced by *in vitro* ascorbate-Fe^{2+} in homogenates and mitochondria has been examined. Lipid peroxidation was maximum in brain, kidney and heart. The higher susceptibilities of brain and liver can be explained by substrate availability and to a lesser extent the level of antioxidants. The differences observed in the tissues studied may reflect their susceptibility to degenerative diseases and xenobiotic toxicity, which are considered as a result of oxidative damage to membranes.[27]

Modification of redox states of vital sulphydryl groups in mitochondria can result in damage to regulatory mechanisms, similar to those suggested to modulate signal transduction cascades. Inactivation of MnSOD in transgenic mice enhances ROS production and results in animal death by dilated cardiomyopathy, with partial inactivation of mitochondrial enzymes containing iron-sulfur centers.[28]

Damage to mtDNA is of special interest since it is extremely susceptible to oxidative damage. Being located in the matrix, it is close to the major source of ROS, moreover lacking introns and devoid of histones and other DNA-associated proteins, the probability of oxidative modification of a coding region of mtDNA is very high.[29] ROS were shown to induce extensive fragmentation and deletions in mtDNA as well as the content of 8-hydroxy-D-guanosine.[30]

Damage to mitochondria inevitably leads to disease. Mitochondrial damage in β-cells causes diabetes. Mitochondrial dysfunction has been implicated in all the major neurodegenerative diseases — Parkinson's, Alzheimer's, motor neuron disease, possibly in multiple sclerosis, cardiomyopathy, multi-organ system failure in sepsis, the process of aging and age-related disease. Some such studies linking mitochondrial oxidative damage to diseases are presented in Table 1. Detailed treatment of this subject will appear as a separate chapter in this book.

Production of free radicals by mitochondria has been considered by many to play a central role in the degradation of cellular function that appears

Table 1. Mitochondrial diseases and the relative parameters studied.

Diseases	Parameters studied	Effects	Reference
Alzheimer's disease and Parkinson's disease	↑Oxidative damage and mitochondrial dysfunction	Progressive supranuclear palsy	Albers *et al.*[117]
Alzheimer's disease	↑Redox transition metals, ↑oxidative stress	↑ROS in diseased neurons	Chao *et al.*[118]
Alzheimer's disease (AD)	↑AD-like pathology in transgenic mice; ↑AbetaPP, 8-OHG COX	Damaged endothelium and perivascular cells of lesioned microvessels in brain	Gjumrakch *et al.*[119]
Neurodegenerative disorders	↑ONOO-induced LP	Mitochondrial oxidative damage	Brooks *et al.*[120]
Cancer — tobacco carcinogenesis	Impaired human circulating lymphocytes	Increased endogenous production of ROS	Miro *et al.*[38]
Hepatocarcinogenesis	Mitochondrial membrane potential (DELTApsim); Levels of ROS by DCFDA and DHR123	Mitochondrial oxidative DNA and protein damage; stimulating formation of ROS leading to cell death	Qu *et al.*[39]
Type 1 and type 2 diabetes	↓Cellular GSH : GSSG ratio, ↑AGEs; ↓insulin secretion by pancreatic β-cells	Progression and pathological complications of diabetes	Green *et al.*[17]
Diabetic hyperglycemia	TBARS and O_2 consumption; coenzyme Q9	Increase in the susceptibility of diabetic heart mitochondria to oxidative stress; ↓coenzyme Q9	Santos *et al.*[121]

Table 1. (*Continued*)

Diseases	Parameters studied	Effects	Reference
Type I diabetes	↓State 3 oxygen consumption in cardiac mitochondria	Dysfunctional cardiomyopathy	Lashin and Romani[122]
Ischemia-reperfusion injury	↓MTT, respiratory control ratio and mitochondrial swelling	↑Phospholipase A2 and phospholipase D	Madesh *et al.*[43]
Heart failure following ischemia-reperfusion	↓Proton gradient; ↓respiration-linked ATP generation	↓Energy conservation and transition to a potent $O_2^{\bullet -}$-radical generator	Nohl *et al.*[45]
Ischemia-reperfusion injury	↓PARP inhibitors, i.e. 3-aminobenzamide, nicotinamide, BGP-15 and 4-hydroxyquinazoline; ↑LP, PO, ss DNA breaks	ROS-induced cardiac dysfunction	Halmosi *et al.*[46]
Coronary artery disease (CAD)	↑DNA damage	Atherosclerosis	Andreassi *et al.*[123]
Uremia	↑mtDNA mutations and oxidative damage in skeletal muscle; ↑8-OHdG	Skeletal myopathy	Lim *et al.*[124]
Arsenic toxicity	↓Pyruvate dehydrogenase (PDH) activity in HL60-cells	Oxidative damage to the protein	Samikkannu *et al.*[48]
Nephrotoxicity of ferric nitrilotriacetate (Fe-NTA)	Iron-induced cell injury	Mitochondrial and nuclear oxidative damage	Zainal *et al.*[49]
Toxicity by non-steroidal anti-inflammatory drugs	Functional impairment and altered lipid composition	Oxidative stress in mitochondria	Basivireddy *et al.*[47]

to underlie the process of aging, whereas some of the genes identified in the control of longevity appear to target mitochondria or at least to alter antioxidant defenses of the cell. In recent years, mitochondria have emerged as central players in the regulation of organized or programmed apoptotic cell death.[7]

Mitochondria play a central role in cell life and cell death. Substantial evidence now suggests that the accumulation of calcium into mitochondrial pathology, especially when that calcium uptake is accompanied by another stressor, in particular nitrosative or oxidative stress. The major process involved is the opening of the mitochondrial permeability transition pore. Hence, mitochondrial function and dysfunction have been implicated in many different aspects of health and disease.[7]

Under normal circumstances, the rate of generation of superoxide from mitochondria is rather low and does little damage, simply because it is efficiently removed by the superoxide dismutases. However, circumstances can arise for a variety of reasons (e.g. ingested chemicals that act as radical amplifiers, medically applied high concentrations of oxygen or during periods of reperfusion of tissues with oxygen following ischemia) where high rates of superoxide production do occur. Superoxide itself is especially damaging to the 4Fe-4S-type of iron-sulfur center.[16] For example, damage to the cytosolic isoenzymes of aconitase evident after exposure to superoxide results in the release of ferrous ions and also sets in motion an important regulatory mechanism: the deactivated enzyme becomes a binding protein for the mRNA for ferritin, prolonging its half-life and ensuring increased ferritin synthesis to bin free iron. The damage to other systems such as mitochondrial aconitase, complex I and succinate dehydrogenase, which also have important functional iron-sulfur centers, becomes very pronounced in MnSOD knockout mice, superoxide produce in the mitochondria is not removed by the normal mechanisms. Damage to these enzymes by superoxide undoubtedly impairs the normal functioning of the citric acid cycle. This, combined with the resulting inactivation of electron transport processes, then results in disordered metabolism with lack of mitochondrial ATP generation, leading to increase flux from glucose to lactate. These mice develop lactic acidonemia, caridomyopathy and degeneration of the basal ganglia, mimicking many of the symptoms seen in children with genetic defects of the respiratory chain. Knockout transgenic mice lacking

CuZn-SOD slowly develop a neuronal axonopathy, but are not affected at birth with the severe phenotypic changes evident in mice lacking MnSOD, which suggests that either the mitochondria are more susceptible to damage from superoxide or that quantitatively intra-mitochondrial superoxide production is more important. On the other hand, *Drosophila* lacking Cu, Zn-SOD, have a short life span.

The production of reactive oxygen species (ROS) by the mitochondrial respiratory chain contributes to a range of pathologies, including neurodegenerative diseases, ischemia-reperfusion injury and aging. There are also indications that mitochondrial ROS production plays a role in damage response and signal transduction pathways. Antioxidants designed to intercept mitochondrial ROS and reagents that specifically label mitochondrial thiol proteins.[31]

Mitochondrial respiratory chain diseases are a highly diverse group of disorders whose main unifying characteristic is the impairment of mitochondrial function. As befits an organelle containing gene products encoded by both mitochondrial DNA (mtDNA) and nuclear DNA (nDNA), these diseases caused by inherited errors in either genome, but the surprising number are sporadic, and a few are even caused by environmental factors.[32]

The mitochondrial genome encodes just a small number of subunits of the respiratory chain. Damaged mitochondrial proteins due to mutation or oxidative damage can be removed in two ways: either through lysosomal autophagy, that can account or an intra-mitochondrial proteinolytic pathway. A number of mitochondrial diseases have been identified whose mechanisms involve proteolytic dysfunction. Similar mechanisms probably play a role in diminished resistance to oxidative stress and in the aging process.[33]

Rat heart mitochondrial membranes exposed to the free radical generating system tert-butylhydroperoxide/Cu^{2+} undergo lipid peroxidation as evidenced by the accumulation of thiobarbituric acid reactive substances. Mitochondrial lipid peroxidation resulted in a marked loss of both cytochrome c oxidase activity and cardiolipin content. The alterations in the properties of cytochrome c oxidase were confined to a decrease in the maximal activity (V_{max}) with no change in the affinity (Km) with respect to the substrate cytochrome c. Various lipid soluble antioxidants could prevent the lipid peroxidation reaction and the associated loss of cytochrome c oxidase activity. External added cardiolipin but no other phospholipids nor peroxidized cardiolipin was able to prevent the loss of cytochrome oxidase activity induced by lipid peroxidation. These results establish a close correlation between oxidative damage to cardiolipin and alterations in the cytochrome oxidase activity and may prove useful in probing the molecular mechanism of free radical-induced peroxidative damage of mitochondria which has been proposed to contribute to aging and to chronic degenerative diseases.[34]

Protein modifications such as carbonylation, nitration and formation of lipid peroxidation adducts, e.g. 4-hydroxynonenal (HNE), are products of oxidative damage attributed to ROS.[35] The mitochondrial respiratory chain complexes I and III have been shown to be a major source of ROS *in vitro*. They showed a basal level of oxidative damage to specific proteins of adult bovine heart submitochondrial particle (SMP) complexes, and that most of these proteins are localized in the mitochondrial matrix. Electron leakage from respiratory chain complexes and subsequent ROS formation may cause damage to specific complex subunits and contribute to long-term accumulation of mitochondrial dysfunction.

Rat liver mitochondria, in different steps of the maturation process, were resolved by differential centrifugation at 1000 g (M1), 3000 g (M3) and 10,000 g (M10), and their characteristics determining susceptibility to stress conditions were investigated by Venditti *et al.*[36] The degree of oxidative damage to lipids and proteins was higher in M1 and not significantly different in M3 and M10 fractions. The order of susceptibility to both oxidative challenge and Ca^{2+}-induced swelling was M1 > M3 > M10. It seems that the swelling is due to permeabilization of oxidatively altered inner membrane and leads to discard mitochondria with high ROS production. If, as previous reports suggest, mitochondrial damage is initiative stimulus to mitochondrial biogenesis, the susceptibility of the M1 mitochondria to stressful conditions could be important to regulate cellular ROS production. In fact, it should favor the substitution of the oldest ROS-overproducing mitochondria with neoformed mitochondria endowed with a smaller capacity to produce free radicals.

Mitochondria constitute a primary locus for the intracellular formation and reactions of peroxynitrite, and these interactions are recognized to contribute to the biological pathological effects of both nitric oxide and peroxynitrite.[37] Extra- or intra-mitochondrially formed peroxynitrite can diffuse through mitochondrial compartments and undergo fast direct and free radical dependent target molecule reactions. These processes result in oxidation, nitration, and nitrosation of critical components in the matrix, inner and outer membrane, and intermembrane space.

4.1. *Mitochondrial damage during cancer and carcinogenesis*

Mitochondria constitute a source of reactive oxygen species. Miro *et al.*[38] tested whether mitochondrial function from human circulating lymphocytes is affected by smoking habit and if this could be associated with an increase in oxidative damage of biological membranes. In smokers, the mitochondrial respiratory chain (MRC) function of lymphocytes is disturbed and correlates with the degree of oxidative damage of membranes. This mitochondrial dysfunction could contribute to increased endogenous production of reactive oxygen species and could play a role in tobacco carcinogenesis.

Peroxisome proliferators have been found to induce hepatocarcinogenesis in rodents, and may cause mitochondrial damage.[39] Consistent with this, clofibrate increased hepatic mitochondrial oxidative DNA and protein damage in mice. The present investigation aimed to study the mechanism by which this might occur by examining the effect of clofibrate on freshly isolated mouse liver mitochondria and a cultured hepatocyte cell line, AML-12. Mitochondrial membrane potential (DELTApsim) was determined by using the fluorescent dye 5,5′,6,6′-tetrachloro-1,1′,3,3′-tetraethyl-benzimidazolylcarbocyanine iodide (JC-1) and tetramethylrhodamine methyl ester (TMRM). Application of clofibrate at concentrations greater than 0.3 mM rapidly collapsed the DELTApsim both in liver cells and in isolated mitochondria. The loss of DELTApsim occurred prior to cell death and appeared to involve the mitochondrial permeability transition (MPT), as revealed by calcein fluorescence studies and the protective effect of cyclosporin A (CsA) on the decrease in DELTApsim. Levels of ROS were measured with the fluorescent probes

5-(and-6)-carboxy-2′,7′-dichlorofluorescein diacetate (DCFDA) and dihydrorhodamine 123 (DHR123). Treatment of the hepatocytes with clofibrate caused a significant increase in intracellular and mitochondrial ROS. Antioxidants such as vitamin C, deferoxamine, and catalase were able to protect the cells against the clofibrate-induced loss of viability, as was CsA, but to a lesser extent. These results suggest that one action of clofibrate might be to impair mitochondrial function, so stimulating formation of ROS, which eventually contribute to cell death.

Oxidative damage to mitochondrial proteins, lipids, and DNA seem to influence the promotion and progression of tumors.[40] High-fat diets and diets high in iron decrease manganese superoxide dismutase activity, a mitochondrial antioxidant, in colon mucosa. Lipid peroxidation products are low in microsomal preparations from colonic mucosa even under peroxide-inducing conditions. However, damage specific to mitochondrial membranes is unknown. This study was designed to investigate dietary lipid and iron effects on fatty acid incorporation and lipid peroxide formation in mitochondrial membranes of colonic mucosa. Peroxidation products in mitochondrial membranes were significantly greater than in microsomal membranes. Dietary treatment significantly affected mitochondrial peroxidation in carcinogen-treated animals. Therefore, mitochondria from colon mucosa are more susceptible to peroxidation than are microsomes, dietary factors influence the degree of peroxidation, and the resulting damage may be important in early colon carcinogenesis.

Studies have indicated that mitochondrial dysfunction is involved in carcinogenesis. Zhou *et al.*[41] examined the possible mechanisms behind mitochondrial impairment in p53-deficient human cancer cells. Their studies have revealed that p53 is involved in the regulation of cytochrome c oxidase II at the protein level but not at the mRNA level. p53 does not affect mtDNA mutation or mitochondrial ultrastructure. Further study by Delsite *et al.*[42] has shown that mitochondrial impairment in breast cancer cells results in altered expression of nuclear genes involved in signaling, cellular architecture, metabolism, cell growth and differentiation, and apoptosis. These genes may mediate the cross talk between mitochondria and the nucleus.

4.2. *Damage during ischemia-reperfusion injury*

Reactive oxygen species have been implicated in cellular injury during ischemia/reperfusion (I/R).[43] Mitochondria are one of the main targets of oxygen free radicals and damage to this organelle leads to cell death. Reports suggest that nitric oxide (NO) may offer protection from damage during I/R. It was observed that I/R of the intestine is associated with functional alterations in mitochondria as suggested by MTT reduction, respiratory control ratio and mitochondrial swelling. Mitochondrial lipid changes suggestive of activation of phospholipase A2 and phospholipase D were also seen after I/R-mediated injury. These changes were prevented by the simultaneous presence of a NO donor in the lumen of the intestine. These studies have suggested that structural and functional alterations of mitochondria are prominent features of I/R injury to the intestine, which can be ameliorated by NO.

Edaravone is a potent free radical scavenger in the prevention of mitochondrial injury induced by hepatic ischemia and reperfusion.[44] Edaravone protects against mitochondrial injury, which prevents mitochondrial oxidative stress and improves I/R-induced hepatic energy metabolism.

Nohl *et al.*[45] elucidated the role of mitochondria in the development of heart failure following I/R. Isolated mitochondria were exposed to metabolic conditions which have developed during I/R in the cell (anoxia, lactogenesis) and their response was studied. Heart mitochondria treated in that way responded with an incomplete collapse of the trans-membranous proton gradient, thereby impairing respiration-linked ATP generation. Mitochondria are likely to play a pathogenic role into the reperfusion injury of the heart both, by an impairment of energy conservation and their transition to a potent $O_2^{\bullet-}$-radical generator. The exogenous NADH-dehydrogenase of heart mitochondria is mainly responsible for functional changes of these organelles during I/R.

Halmosi *et al.*[46] have shown that I/R induces ROS formation, and ROS lead to cardiac dysfunction, in part, via the activation of the nuclear poly (ADP-ribose) polymerase (PARP). PARP inhibitors such as 3-aminobenzamide, nicotinamide, BGP-15 and 4-hydroxyquinazoline significantly decrease the I/R-induced increase of lipid peroxidation, protein oxidation, single strand DNA breaks, and the inactivation of respiratory complexes, which indicate a decreased mitochondrial ROS production in the reperfusion period. Surprisingly, PARP inhibitors, but not the chemically similar 3-aminobenzoic acid, prevented the H_2O_2-induced inactivation of cytochrome oxidase in isolated heart mitochondria, suggesting the presence of an additional mitochondrial target for PARP inhibitors. Therefore, PARP inhibitors, in addition to their important primary effect of decreasing the activity of nuclear PARP and decreasing NAD^+ and ATP consumption, reduce I/R-induced endogenous ROS production and protect the respiratory complexes from ROS-induced inactivation, providing an additional mechanism by which they can protect the heart from oxidative damages.

4.3. *Damage during toxicity by drugs and chemicals*

Non-steroidal anti-inflammatory drugs (NSAIDs) are known to cause small intestinal damage but the pathogenesis of this toxicity is not well established. In isolated mitochondrial preparations from various erythrocyte fractions, significant functional impairment and altered lipid composition were seen mainly in mitochondria from villus cells. Arginine and zinc-pretreatment were found to protect against these effects. These results suggest for the first time that the villus tip cells are more vulnerable to the damaging effects of indomethacin and that oxidative stress in mitochondria is possibly involved in this damage.[47]

Arsenic was shown to inhibit pyruvate dehydrogenase (PDH) activity through binding to vicinal dithiols in pure enzyme and tissue extract. No data are available on how arsenic inhibits PDH activity in human cells. Mitochondrial respiration inhibitors suppressed the As_2O_3-induced H_2O_2 production and As_2O_3 inhibition of PDH activity. Treatment with H_2O_2 plus Fenton metals also decreased the PDH activity in HL60- cells. Therefore, it seems that As_2O_3 elevates H_2O_2 production in mitochondria and this may produce hydroxyl through Fenton reaction and result in oxidative damage to the protein of PDH activity.[48] Study by Zainal *et al.*[49] suggests that the mechanism of acute nephrotoxicity of ferric nitrilotriacetate (Fe-NTA) involves mitochondrial and nuclear oxidative damage, findings that may help to define the mechanisms of iron-induced cell injury.

4.4. *Oxidative damage during normal physiological states — pregnancy*

Pregnancy is a physiological state in which there is increased generation of ROS in various tissues. However, the different maternal tissues are protected against oxidative damage. Progesterone, the gestational steroid elaborated during pregnancy, inhibited lipid peroxidation in brain mitochondria in a dose-dependent manner. The observed temporary decrease in peroxidation potential may be a special adaptation to protect membranes in the brain against oxidative stress during pregnancy.[50]

Decrease in the lipid peroxidation of hepatic mitochondria was observed with the inducers of lipid per oxidation namely the non-enzymatic ascorbate-Fe^{2+} and enzymatic NADPH. Low potential for lipid peroxidation during such a state, besides being a possible factor contributing to the growth of cells, may be an adaptation so as to reduce the chances of unfavorable alterations in the biological membranes involved in biochemical reactions during gestation.[51]

In the renal mitochondria, lipid peroxidation without co-factors and that induced by cumene hydroperoxide, ascorbate and NADPH is decreased during pregnancy.[52] The observed decrease in lipid peroxidation during gestation is reflected by low levels of total lipid and phospholipid. Endogenous inhibitors of lipid peroxidation also increase during pregnancy. Low potential for lipid peroxidation, besides being a possible factor contributing to cell growth, may also be an adaptation so as to reduce the chances of unfavorable alterations in the biological membranes involved in these biochemical reactions.

5. Aging

5.1. *Role of mitochondrial oxidative damage in aging and longevity*

Oxygen enters a mitochondrion and breaks down to ROS. The ROS can attack the membrane, which makes another ROS. The new ROS could attack the mitochondrial DNA, which makes yet another ROS. Eventually the damaged membrane repairs itself but the DNA does not. The destruction continues until an antioxidant molecule destroys the ROS. Injured mitochondria, though, become almost non-functional. The resulting energy shortage inhibits a cell's normal functioning, and tissues start aging.[53]

People spend more time trying to avoid aging than trying to understand it. We deny aging at first and then — seeing its reality in the mirror — grudgingly accept it. Without oxygen, we cannot generate enough energy to live, and we quickly die. Once breathed in, oxygen goes to the mitochondria to help convert the energy from food to a chemical form that is useful to cells. A mitochondrion's lipid membrane and protein enzymes serve as the nearest target for the ROS, but these components can be repaired. Mitochondria, though, are the only cell organelles with their own genetic system, and the one to ten mitochondrial DNA molecules are very vulnerable to irreparable oxidative damage. Injured mitochondria soon become almost non-functional. The resulting energy shortage inhibits a cell's normal functioning, and tissues start aging.

In studies of flies, mice and worms, aging proceeded faster than ever, after inactivating oxidative stress-resistant genes. Apparently, stress-resistance pathways function in a parallel but integrated manner with the insulin-like signaling system. This mitochondrial-free radical theory of aging explains much of what happens in aging laboratory model systems and in humans. Many investigators realized that increasing the level of defense mechanisms against oxidative stress could extend an organism's health span. The lower level of oxidative damage and delayed onset of senescence in those flies arose from decreased production and increased destruction of ROS. However, using genetic engineering techniques to insert extra copies of these oxidative stress resistance genes into mice has not yet resulted in extending longevity.

Mitochondrial oxidative damage increases with aging and this contributes to the decrease in efficiency of oxidative phosphorylation associated with aging. Dietary restriction, which increases life span in mammals, may operate by decreasing mitochondrial damage, supporting a role for mitochondrial oxidative damage in the metabolic decline associated with aging. A large number of inherited and sporadic human diseases are caused by mutations to mitochondrial genes, either those encoded by mtDNA or nuclear DNA. Mitochondrial DNA damage and mutations accumulate with aging and mtDNA defects increase mitochondrial radical production, possibly establishing a destructive spiral of increasing oxidative stress and mtDNA damage.[2]

Oxygen free radicals can contribute in some way to the aging process. Evidence points to a basic aging mechanism, governed by telomere shortening, which can be modulated by the lifetime production rates of oxygen free radicals. The mechanism of influence seems to be mediated through fragility of the telomeric sites predisposing the DNA to single-strand breaks and other damage. When ROS are responsible for such damage, the breaks cannot easily be repaired and telomere shortening is accelerated. The understanding of this relationship between mitochondria, free radical production and the rate of telomere shortening is at an early stage. A new round of experimental work is needed to explain the exact nature of these relationships between mitochondrial metabolism, mitochondrial free radical production, basal metabolic rate, mtDNA mutations and deletion, telomeric damage in chromosomal DNA and the whole complex process of aging.[53]

Birds have a maximum longevity (MLSP) much greater than mammals of similar metabolic rate and body size. Thus they are ideal models to identify longevity characteristics not linked to low metabolic rates. Pamplona *et al.*[54] show that the fatty acid double bond content of total lipids and phosphatidylcholine, phosphatidylethanolamine and cardiolipin fractions of heart mitochondria is intrinsically lower in pigeons (MLSP = 35 years) than in rats (MLSP = 4 years). This is mainly due to the lower content of the most highly unsaturated docosahexaenoic acid ($22:6n-3$) and in some fractions arachidonic acid ($20:4n-6$). The lower double bond content leads to a lower sensitivity to *in vitro* lipid peroxidation and is associated with a lower concentration of lipid peroxidation products *in vivo*, and a lower level of malondialdehyde-lycine protein adducts in heart mitochondria of pigeon than rat. The results also show, for the first time in the physiological model, that lipid peroxidizability is related to lipoxidative protein damage.

In order to ascertain whether lower fatty acid double bond content protects mitochondria by decreasing lipid and protein oxidation and oxygen radical generation, the double bond content of rat heart mitochondrial membranes was manipulated by chronic feeding with semi-purified AIN-93G diets rich in highly unsaturated (UNSAT) or saturated (SAT) oils.[15] UNSAT rat heart mitochondria had significantly higher double bond content and lipid peroxidation than SAT mitochondria. They also showed increased levels of the markers of protein oxidative damage malondialdehyde-lysine, protein carbonyls and (carboxymethyl) lysine adducts. Increasing the degree of fatty acid unsaturation in heart mitochondria increases oxidative damage to their lipids and proteins, and can also increase their rates of mitochondrial oxygen radical generation in situations in which the degree of reduction of Complex III is higher than normal. These observations strengthen the notion that the relatively low double bond content of the membranes of long-lived animals could have evolved to protect them from oxidative damage.

Endogenous antioxidants are negatively correlated with maximum longevity. The same is true for the rates of mitochondrial oxygen radical generation, oxidative damage to mitochondrial DNA, and the degree of fatty acid unsaturation of cellular membranes in postmitotic tissues.[55] The lower rate of mitochondrial oxygen radical generation of long-lived animals in relation to that of short-lived ones can be a primary cause of their slow aging rate. This is secondarily complemented in long-lived animals with low rates of lipid peroxidation due to their low degrees of fatty acid unsaturation. These two traits suggest that the rate of generation of endogenous oxidative damage determines, at least in part, the rate of aging in animals.

Aging-associated respiratory function decline can result in enhanced production of ROS in mitochondria. Within a certain concentration range, ROS may induce stress response of the cells by altering expression of respiratory genes to uphold the energy metabolism to rescue the cell.[56] However, beyond the threshold, ROS may cause a wide spectrum of oxidative damage to various cellular components to result in cell death or elicit apoptosis by induction of mitochondrial membrane permeability transition and release of apoptogenic factors such as cytochrome c. Mitochondria act like a biosensor of oxidative stress and they enable cells to undergo changes in aging and age-related diseases. Work done in the past few years supports the view that oxidative stress and oxidative damage are a result of concurrent accumulation of mtDNA mutations and defective antioxidant enzymes in human aging.

The purpose of study by Yan *et al.*[57] to test the hypothesis that elevation in protein oxidative damage during the aging process is a targeted rather than a stochastic phenomenon. Oxidative damage to proteins in mitochondrial membranes in the flight muscles of the housefly, manifested as carbonyl modifications, was detected immunochemically with anti-dinitrophenyl antibodies. Adenine nucleotide translocase (ANT) was found to be the only protein in the mitochondrial membranes exhibiting a detectable age-associated increase in carbonyls. The age-related elevation in ANT carbonyl content was correlated with a corresponding loss in its functional activity. Senescent flies that had lost the ability to fly exhibited a relatively higher degree of ANT oxidation and a greater loss of functional activity than their cohorts of the same age that were still able to fly. ANT was also the only mitochondrial membrane protein exhibiting adducts of the lipid peroxidation product of 4-hydroxynonenal. Results of this study indicate that proteins in mitochondrial membranes are modified selectively during aging.

Bejma *et al.*[58] examined the effect of an acute bout of exercise on intracellular ROS production, lipid and protein peroxidation, and GSH status in the skeletal muscle of young adult (8 mo, n = 24) and old (24 mo, n = 24) female Fischer 344 rats. This data provided direct evidence that oxidant production in skeletal muscle is increased in old age and during prolonged exercise, with both mitochondrial respiratory chain and NADPH oxidase as potential sources. The alteration of muscle lipid peroxidation and mitochondrial GSH status were consistent with these conclusions.

5.2. *Ischemia-reperfusion injury in the heart and aging*

Cardiac mitochondria exhibit decreased rates of ATP-dependent respiration as a result of ischemia with further declines evident upon reperfusion.[59] Studies indicate that an increase in mitochondrial generation of reactive oxygen radical species contributes to the loss in mitochondrial function observed during ischemia-reperfusion. Alterations in certain electron transport chain components contribute to increased generation of oxygen radicals and studies have identified oxidative modifications that are likely to contribute to loss in mitochondrial function during cardiac ischemia-reperfusion.

The aged heart sustains greater injury during ischemia and reperfusion compared to the adult heart.[60] Aging decreases oxidative phosphorylation and the activity of complexes III and IV only in interfibrillar mitochondria

(IFM) that reside among the myofibrils, whereas subsarcolemmal mitochondria (SSM), located beneath the plasma membrane, remain unaltered. Mitochondria are the major source of the reactive oxygen species that are generated during myocardial ischemia. Complex III is the major site of mitochondrial oxyradical production during ischemia in the adult heart. Ischemic damage to the electron transport chain and release of reactive oxygen species increases from mitochondria in the aged heart, leading to additional damage during reperfusion.

Cardiac reperfusion and aging are associated with increased rates of mitochondrial free radical production.[61] Mitochondria are therefore a likely site of reperfusion-induced oxidative damage, the severity of which may increase with age. 4-Hydroxy-2-nonenal (HNE), a major product of lipid peroxidation, increases in concentration upon reperfusion of ischemic cardiac tissue, can react with and inactivate enzymes, and inhibits mitochondrial respiration *in vitro*. HNE modification of mitochondrial protein(s) might, therefore, be expected to occur during reperfusion and result in loss in mitochondrial function. In addition, this process may be more prevalent in aged animals. Thus, HNE-modified protein was present in only those mitochondria exhibiting reperfusion-induced declines in function. These studies therefore identify mitochondria as a subcellular target of reperfusion damage and a site of age-related increases in susceptibility to injury.

5.3. *Aging and caloric restriction*

Caloric restriction is known to delay aging. The best studied candidate for a caloric restriction mimetic, 2DG (2-deoxy-D-glucose), works by interfering with the way cells process the sugar glucose.[62] It has demonstrated that chemicals can replicate the effects of caloric restriction. By limiting food intake, caloric restriction minimizes the amount of glucose entering cells. Researchers have proposed several explanations for why interruption of glucose processing and ATP production might retard aging. One possibility relates to the ATP-making machinery's emission of free radicals, which are thought to contribute to aging and to such age-related diseases as cancer by damaging cells. Reduced operation of the machinery should limit their production and thereby constrain damage.

5.4. *Aging and DNA damage*

In recent years, oxidative modification and mutation of mtDNA have been found to increase exponentially with age in human and animal tissues.[63] The mutant mtDNA-encoded respiratory enzymes exhibit impaired respiratory function, and thereby increase the production of ROS and free radicals, which further elevate the oxidative stress and oxidative damage to mitochondria.

mtDNA mutations and impaired respiratory function have been demonstrated in various tissues of aged individuals. Lu *et al.*[64] hypothesized that age-dependent increase of ROS and free radicals production in mitochondria are associated with the accumulation of large-scale mtDNA deletions. Their results showed an age-dependent increase of 8-OH-dG level in the total DNA of skin tissues of the subjects above the age of 60 years. The specific content of malondialdehyde, an end-product of lipid peroxidation, was also found to increase with age. The activities of Cu, Zn SOD, catalase, and glutathione peroxidase (GPx) were found to decrease with age. Taken together, they suggest that the functional decline of free radical scavenging enzymes and the elevation of oxidative stress may play an important role in eliciting oxidative damage and mutation of mtDNA during the human aging process.

Respiratory function of mitochondria is compromised in aging human tissues and severely impaired in the patients with mitochondrial disease.[65] A wide spectrum of mtDNA mutations has been established to associate with mitochondrial diseases. Some of these mtDNA mutations also occur in various human tissues in an age-dependent manner. These mtDNA mutations cause defects in the respiratory chain due to impairment of the gene expression and structure of respiratory chain polypeptides that are encoded by the mitochondrial genome. Since defective mitochondria generate more ROS such as $O_2^{\bullet -}$ and H_2O_2 via electron leak, we hypothesized that oxidative stress is a contributing factor for aging and mitochondrial disease. This hypothesis has been supported by the findings that oxidative stress and oxidative damage in tissues and culture cells are increased in elderly subjects and patients with mitochondrial diseases. Another line of supporting evidence is the recent finding that the enzyme activities of Cu, Zn-SOD, catalase and glutathione peroxidase (GPx) decrease with age in skin fibroblasts. The imbalance in the expression of these antioxidant enzymes indicates that the production of ROS is in excess of their removal, which in turn may elicit an elevation of oxidative stress in the fibroblasts. Indeed, it was found that intracellular levels of H_2O_2 and oxidative damage to DNA and lipids in skin fibroblasts from elderly subjects or patients with mitochondrial diseases are significantly increased as compared to those of age-matched controls. Furthermore, Mn-SOD or GPx-1 gene knockout mice were found to display neurological disorders and enhanced oxidative damage similar to those observed in the patients with mitochondrial disease.

5.5. *Antioxidants and aging*

Micronutrients deficiency may explain, in good part, why the quarter of the population that eats the fewest fruits and vegetables (five portions a day is advised) has approximately double the cancer rate for most types of cancer when compared to the quarter with the highest intake.[66] Aging appears to be due to the oxidants produced by mitochondria as by-products of normal metabolism. In old rats, mitochondrial membrane potential, cardiolipin levels, respiratory control ratio, and overall cellular O_2, consumption are lower than in young rats, and the level of oxidants (per unit O_2) is higher. The level of mutagenic aldehydes from lipid peroxidation is also increased. Ambulatory activity declines markedly in old rats. Feeding old rats the normal mitochondrial metabolites acetyl carnitin and lipoic acid for a few weeks restores mitochondrial functions, lowers oxidants to the level of a young rat, and increases ambulatory activity. Thus, these two metabolites can be considered necessary for health in old age and are therefore conditional micronutrients. This restoration suggests a plausible mechanism: age-increased oxidative damage to proteins and lipid membranes causes a deformation of structure of key enzymes, with a consequent lessening of affinity (Km) for the enzyme substrate; an increased level of the substrate restores the velocity of the reaction, and thus restores function.

Mitochondrial dysfunction appears to contribute to some of the loss of function accompanying aging. A high flux of oxidants during aging not only damages mitochondria, but other important cell biomolecules as well.[67] DL-alpha-lipoic acid supplemented aged rats showed a decrease in the levels of lipid peroxidation and oxidized glutathione and an increase in the levels of reduced glutathione, vitamins C and E and the activities of mitochondrial enzymes like isocitrate dehydrogenase, alpha-ketoglutarate dehydrogenase, succinate dehydrogenase, NADH-dehydrogenase and cytochrome-c-oxidase. Thus, lipoic acid reverses the age-associated decline in endogenous low molecular weight antioxidants and mitochondrial enzymes and, therefore, may lower the increased risk of oxidative damage that occurs during aging. It can be concluded that lipoic acid supplementation enhances the activities of mitochondrial enzymes and antioxidant status and thereby protects mitochondria from aging.

Harman first suggested in 1972 that mitochondria might be the biological clock in aging, noting that the rate of oxygen consumption should determine the rate of accumulation of mitochondrial damage produced by free radical reactions[68]. Later in 1980, Miquel and coworkers proposed the mitochondrial theory of cell aging. Mitochondria from post-mitotic cells use O_2 at a high rate, hence releasing oxygen radicals that exceed the cellular antioxidant defenses. The key role of mitochondria in cell aging has been outlined by the degeneration induced in cells microinjected with mitochondria isolated from fibroblasts of old rats, espccially by the inverse relationship reported between the rate of mitochondrial production of hydroperoxide and the maximum life span of species. An important change in mitochondrial lipid composition is the age-related decrease found in cardiolipin content. The concurrent enhancement of lipid peroxidation and oxidative modification of proteins in mitochondria further increases mutations and oxidative damage to mtDNA in the aging process. Treatment with certain antioxidants, such as sulfur-containing antioxidants, vitamins C and E, or the *Ginkgo biloba* extract EGb 761, protects against the age-associated oxidative damage to mtDNA and the oxidation of mitochondrial glutathione.

Although diet supplementation with antioxidants has not been able to increase consistently the species-characteristic maximum life span, it results in significant extension of the mean life span of laboratory animals.[69] Moreover, diets containing high levels of antioxidants such as vitamins C and E seem able to reduce the risk of suffering age-related immune dysfunctions and arteriosclerosis. Presently, the focus of age-related antioxidant research is on compounds such as deprenyl, coenzyme Q10, alpha lipoic acid, and the glutathione-precursors thioproline and N-acetylcyctein, which may be able to neutralize the ROS at their sites of production in the mitochondria. Diet supplementation with these antioxidants may protect the mitochondria against respiration-linked oxygen stress, with preservation of the genetic and structural integrity of these energy-producing organelles and concomitant increase in functional life span.

6. Antioxidants and Mitochondrial Oxidative Damage

A number of antioxidants are shown to protect mitochondria against oxidative damage (see Table 2). These include (1) vitamins and related compounds, (2) other endogenous compounds, (3) natural compounds, (4) synthetic antioxidants, and (5) expression of genes.

6.1. *Vitamins and related compounds*

6.1.1. *Beta-carotene*

Elliott *et al.*[70] investigated the effects of oxidative insult, applied with hydrogen peroxide, on gene transcript levels in a human lymphocyte cell line (Molt-17) using mRNA differential display. Levels of the rarer, larger transcript were consistently reduced in a rapid, sustained and dose-dependent manner following hydrogen peroxide treatment. Prior supplementation of the cells with beta-carotene provided some protection against the reduction levels of this transcript following hydrogen peroxide treatment. It is an incompletely processed product of the mitochondrial genome encompassing ATPase subunits 8 and 6 plus the adjacent gene for cytochrome c oxidase subunit 3. This decrease in one specific mitochondrial transcript may represent a novel mechanism for differential expression of mitochondrially-encoded genes. The aim of this study was to identify genes regulated at the level of transcription in response to oxidative stress that might be of use as markers of oxidative stress or oxidative status *in vivo* in human studies.

6.1.2. *Alpha-tocopherol*

Supplementation with alpha-tocopheryl acetate had little or no impact on the steady-state level of cellular oxidative damage.[71] Zhang *et al.*[72] investigated

Table 2. Various antioxidants and their protective effects on oxidative damage in mitochondria.

Antioxidants	Parameters studied	Effects	References
Lipoic acid	Neutralize ROS in mitochondria of somatic differentiated cells	↑Functional life span	Miquel[64]
Beta-carotene	mRNA differential display in human lymphocyte cell line	Markers oxidative status *in vivo* in human studies	Elliott *et al.*[70]
Alpha-tocopherol	Caloric restriction	Little or no impact on the steady-state level of cellular oxidative damage	Sumien *et al.*[71]
Alpha tocopheryl succinate (TS)	↑LOOH, ↓alpha-tocopherol (T)	Complete protection against ethyl methanesulphonate (EMS)-induced oxidative damage	Zhang *et al.*[72] Fariss *et al.*[73]
2-(2-(triphenylphosphonio) ethyl)-3,4-dihydro-2,5,7,8-tetramethyl-2H-1-benzopyran-6-ol bromide (TPPB)	Coupling to another antioxidant vitamin E	↓Mitochondrial oxidative damage	Smith *et al.*[74]
Vitamins C and E at supra-nutritional doses	Oxidative damage to DNA in skeletal muscle mitochondria	Protect against oxidative damage to skeletal muscle mitochondria caused by AZT	Garcia *et al.*[75]
Tocotrienols in palm oil	LP in hepatic mitochondria	↓LP in hepatic mitochondria in palm oil-fed rats	Nesaretnam *et al.*[76]

(continued)

Table 2. (*Continued*)

Antioxidants	Parameters studied	Effects	References
Tocotrienol-rich fraction (TRF) from palm oil	AAPH, photosensitization, ascorbate-Fe^{2+}-induced damage to lipids and proteins in rat brain mitochondria	More effective than α-tocopherol as natural antioxidant supplement	Kamat and Devasagayam[77]
Tocotrienol-rich fraction (TRF) from palm oil	↓LP	Effectively protects RLM against oxidative damage induced by peroxynitrite an $^1O_2$	Kamat *et al.*[78]
Chlorophyllin (CHL)	γ-Radiation, photosensitization-induced LP, protein oxidation, GSH and SOD	10 μM CHL gives high degree of protection	Boloor *et al.*[89]
Chlorophyllin (CHL)	Cytochrome c oxidase, succinate dehydrogenase and protein carbonyls in rat liver mitochondria	10 μM more effective than ascorbic acid, glutathione, mannitol and tert-butanol	Kamat *et al.*[90]
Vanillin	Protein oxidation and lipid peroxidation in hepatic mitochondria	2.5 mM vanillin prevents oxidative damage	Kamat *et al.*[91]
Caffeine	Modification of oxygen-dependent and independent effects of γ-irradiation in membranes; LP, protein oxidation, GSH and SOD	Effectively protected membranes against the oxic component of damage but may not do so for the anoxic component	Kamat *et al.*[92]

Table 2. (*Continued*)

Antioxidants	Parameters studied	Effects	References
Caffeine	^{60}Co γ-rays (45-600Gy) – induced damage to SOD, SDH, cytochrome c oxidase	1 mM caffeine is effective	Kamat *et al.*[86]
Nicotinamide (vitamin B_3)	Ascorbate-Fe^{2+} and photosensitization-induced LP and protein oxidation systems in rat brain mitochondria	Protection of cellular membranes in brain	Kamat *et al.*[79]
Asparagus racemosus	Gamma radiation-induced damage in rat liver mitochondria	10 μg/ml is comparable to standard antioxidants glutathione and ascorbic acid	Kamat *et al.*[93]
Coenzyme Q (CoQ_{10})	↑CoQ homologues	↓Protein oxidative damage, ↑Antioxidant potential	Kwong *et al.*[80]
Serotonin	Dopamine-induced viability loss in PC12 cells	↓Thiol oxidation	Park *et al.*[82]
Beta-carbolines	Dopamine or 6-hydroxydopamine-induced viability loss in PC12 cell	↓Thiol oxidation	Kim *et al.*[97]

(*continued*)

Table 2. (*Continued*)

Antioxidants	Parameters studied	Effects	References
N-acetylcysteine	GSH	↑Mitochondrial complex I and IV specific activities	Banaclocha[98]
Melatonin	GSH-Px in fetal rat brain	Cell survival	Acuna *et al.*[83] Wakatsuki *et al.*[84]
Carvedilol	Preservation of mitochondrial functions	Cardioprotective effects	Santos and Moreno[99]
Boldine	MDA, carbonyls in pancreas, kidney and liver in STZ-induced diabetic rats	Protects from diabetes mellitus	Jang *et al.*[100]
Curcuma longa	LP in liver mitochondria and microsome membranes in atherosclerotic rabbits	↓LP	Quiles *et al.*[95]
Curcumin	LP induced by methylene blue and Rose Bengal in mitochondria of rat skin	↓LP	Devasagayam *et al.*[96]
Edavarone, a free radical scavenger	Hepatic ischemia-reperfusion injury	Prevents mitochondrial oxidative stress	Okatani *et al.*[44]

the mechanism of alpha-tocopheryl succinate (TS) cytoprotection against mitochondria-derived oxidative damage. Incubation of isolated rat hepatocytes with ethyl methane sulphonate (EMS), a mitochondrial alkylating toxicant, caused mitochondrial dysfunction and necrotic cell death that was dependent on the production of ROS and lipid peroxidation. Mitochondria isolated from these cells showed a three-fold increase in lipid hydroperoxides and a selective depletion of alpha-tocopherol (T), which preceded cell death. The pretreatment of hepatocytes with TS dramatically enriched cells and mitochondria with alpha-tocopherol and provided these membranes with complete protection against EMS-induced oxidative damage. Inhibition of mitochondrial ROS production and lipid peroxidation by T released from TS are the critical events responsible for TS-mediated cytoprotection against toxic oxidative stress derived from both mitochondrial complexes I and III. The findings suggest that TS treatment may prove useful in combating diseases associated with mitochondrial-derived oxidative stress.

Vitamin E succinate (TS) administration may prove useful for the prevention and treatment of oxidative stress-mediated diseases, especially those of mitochondrial origin.[73]

Mitochondrial oxidative damage contributes significantly to a range of human disorders. To prevent this damage, Smith *et al.*[74] have delivered a molecule containing the active antioxidant moiety of vitamin E to mitochondria. This was carried out by covalently coupling the antioxidant moiety to a lipophilic triphenylphosphonium cation. This mitochondrially targeted antioxidant, 2-(2-(triphenylphosphonio) ethyl)-3,4-dihydro-2,5,7,8-tetramethyl-2H-1-benzopyran-6-ol bromide (TPPB), accumulated several hundred-fold within the mitochondrial matrix, driven by the organelle's large membrane potential. The mitochondrially targeted antioxidant TPPB has potential as an antioxidant therapy for disorders involving mitochondrial oxidative damage. It also suggests a new family of mitochondrially targeted antioxidants, redox active and pharmacologically active molecules designed to prevent damage or manipulate mitochondrial function.

AIDS patients who receive zidovudine (AZT) frequently suffer from myopathy. This has been attributed to mitochondrial (mt) damage, and specifically to the loss of mtDNA.[75] Their study examines whether AZT causes oxidative damage to DNA in patients and to skeletal muscle mitochondria in mice, and whether this damage may be prevented by supranutritional doses of antioxidant vitamins. Dietary supplements with vitamins C and E at supranutritional doses protect against oxidative damage to skeletal muscle mitochondria caused by AZT.

6.1.3. *Tocotrienols*

Long term feeding of rats with palm oil as one of the dietary components significantly reduced the peroxidation potential of hepatic mitochondria.[76] As compared to hepatic mitochondria isolated from rats fed control or corn oil rich diet, those from palm oil fed group showed significantly less susceptibility to peroxidation induced by ascorbate and NADPH. *In vitro* studies as well as analyses of co-factors related to peroxidation potential indicated that the observed decrease in palm oil-fed rats may be due to increased amounts of antioxidants in terms of tocotrienol as well as decrease in the availability of substrates for peroxidation.

The tocotrienol-rich fraction (TRF) from palm oil, being tried as a more economical and efficient substitute for α-tocopherol, significantly inhibited oxidative damage *in vitro* to both lipids and proteins in rat brain mitochondria induced by ascorbate-Fe^{2+}, the free radical initiator azobis (2-amidopropane) dihydrochloride (AAPH) and photosensitization.[77] TRF was significantly more effective than α-tocopherol. This fraction from palm oil can be considered as natural antioxidant supplement capable of protecting the brain against oxidative damage and thereby from the ensuing adverse alterations.

Energy absorption process of oxygen generates singlet oxygen ($^1O_2$). Peroxynitrite is a potent oxidant of biological interest; it is produced by endothelial cells, Kupffer cells, neutrophils, and macrophages during phagocytosis. The peroxynitrite mediates oxidation of large numbers of crucial cellular molecules. Studies by Kamat *et al.*[78] have focused attention on palm oil, an edible vegetable oil rich in vitamin E (having both tocotrienol and tocopherol), because of its popularity in human diets in all parts of the world. Their studies showed that TRF from palm oil effectively protects rat liver mitochondria against oxidative damage induced by peroxynitrite. An $^1O_2$ TRF may have potential applications as a dietary supplement in preventing humans against the effect of ROS/RNS.

6.1.4. *Nicotinamide*

Nicotinamide (vitamin B_3) and endogenous metabolite showed significant inhibition of oxidative damage induced by ROS generated by ascorbate-Fe^{2+} and photosensitization systems in rat brain mitochondria.[79] It protected against both protein oxidation and lipid peroxidation at millimolar concentrations. Inhibition was more pronounced against oxidation of proteins than peroxidation of lipids. The protective effect observed, at biologically relevant concentrations, with nicotinamide was more than that of the endogenous antioxidant ascorbic acid and α-tocopherol. Hence, our studies suggest that nicotinamide (vitamin B_3) can be considered as a potent antioxidant capable of protecting the cellular membranes in brain, which is highly susceptible to prooxidants, against oxidative damage induced by ROS.

6.1.5. *Coenzyme Q10*

Coenzyme Q (CoQ_{10}) is a component of the mitochondrial electron transport chain and also a constituent of various cellular membranes. It acts as an important *in vivo* antioxidant.[80] Administration of CoQ10 increased plasma and mitochondria levels of CoQ10 as well as its predominant homologue CoQ9. CoQ supplementation resulted in an elevation of CoQ homologues in tissues and their mitochondria, a selective decrease in protein oxidative damage, and an increase in antioxidative potential in the rat.

6.1.6. *Other antioxidants*

Mitochondria are the major source of superoxide, and are responsible for activating apoptosis and oxidative damage during acute neuronal cell death and neurodegenerative disorders like Alzheimer and Parkinson diseases. Attempts to achieve neuroprotection using antioxidant molecules have been successful in several models of neuronal cell death.[81]

6.2. *Other endogenous compounds*

6.2.1. *Serotonin*

Serotonin may attenuate the oxidative damage of mitochondria and synaptosomes and the dopamine-induced viability loss in PC12 cells by a decomposing action on reactive oxygen species and inhibition of thiol oxidation and shows the effect comparable to melatonin. Serotonin may show a prominent protective effect on the iron-mediated neuronal damage.[82]

6.2.2. *Melatonin*

Melatonin has been reported to exert neuroprotective effects in several experimental and clinical situations involving neurotoxicity and/or excitotoxicity.[83] Additionally, in a series of pathologies in which high production of free radicals is the primary cause of the disease, melatonin is also protective. A common feature in these diseases is the existence of mitochondrial damage due to oxidative stress. The discoveries of new actions of melatonin in mitochondria support a novel mechanism, which explains some of the protective effects of the indoleamine on cell survival.

Administration of melatonin to the pregnant rat may prevent the free radical-induced oxidative mitochondrial damage to fetal rat brain by a direct antioxidant effect and the activation of GSH-Px.[84]

6.2.3. *Thioredoxin and GSH*

While thioredoxin and thioredoxin reductase 1 were found in all subcellular locations in kidney cells, thioredoxin reductase 2 was found predominantly in mitochondria.[85] Thioredoxin reductase 1 was identified in rat plasma, suggesting it is a secreted protein. Peroxiredoxins often had specific subcellular locations, with peroxiredoxins III and V found in mitochondria and peroxiredoxin IV found in lysosomes. Our results emphasize the complex nature of the thioredoxin system, demonstrating unique cell-type and organelle specificity. Within the mitochondrial phospholipid bilayer, the fat-soluble antioxidants vitamin E and coenzyme Q both prevent lipid peroxidation, while coenzyme Q also recycles vitamin E and is itself regenerated by the respiratory chain. The mitochondrial isoform of phospholipid hydroperoxide glutathione peroxidase degrades lipid peroxides within the mitochondrial inner membrane. There are also a range of mechanisms to repair or degrade oxidatively damaged lipid, protein, and DNA.

Mitochondria have a set of defense against oxidative damage. The antioxidant enzyme MnSOD converts superoxide to hydrogen peroxide.[17]

The mitochondria isoform of glutathione peroxidase and the thioredoxin-dependent enzyme peroxiredoxin III both detoxify hydrogen peroxide; alternatively, hydrogen peroxide can diffuse from the mitochondria into the cytoplasm.

6.2.4. *Superoxide dismutase*

Oxidative damage occurs whenever the ROS produced by mitochondria evade detoxification, and the steady-state level of oxidative damage depends on the relative rates of damage accumulation, repair, and degradation. That mitochondrial ROS production occurs at all times is suggested by mice lacking MnSOD, which die within a few days of birth, while those lacking the cytosolic isoform Cu, Zn SOD survive. Further evidence of mitochondrial ROS production under normal conditions is the efflux of hydrogen peroxide from intact mitochondria and from perfused organs, suggesting that mitochondria produce superoxide, which is then converted to hydrogen peroxide *in vivo*. There is also evidence that, under certain conditions, mitochondrial DNA and protein accumulate greater oxidative damage *in vivo* than the rest of the cell. Many other enzymes associated with mitochondria can also produce superoxide or hydrogen peroxide, but even though their contribution to ROS formation *in vivo* is unclear, the current tacit assumption that only complexes I and III produce ROS may have to be re-assessed. Even low concentrations of artificial uncouplers have been shown to lower the rate of superoxide production by mitochondria.[86]

6.2.5. *Bcl-2*

The bcl-2 proto-oncogene product possesses anti-apoptotic properties in neuronal and non-neuronal cells.[87] Recent data suggest that Bcl-2's potency as a survival factor hinges on its ability to suppress oxidative stress, but neither the subcellular site(s) nor the mechanism of its action is known. In this report, electron paramagnetic resonance (EPR) spectroscopy analyses were used to investigate the local effects of Bcl-2 on membrane lipid peroxidation. Using H_2O_2 and amyloid beta peptide as lipoperoxidation initiators, we examined the loss of EPR detectable paramagnetism of nitroxyl stearate (NS) spin labels 5-NS and 12-NS. Collectively, the data suggest that Bcl-2 is localized to mitochondrial and plasma membranes where it can act locally to suppress oxidative damage induced by H_2O_2 and amyloid beta peptide, further highlighting the important role of lipid peroxidation in apoptosis.

6.2.6. *Endogenous antioxidant — isocitrate dehydrogenase*

Production of NADPH required for the regeneration of glutathione in the mitochondria is critical for scavenging mitochondrial ROS through glutathione reductase and peroxidase systems. Jo *et al.*[88] investigated the role of mitochondrial $NADP^+$-dependent isocitrate dehydrogenase (IDPm) in controlling the mitochondrial redox balance and subsequent cellular defense against oxidative damage. They demonstrate in this report that IDPm is induced by ROS and that decreased expression of IDPm markedly elevates the ROS generation, DNA fragmentation, lipid peroxidation, and concurrent mitochondrial damage with a significant reduction in ATP levels. Conversely, overproduction of IDPm protein efficiently protected the cells from ROS-induced damage. The protective role of IDPm against oxidative damage may be attributed to increased levels of a reducing equivalent, NADPH, needed for regeneration of glutathione in the mitochondria. Our results strongly indicate that IDPm is a major NADPH producer in the mitochondria and thus plays a key role in cellular defense against oxidative stress-induced damage.

6.3. *Natural compounds*

6.3.1. *Chlorophyllin*

Using rat liver mitochondria as model systems the mechanisms of damage induced by radiation and photosensitization as well as its possible prevention by chlorophyllin (CHL) have been examined.[89] Peroxidation increases with radiation dose, in the range of 75-600 Gy. A similar observation was also observed with photosensitization, as a function of time. CHL, at a concentration of 10 μM offered a high degree of protection against radiation and photosensitization as indicated by decreased peroxidation, protein oxidation as well as the restoration of GSH and SOD. When compared with the established antioxidants, ascorbic acid and GSH, CHL offered a much higher degree of protection.

CHL, the sodium-copper salt and the water-soluble analogue of the ubiquitous green pigment chlorophyll, has been attributed to have several beneficial properties. Its antioxidant ability, however, has not been examined in detail. Using rat liver mitochondria as a model system and various sources for the generation of ROS, Kamat *et al.*[90] have examined the membrane-protective properties of CHL both under *in vitro and ex vivo* conditions. Oxidative damage to proteins was assessed as inactivation of enzymes, cytochrome c oxidase and succinate dehydrogenase besides formation of protein carbonyls. Damage to membrane lipid was measured by formation of lipid hydroperoxides and thiobarbituric acid reactive substances. Our results show that CHL is highly effective in protecting mitochondria, even at low concentration of 10 μM. The antioxidant activity at equimolar concentration, was more than that observed with ascorbic acid, glutathione, mannitol and tert-butanol. In conclusion, our studies showed that CHL is a highly effective antioxidant, capable of protecting mitochondria against oxidative damage induced by various ROS.

6.3.2. *Vanillin*

Using rat liver mitochondria as model systems, Kamat *et al.*[91] have examined the ability of the natural compound and the food-flavoring agent, vanillin, to protect membranes against oxidative damage induced by photosensitization at concentrations normally used in food preparations. Vanillin, at a concentration of 2.5 mmol/L, has afforded significant protection against protein oxidation and lipid peroxidation in hepatic mitochondria induced by photosensitization with methylene blue plus light. Hence, this flavoring compound, due to its antioxidant ability, may have potential to prevent oxidative damage to membranes in mammalian tissues and thereby the ensuing diseased states.

6.3.3. *Caffeine*

Caffeine in coffee or cola-based soft drinks is being consumed regularly by several million people. The differential modification of oxygen-dependent and independent effects of γ-irradiation by caffeine in membranes was examined, using rat liver mitochondria as a model system.[92] Membrane damage was examined as lipid peroxidation, protein oxidation, and depletion of protein thiols, superoxide dismutase or glutathione. The results suggest that caffeine effectively protected membranes against the oxic component of damage but may not do so for the anoxic component.

Radiation is one of the physical agents that induce oxidative stress. Exposure of rat liver mitochondria to high doses of ^{60}Co γ-rays (45-600Gy) results in the loss of activity of loss of superoxide dismutase (SOD). Presence of caffeine, even in micromolar amounts during exposure prevents loss of SOD activity.[86] Caffeine, at a concentration of 1mM also showed protection against radiation-induced inhibition of two other mitochondrial enzymes, namely succinate dehydrogenase and cytochrome c oxidase. The observed radioprotective activity of caffeine may be due to its ability to scavenge the reactive oxygen species generated by radiation and to inhibit radication-induced membrae damage, as assessed by lipid peroxidation and protein oxidation.

6.3.4. *Medicinal plant — Asparagus racemosus*

The possible antioxidant effects of crude extract and a purified aqueous fraction of *Asparagus racemosus* against membrane damage induced by the free radicals generated during gamma-radiation were examined in rat liver mitochondria.[93] The inhibitory effects of these active principles, at the concentration of 10 μg/ml, are comparable to that of the established antioxidants glutathione and ascorbic acid. Hence, our results indicate that extracts from *A. racemosus* have potent antioxidant properties *in vitro* in mitochondrial membranes of rat liver.

6.3.5. *Herbal formulation*

The effects of Yukmi (decoction of six plants including rehmannia), a herbal formula, were studied on liver oxidant damage induced by paraquat (PQ) administered intravenously in the senescence accelerated mice (SAM-P/8).[94] Yukmi extracts inhibited PQ-induced damage to the hepatic mitochondria and their membranes. Data suggest that Yukmi extracts may be useful in protecting against oxidative damage.

6.3.6. *Turmeric extract*

Atherosclerosis is characterized by oxidative damage which affects lipoproteins, the walls of blood vessels and subcellular membranes. Study by

Quiles *et al.*[95] evaluates the antioxidant capacity of a *Curcuma longa* extract on the lipid peroxidation of liver mitochondria and microsome membranes in atherosclerotic rabbits. The findings suggest that active compounds in curcuma extract may be protective in preventing lipoperoxidation of subcellular membranes in a dosage-dependent manner.

6.3.7. *Curcumin*

Devasagayam *et al.*[96] examined the influence of curcumin on the time course of lipid peroxidation induced by methylene blue and Rose Bengal in mitochondria of rat skin. Rose Bengal induces almost twice the amount of peroxidation compared with mythelene blue. In both cases, significant protection of mitochondria by curcumin was observed against this form of oxidative damage. Curcumin is also a potent inhibitor of lipid peroxidation induced by photosensitization with mythelene blue plus light in rat hepatic mitochondria. Curcumin, the major coloring compound from turmeric, has significant abilities to protect subcellular fractions from peroxidation induced by photosensitization involving type I and type II pathways.

6.4. *Synthetic antioxidants*

6.4.1. *Beta-carbolines*

The study by Kim *et al.*[97] elucidated the protective effect of beta-carbolines (harmaline, harmalol and harmine) against oxidative damage of brain mitochondria, synaptosomes and PC12 cells induced by either dopamine or 6-hydroxydopamine. Beta-carbolines may attenuate the dopamine- or 6-hydroxydopamine-induced alteration of brain mitochondrial and synaptosomal functions, and viability loss in PC12 cells, by a scavenging action on reactive oxygen species and inhibition of thiol oxidation.

6.4.2. *N-Acetylcysteine*

Increasing lines of evidence suggest a key role for mitochondrial damage in neurodegenerative diseases.[98] Brain aging, Parkinson's disease, Alzheimer's disease, Huntington's disease and Friedreich's ataxia have been associated with several mitochondrial alterations including impaired oxidative phosphorylation. Mechanisms of N-acetylcysteine action at the cellular level, and the possible usefulness of this antioxidant for the treatment of age-associated neurodegenerative diseases. It can act as a precursor for glutathione synthesis as well as a stimulator of the cytosolic enzymes involved in glutathione regeneration. It acts by direct reaction between its reducing thiol group and reactive oxygen species and prevent programmed cell death in cultured neuronal cells. N-acetylcysteine also increases mitochondrial complex I and IV specific activities. The potential usefulness of N-acetylcysteine in the treatment of age-associated mitochondrial neurodegenerative diseases deserves investigation.

6.4.3. *Carvedilol*

Carvedilol, a non-selective beta-adrenoreceptor blocker, has been shown to possess a high degree of cardioprotection in experimental models of myocardial damage.[99] Reactive oxygen species have been proposed to be implicated in such situations, and antioxidants have been demonstrated to provide partial protection to the reported damage. The antioxidant properties of carvedilol may contribute to the cardioprotective effects of the compound, namely through the preservation of mitochondrial functions whose importance in myocardial dysfunction is clearly documented. Additionally, its hydroxylated analog BM-910220, with its notably superior antioxidant activity, may significantly contribute to the therapeutic effects of carvedilol.

6.4.4. *Boldine*

Boldine ((s)-2,9-dihydroxy-1,10-dimethoxyaporphine) is a major alkaloid found in the leaves and bark of boldo (*Peumus boldus Molina*), and has been shown to possess antioxidant activity and anti-inflammatory effects. The effect of boldine on the STZ-induced diabetic rats was examined with the formation of malondialdehydes and carbonyls and the activities of endogenous antioxidant enzymes (superoxide dismutase and glutathione peroxidase) in mitochondria of the pancreas, kidney and liver.[100] Boldine may exert an inhibitory effect on STZ-induced oxidative tissue damage and altered antioxidant enzyme activity by the decomposition of reactive oxygen species and inhibition of nitric oxide production and by the reduction of the peroxidation-induced product formation. Boldine may attenuate the development of STZ-induced diabetes in rats and interfere with the role of oxidative stress, one of the pathogeneses of diabetes mellitus.

6.4.5. *Mitochondria-targeted antioxidants*

Too few large-scale double blind trials on the use of antioxidants in diabetes have been carried out for conclusions. However, a few small-scale trials have suggested the efficacy of the natural antioxidants α–tocopherol (vitamin E), ascorbate (vitamin C), coenzyme Q and α–lipoic acid, although in other trials, the efficacy of ascorbate and α–tocopherol were ambiguous. Because these natural antioxidants can be given at high doses and have shown some efficacy in other degenerative diseases, there is a strong rationale for trailing them in diabetes. Many other artificial antioxidants are being developed such as mimetics of sod or peroxidase that may be more potent than natural antioxidants and also have improved bioavailability, pharmacokinetics and stability. Both the natural and artificial antioxidants distribute throughout the body, with only a small proportion reaching the mitochondria, where much of the oxidative damage associated with hyperglycemia may occur. Because mitochondrial oxidative damage is thought to be critical in the pathophysiology of diabetes, antioxidants that accumulate within mitochondria may offer more protection than untargeted antioxidants. A strategy has been developed to deliver antioxidants to mitochondria by covalent attachment to the triphenylphosphonium cation through an alkyl chain.

Experiments *in vitro* showed that the mitochondria–targeted derivative of α-tocopherol (MitoVit E) and the mitochondria–targeted ubiquinone were rapidly and selectively accumulated by isolated cells. Importantly, the accumulation of these antioxidants by mitochondria protected them from oxidative damage far more effectively than untargeted antioxidants, suggesting that the accumulation of antioxidants within mitochondria does increase their efficacy. Most interestingly, these compounds were several hundredfold more effective at preventing cell death in fibroblasts from Friedreich Ataxia patients. Because cell death in this model is due to endogenous mitochondrial oxidative damage, it is suggested that the accumulation of antioxidants by mitochondria within cells blocks mitochondrial oxidative damage and that their uptake into mitochondria makes them far more effective than untargeted antioxidants. Because alkyltriphenylphosphonium cations pass easily through lipid bilayers by non-carrier-mediated transport, they should be taken up by the mitochondria of all the tissues, in contrast to hydrophilic compounds, which rely on the tissue-specific expression of carriers for uptake. Mice were fed mitochondria-targeted antioxidants for several weeks, leading to stable, steady-state concentrations within all tissues assessed including the brain, heart, liver and kidneys. The levels of methyltriphenylphosphonium and MitoVit E that accumulated in mouse tissues *in vivo* after feeding were in the range of 5–20 nmol/g wet wt, or about 5–20 μmol/l in the tissue. Because these compounds accumulate within mitochondria, the intra-mitochondrial concentration will be about millimolar. These concentrations are likely to be in the therapeutically effective range, because mitochondria-targeted antioxidants prevented oxidative damage to isolated mitochondria at 1–2.5 μmol/l.

It seems probable that mitochondrial radical production and consequent oxidative damage contribute to the progression and pathophysiology of diabetes. A first step in developing antioxidant therapies is to give large doses of natural antioxidants such as vitamin E, α–lipoic acid, or coenzyme Q to see if this approach has potential. The advantage of natural antioxidants is their safety and that large oral doses are well tolerated. However, in other degenerative diseases, very large doses have been required to see beneficial effects, possibly because of their poor bioavailability, and pharmacokinetics. Among these, a case can be made for testing mitochondria-targeted antioxidants. To date, mitochondria-targeted versions of coenzyme Q and vitamin E have been made and can be administered safely to mice.

6.5. *Expression of antioxidant genes*

Mitochondria have recently been shown to serve a central role in programmed cell death.[101] In addition, ROS have been implicated in the cell death pathways upon treatment with a variety of agents; however, the specific, cellular source of the ROS generation is unknown. Mitochondrial-mediated ROS generation is a key event by which inhibition of respiration causes cell death, and identifies CPP-32 and the PARP-linked pathway as targets of mitochondrial-derived ROS-induced cell death. Overexpression of Mn SOD protects against mitochondrial initiated poly-(ADP-ribose) polymerase-mediated cell death.

Borras *et al.*[102] examined the differential mitochondrial oxidative stress between males and females to understand the molecular mechanisms enabling females to live longer than males. Those from female rats generate half the amount of peroxides than those of males. This does not occur in ovariectomized animals. Estrogen replacement therapy prevents the effect of ovariectomy. Mitochondria from females have higher levels of reduced glutathione than those from males. Those from ovariectomized rats have similar levels to males, and estrogen therapy prevents the fall in glutathione levels that occurs in ovariectomized animals. Oxidative damage to mitochondrial DNA in males is four-fold higher than that in females. This is due to higher expression and activities of Mn-superoxide dismutase and of glutathione peroxidase in females, which behave as double transgenics overexpressing superoxide dismutase and glutathione peroxidase, conferring protection against free radical-mediated damage in aging. Moreover, 16S rRNA expression, which decreases significantly with aging, is four times higher in mitochondria from females than those from males of the same chronological age. The facts reported here provide molecular evidence to explain the different life span in males and females.

To determine the importance of mitochondrial ROS toxicity in aging and senescence, Kokoszka *et al.*[103] analyzed changes in mitochondrial function with age in mice with partial or complete deficiencies in the mitochondrial antioxidant enzyme manganese superoxide dismutase (MnSOD). Liver mitochondria from homozygous mutant mice, with a complete deficiency in MnSOD, exhibited substantial respiration inhibition and marked sensitization of the mitochondrial permeability transition pore. Mitochondria from heterozygous mice, with a partial deficiency in MnSOD, showed evidence of increased proton leak, inhibition of respiration, and early and rapid accumulation of mitochondrial oxidative damage. Furthermore, chronic oxidative stress in the heterozygous mice resulted in an increased sensitization of the mitochondrial permeability transition pore and the premature induction of apoptosis, which presumably eliminates the cells with damaged mitochondria. Mitochondrial reactive oxygen species production, oxidative stress, functional decline, and the initiation of apoptosis appear to be central components of the aging process.

7. Mitochondria Permeability Transition (MPT) and Apoptosis

Oxidative damage to mitochondria in conjunction with calcium loading leads to induction of the mitochondrial permeability transition (MPT).[2] The MPT is due to the formation of a non-specific pore in the inner membrane which renders the mitochondrial inner membrane permeable to solutes smaller than about 1.5 kDa, thus preventing oxidative phosphorylation. Mitochondria play a central role in both apoptotic and necrotic cell death. Necrotic cell death follows ATP depletion and cellular calcium overloading, consequently extensive mitochondrial damage leads to necrotic cell death in situations such as heart attack and stroke. During apoptotic cell death, an endogenous cell death program is activated that causes the ordered self-destruction of the cell, ending with its phagocytosis by surrounding cells without leakage of damaging contents and thus no inflammatory response. The distinction between apoptotic and necrotic cell death in response to cell death to cell damage is somewhat arbitrary as completion of the apoptotic program requires ATP, and if the ATP level falls below a critical threshold after initiation of apoptotic program is aborted and the cell dies by necrosis.

Mitochondria are critically involved in deciding whether a cell undergoes apoptosis. Cells commit irreversibly to apoptosis by activities caspases. Mitochondria play a critical role in switching on the caspases cascade by releasing cytochrome c from the intermembrane space into the cytoplasm. In the cytoplasm, cytochrome c interacts with Apaf-1 and pro-caspase 9, activating caspases 9, which in turn activates pro-caspase 3 and leads to the induction of apoptosis. How mitochondria release cytochrome c is unclear, but following pro-apoptotic stimuli the mitochondrial outer membrane becomes permeable to cytochrome c and other inter-membrane space proteins, possibly due to mitochondrial matrix swelling following, or associated with, decreased activity of adenine nucleotide carrier.

Mitochondria also induce apoptosis by another pathway involving release of intermembrane space proteins. However, in this case there is an early loss of mitochondrial membrane potential due to induction of the MPT, which leads to mitochondrial swelling and release of intermembrane space proteins into the cytosol. One of these intermembrane space proteins is a 50 kDa protein called apoptosis inducing factor (AIF) which does not directly activate cytoplasmic caspases but instead localizes to the nucleus and induces apoptotic cell death.

Mitochondria accumulate calcium by a membrane potential driven uniporter and release calcium by electroneutral exchange for sodium or protons. Mitochondrial calcium uptake and release is also important in subtly modulating cytoplasmic calcium signaling. Disruption to mitochondrial calcium metabolism both interferes with cellular calcium signaling and renders cells vulnerable to death from calcium overloading.

The production of ROS, induced by tumor necrosis factor-α (TNF-α), ceramide, staurosporine and hypoglycemia, in mitochondria has been proposed as an early event in the induction of apoptosis. Recent evidence suggests that mitochondrion-derived ROS might be involved in the induction of apoptotic death; those antioxidant enzymes in mitochondria might participate in apoptosis and contribute to the modulation of apoptotic signals.[13]

Mitochondria play a role in apoptosis and necrosis through the opening of the mitochondrial permeability transition pore (MPTP).[104] Opening of the MPTP causes swelling and uncoupling of mitochondria, which unrestrained, leads to necrosis. MPTP opening may also be involved in apoptosis, by initially causing swelling and rupture of the outer membrane to release cytochrome c (cyt c), which then activates caspase cascade and sets apoptosis in motion. Subsequent MPTP closure allows ATP levels to be maintained, ensuring that cell death remains apoptotic rather than necrotic. Other apoptotic stimuli such as cytokines or the removal of growth factors also involve mitochondrial cyt c release, but here there is controversy over whether the MPTP is involved. In many cases, cyt c release is seen without any mitochondrial depolarization, suggesting that the MPTP does not open. Recent data have revealed a specific outer-membrane cyt c-release pathway involving porin that does not release other intermembrane proteins such as adenylate kinase. This is opened by pro-apoptotic members of the Bcl-2 family such as BAX and prevented by anti-apoptotic members such as Bcl-x1.

The mechanism of oxidative phosphorylation requires that the mitochondrial inner membrane be impermeable to all but a few selected metabolites and ions. If this permeability barrier is lost, mitochondria become impermeable and hydrolyze ATP rather than synthesizing it leading to cell death. A latent non-specific protein in its inner membrane which when activated causes just such an increase in membrane permeability. The MPTP opens when the mitochondria are exposed to high calcium concentrations, associated with adenine nucleotide depletion and oxidative stress. These are exactly the conditions that accompany many cellular insults that lead to necrotic cell death. The MPTP is non-specific and transports any molecule of $< 1500\,\text{Da}$. Not only does its opening prevent ATP synthesis, it also causes the loss of ions and metabolites from the mitochondrial matrix and induces extensive swelling of the mitochondria as a result of the colloidal osmotic pressure exerted by the matrix proteins. It is well established that mitochondria in necrotic cells are swollen and have greatly impaired respiration and oxidative phosphorylation. MPTP opening causes uncoupling of oxidative phosphorylation, the loss of ions and small molecules from the mitochondrial matrix and extensive swelling of the mitochondria.

In recent years there has been a flood of data implicating the mitochondria in apoptotic cell death. It is now clearly established that in many if not all apoptotic cells an early event is the release of proteins from the intermembrane space of mitochondria. The protein whose release appears more critical in cyt c which in the presence of ATP and dATP, forms a complex with apoptosis activating factor-1 (APAF-1) and procaspase 9. This induces cleavage of procaspase 9 with the release of caspase 9 that cleaves and activates procaspase 3. The active caspase 3 then induces proteolytic cleavage of a range of target proteins responsible for the rearrangements of the cytosol, nucleus and plasma membrane that are characteristic of apoptosis.

7.1. *MPT and toxicity*

Oxidative damage to mitochondria and the permeability transition plays a role in the CYP2E1-dependent toxicity of Fe^{+}AA in HepG2 cells, both in MEM and SMEM.[105] Ca^{+2}-mobilization and activation of calpain contributes to the more rapid onset of mitochondrial damage in MEM, while oxidative damage and lipid peroxidation are involved in the Ca^{2+}-independent later onset of mitochondrial damage.

Anuradha *et al.*[106] have previously reported that fluoride (NaF) induces apoptosis in HL-60 cells by caspase 3 activation. The main focus of this investigation was to arrive at a possible pathway of the apoptosis induced by

NaF upstream of caspase 3, because the mechanism is still unknown. The present study showed that after exposure to NaF, there was an increase in MDA and 4-HNE and a loss of mitochondrial membrane potential (deltaPSIm) was also observed in NaF-treated cells. There was a significant increase in cytosolic cytochrome c, which is released from the mitochondria. They have reported a downregulation of *Bcl*-2 protein in NaF-treated cells. The antioxidants N-acetyl cysteine (NAC) and glutathione (GSH) protected the cells from loss of deltaPSIm, and there was no cytochrome c exit or *Bcl*-2 downregulation, and they suggest that these antioxidants prevent apoptosis induced by NaF. These results suggested that perhaps NaF induced apoptosis by oxidative stress-induced lipid peroxidation, causing loss of deltaPSIm, and thereby releasing cytochrome c into the cytosol and further triggering the caspase cascade leading to apoptotic cell death in HL-60 cells.

7.2. *MPT and ischemia-reperfusion injury*

The study by Berkich *et al.*[107] suggests that the mitochondrial permeability transition plays a role in ischemic cell death but is not triggered by influx of Ca^{2+} through the plasma membrane. When open, the pore permits loss of molecules 100 kDa or smaller. Key cofactors of mitochondria metabolism and substrate oxidation are lost as well as any capacity to maintain the electrochemical gradient of protons across the inner membrane, which couples electron transfer to ATP synthesis.

7.3. *MPT and influence by antioxidant-genistein*

Genistein occurs in plants and has been shown to have anti-tumor, antioxidant and anti-inflammatory effects. It has been proposed that genistein induces apoptosis in RPE-J cells by provoking mitochondrial alterations characteristic of MPT induction, a key phenomenon in cell death by apoptosis and necrosis.[108] Genistein, a natural isoflavone present in soybeans, is a potent agent in the prophylaxis and treatment of cancer. Genistein induces the MPT by the generation of ROS due to its interaction with the respiratory chain at the level of mitochondrial complex III.

8. Mitochondria and Cancer Treatment (Photodynamic Therapy)

Photodynamic therapy (PDT), a treatment for cancer and for certain benign conditions, utilizes a photosensitizer and light to produce reactive oxygen in cells.[109] PDT is primarily employed to kill tumor and other abnormal cells, so it is important to ask how this occurs. Many of the photosensitizers currently in clinical or preclinical studies of PDT localize in or have a major influence on mitochondria, and PDT is a strong inducer of apoptosis in many situations.

The subcellular localization of many photosensitizers and the early responses to light activation indicate that mitochondria play a major role in photodynamic cell death.[110] PDT with many agents, which damage or inhibit different or multiple mitochondrial targets, has many of the desirable characteristics for an effective anticancer therapy. Mitochondrial localized photosensitizers are able to induce apoptosis very rapidly.[111] Lysosomal localized photosensitizers can elicit either a necrotic or an apoptotic response.

Delocalized lipophilic cations (DLCs) are concentrated in mitochondria in response to negative charge inside transmembrane potentials.[112] The higher plasma and/or mitochondrial membrane potentials of carcinoma cells compared to normal epithelial cells account for the selective accumulation of DLCs in carcinoma mitochondria. Since most DLCs are toxic to mitochondria at high concentrations, their selective accumulation in carcinoma mitochondria and consequent mitochondrial toxicity provide a basis for selective carcinoma cell killing.

Using mitochondria isolated from Sarcoma 180 ascites tumor in Swiss mice as a model system, Chatterjee *et al.*[113] have evaluated the ability of a novel porphyrin meso-tetrakis (4(carboxymethylenoxy)phenyl) porphyrin (H2T4CPP), to induce damage on photosensitization. Oxidative damage to mitochondria, one of the primary and crucial targets of the photodynamic effect, is assessed by measuring products of lipid peroxidation such as thiobarbituric acid reactive substances (TBARS) and lipid hydroperoxides (LOOH), besides the loss of activity of the mitochondrial marker enzyme succinate dehydrogenase (SDH). Fluorescence spectroscopy, used to ascertain the binding of this porphyrin to the mitochondrial proteins, shows a rapid association within 0–2 hours and a decline thereafter. Confocal microscopy reveals intracellular localization of this porphyrin in cells *in vitro*. Our overall results suggest that the porphyrin H2T4CPP, due to its ability to bind to mitochondrial protein components and to generate ROS upon photo-excitation, may have potential applications in photodynamic therapy.

With a view to locate porphyrins for use in PDT, the new modality of cancer treatment, Chatterjee *et al.*[114] have evaluated the ability of a novel water soluble porphyrin meso-tetrakis [4-(carboxymethyleneoxy) phenyl] porphyrin (T4CPP) to induce damage to mitochondria during photosensitization. T4CPP, when exposed to visible light, induced lipid peroxidation in rat liver mitochondria. T4CPP plus light also caused significant lipid peroxidation in Sarcoma 180 ascites tumor mitochondria. Our studies indicate that T4CPP has the potential to photoinduce damage in hepatic and ascites mitochondria, a crucial site of damage in PDT.

Among the subcellular organelles, damage to mitochondria is considered crucial and can lead to cytotoxicity and cell death.[115] However, the same damage, if it is selectively induced in cancer tissues can lead to its cure. Hence, analyzing the mechanisms of such damage and its modulation may result in better prevention or cure. Using mitochondria derived from rat brain/liver as well as Sarcoma 180 ascites cells, the mechanisms of damage to lipid was examined, as assessed by different products of lipid peroxidation and to proteins, as determined by loss of enzyme activity and protein oxidation. The mechanisms involved, in terms of scavenging of ROS have been determined using pulse radiolysis for hydroxyl radical and histidine destruction assay for singlet oxygen. Some novel porphyrins, with potential uses in photodynamic therapy were also used as photosensitizers. They showed that ROS can induce significant oxidative damage in mitochondria from both normal and tumor tissues and this can be inhibited by natural antioxidants. Damage can be enhanced by deuteration of the buffer and oxygenation. Their results hence demonstrated that mitochondria were sensitive to damage by ROS and its modulation may have potential uses in prevention of the disease in normal tissues; if damage can be selectively induced in tumor, it can lead to its regression.

9. New Developments and Possible Applications

The rapid advance of proteomic methodologies and their application to large scale studies of protein-protein interactions and protein expression profiles suggest that these methods are well suited to provide the molecular details needed to fully understand oxidative injury.[116] It has been suggested that mitochondria are a desirable pharmacological target, and drugs that modulate mitochondrial function include those that target oxidative stress. One reason why this may be true is the crucial role mitochondria play in energy metabolism and cell death signaling pathways, both of which have links to cancer, neurodegenerative disease, diabetes, and aging.

Given their close proximity to ROS generated in mitochondria, proteins would be expected to be among the most likely targets of oxidative damage. Over the last two decades, considerable progress has been made in identifying individual proteins that are localized to the mitochondria. In particular the 100 or so subunits that constitute the five complexes of the electron transport chain (ETC). Recently, using modern mass spectrometry (MS)-based proteomic strategies, several groups have begun to tackle the larger job of determining the composition of entire mitochondrial proteomes from a number of important model systems as well as from human tissues. Using mitochondria isolated from the human heart, Gibson and coworkers have identified 684 unique proteins from the combined peptide data obtained from over 100,000 mass spectra generated by MALDI-MS and high performance liquid chromatography (HPLC) MS/MS analyses. These data are now part of MitoProteome, a publicly accessible database for the human heart mitochondrial proteome. It seems to be only a matter of time before the mitochondrial proteome is exploited in drug development. Proteomics investigations can also be used to identify proteins that have undergone oxidative modification, as well as the molecular and site-specific details of these oxidative events. Studies in knock-out mice that lack the gene encoding superoxide dismutase 2 indicated there was differential sensitivities of mitochondrial proteins to oxidative stress and the fact that antioxidant treatment could rescue the neuronal cell death phenotype. Obtaining a proteomic analysis of oxidative stress should lead to a better assessment of antioxidant drug therapy.

In conclusion, the present chapter reveals the importance of mitochondria in cellular functions. If free radicals can induce damage to mitochondria it can lead to undesirable consequences possibly in the form of disease development or cell death. There are various strategies adapted to prevent such damage. If damage can be selectively induced in mitochondria of cancer tissue it can lead to cancer treatment. There are several new approaches including that of proteomics that can further throw light on the mechanisms behind mitochondrial damage and its implications.

References

1. Sperelakis N. *Cell Physiology: Source Book*. Academic Press, USA, 1997.
2. Murphy MP, Smith RAJ. Drug delivery to mitochondria: the key to mitochondrial medicine. *Adv. Drug Deliv. Rev.* 41: 235–250 (2000).
3. Frey TG, Mannella CA. The internal structure of mitochondria. *Trends Biochem. Sci.* 25: 319–324 (2000).
4. Rutter GA, Rizzuto R. Regulation of mitochondrial metabolism by ER Ca^{2+} release: an intimate connection. *Trends Biochem. Sci.* 25: 215–221 (2000).
5. Lodish H, Baltimore D, Berk A, Zipursky SL, Matsudaira P, Darnell J. *Molecular Cell Biology*. WH Freeman and Company, New York, 1996.
6. Capaldi RA. The changing face of mitochondrial research. *Trends Biochem. Sci.* 25: 212–214 (2000).
7. Duchen MR. Role of mitochondria in health and disease. *Diabetes* 53: S96–S102 (2004).
8. Shiva S, Brooks PS, Patel RP, Anderson PG, Darley-Usmar VM. Nitric oxide partitioning into mitochondrial membranes and the control of respiration at cytochrome c oxidase. *Proc. Natl. Acad. Sci. USA* 98: 7212–7217 (2001).
9. Bringold U, Ghafourifar P, Richter C. Peroxynitrite formed by mitochondrial NO synthase promotes mitochondrial Ca^{2+} release. *Free Radic. Biol. Med.* 29: 343–348 (2000).
10. Nohl H, Kozlov AV, Gille L, Staniek K. Cell respiration and formation of reactive oxygen species: facts and artifacts. *Biochem. Soc. Trans.* 31: 1308–1311 (2003).
11. Douglas CW, Lott MT. Mitochondria bioenergetics and reactive oxygen species in degenerative diseases and aging. In: Bohr VA, Clark BSC, Stevnsner T (eds.) *Molecular Biology of Aging*. Munksgaard, Copenhagen, 1999, pp. 125–147.
12. Chance B, Sehotner B, Oshino R, Itshka M, Nakase Y. Oxidation-reduction ratio studies of mitochondria in freeze traped sample. NADH and flavoprotein fluorescence signals. *J. Biol. Chem.* 254: 4764–4771 (1979).

13. Yoshikawa T, Toyokuni S, Yamamoto Y, Naito Y (eds.) *Free Radicals in Chemistry Biology and Medicine*. OICA International, London, 2000.
14. Wallace DC. Aging and degenerative diseases: mitochondria paradigm. In: Papa S, Guerrieri F, Tager JN (eds.) *Frontier Cell Bioenergetics*. Kluwer Academic/Plenum Publishers, New York, 1999, pp. 751–771.
15. Herrero A, Portero OM, Bellmunt MJ, Pamplona R, Barja G. Effect of the degree of fatty acid unstauration of rat heart mitochondria on their rates of H_2O_2 production and lipid and protein oxidative damage. *Mech. Ageing Dev.* 122: 427–443 (2001).
16. Raha, Robinson. Mitochondria, oxygen free radicals, disease and ageing. *Trends Biol. Sci.* 25: 502–508 (2000).
17. Green K, Brand MD, Murphy MP, Prevention of mitochondrial oxidative damage as a therapeutic strategy in diabetes. *Diabetes* 53: S110–S118 (2004).
18. Sies H. Biochemistry of Oxidative Stress. *Angew. Chem. Int. Ed. Engl.* 25: 1058–1071 (1986).
19. Ong ASH, Packer L. *Lipid Soluble Antioxidants: Biochemistry and Clinical Applications*. Birkhauser Verlag, 1997.
20. Cadenas E, Packer L (eds.). *Handbook of Antioxidants*. Plenum Publishers, New York, 1996.
21. Ottolenghi A. Interaction of ascorbic acid and mitochondrial lipids. *Arch. Biochem. Biophys.* 79: 355–363 (1959).
22. Hoffsten PE, Hunter FE, Gebicki Jr JM, Weinstein J. Formation of "lipid peroxide" under conditions which lead to swelling and lysis of rat liver mitochondria. *Biochem. Biophys. Res. Commun.* 7: 276–281 (1962).
23. Hunter FE, Weinstein J, Scott AA, Schneider AK. The effect of phosphate on glutathione-induced lipid per oxidation and swelling in rat liver mitochondria. *Biochem. Biophys. Res. Commun.* 11: 456–460 (1963).
24. Wills ED. Lipid peroxide formation in microsomes. *Biochem. J.* 113: 315–324 (1969).
25. Stadtman ER. Metal-ion catalyzed oxidation of proteins: biochemical mechanism and biological consequences. *Free Radic. Biol. Med.* 9: 315–325 (1990).
26. Stadtman ER, Berlett BS. Reactive oxygen mediated protein oxidation in aging and disease. *Chem. Res. Toxicol.* 10: 485–494 (1997).
27. Pushpendran CK, Subramanian M, Devasagayam TPA, Singh BB. Study on lipid peroxidation potential in different tissues induced by ascorbate-Fe^{2+}: possible factors involved in their differential susceptibility. *Mol. Cell Biochem.* 178: 197–208 (1998).

28. Li Y, Huang TT, Carlson EJ, Melov S, Ursell PC, Olson JL, Noble LJ, Yoshimaru MP, Berger C, Chang PH *et al.* Dilated cardiomyopathy and neonatal lethality in mutant mice lacking manganese superoxide dismutase. *Nature Genet.* 11: 376–381 (1995).
29. Wallace DC. Mitochondria DNA mutations in human disease and aging. In: Esser K, Martin GM (eds.) *Molecular Aspects of Aging*. John Wiley & Sons Ltd. USA, 1995, pp. 163–177.
30. Shigenaga MK, Hagen PM, Ames BN. Oxidative damage and mitochondrial decay in ageing. *Proc. Natl. Acad. Sci. USA* 91: 10771–10778 (1994).
31. Smith SJ. Superoxide: production and destruction. *Biochem. Soc. Trans.* 31: 1295–1299 (2003).
32. Schon EA. Mitochondrial genetics and disease. *Trends Biochem. Sci.* 25: 555–560 (2000).
33. Bota DA, Davies KJA. Protein degradation in mitochondria: implications for oxidative stress, aging and disease: a novel etiological classification of mitochondrial proteolytic disorders. *Mitochondrion Kidlington* 1: 33–49 (2001).
34. Paradies G, Ruggiero FM, Petrosillo G, Quagliariello E. Peroxidative damage to cardiac mitochondria: cytochrome oxidase and cardiolipin alterations. *FEBS Lett.* 178: 155–158 (1998).
35. Choksi KB, Boylston WH, Rebek JP, Widger WR, Papaconstantinou J. Oxidatively damaged proteins of heart mitochondrial electron transport complexes. *Biochim. Biophys. Acta* 1688: 95–101 (2004).
36. Venditti P, Costagliola IR, Di MS. H_2O_2 production and response to stress conditions by mitochondrial fractions from rat liver. *J. Bioenerg. Biomem.* 34: 115–125 (2002).
37. Radi R, Cassina A, Hodara R, Quijano C, Castro L. Peroxynitrite reactions and formation in mitochondria. *Free Radic. Biol. Med.* 33: 1451–1464 (2002).
38. Miro O, Alonso JR, Casademont J, Urbano LA, Cardellach F. Smoking disturbs mitochondril respiratory chain function and enhances lipid peroxidation on human circulating lymphocytes. *Carcinogenesis* 20: 1331–1336 (1999).
39. Qu B, Li QT, Wong KP, Tan TMC, Halliwell B. Mechanism of clofibrate hepatotoxicity: mitochondrial damage and oxidative stress in hepatocytes. *Free Radic. Biol. Med.* 31: 659–669 (2001).
40. Kuratko CN. Mitochondrial lipid peroxidation is influenced by dietary factors in early colon carcinogenesis. *J. Nutr. Biochem.* 8: 696–701 (1997).
41. Zhou S, Kachchap S, Singh KK. Mitochondria impairment in p53-deficient human cancer cells. *Mutagenesis* 18: 287–292 (2003).

42. Delsite R, Kachhap S, Anbazhagan R, Gabrielson E, Singh KK. Nuclear genes involved in mitochondria-to-nucleus communication in breast cancer cells. *Mol. Cancer* 1: 6 (2002).
43. Madesh M, Ramachandran A, Pulimood A, Vadranam M, Balsubramanian KA. Attenuation of intestinal ischemia/reperfusion injury with sodium nitroprusside: studies on mitochondrial function and lipid changes. *Biochim. Biophys. Acta* 1500: 204–216 (2000).
44. Okatani Y, Wakatsuki A, Enzan H, Miyahara Y. Edaravone protects against ischemia/reperfusion-induced oxidative damage to mitochondria in rat liver. *Euro. J. Pharmacol.* 465: 163–170 (2003).
45. Nohl H, Koltover V, Stolze K. Ischemia/reperfusion impairs mitochondrila energy conservation and triggers $O_2^{\bullet-}$ release as a byproduct of respiration. *Free Radic. Res. Comm.* 18: 127–137 (1993).
46. Halmosi R, Berente Z, Osz E, Toth K, Literati NP, Sumegi B. Effect of poly (ADP-ribose) polymerase inhibitors on the ischemia reperfusion-induced oxidative cell damage and mitochondrial metabolism in Langendorff heart perfusion system. *Mol. Pharmacol.* 59: 1497–1505 (2001).
47. Basivireddy J, Vasudevan A, Jacob M, Balasubramaniam KA. Indomethacin-induced mitochondrial dysfunction and oxidative stress in villus erythrocytes. *Biochem. Pharmacol.* 64: 339–349 (2002).
48. Samikkannu T, Chen CH, Yih LH, Wang ASS, Lin SY, Chen TC, Jan KY. Reactive oxygen species are involved in arsenic trioxide inhibition of pyruvate dehydrogenase activity. *Chem. Res. Toxicol.* 16: 409–414 (2003).
49. Zainal TA, Weindruch R, Szweda LI, Oberley TD. Localization of 4-hydroxy-2-nonenal-modified proteins in kidney following iron overload. *Free Radic. Biol. Med.* 26: 1181–1193 (1999).
50. Subramanian M, Puspendran CK, Tarachand U, Devasagayam TPA. Gestation confers temporary resistance to peroxidation in the maternal rat brain. *Neurosci. Lett.* 155: 151–154 (1993).
51. Devasagayam TPA, Tarachand U. Pregnancy-associated decrease in lipid peroxidation in rat liver. *Biochem. Int.* 16: 45–52 (1988).
52. Devasagayam TPA, Tarachand U. Decreased lipid peroxidation in rat kidney during gestation. *Biochem. Biophys. Res. Commun.* 145: 134–138 (1987).
53. Arking R. Ageing: a biological perspective. *Am. Sci.* 91: 508–515 (2003).
54. Pamplona R, Portero OM, Requena JR, Thorpe SR, Herrero A, Barja G. A low degree of fatty acid unsaturation leads to lower lipid peroxidation and lipo-oxidation derived protein modification in heart mitochondria of the longevous pegion than in the short lived rat. *Mech. Aging Dev.* 106: 283–296 (1999).

55. Barja G. Rate of generation of oxidative stress-related damage and animal longevity. *Free Radic. Biol. Med.* 33: 1167–1172 (2002).
56. Huei WY, Chen LH. Oxidative stress, mitochondrial DNA mutation and impairment of antioxidant enzymes during ageing. *Exp. Biol. Med. Maywood* 227: 671–682 (2002).
57. Yan LJ, Sohal RS. Mitochondrial adenine nucleotide translocase is modified oxidatively during aging. *Proc. Natl. Acad. Sci. USA* 95: 12896–12901 (1998).
58. Bejma J, Ji LL. Aging and acute exercise enhance free radical generation in rat skeletal muscle. *J. Appl. Physiol.* 87: 465–470 (1999).
59. Sadek HA, Nulton-Pursson AC, Szweda PA, Szweda LI. Cardiac ischemia/reperfusion, ageing, and redox-dependent alterations in mitochondrial functions. *Arch. Bichem. Biophys.* 420: 201–208 (2003).
60. Lesnefsky EJ, Hoppel CL. Ischemia-reperfusion injury in the aged heart: role of mitochondria. *Arch. Biochem. Biophys.* 420: 287–297 (2003).
61. Lucas DT, Szweda LI. Cardiac reperfusion injury: ageing, lipid peroxidation and mitochondrial dysfunction. *Proc. Natl. Acad. Sci. USA* 95: 510–514 (1998).
62. Lane MA, Ingram DK, Roth GS. The serious search for an anti-ageing pill. *Sci. Am.* August 2002, pp. 24–29.
63. Wei YH, Pang CY, Lee HC, Lu CY. Roles of mitochondrial DNA mutation and oxidative damage in human ageing. *Curr. Sci. Bangalore* 74: 887–893 (1998).
64. Lu CY, Lee F, Wei YH. Oxidative damage elicited by imbalance of free radical scavenging enzymes is associated with large scale mtDNA deletions I ageing human skin. *Mutat. Res.* 423: 11–21 (1999).
65. Wei YH, Lu CY, Wei CY, Ma YS, Lee HC. Oxidative stress in human aging and mitochondrial disease: consequences of defective mitochondrial respiration and impaired antioxidant enzyme system. *Chin. J. Physiol.* 44: 1–11 (2001).
66. Ames BN. Micronutrients prevent cancer and delay ageing. *Toxicol. Lett. Shannon* 102–103: 5–18 (1998).
67. Arivazhagan P, Ramanathan K, Panneerselvam C. Effect of DL-alpha-lipoic acid on mitochondrial enzymes in aged rats. *Chem. Biol. Interact.* 138: 189–198 (2001).
68. Sastre J, Pallardo FV, Vina J. Mitochondrial oxidative stress plays a key role in aging and apoptosis. *IUBMB Life* 49: 427–435 (2000).
69. Miquel J. Can antioxidant diet supplementation protect against age-related mitochondrial damage? *Ann. NY Acad. Sci.* 959: 508–516 (2002).

70. Elliott RM, Southon S, Archer DB. Oxidative insult specifically decreases levels of a mitochondrial transcript. *Free Radic. Biol. Med.* 26: 646–655 (1999).

71. Sumien N, Forster MJ, Sohal RS. Supplementation with vitamin E fails to attenuate oxidative damage in aged mice. *Exp. Gerontol.* 38: 699–704 (2003).

72. Zhang JG, Nicholls GFA, Tirmenstein MA, Fariss MW. Vitamin E succinate protects hepatocytes against the toxic effect of reactive oxygen species generated at mitochondrial complexes I and III by alkylating agents. *Chem. Biol. Int.* 138: 267–284 (2001).

73. Fariss MW, Nicholls GFA, Tirmenstein MA, Zhang JG. Enhanced antioxidant and cytoprotective abilities of vitamin E succinate is associated with a rapid uptake advantage in rat hepatocytes and mitochondria. *Free Radic. Biol. Med.* 31: 530–541 (2001).

74. Smith RAJ, Porteous CM, Coulter CV, Murphy MP. Selective targeting of an antioxidant to mitochondria. *Eur. J. Biochem.* 263: 709–716 (1999).

75. Garcia De La AJ, Del OML, Sastre J, Millan A, Pellin A, Pallardo FV, Vina J. AZT treatment induces molecular and ultrastructural oxidative damage to muscle mitochondria: prevention by antioxidant vitamins. *J. Clin. Invest.* 102: 4–9 (1998).

76. Nesaretnam K, Devasagayam TPA, Singh BB, Basiron Y. Influence of palm oil or its tocotrienol-rich fraction on the lipid peroxidation potential of rat liver mitochondria and microsomes. *Biochem. Mol. Biol. Int.* 30: 159–167 (1993).

77. Kamat JP, Devasagayam TPA. Tocotrienols from palm oil as potent inhibitors of lipid peroxidation and protein oxidation in rat brain mitochondria. *Neurosci. Lett.* 195: 179–182 (1995).

78. Kamat JP, Boloor KK, Devasagayam TPA, Nesaretnam K, Basiron Y. Oxidative damage induced by peroxynitrite/singlet oxygen in rat liver mitochondria and its inhibition by tocotrienols from palm oil. In: Nesaretnam K, Packer L (eds.) *Micronutrients and Health: Molecular Biological Mechanisms.* AOCS Press, Champaign IL, USA, 2001.

79. Kamat JP, Devasagayam TPA. Nicotinamide (vitamin B_3) as an effective antioxidant against oxidative damage in rat brain mitochondria. *Redox Rep.* 4: 179–184 (1999).

80. Kwong LK, Kamzalov S, Rebrin I, Bayne ACV, Jana CK, Morris P, Forster MJ, Sohal RS. Effects of coenzyme Q10 administration on its tissue concentrations, mitochondrial oxidant generation, and oxidative stress in the rat. *Free Radic. Biol. Med.* 33: 627–638 (2002).

81. Dessolin J, Schuler M, Quinart A, De GF, Ghosez L, Ichas F. Selective targeting of synthetic antioxidants to mitochondria: towards a mitochondrial medicine for neurodegenerative diseases? *Eur. J. Pharmacol.* 447: 155–161 (2002).
82. Park JW, Youn YC, Kwon OS, Jang YY, Han ES, Lee CS. Protective effect of serotonin on 6-hydroxydopamine- and dopamine-induced oxidative damage of brain mitochondria and synaptosomes and PC12 cells. *Neurochem. Int.* 40: 223–233 (2002).
83. Acuna CD, Martin M, Macias M, Escames G, Leon J, Khaldy H, Reiter RJ. Melatonin, mitochondria, and cellular bioenergetics. *J. Pineal. Res.* 30: 65–74 (2001).
84. Wakatsuki A, Okatani Y, Shinohara K, Ikenoue N, Kaneda C, Fukaya T. Melatonin protects fetal rat brain against oxidative mitochondrial damage. *J. Pineal Res.* 30: 22–28 (2001).
85. Oberley TD, Verwiebe E, Zhong W, Kang SW, Rhee SG. Localization of the thioredoxin system in normal rat kidney. *Free Radic. Biol. Med.* 30: 412–424 (2001).
86. Kamat JP, Boloor KK, Devasagayam TPA, Kesavan PC. Protection of superoxide dismutase by caffeine in rat liver mitochondria against γ-irradiation. *Curr. Sci.* 77: 286–289 (1999).
87. Bruce KAJ, Begley JG, Fu W, Butterfield DA, Bredeson DE, Hutchins JB, Hensley K, Mattson MP. Bcl-2 protects isolated plasma and mitochondrial membranes against lipid peroxidation induced by hydrogen peroxide and amyloid beta peptide. *J. Neurochem.* 70: 31–39 (1998).
88. Jo SH, Son MK, Koh HJ, Lee SM, Song IH, Kim YO, Lee YS, Jeong KS, Kim WB, Park JW, Song BJ, Huhe TL. Control of mitochondrial redox balance and cellular defense against oxidative stress by mitochiondrial $NADP^+$-dependent isocitrate dehydrogenase. *J. Biol. Chem.* 276: 16168–16176 (2001).
89. Boloor KK, Kamat JP, Devasagayam TPA. Chlorophyllin as a protector of mitochondrial membranes against gamma-radiation and photosensitization. *Toxicol.* 155: 63–71 (2000).
90. Kamat JP, Boloor KK, Devasagayam TPA. Chlorophyllin as an effective antioxidant against membrane damage *in vitro* and *ex vivo*. *Biochim. Biophys. Acta* 1487: 113–127 (2000).
91. Kamat JP, Ghosh A, Devasagayam TPA. Vanillin as an antioxidant in rat liver mitochondria: inhibition of protein oxidation and lipid peroxidation induced by photosensitization. *Mol. Cell Biochem.* 209: 47–53 (2000).

92. Kamat JP, Boloor KK, Devasagayam TPA, Jayashree B, Kesavan PC. Differential modification by caffeine of oxygen-dependent and independent effects of γ-irradiation on rat liver mitochonria. *Int. J. Radiat. Biol.* 76: 1281–1288 (2000).
93. Kamat JP, Boloor KK, Devasagayam TPA, Venkatachalam SR. Antioxidant properties of *Asparagus racemosus* against damage induced by gamma-radiation in rat liver mitochondria. *J. Ethnopharmacol.* 71: 425–435 (2000).
94. Kim JS, Na CS, Pak SC, Kim YG. Effects of Yukmi, a herbal formula, on the liver of senescence accelerated mice (SAM) exposed to oxidative stress. *Am. J. Chin. Med.* 28: 343–350 (2000).
95. Quiles JL, Aguilera C, Mesa MD, Ramirez TMC, Baro L, Gil A. An ethanolic-aqueous extract of *Curcuma longa* decreases the susceptibility of liver microsomes and mitochondrial to lipid peroxidation in atherosclerotic rabbit. *Biofactors* 8: 51–57 (1998).
96. Devasagayam TPA, Kamat JP, Sreejayan N. Antioxidant action of curcumin. In: Nesaretnam K, Packer L (eds.) *Micronutrients and Health: Molecular Biological Mechanisms.* AOCS Press, Champaign, USA, 2001.
97. Kim DH, Jang YY, Han ES, Lee CS. Protective effect of harmaline and harmalol against dopamine- and 6-hydroxydopamine-induced oxidative damage of brain mitochondria and synaptosomes, and viability loss of PC12 cells. *Eur. J. Neurosci.* 13: 1861–1872 (2001).
98. Banaclocha MM. Therapeutic potential of N-acetylcysteine in age-related mitochondrial neurodegenerative diseases. *Med. Hypotheses* 56: 472–477 (2001).
99. Santos DJSL, Moreno AJM. Inhibition of heart mitochondrial lipid peroxidation by non-toxic concentrations of carvedilol and its analog BM-910228. *Biochem. Pharmacol.* 61: 155–164 (2001).
100. Jang YY, Song JH, Shin YK, Han ES, Lee CS. Protective effect of boldine on oxidative mitochondrial damage in streptozotocin-induced diabetic rats. *Pharmacol. Res.* 42: 361–371 (2000).
101. Kiningham KK, Oberley TD, Lin SM, Mattingly CA, Clair DKSt. Overexpression of manganese superoxide dismutase protects against mitochondrial-initioated poly(ADP-ribose) polymerase-mediated cell death. *FASEB J.* 13: 1601–1610 (1999).
102. Borras C, Sastre J, Garcia SD, Lloret A, Pallardo FV, Vina J. Mitochondria from females exhibit higher antioxidant gene expression and lower oxidative damage than males. *Free Radic. Biol. Med.* 34: 546–552 (2003).
103. Kokoszka JE, Coskun P, Esposito LA, Wallace DC. Increased mitochondrial oxidative stress in the Sod2 (+/−) mouse results in the age-related decline of

mitochondrial function culminating in increased apoptosis. *Proc. Natl. Acad. Sci. USA* 98: 2278–2283 (2001).

104. Halestrap AP, Doran E, Gillespie JP, O'Toole A. Mitochondria and cell death. *Biochem. Soc. Trans.* 28: 170–177 (2000).
105. Caro AA, Cederbaum AI. Ca^{2+}-dependent and- independent mitochondrial damage in HepG2 cells that overexpress CYP2E1. *Arch. Biochem. Biophys.* 408: 162–170 (2002).
106. Anuradha CD, Kanno S, Hirano S. Oxidative damage to mitochondria is a preliminary step to caspase-3 activation in fluoride-induced apoptosis in HL-60 cells. *Free Radic. Biol. Med.* 31: 367–373 (2001).
107. Berkich DA, Salama G, LaNoue KF. Mitochondrial membrane potentials in ischemic hearts. *Arch. Biochem. Biophys.* 420: 279–286 (2003).
108. Salvi M, Brunati AM, Clari G, Toninello A. Interaction of genistein with the mitochondrial electron transport chain results in opening of the membrane transition pore. *Biochim. Biophys. Acta* 1556: 187–196 (2002).
109. Oleinick NL, Morris RL, Belichenko I. The role of apoptosis in response to photodynamic therapy: what, where, why, and how. *Photochem. Photobiol. Sci.* 1: 1–21 (2002).
110. Morgan J, Oseroff JR. Mitochondria-based photodynamic anti-cancer therapy. *Adv. Drug Deliv. Rev.* 49: 71–86 (2001).
111. Moor AC. Signaling pathways in cell death and survival after photodynamic therapy. *J. Photochem. Photobiol.* 57: 1–13 (2000).
112. Modica-Napolitano JS, Aprille JR. Delocalized lipophilic cations selectively target the mitochondria of carcinoma cells. *Adv. Drug Deliv. Rev.* 49: 63–70 (2001).
113. Chatterjee SR, Possel H, Srivastava TS, Kama JP, Wolf G, Devasagayam TPA. Photodynamic effects induced by meso-tetrakis (4(carboxymethylenoxy)phenyl) porphyrin on isolated Sarcoma 180 ascites mitochondria. *J. Photochem. Photobiol. B-Biol.* 50: 79–87 (1999).
114. Chatterjee SR, Srivastava TS, Kamat JP, Devasagayam TPA. Lipid peroxidation induced by a novel porphyrin plus light in isolated mitochondria: possible implications in photodynamic therapy. *Mol. Cell. Biochem.* 166: 25–33 (1997).
115. Kamat JP, Devasagayam TPA. Oxidative damage to mitochondria in normal and cancer tissues, and its modulation. *Toxicology* 155: 73–82 (2000).
116. Gibson BW. Exploiting proteomics in the discovery of drugs that target oxidative damage. *Science* 304: 176–177 (2004).
117. Albers DS, Augood SJ. New insights into progressive supranuclear palsy. *Trends Neurosci.* 24: 347–352 (2001).

118. Chao M, Zhu X, Raina AK, Aliev G, Takeda A, Peterson RB, Nunomura A, Tabaton M, Perry G, Smith MA. Sources contributing to the initiation and propagation of oxidative stress in Alzheimer's disease. *Proc. Indian Natl. Sci. Acad. Part B-Biol. Sci.* 69: 251–260 (2003).
119. Gjumrakch A, Dilara S, Lamb-Bruce T, Obrenovich ME, Siedlak SL, Vinters HV, Friedland RP, LaManna JC, Smith MA, Perry G. Mitochondria and vascular lesions as a central target for the development of Alzheimer's disease and Alzheimer-disease like pathology in transgenic mice. *Neurol. Res.* 25: 665–674 (2003).
120. Brooks PS, Land JM, Clark JB, Heales SJR. Peroxynitrite and brain mitochondria: evidence for increased proton leak. *J. Neurochem.* 70: 2195–2202 (1998).
121. Santos DL, Palmeira CM, Seica R, Dias J, Mesquita J, Moreno AJ, Santos MS. Diabetes and mitochondrial oxidative stress: a study using heart mitochondria from the diabetic Goto-Kakizaki rat. *Mol. Cell Biochem.* 246: 163–170 (2003).
122. Lashin O, Romani A. Mitochondria respiration and susceptibility to ischemia-reperfusion injury in diabetic hearts. *Arch. Biochem. Biophys.* 420: 298–304 (2003).
123. Andreassi MG. Coronary atherosclerosis and somatic mutations: An overview of the contributive factors for oxidative DNA damage. *Mutat. Res.* 543: 67–86 (2003).
124. Lim PS, Ma YS, Cheng YM, Chai H, Lee CF, Chen TL, Wei YH. Mitochondrial DNA mutations and oxidative damage in skeletal muscle of patients with chronic uremia. *J. Biomed. Sci.* 9: 549–560 (2002).

4 Oxidative Stress and Antioxidant Defenses in Plants

Olga Blokhina and Kurt Fagerstedt

1. Introduction

The scope of this review covers the basic chemistry of reactive oxygen species (ROS) and reactive nitrogen species (RNS), while more stress is placed on different types of low molecular mass antioxidants and genes coding for enzymes involved in their synthesis and turnover with the emphasis on plant-specific compounds. Enzymatic and non-enzymatic sources of ROS/RNS and their possible targets with respect to oxidative stress signaling are discussed. Compartmentalization of oxidative metabolism, its place and interactions with the other well-established constituents of the signaling pathways are also considered.

2. Chemistry of Oxidative Metabolism

2.1. *Types of reactive oxygen species (ROS) and sources of ROS formation*

Generation of reactive oxygen species (ROS) is characteristic for all tissues and cells, and increases under stress conditions. Molecular oxygen is not very reactive as such, as it has two unpaired electrons with parallel spins on the last electron sheath. Such spin orientation puts a restriction on O_2 interaction with most organic molecules.[1] The initial step in oxygen activation (one e^- reduction) requires energy, while the subsequent reduction steps can proceed spontaneously in the presence of appropriate e^- donors. In plants electron transport chains of chloroplasts, mitochondria and, in some cases of the plasma membrane are the main sources of e^- together with transition metal ions (Fe^{2+}, Cu^{2+}) and semiquinones.

Singlet oxygen ($^1O_2$), where one of the electrons on the outer electron sheath has changed its spin, is produced in tissues under UV-exposure and during photoinhibition in chloroplasts. Of the ROS hydrogen peroxide (H_2O_2) and superoxide (O_2^-) are both produced in a number of cellular reactions including the Mehler reaction in the chloroplasts, the iron catalyzed Fenton reaction, photorespiration and by various enzymes such as lipoxygenases, peroxidases, NADPH oxidase and xanthine oxidase.[2] O_2^- is membrane impermeable and is converted to H_2O_2 by compartment specific superoxide dismutase isoforms (SOD).[3]

The H_2O_2 molecule is relatively stable and less reactive than O_2^-, and is able to cross the lipid bilayer, a property which makes it a good candidate as a signaling species. It has been suggested that H_2O_2 passes the membrane through aquaporins.[4] If so, the delivery of H_2O_2 signal to a particular site can be indirectly regulated via aquaporin manipulation and, to some extent can solve the question of ROS signal specificity.

A very reactive oxygen species, the hydroxyl radical OH•, is produced in the decomposition of ozone in the presence of protons in the apoplastic space and also in defense against pathogens,[5] while the perhydroxyl radical O_2H• is produced in a reaction of ozone with hydroxyl ions.

The various types of ROS and their cellular localization are presented in Table 1. Abbreviations for reactive oxygen species and antioxidants are also listed in Table 1.

2.2. *Types of reactive nitrogen species (RNS) and sources of NO•*

The chemical properties of nitric oxide make this gas a good candidate for a signaling molecule. NO can freely penetrate the lipid bilayer and, hence be transported within the cell. NO is quickly produced on demand via inducible enzymatic of non-enzymatic routes. Due to its free radical nature (one unpaired electron) NO has a short half-life (in order of seconds), and can be removed easily when no longer needed.[6–8] Nitric oxide

Table 1. Reactive oxygen species, reactive nitrogen species and antioxidants.

Molecular species	Chemical formula or abbreviation	Cellular localization	Comments
Singlet oxygen	$^1O_2$	Chloroplast, thylakoid, mitochondria, peroxisome	Membrane impermeable, local signal
Superoxide anion radical	$O_2^{-\bullet}$	Chloroplast, thylakoid, mitochondria, peroxisome, apoplast	Membrane impermeable, interacts with $NO^{\bullet}$
Hydrogen peroxide	H_2O_2	Chloroplast, mitochondria, peroxisome, apoplast	Membrane permeable, signalling molecule
Nitric oxide	$NO^{\bullet}$	Mitochondria, cytosol, peroxisome, apoplast	Membrane permeable, can react with O_2^-; SH-groups of proteins
Peroxynitril	$ONOO^-$	Peroxisome, apoplast cytosol	Formed via interaction with O_2^-
Antioxidants			
Ascorbic acid	AA	Mitochondria, chloroplast, cytosol, apoplast, peroxisome	AA-GSH cycle, synthesized in mitochondrial inner membrane, negatively charged at cellular pH
Dehydroascorbic acid	DHA	See AA	Oxidized form of AA, uncharged
Monodehydro ascorbic acid	MDHA	See AA	Unstable radical form, disproportionates to AA and DHA
Glutathione	GSH/GSSG	Chloroplast, cytosol, mitochondria	AA/GSH cycle
Tocopherol	TP	Chloroplast envelope, thylakoids, mitochondria	Regenerated in membranes by AA, synthesis in chloroplast envelope
Thioredoxins	Trx	Chloroplast, mitochondria	H_2O_2 reduction via thiol-disulphide cycle
Phenolic compounds		Apoplast, vacuole	Efficient scavengers of ROS

is represented by three species with different chemical reactivity and physical properties: radical $NO^{\bullet}$, nitrosonium cation NO^{+} and nitroxyl anion NO^{-}.[9] Nitric oxide can have direct or indirect biological effects; the direct effects take place at low NO concentrations ($<1\,\mu M$), while the indirect effects through RNS take place at higher local concentrations ($>1\,\mu M$).[6] The direct effects of NO include reduction of free metal ions or oxidation of metals in protein complexes such as hemoglobin, and Fe-nitrosyl formation resulting in activation of guanylate cyclase and hemoxygenase, inhibition of P450, cytochrome c oxidase and catalase, stimulation of $T_f R$ protein and down-regulation of ferritin.[6] The indirect effects happen through NO reacting either with oxygen or superoxide. The end products, NO_2, N_2O_2, and peroxynitrite $ONOO^{-}$ all have deleterious effects in biological systems.[6] The RNS and their cellular localization are presented in Table 1.

2.2.1. *Enzymatic sources of NO*

In mammalian cells three types of nitric oxide synthases (NOS, EC 1.14.13.39) have been described — a constitutively expressed neuronal (nNOS), an endothelial (eNOS), both under the control of Ca^{2+}-calmodulin, and an inducible (immunological) iNOS. The isoforms are products of different genes with 50–60% homology and share common cofactors and chemistry of NO production.[10] NOS consists of an N-terminal oxygenase domain with binding sites for haem, tetrahydrobiopterin, a calmodulin-binding site and a C-terminal reductase domain with binding sites for NADPH; FAD and FMN. Functional NOS assembles to a dimer and catalyzes oxygen dependent conversion of L-arginine to citrulline (for discussion on mechanism see Alderton *et al.*[11]).

$$\text{L-arginine} + \text{NADPH} + O_2 \rightarrow \text{citrulline} + NO^{\bullet} + \text{NADP}^{+}$$

Occurrence of a mitochondrial isoenzyme, a constitutive mitochondrial NOS (130 kDa), distinct from the nNOS, eNOS and iNOS has been recently reported in NOS knockout mice,[12] and another type of mtNOS, similar to a brain NOS_{α} but post-translationally modified by acylation and phosphorylation at the C terminus, has been found in the mitochondria of rat liver, brain, heart, muscle, kidney, lung, testis and spleen.[13]

The existence of NOS-like proteins in plants has been assessed by biochemical (conversion of L-arginine to citrulline, sensitivity to mammalian

NOS inhibitors) and immunological methods. The latter have proved to be non-conclusive due to the cross-reactivity of mammalian NOS antibodies with NOS-unrelated plant proteins.[14] Furthermore, no plant homologue of mammalian NOS has been found in the *Arabidopsis thaliana* genome[15] supporting the idea that plants have a structurally different enzyme with somewhat similar chemistry to the mammalian counterparts. Analysis of *Arabidopsis Atnos1* mutant with impaired NO production, growth and ABA signalling, has revealed that *AtNOS1* encodes a NOS distinct from mammalian isoforms but nevertheless is capable of using arginine as a substrate, is sensitive to inhibitors of mammalian nNOS and eNOS and is dependent on NADPH, calmodulin and Ca^{2+}.[16] However, other cofactors of mammalian NOS such as tetrahydrobiopterin, FAD and FMN do not exert any effect on the plant enzyme.[16]

Xanthine oxidoreductase, a redox enzyme with Mo cofactor, is another inducible source of NO in the context of stress responses. At low oxygen tensions NO-generating activity of this enzyme is increased. Interestingly, under normoxic conditions xanthine oxidoreductase is capable of both $NO^{\bullet}$ and $O_2^{-\bullet}$ formation with consequent production of $ONOO^-$.[17]

In plants, nitrate reductase (NR) is another important source of $NO^{\bullet}$. Three prosthetic groups of this homodimeric enzyme (FAD, heme and Mo cofactor) normally transfer e^- from NADH to nitrate. NR is controlled by the substrate (nitrate), and induced by light and sugars.[18] Post-translational regulation is achieved by phosphorylation of critical serine residue and by interaction with divalent cations or polyamines and 14-3-3 proteins.[19] In the presence of nitrite and NADH under physiological pH, the plant nitrate reductases are capable of $NO^{\bullet}$ and RNS production *in vivo* and *in vitro* without the presence of O_2.[20,21] Activation of nitrate reductase under hypoxic conditions in barley roots, and accumulation of NO during hypoxic treatment in maize cells have been shown[22,23] and a role for NO as a signal for aerenchyma formation has been hypothesized.[22] Regulation of NO level under oxygen deprivation can be achieved in plants via interaction with stress-induced non-symbiotic hemoglobins (Hb) through several routes: In a reaction with oxyhemoglobin to form nitrate and methemoglobin (Fe^{3+}) with the latter being reduced to hemoglobin (Fe^{2+}) and in a NADH-dependent reaction. Another route is interaction of NO with deoxyhemoglobin to form nitrosylhemoglobin.[23] Under low oxygen tension, nitrosylhemoglobin will represent a significant part of the Hb pool. Reactions of NO with Hb allow the maintenance of NAD^+ levels for the needs of glycolysis under hypoxic conditions.[24] In the apoplastic space of tobacco roots in addition to non-enzymatic route of NO formation a plasma membrane-bound enzyme nitrite: NO reductase has been biochemically characterized. The enzyme uses cytochrome *c* as an e^- donor for reduction of nitrite to NO.[25,26]

Inhibition of nitrite reductase (NiR), a plastidic enzyme which reduces nitrite to ammonium with concurrent activation of NR (e.g. under anoxia) can lead to nitrite accumulation. The protonated form of nitrite (HNO_2) is membrane permeable and can be freely excreted by the cell to the acidic apoplast and provides a source for non-enzymatic NO production.[18]

2.2.2. *Non-enzymatic sources of NO*

The formation of NO via non-enzymatic reduction of exogenous nitrite has been shown in the apoplast of barley (*Hordeum vulgare*) aleurone layers. The process requires acidic pH and its rate is enhanced by phenolic compounds.[27]

$$2HNO_2 \leftrightarrow NO + NO_2 + H_2O$$

Light-dependent reduction of NO_2^- by carotenoids leads to NO release.[28] Non-enzymatic NO production can be a factor under pathological conditions, i.e. hypoxia, which is characterized by cytoplasmic acidosis and accumulation of reducing equivalents in both animal[29] and plant systems.[23]

3. Physiological Roles of ROS and RNS, Oxidative Stress and Signaling

Oxidative stress is defined as "an imbalance between oxidants and antioxidants in favor of the oxidants, potentially leading to damage".[30] ROS are formed constitutively as the byproducts of oxidative metabolism. Imposition of stress results in a disturbance of cellular homeostasis with one major consequence: a shift in redox balance towards oxidation. These changes are brought about by intensified ROS formation and/or by the depletion of antioxidants and inhibition of enzymes of antioxidant synthesis and turnover. Disturbed redox balance can itself be an inducing signal for defense mechanisms. Under particular stress (pathogen defense) or physiological conditions (programmed cell death, stomatal movements) plant cells are capable of controlled production of ROS as a signaling species. Currently oxidative stress, although damaging in its extremes, is viewed as an essential component of plant signalling networks. ROS (and/or oxidative event) have recently been suggested to mediate physiological responses via a ripple effect: local and transient changes in redox status affect an increasing number of downstream mediators (Ca^{2+} release, salicylic acid, GSH) eliciting a sustained response, which in turn modulates the expression of stress-related genes.[31]

3.1. *ROS-mediated signaling*

Implication of ROS and particularly H_2O_2 in signaling has been shown for cell cycle regulation, cell death, wounding response, pathogen defense, and in a number of abiotic stress responses (reviewed in several articles recently.[32–38]

Monitoring the expression of over 14,000 genes in catalase-deficient tobacco (CAT1AS) under H_2O_2-inducing exposure to high light revealed transcriptional response that mimicked that of both biotic and abiotic stresses. Clustering and sequence analysis revealed induction of genes responsible for hormonal biosynthesis, pathogen defense, mitochondrial metabolism, vesicular trafficking, proteolysis and cell death.[39] However, it is not fully understood how H_2O_2 signal is perceived and transduced. It has been shown recently that H_2O_2 is a potent inducer of specific mitogen-activated protein kinase kinase kinase (ANP1) in *Arabidopsis*. ANP1 initiates a phosphorylation cascade by mitogen-activated protein kinases (MAPK) which in turn lead to the induction of stress responsive genes.[40] In another study H_2O_2 exposure of *Arabidopsis* cells lead to changed expression levels of 175 genes, of which 113 coded for proteins with antioxidant functions or were related to stress responses.[41] Although no redox-sensitive transcription factors have as yet been identified in plants, it is likely that such transcription factors (as *E. coli* and yeasts have) exist.[38]

H_2O_2 is known to act as a signaling molecule in defense against pathogens,[42] in programmed cell death (H_2O_2 accumulation triggers cell death),[43] in growth and morphogenesis through the cell cycle[44] and in responses to plant hormones such as salicylic acid,[45] ethylene,[46] abscisic acid,[47] and probably also jasmonic acid.[37] It has also been shown that H_2O_2-induced MAPK cascade in *Arabidopsis* represses auxin-inducible gene expression.[40] However, it is also known that oxidative burst and cognate redox signaling work in a signal network that functions independently of ethylene, SA and Me-JA but is dependent on MAPKK activity.[48]

3.2. *Physiological functions of NO•, molecular targets and interaction with ROS*

Implementation of ROS and RNS formation as stress markers also suggest their participation in signaling cascades. The role of active oxygen species and NO in plant defense responses has been reviewed by Bolwell[49] and Grant.[32] The field of RNS signaling has been thoroughly investigated in mammalian models during the last decade. In plant science the most examined area is biotic stress signaling. Indeed, the burst of NO production during plant–pathogen interaction is associated with induction of iNOS and has been shown in tobacco and *Arabidopsis*.[32,50] A number of investigations have been carried out on NO interactions with plant development.[10,51,52] NO has also been found to slow down plant senescence in pea leaves,[53] in cut flowers[54] and in ripening fruits[55] pointing towards NO and hormone interplay. Furthermore, cytokinins have been shown to induce NO synthesis in tobacco, parsley and *Arabidopsis* cell cultures.[56] Since a NOS-inhibitor has been shown to hinder cytokinin-induced betalaine accumulation in *Amaranthus*, it has been suggested that NO may mediate some cytokinin effects.[57] Hence, NO may also mediate cytokinin-induced programmed cell death.[58] It has also been shown that NO induces apoptosis via hydrogen peroxide.[59] Recently, several new physiological roles for NO have been described such as cGMP-dependent adventitious root formation, activation of mitogen-activated protein kinase cascade, regulation of cell death during xylem differentiation, auxin-dependent gravitropic reaction of roots, stomatal movements, control of flower timing and regulatory genes related to flowering.[26,60,61]

The large number of physiological and developmental effects of NO point towards regulation of gene expression.[8] This has indeed been observed in some occasions, e.g. in TMV-resistant tobacco NOS activity increases after infection.[62,63] In a microarray study on *Arabidopsis* suspension cultures it has been shown that a number of genes are induced by NO and a common induction mechanism has been suggested for some of the genes, although no data on a common regulatory element in the promoter areas of these genes exist as yet.[64]

3.2.1. *NO, free radicals, lipid peroxidation and DNA damage*

Peroxidation of polyunsaturated fatty acids (PUFA) incorporated in membrane lipids is one of the most dangerous consequences of oxidative stress. A reaction of ROS (hydroxyl radical and singlet oxygen) with methylene groups of PUFA results in the rearrangement of the double bond and the formation of conjugated dienes, lipid peroxy (L-OO$^{\bullet}$) and alkoxy (L-O$^{\bullet}$) radicals and lipid hydroperoxides (LOOH). In turn, lipid radical species propagate or initiate (branch) a new chain of peroxidative reactions in membrane lipids.[65] The main chain breaking antioxidant in biological membranes is tocopherol (see below). NO can react with alkoxy and peroxy radicals thus terminating the chain reaction of lipid peroxidation:[6]

$$\mathrm{LOO^{\bullet} + NO \rightarrow LOONO}$$

It has been proposed that NO is responsible for DNA damage through its autooxidation to form RNS (such as N_2O_3 and peroxynitrite) which result in deamination of cytosine, adenine and guanine.[66,67]

4. Antioxidant Defense Systems in Plants

4.1. *Ascorbate*

L-ascorbic acid (l–*threo*-hex-2-enono-1,4-lactone) is a powerful antioxidant, redox regulator and a signaling molecule in plants, which has been implicated in the regulation of cell division, cell elongation and the cell cycle (reviewed in several articles recently[68–73]). Ascorbate is universally distributed *in planta* and has been detected virtually in all compartments of the plant cell: cytoplasm, mitochondria, chloroplasts, peroxisomes and the apoplast. In photosynthesizing tissues reduced form of AA comprises 90% of total AA pool and can build up to 20 mM in the cytosol and 200–300 mM in the chloroplast stroma.[69] The biosynthetic route of AA in plants differs from that of animals and has been elucidated recently.[74] Unlike in animal tissues no inversion of D-glucose carbon skeleton occurs in plants. The synthesis proceeds through D-glucose $\Leftrightarrow$ GDP-D-mannose $\Leftrightarrow$ GDP-L-galactose $\Rightarrow$ L-galactose $\Rightarrow$ L-galactono-1, 4-lactone. In plants the last step of AA biosynthesis i.e. the conversion of L-galactono-1,4-lactone to AA by L-galactono-γ lactone dehydrogenase (GAL, EC 1.3.2.3), is localized to the inner mitochondrial membrane and requires oxidized cytochrome *c* as an electron acceptor.[75,76] Functional and structural association of GAL with mitochondrial complex I suggests the mechanism of AA level manipulation via the redox state of electron transport chain.[77] Other than L-galactono-1, 4-lactone biosynthetic pathways for AA have also been suggested.[78,79]

Due to its ability to donate electrons AA is recruited in a number of cellular redox reactions and serves as a major cellular redox regulator, antioxidant and a cofactor for metal prosthetic groups of enzymes. AA can directly scavenge singlet oxygen, $O_2^{-\bullet}$ and the hydroxyl radical. A cascade of coupled reactions of AA with GSH and NADH (an ascorbate–glutathione cycle) is a main route of H_2O_2 elimination under stress conditions.[69] The ability to interact with other antioxidant molecules adds to the antioxidant properties of AA. Except for participation in AA-GSH cycle; AA is capable of tocopherol reduction from tocopheroxyl in the aqueous phase, providing membrane protection.[80,81] AA serves as an e^- donor in phenoxyl radical regeneration in vacuole-localized elimination of H_2O_2.[82] In chloroplasts AA acts as a cofactor of violaxanthin de-epoxidase sustaining regeneration in the xantophyll cycle, and hence is vital in photoprotection.[71]

Isolation and characterization of AA-deficient *Arabidopsis vtc* mutants, defective in AA biosynthesis, has proved to be a useful tool in studies on oxidative stress and the signaling role of AA. *VTC1* encodes GDP-d-man pyrophosphorylase, an enzyme in AA biosynthetic pathway and the mutant plants contain approximately 30% of AA found in wt.[79] Recent studies of *vtc1* mutant provided the molecular signature of AA deficiency: a differential expression of 171 genes as compared with wt (Col0) and suggest a link with hormone-mediated signaling.[83] The transcripts detected code for putative DNA binding proteins, and proteins connected with the cell cycle, plant development and signaling. Interestingly, the transcripts of defense genes upregulated in *vtc1* include pathogenesis-related proteins but not antioxidant enzymes. In addition, transcript levels of enzymes which regulate carbon, lipid, cell wall and indole metabolism were modified. Retarded growth and flowering in *vtc1* is possibly associated with upregulation of ABA-synthesis and ABA-modulated transcripts which result in metabolic arrest. The upregulation of ethylene-responsive transcription factor in *vtc1* further confirmed close connection between AA level and hormonal control of plant development.[83] Antisense suppression of GAL mRNA in tobacco resulted in decreased AA content and retardation of cell division growth and altered the structure of plant cells.[84]

Localization of AA synthesis in mitochondria, ubiquitous distribution of AA in cellular compartments, and implication of AA in the regulation of cellular metabolism and defense reactions, all emphasize the importance of AA transport mechanisms in the regulation of cellular redox milieu. Under physiological pH AA exists in a negatively charged form and cannot penetrate the lipid bilayer, while DHA is uncharged and more hydrophobic but it is also unlikely to diffuse through the membrane.[85] From the site of synthesis in the inner mitochondrial membrane AA diffuses to the cytoplasm and is further transported to the chloroplast by facilitated diffusion via low affinity (5 mM for ascorbate) carrier. The transporter is trans-stimulated by DHA, indicating the possibility of an exchange mechanism.[70] AA transport across the thylakoid and tonoplast membranes does not show any saturation kinetics and is not carrier-mediated. The existence of specific transporters across plasma membrane for AA and DHA, and electron transport chain for AA regeneration in the apoplast has been suggested.[86] Due to the absence (or very low content) of GSH in the apoplast, AA-GSH cycle is not operational and DHA has to be transported to the cytoplasm for reduction. AA is transported back to the apoplast via the hypothetical AA/DHA carrier.[86] Another route for AA regeneration in the apoplast is $cytb_{556}$-mediated e^- transfer across the plasmalemma coupled with AA oxidation in the cytoplasm and AA re-reduction by plasma membrane NADH-MDHA oxidoreductase.[87,88]

4.2. *Glutathione*

Glutathione is a versatile redox active tripeptide (γ-glutamylcysteinyl glycine) responsible for multiple functions in plant cells.[69,89–91] The nucleophilic cysteine residue with high reductive potential determines the chemical and biological properties of GSH and its non-enzymatic interaction with $O_2^{-\bullet}$, H_2O_2, $^1O_2$, $OH^\bullet$[92] and coupled enzymatic H_2O_2 elimination via the AA-GSH cycle (see Sec. 4.1 and Figs. 1 and 2). As a substrate for phospholipid

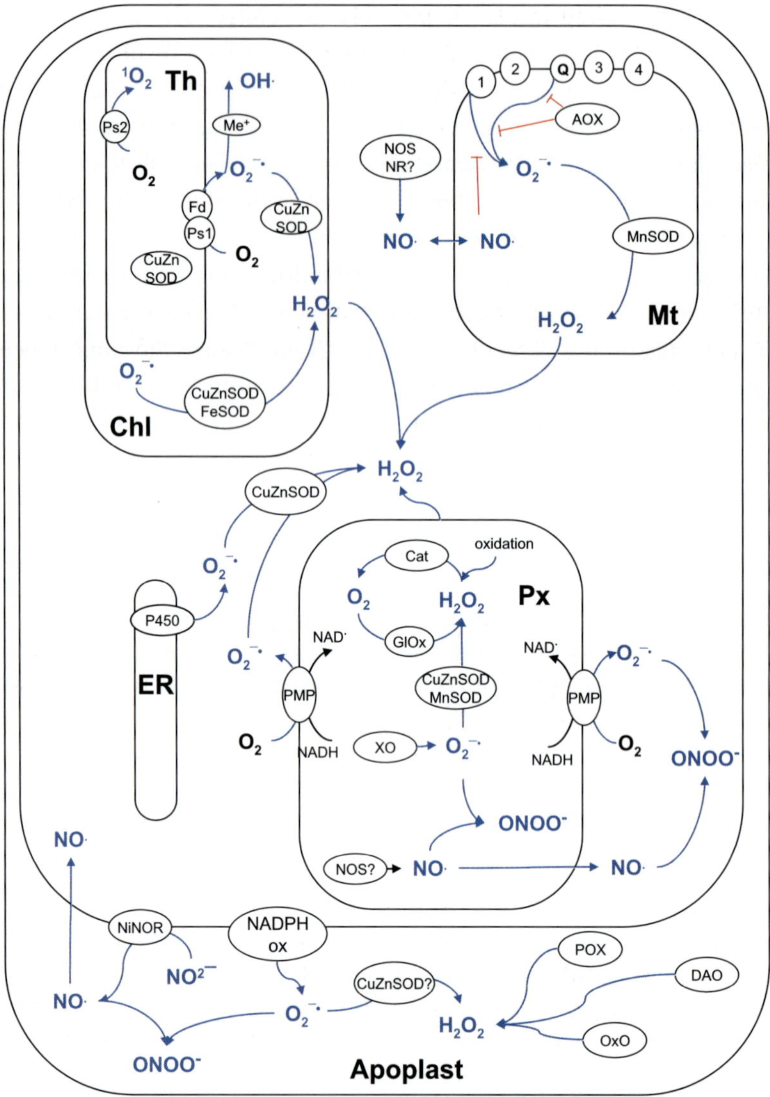

Fig. 1. Reactive oxygen and nitrogen species: Sources and intracellular distribution. In the apoplast NADPH oxidase (NADPH ox) is the main enzyme producing the superoxide anion radical ($O_2^{-\bullet}$), which is dismutated by superoxide dismutase (CuZn-SOD) to H_2O_2. Some of the $O_2^{-\bullet}$ produced can react with nitric oxide ($NO^\bullet$) to form peroxynitrite ($ONOO^-$). $NO^\bullet$ in the apoplast can be reduced from nitrite (NO_2^-) non-enzymatically or via plasma membrane-bound nitrite: NO reductase (NiNOR). Several apoplastic enzymes such as

(*continued on facing page*)

hydroperoxide glutathione peroxidase (Table 2) GSH protects membranes from lipid peroxidation. Conjugation with GSH is the main process for the detoxification of herbicides, heavy metals and cytotoxic products resulted from oxidative stress and pathogen attack.[93] GSH is the main source of non-protein sulphur and provides protection for –SH groups in proteins under oxidative stress. Above all GSH exerts a number of signaling functions: transition in the cell cycle from G1 to S phase and regulation of expression of many genes.

Leguminous plants are able to synthesize a GSH homologue homoglutathione (γ-glutamylcysteine β-alanine). Together with GSH homoglutathione maintains redox state and controls senescence in nitrogen-fixing nodules. Homoglutathione synthetase from pea nodules has been recently cloned and characterized.[94]

Fig. 1. *(continued from previous page)*
pH-dependent peroxidases (POX), diaminooxidase (DAO) and germin-like oxalate oxidase (OxO) add to H_2O_2 formation in the apoplast. Inside the cell chloroplastic and mitochondrial electron transport chains are the main sites of O_2 reduction. In the thylakoid membranes photosystem 1 (PS1) donates e^- to oxygen with the formation of $O_2^{-\bullet}$. The fate of $O_2^{-\bullet}$ in the thylakoid can vary: i) Dismutation by CuZn-SOD to yield H_2O_2; or ii) Interaction with transition metal ions (Me^+) to form hydroxyl radicals (OH•) in the Fenton reaction. Under excess light photosystem 2 (PS2) is able to generate singlet oxygen ($^1O_2^-$). In mitochondria reduction of O_2 can occur at the matrix side of complex 1 (1, 2, 3, 4 and Q — respiratory complexes one to four and ubiquinone) and at Q site. Alternative oxidase (AOX) prevents ROS formation via competition for electrons. $NO^\bullet$ production has been shown in plant mitochondria, but the mechanism is unknown. $NO^\bullet$ inhibits ROS accumulation by mitochondria. Peroxisomes produce H_2O_2 as a result of fatty acid β-oxidation and glycolate oxidation. Catalase (CAT) is responsible for H_2O_2 elimination. Xanthine oxidase (XOD) catalyzed formation of $O_2^{-\bullet}$ leads to H_2O_2 accumulation via a SOD-dependent reaction. Interaction of $O_2^{-\bullet}$ and $NO^\bullet$ results in $ONOO^-$. In peroxisomes $NO^\bullet$ is enzymatically produced presumably by nitric oxide synthase (NOS). Integral peroxisomal membrane protein (PMP) reduces O_2 to $O_2^{-\bullet}$ on the outer surface of the membrane in a NADPH-dependent reaction. Cytochrome P450 localized in the endoplasmic reticulum (ER) and cytoplasm produce $O_2^{-\bullet}$ during catalytic action, and the radical disproportionates to H_2O_2 by cytoplasmic CuZn-SOD. For the clarity of the picture and due to space limitation most enzymatic reactions are not fully presented. Consult Table 2 for the full reactions and enzyme code (EC) numbers. Blue lines denote routes of ROS formation. Chl — chloroplast; Th — thylakoid; Mt — mitochondria; Px — peroxisome.

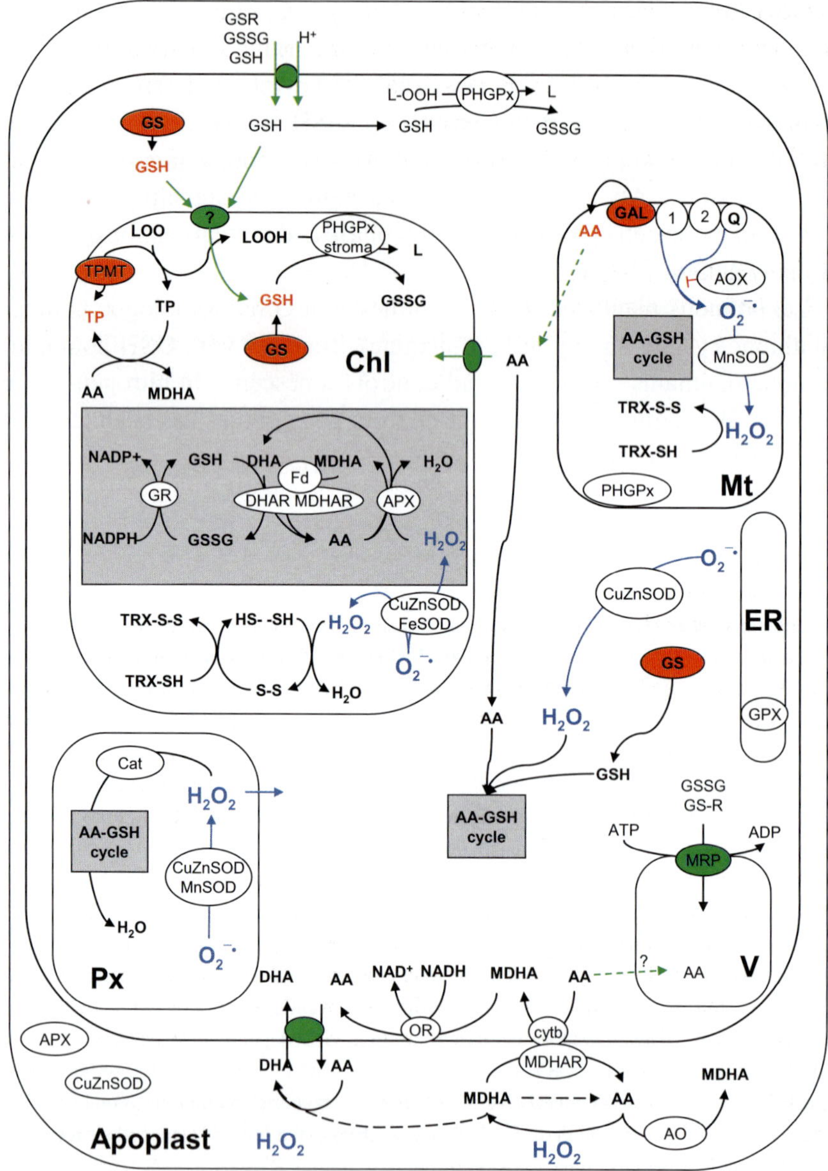
GSR
GSSG
GSH
H+
L-OOH
PHGPx
L
GSH
GSH
GSSG
GS
GSH
?
LOO
LOOH
PHGPx stroma
L
TPMT
TP
TP
GSH
GSSG
GS
Chl
AA
MDHA
NADP+
GSH
DHA
MDHA
H_2O
Fd
GR
DHAR MDHAR
APX
NADPH
GSSG
AA
H_2O_2
CuZnSOD
FeSOD
TRX-S-S
HS- -SH
H_2O_2
TRX-SH
S-S
H_2O
$O_2^{-\cdot}$
GAL
1
2
Q
AA
AOX
$O_2^{-\cdot}$
AA-GSH cycle
MnSOD
AA
TRX-S-S
H_2O_2
TRX-SH
PHGPx
Mt
$O_2^{-\cdot}$
CuZnSOD
ER
GS
AA
H_2O_2
GPX
GSH
Cat
H_2O_2
AA-GSH cycle
AA-GSH cycle
GSSG
GS-R
ATP
ADP
MRP
CuZnSOD MnSOD
H_2O
$O_2^{-\cdot}$
Px
DHA
AA
NAD+
NADH
MDHA
AA
?
AA
V
OR
cytb
APX
DHA
AA
MDHAR
MDHA
CuZnSOD
MDHA
AA
AO
Apoplast
H_2O_2
H_2O_2

GSH homeostasis in plant cells is tightly controlled on multiple levels: synthesis, transport, partitioning, conjugation and degradation.[90,91,93] The synthetic route for GSH is similar in animals and plants: it is an ATP- and Mg^{2+}-dependent two-step process involving γ-glutamylcysteine synthetase (γ-ECS)-catalyzed formation of γ-glutamylcysteine from

---

Fig. 2. Synthesis, transport and subcellular localisation of the main antioxidants and antioxidative enzymatic systems. The last step of AA biosynthesis is catalyzed by L-galactono-γ lactone dehydrogenase (GAL) and is localized to inner mitochondrial membrane. AA diffuses from mitochondria and can enter the chloroplast (Chl) via a low affinity AA carrier. AA-DHA carrier localized on the plasma membrane supports DHA transport and regeneration of apoplastic ascorbate in the cytoplasm. Regeneration of AA can also occur in the apoplast by cytochrome b_{551} e^- transport system (cyt b) coupled to NADH-dependent oxidoreductase (OR). GSH is synthesized in chloroplast stroma and cytosol by glutathione synthetase (GS). GSH is actively taken up by chloroplasts through an unidentified transporter. Glutathione exchange between apoplast and cytosol is mediated by H^+-gradient driven transporter with preference for GSSG and glutathione conjugates (GSR). For degradation these oxidized species can be transported to the vacuole (V) by ATP-dependent multidrug-resistance-associated protein (MRP) localized on the tonoplast. The last step of tocopherol (TP) biosynthesis takes place in the inner membrane of chloroplast envelope and is catalyzed by γ-tocopherol methyltransferase (TPMT). TP directly interacts with lipid peroxyl radicals ($LOO^\bullet\cdot$) terminating lipid peroxidation. The resulting tocopheroxyl radical ($TO^\bullet$) is regenerated to TP by AA. Superoxide dismutases (SOD, see also Fig. 1) operate in all cellular compartments and provide protection by scavenging superoxide anion-radical ($O_2^{\bullet-}$). H_2O_2 derived from SOD reaction is effectively eliminated in ascorbate-glutathione cycle (gray rectangles), which is operational in Chl, mitochondria (Mt), peroxisomes (Px) and cytosol. In Chl and Mt oxidative damage to –SH groups of proteins caused by H_2O_2 escaped from AA-GSH cycle is repaired by thioredoxin system (TRX). Phospholipid-hydroperoxide glutathione peroxidase (PHGPx) protects membrane lipids from lipid peroxidation via the reduction of lipid hydroperoxides (LOOH) at the expense of GSH. PHGPx is localized to Chl stroma, where it acts synergetically with TP, and to plasma membrane and putatively to Mt. Protective enzymes specific to particular organelle are represented by catalase (CAT) in peroxisomes and alternative oxidase (AOX) in mitochondria. Catalase removes H_2O_2 derived from photorespiration and Px metabolism. AOX acts as e^- sink in Mt, thus indirectly preventing ROS formation via Mt electron transport chain. In the apoplast ascorbate peroxidase (APX), monodehydroascorbate reductase (MDHAR) and ascorbate oxidase (AO) regulate AA redox state in concert with plasma membrane DHA-AA exchanger. Monodehydroascorbic acid (MDHA) is unstable and disproportionates to AA and DHA (dashed lines). Biosynthetic sites are marked in red, transporters are marked in green. Blue lines denote routes of ROS formation.

Table 2. ROS–related enzymes: formation, scavenging and detoxification.

Enzyme	EC number	Reaction catalyzed	Comment
Superoxide dismutase	1.15.1.1	$O_2^{-\bullet} + O_2^{-\bullet} + 2H^+ \Leftrightarrow 2H_2O_2 + O_2$	
Catalase	1.11.1.6	$2H_2O_2 + \Leftrightarrow O_2 + 2H_2O$	
Glutathione S-transferases	2.5.1.18	$RX + GSH \Leftrightarrow HX + GS\text{-}R$	R may be an aliphatic, aromatic or heterocyclic group; X may be a sulphate, nitrite or halide group; role in detoxification of LP products
Glutathione peroxidase	1.11.1.9	$2GSH + ROOH \Leftrightarrow GSSG + ROH + 2H_2O$	
Glycolate oxidase	1.1.3.15	glycolate + O_2 = glyoxylate + H_2O_2	Functions in photorespiration, flavoprotein, localized to peroxisomes
Phospholipid-hydroperoxide Glutathione peroxidase	1.11.1.12	$2GSH + PUFA\text{-}OOH\ (H_2O_2) \Leftrightarrow GSSG + PUFA + 2H_2O$	Reaction with H_2O_2 is slow; location: cytoplasm, chloroplast stroma, mitochondria (potential site in *Arabidopsis*)
Ascorbate oxidase	1.10.3.3	$2AA + O_2 \Leftrightarrow 2MDHA \Leftrightarrow DHA + AA + 2H_2O$	No clear biological function, in the apoplast believed to regulate AA cycling
Ascorbate peroxidase	1.11.1.11	$AA + H_2O_2 \Leftrightarrow DHA + 2H_2O$	Localized to mitochondrial inner membrane and matrix, apoplast, chloroplast and cytosol

Table 2. (*Continued*)

Enzyme	EC number	Reaction catalyzed	Comment
Guaiacol type peroxidase	1.11.1.7	Donor + H_2O_2 ⇔ oxidized donor + $2H_2O$	
Monodehydroascorbate reductase	1.6.5.4	NADH + 2MDHA ⇔ NAD^+ + 2AA	
Dehydroascorbate reductase	1.8.5.1	2GSH + DHA ⇔ GSSG + AA	
Glutathione reductase	1.6.4.2	NADPH + GSSG ⇔ $NADP^+$ + 2GSH	
NADPH:cytochrome P450 oxidoreductase	1.6.2.4	RH + NADPH + O_2 = ROH + NAD^+ + H_2O	Catalytic cycle involves $O_2^{-\bullet}$ formation
L-Galactono-γ lactone dehydrogenase	1.3.2.3	L-galactono-γ lactone + 2 ferricytochrome c = L-ascorbate + 2 ferrocytochrome c	AA synthesis, localized to the inner mitochondrial membrane
γ-Glutamylcysteine synthetase	6.3.2.2	ATP + L-Glu + L-Cys = ADP + Pi + γ-L-Glu-L-Cys	GSH biosynthesis, localized in chloroplast and cytosol
GSH synthetase	6.3.2.3	ATP + γ-L-Glu-L-Cys = ADP + Pi + GSH	GSH biosynthesis, localized in chloroplast and cytosol
Xanthine oxidoreductase	1.1.3.22	Xanthine + H_2O + O_2 = urate + H_2O_2	

glutamate and cysteine, and glutathione synthetase (GSH-S)-catalyzed addition of glycine. Both genes (*gsh1* for γ-ECS and *gsh2* for GSH-S) have been cloned from *Arabidopsis* by complementation of *E. coli* mutants deficient in corresponding enzyme activities. The studies of Arabidopsis *gsh1* mutant and overexpression of γ-ECS and GSH-S in poplar and tobacco, have shown that regulation of GSH biosynthesis is achieved via feedback inhibition by GSH, cysteine availability and transcriptional/translational control of γ-ECS activity.[91] Heavy metals and jasmonic acid lead to increased *gsh1* and *gsh2* transcript abundance, however the additional redox signal (H_2O_2 or altered GSH/GSSH) is required for translation, providing an additional point for the regulation of GSH homeostasis.[95] GSH synthesis has been shown to occur in the chloroplast stroma and in the cytosol in both photosynthesizing and non-photosynthesizing tissues. Gradients in GSH distribution over different cellular compartments imply the existence of a coordinated intracellular transport system, necessary to maintain a compartment-specific redox milieu. The apoplast and the vacuole, compartments deprived of GSH synthesizing capacity, have to exchange GSH species with their intra- and extracellular environment. The proton gradient across plasmalemma drives H^+-glutathione symport into the cytoplasm, with a clear preference for GSSG and GS-conjugates over GSH. Such selectivity of transport makes sense under oxidative stress, when GSH is in great demand in the apoplast and GSSG has to be re-reduced in the cytosol. However, GSH transport into plant cells show different affinities, and, in some cases is distinct from GSSG transport. Cloning and characterization of high affinity glutathione transporter HGT1 from yeast has led to identification of nine *Arabidopsis Hgt 1* homologues[96,97] and a broad specificity rice GSH transporter.[98] Plant cells actively transport GSH across the chloroplast envelope by an unknown mechanism, showing saturation kinetics and inhibition by GSSG.[91] A multidrug-resistance-associated protein (MRP) localized on the tonoplast membrane transports GSSG and GS-R from the cytoplasm to the vacuole sustaining the detoxification of stress-related products (see Sec. 5.2) and cytotoxins. These findings are consistent with the existence of several glutathione transport systems on the plasma membrane and endomembranes of the plant cells. The reliance of GSH transport on trans-membrane potential, H^+ symport, ATP dependence and competitiveness between glutathione species present an opportunity for indirect tuning of GSH/GSSG redox ratio in different cellular compartments.

4.3. *Tocopherols*

Tocopherols (TP, vitamin E) and tocotrienols are the main chain-breaking antioxidants in biological membranes. The chemical structure of TP, i.e. the polar chroman head group and hydrophobic prenyl tail determine the amphipathic character of the molecule, its orientation in the membrane and mode of action on radical species. TPs are reported to be under certain conditions less effective as antioxidants than tocotrienols, the derivatives with an unsaturated hydrophobic tail.[99] Antioxidative activity among four TP isomers increases in the range: $\alpha > \beta > \gamma > \delta$, depending on the methylation pattern and on the number of methyl groups at the phenol ring of the chroman head group. Three methyl substituents of α-TP sustain the highest antioxidative activity of this isomer.[100] TP prevents the propagation of lipid peroxidation by direct interaction with lipid radicals, the alkoxy radicals (LO•), lipid peroxyl radicals (LOO•) and with alkyl radicals (L•), derived from the oxidation of polyunsaturated fatty acids:

$$\text{TP–OH} + \text{L–OO}^{\bullet} \rightarrow \text{L–OOH} + \text{TO}^{\bullet}$$

The reaction occurs in the lipid/water interphase and results in the formation of lipid hydroperoxides (L–OOH) and the tocopheroxyl radical ($TO^{\bullet}$) which can be re-reduced by AA, GSH[74] or coenzyme Q.[101] In addition, TPs react directly with $OH^{\bullet}$, quench triplet state of chlorophylls in thylakoid membranes, chemically scavenge $O_2^{-\bullet}$ by irreversible oxidation of TP and can also act as physical deactivators of $O_2^{-\bullet}$ by a charge transfer mechanism.[80,99] The estimated ratio of TP to polyunsaturated fatty acid is 1:1000,[65] but TPs are not evenly distributed in cell membranes. TPs accumulated in the fluid membrane domains with the highest content of unsaturated fatty acids. There are two proposed mechanisms which compensate the low TP concentration in cell membranes. First, the accumulation of TPs into the most fluid membrane domains supports PUFA protection against lipid peroxidation. Secondly, TPs move rapidly in the lateral plane of the lipid bilayer, hence providing protection to the parts of the membranes under oxidative pressure.[102]

TP is synthesized only by plants, photosythetic bacteria and some oxygenic cyanobacteria. Other organisms rely on the dietary intake of this essential vitamin. Biosynthetic route of TP is characterized and the enzymes of TP biosyntesis are localized to the inner chloroplast envelope (for details on TP biosynthesis see Munne-Bosch and Alegre,[99] Hofius and Sonnewald[103] and Ajjawi and Shintani[104]). A number of attempts have been made to manipulate TP biosynthesis in order to increase its content, and particularly α-TP, in plant organs. A gene coding for γ-tocopherol methyltransferase (an enzyme catalyzing the final methylation step in the biosynthesis of TP species) has been isolated from the cyanobacteria *Synechocystis* and a ninefold increase in vitamin E activity and improved ratio of α- to γ-TP in *Arabidopsis* seeds has been achieved by overexpression of the *Arabidopsis* orthologue.[105] Seed-specific overexpression of the upstream enzyme homogentisate prenyltransferase has resulted in a twofold increase in the TP pool in *Arabidopsis*.[106] The vitamin E-deficient *vte1* mutant isolated from *Arabidopsis* by Porfirova *et al.*[107] lacks four TP species and tocopherol cyclase activity. Interestingly, this mutant showed no altered phenotype but is identical to *sxd1* (sucrose export defective 1) mutant of maize and *Synechocystis* with disturbed plasmodesmatal function. Deterioration of cellular functions which are not directly related to oxidative stress by TP deficiency suggests that in plant cells TP executes also other than antioxidative functions.

Such non-antioxidant functions of TP are relatively well characterized in animal cells and briefly include: modulation of membrane fluidity and permeability, complexation of free fatty acids and lysophospholipids, and inhibition of protein kinase C. The last results in an incorrect assembly of NADPH oxidase complex with a consequent decrease in $O_2^{-\bullet}$ production. Non-antioxidant effects are specific to α-TP but not β-TP.[108] In plant cells α-TP has been suggested to affect signalling via regulation of ROS levels and via the control of secondary oxidation product formation such as jasmonic acid.[99]

4.4. *Thioredoxins*

Thioredoxins (Trx) are ubiquitous small proteins which are found in all organisms from prokaryotes to higher eukaryotes, and they control the cellular redox state. Thioredoxins and their action in plants has been reviewed recently by Schürman and Jacquot.[109] Trxs can be divided into two families according to their amino acid sequence: Family I proteins contain only one Trx domain while family two proteins contain one or more Trx domains and additional protein domains. The Trx family I is prevalent in plants with at least 20 genes found in *Arabidopsis thaliana* while in mammals only two genes are known.[110] In higher plants the Trxs are divided into six groups: Trxs *f, m, o, x* and *y*. Of these *f*, *h* and *o* are specific to eukaryotes. Trxs *f*, *m*, *x* and *y* are found in the chloroplasts while *o* is present in mitochondria.[111] Trx *h* is encoded by a multigene family in higher plants with at least three different subgroups of variable primary structures and cellular localization.[111]

The main function of Trxs is to control the reduction status of disulphur bridges in proteins. The catalytic activity of many proteins depends on the presence of free –SH-groups or disulphide bridges, e.g. the plant mitochondrial alternative oxidase activity is controlled in this way.[112] In the chloroplasts Trxs are in turn reduced by the ferredoxin-thioredoxin system catalyzed by ferredoxin-thioredoxin reductase (FTR), which is important in the regulation of the photosynthetic Calvin cycle.[113]

The mitochondrial Trx *o*, and an associated flavoenzyme, NADP/Trx reductase, provide a link to NADPH in this organelle. Unlike animal and yeast counterparts, the function of Trx in plant mitochondria is largely unknown. Balmer[114] has recently applied proteomic approaches to identify soluble Trx-linked proteins in plant mitochondria isolated from photosynthetic and heterotrophic sources, and identified 50 potential Trx-linked proteins functional in various aspects of plant metabolism: photorespiration, citric acid cycle and associated reactions, lipid metabolism, electron transport, ATP synthesis/transformation, membrane transport, translation, protein assembly/folding, nitrogen metabolism, sulphur metabolism, hormone synthesis, and stress-related reactions. The results are in favor of the view that Trx acts as a sensor and enables mitochondria to adjust key reactions in accord with the prevailing redox state. These and earlier findings further suggest that, by sensing redox in chloroplasts and mitochondria, Trx enables the two organelles of photosynthetic tissues to communicate by means of a network of transportable metabolites such as dihydroxyacetone phosphate, malate, and glycolate.[114]

4.5. *Carotenoids*

Many carotenoids can act as antioxidants even though their main function in plants is to gather light energy in the photosynthetic apparatus. A large array of different carotenoids such as lycopene, lutein, zeaxanthin, and beta-carotene are known.[115] Plants deficient in carotenoid biosynthesis at phytoene desaturation step show a variegated phenotype due to chlorophyll bleaching under high light (ROS inducing conditions). Cloning of the gene responsible for this phenotype in *Arabidopsis* Immutans (*Im*) has revealed that the corresponding protein is involved in phytoene desaturation and shares homology with plant mitochondrial alternative oxidase (see below). Presumably *Im* protein acts as plastoquinol oxidase, transferring electrons from phytoene desaturation reaction to molecular oxygen.[116]

4.6. *Phenolic compounds as antioxidants*

Plants produce a wide array of secondary metabolites with the phenol-group which are characteristically called plant phenolics. These compounds are chemically variable and in the plant kingdom c. 10,000 of these are known. They vary in their properties and functions: some are water-soluble and others form crystals only dissolved in organic solvents while some polymerize into large insoluble polymers such as the lignin polymer prevalent in wood. Plant phenolics are end products of two metabolic pathways: the shikimic acid pathway and the malonic acid pathway, and they can roughly be divided into the following groups: hydrolysable tannins, simple phenolics and their polymers, flavonoids and condensed tannins and miscellaneous phenolics.[117] Polyphenols possess ideal structural chemistry for free radical scavenging activity, and they have been shown to be more effective antioxidants *in vitro* than tocopherols and ascorbate. Antioxidative properties of polyphenols arise from their high reactivity as hydrogen or electron donors, and from the ability of the polyphenol-derived radical to stabilize and delocalize the unpaired electron (chain-breaking function), and from their ability to chelate transition metal ions (termination of the Fenton reaction).[118] Plant phenols may exert their protective effects by scavenging superoxide, and especially phenolics with pyrogallol or catechol moieties have been revealed as the most rapid superoxide scavengers.[119]

Another mechanism underlying the antioxidative properties of phenolics is the ability of flavonoids to alter peroxidation kinetics by modification of the lipid packing order and to decrease fluidity of the membranes.[120] These changes could sterically hinder diffusion of free radicals and restrict peroxidative reactions. Moreover, it has been shown recently that phenolic compounds can be involved in the hydrogen peroxide scavenging cascade in plant cells.[121] During the last decade an image on the significance of plant derived phenolics in dietary antioxidants in mammals has begun to emerge.[122–124] Naturally, many phenolics protect plant tissues from oxidative damage and this seems to be very important under stress conditions and in defense against micro-organisms and herbivores.[125] According to our unpublished results the content of condensed tannins (flavonols) as measured by HPLC, was 100 times higher in oxygen stressed Yellow flag iris (*Iris pseudacorus*) rhizomes in comparison with that of the garden Iris (*I. germanica*), a results which suggests flavonol participation in the antioxidative defense of tissues.

4.7. *Enzymes of ROS-detoxification and antioxidant turnover*

4.7.1. *Superoxide dismutase*

The scavenging of $O_2^{\bullet -}$ is achieved with superoxide dismutase (SOD, EC 1.15.1.1) which catalyzes the dismutation of superoxide to H_2O_2. This reaction has a 10,000-fold faster rate than spontaneous dismutation.[3] The enzyme is present in all aerobic organisms and in all subcellular compartments susceptible of oxidative stress.[3] A new type of SOD with Ni in the active center, structurally different from already known SOD types, has been described in Streptomyces.[126] The other three types of this enzyme, classified by their metal cofactor, can be found in all living organisms, and they are the structurally similar FeSOD (prokaryotic organisms, chloroplast stroma) and MnSOD (prokaryotic organisms and the mitochondrion of eukaryotes); and the structurally unrelated Cu/ZnSOD (cytosolic and chloroplast enzyme, gram-negative bacteria). These isoenzymes differ in their sensitivity to H_2O_2 and KCN.[127] All three enzymes are nuclear encoded, and SOD genes have been shown to be sensitive to environmental stresses, presumably as a consequence of increased ROS formation.[128,129] For example an increase in total SOD activity has been detected in wheat roots under anoxia but not under hypoxia.[130] However, biochemical studies on SOD activity under diverse abiotic stresses do not always show elevation of SOD activity in concert with oxidative stress.[34] The reasons can lie in diversification of ROS-forming pathways, compartmentalization of ROS and/or antioxidants. The formation of a strong pro-oxidant, which is neither $O_2^{\bullet -}$, nor H_2O_2 has been suggested to explain SOD activity pattern under water deficit.[131] Besides, some unknown factors can regulate the availability of substrate for SOD. Experiments on overexpression of different SODs targeted to chloroplast, mitochondria and cytosol to improve oxidative stress tolerance have lead to contradictory results.[129] In general, successful protection has been achieved when SOD overexpression is reinforced by other AO enzymes, e.g. when increased SOD activity and ROS-inducing treatment were co-localized in the same compartment (e.g. chloroplastic SOD and ROS induction by high light or methyl viologen).

4.7.2. *Catalase*

The intracellular level of H_2O_2 is regulated by a wide range of enzymes, the most important being catalase (EC 1.11.1.6)[132] and peroxidases. Catalases in plants are presented by multiple isoforms and are generally found in peroxysomes, glyoxysomes and one isoform in maize mitochondria.[133] There are three main isoform classes: CAT1, a light-dependent type, highly expressed in photosynthesizing tissues and representing 80% of catalase activity in leaves. It removes H_2O_2 derived from photorespiration. CAT2 is expressed in vascular tissues and is possibly connected with lignification. CAT3 is a seed-specific isoform which utilizes H_2O_2 originated from fatty acid oxidation during seed germination.[33,132] Catalase functions through an intermediate catalase-H_2O_2 complex (Compound I) and produces water and dioxygen (catalase action) or can decay to an inactive Compound II. In the presence of an appropriate substrate Compound I drives the peroxidatic reaction. Compound I is a much more effective oxidant than H_2O_2 itself, thus the reaction of Compound I with another H_2O_2 molecule (catalase action) represents a one-electron transfer, which splits peroxide and produces another strong oxidant, the hydroxyl radical ($OH^{\bullet}$).[1] $OH^{\bullet}$ is a very strong oxidant and can initiate radical chain reactions with organic molecules, particularly with PUFA in membrane lipids.

Catalases do not require the supply of reducing equivalents for functioning, hence they can be insensitive to the changes in the redox status of the cell under stress conditions.[35] Indeed, only catalase transcripts out of 495 transcripts with altered abundance were not affected by changes in AA redox state in *vtc1 Arabidopsis* mutant[134] and in knockout-APX plants.[135]

Catalase-deficient *Nicotiana tabacum* plants engineered by sense and antisense technology have been used to unravel the role of antioxidant systems under photooxidative stress. Transgenic plants showed no altered phenotype under low light conditions, but developed necrotic lesions when exposed to high light. Catalase deficiency was compensated by the addition of exogenous catalase and increased APX and GR activities. Altered redox state of ascorbate and glutathione pools suggests that catalase and APX systems of H_2O_2 removal are not mutually replaceable and that catalase function supports high redox state of AA-GSH system.[136] Recognition of H_2O_2 as a universal signal under diverse stress situations makes catalase deficient plants an essential tool in oxidative stress studies.[137]

4.7.3. *Peroxidases*

Common plant peroxidases (EC 1.11.1.7) are divided into three classes: Class I which are of procaryotic origins, Class II of typical fungal peroxidases, and Class III which are secretable plant peroxidases. It is generally accepted that plant peroxidases are present in the Golgi apparatus, in peroxisomes, in the endoplasmic reticulum and in vacuoles, while the more substrate specific peroxidases are found in the chloroplast and mitochondria.

Ascorbate peroxidase (APX, EC 1.11.1.11) acts in the chloroplast thylakoid membranes and protects them against hydrogen peroxide using ascorbate to form monodehydroascorbate, which in turn is spontaneously reconverted to ascorbate by reduced ferredoxin in photosystem I. This conversion can also be executed by NAD(P)H monodehydroascorbate reductase present in the chloroplast stroma and cytosol. Multiple isoforms of APX (stromal, thylakoid membrane-bound, microbody membrane-bound, mitochondrial and cytosolic) are characterized by high specificity to AA.[138] The expression of cytosolic *APX 2* in *Arabidopsis* bundle sheath cells has been shown to be regulated by a pleiotropic action of H_2O_2 and ABA. Indeed, under stimulating conditions in ABA-insensitive mutants *APX 2* expression is reduced.[139] *Arabidopsis* knockout plants deficient in cytosolic APX 1 are characterized by high level of H_2O_2, altered growth, flowering and stomatal responses. Under oxidative stress the expression of *APX 1* requires the zinc finger protein Zat12, which exhibits stress-specific expression.[140] Isolation and characterization of *Arabidopsis* mutant deficient in *apx1* gene has revealed normal growth of the mutant and compensation by other antioxidant systems.[141]

Peroxiredoxins (Prx) form a ubiquitous group of peroxidases found in bacteria, yeast, animals and higher plants.[142–144] Prxs are abundant low-efficiency peroxidases located in distinct cell compartments including the chloroplast and mitochondrion. The catalytic center contains a cysteinyl residue that reduces diverse peroxides and is regenerated via intramolecular or intermolecular thiol-disulfide-reactions and finally by electron donors such as thioredoxins and glutaredoxins. Prxs are regulated by endogenous and environmental stimuli at the transcript and protein levels. In addition to their role in antioxidant defense in photosynthesis, respiration, and stress response, they may also be involved in modulating redox signaling during development and adaptation.[143] Antisense suppression of 2-cys peroxiredoxin in *Arabidopsis* chloroplasts caused a decrease in AA redox state and concomitant elevation in the activity and transcript levels of the enzymes involved in AA turnover: stroma and thylakoid APX, and monodehydroascorbate reductase, but not in the enzymes of GSH metabolism. These findings indicate that 2-cys peroxiredoxins are the integral part of chloroplast defense machinery and interact directly with antioxidant systems via the ascorbate pool.[145]

4.7.4. *Glutathione peroxidase*

Glutathione peroxidases (GPX) are not haem-containing proteins as are other plant peroxidases. At the active site plant GPX contains cysteine instead of selenocysteine as is the case in the animal protein. This substitution reduces nucleophilic interactions of the enzyme and results in lower activity towards H_2O_2.[146] Putative plant GPX proteins, when expressed in *E. coli*, showed both PHGPX activity and thioredoxin peroxidase activity but not H_2O_2-reducing activity.[147] These results suggest different enzymatic properties for the plant protein and mammalian GPX and a connection between GSH and thioredoxin antioxidant systems in plants. Several plant GPX cDNAs have been isolated from a number of species. Recently, seven genes of GPX family have been identified in *Arabidopsis* (AtGPX1-AtGPX7). It has been shown that the corresponding proteins are putatively localized to cytosol, chloroplast, mitochondria and endoplasmic reticulum. Under abiotic stress these genes are differentially expressed and regulated by multiple signaling pathways as judged by plant hormone treatment. Upstream region of AtGPX genes contains conserved motifs with similarity to antioxidant-responsive elements.[148]

Phospholipid-hydroperoxide glutathione peroxidase (PHGPX, EC 1.11.1.12) belongs to the glutathione peroxidase family and functions to remove hydroperoxides of unsaturated fatty acids at the expense of GSH (Table 2). The PHGPX is stress-inducible and protects membranes from excessive lipid peroxidation under oxidative stress. In plant tissues PHGPX is localized to the cytosol, chloroplast stroma and putatively to mitochondria. Transgenic tobacco plants expressing glutathione peroxidase-like protein in the cytosol and chloroplasts, have shown suppressed lipid peroxidation and enhanced tolerance to oxidative stress caused by a number of treatments.[149] The PHGPX protein and its encoding gene *csa* have been isolated and characterized in citrus. It has been shown that *csa* is directly induced by the substrate of PHGPX under heat, cold and salt stresses, and that this induction occurs mainly via the production of ROS.[150] A cDNA homologous to PHGPX has been isolated from tobacco, maize, soybean, pea and *Arabidopsis*.[151,152] Accumulating evidence suggests that in plant cells PHGPX is a ubiquitous enzyme maintaining the membrane structure and function via regeneration of phospholipid hydroperoxides, and that it can act synergetically with tocopherol.

4.7.5. *Glutathione-S-transferase*

Glutathione-S-transferase (GST, 2.5.1.18, Table 2) catalyzes the conjugation of GSH to cytotoxic compounds arising from oxidative stress, to plant secondary metabolites (e.g. anthocyanins) and mediates the detoxification of herbicides and heavy metals in concert with ATP-dependent ABC transporters[93,153] (see Sec. 5.2).

4.7.6. *Glutathione reductase*

Glutathione reductase (GR) is a flavoprotein oxidoreductase catalyzing the regeneration of GSSG to the reduced form GSH using NADPH for reducing power. The importance of the maintenance of the GSH pool in reduced state cannot be overestimated due to the numerous functions of GSH in cellular metabolism (see Sec. 4.2). It is a component of the AA-GSH cycle and plays an important role in the regulation of AA redox state. Manipulation of GR and glutathione synthetase has pointed out the importance of GSH cycling rather than the size of the GSH pool.[90] GR-overexpressing poplar has been found more resistant to oxidative stress when GR is targeted to the chloroplast (with accompanying increase in foliar GSH and AA levels).[154] A recent study on tobacco plants expressing *E. coli* GR demonstrated increased lipid peroxidation, but the plants were more resistant to paraquat and H_2O_2. Altering of the AO system by GR overexpression was reflected in significant reduction of transcript levels for violaxanthin deepoxidase and cytosolic CuZn-SOD.[155]

4.7.7. *Dehydroascorbate reductase*

During oxidative stress AA is oxidized to MDHA, an unstable radical compound which quickly disproportionates to AA and DHA. Dehydroascorbate reductase (DHAR) carries out the reduction of DHA to AA at the expense of GSH. The enzyme is vital for protection against oxidative stress and elevation of DHAR activity has been documented under diverse stresses.[156] Several other enzymes are reported to have DHAR activity: glutaredoxin, protein disulphide isomerase[157] and Kunitz-type trypsin inhibitor.[158] Chloroplast DHAR has been purified and a corresponding gene cloned from spinach[159] and rice.[160] The metabolic model on chloroplast AO fluxes predicts that DHAR activity is insignificant in DHA reduction and the flux via slow chemical reduction of DHA by GSH is enough to maintain AA at the reduced state.[161] However, transgenic tobacco and maize overexpressing wheat DHAR have showed increases in both AA level and ascorbate redox state in both plants.[162] The crucial role of DHAR in AA cycling has been confirmed in plants overexpressing DHAR with associated increases in AA redox state and decline in H_2O_2 in guard cells.[163] Interestingly, transgenic plants were less responsive to H_2O_2 and abscisic acid signaling and demonstrated decreased drought tolerance. This finding is an extra evidence of the regulatory role of AA redox state.

4.7.8. *Ascorbate oxidase*

Ascorbate oxidase (AO, EC 1.10.3.3.) is an apoplastic enzyme which converts AA to MDHA which readily disproportionates to DHA and AA. Although its biological functions are far from clear, it seems to play a role in cell elongation and regulation of AA cycling in the apoplast.[73,164] In sense and antisense transformed tobacco plants very little change in whole leaf AA levels took place, while apoplastic AA levels were much reduced in AO enhanced plants while the contrary happened when AO activity was reduced.[164] It has been concluded that there is an interaction between hormone, redox and light signals in the apoplast and this is connected with apopalstic AA levels.[164]

5. Antioxidant Network in Defence Against Oxidative Stress in Various Cellular Compartments

5.1. *Apoplast and plasma membrane*

Apoplast is the "inter protoplast compartment" of plant cells which exerts vital transport and metabolic functions and encompasses all compartments outside the plasma membrane including the plant cell wall and intercellular spaces. The apoplast acts as a sensor for environmental challenges, transfers information to the protoplast and sustains defense reactions initiated within the cell. Easily perturbed apoplast homeostasis provides mechanisms of stress perception on the cellular level: changes in ion concentrations, pH fluctuation and associated ROS production.[73] Apoplast–based redox signaling represents a complex network of plasma membrane receptors (elicitor recognition in pathogen attack), transport mechanisms for redox-active compounds (AA, DHA), enzymatic sources of ROS (NADPH oxidase, peroxidases), and such physiological factors as pH. The latter has been shown to regulate the activity of peroxidases (alkalinization favors peroxidase-dependent oxidative burst)[165] and facilitation of nonenzymatic production of NO due to acidification.[27]

Apoplastic ROS elevation under stress is tightly controlled by enzymatic systems in the apoplast and plasma membrane and serves for both defense and signaling. Pathogen invasion accompanied by oxidative burst is the most studied example of this concerted action, where the main player is plasma membrane NADPH oxidase.[5] The plant enzyme is homologous to *gp91*^{phox} subunit of mammalian respiratory burst oxidase, a transmembrane protein, responsible for e^- transfer from NADPH to O_2 resulting in extracellular $O_2^{-\bullet}$ formation. The fine tuning of ROS production is allowed by the several points of regulation of the enzyme such as direct stimulation by Ca^{2+}, control by small GTP-binding protein Rac,[166] and responsiveness to plant hormones salicylic acid and abscisic acid.[167]

Ascorbate oxidase (AO; Table 2) is the main apoplastic enzyme of AA cycling and a control point of redox regulation. Ascorbate peroxidase (APX, Table 2) is the major H_2O_2 eliminator in the apoplast. The enzyme uses AA as an e^- donor, however the recycling of the resulting DHA, an oxidized form of AA, via AA-GSH cycle is restricted due to absence (or very low content) of GSH and lack of NAD(P)H in the apoplast. The reduction cycle operates via transport and recycling of AA via PM transporters and e^- flow across plasmalemma (see Sec. 4.1 and Fig. 2).

5.2. *Endoplasmic reticulum and vacuole*

It has become increasingly evident that the plant vacuole plays an important role in cellular redox homeostasis. Redox coupling between cytoplasm and vacuole has been suggested: H_2O_2 diffused to vacuole is reduced by peroxidases which use phenolic compounds as primary e^- donors. The resulting phenoxyl radicals can be reduced by both AA and monodehydroascorbate radicals. Regeneration of AA in the cytoplasm completes the peroxidase-phenolics-AA cycle.[82] Presence of AA-reducible b-type cytochrome in tonoplast membrane revealed by expression in yeast of putative *Arabidopsis* cytochrome b561 gene (CYBASC1), provides evidence of a transmembrane redox system in the tonoplast. Such a system indicates coupling between cytoplasm and vacuole via the AA redox system.[168]

Another important role for vacuole under stress conditions is sequesterization of stress-related metabolites conjugated to GSH. The reaction is catalyzed by glutathione-S-transferase (Table 2 and Sec. 4.6). Products of lipid peroxidation such as membrane lipid hydroperoxides (e.g. 4-hydroxyalkenals), epoxides, organic hydroperoxides[169] and oxidative products of DNA degradation (base propanols) are the substrates for GST; they can be conjugated to GSH and detoxified.[93,170] The uptake of GSSG and GS-R (a product of glutathione-S-transferase) across tonoplast membrane is mediated by multidrug-resistance-associated protein (MRP, an ABC transporter).[171,172] Conjugation to GSH serves as a specific "tag" for recognition, transport and sequestration of endogenous and stress-specific metabolites.[97]

Another possible source of ROS in cytoplasm, ER and possibly chloroplasts is cytochrome P450 system (CYP). It plays a major role in catabolic, detoxification and phenylpropanoid biosynthetic reactions in plants (in plants most of mono-oxygenase reactions are accomplished by NADPH:cytochrome P450 oxidoreductase. EC 1.6.2.4). Generally CYPs catalyze the reaction:

$$\mathrm{RH} + 2\mathrm{NADPH} + \mathrm{O_2} = \mathrm{ROH} + 2\mathrm{NAD^+} + \mathrm{H_2O}$$

The catalytic mechanism involves reductive activation of O_2 and hence leads to the formation of the superoxide radical.[173]

5.3. *Peroxisomes*

Peroxisomes are morphologically simple, single membrane-bound organelles with predominantly oxidative type of metabolism. In plant cells they accomplish several functions: photorespiration, glyoxylate cycle and fatty acid β-oxidation. Many ROS-processing and antioxidant turnover enzymes have been localized to peroxisomes: Mn-SOD, CuZn-SOD, xanthine oxidoreductase, glutathione reductase, dehydroascorbate reductase, monodehydroascorbate reductase, ascorbate peroxidase and catalase[174] along with the low molecular mass antioxidants ascorbate and glutathione. Two distinct sites are responsible for $O_2^{-\bullet}$ formation in peroxisomes: xanthine oxidoreductase in the matrix and a NAD(P)H-dependent integral membrane system. Recently, the production of yet another signaling molecule — NO has been localized to peroxisomes.[174,175] Simple morphology of the organelle which handles metabolite fluxes from the chloroplast and mitochondria and accomplishes ROS-detoxifying functions requires microcompartmentalization — a peroxisomal matrix. Organization of enzymes into multienzyme complexes provides the possibility for substrate channeling:

transfer of metabolites from one enzyme to another in sequential steps without release into the bulk phase.[176,177] Such microcompartmentalization provides additional protection against oxidative damage by H_2O_2 — an abundant peroxisomal metabolite.

Interestingly, *PEX* genes responsible for peroxisome biogenesis and import of peroxisomal proteins, are induced by elevated H_2O_2 levels, suggesting one more possibility for the regulation of cellular redox balance.[178]

On the basis of a differential response to senescence of the mitochondrial and peroxisomal ascorbate-glutathione cycle, it has been suggested that mitochondria may senesce earlier that peroxisomes, which may participate in the cellular oxidative mechanism of leaf senescence longer than mitochondria.[179] There is also an emerging idea of mitochondria-peroxisome interaction in respect to ROS/NO signaling.[175,180]

5.4. *Mitochondria*

Mitochondria have long been recognized as a site of ROS production. They are able to produce ROS (superoxide anion O^{2-} and the succeeding H_2O_2) due to electron leakage at the ubiquinone site — ubiquinone: cytochrome b region[181] — and at the matrix side of complex I (NADH dehydrogenase).[182,183] Hydrogen peroxide generation by higher plant mitochondria and its regulation by uncoupling of electron transport chain and oxidative phosphorylation have been demonstrated.[184] The alternative oxidase (AOX) present in plant mitochondria catalyzes four-electron reduction of O_2 by ubiquinone and, hence, competes for the electrons with the main respiratory chain. Control of H_2O_2 formation in mitochondrial ETC is one of the functions suggested for AOX. Antisense suppression of AOX in tobacco has resulted in ROS accumulation, while overexpression lead to decreased ROS levels.[185] In the same study coordinated changes have been observed in antioxidative enzymes: lower expression of SodA, SodB and glutathione peroxidase genes were detected.

An antioxidant role has recently been suggested for mitochondrial uncoupling protein (UCP) which transports fatty acid anions from the inner to the outer leaflet of the membrane. Fatty acids become protonated in the intermembrane space and by a flip-flop mechanism transport H^+ to the matrix providing an uncoupling effect. First, uncoupling itself lowers mitochondrial ROS production; and second, it is hypothesized that UCP is able to electrophoretically transport fatty acid hydroperoxides from mitochondrial matrix to the intermembrane space.[186] Such extrusion preserves mtDNA and matrix proteins from contact with intermediates of lipid peroxidation. Indeed, overexpression of *Arabidopsis* uncoupling protein encoded by AtUCP1 leads to increased oxidative stress tolerance in tobacco.[187]

Oxidative stress elicits a significant effect on mitochondrial proteome. Treatment of *Arabidopsis* cell culture with H_2O_2 or antimycin A resulted in degradation of key mitochondrial proteins: ATP synthase subunits, complex I, succinyl CoA ligase, aconitase, and lead to decreased abundance of TCA cycle proteins, two subunits of complex I, β-subunit of ATP synthase, Fe-SOD and an array of other metabolically competent proteins.[188] At the same time two out of nine proteins induced by H_2O_2 appeared to be novel putative mitochondrial antioxidants. At3g06050 homologous to bacterial peroxiredoxins is suggested to participate in the reduction of H_2O_2 to water via mitochondrial Trx system and the second one, At5g60640 belongs to a protein disulphide isomerase family. These proteins can be responsible for the removal of anomalous disulphides brought about by oxidative stress and for the reduction of disulphide bridges in proteins to restore their activity (e.g. the AOX, which is inactive upon disulphide bridge formation).[189] Inner membrane of plant mitochondria is the site of AA biosynthesis (see Sec. 4.1) and, most importantly, mitochondria have been shown to accommodate the enzymes of AA-GSH cycle, a powerfull cascade for efficient H_2O_2 removal.[190]

5.5. *Chloroplasts*

Due to the very nature of plant chloroplasts as photosynthesizing and water splitting organelles, ROS are produced and this production increases in stress situations such as cold, high light and drought.[139,148] This is why the chloroplast is heavily protected against oxidative damage. Apart from ascorbate and glutathione, the most important small molecular antioxidants in the chloroplasts, also some of the light absorbing pigments, the carotenoids, can act as antioxidants. In addition, large amounts of α-tocopherol, the very powerful lipid-soluble antioxidant, are synthesized on the inner chloroplasts envelope membranes.[191,192] Some antioxidants of phenolic origin such as chlorogenic acid are also present in the chloroplasts.[193,194] Chloroplasts have a high antioxidative capacity and even in severe oxidative stress accumulation of superoxide or hydrogen peroxide to levels above those of healthy tissues hardly occurs. This has been tested with metabolic modeling of the superoxide dismutase–ascorbate peroxidase–glutathione pathway in chloroplasts.[161] This does not mean though, that ROS-levels would not have to be constantly sensed and regulated.[133] In the chloroplasts a specific Mehler-peroxidase reaction sequence takes place: APX and stromal/thylakoid SOD eliminate $O_2^{-\bullet}$ and H_2O_2 produced in photosynthesis. MDHA, the product of AA oxidation by APX can be reduced directly by ferredoxin. Additionally AA can be regenerated in the chloroplast by the enzymes of AA-GSH cycle (see Sec. 4.1 and Fig. 1), providing a second regulatory system of AA redox state.[69,133,195] Thioredoxin also plays an important role in plant chloroplasts (see Sec. 4.4).[196]

6. Concluding Remarks

Recent developments made possible by mutagenesis and transformation techniques have extended our knowledge on the mechanisms of control and regulation of the antioxidant networks beyond the limitations of biochemical and cell biological studies. New techniques have shown us how the intricate antioxidant network is coordinated in its fine detail and synchronized with metabolic ROS-producing events, which especially in photosynthesizing tissues is of vital importance.

Several spatial factors affect the antioxidant (AO) system efficiency under normal and oxidative stress conditions. Stress-specific localized ROS production imposes an oxidative load on a particular cellular compartment as it occurs e.g. under high light conditions in the chloroplast or in the apoplast during plant-pathogen interactions. The degree of antioxidant protection will be determined by AO gradients existing in cellular compartments. The latter are under control of multiple factors: ROS-induced local depletion of antioxidants; restrictions imposed by AO transport and non-enzymatic chemical interactions; inhibition or metabolic control of AO synthesis (e.g. feedback regulation of GSH biosynthesis); differences in the expression or post-translational control of AO-related enzymes (e.g. γ-ECS in GSH biosynthesis). Under a developing stress situation direct interactions (e.g. AA and TP) and coupling (e.g. AA-GSH) between different AO systems become extremely important in terms of coping with ROS and, perhaps, for amplification and transduction of redox signals.[194] Moreover, local changes in AO levels and shift in their redox state can affect non-antioxidant signaling functions exerted by AO. Such functions have been described at least for the main cellular antioxidants: AA, GSH and TP. To make things more complicated AO-induced changes in gene expression, signal transduction, and the cell cycle can interfere with ROS-mediated signaling. Development of any stress reaction occurs in a certain timescale ranging, in case of oxidative stress, from several microseconds (half-life of singlet oxygen and superoxide anion) and milliseconds (half-life of H_2O_2) to minutes required for protein synthesis. Superimposition of spatial and temporal patterns of ROS and AO, interference with ROS signaling, multiplicity of AO functions and intrinsic redox sensitivity of cell metabolism create a complicated network, where redox balance is a key factor determining the cell fate: cell death or acclimatory responses.

Due to the wealth and variability of the plant kingdom, there is large diversity in the small molecular antioxidants of plants and especially in the phenolics. This naturally gives a great opportunity for animals to utilize this wealth and at the same time avoid the expense of actually synthesizing these antioxidants themselves. Plant-derived antioxidative compounds have been and will be still of great importance in human nutrition, medication and well-being.

References

1. Elstner EF. Metabolism of activated oxygen species. In: Davies DD (ed.) *Biochemistry of Plants*. Academic Press, London, 1987, Vol. 11, pp. 253–315.
2. Bolwell GP, Wojtaszek P. Mechanisms for the generation of reactive oxygen species in plant defence — a broad perspective. *Physiol. Mol. Plant Pathol.* 51: 347–366 (1997).
3. Bowler C, van Montagu M, Inze D. Superoxide dismutase and stress tolerance. *Annu. Rev. Plant Physiol. Plant Mol. Biol.* 43: 83–116 (1992).
4. Henzler T, Steudle E. Transport and metabolic degradation of hydrogen peroxide in *Chara corallina*: model calculations and measurements with the

pressure probe suggest transport of H_2O_2 across water channels. *J. Exp. Bot.* 51: 2053–2066 (2000).
5. Bolwell GP *et al.* The apoplastic oxidative burst in response to biotic stress in plants: a three-component system. *J. Exp. Bot.* 53: 1367–1376 (2002).
6. Wink DA, Mitchell JB. Chemical biology of nitric oxide: insights into regulatory, cytotoxic, and cytoprotective mechanisms of nitric oxide. *Free Radic. Biol. Med.* 25: 434–456 (1998).
7. Lamattina L, Garcia-Mata C, Graziano M, Pagnussat G. Nitric oxide: the versatility of an extensive signal molecule. *Annu. Rev. Plant Biol.* 54: 109–136 (2003).
8. Neill SJ, Desikan R, Hancock JT. Nitric oxide signalling in plants. *New Phytol.* 159: 11–35 (2003).
9. Wojtaszek P. Nitric oxide in plants. To NO or not to NO. *Phytochemistry* 54: 1–4 (2000).
10. Wendehenne D, Lamotte O, Pugin A. Plant iNOS: conquest of the Holy Grail. *Trends Plant Sci.* 8: 465–468 (2003).
11. Alderton WK, Cooper CE, Knowles RG. Nitric oxide synthases: structure, function and inhibition. *Biochem. J.* 357: 593–615 (2001).
12. Lacza Z *et al.* Mitochondrial nitric oxide synthase is not eNOS, nNOS or iNOS. *Free Radic. Biol. Med.* 35: 1217–1228 (2003).
13. Elfering SL, Sarkela TM, Giulivi C. Biochemistry of mitochondrial nitric-oxide synthase. *J. Biol. Chem.* 277: 38079–38086 (2002).
14. Butt YK, Lum JH, Lo SC. Proteomic identification of plant proteins probed by mammalian nitric oxide synthase antibodies. *Planta* 216: 762–771 (2003).
15. Arabidopsis Genome Initiative. Analysis of the genome sequence of the flowering plant *Arabidopsis thaliana*. *Nature* 408: 796–815 (2000).
16. Guo F, Okamoto M, Crawford NM. Identification of a plant nitric oxide synthase gene involved in hormonal signaling. *Science* 302: 100–103 (2003).
17. Godber BL *et al.* Reduction of nitrite to nitric oxide catalyzed by xanthine oxidoreductase. *J. Biol. Chem.* 275: 7757–7763 (2000).
18. Meyer K, Lea US, Provan F, Kaiser WM, Lillo C. Is nitrate reductase a major player in the plant NO (nitric oxide) game? *Photosynth. Res.* 83: 181–189 (2005).
19. Lillo C, Meyer C, Lea US, Provan F, Oltedal S. Mechanism and importance of post-translational regulation of nitrate reductase. *J. Exp. Bot.* 55: 1275–1282 (2004).
20. Yamasaki H, Sakihama Y. Simultaneous production of nitric oxide and peroxynitrite by plant nitrate reductase: *in vitro* evidence for the NR-dependent formation of active nitrogen species. *FEBS Lett.* 468: 89–92 (2000).

21. Rockel P, Strube F, Rockel A, Wildt J, Kaiser WM. Regulation of nitric oxide (NO) production by plant nitrate reductase *in vivo* and *in vitro*. *J. Exp. Bot.* 53: 103–110 (2002).
22. Drew MC. Oxygen deficiency and root metabolism: injury and acclimation under hypoxia and anoxia. *Annu. Rev. Plant Physiol. Plant Mol. Biol.* 48: 223–250 (1997).
23. Dordas C, Rivoal J, Hill RD. Plant haemoglobins, nitric oxide and hypoxic stress. *Ann. Bot. (Lond.)* 91: 173–178 (2003).
24. Igamberdiev AU, Hill RD. Nitrate, NO and haemoglobin in plant adaptation to hypoxia: an alternative to classic fermentation pathways. *J. Exp. Bot.* 55: 2473–2482 (2004).
25. Stöhr C, Strube F, Marx G, Ullrich WR, Rockel P. A plasma membrane-bound enzyme of tobacco roots catalyses the formation of nitric oxide from nitritre. *Planta* 212: 835–841 (2001).
26. Lamotte O, Courtois C, Barnavon L, Pugin A, Wendehenne D. Nitric oxide in plants: the biosynthesis and cell signalling properties of a fascinating molecule. *Planta* 221: 1–4 (2005).
27. Bethke PC, Badger MR, Jones RL. Apoplastic synthesis of nitric oxide by plant tissues. *Plant Cell* 16: 332–341 (2004).
28. Cooney RV, Harwood PJ, Custer LJ, Franke AA. Light-mediated conversion of nitrogen dioxide to nitric oxide by carotenoids. *Environ. Health Perspect.* 102: 460–462 (1994).
29. Zweier JL, Samouilov A, Kuppusamy P. Non-enzymatic nitric oxide synthesis in biological systems. *Biochimica Et Biophysica Acta (BBA) — Bioenergetics* 1411: 250–262 (1999).
30. Sies H. Oxidative stress: oxidants and antioxidants. *Exp. Physiol.* 82: 291–295 (1997).
31. Foyer CH, Noctor G. Oxidant and antioxidant signalling in plants; a re-evaluation of the concept of oxidative stress in a physiological context. *Plant Cell Env.* 28: 1056–1071 (2005).
32. Grant JJ, Loake GJ. Role of reactive oxygen intermediates and cognate redox signaling in disease resistance. *Plant Physiol.* 124: 21–29 (2000).
33. Van Breusegem F, Vranova E, Dat JF, Inze D. The role of active oxygen species in plant signal transduction [Review]. *Plant Science* 161: 405–414 (2001).
34. Blokhina O, Virolainen E, Fagerstedt KV. Antioxidants, oxidative damage and oxygen deprivation stress: a review. *Ann. Bot. (Lond.)* 91: 179–194 (2002).

35. Mittler R. Oxidative stress, antioxidants and stress tolerance. *Trends Plant Sci.* 7: 405–410 (2002).
36. Vranova E, Inze D, Van Breusegem F. Signal transduction during oxidative stress. *J. Exp. Bot.* 53: 1227–1236 (2002).
37. Overmyer K, Brosche M, Kangasjarvi J. Reactive oxygen species and hormonal control of cell death. *Trends Plant Sci.* 8: 335–342 (2003).
38. Apel K, Hirt H. Reactive oxygen species: metabolism, oxidative stress, and signal transduction. *Annu. Rev. Plant Biol.* 55: 373–399 (2004).
39. Vandenabeele S *et al.* A comprehensive analysis of hydrogen peroxide-induced gene expression in tobacco. *Proc. Natl. Acad. Sci. USA* 100: 16113–16118 (2003).
40. Kovtun Y, Chiu W, Tena G, Sheen J. Functional analysis of oxidative stress-activated mitogen-activated protein kinase cascade in plants. *PNAS* 97: 2940–2945 (2000).
41. Desikan R, Mackerness S, Hancock JT, Neill SJ. Regulation of the *Arabidopsis* transcriptome by oxidative stress. *Plant Physiol.* 127: 159–172 (2001).
42. Levine A, Tenhake R, Dixon R, Lamb C. H_2O_2 from the oxidative burst orchestrates the plant hypersensitive disease resistance response. *Cell* 79: 583–593 (1994).
43. Jabs T. Reactive oxygen intermediates as mediators of programmed cell death in plants and animals. *Biochem. Pharmacol.* 57: 231–245 (1999).
44. Reichheld J, Vernoux T, Lardon F, Van Montagu M, Inze D. Specific checkpoints regulate plant cell cycle progression in response to oxidative stress. *Plant J.* 17: 647 (1999).
45. Durner J, Shah J, Klessig DF. Salicylic acid and disease resistance in plants. *Trends Plant Sci.* 2: 266–274 (1997).
46. Ievinsh G, Tillberg E. Stress-induced ethylene biosynthesis in pine needles: a search for the putative 1-aminocyclopropane-1-carboxylic-independent pathway. *J. Plant Physiol.* 145: 308–314 (1995).
47. Prasad TK, Anderson MD, Stewart CR. Acclimation, hydrogen peroxide, and abscisic acid protect mitochondria against irreversible chilling injury in maize seedlings. *Plant Physiol.* 105: 619–627 (1994).
48. Grant JJ, Yun BW, Loake GJ. Oxidative burst and cognate redox signalling reported by luciferase imaging: identification of a signal network that functions independently of ethylene, SA and Me-JA but is dependent on MAPKK activity. *Plant J.* 24: 569–582 (2000).
49. Bolwell GP. Role of active oxygen species and NO in plant defence responses. *Curr. Opin. Plant Biol.* 2: 287–294 (1999).

50. Delledonne M, Xia Y, Dixon RA, Lamb C. Nitric oxide functions as a signal in plant disease resistance. *Nature* 394: 585–588 (1998).
51. Beligni MV, Lamattina L. Nitric oxide: a non-traditional regulator of plant growth. *Trends Plant Sci.* 6: 508–509 (2001).
52. Wendehenne D, Pugin A, Klessig DF, Durner J. Nitric oxide: comparative synthesis and signaling in animal and plant cells. *Trends Plant Sci.* 6: 177–183 (2001).
53. Leshem YY, Haramaty E. The characterization and contrasting effects of the nitric oxide free radical in vegetative stress and senescence in *Pisum sativum* Linn. foliage. *J. Plant Physiol.* 148: 258–263 (1996).
54. Leshem Y. *Nitric Oxide in Plants.* Kluwer Academic Publishers, London, 2001.
55. Leshem YY, Pinchasov Y. Non-invasive photoacoustic spectroscopic determination of relative endogenous nitric oxide and ethylene content stoichiometry during the ripening of strawberries *Fragaria ananassa* (Duch.) and avocados *Persea americana* (Mill.). *J. Exp. Bot.* 51: 1471–1473 (2000).
56. Tun NN, Holk A, Scherer GF. Rapid increase of NO release in plant cell cultures induced by cytokinin. *FEBS Lett.* 509: 174–176 (2001).
57. Scherer GFE, Holk A. NO donors mimic and NO inhibitors inhibit cytokinin action in betalaine accumulation in *Amaranthus caudatus*. *Plant Growth Regul.* 32: 345–350 (2000).
58. Carimini F, Zottini M, Formentin E, Terzi M, Lo Schiavo F. Cytokinins, new apoptotic inducers in plants. *Planta* 216: 413–421 (2002).
59. Borutaite V, Brown GC. Nitric oxide induces apoptosis via hydrogen peroxide, but necrosis via energy and thiol depletion. *Free Radic. Biol. Med.* 35: 1457–1468 (2003).
60. Delledonne M. NO news is good news for plants (Review). *Curr. Opin. Plant Biol.* 8: 390–396 (2005).
61. Crawford NM, Guo F-Q. New insights into nitric oxide metabolism and regulatory functions. *Trends Plant Sci.* 10: 195–200 (2005).
62. Durner J, Wendehenne D, Klessig DF. Defense gene induction in tobacco by nitric oxide, cyclic GMP, and cyclic ADP-ribose. *Proc. Natl. Acad. Sci. USA* 95: 10328–10333 (1998).
63. Klessig DF *et al.* Nitric oxide and salicylic acid signaling in plant defense. *Proc. Natl. Acad. Sci. USA* 97: 8849–8855 (2000).
64. Huang X, von Rad U, Durner J. Nitric oxide induces transcriptional activation of the nitric oxide-tolerant alternative oxidase in Arabidopsis suspension cells. *Planta* 215: 914–923 (2002).

65. Buettner GR. The pecking order of free radicals and antioxidants: lipid peroxidation, alpha-tocopherol, and ascorbate. *Arch. Biochem. Biophys.* 300: 535–543 (1993).
66. Wink DA *et al.* DNA deaminating ability and genotoxicity of nitric oxide and its progenitors. *Science* 254: 1001–1003 (1991).
67. Nguyen T, Brunson D, Crespi CL, Penman BW, Wishnok JS, Tannenbaum SR. DNA damage and mutation in human cells exposed to nitric oxide *in vitro*. *Proc. Natl. Acad. Sci. USA* 89: 3030–3034 (1992).
68. Conklin PL. Vitamin C: a new pathway for an old antioxidant. *Trends Plant Sci.* 3: 329–330 (1998).
69. Noctor G, Foyer CH. Ascorbate and glutathione: keeping active oxygen under control. *Annu. Rev. Plant Physiol. Plant Mol. Biol.* 49: 249–279 (1998).
70. Horemans N, Foyer CH, Potters G, Asard H. Ascorbate function and associated transport systems in plants. *Plant Physiol. Biochem.* 38: 531–540 (2000).
71. Smirnoff N. Ascorbic acid: metabolism and functions of a multi-facetted molecule. *Curr. Opin. Plant Biol.* 3: 229–235 (2000).
72. Arrigoni O, De Tullio MC. Ascorbic acid: much more than just an antioxidant. *Biochim. Biophys. Acta* 1569: 1–9 (2002).
73. Pignocchi C, Foyer CH. Apoplastic ascorbate metabolism and its role in the regulation of cell signalling. *Curr. Opin. Plant Biol.* 6: 379–389 (2003).
74. Wheeler GL, Jones MA, Smirnoff N. The biosynthetic pathway of vitamin C in higher plants. *Nature* 393: 365–369 (1998).
75. Siendones E, Gonzalez-Reyes JA, Santos-Ocana C, Navas P, Cordoba F. Biosynthesis of ascorbic acid in kidney bean. L-galactono-gamma-lactone dehydrogenase is an intrinsic protein located at the mitochondrial inner membrane. *Plant Physiol.* 120: 907–912 (1999).
76. Bartoli CG, Pastori GM, Foyer CH. Ascorbate biosynthesis in mitochondria is linked to the electron transport chain between complexes III and IV. *Plant Physiol.* 123: 335–344 (2000).
77. Millar AH *et al.* Control of ascorbate synthesis by respiration and its implications for stress responses. *Plant Physiol.* 133: 443–447 (2003).
78. Davey MW *et al.* Ascorbate biosynthesis in Arabidopsis cell suspension culture. *Plant Physiol.* 121: 535–543 (1999).
79. Smirnoff N, Conklin PL, Loewus FA. Biosynthesis of ascorbic acid in plants: a renaissance. *Annu. Rev. Plant Physiol. Plant Mol. Biol.* 52: 437–467 (2001).
80. Fryer MJ. The antioxidant effects of thylakoid vitamin E (a-tocopherol). *Plant Cell Env.* 15: 381–392 (1992).

81. Thomas CE, McLean LR, Parker RA, Ohlweiler DF. Ascorbate and phenolic antioxidant interactions in prevention of liposomal oxidation. *Lipids* 27: 543–550 (1992).
82. Yamasaki H, Grace SC. EPR detection of phytophenoxyl radicals stabilized by zinc ions: evidence for the redox coupling of plant phenolics with ascorbate in the H_2O_2-peroxidase system. *FEBS Lett.* 422: 377–380 (1998).
83. Pastori GM *et al.* Leaf vitamin C contents modulate plant defense transcripts and regulate genes that control development through hormone signaling. *Plant Cell* 15: 939 (2003).
84. Tabata K, Oba K, Suzuki K, Esaka M. Generation and properties of ascorbic acid-deficient transgenic tobacco cells expressing antisense RNA for L-galactono-1,4-lactone dehydrogenase. *Plant J.* 27: 139–148 (2001).
85. Rose RC. Transport of ascorbic acid and other water-soluble vitamins. *Biochim. Biophys. Acta* 947: 335–366 (1988).
86. Horemans N, Foyer CH, Asard H. Transport and action of ascorbate at the plant plasma membrane. *Trends Plant Sci.* 5: 263–267 (2000).
87. Horemans N, Asard H, Caubergs RJ. The role of ascorbate free radical as an electron acceptor to cytochrome b-mediated trans-plasma membrane electron transport in higher plants. *Plant Physiol.* 104: 1455–1458 (1994).
88. Berczi A, Moller IM. NADH-monodehydroascorbate oxidoreductase is one of the redox enzymes in spinach leaf plasma membranes. *Plant Physiol.* 116 1029–1036 (1998).
89. May M, Vernoux T, Leaver C, Van Montagu M, Inze D. Review article. Glutathione homeostasis in plants: implications for environmental sensing and plant development. *J. Exp. Bot.* 49: 649–667 (1998).
90. Noctor G, Arisi A, Jouanin L, Kunert K, Rennenberg H, Foyer CH. Review article. Glutathione: biosynthesis, metabolism and relationship to stress tolerance explored in transformed plants. *J. Exp. Bot.* 49: 623–647 (1998).
91. Noctor G, Gomez L, Vanacker H, Foyer CH. Interactions between biosynthesis, compartmentation and transport in the control of glutathione homeostasis and signalling. *J. Exp. Bot.* 53: 1283–1304 (2002).
92. Larson RA. The antioxidants of higher plants. *Phytochemistry* 27: 969–978 (1988).
93. Marrs KA. The functions and regulation of glutathione S-transferases in plants. *Annu. Rev. Plant Physiol. Plant Mol. Biol.* 47: 127–158 (1996).
94. Iturbe-Ormaetxe I, Heras B, Matamoros MA, Ramos J, Moran JF, Becana M. Cloning and functional characterization of a homoglutathione synthetase from pea nodules. *Physiol. Plantarum* 115: 69–73 (2002).

95. Xiang C, Oliver DJ. Glutathione metabolic genes coordinately respond to heavy metals and jasmonic acid in Arabidopsis. *Plant Cell* 10: 1539–1550 (1998).
96. Bourbouloux A, Shahi P, Chakladar A, Delrot S, Bachhawat AK. Hgt1p, a high affinity glutathione transporter from the yeast *Saccharomyces cerevisiae*. *J. Biol. Chem.* 275: 13259–13265 (2000).
97. Foyer CH, Theodoulou FL, Delrot S. The functions of inter- and intracellular glutathione transport systems in plants. *Trends Plant Sci.* 6: 486–492 (2001).
98. Zhang M *et al.* A novel family of transporters mediating the transport of glutathione derivatives in plants. *Plant Physiol.* 134: 482–491 (2004).
99. Munne-Bosch S, Alegre L. The function of tocopherols and tocotrienols in plants. *Crit. Rev. Plant Sci.* 21: 31–57 (2002).
100. Kamal-Eldin A, Appelqvist LA. The chemistry and antioxidant properties of tocopherols and tocotrienols. *Lipids* 31: 671–701 (1996).
101. Kagan VE, Fabisiak JP, Quinn PJ. Coenzyme Q and vitamin E need each other as antioxidants. *Protoplasma* 214: 11–18 (2000).
102. Gomez-Fernandez JC *et al.* Localization of a-tocopherol in membranes. *Ann. New York Acad. Sci.* 570: 109–120 (1989).
103. Hofius D, Sonnewald U. Vitamin E biosynthesis: biochemistry meets cell biology. *Trends Plant Sci.* 8: 6–8 (2003).
104. Ajjawi I, Shintani D. Engineered plants with elevated vitamin E: a nutraceutical success story. *Trends Biotechnol.* 22: 104–107 (2004).
105. Shintani D, DellaPenna D. Elevating the vitamin E content of plants through metabolic engineering. *Science* 282: 2098–2100 (1998).
106. Savidge B *et al.* Isolation and characterization of homogentisate phytyltransferase genes from *Synechocystis* sp. PCC 6803 and Arabidopsis. *Plant Physiol.* 129: 321–332 (2002).
107. Porfirova S, Bergmuller E, Tropf S, Lemke R, Dormann P. Isolation of an Arabidopsis mutant lacking vitamin E and identification of a cyclase essential for all tocopherol biosynthesis. *Proc. Natl. Acad. Sci. USA* 99: 12495–12500 (2002).
108. Azzi A *et al.* Specific cellular responses to alpha-tocopherol. *J. Nutr.* 130: 1649–1652 (2000).
109. Schurmann P, Jacquot JP. Plant thioredoxin systems revisited. *Annu. Rev. Plant Physiol. Plant Mol. Biol.* 51: 371–400 (2000).
110. Meyer Y, Vignols F, Reichheld JP. Classification of plant thioredoxins by sequence similarity and intron position. *Methods Enzymol.* 347: 394–402 (2002).

111. Gelhaye E, Rouhier N, Jacquot JP. The thioredoxin h system of higher plants. *Plant Physiol. Biochem.* 42: 265–271 (2004).
112. Day DA, Whelan J, Millar AH, Siedow JN, Wiskich JT. Regulation of the alternative oxidase in plants and fungi. *Aust. J. Plant Physiol.* 22: 497–509 (1995).
113. Schuermann P, Buchanan BB. The structure and function of the ferredoxin/thioredoxin system in photosynthesis. In: Aro E-M, Andersson B (eds.) *Regulation of Photosynthesis*. Kluwer Academic Publishers, Dordrecht, Boston, London, 2001, Vol. 11, pp. 331–361.
114. Balmer Y *et al.* Thioredoxin links redox to the regulation of fundamental processes of plant mitochondria. *PNAS* 101: 2642–2647 (2004).
115. Sies H, Stahl W. Non-nutritive bioactive constituents of plants: lycopene, lutein and zeaxanthin. *Int. J. Vitam. Nutr. Res.* 73: 95–100 (2003).
116. Berthold DA, Andersson ME, Nordlund P. New insight into the structure and function of the alternative oxidase. *Biochim. Biophys. Acta* 1460: 241–254 (2000).
117. Grace S, Logan BA. Energy dissipation and radical scavenging by the plant phenylpropanoid pathway. *Trans. R. Soc. Lond. B* 355: 1499–1510 (2000).
118. Rice-Evans CA, Miller NJ, Paganga G. Antioxidant properties of phenolic compounds. *Trends Plant Sci.* 2: 152–159 (1997).
119. Taubert D *et al.* Reaction rate constants of superoxide scavenging by plant antioxidants. *Free Radic. Biol. and Med.* 35: 1599–1607 (2003).
120. Arora A, Byrem TM, Nair MG, Strasburg GM. Modulation of liposomal membrane fluidity by flavonoids and isoflavonoids. *Arch. Biochem. Biophys.* 373: 102–109 (2000).
121. Takahama U, Oniki T. A peroxide/phenolics/ascorbate system can scavenge hydrogen peroxide in plant cells. *Physiol. Plant.* 101: 845–852 (1997).
122. Decker EA. The role of phenolics, conjugated linoleic acid, carnosine and pyrroloquinoline as non-essential dietary antioxidants. *Nutr. Rev.* 53: 49–58 (1995).
123. Grassmann J, Hippeli S, Elstner EF. Plant's defence and its benefits for animals and medicine: role of phenolics and terpenoids in avoiding oxygen stress. *Plant Physiol. Biochem.* 40: 471–478 (2002).
124. Miranda-Rothmann S, Aspillaga AA, Perez DD, Vasquez L, Martinez ALF, Leighton F. Juice and phenolic fractions of the berry *Aristotelia chilensis* inhibit LDL oxidation *in vitro* and protect human endothelial cells against oxidative stress. *J. Agric. Food Chem.* 50: 7542–7547 (2002).

125. Beckman CH. Phenolic-storing cells: key to prgrammed cell death and periderm formation in wilt disease resistance and in general defense responses in plants? *Phys. Mol. Plant Pathol.* 57: 101–110 (2000).
126. Youn HD, Kim EJ, Roe JH, Hah YC, Kang SO. A novel nickel-containing superoxide dismutase from *Streptomyces* spp. *Biochem. J.* 318 (Pt 3): 889–896 (1996).
127. Bannister JV, Bannister WH, Rotilio G. Aspects of the structure, function, and applications of superoxide dismutase. *CRC Crit. Rev. Biochem.* 22: 111–180 (1987).
128. Monk LS, Fagerstedt KV, Crawford RMM. Superoxide dismutase as an anaerobic polypeptide — a key factor in recovery from oxygen deprivation in *Iris pseudacorus*? *Plant Physiol.* 85: 1016–1020 (1987).
129. Alscher RG, Erturk N, Heath LS. Role of superoxide dismutases (SODs) in controlling oxidative stress in plants. *J. Exp. Bot.* 53: 1331–1341 (2002).
130. Biemelt S, Keetman U, Albrecht G. Re-aeration following hypoxia or anoxia leads to activation of the antioxidative defense system in roots of wheat seedlings. *Plant Physiol.* 116: 651–658 (1998).
131. Boo YC, Jung J. Water deficit-induced oxidative stress and antioxidative defenses in rice plants. *J. Plant Physiol.* 155: 255–261 (1999).
132. Willekens H, Inze D, Van Montagu M, Van Camp W. Catalase in plants. *Mol. Breeding* 1: 207–228 (1995).
133. Foyer CH, Noctor G. Tansley Review No. 112. Oxygen processing in photosynthesis: regulation and signalling. *New Phytol.* 146: 359–388 (2000).
134. Kiddle G *et al.* Effects of leaf ascorbate content on defense and photosynthesis gene expression in *Arabidopsis thaliana*. *Antioxid. Redox Signal.* 5: 23–32 (2003).
135. Pnueli L, Liang H, Rozenberg M, Mittler R. Growth suppression, altered stomatal responses, and augmented induction of heat shock proteins in cytosolic ascorbate peroxidase (Apx1)-deficient Arabidopsis plants. *Plant J.* 34: 187–203 (2003).
136. Willekens H *et al.* Catalase is a sink for H_2O_2 and is indispensable for stress defence in C_3 plants. *EMBO J.* 16: 4806–4816 (1997).
137. Dat JF, Inze D, Van Breusegem F. Catalase-deficient tobacco plants: tools for in planta studies on the role of hydrogen peroxide. [Review] [54 refs]. *Redox Report* 6: 37–42 (2001).
138. Shigeoka S *et al.* Regulation and function of ascorbate peroxidase isoenzymes. *J. Exp. Bot.* 53: 1305–1319 (2002).
139. Fryer MJ, Ball L, Oxborough K, Karpinski S, Mullineaux PM, Baker NR. Control of ascorbate peroxidase 2 expression by hydrogen peroxide and leaf

water status during excess light stress reveals a functional organization of Arabidopsis leaves. *Plant J.* 33: 691–705 (2003).

140. Rizhsky L, Davletova S, Liang H, Mittler R. The zinc finger protein Zat12 is required for cytosolic ascorbate peroxidase 1 expression during oxidative stress in Arabidopsis. *J. Biol. Chem.* 279: 11736–11743 (2004).
141. Asai N *et al.* Compensation for lack of a cytosolic ascorbate peroxidase in an Arabidopsis mutant by activation of multiple antioxidative systems. *Plant Sci.* 166: 1547–1554 (2004).
142. Baier M, Dietz KJ. Primary structure and expression of plant homologues of animal and fungal thioredoxin-dependent peroxide reductases and bacterial alkyl hydroperoxide reductases. *Plant Mol. Biol.* 31: 553–564 (1996).
143. Dietz K. Plant peroxiredoxins. *Annu. Rev. Plant Biol.* 54: 93–107 (2003).
144. Wood ZA, Schroder E, Harris JR, Poole LB. Structure, mechanism and regulation of peroxiredoxins. *Trends Biochem. Sci.* 28: 32–40 (2003).
145. Baier M, Noctor G, Foyer CH, Dietz KJ. Antisense suppression of 2-cysteine peroxiredoxin in arabidopsis specifically enhances the activities and expression of enzymes associated with ascorbate metabolism but not glutathione metabolism. *Plant Physiol.* 124: 823–832 (2000).
146. Baier M, Dietz KJ. Alkyl hydroperoxide reductases: the way out of the oxidative breakdown of lipids in chloroplasts. *Trends Plant Sci.* 4: 166–168 (1999).
147. Herbette S, Lenne C, Leblanc N, Julien JL, Drevet JR, Roeckel-Drevet P. Two GPX-like proteins from *Lycopersicon esculentum* and *Helianthus annuus* are antioxidant enzymes with phospholipid hydroperoxide glutathione peroxidase and thioredoxin peroxidase activities. *Eur. J. Biochem.* 269: 2414–2420 (2002).
148. Milla MAR, Maurer A, Huete AR, Gustafson JP. Glutathione peroxidase genes in *Arabidopsis* are ubiquitous and regulated by abiotic stresses through diverse signaling pathways. *Plant J.* 36: 602–615 (2003).
149. Yoshimura K *et al.* Enhancement of stress tolerance in transgenic tobacco plants overexpressing Chlamydomonas glutathione peroxidase in chloroplasts or cytosol. *Plant J.* 37: 21–33 (2004).
150. Avsian-Kretchmer O, Eshdat Y, Gueta-Dahan Y, Ben-Hayyim G. Regulation of stress-induced phospholipid hydroperoxide glutathione peroxidase expression in citrus. *Planta* 209: 469–477 (1999).
151. Sugimoto M, Furui S, Suzuki Y. Molecular cloning and characterization of a cDNA encoding putative phospholipid hydroperoxide glutathione peroxidase from spinach. *Biosci. Biotechnol. Biochem.* 61: 1379–1381 (1997).

152. Mullineaux PM, Karpinski S, Jiménez A, Cleary SP, Robinson C, Creissen GP. Identification of cDNAS encoding plastid-targeted glutathione peroxidase. *Plant J.* 13: (1998).
153. Martinoia E, Massonneau A, Frangne N. Transport processes of solutes across the vacuolar membrane of higher plants. *Plant Cell Physiol.* 41: 1175–1186 (2000).
154. Foyer CH *et al.* Overexpression of glutathione reductase but not glutathione synthetase leads to increases in antioxidant capacity and resistance to photoinhibition in poplar trees. *Plant Physiol.* 109: 1047–1057 (1995).
155. Lederer B, Boger P. Antioxidative responses of tobacco expressing a bacterial glutathione reductase. *Z. Naturforsch. [C].* 58: 843–849 (2003).
156. Foyer CH, Mullineaux PM. The presence of dehydroascorbate and dehydroascorbate reductase in plant tissues. *FEBS Lett.* 425: 528–529 (1998).
157. Wells WW, Xu DP, Yang YF, Rocque PA. Mammalian thioltransferase (glutaredoxin) and protein disulfide isomerase have dehydroascorbate reductase activity. *J. Biol. Chem.* 265: 15361–15364 (1990).
158. Trumper S, Follmann H, Haberlein I. A novel-dehydroascorbate reductase from spinach chloroplasts homologous to plant trypsin inhibitor. *FEBS Lett.* 352: 159–162 (1994).
159. Shimaoka T, Yokota A, Miyake C. Purification and characterization of chloroplast dehydroascorbate reductase from spinach leaves. *Plant Cell Physiol.* 41: 1110–1118 (2000).
160. Urano J *et al.* Molecular cloning and characterization of a rice dehydroascorbate reductase. *FEBS Lett.* 466: 107–111 (2000).
161. Polle A. Dissecting the superoxide dismutase-ascorbate-glutathione-pathway in chloroplasts by metabolic modeling. Computer simulations as a step towards flux analysis. *Plant Physiol.* 126: 445–462 (2001).
162. Chen Z, Young TE, Ling J, Chang SC, Gallie DR. Increasing vitamin C content of plants through enhanced ascorbate recycling. *Proc. Natl. Acad. Sci. USA* 100: 3525–3530 (2003).
163. Chen Z, Gallie DR. The ascorbic acid redox state controls guard cell signaling and stomatal movement. *Plant Cell* 16: 1143–1162 (2004).
164. Pignocchi C, Fletcher JM, Wilkinson JE, Barnes JD, Foyer CH. The function of ascorbate oxidase in tobacco. *Plant Physiol.* 132: 1631–1641 (2003).
165. Roos W, Evers S, Hieke M, Tschope M, and Schumann B. Shifts of intracellular pH distribution as a part of the signal mechanism leading to the elicitation of benzophenanthridine alkaloids. Phytoalexin biosynthesis in cultured cells of *Eschscholtzia californica. Plant Physiol.* 118: 349–364 (1998).

166. Moeder W, Yoshioka K, Klessig DF. Involvement of the small GTPase Rac in the defence responses of tobacco to pathogens. *Mol. Plant Microbe Interact.* 18: 116–124 (2005).
167. Torres MA, Dangl JL. Functions of the respiratory burst oxidase in biotic interactions, abiotic stress and development. *Curr. Opin. Plant Biol.* 8: 397–403 (2005).
168. Griesen D, Su D, Berczi A, Asard H. Localization of an ascorbate-reducible cytochrome b561 in the plant tonoplast. *Plant Physiol.* 134: 726–734 (2004).
169. Alin P, Jensson H, Guthenberg C, Danielson UH, Tahir MK, Mannervik B. Purification of major basic glutathione transferase isoenzymes from rat liver by use of affinity chromatography and fast protein liquid chromatofocusing. *Anal. Biochem.* 146: 313–320 (1985).
170. Dixon DP, Cummings I, Cole DJ, Edwards R. Glutathione-mediated detoxification systems in plants. *Curr. Opin. Plant Biol.* 1: 258–266 (1998).
171. Rea PA, Li Z, Lu Y, Drozdowicz YM, Martinoia E. From vacuolar GS-X pumps to multispecific ABC transporters. *Annu. Rev. Plant Physiol. Plant Mol. Biol.* 49: 727–760 (1998).
172. Jasinski M, Ducos E, Martinoia E, Boutry M. The ATP-binding cassette transporters: structure, function, and gene family comparison between rice and arabidopsis. *Plant Physiol.* 131: 1169–1177 (2003).
173. Halkier BA. Catalytic reactivities and structure/function relationships of cytochrome P450 enzymes. *Phytochem.* 43: 1–21 (1996).
174. Corpas FJ, Barroso JB, del Rio A. Peroxisomes as a source of reactive oxygen species and nitric oxide signal molecules in plant cells. *Trends Plant Sci.* 6: 145–150 (2001).
175. del Rio LA, Corpas FJ, Sandalio LM, Palma JM, Gomez M, Barroso JB. Reactive oxygen species, antioxidant systems and nitric oxide in peroxisomes. *J. Exp. Bot.* 53: 1255–1272 (2002).
176. Miles EW, Rhee S, Davies DR. The molecular basis of substrate channeling. *J. Biol. Chem.* 274: 12193–12196 (1999).
177. Reumann S. The structural properties of plant peroxisomes and their metabolic significance. *Biol. Chem.* 381: 639–648 (2000).
178. Lopez-Huertas E, Charlton WL, Johnson B, Graham IA, Baker A. Stress induces peroxisome biogenesis genes. *EMBO J.* 19: 6770–6777 (2000).
179. Jimenez A, Hernandez JA, Pastori G, del Rio LA, Sevilla F. Role of the ascorbate-glutathione cycle of mitochondria and peroxisomes in the senescence of pea leaves. *Plant Physiol.* 118: 1327–1335 (1998).
180. Nisoli E, Clementi E, Moncada S, Carruba MO. Mitochondrial biogenesis as a cellular signaling framework. *Biochem. Pharmacol.* 67: 1–15 (2004).

181. Gille L, Nohl H. The ubiquinol/bc1 redox couple regulates mitochondrial oxygen radical formation. *Arch. Biochem. Biophys.* 388: 34–38 (2001).
182. Chakraborti T, Das S, Mondal M, Roychoudhury S, Chakraborti S. Oxidant, mitochondria and calcium: an overview. *Cell. Signal.* 11: 77–85 (1999).
183. Moller IM. Plant mitochondria and oxidative stress: Electron transport, NADPH turnover, and metabolism of reactive oxygen species. *Annu. Rev. Plant Physiol. Plant Mol. Biol.* 52: 561–591 (2001).
184. Braidot E, Petrussa E, Vianello A, Macri F. Hydrogen peroxide generation by higher plant mitochondria oxidizing complex I or complex II substrates. *FEBS Lett.* 451: 347–350 (1999).
185. Maxwell DP, Wang Y, McIntosh L. The alternative oxidase lowers mitochondrial reactive oxygen production in plant cells. *Proc. Natl. Acad. Sci. USA.* 96: 8271–8276 (1999).
186. Goglia F, Skulachev VP. A function for novel uncoupling proteins: antioxidant defense of mitochondrial matrix by translocating fatty acid peroxides from the inner to the outer membrane leaflet. *FASEB J.* 17: 1585–1591 (2003).
187. Brandalise M, Maia IG, Borecký J, Vercesi ABE, Arruda P. Overexpression of plant uncoupling mitochondrial protein in transgenic tobacco increases tolerance to oxidative stress. *J. Bioenerg. Biomembr.* 35: 203–209 (2003).
188. Sweetlove LJ *et al.* The impact of oxidative stress on Arabidopsis mitochondria. *Plant J.* 32: 891–904 (2002).
189. Millenaar FF, Lambers H. The alternative oxidase: *in vivo* regulation and function [Review]. *Plant Biol.* 5: 2–15 (2003).
190. Jimenez A, Hernandez JA, Del Rio LA, Sevilla F. Evidence for the presence of the ascorbate-glutathione cycle in mitochondria and peroxisomes of pea leaves. *Plant Physiol.* 114: 275–284 (1997).
191. Audran C *et al.* Expression studies of the zeaxanthin epoxidase gene in *Nicotiana plumbaginifolia. Plant Physiol.* 118: 1021–1028 (1998).
192. Joyard J *et al.* The biological machinery of plastid envelope membranes. *Plant Physiol.* 118: 715–723 (1998).
193. Grace SC, Logan BA, Adams WW. Seasonal differences in foliar content of chlorogenic acid, a phenylpropanoid antioxidant, in *Mahonia repens. Plant Cell Environ.* 21: 513–521 (1998).
194. Foyer CH. Ascorbate and glutathione metabolism in plants: H_2O_2 processing and signaling. In: Gitler C, Danon A (eds.) *Cellular Implications of Redox Signaling*. Imperial College Press, London, 2003, pp. 191–212.

195. Asada K. The water-water cycle in chloroplasts: scavenging of active oxygens and dissipation of excess photons. *Annu. Rev. Plant Physiol. Plant Mol. Biol.* 50: 601–639 (1999).
196. Foyer CH, Lopez-Delgado H, Dat JF, Scott IM. Hydrogen peroxide- and glutathione-associated mechanisms of acclimatory stress tolerance and signalling. *Physiol. Plantarum* 100: 241–254 (1997).

5 Lipid- and Protein-Mediated Oxidative Damage to DNA

Mark D. Evans and Marcus S. Cooke

1. Introduction

Oxidative stress was defined in 1991 by Helmut Sies as "an imbalance of oxidants and antioxidants in favor of the former." Under conditions of oxidative stress all cellular biomolecules are potential targets for reactive oxygen species (ROS). The ROS comprise a group of radical and non-radical oxygen-containing chemical species with the ability to permanently alter the structure, and in many cases the function, of biomolecules. These ROS have differing reactivities and differing abilities to diffuse to, and react with, a target. Protein, lipid and DNA have received the most study in terms of oxidative damage. These cellular components are potentially exposed to oxidants derived from both endogenous sources (e.g. electron transport chains, the respiratory burst) and exogenous sources (e.g. radiation, redox cycling xenobiotics). A common protective mechanism for all biomolecules is the interception of oxidants at various stages of formation by high and low molecular weight antioxidants. Low molecular weight antioxidants include ascorbic acid, vitamin E (comprising a group of structurally related tocopherols and tocotrienols), carotenoids, urate and glutathione. These can intercept oxidants and free radicals in hydrophilic and hydrophobic environments. Sacrificial oxidation of these antioxidants thus prevents damage to more important targets. Furthermore, some of these antioxidants, e.g. glutathione and tocopherols, have the potential to be regenerated. High molecular weight antioxidant proteins include those with catalytic functions, e.g. superoxide dismutase (dismutation of superoxide, the product of one-electron reduction of oxygen, to hydrogen peroxide and oxygen), catalase (degradation of hydrogen peroxide to water and oxygen), glutathione peroxidase (reduction of hydrogen peroxide to water with concomitant oxidation of glutathione). There have also been proposals that highly abundant proteins such as serum albumin may also act as sacrificial targets for oxidants. Whilst these broad-ranging antioxidant species can prevent the induction of oxidative damage, some damage still occurs, accounting for background levels of lesions, which become elevated under oxidative stress. Once formed, such damage may be reversed by specific repair processes, which are highly conserved throughout evolution.

Many studies have focused upon the oxidative modification of individual types of biomolecule in isolation, but it is evident that biological systems are complex and interactive, and modification of one molecule can impact upon another. Oxidative damage to DNA would seem to be particularly important in terms of carcinogenesis, many oxidative modifications being mutagenic, for example. However, nuclear DNA is not an isolated entity, but exists in complexes with protein, as chromatin, is surrounded by other nuclear proteins and is encased in a lipid membrane. It would therefore seem entirely reasonable that modification of one type of biomolecule can affect another.

In this chapter we propose to discuss briefly DNA, lipid and protein oxidation in isolation, and then focus upon the damaging interactions between these biomolecules. We conclude the chapter with a discussion of the occurrence and biological consequences of the adducts.

2. DNA, Lipid and Protein: Oxidative Damage, Protection and Repair

2.1. *Oxidative damage to DNA*

Virtually all the structural components that comprise DNA can be oxidatively modified, yielding alterations of deoxyribose, the constituent bases and induction of strand breaks. The oxidation of both purines and pyrimidines generates a large array of products, of which some 20–30 have been identified. An even smaller set of lesions have been the focus of analysis as markers of oxidative damage to DNA, particularly 8-hydroxy-7,8-dihydroguanine, thymine glycol and 5-(hydroxymethyl)uracil.[1] Mechanistically, particular attention has been paid to the reaction of hydroxyl radicals with DNA, which can undergo addition or hydrogen abstraction reactions with bases yielding carbon- or nitrogen-centered radicals that then undergo further reactions to yield an array of end-products. Specific information regarding the mechanism of formation of various representative base products arising from DNA oxidation have been covered in recent review articles and oxidative DNA damage is discussed in more detail in this volume.[1] The 2′-deoxyribose moiety is also a target for oxidation, leading to the liberation of oxidatively-modified sugar products or the generation of sugar remnants still attached to DNA as end groups on DNA strand breaks. At this point it should also be noted that the various types of RNA may also be oxidatively damaged. However, studies of the occurrence and consequences of such damage are at a more poorly developed level of understanding compared to DNA.[2]

Certainly, the most highly developed and extensive biomolecule repair process is that for DNA, reflective of the biological importance of preserving the integrity of this molecule. Other chapters in this volume discuss DNA repair in more detail and we will only provide an overview here, as much of this material has also been covered in recent review articles.[1] Broadly, there are two main repair processes for oxidative DNA damage, base excision repair (BER) and nucleotide excision repair (NER). The former involves the use of glycosylases, with a defined substrate range, which excise the damaged base. The resultant apurininc or apyrimidinic site is then processed and the gap filled with undamaged nucleotides to yield the original sequence. A range of glycosylases are present in mammalian cells excising specific oxidized purines (e.g. 8-oxo-guanine glycosylase [Ogg1]) or several oxidized pyrimidines (e.g. NTH1). Evidence that endonucleases removing the base and sugar as a single entity to yield a damaged base-containing 2′-deoxynucleoside is rather limited at present.[3] A feature of this DNA repair machinery is the high element of redundancy, so that cells are often able to compensate for the physical or functional absence of a particular repair protein. Nucleotide excision repair involves the removal of a small nucleotide patch containing the lesion from one strand of DNA and the gap is then filled. This process involves a larger number of DNA recognition and excision proteins than for base excision repair and is often associated with the removal of helix-distorting, "bulky," DNA adducts. It seems reasonable that certain products of oxidative DNA damage, for example tandem DNA lesions formed via intramolecular cyclisation between a sugar radical and purine base (e.g. 8,5′-cyclo-2′-deoxyguanosine) would be substrates for NER, but there is still some debate as to the extent that smaller oxidized bases such as thymine glycol or 8-oxo-guanine are substrates. The removal of oxidized DNA polymerase substrates, such as 8-oxo-2′-deoxyguanosine triphosphate, by MTH1 provides an additional protective mechanism to limit the presence of oxidatively modified bases in DNA.[4] Processes such as the preferential repair of lesions in actively transcribed strands (transcription-coupled repair; TCR) and the direction of repair processes to nascent DNA strands are also understood to occur.

2.2. *Lipid peroxidation*

The ubiquitous nature of lipids, particularly in biomembranes, makes them a primary target for both extra- and intracellularly generated oxidants. The oxidative degradation of polyunsaturated fatty acids (PUFA) is a complex autocatalytic process (lipid peroxidation; LPO) requiring initiation, often by free radical species. Initiators may include the hydroxyl radical, which is able to abstract a hydrogen from a lipid methylene group; oxygen can then add to the subsequent lipid alkyl radical to form a lipid peroxyl radical. These newly formed radical species provide routes to sustain LPO by acting as further initiators. The PUFA are particularly liable to LPO because the radicals can be stabilized by electron delocalization across the methylene-interrupted double bonds. Initial products of LPO include lipid hydroperoxides, which can form reactive radicals, via homolytic bond scission in the presence of reduced transition metal ions. This allows for the propagation of LPO. The relative instability and hydrophobicity of lipid hydroperoxides implies that they may present an oxidative threat to proteins embedded in lipid membranes. However, lipid hydroperoxides are only one product of LPO which, via a number of intermediates, can generate numerous end-products, many of which exert biological activity. Of particular significance, with regard to extra-membrane protein and DNA damage, are reactive, yet diffusible, unsaturated aldehyde species, for example 4-hydroxy-2-alkenals, e.g. 4-hydroxy-nonenal (HNE), acrolein and crotonaldehyde, and dicarbonyls, e.g. malondialdehyde (MDA) and glyoxal. The primary targets for the modification of DNA bases by reactive aldehydes are amino groups, which in the case of HNE, acrolein and crotonaldehyde leads to the production of cyclic propano- and etheno-adducts.

In addition to vitamin E, which can act as a chain-breaking antioxidant, enzyme activities exist to inhibit LPO. Limiting the levels of lipid hydroperoxides is important from the perspective of their possible damaging and LPO-potentiating properties. Cytosolic and mitochondrial glutathione peroxidase, usually associated with the decomposition of hydrogen peroxide, can also use lipid hydroperoxides as substrates, at least in a non-membrane bound form.[5] Another selenium-containing phospholipid hydroperoxide glutathione peroxidase (GPX4) can directly reduce membrane-bound phospholipid hydroperoxides.[5] The importance of GPX4 in limiting cellular oxidative stress has been noted in the increased sensitivity of $Gpx4^{+/-}$ cell lines to various oxidative insults.[6] Additionally, a non-selenium dependent glutathione peroxidase activity is associated, in humans, with cationic alpha-class glutathione-S-transferases (α-GST) of cytosolic and microsomal origin and can degrade fatty acid and phospholipid hydroperoxides.[7,8] Interception and detoxification of reactive carbonyls is an additional protective mechanism against LPO-mediated damage. For example, HNE is reported to be metabolized in particular via alcohol dehydrogenases, aldehyde dehydrogenases and glutathione S-transferases, to yield 2-nonene-1,4-diol, 4-hydroxy-2-nonenoic acid and glutathione conjugates (which may then be subject to further metabolism).[9–11]

2.3. *Protein oxidation*

Quantitatively, proteins represent the majority of the dry weight of a typical cell, and as such are likely to be a major target for ROS attack. The preponderance of proteins itself serves an antioxidant function, mopping up various free radical species. Indeed, some amino acids, such as methionine, appear to have a specific antioxidant function, interacting with ROS with no detrimental consequences to protein activity.[12] However, for many proteins, modification by ROS significantly alters their function as a consequence of side-chain group oxidation, backbone fragmentation, cross-linking, unfolding, changes in hydrophobicity and conformation, along with altered susceptibility to proteolysis. In addition, new reactive species may be formed, such as protein carbonyls, hydroperoxides[13] and chloramines.[14] In the presence of exogenous catalysts, such as transition metal ions, hydroperoxides undergo decomposition to various free radicals, such as alkoxyl ($RO^{\bullet}$), peroxyl ($ROO^{\bullet}$) and carbon-centred ($R^{\bullet}$) species.[15,16] These further reactive groups perpetuate the initial damage to protein by interacting with other cellular molecules, including lipids, generating lipid hydroperoxides and conjugated dienes,[17] and DNA, forming DNA-protein crosslinks[18] (DPC), oxidized nucleobases[19] and single strand breaks.[16]

The presence of oxidized proteins appears to have relevance to a number of diseases (reviewed in Dean *et al.*[20]) and their accumulation in the cell should be avoided. To this end, the cell possesses several strategies to remove protein damage. Some damage may be chemically reversed, for example, methionine sulphoxide can be reduced back to methionine, catalyzed by methionine sulphoxide reductase. However, mammalian cells have only a limited capacity to undertake this form of direct repair.[21] Furthermore, it seems that ROS damage to other amino acids is irreversible and the modified amino acid, or protein, needs to be removed from the cell. To this end, such modified proteins are rapidly degraded by proteolytic enzymes, in the form of the proteasome complex, with new enzymes then being synthesized *de novo*.[21] The impacts, in terms of structural modification, on DNA by lipid and protein oxidation are outlined in Table 1.

Table 1. Products of DNA base interaction with lipid peroxidation and protein oxidation.

Process	Product	Adducts*
Lipid peroxidation	Lipid hydroperoxides	Strand breaks; simple oxidized bases
	MDA	e.g. M_1G, M_1A, M_1C
	HNE, acrolein, crotonaldehyde	Propano-adducts with dG, dA and dC
	HNE, via 2,3-epoxy-4-hydroxynonanal	Etheno-adducts (εA, εC, εG)
	Glyoxal	Glyoxal-dG; glyoxal-dC
Protein oxidation	Protein hydroperoxides	DNA-protein crosslinks; simple oxidized bases

*Further information on the nature and abbreviations for these adducts is provided in the text.

3. Lipid Peroxidation: DNA Damage and Repair

3.1. *Induction of DNA damage by lipid peroxidation products*

Whilst it would seem that physical contact between DNA and lipid hydroperoxides in a nucleus may be limited, there are studies implying, at least *in vitro*, that lipid hydroperoxides can cause oxidative DNA damage, such as strand breaks and oxidized bases.[22] Treatment of cells in culture with lipid hydroperoxide, does generate DNA base oxidation, implying that either these species are able to access DNA or act as sources of initiation of peroxidation of endogenous lipids which then produce the ultimate DNA-damaging species.[23] The types of adducts generated by hydroperoxides are of the small oxidative type mentioned in Sec. 2.1.

Of notable importance with relevance to DNA damage arising from LPO is the interaction of reactive carbonyls with DNA bases to form covalent adducts. DNA adduct formation has been noted for several of the reactive carbonyl end-products of LPO (examples illustrated in Fig. 1) including MDA, HNE, glyoxal, acrolein, crotonaldehyde and 4-oxo-2-alkenals (e.g. 4-oxo-nonenal). The particular chemical identity of the PUFA undergoing peroxidation [ω-3 or ω-6] determines the likely DNA adducts produced, for example acrolein is an end-product of both ω-3 and ω-6 PUFA oxidation, whereas crotonaldehye is derived from ω-3 PUFA and HNE from ω-6 PUFA.[24,25] Furthermore, these species, because of their relative stability compared to hydroperoxides, have a greater ability to diffuse to and react with DNA. Additionally, oxidative degradation of deoxyribose can lead to the formation of glyoxal and MDA, enabling *in situ* production of reactive carbonyls close to DNA. Amino groups in the DNA bases are important sites of interaction with reactive carbonyls, thus adenine, cytosine and guanine are all substrates for adduct formation. However, the relative propensity of the base for modification varies, depending on the identity of the reactive carbonyl, with adenine a little less reactive than guanine and cytosine.

The interaction of reactive carbonyls with DNA bases in many cases produces adducts with additional heterocyclic ring structures; the adducts classified into three main groups — etheno, propano and MDA adducts. The resulting adduct, etheno or propano, is named on the basis of the new ring structure containing two or three new carbon atoms (exocyclic

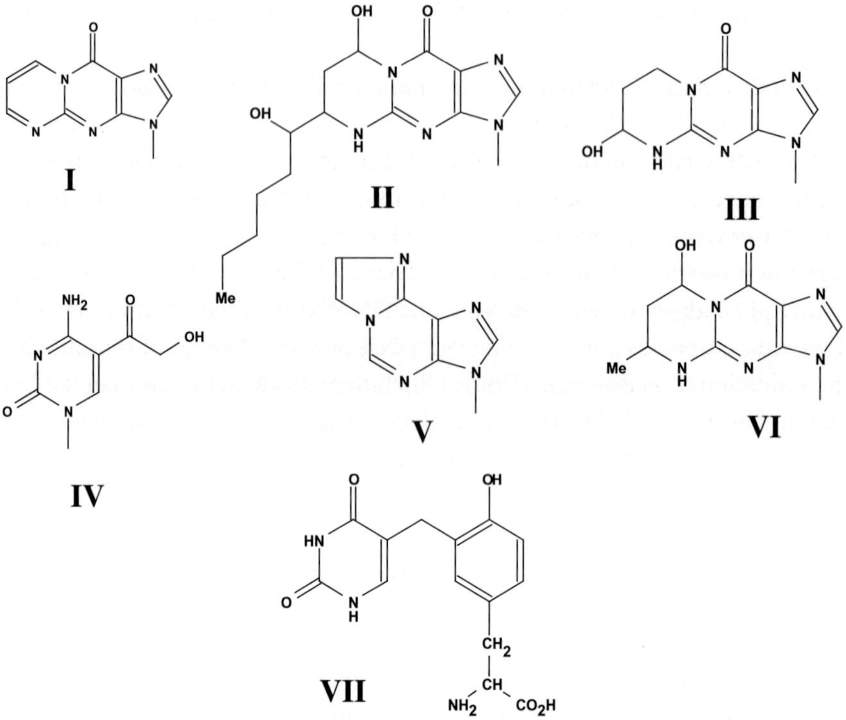

Fig. 1. Examples of DNA adducts arising from interaction of lipid peroxidation and protein oxidation products with DNA. I, M_1dG; II, HNE-dG; III, acrolein-dG; IV, glyoxal-dC; V, etheno-dA; VI, crotonaldehyde-dG; VII, Thy-Tyr crosslink. (Structures II, III and VI represent propano-dG adducts.)

ring). The propano adducts are formed from α,β-unsaturated aldehydes such as HNE, acrolein and crotonaldehyde; 1,N^2-propanodeoxyguanosine (PdG) represents a generic propano adduct structure with differing positions of alkyl and/or hydroxyl substitution on the exocyclic ring dependent on the identity of the reactive aldehyde (see Fig. 1). The MDA adducts arise from MDA produced during LPO or base propenals formed during DNA oxidation and etheno adducts from a metabolite of HNE (2,3-epoxy-4-hydroxynonanal produced via oxidative metabolism). The PdG adducts have been more widely studied, but dA and dC are also able to form propano-adducts.[26,27] Glyoxal reacts primarily with dG and dC, in the case of the former to form a new five-membered heterocyclic ring. Reaction with dC yields 5-hydroxyacetyl-dC or deoxyuridine via a deamination reaction.[28]

The stability of the former adduct is enhanced in the context of single or double-stranded DNA.

Another property shared by several of the LPO products is the induction of crosslinks, either between bases or between DNA and protein. Glyoxal can induce inter- and intra-strand crosslinking; *in vitro* treatment of DNA with glyoxal predominantly induces G-C and G-A crosslinks.[28]

Acrolein, crotonaldehyde and MDA also induce inter- and intra-strand DNA crosslinks.[29–32] In the case of acrolein, DNA-DNA and DNA-protein crosslinks can form via a ring-opened exocyclic adduct intermediate.[33] Crosslinking of DNA to histones under physiologically relevant conditions by MDA forms relatively stable DNA-protein crosslinks because of the bi-functional nature of the MDA. Initial reaction of MDA with histone, e.g. with the ε-amino group of lysine, to form a protein adduct is then followed by reaction with exocyclic amino groups on DNA to form the crosslink.[34] The reverse, i.e. initial adduct formation between MDA and DNA followed by crosslinking to protein does not appear to be as favorable a route.

3.2. *Repair of lipid peroxidation-induced DNA damage*

Studies on the repair of DNA adducts derived from LPO is not as advanced as that for the "smaller" DNA oxidation products described in Sec. 2.1, however, notable advances are being made. As is the case with these smaller lesions, the existence of repair processes for these lesions would indicate they have some biological importance. A summary of the major known repair processes for the LPO-derived lesions in mammalian cells is outlined in Table 2. Both BER and NER are involved in the repair of these lesions. Two enzymes dominate in the BER pathway for the repair of the etheno adducts, alkylpurine-DNA-N-glycosylase (ANPG) and mismatch-specific thymine-DNA glycosylase (TDG). It is probable that other enzymes may excise these lesions, but this is awaiting more detailed study, for example single-stranded monofunctional uracil DNA glycosylase (SMUG1) and methyl-CpG binding domain protein (MBD4/MED1) are also reported to excise εC, but less efficiently than for TDG.[35] In fact, redundancy in the repair of LPO-derived DNA adducts should not be unexpected, given the observations for the repair of "smaller" DNA oxidation products. In contrast to the etheno adducts, M_1dG and PdG are substrates for NER; by

Table 2. Repair processes for products of lipid peroxidation-induced DNA base damage.

Lesion	Pathway/Enzyme	Ref.
εA	ANPG	[38, 39]
εC	TDG	[40]
1,N^2-εG	ANPG	[41]
M_1dG	NER; TCR	[32, 37]
PdG	NER; TCR	[36, 37, 42, 43]

Notes: εA, 1,N^6-ethenoadenine; εC, 3,N^4-ethenocytosine; 1,N^2-εG, 1,N^2-ethenoguanine; M_1G, pyrimidino[1,2-a]purin-10(3H)-one; PdG, 1,N^2-propanodeoxyguanosine; ANPG, alkylpurine-DNA-N-glycosylase; TDG, mismatch-specific thymine-DNA glycosylase.

implication the adducts derived from acrolein and crotonaldehyde are also probable substrates for NER.[36] Additionally M_1dG and PdG are likely substrates for TCR, based on their ability to block the transcribing activity of RNA polymerase II.[37]

4. Protein Oxidation: DNA Damage and Repair

The role nucleohistones play in the packaging of DNA (reviewed in Evans and Cooke[2]) may, in part, have a protective function.[44] However, this close physical proximity to DNA, would suggest that these proteins may also be a source of various forms of damage to DNA.

4.1. *DNA protein crosslinks*

Covalent bonds between DNA and protein, are known as DNA-protein crosslinks (DPC). The involvement of basic amino acids, such as lysine (Lys), in DPC is of particular interest, as they constitute a large proportion of the amino acids in nucleohistones.[45] Whilst DPC may be produced from the action of reactive aldehydes,[46] some of which may arise from LPO (see above[34]), these are largely outside the remit of this section, as we will focus upon DPC arising from free radical damage to proteins.

For the most part, it would appear that, in the case of $^{\bullet}$OH-derived DPC, radicals are required to be present on both the DNA and protein, and in close proximity to each other.[47] This may be achieved, and provide preference for particular amino acids and DNA bases, as a result of the unique hydrogen bonding between Lys and adjacent thymine (Thy) moieties.[48] Similarly, crosslinking of Thy and tyrosine (Tyr) may occur, again facilitated by hydrogen bonding between Thy and Tyr,[48] although not necessarily requiring a radical to be present on the amino acid, only the DNA base.[49] The actual mechanism of formation appears to be dependent upon the source of the oxidant, e.g. γ radiation or H_2O_2, although neither pathway may be mutually exclusive.[50]

When oxygen is present in the system, conversion of the Thy or Tyr radical to a peroxyl radical is expected to largely prevent Thy-Tyr crosslink formation.[49] However, the presence of oxygen does not appear to affect Thy-Tyr crosslink formation in isolated chromatin, exposed *in vitro* to γ radiation or H_2O_2/metal ions,[51] and does not prevent, at least not entirely, their formation in cells treated similarly. In contrast, the formation of DPC involving thymine and glycine, alanine, valine, leucine, isoleucine and threonine, all previously reported to occur[52] as well as cytosine and tyrosine, are inhibited by oxygen, and quantitatively Thy-Tyr crosslinks predominate.[50]

Another route by which DPC may be formed appears to be $^{\bullet}$OH-independent, involving protein hydroperoxides (Pr-OOH). Davies *et al.*[15] demonstrated that metal-catalyzed decomposition of Pr-OOH generated $R^{\bullet}$, $ROO^{\bullet}$, $O_2^{\bullet-}$, and $CO^{\bullet-}$ radicals. The proposed mechanism for DNA crosslinking by Pr-OOH is[53]:

(a) DNA-bound metal mediated formation of alkoxyl radicals:

$$\text{DNA-M}^{n+} + \text{Pr-OOH} \rightarrow \text{DNA-M}^{(n+1)+} + \text{Pr-O}^{\bullet} + \text{OH}^{-}$$

(b) Interaction of protein radical with DNA

$$\text{Pr-O}^{\bullet} + \text{DNA} \rightarrow \text{Pr-O-DNA}^{\bullet}$$

resulting in a DPC radical. From the above equation, the presence of metal ions appears to be an obligate requirement; indeed scavenging and chelating experiments have failed to rule out their involvement.[53] The potential for proteins to contain multiple -OOH groups, each one capable of participating in the above reaction, represents a major source of Pr-O$^{\bullet}$, and hence damage. Furthermore, protein hydroperoxides have an appreciably greater half life than $^{\bullet}$OH, and they are more mobile than base and amino acid radicals in their macromolecule context which, taken together, would suggest this to be a significant route to DPC formation.

A third route for DPC formation, involves protein chloramines, derived from the interaction of HOCl with amino acids (both free and protein-bound[54]). The presence of HOCl arises from the reaction of H_2O_2 with physiological concentrations of Cl^-, a reaction catalyzed by myeloperoxidase, following phagocytic cell activation.[55] Reaction of HOCl with proteins forms short-lived chloramines, decomposing to protein-derived, nitrogen-centered radicals.[56] Whilst HOCl may react directly with DNA, forming chlorinated bases, these do not appear to arise from the reaction of amino acid or protein chloramines with DNA.[57] The Arg- and Lys-rich histone proteins are likely to be more favorable targets for HOCl, compared to DNA.[14] Interaction of Lys, for example, with HOCl will form Lys chloramine, thermal decomposition of which will release Cl^-, resulting in a Lys radical. This radical may subsequently add to the C5-C6 double bond of pyrimidine bases, resulting in C5-yl and C6-yl radical adducts respectively.[57]

In general, little appears to be known about the levels of DPC derived via the above routes *in vivo*, and consideration of other sources of DPC need to be taken into account and inferences made. For MDA-derived DPC, background levels in human white blood cells range from 0.5 to 4.5 per 10^7 bases,[34] suggesting a certain prevalence. Equally very little is known about the repair of these lesions. It has been proposed that NER is the pathway primarily responsible for the removal of aldehyde-derived DPC,[46,58] perhaps coupled with the proteolytic degradation of crosslinked proteins.[58] Indeed, poly-ADP ribose polymerase (PARP), an enzyme closely associated with DNA repair, has been shown to activate nuclear 20S proteasome to degrade oxidatively damaged histones,[59] implying a coupling of DNA and protein repair pathways in cellular defence. However, findings with formaldehyde-derived DPC would suggest that NER has a limited role (if any) in the repair of these DPC.[46,58] Nevertheless, evidence still remains which suggests that at least a certain sub-group of DPC are repaired by NER,[60] and these may include those derived from free radical damage to protein.

4.2. *Oxidative DNA base damage*

Hydroxyl radical addition to tyrosine generates 3,4-dihydroxyphenylalanine (DOPA), a major, long-lived, reactive intermediate product of the interaction of free radicals with proteins. In the context of protein, or peptides, DOPA is often referred to as protein-, or peptide-bound DOPA (PB-DOPA[61]). PB-DOPA has been shown to catalyze Cu and Fe ion-mediated damage to DNA, via $^{\bullet}OH$ formation.[61] Indeed, Morin *et al.*[61] demonstrated the formation of 8-OHGua and 5-hydroxy-2′-deoxycytidine in calf thymus DNA following incubation with DOPA or PB-DOPA, proposing the following reactions:

(a) $Cu^{+} + H_2O_2 \rightarrow Cu^{2+} + HO^{-} + ^{\bullet}OH$
(b) $Cu^{2+} + DOPA \rightarrow Cu^{+} + DOPA^{\bullet -}$
(c) $Cu^{+} + O_2 \rightarrow Cu^{2+} + O_2^{\bullet -}$
(d) $DOPA^{\bullet -} + O_2 \rightarrow DOPA + O_2^{\bullet}$

DNA may be damaged directly by $^{\bullet}OH$, whereas $O_2^{\bullet -}$ would need to go through the Haber-Weiss reaction before producing a species which could damage DNA (again $^{\bullet}OH$). In addition to the above reactions, oxidative damage to DNA and RNA may also be mediated via histone hydroperoxides, in conjunction with transition metal ions, acting through $RO^{\bullet}$, $ROO^{\bullet}$, or $R^{\bullet}$,[62] although it is not clear which radical reacts with the nucleobases.[19]

Protein hydroperoxides and PB-DOPA represent an additional route by which ROS may generate potentially mutagenic lesions in DNA without the formation of DNA-protein adducts.[61] Furthermore, it may be postulated that, given the protective role of histone proteins, and the likelihood that they are the first target for radicals generated in the cytoplasm and nucleoplasm, a significant proportion of oxidative DNA base damage may be secondary to radical damage to proteins. This would certainly appear to be the case for radiation-induced ROS.[62]

Repair of oxidatively damaged DNA has been the subject of intense research, and has been outlined in Sec. 2.1 above, in addition to being detailed elsewhere in this volume.

4.3. *Single-strand breaks*

There appears to be little evidence for protein hydroperoxide-induced DNA strand breaks, other than those produced by γ-irradiated lysine.[16] In contrast, isolated lysine, histidine, peptide and protein chloramines have all been shown to generate DNA strand breaks, either via DNA-derived radicals, carbon-centered radicals or peroxyl radicals, when in the presence of oxygen.[14] As with oxidatively modified DNA, the repair of single-strand breaks (SSB) is well-established in the literature (reviewed in Caldecott[63]). Briefly, SSB appear to be detected by PARP, which may also recruit repair proteins to the site. The "damaged" termini of SSB are characterized by their lack of 3′-hydroxy and/or 5′-phosphate end groups, which prevent DNA polymerase or ligase activity. With the repair enzymes recruited, PARP leaves the SSB site and allows the processing of the damaged termini by the apurinic/apyrimidinic (AP) lyase activity of polymerase β, and AP endonuclease 1. The continued proximity of pol β then facilitates gap filling.

5. Biological Consequences and Occurrence of Protein-DNA and Lipid-DNA Adducts

The mutagenic properties of the various etheno adducts were, relatively speaking, the earliest examined, possibly because of their proposed involvement in the carcinogenic properties of various industrial (vinyl halides) or environmental (urethanes) carcinogens. In mammalian cells εC produces predominantly C:G to A:T transversions and C:G to T:A transitions[64,65] and the mispairing in replicating DNA appears to depend on the identity of the DNA polymerase. The εA adduct induces A:T to G:C transitions predominantly, but also a smaller contribution from A:T to T:A transversions when examined in simian kidney cells.[66] In human cells, A:T to T:A transversions appeared to predominate, consistent with the high frequency of detection of this mutation *ras* and *p53* genes from vinyl chloride-induced tumors.[67] 1,N^2-ε G induces predominantly G:C to A.T transitions, but is also reported to block DNA polymerase activity.[68,69] Some of these studies also showed that the mutagenic potency or identity of the predominant mutagenic event depends on the test system; in order to assess the mutagenic impact of these lesions in mammals it is important to use mammalian cell lines, since the transfer of information from bacterial strains is often inappropriate.

The genotoxicity of HNE has proven difficult to examine in some instances because of its potent cytotoxicity, but HNE treatment of DNA induces a relatively high frequency of tandem mutations (substitution of two adjacent guanines for example); a similar situation occurring for acrolein and crotonaldehyde-modified DNA. These mutations are thought to arise primarily via the DNA crosslinking properties of these compounds.[43] The propano adduct HNE-dG induces predominantly G:C to T:A transversions in human cells. The reaction of HNE with dG generates four PdG stereoisomers and of the four, two are particularly promutagenic, while the other two show minimal mutagencity.[70] A similar situation exists for acrolein, of which there are two adduct isomers (α-OHPdG and γ-OHPdG, the latter of which is more prevalent) with differing position of a hydroxyl moiety in the exocyclic ring. The α-adduct is reported to be more genotoxic, being able to block DNA synthesis and induce largely G:C to T:A transversions.[71] In the context of DNA, the exocyclic ring of γ-OHPdG may open, enabling the adduct to adopt a normal Watson-Crick conformation which is thought to confer the minimal miscoding properties on the lesion.[33,72,73]

The M_1dG adduct has also recently been reported to be mutagenic in mammalian cells, inducing point mutations, G:C to T:A transversions and G:C to A:T transitions.[32] Additionally, consistent with its interstrand crosslinking ability, MDA is also able to induce large insertions and deletions in DNA.[32] The induction of frameshift mutations in repetitive sequences (microsatellites) implies that MDA (perhaps via M_1dG) may induce microsatellite instability, even in the presence of functional mismatch repair, a phenomenon often associated with carcinogenesis.[74] Glyoxal induces not only point mutations, predominantly G:C to T:A transversions, but also G:C to C:G transversions and G:C to A:T transitions.

Lipid peroxidation has been associated with carcinogenesis in a number of instances, co-incident with the formation of LPO-derived DNA adducts[75,76] and some additional evidence comes from associations between DNA adduct formation, dietary PUFA (quality as well as quantity of PUFA) and the occurrence of malignancies associated with the breast and colorectum.[77] Since the etheno adducts can also form via exposure to specific environmental agents, dissociating the formation of sporadic cancers from such exposures is difficult. Despite this, evidence does indicate that increased etheno adduct levels are detected in some pre-malignant conditions, e.g. familial adenomatous polyposis coli, cirrhotic liver and metal storage diseases, primary hemochromatosis and Wilson's disease.[76,78] In contrast to the etheno adducts, the PdG adducts, formed from HNE, are most likely to arise from endogenous LPO, and have been detected as endogenous lesions in a similar manner to etheno and malondialdehyde adducts.[79–82] Demonstration that many of the reactive aldehyde-DNA adducts have miscoding potential and the existence of repair processes for these lesions further suggests they could have important roles in carcinogenesis. The occurrence of LPO-derived DNA adducts at background levels, in healthy tissues obtained in the absence of deliberate carcinogen exposure also points towards an endogenous source for a portion of the adducts and a possible role in sporadic carcinogenesis. The detection of elevated lesion levels in transformed cells is possibly too late in the carcinogenic process to be of consequence, unless this is a process maintaining genome instability in tumor cells. Detection of elevated levels of these lesions in certain premalignant conditions, mentioned earlier could point to a role in the initiation phase of carcinogenesis.

The role of oxidative damage to DNA bases has recently been thoroughly reviewed, with elevated levels of damage being associated with numerous malignant and non-malignant diseases, although exact mechanisms appear far from clear.[83] An important conclusion by the authors was that despite the large number of DNA adducts identified, which would include those derived from lipids and protein described here, the main focus has been upon 8-OHdG, with little consideration for the biological significance of other lesions. This is evident from the literature in which a search revealed only one report of a study associating DPC with disease. In this study skin fibroblasts from patients with the autoimmune disease, systemic lupus erythematosus (SLE), were shown to possess abnormalities in the formation and repair of DPC and DNA single-strand breaks (SSB), following exposure to simulated sunlight.[84] Similarly, the cellular consequences of DPC appear unclear. In contrast, there are many studies linking protein oxidation with pathologies such as aging, diabetes, atherosclerosis and neurodegenerative disease (reviewed in Dean *et al.*[20]); a role for DPC in these conditions is likely, but can only be inferred.

6. Conclusions

Although direct oxidative damage to DNA shares some common features with LPO- and protein-derived damage to DNA, these latter interactions appear to produce a range of more distinctive and complex lesions. The formation of DNA damage from ROS-modified proteins has not, to date, received much attention, although this would appear to be an important area to study, given the close interaction between DNA and certain proteins. The situation for lipid-peroxidation-derived DNA damage is somewhat clearer and the identity of the lesions, their formation and chemistry is becoming understood. The potential mutagenic properties of selected lesions are also being unraveled in some detail, along with their repair processes. However, mutagenicity in human cells remains to be defined more thoroughly, as does their endogenous formation, occurrence and in some cases biological importance. When considering DNA damage it is important to remember that DNA does not exist on its own and a simplistic view of DNA oxidation, that does not account for the likely interactions with its more abundant molecular neighbors, is probably naïve.

Acknowledgments

The authors acknowledge the following agencies for financial support: UK Food Standards Agency, Arthritis Research Campaign, Lupus UK, Leicester Dermatology Fund.

References

1. Cooke MS, Evans MD, Dizdaroglu M, Lunec J. *FASEB J.* 17: 1195–1214 (2003).
2. Evans MD, Cooke MS. *Bioessays* 26: 533–542 (2004).
3. Bessho T, Tano K, Kasai H, Ohtsuka E, Nishimura S. *J. Biol. Chem.* 268: 19416–19421 (1993).
4. Sekiguchi M, Tsuzuki T. *Oncogene* 21: 8895–8904 (2002).
5. Ursini F, Bindoli A. *Chem. Phys. Lipids* 44: 255–276 (1987).
6. Yant LJ, Ran Q, Rao L, Van Remmen H, Shibatani T, Belter JG, Motta L, Richardson A, Prolla TA. *Free Radic. Biol. Med.* 34: 496–502 (2003).

7. Yang Y, Cheng JZ, Singhal SS, Saini M, Pandya U, Awasthi S, Awasthi YC. *J. Biol. Chem.* 276: 19220–19230 (2001).
8. Sandeep Prabhu K, Reddy PV, Jones EC, Liken AD, Channa Reddy C. *Arch. Biochem. Biophys.* 424: 72–80 (2004).
9. Hartley DP, Ruth JA, Petersen DR. *Arch. Biochem. Biophys.* 316: 197–205 (1995).
10. Srivastava S, Dixit BL, Cai J, Sharma S, Hurst HE, Bhatnagar A, Srivastava SK. *Free Radic. Biol. Med.* 29: 642–651 (2000).
11. Canuto RA, Ferro M, Muzio G, Bassi AM, Leonarduzzi G, Maggiora M, Adamo D, Poli G, Lindahl R. *Carcinogenesis* 15: 1359–1364 (1994).
12. Levine RL, Berlett BS, Moskovitz J, Mosoni L, Stadtman ER. *Mech. Ageing Dev.* 107: 323–352 (1999).
13. Headlam HA, Davies MJ. *Free Radic. Biol. Med.* 36: 1175–1184 (2004).
14. Hawkins CL, Pattison DI, Davies MJ. *Biochem. J.* 365: 605–615 (2002).
15. Davies MJ, Fu S, Dean RT. *Biochem. J.* 305 (Pt 2): 643–649 (1995).
16. Luxford C, Dean RT, Davies MJ. *Biogerontology* 3: 95–102 (2002).
17. Ostdal H, Davies MJ, Andersen HJ. *Free Radic. Biol. Med.* 33: 201–209 (2002).
18. Dizdaroglu M, Simic MG. *Int. J. Radiat. Biol. Relat. Stud. Phys. Chem. Med.* 47: 63–69 (1985).
19. Luxford C, Morin B, Dean RT, Davies MJ. *Biochem. J.* 344 (Pt 1): 125–134 (1999).
20. Dean RT, Fu S, Stocker R, Davies MJ. *Biochem. J.* 324 (Pt 1): 1–18 (1997).
21. Davies KJ. *Biochimie.* 83: 301–310 (2001).
22. Termini J. *Mutat. Res.* 450: 107–124 (2000).
23. Kaneko T, Tahara S. *Lipids* 35: 961–965 (2000).
24. Pan J, Chung FL. *Chem. Res. Toxicol.* 15: 367–372 (2002).
25. Chung FL, Pan J, Choudhury S, Roy R, Hu W, Tang MS. *Mutat. Res.* 531: 25–36 (2003).
26. Smith RA, Williamson DS, Cohen SM. *Chem. Res. Toxicol.* 2: 267–271 (1989).
27. Smith RA, Williamson DS, Cerny RL, Cohen SM. *Cancer Res.* 50: 3005–3012 (1990).
28. Kasai H, Iwamoto-Tanaka N, Fukada S. *Carcinogenesis* 19: 1459–1465 (1998).
29. Kawanishi M, Matsuda T, Nakayama A, Takebe H, Matsui S, Yagi T. *Mutat. Res.* 417: 65–73 (1998).
30. Kozekov ID, Nechev LV, Sanchez A, Harris CM, Lloyd RS, Harris TM. *Chem. Res. Toxicol.* 14: 1482–1485 (2001).
31. Kozekov ID, Nechev LV, Moseley MS, Harris CM, Rizzo CJ, Stone MP, Harris TM. *J. Am. Chem. Soc.* 125: 50–61 (2003).

32. Niedernhofer LJ, Daniels JS, Rouzer CA, Greene RE, Marnett LJ. *J. Biol. Chem.* 278: 31426–31433 (2003).
33. Sanchez AM, Minko IG, Kurtz AJ, Kanuri M, Moriya M, Lloyd RS. *Chem. Res. Toxicol.* 16: 1019–1028 (2003).
34. Voitkun V, Zhitkovich A. *Mutat. Res.* 424: 97–106 (1999).
35. Gros L, Ishchenko AA, Saparbaev M. *Mutat. Res.* 531: 219–229 (2003).
36. Johnson KA, Fink SP, Marnett LJ. *J. Biol. Chem.* 272: 11434–11438 (1997).
37. Cline SD, Riggins JN, Tornaletti S, Marnett LJ, Hanawalt PC. *Proc. Natl. Acad. Sci. USA* 101: 7275–7280 (2004).
38. Asaeda A, Ide H, Asagoshi K, Matsuyama S, Tano K, Murakami A, Takamori Y, Kubo K. *Biochemistry* 39: 1959–1965 (2000).
39. Saparbaev M, Kleibl K, Laval J. *Nucleic Acids Res.* 23: 3750–3755 (1995).
40. Saparbaev M, Laval J. *Proc. Natl. Acad. Sci. USA* 95: 8508–8513 (1998).
41. Saparbaev M, Langouet S, Privezentzev CV, Guengerich FP, Cai H, Elder RH, Laval J. *J. Biol. Chem.* 277: 26987–26993 (2002).
42. Choudhury S, Pan J, Amin S, Chung FL, Roy R. *Biochemistry* 43: 7514–7521 (2004).
43. Feng Z, Hu W, Amin S, Tang MS. *Biochemistry* 42: 7848–7854 (2003).
44. Nygren J, Ljungman M, Ahnstrom G. *Int. J. Radiat. Biol.* 68: 11–18 (1995).
45. Elgin SC, Weintraub H. *Annu. Rev. Biochem.* 44: 725–774 (1975).
46. Speit G, Schutz P, Merk O. *Mutagenesis* 15: 85–90 (2000).
47. Dizdaroglu M, Gajewski E. *Cancer Res.* 49: 3463–3467 (1989).
48. Hendry LB, Bransome Jr. ED, Hutson MS, Campbell LK. *Proc. Natl. Acad. Sci. USA* 78: 7440–7444 (1981).
49. Dizdaroglu M, Gajewski E, Reddy P, Margolis SA. *Biochemistry* 28: 3625–3628 (1989).
50. Olinski R, Nackerdien Z, Dizdaroglu M. *Arch. Biochem. Biophys.* 297: 139–143 (1992).
51. Nackerdien Z, Rao G, Cacciuttolo MA, Gajewski E, Dizdaroglu M. *Biochemistry* 30: 4873–4879 (1991).
52. Gajewski E, Fuciarelli AF, Dizdaroglu M. *Int. J. Radiat. Biol.* 54: 445–459 (1988).
53. Gebicki S, Gebicki JM. *Biochem. J.* 338 (Pt 3): 629–636 (1999).
54. Kulcharyk PA, Heinecke JW. *Biochemistry* 40: 3648–3656 (2001).
55. Weiss SJ, LoBuglio AF. *Lab. Invest.* 47: 5–18 (1982).
56. Hawkins CL, Davies MJ. *Biochem. J.* 332 (Pt 3): 617–625 (1998).
57. Hawkins CL, Davies MJ. *Chem. Res. Toxicol.* 14: 1071–1081 (2001).
58. Quievryn G, Zhitkovich A. *Carcinogenesis* 21: 1573–1580 (2000).
59. Ullrich O, Reinheckel T, Sitte N, Hass R, Grune T, Davies KJ. *Proc. Natl. Acad. Sci. USA* 96: 6223–6228 (1999).

60. Minko IG, Zou Y, Lloyd RS. *Proc. Natl. Acad. Sci. USA* 99: 1905–1909 (2002).
61. Morin B, Davies MJ, Dean RT. *Biochem. J.* 330 (Pt 3): 1059–1067 (1998).
62. Luxford C, Dean RT, Davies MJ. *Chem. Res. Toxicol.* 13: 665–672 (2000).
63. Caldecott KW. *Biochem. Soc. Trans.* 31: 247–251 (2003).
64. Moriya M, Zhang W, Johnson F, Grollman AP. *Proc. Natl. Acad. Sci. USA* 91: 11899–11903 (1994).
65. Shibutani S, Suzuki N, Matsumoto Y, Grollman AP. *Biochemistry* 35: 14992–14998 (1996).
66. Pandya GA, Moriya M. *Biochemistry* 35: 11487–11492 (1996).
67. Levine RL, Yang IY, Hossain M, Pandya GA, Grollman AP, Moriya M. *Cancer Res.* 60: 4098–4104 (2000).
68. Akasaka S, Guengerich FP. *Chem. Res. Toxicol.* 12: 501–507 (1999).
69. Langouet S, Muller M, Guengerich FP. *Biochemistry* 36: 6069–6079 (1997).
70. Fernandes PH, Wang H, Rizzo CJ, Lloyd RS. *Environ. Mol. Mutagen.* 42: 68–74 (2003).
71. Yang IY, Chan G, Miller H, Huang Y, Torres MC, Johnson F, Moriya M. *Biochemistry* 41: 13826–13832 (2002).
72. Yang IY, Johnson F, Grollman AP, Moriya M. *Chem. Res. Toxicol.* 15: 160–164 (2002).
73. de los Santos C, Zaliznyak T, Johnson F. *J. Biol. Chem.* 276: 9077–9082 (2001).
74. VanderVeen LA, Hashim MF, Shyr Y, Marnett LJ. *Proc. Natl. Acad. Sci. USA* 100: 14247–14252 (2003).
75. Yang Y, Nair J, Barbin A, Bartsch H. *Carcinogenesis* 21: 777–781 (2000).
76. Frank A, Seitz HK, Bartsch H, Frank N, Nair J. *Carcinogenesis* 25: 1027–1031 (2004).
77. Bartsch H, Nair J, Owen RW. *Carcinogenesis* 20: 2209–2218 (1999).
78. Schmid K, Nair J, Winde G, Velic I, Bartsch H. *Int. J. Cancer* 87: 1–4 (2000).
79. Nath RG, Chung FL. *Proc. Natl. Acad. Sci. USA* 91: 7491–7495 (1994).
80. Chung FL, Nath RG, Nagao M, Nishikawa A, Zhou GD, Randerath K. *Mutat. Res.* 424: 71–81 (1999).
81. Nair J, Barbin A, Velic I, Bartsch H. *Mutat. Res.* 424: 59–69 (1999).
82. Zhang Y, Chen SY, Hsu T, Santella RM. *Carcinogenesis* 23: 207–211 (2002).
83. Evans M, Dizdaroglu M, Cooke MS. *Rev. Mutat. Res.* 567: 1–61 (2004).
84. Rosenstein BS, Rosenstein RB, Zamansky GB. *J. Invest. Dermatol.* 98: 469–474 (1992).

6 Oxidative Damage to Nucleotide: Consequences and Preventive Mechanisms

Yoshimichi Nakatsu and Mutsuo Sekiguchi

1. Introduction

Reactive oxygen species (ROS), such as superoxide, hydrogen peroxide, hydroxyl radicals and singlet oxygen, are produced through normal cellular metabolism, and the formation of such radicals is further enhanced by ionizing radiation and various chemicals.[1,2] Nucleic acids exposed to oxygen radicals generate various modified bases, and more than 20 different types of oxidatively altered purines and pyrimidines have been detected.[3,4] Among them, 8-oxo-7, 8-dihydroguanine (8-oxoguanine) is the most abundant, and it seems to play a critical role in mutagenesis and in carcinogenesis.[5,6] Unlike other types of oxidative DNA damage, such as thymine glycol and 5′,8-purine cyclodeoxynucleoside,[7–9] 8-oxoguanine does not block DNA synthesis, rather it induces base mispairing. 8-Oxoguanine can pair with both cytosine and adenine during DNA synthesis, and this mispairing is considered to contribute significantly to the spontaneous mutations in genomic DNA.[10,11]

Studies on *Escherichia coli* mutator mutants revealed that cells possess elaborate mechanisms that can prevent mutations caused by oxidation of guanine residues of DNA. 8-Oxoguanine residues in DNA can be removed by MutM,[12–15] while MutY removes adenine mispaired with 8-oxoguanine.[16–19] As a result, MutM and MutY cooperatively act to prevent the mutagenesis caused by 8-oxoguanine.[20] In higher organisms, similar enzyme activities have been detected, which may account for the rapid elimination of 8-oxoguanine from chromosomal DNA. MUTYH has been identified as a mammalian MutY homolog.[21,22] MUTYH excises adenine and 2-hydroxyadenine, a form of oxidized adenine, paired with either guanine or 8-oxoguanine. Hirano *et al.*[22] generated *MUTYH*-null mouse embryonic stem (ES) cells carrying no adenine DNA glycosylase activity. The spontaneous mutation rate in the *MUTYH*-deficient ES cells increased twofold in comparison with wild type cells. There is no MutM homolog in either the human or mouse genome. However, an ortholog for yeast 8-oxoguanine DNA glycosylase, Ogg1, which is a functional counterpart of *E. coli* MutM, has been identified in both humans and mice. *OGG1*-deficient mice have been generated.[23–25] The animals accumulate abnormal levels of 8-oxoguanine in their genomes, and exhibit a moderately, but significantly, elevated spontaneous mutation rate.

The oxidation of guanine also occurs in the cellular nucleotide pool, and 8-oxo-dGTP, the oxidized form of dGTP, is the mutagenic substrate for DNA synthesis. It can be incorporated opposite either the adenine or cytosine residues of template DNA, thus resulting in A:T to C:G and G:C to T:A transversions.[26,27] However, in normally growing cells, the frequency of these types of mutations remains low, owing to the action of such enzymes degrading mutagenic substrates.[28,29] *E. coli* MutT hydrolyzes 8-oxo-dGTP to 8-oxo-dGMP, thereby preventing the misincorporation of 8-oxoguanine into DNA.[26] A similar enzyme activity has been detected in mammalian cells, and the protein responsible was named MTH1.[30–32] As the expression of human *MTH1* cDNA in *E. coli mutT*$^{-}$ cells significantly suppressed the frequency of spontaneous mutations in these cells, MTH1 may have the same antimutagenic ability as MutT. In order to elucidate the function of MTH1 in mammals, a targeted disruption of the *MTH1* gene has been performed.[33] The spontaneous mutation rate in the *MTH1*-deficient ES cells increased twofold in comparison with wild type cells and an elevated incidence of tumor formation was also observed in the liver, lung and stomach of the *MTH1*-deficient mice.[33] Therefore, MTH1 is considered to have an antimutagenic ability, to some degree, thus resulting in the suppression of spontaneous tumorigenesis in animals.

The spontaneous mutation rate observed in the *MTH1*-deficient cells is considerably lower than that in *E. coli mutT*$^{-}$ cells, in which the rate increased up to 1000-fold that seen in wild type cells.[34–36] This difference may be attributed to the difference in the mechanism for avoiding mutations caused by 8-oxoguanine incorporated into DNA between animals and bacteria. Alternatively, mammalian cells may have another mechanism that is able to efficiently eliminate 8-oxoguanine-containing nucleotides from the precursor pool. The human genome encodes at least 15 proteins that have a sequence, which is called the "MutT-signature", and is conserved through MutT-related proteins. Recently, Ishibashi *et al.*[37] found that human NUDT5, one of the MutT-related proteins, prevents mutations, caused by the oxidation of guanine nucleotides, by specifically degrading 8-oxo-dGDP to 8-oxo-dGMP. These findings have provided us with important insight into the mechanisms for removing mutagenic substrates from the nucleotide pool in mammalian cells.

2. Damage of Nucleotides by ROS

Free radicals attack the purine and pyrimidine bases primarily by the addition of •OH to the π bond of the bases, thus giving rise to the C4-OH-, C8-OH-adducts of purines, and the C-5-OH-, C-6-OH-adducts of pyrimidines, and resulting in a wide variety of modified bases. Some of them are unstable and breakdown to more stable products.[38]

The biological consequences of DNA lesions are determined by following factors; (1) the repair efficiency of an individual DNA lesion, (2) whether or not DNA polymerases can bypass a individual lesion (translesion synthesis), (3) whether a correct or incorrect base is inserted opposite the lesion in the DNA if translesion synthesis occurs. When DNA lesions are introduced by ROS, the lesions are primarily removed by cellular enzymes, thereby restoring the original nucleotide sequences. However, when DNA replication occurs before the lesion is removed, the blockage of the DNA replication fork by the lesion or translesion synthesis at the site of the lesion occurs. If the lesion completely blocks the progression of the DNA replication fork, it thus becomes a potentially lethal lesion. If the lesion can be bypassed by the DNA polymerase in the replication fork and an incorrect base is incorporated opposite the lesion, then such a lesion is potentially mutagenic.

In the case of damaged DNA precursors, another factor should be considered in order to determine the biological consequences of the damage. Damaged nucleotides appear to have no biological effect if they are not incorporated into DNA by DNA polymerases. Since a damaged nucleotide competes with the normal nucleotides and much larger amounts of normal nucleotides exist in cell, the incorporation efficiency of the damaged nucleotides is a key factor for evaluating their biological consequences. Therefore, the mutagenic potential of oxidized DNA precursors may be evaluated by determining the relative incorporation frequency in comparison to the normal pairing event which occurs during *in vitro* DNA synthesis using several types of DNA polymerases.

Maki and Sekiguchi[26] examined the incorporation of 8-oxo-dGTP by the *E. coli* DNA pol III using synthetic oligomers as templates. 8-Oxoguanine was inserted opposite adenine and cytosine with almost equal efficiency. A kinetic analysis showed that the incorporations of 8-oxoguanine opposite adenine were 30-fold less efficient than those of the normal pairing. Kinetic analyses of the incorporation of 8-oxo-dGTP were also performed with several other DNA polymerases including the *E. coli* DNA pol I, pol II, T7 DNA polymerase and HIV reverse transcriptase.[39,40] The misincorporation opposite adenine depended upon the DNA polymerase, and the ratio of the incorporation of 8-oxoguanine opposite adenine to that opposite cytosine also varied.

Cheng *et al.*[27] added 8-oxo-dGTP to the deoxyribonucleotides used for the gap-filling reaction by *E. coli* pol I Klenow fragment, and transfected the synthesized DNA into *E. coli* to analyze the mutations caused by 8-oxoguanine misincorporation. In this case, A to C transversions were almost exclusively detected. Similar results were obtained when the *E. coli* DNA pol III holoenzyme were used.[41] To determine whether the A:8-oxoguanine mispair can be proofread, Pavlov *et al.*[42] compared the fidelity of proofreading-proficient and proofreading-deficient Klenow and T4 DNA polymerases. Although the exonuclease activity of Klenow polymerase did not substantially reduce the overall misincorporation of 8-oxoguanine, the degree of misincorporation was lower for the proofreading-proficient T4 enzyme as compared to its proofreading-deficient derivative. These data suggest that the A:8-oxoguanine mispair can thus be proofread. They also examined the mutagenic potential of 8-oxo-dGTP with eukaryotic systems. The misincorporation of 8-oxoguanine opposite adenine was observed during the SV40 origin-dependent replication of double-stranded DNA in HeLa cell extracts. In these experiments, the replicated DNA was transfected into *E. coli* and the induced mutations were analyzed. When present during replication at a concentration equal to those for the four normal dNTPs, 8-oxo-dGTP was at least 13-fold more mutagenic for A:T to C:G transversions than a 100-fold excess of normal dGTP.

Inoue *et al.*[43] developed a new evaluation method using *E. coli* as a host. This method involves the direct incorporation of a damaged nucleotide into $CaCl_2$-treated *E. coli* cells, followed by the detection of *lacI*$^-$ and *lacO*^{c} mutants. The treatment with 8-oxo-dGTP increased the frequency of substitution mutations, in comparison to the treatment with either dGTP or dATP. An A:T to C:G transversion was most frequently found in the 8-oxo-dGTP-induced substitution mutations (90% of the substitution mutations).

The same type of analyses were performed to evaluate the mutagenic potentials of other oxidatively damaged DNA precursors.[39,41,44–48] Deoxyribonucleoside triphosphate forms containing damaged bases depicted in Fig. 1 were shown to be incorporated into DNA, to some extent, and some of them are potentially mutagenic. Among them, 8-oxo-dGTP is most abundant and highly mutagenic. In addition, the biological significance of 8-oxo-dGTP has been well established in *E. coli* and the defense systems against mutagenesis caused by this damaged nucleotide have been well characterized. Furthermore, recent studies have provided evidence that 8-oxo-dGTP is involved in mutagenesis as well as carcinogenesis in mammals. In the following section, therefore, we will focus upon the avoidance mechanisms for 8-oxoguanine-related mutagenesis.

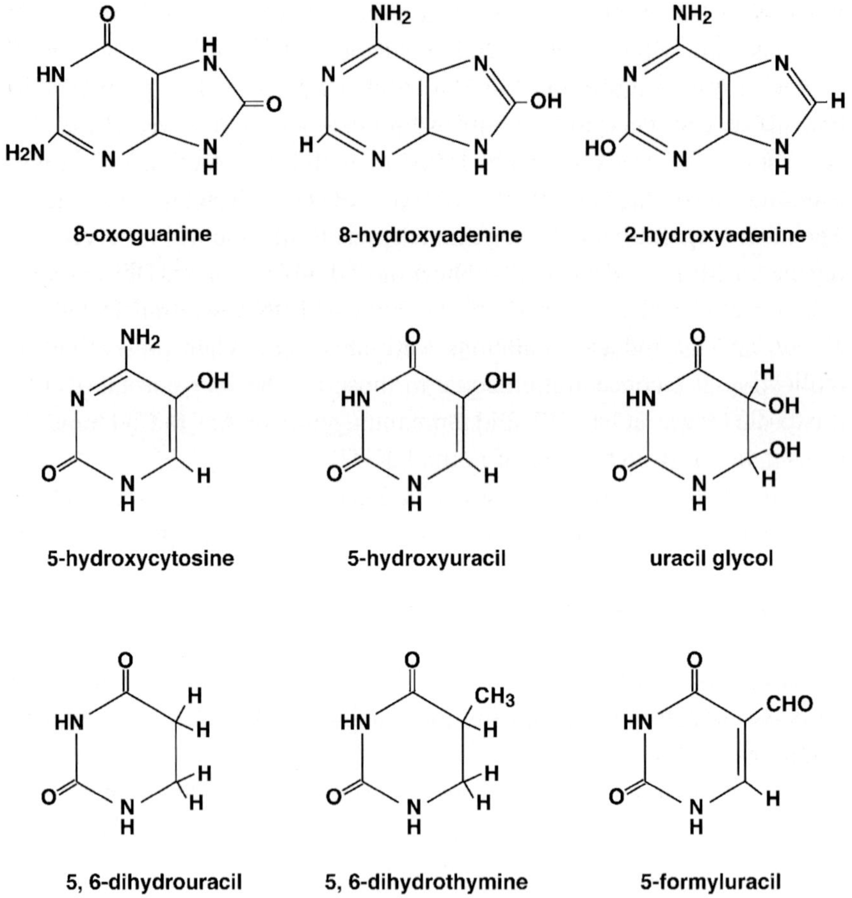

8-oxoguanine 8-hydroxyadenine 2-hydroxyadenine

5-hydroxycytosine 5-hydroxyuracil uracil glycol

5, 6-dihydrouracil 5, 6-dihydrothymine 5-formyluracil

Fig. 1. The structure of oxidized purines and pyrimidines. Deoxyribonucleoside-5′-triphosphate derivatives of these modified bases can be incorporated into DNA by DNA poymerases. The nucleotides containing these modified bases, except for 5,6-dihydrothymine, cause base-mispairing during DNA replication.

3. Error Avoidance Mechanism from Oxidative Damage

3.1. *Role of E. coli MutT in error avoidance*

The mutation frequency in *E. coli mutT*$^{-}$ cells is 1000 times greater than that of wild-type cells. *MutT* is one of the first mutators found in organisms[49] and specifically induces A:T to C:G transversion mutations.[34] As a consequence of this unidirectional mutator activity, *mutT*$^-$ cells have increased the GC content in the chromosomal DNA.[50] Akiyama *et al.*[51] cloned the *mutT* gene and, based on a sequence analysis, identified a protein with 129 amino acid residues. MutT protein was purified to physical homogeneity and it was shown to have nucleoside triphosphatase activity.[52] Using an *in vitro* DNA synthesis system, Akiyama *et al.*[35] demonstrated that MutT specifically prevents the misincorporation of dGMP onto the poly(dA)/oligo$(dT)_{20}$ template-primer. Subsequently Maki and Sekiguchi[26] found that the nucleotide misincorporated opposite the adenine residue of the template is not dGMP but rather its oxidized form, 8-oxo-dGMP. When 8-oxo-dGTP was added to an *in vitro* DNA replication system, 8-oxo-dGMP was incorporated opposite the cytosine and adenine residues of the template, with almost equal frequencies. MutT therefore prevents the misincorporation of 8-oxoguanine into DNA, by degrading 8-oxo-dGTP to 8-oxo-dGMP, an unusable form for DNA synthesis.

Figure 2 shows the preventive mechanisms for the occurrence of mutations and phenotypic alterations caused by guanine oxidation in *E. coli.* Principally, MutT can prevent both A:T to C:G and G:C to T:A transversions by eliminating 8-oxo-dGTP from the nucleotide pool. For the control of spontaneous mutagenesis in *E. coli* cells, MutM and MutY also play a role, but their functions in the A:T to C:G pathway differ from those in the G:C to T:A pathway.[36,53] When 8-oxo-dGTP is incorporated opposite cytosine, MutM removes 8-oxoguanine and MutY removes adenine from the A: 8-oxoguanine pair that may be formed in the next round of DNA replication. The cooperative action of MutM and MutY suppresses the G:C to T:A transversion caused by 8-oxoguanine misincorporation, as in the case of the direct oxidation of guanine in DNA. The MutY protein tends to instead promote the fixation of A:T to C:G transversion when 8-oxo-dGTP is incorporated opposite adenine. As a result, A:T to C:G transversion predominantly occurs in *MutT*-deficient bacterial cells.

The *E. coli* MutT protein cleaves 8-oxo-GTP as efficiently as does 8-oxo-dGTP. MutT, indeed, suppresses the misincorporation of 8-oxo-GTP into RNA, thus avoiding the production of abnormal proteins.[54] In the case of the direct oxidation of guanine in RNA, cells must have another mechanism to eliminate oxidized RNA. *E. coli* polynucleotide phosphorylase

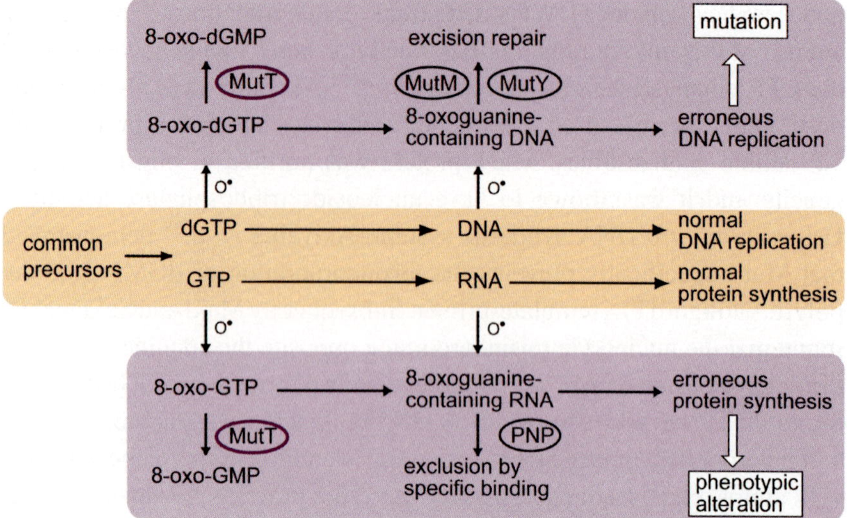

Fig. 2. Preventive mechanisms for the occurrence of mutation and phenotypic alteration caused by guanine oxidation in *E. coli*. This scheme is based on the results of Michaels *et al.*[53] Tajiri *et al.*[36] Taddei *et al.*[54] and Hayakawa *et al.*[55] O• denotes an oxidative reaction. The reactions in the yellow-colored area represent those occurring in normal cells while the reactions in the purple-colored area show those for an oxidized state.

(Pnp) has been shown to bind specifically to 8-oxoguanine-containing RNA.[55] *Pnp*-deficient *E. coli* cells exhibit a hyper-resistance to the killing effect of paraquot, a strong oxidizing reagent. The binding of Pnp protein to 8-oxoguanine-containing RNA is thus considered to inhibit cell growth, probably due to withdrawal of such RNA from the translational machinery. The Pnp may thus play a role in distinguishing oxidized RNA molecules from normal ones, thus contributing to a high fidelity of translation.

3.2. *Mammalian MTH1 with 8-oxo-dGTPase activity*

An enzyme with an activity similar to *E. coli* MutT was purified to apparent physical homogeneity from Jurkat cells, a human T-cell leukemia cell line.[30,31] The substrate specificity of the enzyme was examined using various forms of ^{32}P-labeled dNTPs. Although dGTP and dATP can also be hydrolyzed to the corresponding nucleoside monophosphates, the product yields were only about 5% of those with 8-oxo-dGTP. Neither TTP nor dCTP was hydrolyzed by the enzyme. The apparent *K*m of this enzyme for hydrolysis of 8-oxo-dGTP was 70 times lower than that for the degradation of dGTP, whereas the maximal reaction rates observed with both substrates were similar. Based on the partial amino acid sequence determined with the purified human 8-oxo-dGTPase protein, a cDNA for human enzyme was cloned and the nucleotide sequence was determined.[31] The molecular mass of the protein, as calculated from the predicted amino acid sequence, was 17.9 kDa, a value close to that estimated from an analysis of SDS-PAGE. After the cDNA was expressed in *E. coli* $mutT^-$ cells the increased spontaneous mutation frequency decreased considerably. Similar but more striking suppressive effects were observed when mouse or rat cDNA was expressed in the $mutT^-$ cells.[56,57] Therefore, mammalian 8-oxo-dGTPase functions in *E. coli* cells to prevent mutations caused by the accumulation of 8-oxo-dGTP in the nucleotide pool.

The mammalian gene for 8-oxo-dGTPase has been named *MTH1* for **m**ut**T h**omolog **1** (Fig. 3). The transfection of human *MTH1* cDNA caused a significant reduction in the 8-oxoguanine content of DNA in mouse embryonic fibroblasts as well as in tumor cells, with or without H_2O_2 treatment.[58–60] As MTH1 decreases both the steady-state and oxidant-induced 8-oxoguanine levels in DNA, the endogenous oxidation of the deoxynucleotide pool is a definite source of DNA damage and the deoxynucleotide pool is a significant target for exogenous oxidative damage.

4. Structure and Function of MTH1

4.1. *Structure of MTH1*

Human MTH1 and *E. coli* MutT proteins are similar in size and there is a certain degree of sequence homology in these proteins. The genes for analogous functions were isolated from *Proteus vulgaris* and *Streptococcus pneumoniae*, bacteria distantly related to *E. coli*.[61,62] The products of the latter two genes possess an enzyme activity which can specifically degrade dGTP to dGMP and they are also structurally and functionally related to the *E. coli* MutT protein. Most of the identical residues are in a region corresponding to the 23 residues from G37 to G59 of *E. coli* MutT, known as the MutT signature.[63] Homologs of human MTH1

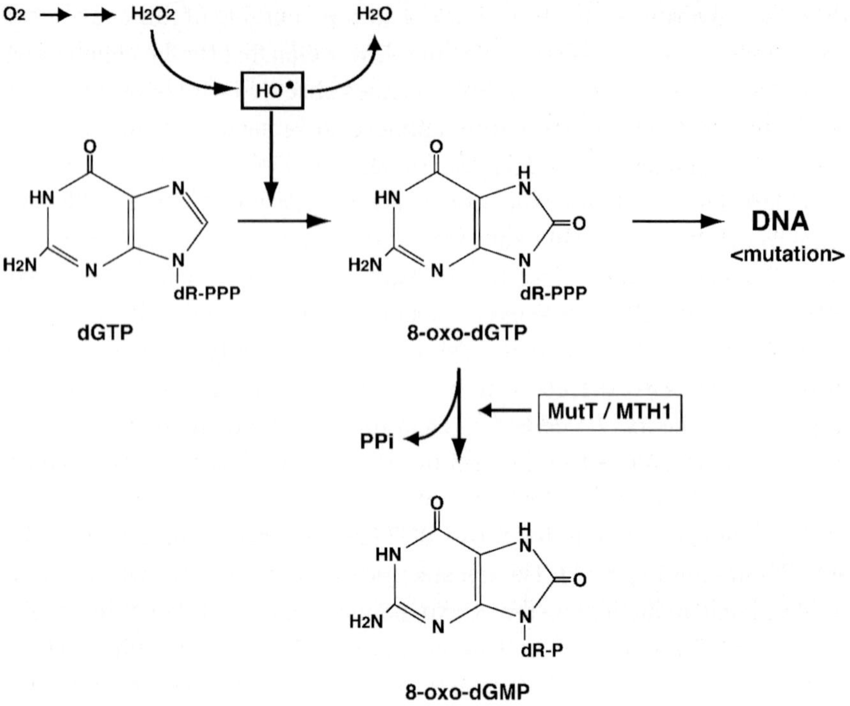

Fig. 3. Action of *E. coli* MutT and mammalian MTH1. Hydroxyl radicals ($OH^{\bullet}$) attack dGTP, thus resulting in the generation of 8-oxo-dGTP in DNA precursor pool. 8-Oxo-dGTP can be hydrolyzed to 8-oxo-dGMP by MutT and MTH1 in *E. coli* and mammalian cells, respectively.

protein were identified in the mouse and rat based on the isolation of cDNAs.[56,57] Both proteins comprise 156 amino acid residues, as was the case for the human MTH1 protein, and amino acid sequences are highly conserved. The alignment of the sequences of these six proteins shows that all carry a highly conserved sequence in nearly the same region, thus corresponding to amino acids 36 to 58 for human MTH1. Ten of 23 amino acid residues in this region are identical, hence this probably constitutes an active center for the enzyme. The 23-residue sequence is a sole conserved sequence among all MutT and MTH1 homologs with 8-oxo-dGTPase, and of the many other proteins with the MutT signature so far identified, some hydrolyze various nucleotide derivatives, such as dATP, diadenosine oligophosphates, NADH, ADP-ribose, and GDP-mannose.[64–66] Furthermore, a diphosphoinositol polyphosphate phosphohydrolase, which hydrolyzes a non-related polyphosphate, also contains the 23-residue sequence.[67] A chimeric protein, in which the 23-residue sequence of MTH1 was replaced with that of MutT, retains its capacity to hydrolyze 8-oxo-dGTP,[68] thereby indicating that the 23-residue sequences of MTH1 and MutT are functionally and structurally equivalent and thus constitute functional modules.

The secondary structure of *E. coli* MutT and human MTH1 has been determined by multidimensional heteronuclear NMR spectroscopy.[69–73] Figure 4 shows the amino acid sequence alignment and the secondary structure of MTH1 and MutT. Although the sequence identity between the two proteins is less than 10% outside the MutT signature, the overall folds of these proteins are quite similar. In particular, the central part of MTH1, comprising β-strands A, D, C and α-helix I, highly resembles the corresponding part of MutT. The largest difference is the presence of β-hairpin comprising strands F, G and their connecting loop in MTH1, which is absent in MutT. The β-strand F is connected to β-strand C through a main-chain hydrogen bond network, thus resulting in the formation of a continuous five-stranded β-sheet (β-strand A, D, C, F and G). The additional β-strands in MTH1 interact with α-helix II, thus leading to differences in the orientation of the αII and N-terminal half of loop L1, in comparison to those of MutT.[73] The deletion of the β-strand G totally abolished the enzymatic activity of MTH1,[74] thus indicating that this structure is essential for the enzyme activity of MTH1. Chemical shift perturbation experiments with 8-oxo-dGDP suggested that the nucleotide-binding site resides in a pocket that is formed between the five-stranded β-sheet, α-helix II and the hairpin loop.[73] The nucleotide-binding pocket is juxtaposed to exposed residues (R51, E52, E53, E56) in the MutT signiture, which probably binds to the phosphate groups of the substrate.[75] The pocket of MTH1 is much deeper and narrower than that of MutT because of the presence in part of the pocket wall defined by residues F27, N33 from loop L1 and W117, D119 from loop L4. These residues make contact with the residues from β-hairpin composed of βF-loop-βG. Therefore, the different shape of the MTH1 pocket can be attributed, at least in part, to the presence of the β-hairpin.[73]

Unlike *E. coli* MutT, MTH1 efficiently hydrolyzes two forms of oxidized dATP, 2-hydroxy (OH)-dATP and 8-oxo-dATP, as well as 8-oxo-dGTP.[76]

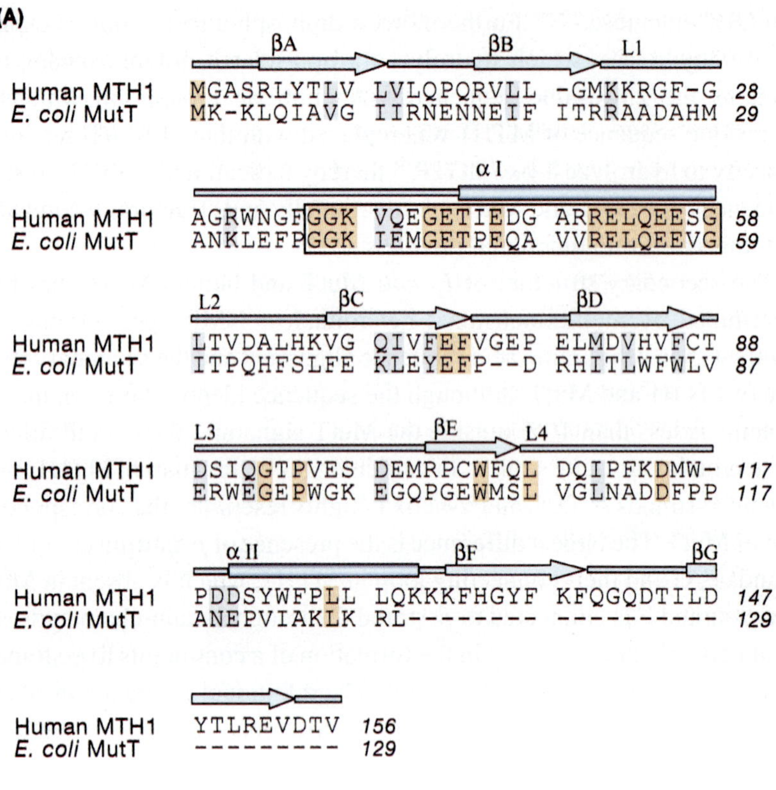

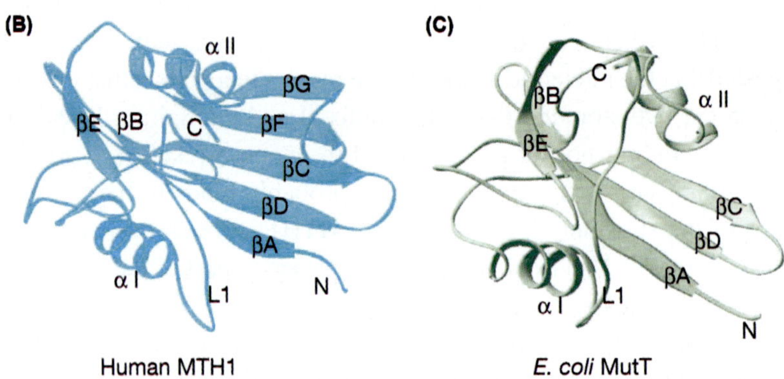

Fig. 4. The sequence alignment and structures of MTH1 and MutT. The amino acid sequence alignment of human MTH1 and *E. coli* MutT is shown in (A). Conserved residues are shown in yellow, homologus residues in gray. The secondary structure elements of MTH1 are indicated on the top and MutT-signature is boxed. Ribbon representations of MTH1 and MutT are shown in B and C, respectively.

MTH1 also hydrolyzes oxidized ribonucleotides, 2-OH-ATP, 8-oxo-ATP, and 8-oxo-GTP.[77] The substrate specificity of MTH1 for oxidized purine nucleoside triphosphates was investigated by mutation analyses based on sequence and structural comparison with the *E. coli* MutT, which hydrolyzes only 8-oxo-dGTP and 8-oxoGTP but not oxidized forms of dATP or ATP.[73,74] W117A mutation significantly increased the *K*m for both 8-oxo-dGTP and 2-OH-dATP. However, the W117Y mutant exhibited the wild-type level of 2-OH-dATPase activity but drastically decreased the activity for 8-oxo-dGTP. The D119A mutant had about half of the wild-type activity for 8-oxo-dGTP, but it showed almost no activity for 2-OH-dATP.[74] The N33A mutation decreased the activity for 2-OH-dATP to 5% of that seen for the wild-type activity, whereas the N33E mutant showed a relative activity of 53%. The N33A mutant showed 14% of the wild-type 8-oxo-dGTPase activity, whereas the N33E mutation totally abolished the activity.[73] These results suggested that three of the pocket-forming residues (N33, W117, and D119) of MTH1 thus appeared to contribute to substrate recognition.

4.2. *Tumorigenesis and mutagenesis in mice lacking MTH1*

Mouse lines defective in the *MTH1* gene have been established to investigate the role of MTH1 in spontaneous tumorigenesis as well as in mutagenesis. The mouse *MTH1* gene is composed of five exons and spans about 10 kb.[78] The third exon containing the initiation codon and the adjacent intron regions were replaced with a *neo* cassette.[33] $MTH1^{-/-}$ mice are apparently normal, but have a high susceptibility for spontaneous tumorigenesis.[33] At the age of 18 months, more tumors were found in the lungs, livers and stomach of $MTH1^{-/-}$ mice than in $MTH1^{+/+}$ mice (Fig. 5). The elevated incidence of tumor formation in the liver of $MTH1^{-/-}$ mice correlated well with the highest content of MTH1 protein in this organ of the wild-type mouse.[57] These observations indicate that the intracellular level of MTH1 is an important factor in determining the susceptibility of mice to tumor induction by endogenous oxidative damage.

$MTH1^{-/-}$ ES cell lines exhibited an approximately twofold higher mutation rate, as compared with the parental ES cells, when scoring mutations in the *Hprt* gene in the mouse genome. Using a transgenic mouse

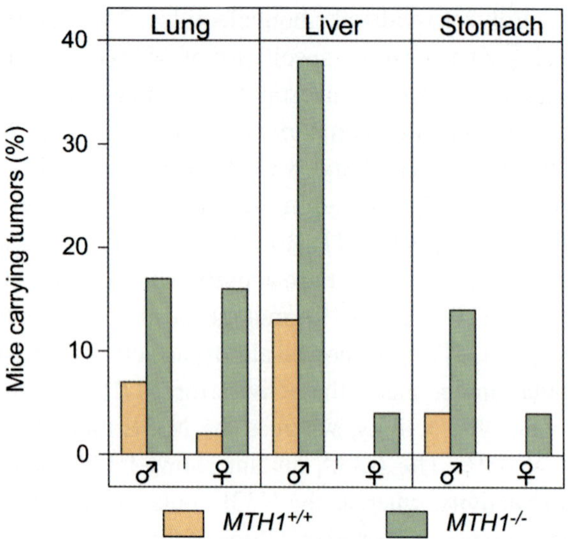

Fig. 5. Comparison of tumor incidences of wild-type and *MTH1*-deficient mice. The histogram shows tumor incidence of $MTH1^{+/+}$ and $MTH1^{-/-}$ mice.[33]

harboring *E. coli rpsL* gene as a reporter, Egashira *et al.*[79] measured mutation frequency of $MTH1^{-/-}$ mice. In this case, the net frequency of mutation showed no apparent increase in $MTH1^{-/-}$ mice, in comparison to the $MTH1^{+/+}$ mice. However, some differences exist between these two genotypes in class- and site-distributions of the $rpsL^{-}$ mutations recovered from the mice. The frequency of single-base frameshifts at mononucleotide runs (a sequence composed of single nucleotide) was 3.4-fold higher in the spleens of the $MTH1^{-/-}$ mice than in those of wild-type mice. Since the elevated incidence of single-base frameshifts at the mononucleotide runs is a hallmark of the defect in MSH2-dependent mismatch repair system, this weak site-specific mutator effect of $MTH1^{-/-}$ mutation could be attributed to a partial sequestration of the mismatch repair function that may act to correct mispairs with the oxidized nucleotides. Interestingly, in a mismatch repair-deficient background, a significant increase in the frequency of G:C to T:A transversions was observed in $MTH1^{-/-}$ mice, thus suggesting an involvement of mismatch repair in the suppression of G:C to T:A transversions in a *MTH1*-deficient condition. Consistent with these observations, Russo *et al.*[60] demonstrated that an overexpression of human MTH1 brought about a significant reduction in the genetic instability of mismatch repair-deficient mouse embryonic fibroblasts and human tumor cell lines. These observations imply that MTH1 thus plays a role in preventing the occurrence of mutations in mammalian cells.

MTH1 hydrolyzes 8-oxo-dGTP and 2-OH-dATP to prevent the incorporation of these mutagenic substrates into DNA, thus avoiding transversion mutations in mammalian cells. Unlike *MutT*-deficient *E. coli*, an increase in frequency of A:T to C:G transversion was not evident in $MTH1^{-/-}$ mice. An excess of A:T to C:G transversion in MutT-deficient *E. coli* is attributed to MutY function, by which mispaired adenine in either template or nascent DNA strand is removed.[36,53] MUTYH, a mammalian counterpart of MutY, has been shown to be associated with PCNA and it could only remove mispaired adenine in the nascent DNA strand in mammalian cells.[80] It is possible that other DNA repair enzyme(s), which are as yet still unidentified, may remove the 8-oxoguanine incorporated opposite adenine in mammalian cells.

4.3. *Function of MTH1 in mitochondria*

In human cells, MTH1 is mostly localized in the cytoplasm with approximately 17% in the mitochondria.[81] In eukaryotic cells, a pool of dNTP for nuclear DNA replication is mainly present in the cytosol.[82] Mitochondria, which preserve a pool of dNTP for mitochondrial DNA synthesis, consist of more than 10% of the total intracellular dNTP. The mitochondrial respiratory chain located on inner membranes is a major site for the initiation of lipid peroxidation, which can lead to oxidation of the guanine to 8-oxoguanine. DNA and dNTP in the mitochondrial pool may thus be exposed to a greater degree of oxidative stress than is the case in the nucleus. MTH1, localized in the matrix of the mitochondria, may thus help to maintain the integrity of the mitochondrial genome.

MTH1-null mouse embryo fibroblasts are highly susceptible to cell dysfunction and death caused by exposure to H_2O_2.[59] The insulted cells showed morphological features of pyknosis and an accumulation of electron-dense deposits was observed in their mitochondria, thus indicating mitochondrial dysfunction. A high performance liquid chromatography-tandem mass spectrometry analysis and immunofluorescence microscopy revealed a continuous accumulation of 8-oxoguanine both in nuclear and mitochondrial DNA after exposure to H_2O_2. The mitochondria dysfunction as well as cell death caused by the H_2O_2 treament were effectively suppressed by the expression of wild type human MTH1. Interestingly, the expression of mutant MTH1, defective in either 8-oxo-dGTPase or 2-OH-dATPase activity, partially suppressed such cell death. MTH1 may thus protect cells from H_2O_2-induced mitochondrial dysfunction and cell death by hydrolyzing oxidized purine nucleotides including 8-oxo-dGTP and 2-OH-dATP.

5. MTH1-Related Proteins in Mammalian Cells

As described above, the levels of the increase in the frequency of spontaneous mutations due to the lack of MutT-related functions considerably differ in *E. coli* and mammalian cells. The frequency of spontaneous mutations detected in mouse *MTH1*$^{-/-}$ cells is approximately twice that detected in *MTH1*$^{+/+}$ cells,[33] whereas the mutation frequency in *E. coli mutT*$^-$ cells is 1000 times greater than that of wild-type cells.[34–36] These facts give rise to the idea that mammalian cells may have additional enzyme(s) or mechanism(s) which are able to efficiently eliminate 8-oxoguanine-containing nucleotides from the precursor pool. 8-Oxo-dGMP, which is formed by the action of MTH1, cannot be used for DNA synthesis, as the cellular guanylate kinase enzyme is completely inactive for 8-oxoguanine-containing nucleotides.[83] However, 8-oxo-dGDP, which is produced by the direct oxidation of dGDP, and also by the enzymatic cleavage of 8-oxo-dGTP, is readily phosphorylated by nucleoside diphosphate kinase to generate 8-oxo-dGTP. In addition, 8-oxo-dGDP inhibits the MTH1 reaction to hydrolyze 8-oxo-dGTP. Considering these facts, it seems important for mammalian cells to be able to degrade 8-oxo-dGDP to monophosphate.

Recently, two proteins have been identified to considerably suppress the high mutability of *E. coli mutT*$^-$ cells when expressed in such bacterial cells.[37,84]

5.1. *NUDT5 with 8-oxo-dGDPase*

Based on the 23-amino acid sequence that is conserved in MutT-related proteins,[63,68] Ishibashi *et al.*[37] isolated cDNA clones using the BLAST programme. Among several candidates, NUDT5 was found to have the highest level of similarity to MutT-related proteins. Thirty (23.2%) and 27 (17.3%) amino acid residues of NUDT5 are identical to those of MutT and MTH1, respectively. The amino acid residues that are conserved in these three proteins were found to be located almost exclusively in the 23-residue conserved sequence, which is essential for the hydrolysis of a phosphodiester bond in Nudix (nucleotide diphosphate linked moiety X) and in diphosphoinositol derivatives.[63,68,73] A comparison of the amino acid sequences of *E. coli* MutT, human MTH1 and NUDT5 proteins is shown in Fig. 6. In the highly conserved regions, two of the amino acid residues of NUDT5 (A96 and L98) differ from those of MutT and MTH1. The glycine residue (G37) of MutT, which corresponds to A96 of NUDT5, is essential for the 8-oxo-dGTPase activity, as exchanges of this residue to any of the other 19 amino acids resulted in a loss of enzyme activity.[85] These amino acid residues may be required for the substrate specificities of the enzymes.

NUDT5 was purified as a His-tagged protein expressed in *E. coli*, and the enzyme activities were measured using 8-oxo-dGDP and 8-oxo-dGTP. When the products were analyzed by high-performance liquid chromatography, it was found that NUDT5 efficiently degrades 8-oxo-dGDP to

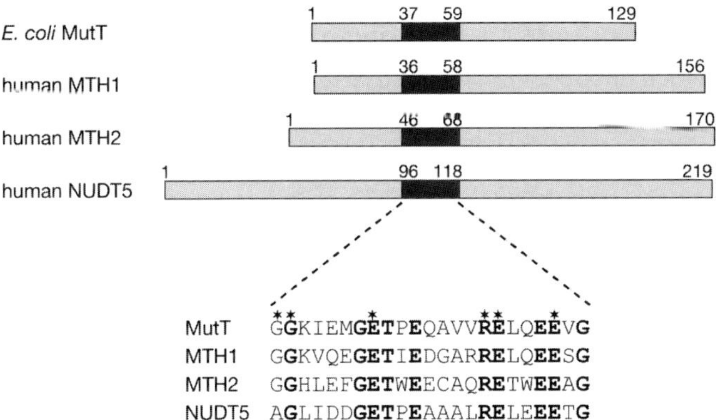

Fig. 6. MutT-related proteins. Comparison of the amino acid sequences of *E. coli* MutT and human MTH1, MTH2, and NUDT5 is shown. The 23-residue of the MutT signatures from these proteins are shown. The residues conserved in all four proteins are indicated in bold letters. The essential residues for MutT catalytic activities are indicated by asterisks above the columns.[68,85]

Table 1. Substrate specificity of human NUDT5 protein.

Substrate	*K*m (μM)	Vmax*	Vmax/*K*m*
8-Oxo-dGDP	0.77	1.0	100
dGDP	7.1	3.1	32
8-Oxo-dGTP	63	0.06	0.07
dGTP	120	0.55	0.35
dADP	11	0.70	4.9
dTDP	13	0.34	2.0
dCTP	130	0.12	0.07

*Relative values are shown. These data were taken from Ishibashi *et al.*[37]

its monophosphate form. Similar results were obtained with an authentic NUDT5 protein, which was affinity-purified with anti-NUDT5 IgG. The kinetic parameters of the NUDT5 enzyme were determined for the hydrolysis of several nucleotides (Table 1). The *K*m for the hydrolysis of 8-oxo-dGDP is ten times lower than that for dGDP, which is the second best substrate for the enzyme. 8-Oxo-dGTP is hydrolyzed by NUDT5 only at very low levels under these conditions, but when a large amount of NUDT5 was used in the reaction, the cleavage of 8-oxo-dGTP was detected, for which the apparent *K*m was 63 μM. It should be noted that NUDT5 has a *K*m of 0.77 μM for 8-oxo-dGDP, which is considerably lower than those for ADP sugars (32 μM for ADP-ribose, and higher values for other ADP sugars), which have previously been identified as substrates.[86] These results indicated that 8-oxo-dGDP is a specific substrate for NUDT5.

To examine the biological significance of the cleavage of 8-oxo-dGDP, Ishibashi *et al.*[37] expressed the *NUDT5* cDNA in *mutT*-deficient tester strain (CC101T), in which A:T to C:G transversion can be specifically detected.[32] Numerous papillae were formed in the cells that carried the vector plasmid without cDNA, and this formation of papillae was then almost completely suppressed when a plasmid carrying the *NUDT5* cDNA was introduced into these cells. A fluctuation test indicated that the mutation rate in $mutT^-$ cells is almost 1000-fold higher than that in wild-type cells. This increased mutation rate was then reduced to the wild-type level by the introduction of *NUDT5* cDNA into $mutT^-$ cells (Fig. 7). These results show that human NUDT5 can function in *E. coli* to clean up the nucleotide pool.

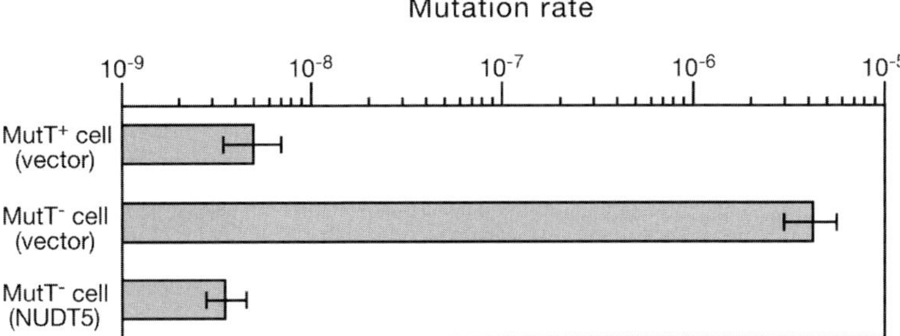

Fig. 7. A suppression of mutation by the expression of human NUDT5. Mutation rates, as determined by *lacZ* reversion, in three independent experiments. $MutT^+$ and $MutT^-$ cells are *E. coli* strains CC101 and CC101T, respectively, and carry either pQE30 (vector) or PQE30::NUDT5 (cDNA).

5.2. *MTH2 with 8-oxo-dGTPase*

Cai *et al.*[84] found a mouse cDNA clone with a 510-base open reading frame (ORF), potentially encoding a 170 amino acid residue sequence. This ORF had a 24% and 26% amino acid sequence identity with mMTH1 and MutT, respectively. The cloned mouse MTH2 (mMTH2) cDNA was expressed in *E. coli mutT*$^-$ cells and the protein was purified. The purified mMTH2 protein hydrolyzes 8-oxo-dGTP to 8-oxo-dGMP, with apparent *K*m of 32 μM. The expression of the cDNA reduced significantly the elevated level of spontaneous mutation frequency of *E. coli mutT*$^-$ cells. MTH2 thus has a potential to protect the genetic material from the untoward effects of endogenous oxygen radicals. MTH2 may therefore act as an MTH1 redundancy factor.

6. Exclusion of Mutagenic Nucleotides from the DNA Precursor Pool

In mammalian cells, at least three proteins have been identified to degrade 8-oxoguanine-containing deoxyribonucleotides, the mutagenic substrate for DNA synthesis. The substrate specificities of these MutT-related proteins are listed in Table 2. In *E. coli* cells, MutT protein, which has a potent 8-oxo-dGTPase activity, is almost solely responsible for reducing the mutagenic nucleotide level, on the basis of the finding that *mutT*$^-$ mutants show

Table 2. Substrate specificities of MutT-related proteins.

Enzyme	Substrate	*K*m (μM)	Reference
E. coli MutT	8-Oxo-dGTP	0.081	(1)
	dGTP	1100	
Human MTH1	8-Oxo-dGTP	12.5	(2)
	dGTP	870	
	2-OH-dATP	8.3	(3)
	8-OH-dATP	13.9	
Human MTH2	8-Oxo-dGTP	32	(4)
	dGTP	75	
Human NUDT5	8-Oxo-dGTP	63	(5)
	8-Oxo-dGDP	0.77	
	dGTP	120	

These values were taken from (1) Ito *et al.*,[87] (2) Mo *et al.*,[30] (3) Fujikawa *et al.*,[76] (4) Cai *et al.*,[84] and (5) Ishibashi *et al.*[37]

a 1000-fold higher frequency of spontaneous mutations, as compared with wild-type cells. In contrast, *MTH1*$^{-/-}$ ES cell lines exhibited an approximately twofold higher mutation rate, as compared with the parental ES cells. This difference may be due to the ability of the two types of enzymes to cleave 8-oxo-dGTP. The *K*m values of MutT and MTH1 for 8-oxo-dGTP cleavage are 0.081 and 12.5, respectively.[30,87]

MTH1 has a broader substrate specificity than *E. coli* MutT. MTH1 hydrolyzes 8-oxo-dATP, 2-OH-dATP and 2-OH-ATP as well as 8-oxo-dGTP, and exhibits a higher affinity to 2-hydroxyadenine-containing nucleotides.[76,77] This is in contrast to MutT, which acts on 8-oxoguanine-containing nucleotides alone. Therefore, MTH1 with a broader substrate specificity and NUDT5, which has a higher affinity to the 8-oxoguanine-containing nucleotides substrate, may have overlapping but somewhat different roles for cleaning up the precursor pool in mammalian cells. MTH2 may participate, to some extent, in reducing the amount of 8-oxoguanine-containing deoxyribonucleotides in the DNA precursor pool.

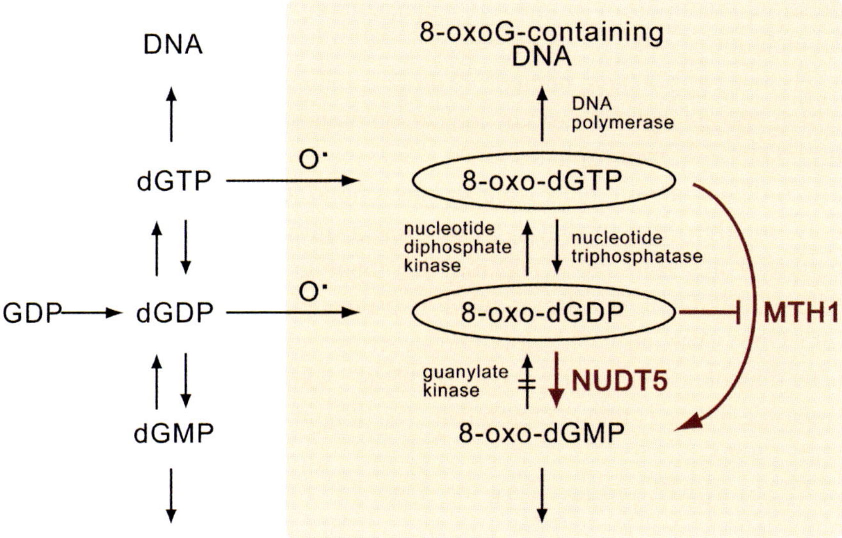

Fig. 8. A model for the exclusion of 8-oxoguanine-containing deoxyribonucleotides from the DNA precursor pool in mammalian cells. 8-Oxo-dGTP and 8-oxo-dGDP, which are produced by the oxidation of dGTP and dGDP, respectively, are interconverted by the actions of nucleoside diphosphate kinase and nucleoside triphosphatase. 8-Oxo-dGTP is misincorporated into DNA by DNA polymerase to yield mutations. NUDT5 and MTH1 degrade 8-oxo-dGDP and 8-oxo-dGTP, respectively, thus producing 8-oxo-dGMP, which is an unusable form for DNA synthesis. As the activity of MTH1 is inhibited by 8-oxo-dGDP, NUDT5 works in two ways: first, to reduce the amount of substrate for 8-oxo-dGTP synthesis and, second, to promote the cleavage of 8-oxo-dGTP by MTH1. O• denotes an oxidative reaction.

Figure 8 shows a model for the exclusion of 8-oxoguanine-containing deoxyribonucleotides from the DNA precursor pool in mammalian cells. The enzymatic conversion of ribonucleotides to deoxyribonucleotides occurs at the level of nucleoside diphosphate, and ribonucleotide reductase, the enzyme responsible, has a relatively broad substrate specificity. Four types of naturally occurring ribonucleotides, ADP, GDP, CDP and UDP, are converted to the corresponding deoxyribonucleotides by a single species of reductase enzyme.[88] However, this enzyme is inactive on the 8-oxoguanine-containing nucleotide, as revealed with mouse ribonucleotide reductase.[89] This implies that 8-oxoguanine-containing deoxyribonucleotides must be generated at the site of formation for deoxyribonucleotides or in the deoxyribonucleotide pool.

Human cells contain nucleoside diphosphate kinase, an enzyme activity which phosphorylates various nucleoside diphosphates to the corresponding nucleoside triphosphates.[90] This enzyme can convert 8-oxo-dGDP to 8-oxo-dGTP, although the rate of phosphorylation of 8-oxo-dGDP was only one-third that of dGDP.[83] As a result, in addition to the direct oxidation of dGTP, 8-oxo-dGTP may be generated by the phosphorylation of 8-oxo-dGDP. Once 8-oxo-dGTP is produced, this can be incorporated into DNA. Various DNA polymerases from eukaryotes and prokaryotes have the potential to utilize 8-oxo-dGTP as a substrate.[26,27,42] The action of 8-oxo-dGTPase is thus a prerequisite for obtaining a high fidelity of DNA replication.

8-Oxo-dGMP, produced by the action of 8-oxo-dGTPase, cannot be rephosphorylated by cellular enzymes. Human guanylate kinase, which phosphorylates both GMP and dGMP to the corresponding nucleoside diphosphates, is totally inactive for 8-oxo-dGMP.[83] This would provide another basis for excluding this mutagenic substrate from the DNA precursor.

8-Oxo-dGMP is dephosphorylated to yield the corresponding nucleoside, 8-oxodeoxyguanosine. Nucleosides are readily transported through the cell membrane, and extracellular nucleosides can be excreted into the urine. The dephosphorylation of 8-oxo-dGMP may therefore be an essential step for the excretion of 8-oxoguanine-containing compounds. The enzyme that catalyzes this reaction, 8-oxo-dGMPase, was partially purified from an extract of human Jurkat cells, and the mode of action was elucidated.[83] 8-Oxo-dGMP is the preferred substrate of the enzyme, and other nucleoside monophosphates are cleaved albeit at significantly lower rates.

MTH1 and NUDT5 have opposite preferences for substrates; MTH1 degrades 8-oxo-dGTP, but not 8-oxo-dGDP, whereas NUDT5 cleaves 8-oxo-dGDP, but not 8-oxo-dGTP. As these nucleotides are interconvertible within a cell, NUDT5 can replace MutT function. 8-Oxo-dGDP can be phosphorylated to 8-oxo-dGTP by nucleoside diphosphate kinase, and 8-oxo-dGTP is cleaved to 8-oxo-dGDP by nucleoside triphosphatase.[30] Therefore, two types of enzymes seem to function; MTH1 specifically hydrolyses 8-oxo-dGTP, and NUDT5 cleaves 8-oxo-dGDP. Taking into account the kinetic parameters for these enzymatic reactions, NUDT5 may thus play a greater role in removing the 8-oxoguanine nucleotides from the precursor pool than MTH1. In addition, 8-oxo-dGDP is a potent inhibitor of the MTH1 reaction.[76,91] NUDT5 thus plays another role in promoting the MTH1 reaction, namely by removing its inhibitor, 8-oxo-dGDP. In this respect, it is important to elucidate the levels of 8-oxo-dGDP and 8-oxo-dGTP in the nucleotide pools, as well as their intracellular localization.

Recent studies of *Mth1*-deficient mice revealed that MTH1 is involved, to some extent, in the suppression of spontaneous tumorigenesis.[33] More definite conclusions regarding the biological significance of NUDT5 and MTH1 proteins in maintaining the integrity of genetic information might be obtained by producing mice deficient in NUDT5, as well as those lacking both proteins.

7. Exclusion of Oxidized Guanine Nucleotides from the RNA Precursor Pool

8-Oxoguanine can be formed in RNA by direct oxidation of their bases and also by incorporation of the oxidized base into RNA.[54] Once 8-oxoguanine is formed in RNA, it cannot be eliminated, contrary to the case of DNA, in which damaged bases are excised by specific glycosylases and repaired.[16,53] Thus, organisms must be equipped with other mechanisms to keep the high quality of RNA against oxidative stress. Proteins which specifically bind to oxidized RNA are implicated in a mechanism to scavenge damaged RNA. *E. coli* polynucleotide phosphorylase (PNP) protein and human YB1 protein have been related to such mechanisms.[55,92]

Another mechanism to prevent transcriptional errors caused by oxidative damage is the sanitization of nucleotide pools. As described in preceding sections, the *E. coli* MutT protein is capable of degrading 8-oxoguanine-containing deoxyribo- and ribonucleoside triphosphates to corresponding nucleoside monophosphates. Recently, additional activities of the MutT to sanitize the nucleotide pool were found.[87] It hydrolyzes 8-oxo-dGDP to 8-oxo-dGMP with a *Km* of 0.058 mM, a value considerably lower than that for its normal counterpart, dGDP (170 mM). Furthermore, the MutT possesses an activity to degrade 8-oxo-GDP to the related nucleoside monophosphate, with a *Km* value 8000 times lower than that for GDP (*Km* for 8-oxo-GDP: 0.045 μM, *Km* for GDP: 350 μM). Thus, the MutT protein has an ability to degrade all four forms of 8-oxoguanine-containing nucleotides for facilitating the high fidelity of RNA synthesis as well as of DNA replication.

In mammalian cells, there are at least three enzymes with different degrees of preference for 8-oxo-dGTP and 8-oxo-dGDP. It is of interest to see if some of these enzymes act on ribonucleotide counterparts, 8-oxo-GTP and 8-oxo-GDP, or whether mammalian cells possess an enzyme(s) specific for 8-oxoguanine-containing ribonucleotides. Recent studies have revealed that among human MutT-related proteins, MTH1 and NUDT5 have abilities to prevent translational errors caused by oxidative damage.[93] Expression of cDNA for NUDT5 or MTH1 in *E. coli* MutT-deficient cells reduced the level of production of erroneous proteins to the wild type one. NUDT5 and MTH1 hydrolyze 8-oxo-GDP to 8-oxo-GMP with *Vmax/Km* values of 1.3×10^{-3} and 1.7×10^{-3}, respectively, values considerably higher than those for its normal counterpart, GDP ($0.1 - 0.5 \times 10^{-3}$). MTH1, but not NUDT5, possesses an additional activity to degrade 8-oxo-GTP to the monophosphate. These results indicate that the elimination of 8-oxoguanine-containing ribonucleotides from the RNA precursor pool is important to secure the accurate protein synthesis and that both NUDT5 and MTH1 may be involved in this process in human cells.

Acknowledgments

We extend our special thanks to Dr. Masahiro Shirakawa for kindly supplying the pictures used in Figs. 4(B) and (C), and to Dr. Brian Quinn for useful comments on the manuscript.

References

1. Ames BN, Gold LS. Endogenous mutagens and the causes of aging and cancer. *Mutat. Res.* 250: 3–16 (1991).
2. Henle ES, Linn S. Formation, prevention, and repair of DNA damage by iron/hydrogen peroxide. *J. Biol. Chem.* **272**: 19095–19098 (1997).

3. Gajewski E, Rao G, Nackerdien Z, Dizdaroglu M. Modification of DNA bases in mammalian chromatin by radiation-generated free radicals. *Biochemistry* 29: 7876–7882 (1990).
4. Demple B, Harrison L. Repair of oxidative damage to DNA: enzymology and biology. *Annu. Rev. Biochem.* 63: 915–948 (1994).
5. Kasai H, Nishimura S. Hydroxylation of deoxyguanosine at the C-8 position by ascorbic acid and other reducing agents. *Nucleic Acids Res.* 12: 2137–2145 (1984).
6. Fraga CG, Shigenaga MK, Park JW, Degan P, Ames BN. Oxidative damage to DNA during aging: 8-hydroxy-2′-deoxyguanosine in rat organ DNA and urine. *Proc. Natl. Acad. Sci. USA* 87: 4533–4537 (1990).
7. Evans J, Maccabee M, Hatahet Z, Courcelle J, Bockrath R, Ide H, Wallace S. Thymine ring saturation and fragmentation products: lesion bypass, misinsertion and implications for mutagenesis. *Mutat. Res.* 299: 147–156 (1993).
8. Brooks PJ, Wise DS, Berry DA, Kosmoski JV, Smerdon MJ, Somers RL, Mackie H, Spoonde AY, Ackerman EJ, Coleman K, Tarone RE, Robbins JH. The oxidative DNA lesion 8,5′-(S)-cyclo-2′-deoxyadenosine is repaired by the nucleotide excision repair pathway and blocks gene expression in mammalian cells. *J. Biol. Chem.* 275: 22355–22362 (2000).
9. Kuraoka I, Bender C, Romieu A, Cadet J, Wood RD, Lindahl T. Removal of oxygen free-radical-induced 5′,8-purine cyclodeoxynucleosides from DNA by the nucleotide excision-repair pathway in human cells. *Proc. Natl. Acad. Sci. USA* 97: 3832–3837 (2000).
10. Shibutani S, Takeshita M, Grollman AP. Insertion of specific bases during DNA synthesis past the oxidation-damaged base 8-oxodG. *Nature* 349: 431–434 (1991).
11. Smith KC. Spontaneous mutagenesis: experimental, genetic and other factors. *Mutat. Res.* 277: 139–162 (1992).
12. Cabrera M, Nghiem Y, Miller JH. *mutM*, a second mutator locus in *Escherichia coli* that generates G.C→T.A transversions. *J. Bacteriol.* 170: 5405–5407 (1988).
13. Chung MH, Kasai H, Jones DS, Inoue H, Ishikawa H, Ohtsuka E, Nishimura S. An endonuclease activity of *Escherichia coli* that specifically removes 8-hydroxyguanine residues from DNA. *Mutat. Res.* 254: 1–12 (1991).
14. Michaels ML, Pham L, Cruz C, Miller JH. MutM, a protein that prevents G.C→T.A transversions, is formamidopyrimidine-DNA glycosylase. *Nucleic Acids Res.* 19: 3629–3632 (1991).
15. Bessho T, Tano K, Kasai H, Nishimura S. Deficiency of 8-hydroxyguanine DNA endonuclease activity and accumulation of the 8-hydroxyguanine in

mutator mutant (*mutM*) of *Escherichia coli*. *Biochem. Biophys. Res. Commun.* 188: 372–378 (1992).

16. Au KG, Cabrera M, Miller JH, Modrich P. *Escherichia coli mutY* gene product is required for specific A-G→CG mismatch correction. *Proc. Natl. Acad. Sci. USA* 85: 9163–9166 (1988).
17. Nghiem Y, Cabrera M, Cupples CG, Miller JH. The *mutY* gene: a mutator locus in *Escherichia coli* that generates G.C→T.A transversions. *Proc. Natl. Acad. Sci. USA* 85: 2709–2713 (1988).
18. Au KG, Clark S, Miller JH, Modrich P. *Escherichia coli mutY* gene encodes an adenine glycosylase active on G-A mispairs. *Proc. Natl. Acad. Sci. USA* 86: 8877–8881 (1989).
19. Michaels ML, Tchou J, Grollman AP, Miller JH. A repair system for 8-oxo-7,8-dihydrodeoxyguanine. *Biochemistry* 31: 10964–10968 (1992).
20. Tchou J, Grollman AP. Repair of DNA containing the oxidatively-damaged base, 8-oxoguanine. *Mutat. Res.* 299: 277–287 (1993).
21. Slupska MM, Baikalov C, Luther WM, Chiang JH, Wei YF, Miller JH. Cloning and sequencing a human homolog (*hMYH*) of the *Escherichia coli mutY* gene whose function is required for the repair of oxidative DNA damage. *J. Bacteriol.* 178: 3885–3892 (1996).
22. Hirano S, Tominaga Y, Ichinoe A, Ushijima Y, Tsuchimoto D, Honda-Ohnishi Y, Ohtsubo T, Sakumi K, Nakabeppu Y. Mutator phenotype of MUTYH-null mouse embryonic stem cells. *J. Biol. Chem.* 278: 38121–38124 (2003).
23. Klungland A, Rosewell I, Hollenbach S, Larsen E, Daly G, Epe B, Seeberg E, Lindahl T, Barnes DE. Accumulation of premutagenic DNA lesions in mice defective in removal of oxidative base damage. *Proc. Natl. Acad. Sci. USA* 96: 13300–13305 (1999).
24. Minowa O, Arai T, Hirano M, Monden Y, Nakai S, Fukuda M, Itoh M, Takano H, Hippou Y, Aburatani H, Masumura K, Nohmi T, Nishimura S, Noda T. *Mmh/Ogg1* gene inactivation results in accumulation of 8-hydroxyguanine in mice. *Proc. Natl. Acad. Sci. USA* 97: 4156–4161 (2000).
25. Sakumi K, Tominaga Y, Furuichi M, Xu P, Tsuzuki T, Sekiguchi M, Nakabeppu Y. *Ogg1* knockout-associated lung tumorigenesis and its suppression by *Mth1* gene disruption. *Cancer Res.* 63: 902–905 (2003).
26. Maki H, Sekiguchi M. MutT protein specifically hydrolyses a potent mutagenic substrate for DNA synthesis. *Nature* 355: 273–275 (1992).
27. Cheng KC, Cahill DS, Kasai H, Nishimura S, Loeb LA. 8-Hydroxyguanine, an abundant form of oxidative DNA damage, causes G→T and A→C substitutions. *J. Biol. Chem.* 267: 166–172 (1992).

28. Mo JY, Maki H, Sekiguchi M. Mutational specificity of the *dnaE173* mutator associated with a defect in the catalytic subunit of DNA polymerase III of *Escherichia coli*. *J. Mol. Biol.* 222: 925–936 (1991).
29. Schaaper RM, Danforth BN, Glickman BW. Mechanisms of spontaneous mutagenesis: an analysis of the spectrum of spontaneous mutation in the *Escherichia coli* lacI gene. *J. Mol. Biol.* 189: 273–284 (1986).
30. Mo JY, Maki H, Sekiguchi M. Hydrolytic elimination of a mutagenic nucleotide, 8-oxodGTP, by human 18-kilodalton protein: sanitization of nucleotide pool. *Proc. Natl. Acad. Sci. USA* 89: 11021–11025 (1992).
31. Sakumi K, Furuichi M, Tsuzuki T, Kakuma T, Kawabata S, Maki H, Sekiguchi M. Cloning and expression of cDNA for a human enzyme that hydrolyzes 8-oxo-dGTP, a mutagenic substrate for DNA synthesis. *J. Biol. Chem.* 268: 23524–23530 (1993).
32. Furuichi M, Yoshida MC, Oda H, Tajiri T, Nakabeppu Y, Tsuzuki T, Sekiguchi M. Genomic structure and chromosome location of the human *mutT* homologue gene *MTH1* encoding 8-oxo-dGTPase for prevention of A:T to C:G transversion. *Genomics* 24: 485–490 (1994).
33. Tsuzuki T, Egashira A, Igarashi H, Iwakuma T, Nakatsuru Y, Tominaga Y, Kawate H, Nakao K, Nakamura K, Ide F, Kura S, Nakabeppu Y, Katsuki M, Ishikawa T, Sekiguchi M. Spontaneous tumorigenesis in mice defective in the *MTH1* gene encoding 8-oxo-dGTPase. *Proc. Natl. Acad. Sci. USA* 98: 11456–11461 (2001).
34. Yanofsky C, Cox EC, Horn V. The unusual mutagenic specificity of an *E. coli* mutator gene. *Proc. Natl. Acad. Sci. USA* 55: 274–281 (1966).
35. Akiyama M, Maki H, Sekiguchi M. Horiuchi T. A specific role of MutT protein: to prevent dG.dA mispairing in DNA replication. *Proc. Natl. Acad. Sci. USA* 86: 3949–3952 (1989).
36. Tajiri T, Maki H, Sekiguchi M. Functional cooperation of MutT, MutM and MutY proteins in preventing mutations caused by spontaneous oxidation of guanine nucleotide in *Escherichia coli*. *Mutat. Res.* 336: 257–267 (1995).
37. Ishibashi T, Hayakawa H, Sekiguchi M. A novel mechanism for preventing mutations caused by oxidation of guanine nucleotides. *EMBO Rep.* 4: 479–483 (2003).
38. Dizdaroglu M, Jaruga P, Birincioglu M, Rodriguez H. Free radical-induced damage to DNA: mechanisms and measurement. *Free Radic. Biol. Med.* 32: 1102–1115 (2002).
39. Purmal AA, Kow YW, Wallace SS. 5-Hydroxypyrimidine deoxynucleoside triphosphates are more efficiently incorporated into DNA by exonuclease-free

Klenow fragment than 8-oxopurine deoxynucleoside triphosphates. *Nucleic Acids Res.* 22: 3930–3935 (1994).

40. Einolf HJ, Schnetz-Boutaud N, Guengerich FP. Steady-state and pre-steady-state kinetic analysis of 8-oxo-7,8-dihydroguanosine triphosphate incorporation and extension by replicative and repair DNA polymerases. *Biochemistry* 37: 13300–13312 (1998).
41. Kamiya H, Kasai H. 2-Hydroxy-dATP is incorporated opposite G by *Escherichia coli* DNA polymerase III resulting in high mutagenicity. *Nucleic Acids Res.* 28: 1640–1646 (2000).
42. Pavlov YI, Minnick DT, Izuta S, Kunkel TA. DNA replication fidelity with 8-oxodeoxyguanosine triphosphate. *Biochemistry* 33: 4695–4701 (1994).
43. Inoue M, Kamiya H, Fujikawa K, Ootsuyama Y, Murata-Kamiya N, Osaki T, Yasumoto K, Kasai H. Induction of chromosomal gene mutations in *Escherichia coli* by direct incorporation of oxidatively damaged nucleotides. New evaluation method for mutagenesis by damaged DNA precursors *in vivo*. *J. Biol. Chem.* 273: 11069–11074 (1998).
44. Kamiya H, Kasai H. Formation of 2-hydroxydeoxyadenosine triphosphate, an oxidatively damaged nucleotide, and its incorporation by DNA polymerases. Steady-state kinetics of the incorporation. *J. Biol. Chem.* 270: 19446–19450 (1995).
45. Fujikawa K, Kamiya H, Kasai H. The mutations induced by oxidatively damaged nucleotides, 5-formyl-dUTP and 5-hydroxy-dCTP, in *Escherichia coli*. *Nucleic Acids Res.* 26: 4582–4587 (1998).
46. Purmal AA, Bond JP, Lyons BA, Kow YW, Wallace SS. Uracil glycol deoxynucleoside triphosphate is a better substrate for DNA polymerase I Klenow fragment than thymine glycol deoxynucleoside triphosphate. *Biochemistry* 37: 330–338 (1998).
47. Kamiya H, Maki H, Kasai H. Two DNA polymerases of *Escherichia coli* display distinct misinsertion specificities for 2-hydroxy-dATP during DNA synthesis. *Biochemistry* 39: 9508–9513 (2000).
48. Kamiya H, Murata-Kamiya N, Karino N, Ueno Y, Matsuda A, Kasai H. Induction of T→G and T→A transversions by 5-formyluracil in mammalian cells. *Mutat. Res.* 513: 213–222 (2002).
49. Treffers HP, Spinelli V, Belser NO. A factor (or mutator gene) influencing mutation rates in *E. coli*. *Proc. Natl. Acad. Sci. USA* 40: 1064–1071 (1954).
50. Cox EC, Yanofsky C. Altered base ratios in the DNA of an *Escherichia coli* mutator strain. *Proc. Natl. Acad. Sci. USA* 58: 1895–1902 (1967).

51. Akiyama M, Horiuchi T, Sekiguchi M. Molecular cloning and nucleotide sequence of the *mutT* mutator of *Escherichia coli* that causes A:T to C:G transversion. *Mol. Gen. Genet.* 206: 9–16 (1987).
52. Bhatnagar SK, Bessman MJ. Studies on the mutator gene, *mutT* of *Escherichia coli*. Molecular cloning of the gene, purification of the gene product, and identification of a novel nucleoside triphosphatase. *J. Biol. Chem.* 263: 8953–8957 (1988).
53. Michaels ML, Cruz C, Grollman AP, Miller JH. Evidence that *MutY* and *MutM* combine to prevent mutations by an oxidatively damaged form of guanine in DNA. *Proc. Natl. Acad. Sci. USA* 89: 7022–7025 (1992).
54. Taddei F, Hayakawa H, Bouton M, Cirinesi A, Matic I, Sekiguchi M, Radman M. Counteraction by MutT protein of transcriptional errors caused by oxidative damage. *Science* 278: 128–130 (1997).
55. Hayakawa H, Kuwano M, Sekiguchi M. Specific binding of 8-oxoguanine-containing RNA to polynucleotide phosphorylase protein. *Biochemistry* 40: 9977–9982 (2001).
56. Cai JP, Kakuma T, Tsuzuki T, Sekiguchi M. cDNA and genomic sequences for rat 8-oxo-dGTPase that prevents occurrence of spontaneous mutations due to oxidation of guanine nucleotides. *Carcinogenesis* 16: 2343–2350 (1995).
57. Kakuma T, Nishida J, Tsuzuki T, Sekiguchi M. Mouse MTH1 protein with 8-oxo-7,8-dihydro-2′-deoxyguanosine 5′-triphosphatase activity that prevents transversion mutation, cDNA cloning and tissue distribution. *J. Biol. Chem.* 270: 25942–25948 (1995).
58. Colussi C, Parlanti E, Degan P, Aquilina G, Barnes D, Macpherson P, Karran P, Crescenzi M, Dogliotti E, Bignami M. The mammalian mismatch repair pathway removes DNA 8-oxodGMP incorporated from the oxidized dNTP pool. *Curr. Biol.* 12: 912–918 (2002).
59. Yoshimura D, Sakumi K, Ohno M, Sakai Y, Furuichi M, Iwai S, Nakabeppu Y. An oxidized purine nucleoside triphosphatase, MTH1, suppresses cell death caused by oxidative stress. *J. Biol. Chem.* 278: 37965–37973 (2003).
60. Russo MT, Blasi MF, Chiera F, Fortini P, Degan P, Macpherson P, Furuichi M, Nakabeppu Y, Karran P, Aquilina G, Bignami M. The oxidized deoxynucleoside triphosphate pool is a significant contributor to genetic instability in mismatch repair-deficient cells. *Mol. Cell Biol.* 24: 465–474 (2004).
61. Kamath AV, Yanofsky C. Sequence and characterization of *mutT* from *Proteus vulgaris*. *Gene* 134: 99–102 (1993).
62. Bullions LC, Mejean V, Claverys JP, Bessman MJ. Purification of the MutX protein of *Streptococcus pneumoniae*, a homologue of *Escherichia coli*

MutT. Identification of a novel catalytic domain for nucleoside triphosphate pyrophosphohydrolase activity. *J. Biol. Chem.* 269: 12339–12344 (1994).

63. Bessman MJ, Frick DN, O'Handley SF. The MutT proteins or "Nudix" hydrolases, a family of versatile, widely distributed, "housecleaning" enzymes. *J. Biol. Chem.* 271: 25059–25062 (1996).
64. O'Handley SF, Frick DN, Bullions LC, Mildvan AS, Bessman MJ. *Escherichia coli orf17* codes for a nucleoside triphosphate pyrophosphohydrolase member of the MutT family of proteins. Cloning, purification, and characterization of the enzyme. *J. Biol. Chem.* 271: 24649–24654 (1996).
65. O'Handley SF, Frick DN, Dunn CA, Bessman MJ. Orf186 represents a new member of the Nudix hydrolases, active on adenosine(5′)triphospho(5′)adenosine, ADP-ribose, and NADH. *J. Biol. Chem.* 273: 3192–3197 (1998).
66. Sheikh S, O'Handley SF, Dunn CA, Bessman MJ. Identification and characterization of the Nudix hydrolase from the *Archaeon, Methanococcus jannaschii*, as a highly specific ADP-ribose pyrophosphatase. *J. Biol. Chem.* 273: 20924–20928 (1998).
67. Safrany ST, Caffrey JJ, Yang X, Bembenek ME, Moyer MB, Burkhart WA, Shears SB. A novel context for the 'MutT' module, a guardian of cell integrity, in a diphosphoinositol polyphosphate phosphohydrolase. *EMBO J.* 17: 6599–6607 (1998).
68. Fujii Y, Shimokawa H, Sekiguchi M, Nakabeppu Y. Functional significance of the conserved residues for the 23-residue module among MTH1 and MutT family proteins. *J. Biol. Chem.* 274: 38251–38259 (1999).
69. Abeygunawardana C, Weber DJ, Frick DN, Bessman MJ, Mildvan AS. Sequence-specific assignments of the backbone 1H, 13C, and 15N resonances of the MutT enzyme by heteronuclear multidimensional NMR. *Biochemistry* 32: 13071–13080 (1993).
70. Weber DJ, Abeygunawardana C, Bessman MJ, Mildvan AS. Secondary structure of the MutT enzyme as determined by NMR. *Biochemistry* 32: 13081–13088 (1993).
71. Abeygunawardana C, Weber DJ, Gittis AG, Frick DN, Lin J, Miller AF, Bessman MJ, Mildvan AS. Solution structure of the MutT enzyme, a nucleoside triphosphate pyrophosphohydrolase. *Biochemistry* 34: 14997–15005 (1995).
72. Frick DN, Weber DJ, Abeygunawardana C, Gittis AG, Bessman MJ, Mildvan AS. NMR studies of the conformations and location of nucleotides bound to the *Escherichia coli* MutT enzyme. *Biochemistry* 34: 5577–5586 (1995).

73. Mishima M, Sakai Y, Itoh N, Kamiya H, Furuichi M, Takahashi M, Yamagata Y, Iwai S, Nakabeppu Y, Shirakawa M. Structure of human MTH1, a Nudix family hydrolase that selectively degrades oxidized purine nucleoside triphosphates. *J. Biol. Chem.* 279: 33806–33815 (2004).
74. Sakai Y, Furuichi M, Takahashi M, Mishima M, Iwai S, Shirakawa M, Nakabeppu Y. A molecular basis for the selective recognition of 2-hydroxy-dATP and 8-oxo-dGTP by human MTH1. *J. Biol. Chem.* 277: 8579–8587 (2002).
75. Lin J, Abeygunawardana C, Frick DN, Bessman MJ, Mildvan AS. Solution structure of the quaternary MutT-M^{2+}-AMPCPP-M^{2+} complex and mechanism of its pyrophosphohydrolase action. *Biochemistry* 36: 1199–1211 (1997).
76. Fujikawa K, Kamiya H, Yakushiji H, Fujii Y, Nakabeppu Y, Kasai H. The oxidized forms of dATP are substrates for the human MutT homologue, the hMTH1 protein. *J. Biol. Chem.* 274: 18201–18205 (1999).
77. Fujikawa K, Kamiya H, Yakushiji H, Nakabeppu Y, Kasai H. Human MTH1 protein hydrolyzes the oxidized ribonucleotide, 2-hydroxy-ATP. *Nucleic Acids Res.* 29: 449–454 (2001).
78. Igarashi H, Tsuzuki T, Kakuma T, Tominaga Y, Sekiguchi M. Organization and expression of the mouse *MTH1* gene for preventing transversion mutation. *J. Biol. Chem.* 272: 3766–3772 (1997).
79. Egashira A, Yamauchi K, Yoshiyama K, Kawate H, Katsuki M, Sekiguchi M, Sugimachi K, Maki H, Tsuzuki T. Mutational specificity of mice defective in the *MTH1* and/or the *MSH2* genes. *DNA Repair (Amst.)* 1: 881–893 (2002).
80. Hayashi H, Tominaga Y, Hirano S, McKenna AE, Nakabeppu Y, Matsumoto Y. Replication-associated repair of adenine: 8-oxoguanine mispairs by MYH. *Curr. Biol.* 12: 335–339 (2002).
81. Kang D, Nishida J, Iyama A, Nakabeppu Y, Furuichi M, Fujiwara T, Sekiguchi M, Takeshige K. Intracellular localization of 8-oxo-dGTPase in human cells, with special reference to the role of the enzyme in mitochondria. *J. Biol. Chem.* 270: 14659–14665 (1995).
82. Bestwick RK, Moffett GL, Mathews CK. Selective expansion of mitochondrial nucleoside triphosphate pools in antimetabolite-treated HeLa cells. *J. Biol. Chem.* 257: 9300–9304 (1982).
83. Hayakawa H, Taketomi A, Sakumi K, Kuwano M, Sekiguchi M. Generation and elimination of 8-oxo-7,8-dihydro-2′-deoxyguanosine 5′-triphosphate, a mutagenic substrate for DNA synthesis, in human cells. *Biochemistry* 34: 89–95 (1995).

84. Cai JP, Ishibashi T, Takagi Y, Hayakawa H, Sekiguchi M. Mouse MTH2 protein which prevents mutations caused by 8-oxoguanine nucleotides. *Biochem. Biophys. Res. Commun.* 305: 1073–1077 (2003).
85. Shimokawa H, Fujii Y, Furuichi M, Sekiguchi M, Nakabeppu Y. Functional significance of conserved residues in the phosphohydrolase module of *Escherichia coli* MutT protein. *Nucleic Acids Res.* 28: 3240–3249 (2000).
86. Yang H, Slupska MM, Wei YF, Tai JH, Luther WM, Xia YR, Shih DM, Chiang JH, Baikalov C, Fitz-Gibbon S, Phan IT, Conrad A, Miller JH. Cloning and characterization of a new member of the Nudix hydrolases from human and mouse. *J. Biol. Chem.* 275: 8844–8853 (2000).
87. Ito R, Hayakawa H, Sekiguchi M, Ishibashi T. Multiple enzyme activities of *Escherichia coli* MutT protein for sanitization of DNA and RNA precursor pools. *Biochemistry* 44: 6670–6674 (2005).
88. Thelander L, Reichard P. Reduction of ribonucleotides. *Annu. Rev. Biochem.* 48: 133–158 (1979).
89. Hayakawa H, Hofer A, Thelander L, Kitajima S, Cai Y, Oshiro S, Yakushiji H, Nakabeppu Y, Kuwano M, Sekiguchi M. Metabolic fate of oxidized guanine ribonucleotides in mammalian cells. *Biochemistry* 38: 3610–3614 (1999).
90. Kornberg A, Baker TA. *DNA Replication*, 2nd edn. WH Freeman and Company, New York, 1992, pp. 53–100.
91. Bialkowski K, Kasprzak KS. A novel assay of 8-oxo-2′-deoxyguanosine-5′-triphosphate pyrophosphohydrolase (8-oxo-dGTPase) activity in cultured cells and its use for evaluation of cadmium(II) inhibition of this activity. *Nucleic Acids Res.* 26: 3194–3201 (1998).
92. Hayakawa H, Uchiumi T, Fukuda T, Ashizuka M, Kohno K, Kuwano M, Sekiguchi M. Binding capacity of human YB-1 protein for RNA containing 8-oxoguanine. *Biochemistry* 41: 12739–12744 (2002).
93. Ishibashi T, Hayakawa H, Ito R, Miyazawa M, Yamagata Y, Sekiguchi M. Mammalian enzymes for preventing transcriptional errors caused by oxidative damage. *Nucleic Acids Res.* 33: 3779–3784 (2005).

7 Oxidative Damage to DNA and Its Repair

Lene Juel Rasmussen

1. Introduction

During DNA replication errors may occur as a result of misincorporation of nucleotides opposite modified DNA bases or by incorporation of modified nucleotides. Furthermore, DNA is constantly exposed to damaging agents from both endogenous and exogenous sources. If these lesions are not repaired they can lead to mutations and result in cellular dysfunction including uncontrolled cell proliferation and defective apoptosis. Thus, in order to maintain the integrity of the genome, a complicated network of DNA repair pathways remove the majority of deleterious lesions. However, DNA repair may occasionally fail or become limited due to excess of DNA damage resulting in DNA damage accumulation. In such situations, DNA damage is pathogenic and one of the very serious symptoms of DNA repair deficiency is the development of cancer.

2. Generation and Types of Oxidative Damage

Normal cellular metabolism is well known as the source of endogenous reactive oxygen species (ROS) and it is these usually non-pathogenic cellular processes that account for the background levels of oxidative DNA damage detected in normal tissue. Pathways and events that produce ROS include mitochondrial and peroxisomal metabolism, enzymatic synthesis of nitric oxide (NO), phagocytic leukocytes, heat, radiation, therapeutic drugs, oxidizing agents, and redox-cycling compounds. The reaction of

ROS with pyrimidines and purines produces a variety of different DNA lesions[1] where 8-oxoguanine (8-oxoG) is the far most studied, but not necessarily the most important, DNA lesion when it comes to repair. If cells did not have cellular defenses, such as low molecular weight antioxidants, enzymatic antioxidants, and DNA repair, levels of oxidized bases would quickly represent the majority of bases in DNA.

Superoxide radicals are normally eliminated by superoxide dismutase (SOD), which generates the less reactive hydrogen peroxide (H_2O_2) and O_2. The H_2O_2 is further converted to H_2O and O_2 by catalase. SOD activities are present in both mitochondria (SOD2, Mn-SOD), cytoplasm (SOD1, CuZn-SOD), and extracellularly (SOD3, EC-SOD).[2] A large number of other factors also contributes to cellular defense against ROS, for example antioxidants (arginine, vitamins A, C, and E), thiols (glutathione), polyphenols (tea), enzyme-bound minerals (selenium and zinc), and antioxidant enzymes (glutathione reductase, glutathione peroxidases). All these are important for the repair of amino acids, proteins, and lipids.[3] However, none of these cellular systems repair DNA damage and, therefore does not prevent permanent genetic alterations.

Mitochondrial respiration is the major source of endogenous ROS, including superoxide ($O_2^{\bar{}}$), H_2O_2, and hydroxyl radical ($HO^{\bullet}$). Under normal physiological conditions electrons leak from the electron transport chain converting about 1–2% of oxygen molecules into $O_2^{\bar{}}$.[4–7] Thus, increased mitochondrial metabolism generates higher than normal levels of ROS. However, inhibition of mitochondrial metabolism can also increase ROS production[8–10] suggesting that correct mitochondrial function is important for prevention of excess oxidative DNA damage. The importance of accurate mitochondrial function in preventing mitochondrial-mediated oxidative DNA damage was supported by several studies showing that mitochondrial dysfunction is mutagenic and multiple pathways are involved in this phenotype.[11–13] However, mitochondria are not only involved in the generation of oxidative damage they also have an effect on the repair of DNA lesions. It was shown that a human cell line depleted of the mitochondrial genome showed impaired repair of DNA damage induced by exogenous added H_2O_2.[14] Along these lines, it was reported that pre-exposure of human cells to H_2O_2 suppress DNA repair of alkylation damage[15] suggesting that extensive oxidative damage inhibits cellular repair systems. Explanations for these phenotypes could be oxidative damage of proteins safeguarding the genome[16] or depletion of repair activities caused by excessive oxidative damage of DNA. Overall, these results indicate that correct mitochondrial function is important for both optimal repair of oxidative DNA damage as well as for prevention of excess oxidative damage.

3. Repair of Oxidative Damage

Since oxidized bases are a part of normal cellular metabolism the question is: when is oxidative damage normal and when is it pathogenic? The answer to this question is that if the removal of oxidative DNA lesions becomes limited and the outcome is genetic changes, cytostasis or cytotoxicity; it is pathogenic otherwise oxidative damage must be considered normal. Therefore, it is highly relevant to look at the prevention and repair of oxidative DNA lesions in normal cells to be able to say what went wrong in anomalous cells. In this chapter, the focus is on the repair of oxidative DNA lesions, which in most cases are subject to multiple, overlapping repair processes. The redundancy presents a safety element to DNA repair such that reduction or elimination of one repair pathway does not necessarily prevent repair of a particular DNA lesion. However, this scenario also suggests a competition between the various DNA repair pathways where the outcome (repair of the DNA lesion) depends on how fast and efficiently a specific DNA lesion is recognized and repaired by the individual repair systems.

So far most effort has been put into characterizing repair of the nuclear genome. However, in recent years DNA repair in mitochondria has caught interest and it has turned out to be quite interesting. It seems that several DNA repair proteins are functional both in the nucleus and in the mitochondria whereas others are organelle specific.

4. Base Excision Repair (BER)

Like most repair processes the BER system is highly conserved among organisms from bacteria to humans, and this repair system is believed to be the main repair pathway when it comes to the repair of oxidative DNA damage.[17–20] Traditionally, the BER process has been divided into two mechanistically different subpathways known as the short- and long-patch repair pathways, respectively. Common for both these repair processes is that they are initiated by a DNA lesion-specific glycosylase. The difference between the two repair processes is the downstream reactions (Fig. 1).[21] Generally, the first step of BER is performed by a DNA glycosylase that recognizes and removes the abnormal base by hydrolysis of the N-glycosylic bond between the sugar-phosphate backbone and the base. This results in an abasic site (AP site) that is recognized and cleaved by an AP endonuclease, which introduces a DNA strand break 5′ to the baseless sugar. Alternatively, the AP site is processed by the AP lyase activity of the bifunctional glycosylases creating a 3′-fragmented deoxyribose. Finally, a DNA polymerase fills the gap, and the nick is sealed by

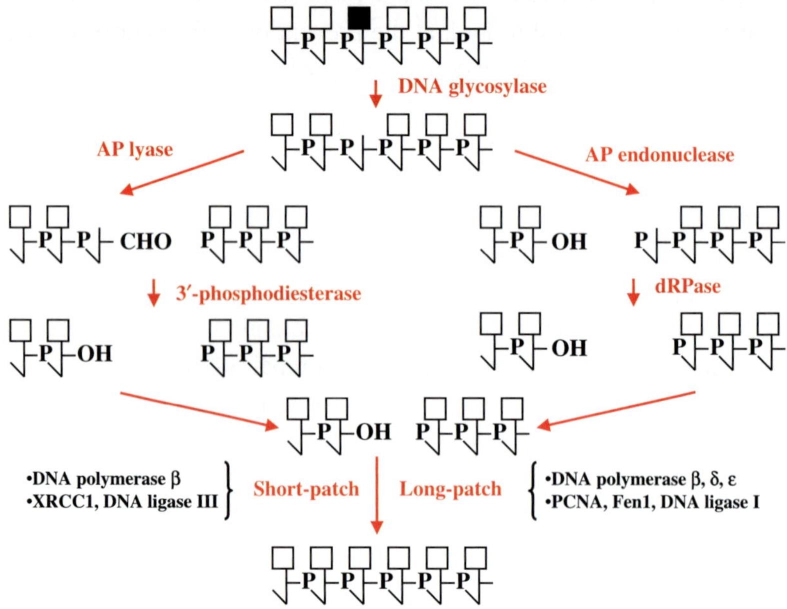

Fig. 1. Base Excision Repair Pathway. The first step in BER is recognition and removal of the DNA lesion by a DNA glycosylase. The abasic site is processed by AP lyase or AP endonuclease activities followed by further processing mediated by 3′-phosphodiesterases or dRPase. In short-patch repair the XRCC1, DNA polymerase β, and DNA ligase III proteins complete the repair processes whereas this is carried out by DNA polymerase β, δ, ε as well as PCNA, Fen1, and DNA ligase I in long-patch repair. (Adapted from Dianov *et al.*[21])

DNA ligase (Fig. 1).[20] Several DNA glycosylases responsible for the repair of oxidized bases participate in both short- and long-patch repair.[22,23] As mentioned earlier, the far best studied oxidative DNA lesion is 8-oxoG, which base pair equally well with both adenine and cytosine during DNA replication. The misincorporation of adenine induces G/C to T/A transversion mutations, which are potentially pathogenic mutations. The 8-oxoG DNA lesions are primarily repaired by the GO-system, which belongs to the short-patch repair pathway of BER (Fig. 2). Bacteria contain complex mechanisms to counteract the mutagenic effect of 8-oxoG namely the two DNA glycosylases MutM (Fpg) and MutY that repair 8-oxoG integrated into DNA. The MutM protein removes 8-oxoG paired with cytosine and

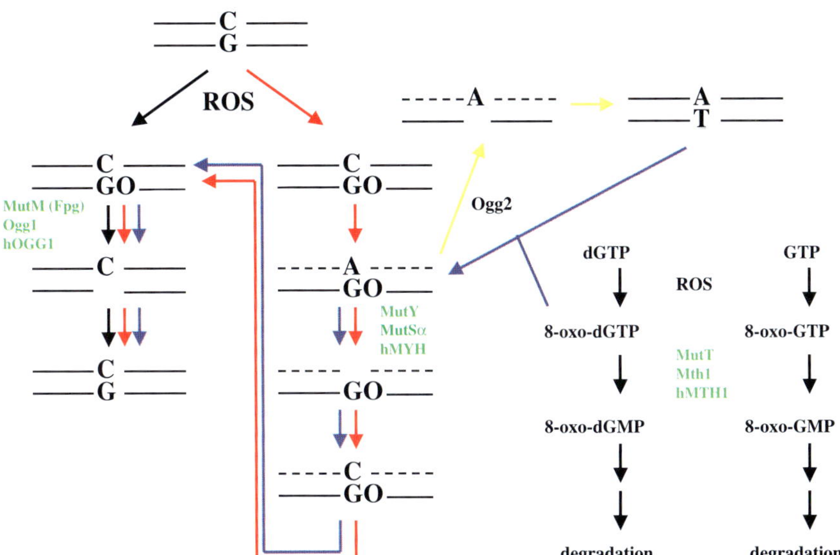

Fig. 2. GO-Repair. The oxidation of guanine in perfectly matched DNA gives rise to 8-oxoG/C mispairs that are substrates for repair by the MutM proteins (MutM (Fpg), Ogg1, and hOGG1). The incorporation of adenine opposite 8-oxoG or the incorporation of 8-oxodGTP opposite adenine during DNA replication result in 8-oxoG/A mispairs. These mispairs are processed by the MutY proteins (MutY, hMYH) or the MMR proteins MutSα as well as by the Ogg2 glycosylase in mitochondria. The MutT proteins (MutT, Mth1, hMTH1) sanitize the oxidized nucleotide pools preventing incorporation of this modified nucleotide into DNA. The color of the arrows indicates the specific routes of repair within the GO-repair system. (Adapted from Gu *et al.*[24])

MutY removes adenine paired with 8-oxoG in DNA. The MutM protein also excises ring-opened purine (fapy), another oxidatively damaged base, and for this reason MutM is also called Fpg protein (Fig. 2). The conservation of this repair process is emphasized by the fact that homologs from other species functionally complement the enzymatic activities of the bacterial proteins. One example is the yeast *OGG1* gene, which encodes a DNA glycosylase that functionally complements the *Escherichia coli* MutM deficiency[25] and is present in both nucleus and mitochondria.[26] The human homolog of yeast Ogg1 (hOGG1) has been cloned and seven splice variants of hOGG1 have been identified.[27] Among them, types 1a and 2a are the major splice variants, which are transported to nucleus and mitochondria, respectively. The nuclear form of hOGG1 (type 1a) contains a mitochondrial-targeting signal (MTS) at the NH_2-terminus and a nuclear localization signal (NLS) at the COOH-terminus whereas the mitochondrial form (type 2a) lacks the COOH-terminal NLS. Another DNA glycosylase Ntg1 (Ogg2, Nth1) also repairs 8-oxoG DNA lesions but in contrast to Ogg1 it preferentially removes 8-oxoG from 8-oxoG/A mispairs and it is localized in mitochondria.[28] Oxidative mtDNA damage is elevated in strains lacking the mitochondrial Ntg1. However, *NTG1* null strains did not exhibit a mitochondrial respiration-deficient (petite) phenotype, suggesting that mtDNA damage is coped with by the joint actions of multiple damage repair pathways.[29] The human MutY gene *hMYH* has been cloned and several splice variant have been identified. In human cell extracts three proteins of 52, 53, and 57 kDa were detected.[30] The 52 and 53 kDa proteins were detected in nucleus whereas the 57 kDa protein was found in mitochondria. Inactivation of mouse mMyh results in a minor two-fold mutator phenotype.[31] Nevertheless, it has been suggested that mutations in hMYH predispose to colorectal cancer based on findings that missense mutations in this gene were identified in individuals with high occurrence of multiple adenomas and colorectal carcinoma.[32–34] The missense mutation in the murine gene *mMYH G365D* corresponding to one of the human germline mutations G382D found in cancer patients was shown to be defective in 8-oxoG/A but not 8-oxoG/C activity *in vitro*.[31] These results suggest that the human G382D missense mutation affect glycosylase activity indicating that these individuals might be more sensitive to genetic changes caused by oxidative DNA damage.

Phosphorylation of repair proteins is a rather unexploited area but might play an important role for repair activity. It has been shown that defective repair of 8-oxoG/A may be partly due to lack of phosphorylation of the hMYH protein. It was shown that hMYH is serine-phosphorylated by protein kinase C (PKC) and that this phosphorylation increases the level of hMYH catalyzed 8-oxoG/A repair.[35]

Nitric oxide is a signaling and effector molecule that contributes to multiple physiological and pathophysiological processes in cells. Both NO and peroxynitrite were capable of inhibiting hOGG1 activity indicating that NO directly inhibits a key BER enzyme responsible for the repair of 8-oxoG.[36] NO-mediated inhibition of base excision DNA repair may generate oxidative DNA damage and contribute to mutagenesis.

Interestingly, an enzyme with MutY-like specificity has not been found in *Saccharomyces cerevisiae*. Instead, it was shown that the mismatch repair (MMR) protein complex Msh2-Msh6 (MutSα) bound 8-oxoG/A base-pairs and mutations in *MSH2* and *MSH6* in combination with mutation in *OGG1* caused a synergistic increase in G/C to T/A transversion mutations.[37] These results suggest that MMR can act as a functional homolog of MutY in *S. cerevisiae* and perhaps also in other organisms which lack MutY enzymes.

Other enzymes involved in the repair of 8-oxoG DNA lesions are *E. coli* MutT and its homologs in eukaryotic cells (Mth1 and hMTH1). The yeast homolog of MutT (Mth1) acts to inhibit erroneous incorporation of 8-oxoG into DNA by converting 8-oxodGTP to 8-oxodGMP (Fig. 2). Similar to 8-oxodGTP Mth1 (MutT) can also convert 8-oxodATP to limit misincorporation of this modified nucleotide into DNA.[38] A role for MutT homologs in cancer development is supported by experimental data using *MTH1* knock-out cell lines as well as mice. The Mth1-deficient mice showed a greater number of tumors in lung, liver, and stomach compared to wild-type mice.[39]

One characteristic of BER is the redundancy of DNA glycosylases in the initial step of this repair process. In addition to the above-mentioned MutM and MutY several other DNA glycosylases have been shown to recognize oxidative damage.[23] The NEIL1 glycosylase removes 8-oxoG in 8-oxoG/G and 8-oxoG/A mispairs as well as fapyGua, fapyAde, and thymine glycols.[40,41] The NTG1 DNA glycosylase has been shown to repair 5-formyluracil, 5-hydroxycytosine, and 5,6-dihydroxycytosine.[41–44] The former lesion is also repaired by NEIL2.[45] The 5-hydroxymethyluracil DNA glycosylase has been shown to repair 5-hydroxymethyluracil[46] in both dsDNA and ssDNA. This DNA glycosylase has only been identified in higher organisms, particularly in those that use 5-methylcytosine in regulation of gene expression. It is unclear if 5-hydroxymethyluracil DNA glycosylase is identical to hSMUG1.[47–49] The uracil DNA glycosylase (UNG or UDG) has been reported to repair oxidized cytosine products such as 5,6-dihydroxycytosine.[50,51] The above-mentioned DNA glycosylases are just some examples of enzymes acting on oxidized DNA and it is very likely that many more will be identified in the future and added to the growing list of BER enzymes.

Interestingly, a DNA glycosylase-independent incision activity of oxidative DNA damage by Nfo/Apn1-like enzymes has been identified and provides an alternative pathway to traditional BER.[52,53] This repair activity has been named nucleotide incision repair (NIR) pathway and provides an explanation for the DNA repair proficiency of DNA glycosylase-deficient mutants as a back-up repair pathway.

In contrast to 8-oxoG the repair of 8-oxoA is poorly understood. However, it has been shown that this lesion is incised by nuclear extracts when paired with cytosine and guanine. In contrast, mitochondrial protein extracts only recognized 8-oxoA when paired with cytosine. It was also shown that mOgg1 is responsible for the incision of 8-oxoA/C in both mitochondria and nucleus whereas another, yet unidentified, glycosylase recognizes 8-oxoA/G mispairs in the nucleus.[54]

The *Xenopus laevis* mitochondrial DNA polymerase γ can replicate past 8-oxoG DNA lesions and it was shown that the polymerase inserted adenine opposite 8-oxoG in approximately one-third of the extended products. However, the 3′-5′ exonuclease proofreading activity of DNA polymerase γ excised these 8-oxoG/A mispairs suggesting that proofreading by DNA polymerases also plays a role in the repair of 8-oxoG residues.[55]

5. Recombinational Repair (RER)

The repair of double-strand DNA breaks (DSB) by homologous recombination is essential for the maintenance of genome stability.[56] The DSBs may arise as a consequence of replication fork collapse at the sites of oxidative damage, and increased levels of DSBs may induce hyper-recombination leading to deleterious genetic changes.[57–60]

It was shown that in a *RAD52* mutant reduced level of Frataxin protein, involved in the human disease Friedreich's ataxia, caused oxidative damage to mitochondrial proteins, mitochondrial dysfunctions as well as nuclear DNA damage. These results suggest that mitochondrial dysfunction generates damage to both mitochondrial and nuclear DNA and that these lesions are converted into DSB that are substrates for repair by the Rad52 protein.[61]

Another protein suggested to be involved in the repair of oxidative damage is the *S. cerevisiae* Tpp1 protein, which is a DNA 3′-phosphatase that is assumed to act during strand break repair.[62–64] Deletion of *TPP1* in an AP-endonuclease deficient *APN1 APN2* mutant background dramatically increased the sensitivity of the double mutant cells to DNA damage caused by H_2O_2 and bleomycin but not to damage caused by methyl methanesulfonate (MMS). The *TPP1 APN1 APN2* triple mutant strain displayed synthetic lethality in combination with *RAD52* suggesting a role for Tpp1, in the repair of DNA strand breaks.[63]

The *S. cerevisiae* MMR proteins Msh2, Msh3, Msh6, Pms1, Mlh1, and Exo1 correct replication errors as well as prevent recombination between homeologous (nonidentical) sequences.[65] Yeast mitochondria are very active in recombination and some of the deletions of mitochondrial DNA observed in rho$^-$ cells could be caused by homeologous recombination between imperfect repeats.[66,67] Another interesting link to mitochondrial recombination is the observation that cells deficient in the mitochondrial MutS homolog Msh1 reveal a phenotype that might suggest altered mtDNA as well as mitochondrial distribution.[68] The same group also suggested a role for Msh1 in homeologous recombination.[69]

Another protein involved in mitochondrial recombination is the Pif DNA helicase, which exists in two forms generated through the alternative use of two AUG codons where the longer form localizes to mitochondria.[70] However, it still remains to be shown if this protein is involved in oxidative damage induced recombination. One more mitochondrial protein involved in recombination is Mhr1 that encodes a protein of unknown function. *S. cerevisiae* cells deficient in *MHR1* are defective in mitochondrial recombination and an active Mhr1 protein is required for mitochondrial function by reducing the level of spontaneous oxidative damage in mtDNA.[71] These results link recombination to repair of oxidative damage in mitochondria.

The *Drosophila melanogaster* recombination repair protein 1 (Rrp1) is a homolog of *E. coli* exonuclease III that repairs oxidative and alkylation induced DNA damage.[72,73] The nuclease activities of Rrp1 include apurinic/apyrimidinic endonuclease, 3′-phosphodiesterase, 3′-phosphatase, and 3′-exonuclease.[73–76]

6. Mismatch Repair (MMR)

The best understood MMR system is the *E. coli* MMR pathway.[77] A model for the initiation of MMR immediately after passage of a DNA replication fork has been developed based on genetics as well as biochemical studies with cell-free extracts of bacteria. On the basis of these studies, a model for eukaryotic MMR has been proposed.[78] In this model, a mismatch is first recognized and bound by either the hMSH2-hMSH6 (hMutSα, MutS homologs) or the hMSH2-hMSH3 (hMutSβ, MutS homologs) complex. The hMLH1-hPMS2 (hMutLα, MutL homologs) complex is believed to create a contact between an endonuclease (MutH homolog) and the hMutSα/hMutSβ complexes. The endonuclease activity is thereby activated and a single nick is introduced into the newly synthesized strand. The DNA double helix is unwound by helicases and exonucleases remove the bases on the newly synthesized strand in the presence of PCNA and RPA. Finally, DNA polymerase fills in the excision tract and DNA ligase closes the nick. The final step in the repair process is marking of the newly synthesized strand, perhaps in an analogous manner as mediated by *E. coli* Dam methyltransferase, but the actual mechanism of DNA strand discrimination in eukaryotes remains an enigma because of the absence of MutH and Dam methyltransferase homologs. When the DNA template is marked, the repair of the newly synthesized strand is inhibited.[79,80] To date, it is still unclear whether mammalian mitochondria harbor a similar MMR system. However, recent data[81] show that the proteasome of *S. cerevisiae* contains several components of the MMR pathway such as Msh1 (MutS homolog) and Mlh1 (MutL homolog). The Msh1 protein has previously been shown to localize to mitochondria and inactivation of the *MSH1* gene resulted in large scale mtDNA rearrangements suggesting that Msh1 is indeed involved in repair of mtDNA.[68] A homolog to yeast Msh1 has not been identified in humans suggesting that other proteins are responsible for this repair activity in humans. Interestingly, Chen *et al.*[82] have identified the MSH2 protein, a central player of the MMR system, in rat mitochondrial lysate. Further support for MMR activity in mitochondria came from Mason *et al.*[83] who showed that purified mammalian mitochondria possess an activity that repairs mismatched substrates *in vitro*.

The MMR pathway has been shown to play a role in mutation avoidance caused by oxidative damage.[37,84,85] Interestingly, Ni *et al.*[37] showed that when MMR-deficient yeast strains are grown anaerobically the mutation frequencies are greatly reduced. The fact that MMR acts on oxidative DNA damage suggests an interaction and competition between BER and MMR, which is supported by results showing that there is a synergistic increase in mutation rates in *MLH1 OGG1*, *MSH2 OGG1* and *MSH6 OGG1* double mutant strains compared to the single mutants.[84,86] One characteristic of MMR-deficiency is microsatellite instability (MSI), which can be caused by oxidative damage.[87,88] There are two obvious explanations for this: (1) the MMR pathways repairs oxidative DNA lesions and/or (2) the MMR pathway is inactivated by oxidative damage, for instance the mitochondrial DNA polymerase γ.[16] In support of the latter, it was shown that low levels of H_2O_2 inactivate MMR activity and that this is most likely due to oxidative damage to the MMR protein complexes hMutSα, hMutSβ, and hMutLα.[89] However, other studies have shown that cells treated with H_2O_2 showed decreased or no effect on mutation frequencies of mononucleotide repeats. A small increase in mutation frequency was observed in CA repeats.[90] Another study showed that in human cells, H_2O_2 treatment caused less cytotoxicity in MMR-deficient cells than in those proficient in MMR and that growth of MMR-defective cells in the presence of the antioxidant ascorbate reduced both the spontaneous mutation rate as well as microsatellite instability. The induction of mutations by exogenously added H_2O_2 was significantly suppressed by antioxidant treatment suggesting that oxidative damage contributes significantly to the spontaneous mutator phenotype in MMR-defective cells.[91]

The MMR system also acts on oxidized bases such as 8-oxoG/A and 8-oxoG/C mispairs.[24,37,84,85,92] The hMutSα complex hydrolyzes ATP in the presence of 8-oxoG/A mispair indicating that MMR processes this lesion.[85] However, it is unclear if the oxidized bases are repaired by the MMR pathway or if the lesions are recognized and marked for repair by other pathways. This would be an interesting question to address in the future. The fact that hMYH and hMSH6 physically interact[24] suggests a direct interaction between BER and MMR at least under certain conditions. Since both are involved in recognition and/or repair of 8-oxoG/A, it is tempting to speculate that these repair proteins play complementary roles in repair of 8-oxoG depending on when in cell cycle the 8-oxoG/A mispair occurs. If the human MMR system was analogous to the bacterial, one would expect that it is only actively repairing during DNA replication, thus, in S-phase. If an 8-oxoG/A mispair is generated due to incorporation of 8-oxodGTP opposite adenine during DNA replication the 8-oxoG lesion would be present in the newly synthesized strand and, therefore, substrate for removal by MMR (Fig. 3). In this case, a thymidine would be inserted and the repair process completed. In this scenario, there would be no need for hMYH to act on this lesion. In contrast, it has been shown that 8-oxoG/A mispairs, where 8-oxoG is present in the parent strand, are not substrate for repair by the MMR system.[93] Instead, when adenine is incorporated opposite an 8-oxoG DNA lesion present in the template strand the adenine needs to be replaced by cytosine to avoid mutation (Fig. 3). In this scenario, there would be a need for hMYH to replace the adenine with a cytosine in the newly synthesized strand to avoid mutations.[94] The question is when would there be a need for hMYH and why is there a physical interaction between hMYH and hMSH6? One explanation is that the 8-oxoG/A mispairs that are substrates for hMYH are not formed during DNA replication but rather during repair synthesis or recombination.[60] During recombination MMR proteins play a major role in preventing recombination between substrates that contain numerous mismatches (homeologous recombination) and, therefore, one could also speculate that MMR could block recombination between substrates containing abnormal bases like 8-oxoG. The importance of hMYH in this situation would be to initiate repair (Figs. 2 and 3) and generate a DNA template, which is error-free after recombination. The protein-protein interaction between hMYH and hMSH6 could serve either to make sure that

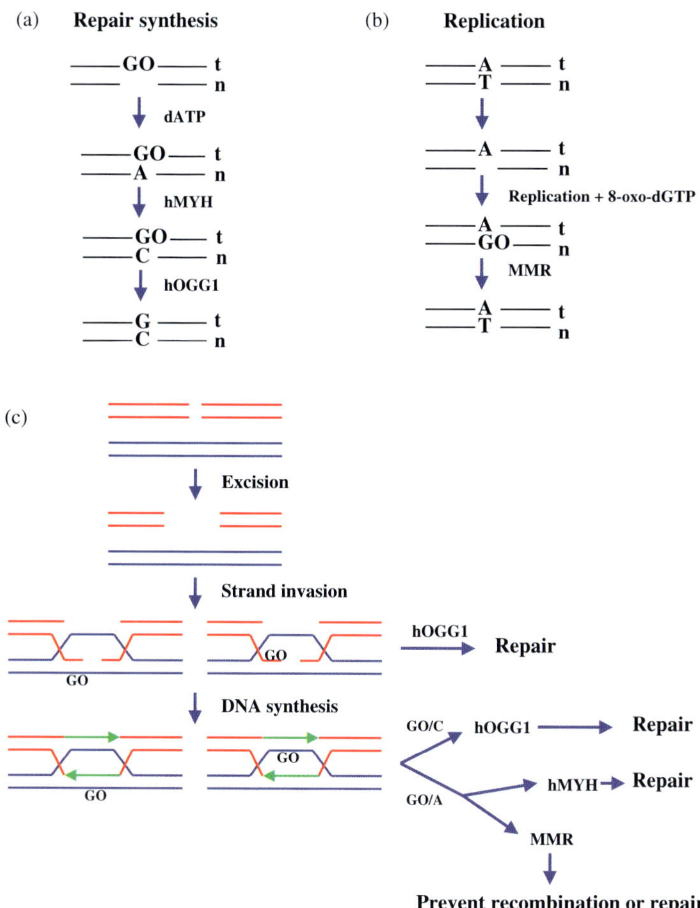

Fig. 3. Mismatch repair processing of oxidative DNA damage. (a) Incorporation of adenine opposite 8-oxoG during repair synthesis results in 8-oxoG/A mispairs that are substrates for repair by the MutY (MutY, hMYH) and MutM (MutM (Fpg), Ogg1, and hOGG1) glycosylases. (b) Incorporation of 8-oxodGTP during DNA replication results in 8-oxoG/A mispairs containing the 8-oxoG in the newly synthesized strand (n) and the adenine in the template strand (t). These mispairs are substrates for repair by the MMR pathway. (c) Model for the role of MMR and BER in recombination. If 8-oxoG/C mispairs are formed during strand invasion these lesions are substrates for repair by the MutM proteins (MutM (Fpg), Ogg1, and hOGG1). If 8-oxoG/C or 8-oxoG/A mispairs are formed during DNA synthesis these can be processed by either the MutM proteins (MutM (Fpg), Ogg1, and hOGG1) or the MutY (MutY, hMYH) and the MMR proteins, respectively. Alternatively, the MMR proteins can prevent recombination if the oxidized bases are not repaired.

the two proteins are physically close to each other and/or to regulate the enzymatic activity of one or both enzymes. On the other hand, if 8-oxoG/A is generated during repair synthesis MMR would not be active and hMYH would be the sole enzyme to initiate removal of the oxidized DNA lesion. Interestingly, Mlh1 has been shown to interact with Ntg2.[95] The Ntg2 is a nuclear thymidine glycol DNA glycosylase that has a broad spectrum of DNA lesions as substrates.[23] The interaction between these repair proteins could be explained as above, for hMYH and hMSH6, suggesting a model where "repair factories" are present in the cell. Interestingly, the closely related Ntg1 glycosylase, which is present both in nucleus and mitochondria, as well as Mlh1 have been found in mitochondria isolated from yeast.[81] However, no physical interaction could be detected between these proteins using the two-hybrid assay.[95] It is nevertheless tempting to speculate that both these enzymes play a role in mitochondrial repair perhaps as a "united" BER-MMR repair system.

7. Nucleotide Excision Repair (NER)

The NER pathway can be divided into two distinct processes, general genomic repair (GGR) and transcription-coupled repair (TCR). The repair of DNA lesions by these two subpathways depends on the localization of the DNA lesion. The GGR subpathway detects and repairs DNA lesions in the entire genome whereas TCR normally is restricted to repair of DNA lesions in actively transcribed genes.[96] Damage recognition in GGR requires the XPC/hHR23B (human homolog of yeast Rad23) followed by helix unwinding by the transcription factor TFIIH, a nine-subunit protein complex including XPB and XPD both of which show helicase activity.[96] The TFIIH protein is involved in the initiation of transcription by RNA polymerase II but is also essential for NER.[97] After initial melting of the helix, the open complex must be stabilized and this is achieved by XPA and RPA. Incision of the damaged DNA is mediated by two endonucleases. XPG initiates incision 3′ to the open complex followed by 5′ incision by ERCC1-XPF. Resynthesis of the repair track is mediated by DNA polymerases δ and ε, PCNA, and RFC and the nick is sealed by DNA ligase I.[98]

The mechanism of DNA damage recognition by TCR is less well established but is believed to involve RNA polymerase II, CSA, and CSB. The role of CSA and CSB in TCR is still unclear but models suggest a role in displacing RNA polymerase II after recruitment of TFIIH.[96] The GGR and TCR subpathways only differ in the initial recognition step. The downstream players are common for these two pathways (TFIIH, XPA, RPA, XPG, ERCC1-XPF, DNA polymerases δ and ε, PCNA, RFC, and DNA ligase I).

NER is best known for the repair of bulky DNA lesions such as pyrimidine dimers.[99] However, it has been reported that 8-oxoG, 5-hydroxycytosine, Cyclo-dA, FapyGua, and thymine glycol are substrates for this repair pathway.[37,86,100–104] In yeast, NER mutants such as *RAD1*, *RAD2*, *RAD10*, and *RAD14* are weak spontaneous mutators suggesting that NER has a significant impact on the correction of endogenous generated DNA damage, for instance oxidative damage. This also suggests both competition as well as interaction between BER and NER for the repair of oxidative DNA damage, though BER is the major contributor. This is supported by results showing that *RAD1 OGG1* double mutants exhibit synergistic increase in spontaneous mutation frequencies when compared to the single mutants.[86] So far, NER activity has only been described in the nucleus and not the mitochondria although these organelles repair DNA lesions that are substrates for nuclear NER proteins.

8. Translesion Synthesis (TLS)

The TLS repair pathway is yet another system that enables cells to repair oxidative and other DNA lesions that escape the generally efficient DNA repair systems.[105–107] Spontaneous mutation rates are decreased in cells deficient in TLS and, therefore, it can be speculated that spontaneous mutations in nuclear DNA of yeast and mammalian cells are attributed to the activity of the TLS pathway.[108] TLS occurs when the replication machinery, upon encountering a lesion, has, or somehow acquires, the ability to copy the damaged template directly by incorporating a nucleotide opposite the modified base. TLS is potentially mutagenic because it often incorporates incorrect nucleotides and is described as an error-prone DNA repair pathway.[109] In *S. cerevisiae* the three proteins, Rev1, Rev3 and Rev7 constitute the major components of TLS. The *REV1* gene product possesses deoxycytidyl transferase activity whereas Rev3 and Rev7 proteins are the subunits of DNA polymerase ζ. The function of these proteins is conserved across the species.[106] The yeast TLS polymerases Polη and Polι are both able to insert a C opposite 8-oxoG and in Polη Ogg1 deficient cells there is a synergistic increase in spontaneous mutations.[110,111] The human and mouse DNA polymerase κ (DINB) can also support TLS across oxidative DNA damage.[112–115] and it has been shown that human POLη (XPV) is not essential for the bypass reaction but when present, it is involved in bypass of 8-oxoG *in vivo*.[116] Not all the TLS polymerases bypass 8-oxoG; some only extend from nucleotides inserted opposite this lesion suggesting a concerted action of the various TLS polymerases in bypassing oxidized DNA lesions.[117] The mechanism underlying the choice of polymerase is not yet clear.

As mentioned, mitochondria are a major source of ROS production and dysfunction of this organelle is implicated in mitochondria-mediated nuclear DNA mutagenesis.[13] It has been demonstrated that inactivation of the yeast *REV1, REV3* and *REV7* genes suppressed the rho^0-mediated mutator phenotype suggesting that rho^0 cells generate DNA damage, which is converted into mutations by the TLS pathway. The *REV1, REV3* and *REV7* genes are conserved between yeast and humans and it is, therefore, tempting to speculate that the human REV1, REV3 and REV7 proteins may also be involved in mitochondria-mediated mutagenesis. While the TLS pathway generates mutations in cells with dysfunctional mitochondria, it does not generate mutations in antimycin A-treated cells.[13] This drug is a specific inhibitor of the quinone reduction site; it binds to the bc_1 complex, and blocks electron flow at complex III. These data suggest that DNA damage arising from mitochondrial dysfunction is complex and is converted into mutations by mechanistically different routes.

9. Interaction and Redundancy Between Repair Pathways for Repair of Oxidative Damage

The removal of oxidative DNA damage from the genome is thought to occur primarily via the BER pathway in a process initiated by several DNA glycosylases. However, yeast strains containing multiple disruptions of BER genes are not hypersensitive to killing by oxidizing agents, but show a spontaneous hyper-recombinogenic and mutator phenotype. Eliminating the NER, TLS, and RER pathways further enhances this phenotype and sensitivity to oxidizing agents is not observed unless multiple pathways are eliminated simultaneously. These data strongly suggest that the BER, NER, RER, and TLS have overlapping specificities in the removal of oxidative DNA damage.[118] Furthermore, it appears likely that BER, NER, and MMR proteins exist in both distinct but also in united complexes in cells, at least transiently. These united complexes or "repair factories" probably consist of different subsets of proteins and each has a specialized repair function. For example, it has been proposed that the interaction between *S. cerevisiae* proteins Ntg2 and Mlh1 is important for BER during chromosomal DNA replication.[95] The finding that both Ntg1 and Mlh1 are present in mitochondria suggests an interaction between BER and MMR in this organelle as well. Another explanation is that this interaction is important for mitochondrial DNA repair and represents an example of an integrated simplified repair activity in mitochondria. This new way of thinking reveals that repair complexes are not unique to a certain pathway.

References

1. Cooke MS, Evans MD, Dizdaroglu M, Lunec J. Oxidative DNA damage: mechanisms, mutation, and disease. *FASEB J.* 17: 1195–1214 (2003).
2. Zelko IN, Mariani TJ, Folz RJ. Superoxide dismutase multigene family: a comparison of the *CuZn-SOD* (*SOD1*), *Mn-SOD* (*SOD2*), and *EC-SOD* (*SOD3*) gene structures, evolution, and expression. *Free Radic. Biol. Med.* 33: 337–349 (2002).
3. Fang YZ, Yang S, Wu G. Free radicals, antioxidants, and nutrition. *Nutrition* 18: 872–879 (2002).
4. Boveris A, Cadenas E. Mitochondrial production of superoxide anions and its relationship to the antimycin insensitive respiration. *FEBS Lett.* 54: 311–314 (1975).
5. Boveris A. Mitochondrial production of superoxide radical and hydrogen peroxide. *Adv. Exp. Med. Biol.* 78: 67–82 (1977).
6. Loft S, Poulsen HE. Cancer risk and oxidative DNA damage in man. *J. Mol. Med.* 74: 297–312 (1996).

7. Papa S. Mitochondrial oxidative phosphorylation changes in the life span. Molecular aspects and physiopathological implications. *Biochim. Biophys. Acta* 1276: 87–105 (1996).
8. Bai J, Rodriguez AM, Melendez JA, Cederbaum AI. Overexpression of catalase in cytosolic or mitochondrial compartment protects HepG2 cells against oxidative injury. *J. Biol. Chem.* 274: 26217–26224 (1999).
9. Esposito LA, Melov S, Panov A, Cottrell BA, Wallace DC. Mitochondrial disease in mouse results in increased oxidative stress. *Proc. Natl. Acad. Sci. USA* 96: 4820–4825 (1999).
10. Raha S, McEachern GE, Myint AT, Robinson BH. Superoxides from mitochondrial complex III: the role of manganese superoxide dismutase. *Free Radic. Biol. Med.* 29: 170–180 (2000).
11. Karthikeyan G, Lewis LK, Resnick MA. The mitochondrial protein frataxin prevents nuclear damage. *Hum. Mol. Genet.* 11: 1351–1362 (2002).
12. Mandavilli BS, Santos JH, Van Houten B. Mitochondrial DNA repair and aging. *Mutat. Res.* 509: 127–151 (2002).
13. Rasmussen AK, Chatterjee A, Rasmussen LJ, Singh KK. Mitochondria-mediated nuclear mutator phenotype in *Saccharomyces cerevisiae*. *Nucleic Acids Res.* 31: 3909–3917 (2003).
14. Delsite RL, Rasmussen LJ, Rasmussen AK, Kalen A, Goswami PC, Singh KK. Mitochondrial impairment is accompanied by impaired oxidative DNA repair in the nucleus. *Mutagenesis* 18: 497–503 (2003).
15. Hu JJ, Dubin N, Kurland D, Ma BL, Roush GC. The effects of hydrogen peroxide on DNA repair activities. *Mutat. Res.* 336: 193–201 (1995).
16. Graziewicz MA, Day BJ, Copeland WC. The mitochondrial DNA polymerase as a target of oxidative damage. *Nucleic Acids Res.* 30: 2817–2824 (2002).
17. Mitra S, Hazra TK, Roy R, Ikeda S, Biswas T, Lock J, Boldogh I, Izumi T. Complexities of DNA base excision repair in mammalian cells. *Mol. Cells* 7: 305–312 (1997).
18. Wilson SH. Mammalian base excision repair and DNA polymerase beta. *Mutat. Res.* 407: 203–215 (1998).
19. Mitra S, Boldogh I, Izumi T, Hazra TK. Complexities of the DNA base excision repair pathway for repair of oxidative DNA damage. *Environ. Mol. Mutagen.* 38: 180–190 (2001).
20. Izumi T, Wiederhold LR, Roy R, Jaiswal A, Bhakat KK, Mitra S, Hazra TK. Mammalian DNA base excision repair proteins: their interactions and role in repair of oxidative DNA damage. *Toxicology* 193: 43–65 (2003).

21. Dianov GL, Sleeth KM, Dianova II, Allinson SL. Repair of abasic sites in DNA. *Mutat. Res.* 531: 157–163 (2003).
22. Bjelland S, Seeberg E. Mutagenicity, toxicity and repair of DNA base damage induced by oxidation. *Mutat. Res.* 531: 37–80 (2003).
23. Slupphaug G, Kavli B, Krokan HE. The interacting pathways for prevention and repair of oxidative DNA damage. *Mutat. Res.* 531: 231–251 (2003).
24. Gu Y, Parker A, Wilson TM, Bai H, Chang DY, Lu AL. Human MutY homolog, a DNA glycosylase involved in base excision repair, physically and functionally interacts with mismatch repair proteins human MutS homolog 2/human MutS homolog 6. *J. Biol. Chem.* 277: 11135–11142 (2002).
25. van der Kemp PA, Thomas D, Barbey R, de Oliveira R, Boiteux S. Cloning and expression in *Escherichia coli* of the OGG1 gene of *Saccharomyces cerevisiae*, which codes for a DNA glycosylase that excises 7,8-dihydro-8-oxoguanine and 2,6-diamino-4-hydroxy-5-N-methylformamidopyrimidine. *Proc. Natl. Acad. Sci. USA* 93: 5197–5202 (1996).
26. Singh KK, Sigala B, Sikder HA, Schwimmer C. Inactivation of *Saccharomyces cerevisiae OGG1* DNA repair gene leads to an increased frequency of mitochondrial mutants. *Nucleic Acids Res.* 29: 1381–1388 (2001).
27. Nishioka K, Ohtsubo T, Oda H, Fujiwara T, Kang D, Sugimachi K, Nakabeppu Y. Expression and differential intracellular localization of two major forms of human 8-oxoguanine DNA glycosylase encoded by alternatively spliced OGG1 mRNAs. *Mol. Biol. Cell* 10: 1637–1652 (1999).
28. Hazra TK, Izumi T, Maidt L, Floyd RA, Mitra S. The presence of two distinct 8-oxoguanine repair enzymes in human cells: their potential complementary roles in preventing mutation. *Nucleic Acids Res.* 26: 5116–5122 (1998).
29. O'Rourke TW, Doudican NA, Mackereth MD, Doetsch PW, Shadel GS. Mitochondrial dysfunction due to oxidative mitochondrial DNA damage is reduced through cooperative actions of diverse proteins. *Mol. Cell. Biol.* 22: 4086–4093 (2002).
30. Nakabeppu Y. Regulation of intracellular localization of human MTH1, OGG1, and MYH proteins for repair of oxidative DNA damage. *Prog. Nucleic Acid Res. Mol. Biol.* 68: 75–94 (2001).
31. Hirano S, Tominaga Y, Ichinoe A, Ushijima Y, Tsuchimoto D, Honda-Ohnishi Y, Ohtsubo T, Sakumi K, Nakabeppu Y. Mutator phenotype of MUTYH-null mouse embryonic stem cells. *J. Biol. Chem.* 278: 38121–38124 (2003).
32. Al-Tassan N, Chmiel NH, Maynard J, Fleming N, Livingston AL, Williams GT, Hodges AK, Davies DR, David SS, Sampson JR, Cheadle JP. Inherited

variants of *MYH* associated with somatic G:C → T:A mutations in colorectal tumors. *Nat. Genet.* 30: 227–232 (2002).

33. Lipton L, Halford SE, Johnson V, Novelli MR, Jones A, Cummings C, Barclay E, Sieber O, Sadat A, Bisgaard ML, Hodgson SV, Aaltonen LA, Thomas HJ, Tomlinson IP. Carcinogenesis in MYH-associated polyposis follows a distinct genetic pathway. *Cancer Res.* 63: 7595–7599 (2003).
34. Sieber OM, Lipton L, Crabtree M, Heinimann K, Fidalgo P, Phillips RK, Bisgaard ML, Orntoft TF, Aaltonen LA, Hodgson SV, Thomas HJ, Tomlinson IP. Multiple colorectal adenomas, classic adenomatous polyposis, and germ-line mutations in *MYH*. *N. Engl. J. Med.* 348: 791–799 (2003).
35. Parker AR, O'Meally RN, Sahin F, Su GH, Racke FK, Nelson WG, DeWeese TL, Eshleman JR. Defective human MutY phosphorylation exists in colorectal cancer cell lines with wild-type *MutY* alleles. *J. Biol. Chem.* 278: 47937–47945 (2003).
36. Jaiswal M, LaRusso NF, Nishioka N, Nakabeppu Y, Gores GJ. Human Ogg1, a protein involved in the repair of 8-oxoguanine, is inhibited by nitric oxide. *Cancer Res.* 61: 6388–6393 (2001).
37. Ni TT, Marsischky GT, Kolodner RD. MSH2 and MSH6 are required for removal of adenine misincorporated opposite 8-oxo-guanine in *S. cerevisiae*. *Mol. Cell* 4: 439–444 (1999).
38. Dherin C, Radicella JP, Dizdaroglu M, Boiteux S. Excision of oxidatively damaged DNA bases by the human alpha-hOgg1 protein and the polymorphic alpha-hOgg1(Ser326Cys) protein which is frequently found in human populations. *Nucleic Acids Res.* 27: 4001–4007 (1999).
39. Tsuzuki T, Egashira A, Igarashi H, Iwakuma T, Nakatsuru Y, Tominaga Y, Kawate H, Nakao K, Nakamura K, Ide F, Kura S, Nakabeppu Y, Katsuki M, Ishikawa T, Sekiguchi M. Spontaneous tumorigenesis in mice defective in the *MTH1* gene encoding 8-oxo-dGTPase. *Proc. Natl. Acad. Sci. USA* 98: 11456–11461 (2001).
40. Hazra TK, Izumi T, Boldogh I, Imhoff B, Kow YW, Jaruga P, Dizdaroglu M, Mitra S. Identification and characterization of a human DNA glycosylase for repair of modified bases in oxidatively damaged DNA. *Proc. Natl. Acad. Sci. USA* 99: 3523–3528 (2002a).
41. Takao M, Kanno S, Kobayashi K, Zhang QM, Yonei S, van der Horst GT, Yasui A. A back-up glycosylase in Nth1 knock-out mice is a functional Nei (endonuclease VIII) homologue. *J. Biol. Chem.* 277: 42205–42213 (2002).
42. Dizdaroglu M, Karahalil B, Senturker S, Buckley TJ, Roldan-Arjona T. Excision of products of oxidative DNA base damage by human NTH1 protein. *Biochemistry* 38: 243–246 (1999).

43. Eide L, Luna L, Gustad EC, Henderson PT, Essigmann JM, Demple B, Seeberg E. Human endonuclease III acts preferentially on DNA damage opposite guanine residues in DNA. *Biochemistry* 40: 6653–6659 (2001).
44. Miyabe I, Zhang QM, Kino K, Sugiyama H, Takao M, Yasui A, Yonei S. Identification of 5-formyluracil DNA glycosylase activity of human hNTH1 protein. *Nucleic Acids Res.* 30: 3443–3448 (2002).
45. Hazra TK, Kow YW, Hatahet Z, Imhoff B, Boldogh I, Mokkapati SK, Mitra S, Izumi T. Identification and characterization of a novel human DNA glycosylase for repair of cytosine-derived lesions. *J. Biol. Chem.* 277: 30417–30420 (2002b).
46. Rusmintratip V, Sowers LC. An unexpectedly high excision capacity for mispaired 5-hydroxymethyluracil in human cell extracts. *Proc. Natl. Acad. Sci. USA* 97: 14183–14187 (2000).
47. Haushalter KA, Stukenberg T, Kirschner MW, Verdine GL. Identification of a new uracil-DNA glycosylase family by expression cloning using synthetic inhibitors. *Curr. Biol.* 9: 174–185 (1999).
48. Boorstein RJ, Cummings A Jr, Marenstein DR, Chan MK, Ma Y, Neubert TA, Brown SM, Teebor GW. Definitive identification of mammalian 5-hydroxymethyluracil DNA N-glycosylase activity as SMUG1. *J. Biol. Chem.* 276: 41991–41997 (2001).
49. Baker D, Liu P, Burdzy A, Sowers LC. Characterization of the substrate specificity of a human 5-hydroxymethyluracil glycosylase activity. *Chem. Res. Toxicol.* 15: 33–39 (2002).
50. Dizdaroglu M, Karakaya A, Jaruga P, Slupphaug G, Krokan HE. Novel activities of human uracil DNA N-glycosylase for cytosine-derived products of oxidative DNA damage. *Nucleic Acids Res.* 24: 418–422 (1996).
51. Fujimoto J, Tran L, Sowers LC. Synthesis and cleavage of oligodeoxynucleotides containing a 5-hydroxyuracil residue at a defined site. *Chem. Res. Toxicol.* 10: 1254–1258 (1997).
52. Ischenko AA, Saparbaev MK. Alternative nucleotide incision repair pathway for oxidative DNA damage. *Nature* 415: 183–187 (2002).
53. Gros L, Ishchenko A, Hiroshi I, Elder RH, Saparbaev MK. The major human AP endonuclease (Ape1) is involved in the nucleotide incision repair pathway. *Nucleic Acids Res.* 32: 73–83 (2004).
54. Jansen JG, de Wind N. Biological functions of translesion synthesis proteins in vertebrates. *DNA Repair* 2: 1075–1085 (2003).
55. Pinz KG, Shibutani S, Bogenhagen DF. Action of mitochondrial DNA polymerase gamma at sites of base loss or oxidative damage. *J. Biol. Chem.* 270: 9202–9206 (1995).

56. Helleday T. Pathways for mitotic homologous recombination in mammalian cells. *Mutat. Res.* 532: 103–115 (2003).
57. Valyi-Nagy T, Olson SJ, Valyi-Nagy K, Montine TJ, Dermody TS. Herpes simplex virus type 1 latency in the murine nervous system is associated with oxidative damage to neurons. *Virology* 278: 309–321 (2000).
58. Milatovic D, Zhang Y, Olson SJ, Montine KS, Roberts LJ 2nd, Morrow JD, Montine TJ, Dermody TS, Valyi-Nagy T. Herpes simplex virus type 1 encephalitis is associated with elevated levels of F2-isoprostanes and F4-neuroprostanes. *J. Neurovirol.* 8: 295–305 (2002).
59. Nimonkar AV, Boehmer PE. Reconstitution of recombination-dependent DNA synthesis in herpes simplex virus 1. *Proc. Natl. Acad. Sci. USA* 100: 10201–10206 (2003).
60. Winn LM, Kim PM, Nickoloff JA. Oxidative stress-induced homologous recombination as a novel mechanism for phenytoin-initiated toxicity. *J. Pharmacol. Exp. Ther.* 306: 523–527 (2003).
61. Karthikeyan G, Santos JH, Graziewicz MA, Copeland WC, Isaya G, Van Houten B, Resnick MA. Reduction in frataxin causes progressive accumulation of mitochondrial damage. *Hum. Mol. Genet.* 12: 3331–3342 (2003).
62. Vance JR, Wilson TE. Repair of DNA strand breaks by the overlapping functions of lesion-specific and non-lesion-specific DNA 3′ phosphatases. *Mol. Cell. Biol.* 21: 7191–7198 (2001a).
63. Vance JR, Wilson TE. Uncoupling of 3′-phosphatase and 5′-kinase functions in budding yeast. Characterization of *Saccharomyces cerevisiae* DNA 3′-phosphatase (TPP1). *J. Biol. Chem.* 276: 15073–15081 (2000b).
64. Karumbati AS, Deshpande RA, Jilani A, Vance JR, Ramotar D, Wilson TE. The role of yeast DNA 3′-phosphatase Tpp1 and Rad1/Rad10 endonuclease in processing spontaneous and induced base lesions. *J. Biol. Chem.* 278: 31434–31443 (2003).
65. Nicholson A, Hendrix M, Jinks-Robertson S, Crouse GF. Regulation of mitotic homeologous recombination in yeast. Functions of mismatch repair and nucleotide excision repair genes. *Genetics* 154: 133–146 (2000).
66. Dujon B, Slonimski PP, Weill L. Mitochondrial genetics IX: A model for recombination and segregation of mitochondrial genomes in *Saccharomyces cerevisiae*. *Genetics* 78: 415–437 (1974).
67. Contamine V, Picard M. Maintenance and integrity of the mitochondrial genome: a plethora of nuclear genes in the budding yeast. *Microbiol. Mol. Biol. Rev.* 64: 281–315 (2000).

68. Reenan RA, Kolodner RD. Characterization of insertion mutations in the *Saccharomyces cerevisiae* MSH1 and MSH2 genes: evidence for separate mitochondrial and nuclear functions. *Genetics* 132: 975–985 (1992).
69. Chi NW, Kolodner RD. Purification and characterization of MSH1, a yeast mitochondrial protein that binds to DNA mismatches. *J. Biol. Chem.* 269: 29984–29992 (1994).
70. Lahaye A, Stahl H, Thines-Sempoux D, Foury F. PIF1: a DNA helicase in yeast mitochondria. *EMBO J.* 10: 997–1007 (1991).
71. Ling F, Morioka H, Ohtsuka E, Shibata T. A role for *MHR1*, a gene required for mitochondrial genetic recombination, in the repair of damage spontaneously introduced in yeast mtDNA. *Nucleic Acids Res.* 28: 4956–4963 (2000).
72. Gu L, Huang SM, Sander M. Single amino acid changes alter the repair specificity of *Drosophila* Rrp1. Isolation of mutants deficient in repair of oxidative DNA damage. *J. Biol. Chem.* 269: 32685–32692 (1994).
73. Szakmary A, Huang SM, Chang DT, Beachy PA, Sander M. Overexpression of a Rrp1 transgene reduces the somatic mutation and recombination frequency induced by oxidative DNA damage in *Drosophila melanogaster*. *Proc. Natl. Acad. Sci. USA* 93: 1607–1612 (1996).
74. Nugent M, Huang SM, Sander M. Characterization of the apurinic endonuclease activity of *Drosophila* Rrp1. *Biochemistry* 32: 11445–11452 (1993).
75. Sander M, Carter M, Huang SM. Expression of *Drosophila* Rrp1 protein in *Escherichia coli*. Enzymatic and physical characterization of the intact protein and a carboxyl-terminally deleted exonuclease-deficient mutant. *J. Biol. Chem.* 268: 2075–2082 (1993).
76. Sander M, Huang SM. Characterization of the nuclease activity of *Drosophila* Rrp1 on phosphoglycolate- and phosphate-modified DNA 3′-termini. *Biochemistry* 34: 1267–1274 (1995).
77. Rasmussen LJ, Samson L, Marinus MG. Dam-directed DNA mismatch repair. In: Hoekstra MF, Nickoloff (eds.) *DNA Damage and Repair: Molecular and Cell Biology*. The Humana Press Inc., pp. 205–228, 1998.
78. Genschel J, Modrich P. Mechanism of 5′-directed excision in human mismatch repair. *Mol. Cell* 12: 1077–1086 (2003).
79. Hsieh P. Molecular mechanisms of DNA mismatch repair. *Mutat. Res.* 486: 71–87 (2001).
80. Jiricny J, Marra G. DNA repair defects in colon cancer. *Curr. Opin. Genet. Dev.* 13: 61–69 (2003).

81. Sickmann A, Reinders J, Wagner Y, Joppich C, Zahedi R, Meyer HE, Schonfisch B, Perschil I, Chacinska A, Guiard B, Rehling P, Pfanner N, Meisinger C. The proteome of *Saccharomyces cerevisiae* mitochondria. *Proc. Natl. Acad. Sci. USA* 100: 13207–13212 (2003).
82. Chen Z, Felsheim R, Wong P, Augustin LB, Metz R, Kren BT, Steer CJ. Mitochondria isolated from liver contain the essential factors required for RNA/DNA oligonucleotide-targeted gene repair. *Biochem. Biophys. Res. Commun.* 285: 188–194 (2001).
83. Mason PA, Matheson EC, Hall AG, Lightowlers RN. Mismatch repair activity in mammalian mitochondria. *Nucleic Acids Res.* 31: 1052–1058 (2003).
84. Earley MC, Crouse GF. The role of mismatch repair in the prevention of base pair mutations in *Saccharomyces cerevisiae*. *Proc. Natl. Acad. Sci. USA* 95: 15487–15491 (1998).
85. Mazurek A, Berardini M, Fishel R. Activation of human MutS homologs by 8-oxo-guanine DNA damage. *J. Biol. Chem.* 277: 8260–8266 (2002).
86. Boiteux S, Gellon L, Guibourt N. Repair of 8-oxoguanine in *Saccharomyces cerevisiae*: interplay of DNA repair and replication mechanisms. *Free Radic. Biol. Med.* 32: 1244–1253 (2002).
87. Jackson AL, Chen R, Loeb LA. Induction of microsatellite instability by oxidative DNA damage. *Proc. Natl. Acad. Sci. USA* 95: 12468–12473 (1998).
88. Turker MS, Gage BM, Rose JA, Elroy D, Ponomareva ON, Stambrook PJ, Tischfield JA. A novel signature mutation for oxidative damage resembles a mutational pattern found commonly in human cancers. *Cancer Res.* 59: 1837–1839 (1999).
89. Chang CL, Marra G, Chauhan DP, Ha HT, Chang DK, Ricciardiello L, Randolph A, Carethers JM, Boland CR. Oxidative stress inactivates the human DNA mismatch repair system. *Am. J. Physiol. Cell Physiol.* 283: C148–C154 (2002).
90. Yamada NA, Parker JM, Farber RA. Mutation frequency analysis of mononucleotide and dinucleotide repeats after oxidative stress. *Environ. Mol. Mutagen.* 42: 75–84 (2003).
91. Glaab WE, Hill RB, Skopek TR. Suppression of spontaneous and hydrogen peroxide-induced mutagenesis by the antioxidant ascorbate in mismatch repair-deficient human colon cancer cells. *Carcinogenesis* 22: 1709–1713 (2001).
92. Colussi C, Parlanti E, Degan P, Aquilina G, Barnes D, Macpherson P, Karran P, Crescenzi M, Dogliotti E, Bignami M. The mammalian mismatch repair pathway removes DNA 8-oxodGMP incorporated from the oxidized dNTP pool. *Curr. Biol.* 12: 912–918 (2002).

93. Larson, ED Iams K, Drummond JT. Strand-specific processing of 8-oxoguanine by the human mismatch repair pathway: inefficient removal of 8-oxoguanine paired with adenine or cytosine. *DNA Repair* 2: 1199–1210 (2003).
94. Slupska MM, Luther WM, Chiang JH, Yang H, Miller JH. Functional expression of hMYH, a human homolog of the *Escherichia coli* MutY protein. *J. Bacteriol.* 181: 6210–6213 (1999).
95. Gellon L, Werner M, Boiteux S. Ntg2p, a *Saccharomyces cerevisiae* DNA N-glycosylase/apurinic or apyrimidinic lyase involved in base excision repair of oxidative DNA damage, interacts with the DNA mismatch repair protein Mlh1p. Identification of a Mlh1p binding motif. *J. Biol. Chem.* 277: 29963–29972 (2002).
96. van Hoffen A, Balajee AS, van Zeeland AA, Mullenders LH. Nucleotide excision repair and its interplay with transcription. *Toxicology* 193: 79–90 (2003).
97. Drapkin R, Reardon JT, Ansari A, Huang JC, Zawel L, Ahn K, Sancar A, Reinberg D. Dual role of TFIIH in DNA excision repair and in transcription by RNA polymerase II. *Nature* 368: 769–772 (1994).
98. de Boer J, Hoeijmakers JH. Nucleotide excision repair and human syndromes. *Carcinogenesis* 21: 453–460 (2000).
99. Hoeijmakers JH. Genome maintenance mechanisms for preventing cancer. *Nature* 411: 366–374 (2001).
100. Lin JJ, Sancar A. A new mechanism for repairing oxidative damage to DNA: (A)BC excinuclease removes AP sites and thymine glycols from DNA. *Biochemistry* 28: 7979–7984 (1989).
101. Czeczot H, Tudek B, Lambert B, Laval J, Boiteux S. *Escherichia coli* Fpg protein and UvrABC endonuclease repair DNA damage induced by methylene blue plus visible light *in vivo* and *in vitro*. *J. Bacteriol.* 173: 3419–3424 (1991).
102. Reardon JT, Bessho T, Kung HC, Bolton PH, Sancar A. *In vitro* repair of oxidative DNA damage by human nucleotide excision repair system: possible explanation for neurodegeneration in xeroderma pigmentosum patients. *Proc. Natl. Acad. Sci. USA* 94: 9463–9468 (1997).
103. Scott AD, Neishabury M, Jones DH, Reed SH, Boiteux S, Waters R. Spontaneous mutation, oxidative DNA damage, and the roles of base and nucleotide excision repair in the yeast *Saccharomyces cerevisiae*. *Yeast* 15: 205–218 (1999).
104. Swanson RL, Morey NJ, Doetsch PW, Jinks-Robertson S. Overlapping specificities of base excision repair, nucleotide excision repair, recombination,

and translesion synthesis pathways for DNA base damage in *Saccharomyces cerevisiae*. *Mol. Cell. Biol.* 19: 2929–2935 (1999).

105. Kusumoto R, Masutani C, Iwai S, Hanaoka F. Translesion synthesis by human DNA polymerase eta across thymine glycol lesions. *Biochemistry* 41: 6090–6099 (2002).

106. Jensen A, Calvayrac G, Karahalil B, Bohr VA, Stevnsner T. Mammalian 8-oxoguanine DNA glycosylase 1 incises 8-oxoadenine opposite cytosine in nuclei and mitochondria, while a different glycosylase incises 8-oxoadenine opposite guanine in nuclei. *J. Biol. Chem.* 278: 19541–19548 (2003).

107. Kozmin SG, Pavlov YI, Kunkel TA, Sage E. Roles of *Saccharomyces cerevisiae* DNA polymerases Poleta and Polzeta in response to irradiation by simulated sunlight. *Nucleic Acids Res.* 31: 4541–4552 (2003).

108. Glassner BJ, Rasmussen LJ, Najarian MT, Posnick LM, Samson LD. Generation of a strong mutator phenotype in yeast by imbalanced base excision repair. *Proc. Natl. Acad. Sci. USA* 95: 9997–10002 (1998).

109. Kunz BA, Straffon AF, Vonarx EJ. DNA damage-induced mutation: tolerance via translesion synthesis. *Mutat. Res.* 451: 169–185 (2000).

110. Haracska L, Yu SL, Johnson RE, Prakash L, Prakash S. Efficient and accurate replication in the presence of 7,8-dihydro-8-oxoguanine by DNA polymerase eta. *Nat. Genet.* 25: 458–461 (2000).

111. Vaisman A, Woodgate R. Unique misinsertion specificity of poliota may decrease the mutagenic potential of deaminated cytosines. *EMBO J.* 20: 6520–6529 (2001).

112. Fischhaber PL, Gerlach VL, Feaver WJ, Hatahet Z, Wallace SS, Friedberg EC. Human DNA polymerase kappa bypasses and extends beyond thymine glycols during translesion synthesis *in vitro*, preferentially incorporating correct nucleotides. *J. Biol. Chem.* 277: 37604–37611 (2002).

113. Schenten D, Gerlach VL, Guo C, Velasco-Miguel S, Hladik CL, White CL, Friedberg EC, Rajewsky K, Esposito G. DNA polymerase kappa deficiency does not affect somatic hypermutation in mice. *Eur. J. Immunol.* 32: 3152–3160 (2002).

114. Guo C, Fischhaber PL, Luk-Paszyc MJ, Masuda Y, Zhou J, Kamiya K, Kisker C, Friedberg EC. Mouse Rev1 protein interacts with multiple DNA polymerases involved in translesion DNA synthesis. *EMBO J.* 22: 6621–6630 (2003).

115. Velasco-Miguel S, Richardson JA, Gerlach VL, Lai WC, Gao T, Russell LD, Hladik CL, White CL, Friedberg EC. Constitutive and regulated expression of the mouse Dinb (Polkappa) gene encoding DNA polymerase kappa. *DNA Repair* 2: 91–106 (2003).

116. Avkin S, Livneh Z. Efficiency, specificity and DNA polymerase-dependence of translesion replication across the oxidative DNA lesion 8-oxoguanine in human cells. *Mutat. Res.* 510: 81–90 (2002).
117. Haracska L, Prakash S, Prakash L. Yeast DNA polymerase zeta is an efficient extender of primer ends opposite from 7,8-dihydro-8-oxoguanine and O6-methylguanine. *Mol. Cell. Biol.* 23: 1453–1459 (2003).
118. Doetsch PW, Morey NJ, Swanson RL, Jinks-Robertson S. Yeast base excision repair: interconnections and networks. *Prog. Nucleic Acid Res. Mol. Biol.* 68: 29–39 (2001).

8 Cellular Responses to Reactive Oxygen Species

Ian W. Dawes

1. Introduction

With the evolution of efficient systems for generating energy that are based on respiration, came the production of reactive species based on the interesting chemistry of oxygen. These species are summarized in Fig. 1.

They are generated mainly as a result of metabolism, primarily through the leakage of electrons from the respiratory chain during the reduction of molecular oxygen to water. This leads to generation of the superoxide anion, $O_2^{\bullet -1}$ which is also generated in microsomal metabolism and during the respiratory burst produced by phagocytes as part of the process of killing bacteria. H_2O_2 is produced from the dismutation of $O_2^{\bullet -}$ catalyzed by superoxide dismutase (SOD) enzymes, as well as from oxidases and β-oxidation of fatty acids in peroxisomes. During phagocytosis, neutrophils produce hypochlorite from H_2O_2 via the action of myeloperoxidase, and this can act on free amines to form chloramines that are also toxic to cells. More serious for the cell, however, is the generation from H_2O_2 of the much more highly reactive hydroxyl radical, $^{\bullet}OH$, which can react indiscriminately with most cellular constituents.[2,3] Generation of $^{\bullet}OH$ is catalyzed by reduced transition metal ions such as Fe^{2+}, which are oxidized in the process in the Fenton reaction, and this reaction is enhanced by the simultaneous presence of $O_2^{\bullet -}$ or other reductants which can reduce the Fe^{3+} to Fe^{2+}. The mechanisms involved metal ion homeostasis for Cu and Fe ions in particular are therefore also of considerable importance in the

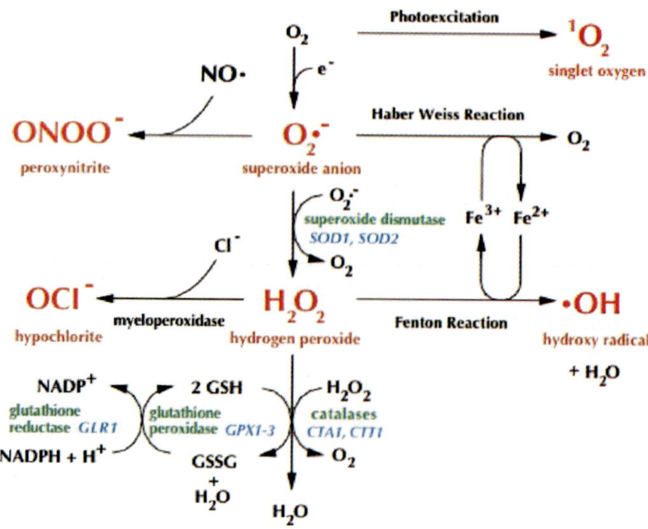

Fig. 1. Reactive oxygen species in biological systems. The reactive species generated from oxygen are indicated in red. Enzymic defences are in green, with genes encoding these in *Saccharomyces cerevisiae* given in blue. Hypochlorite is generated in neutrophils as part of the respiratory burst, while peroxynitrate is produced in those organisms that produce the nitric oxide radical.

cellular defences to minimize formation of reactive oxygen species. Singlet oxygen is formed by fungal metabolites and air pollutants in the presence of light, and in plants by photo-excited chlorophyll, and can cause membrane lipid peroxidation, photo-oxidation of amino acids and DNA damage.[3] In plants there are two organelles (chloroplast and mitochondrion) in which free radical reactions can lead to the generation of reactive oxygen species, and of these the chloroplast may be the more active.

A plethora of secondary ROS and other radicals are formed from reaction of these species with cellular metabolites, and these make molecular analysis of the outcomes of reactive oxygen species generation very difficult. These species differ considerably in reactivity.[4,5] Unsaturated fatty acyl groups are a major target of $^{\bullet}OH$ and the protonated form of $O_2^{\bullet-\bullet}$ These initiate autocatalytic lipid peroxidation to form reactive lipid radicals and lipid hydroperoxides.[6,7] These are very toxic to some cells and can initiate membrane damage.[8] Breakdown of lipid hydroperoxides also leads to the formation of reactive aldehydes such as malondialdehyde and 4-hydroxynonenal which can cause carbonylation of proteins.[9] These modified proteins increase when cells are starved for carbon or nitrogen sources and as cells age.[10,11]

•OH damage to proteins leads to cross-linking, fragmentation and oxidation of amino acyl residues, particularly aromatic side chains and cysteine.[12] The protein hydroperoxides formed are reactive and decompose to free radicals leading to further protein modification and unfolding.[13] Hydroxylated derivatives are formed from damage to amino acids, while oxidation of aromatic amino acid residues can produce reactive phenoxy radicals.[14,15]

DNA damage has been noted following treatment of cells with ROS, and these have been implicated in mutagenesis and carcinogenesis[16,17] as discussed in detail in Chapter 24. In yeast, paraquat (which leads to $O_2^{\bullet-}$) and H_2O_2 cause intra-chromosomal recombination, and also significant levels of inter-chromosomal recombination at high doses.[18] Cells also generate reactive nitrogen species from reaction of the nitric oxide radical $NO^{\bullet}$ with the superoxide anion forming reactive peroxynitrite $ONOO^-$ and the nitrogen dioxide radical ($NO_2^{\bullet}$). These species can nitrate aromatic amino acid residues,[19] damage DNA[6] and oxidize thiols.[20] There is extensive literature on how cells are affected by oxidative stress induced by a variety of reactive oxygen species. Despite this, recent developments in genomic analysis have led to a much more detailed insight into how cells respond to oxidants. This is particularly the case for the yeast *Saccharomyces cerevisiae*. This is due to the speed and ease of biochemical and genetic analyses in this organism coupled with the development of advanced genomic techniques including DNA microarray for analysis of transcription of all genes in the genome,[21,22] deletion mutants for every non-essential gene,[23] and extensive data on protein-protein interactions,[24,25] GST-fusion constructs for expressing every ORF,[26] synthetic lethality of mutations,[27] and transcription factor binding.[28]

2. Cells Have a Range of General Responses to Reactive Oxygen Species

As unicellular microorganisms, yeast cells grown aerobically are exposed to continuous oxidative stress. Since this is probably one of the more ancient stresses with the appearance of oxygen in the atmosphere approximately three billion years ago, and there are many different ROS generated in aerobic cells, organisms have evolved a wide variety of systems and responses to provide defences against the deleterious effects and deal with the ROS. Many of these defence systems are conserved from yeast to human.

In general terms, these include the presence of constitutive functions which protect against sudden exposure as well as the ability to modulate gene expression and metabolism to up-regulate antioxidant and repair systems and down-regulate growth functions to allow the cells time to repair damage.[22,29] The systems involved in maintaining antioxidant functions in yeast include low molecular mass redox-active molecules such as glutathione, D-erythroascorbate (the 5C analogue of ascorbate), ubiquinol and (for hypochlorite stress) urate. The enzymic antioxidants include two superoxide dismutases (Sod1 is mainly cytosolic, Sod2 is mitochondrial), catalases (cytosolic Ctt1 and peroxisomal Cta1), thioredoxins (Trx1 and Trx2) and glutaredoxins (Grx1 and Grx2) glutathione peroxidases (Gpx1, Gpx2 and Gpx3) and thioredoxin peroxidases (periredoxins — encoded by five genes including Tpa1, Tpa2 and Ahp1). These have been discussed in more detail elsewhere.[29] The two Cu-ion scavenging metalothioneins, Cup1 and Crs5, are important, as are many other genes associated with Fe and Cu homeostasis.[30]

As part of the regulation of gene expression in response to ROS cells can adapt to become more resistant to subsequent challenge with a range of ROS[8,31–34] and delay cell division, possibly to increase the opportunity for the cells to repair damage before further proliferation leads to irreparable fixing of the damage if the cells progress in the cell cycle.[35–38] Like higher organisms, when the damage is beyond that which can be repaired they can initiate a form of programmed cell death that resembles apoptosis.[39,40]

3. Adaptation to Resistance

Yeast cells are capable of adapting to treatment with a low dose of a range of ROS such that they become resistant to a subsequent higher dose that would lead to extensive killing of untreated cells. This is illustrated for H_2O_2 in Fig. 2.

Cells are capable of adapting to a wide range of ROS and their breakdown products, including the $O_2^{\bullet -}$ generators paraquat and menadione, linoleate

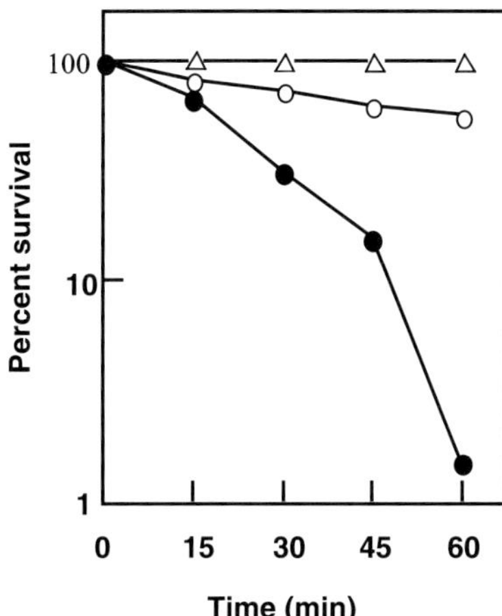

Fig. 2. Adaptation of yeast cells to H_2O_2. Exponential phase cells were treated with either buffer (closed circles) or with 0.2 mM hydrogen peroxide (open circles) in buffer for 1 h then exposed to 2 mM hydrogen peroxide at zero time. The percentage survival was determined at intervals by plating on rich medium. The control data (open triangles) were for cells treated in buffer and resuspended in the buffer.

hydroperoxide (LoaOOH), and malondialdehyde and in all cases adaptation to H_2O_2 depends to a large extent on *de novo* gene expression. For most ROS petite strains lacking a mitochondrial genome are much more sensitive to the oxidant, but adaptation still occurs in petites.[8,31–34] The one exception to the sensitivity of petites is that they are much more resistant to LoaOOH than the wild-type strain.[8] Adaptation is fairly rapid, but is transient lasting only about four hours under normal growth conditions.[41] It has recently been shown that yeast cells are rather less permeable to H_2O_2 than was previously thought, and part of the adaptive process involves regulation of the permeability of the plasma membrane to H_2O_2.[42]

There are differences between the various ROS in the adaptive responses that they elicit and these are highlighted from cross adaptation studies. Heat shock confers adaptation to most ROS treatments, as does H_2O_2, but H_2O_2 does not confer thermotolerance. H_2O_2 leads to superoxide tolerance but not vice versa. Clearly there are distinct, but overlapping pathways involved in these adaptive responses. Despite the relatively early discovery of yeast adaptation, the mechanisms involved are still not fully understood. Most work has been done on H_2O_2. From secondary screening of $\sim$270

H_2O_2-sensitive mutants identified in a genome-wide analysis of the set of deletion mutants (see Sec. 4) we have identified only seven genes that when deleted lead to a marked reduction in the adaptive response to H_2O_2. These fall into two groups; the first encode transcription factors including: Yap1 which is the major oxidative stress transcription factor in yeast;[43] Skn7 which partners Yap1 to regulate genes encoding antioxidant systems rather than NADPH generation;[44] and, the more general transcriptional co-activator Gal11. The second set of genes included ones that may be involved in the generation of NADPH via the pentose phosphate pathway and in the mitochondrion (Ng, personal communication). In previous studies Yap1 and Yap2 were shown to play a role in adaptation to H_2O_2, but not to $O_2^{\bullet -}$.[45] Inhibition of glutathione metabolism has been reported to reduce adaptation,[46] but we and others have not found mutants that are unable to synthesize glutathione to have lost adaptation.[47]

The adaptive response to linoleic acid hydroperoxide is almost completely abolished in mutants that lack the glutathione peroxidases encoded by *GPX1* and *GPX2*, but not in strains lacking *GPX3* (Israel, personal communication). This is interesting in light of the role played by Gpx3 in sensing H_2O_2-induced stress,[48,49] and it is possible that Gpx1 and/or Gpx2 plays a similar role in sensing lipid hydroperoxide-induced damage in membranes. The three *GPX* genes, encoding phospholipid hydroperoxide glutathione peroxidases[50] are regulated differently. *GPX3* is relatively highly expressed and has been reported to be constitutively expressed,[51] although data from this laboratory show that it is subject to the oleate-response system controlled by the Pip1 and Oaf1 transcription factors. Regulation by the system controlling fatty acid breakdown would be consistent with the generation of H_2O_2 during the catabolism of fatty acids in the peroxisome and the role of Gpx3 in sensing this ROS. *GPX1* is up-regulated by glucose starvation via the Msn2/Msn4 transcription factor, while *GPX2* is up-regulated by treatment with ROS, largely under the control of Yap1[51] (Israel, personal communication).

4. Gene Expression Responses to ROS

There is a major dependence on new gene expression for adaptation, and also for the subsequent recovery from oxidative damage since a number of antioxidant and repair systems are up-regulated following ROS exposure. These include Sod1 and Sod2 (cytoplasmic and mitochondrial SODs), Glr1 (glutathione reductase), Ctt1 (cytosolic catalase), Trr1 (thioredoxin reductase) and Trx2 (thioredoxin), Tsa1 (periredoxin or thioredoxin peroxidase), Ssa1 (stress-inducible heat shock protein 70) and Ahp1. Unlike some other response systems in yeast, many of the regulatory changes were found to be relatively low, of the order of four-fold or less. This may reflect the fact that some antioxidant functions can be deleterious when over-expressed, and that cells have evolved a wide range of defences that are each only subtly up-regulated in response to oxidative damage.

The transcription factors that are important in response to ROS stress include the fairly specific oxidative stress-response factor Yap1 (one of the eight homologues of the human AP-1 family of proteins), Skn7 (which plays an auxiliary role with Yap1 the more general stress responsive Msn2 and Msn4, and the Hap1 and the multimeric Hap2,3,4,5 factors that activate genes mainly in response to the switch to respiratory metabolism. The Ace1 and Mac1 transcription factors involved in copper ion homeostasis and Aft1 that regulates iron uptake are also critical to oxidative stress resistance. The promoters of a few of these genes have been studied in detail. It is clear that they have multiple elements responding to a set of stress-related transcription factors. Each gene has its own mix of motifs for binding of transcription factors that activate transcription in different phases of growth or different stress conditions. For example the *SOD2* gene is up-regulated by the Msn2/4 transcription factor in response to the shift from fermentation to respiratory conditions,[52] but in response to superoxide generating agents it is induced through the action of the Hap1 factor.[53]

Genome-wide transcriptional analyses of the response of *Saccharomyces cerevisiae* have been done for a broad range of different stresses, including: heat shock; exposure to H_2O_2, diamide and menadione and the reducing agent dithiothreitol; hypo- and hyper-osmotic shock; amino acid starvation; nitrogen-source depletion; and, progression to stationary phase.[22] A very large group of genes ($\sim$900) were similarly and transiently responsive across most of these stresses, with the exception of starvation conditions, although no two stress conditions elicited an identical pattern of gene expression. This general response has been described as an environmental stress response (ESR). Of the $\sim$600 genes that were repressed, many were involved in growth-related processes, including aspects of RNA metabolism, translation, nucleotide metabolism and ribosomal protein synthesis, indicating that at fairly high doses cellular growth is slowed presumably to allow diversion of energy generation to repair processes. Of the genes that were induced following the shocks, there were representatives of a range of functions including carbohydrate metabolism, detoxification of ROS, cellular redox processes, cell wall modification, protein folding and degradation, DNA damage repair, fatty acid metabolism, metabolite transport, vacuolar and mitochondrial functions, autophagy and signaling. Many of the genes identified had previously been reported to be involved in protecting cells from various stresses, and they included one large group that were known to be controlled via the Msn2/4 transcription factor.

By using *yap1* and *msn2 msn4* mutants, it was shown that this response is not under the control of a single regulatory system, since some genes (e.g. those involved in the redox systems) were controlled by one of these factors under one condition, and another factor under another stress. For example, genes in the *TRX2* cluster (which includes many antioxidant functions) are regulated by Msn2/4 following heat shock, but by Yap1 when cells are treated with H_2O_2.

Since many of the genes that are regulated by the ESR were known to be controlled by the protein kinase A (PKA) signaling pathway in response to nutritional signals, and the protein kinase C (PKC) pathway following inhibition of secretion, it has been suggested that the ESR regulation may be an integration of the PKA response to nutritional signals and the PKC response when secretion is impaired.[22]

Detailed proteomic analysis of the responses of cells to H_2O_2, has identified similar sets of genes to those identified in the transcriptomics, especially those involved in induction of Yap1-regulated genes.[44,54] This also showed that there were two sets of genes in the H_2O_2 stimulon, one set of genes mainly involved in the synthesis of enzymes with antioxidant activity and redox control required Yap1 acting in conjunction with the auxiliary transcription factor Skn7, while others that were needed for NADPH regeneration only depended on Yap1.

In addition to the ESR response, each individual ROS leads to specific induction of genes not commonly induced by other ROS.[55] This is illustrated in Fig. 3, which shows the transcriptional response of cells to relatively high doses of linoleic acid hydroperoxide (LoaOOH) in comparison with the data

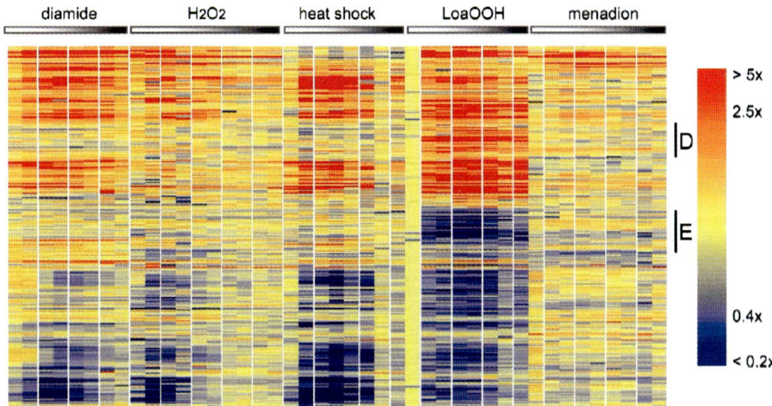

Fig. 3. Hierarchical clustering of transcriptional responses induced by various ROS and heat shock in *Saccharomyces cerevisiae*. The data are the result of time-course studies of the response of cells to a challenge with each stress indicated, and are a composite of those from Gasch *et al.*[22] and Alic *et al.*[55] Each horizontal line represents the expression pattern of a gene that is significantly up-regulated by treatment with 30 micromolar LoaOOH. D indicates the set of genes that are uniquely up-regulated by LoaOOH, and E to those that are specifically down-regulated.

from Gasch *et al.*[22] In addition to the ESR group of genes, there is a set of genes induced only by the LoaOOH, and a specific set of repressed genes. The genes induced encoded proteins associated with membrane functions, as well as the signaling molecule Ste20 that is involved in two MAPK pathways in yeast. Interestingly, in this case a number of the specifically induced genes appear to be regulated by the Pdr1 and Pdr3 transcription factors that mediate the metabolism of xenobiotics and multi-drug resistance transport systems in yeast. These are homologues of the human *mrd* multi-drug resistance transcription factors.

5. Cell Transcriptional Response Patterns are very Concentration Dependent

High-dose treatment of cells with LoaOOH led to a switch in transcription from biosynthetic to protective functions, and to repression of growth functions (Fig. 3)[55] as found by other microarray and proteomic analyses.[22,54,56] This study was extended, with interesting results, to determine the changes

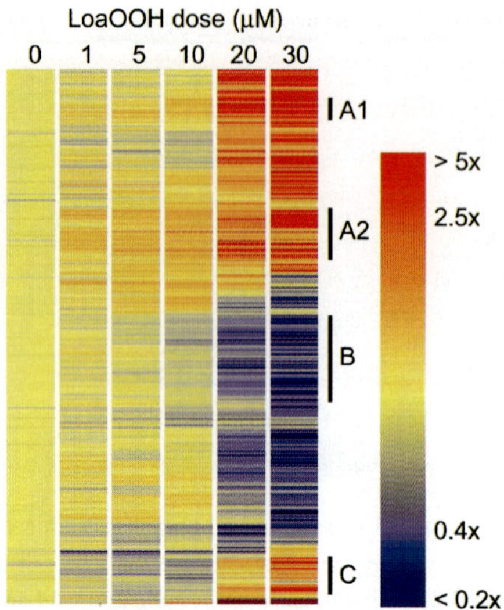

Fig. 4. Dose dependence of the pattern of transcriptional changes in response to LoaOOH. Exponential cells were treated with the concentration indicated for 1 h prior to microarray analysis and the data obtained analyzed by hierarchical clustering. A1 and A2 indicate the genes that are up-regulated even at low doses; B those that are down-regulated at low doses, while C (which contains many involved in oxidative stress defences) indicates the set of genes that are down-regulated at low dose and up-regulated at higher doses. Modified from Alic *et al.*[55]

in transcripts across a wide range of doses, from very low ones that were known to lead to stimulation of the Mpk1 protein in the cell integrity MAPK pathway,[57] to low doses that led to adaptation,[8,55] to higher doses that cause cell cycle delay[38] and to high doses that cause loss of viability of some of the population. The gene clustering data from these experiments are shown in Fig. 4.

Adaptive doses elicited a more subtle response that affected metabolic functions, increasing the capacity for export of LoaOOH from the cell and regeneration of NADPH — these were among the functions that were uniquely up-regulated by LoaOOH relative to other ROS. These changes are relevant since protein synthesis is required for adaptation to LoaOOH.[8]

Surprisingly, the major oxidant defence functions of the cell were down-regulated at these doses, and were only induced when a threshold level of cell tolerance was exceeded at doses leading to cell cycle delay and some cell death. Since two of these genes (*TRX2* and *GRX1*) are involved in maintenance of redox homeostasis[58] it was speculated that this threshold may be the redox buffering capacity of the cell. Alic *et al.*[55] have also suggested that there may be coupling of the broad defence systems of the general stress[59] and the environmental stress responses[22,60] with cell cycle progression since these are mediated by the same branch of the PKA pathway through the Msn2 and Msn4 transcription factors. This coupling of the induction of broad induction of cellular defence systems to cell cycle delay may explain why these are excluded from the responses to low doses of LoaOOH since the aerobic cell needs to continuously cope with such doses without impairing its capacity to replicate.

Regardless of the explanation, it is clear that the many studies on cellular responses to ROS (and other environmental stresses) that are based on use of a single treatment concentration (usually these are extreme) may be missing important physiological cues.

6. Cells Have Different Constitutive Systems for Protection Against Different ROS: There is No One Oxidant That is Representative of a General Oxidative Stress

Transcriptional responses do not give a clear indication of which functions are essential for survival of exposure to a given ROS since some genes may be induced or repressed without having an important role in stress responses. Previously genetic approaches have been used to assess the role of specific gene products in defence and many antioxidant and repair functions were identified by isolating mutants that are sensitive or resistant to specific ROS, or identifying genes that confer altered sensitivity when over-expressed. This has led to the identification of a range of transcription factors that are important in the stress response, plus genes encoding enzymic detoxification systems including the catalases, superoxide dismutases, glutaredoxins and thioredoxins, glutathione and thioredoxin peroxidases, and those involved in the synthesis of antioxidants such as glutathione, ubiquinol, and D-erythroascorbic acid.[29,30] Others have been identified by mutation of genes that are involved in the synthesis of antioxidants or known repair functions.

The availability of the genome-wide set of deletion strains which cover almost all of the non-essential genes in yeast[23] has led to comprehensive screenings of the involvement of cellular functions in the response to a range of oxidants or species generating ROS.[61–63] The most comprehensive of these studies used diamide, cumene hydroperoxide, H_2O_2, linoleic acid hydroperoxide and menadione.[62] Recently this has been extended to hypochlorite (Kirsch, personal communication). While this approach may miss some important genes for which there is functional redundancy or compensatory parallel pathways, it has been observed for several homologous gene sets that a phenotype is observed when only one of the genes is deleted. A good example of redundancy and parallel pathways is seen with the two glutaredoxin (*GRX1* and *GRX2*) and two thioredoxin (*TRX1* and *TRX2*) genes. Deletion of any three of the four does not lead to cell death, but each separate deletion has a detectable, if subtle, oxidant-sensitive phenotype.[64]

The power of this genome-wide approach relies on the sheer number of genes under study, since even when there is redundancy of genes in a particular pathway or function, there are usually some mutants affecting the function that will show a phenotype of sensitivity or resistance.

The results of these studies were striking — for the more extensive screen, at least 657 deletant strains (~14% of all the non-essential genes screened) showed sensitivity to at least one of the five reagents used.[62] The genes identified included many involved in known antioxidant functions including *GPX3*, *TRX2*, *CCP1* (encoding cytochrome c peroxidase), *GND1* and *RPE1* (pentose phosphate pathway enzymes) and *YAP1* and *SKN7* (oxidative stress response transcription factors). Many hundreds of other genes of equal or greater importance (based on the deletion phenotype) that had not previously been associated with oxidative stress resistance were identified, representing functions not previously known to be associated with tolerance of ROS. These functions included vacuolar protein sorting, vacuolar acidification and ergosterol metabolism. Subsequently it was shown that viable *ERG* mutants affected in the terminal steps of ergosterol biosynthesis are sensitive to various forms of oxidative stress, especially those that are more likely to affect membranes.[65] These mutants incorporate sterols other than ergosterol in their membranes.

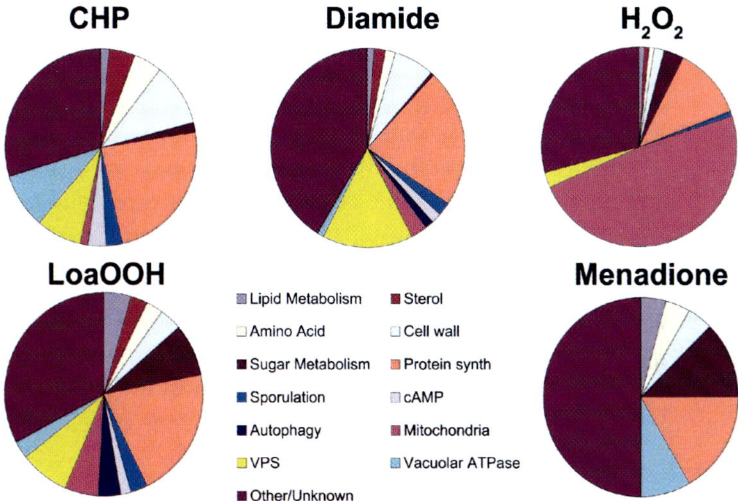

Fig. 5. Functions that are represented in the deletion mutants that are sensitive to each of the five ROS or compounds used. Sensitive strains were categorized in functional groups based on gene categories in the MIPS and SGD databases combined with visual inspection. The relative contribution of each color-coded functional group to sensitivity is shown for cumene hydroperoxide (CHP), diamide, H_2O_2, linoleic acid hydroperoxide (LoaOOH) and the superoxide generating agent menadione. Data adapted from Thorpe *et al.*[62]

Other surprising features of these results were that no two oxidants of the five tested (six including hypochlorite) gave the same, or even similar profile of sensitivity (Fig. 5), and the majority of mutants were sensitive to only one oxidant. "Oxidative stress" therefore encompasses a broad range of cellular insults that have profoundly different and very specific physiological outcomes. This has important implications for those studying the pathophysiology of conditions in which ROS are thought to be involved, since clearly the effects on the cell will be very different for each different ROS — there is no single oxidant that is representative of oxidative stress, and there is no one general "oxidative stress" condition. This is consistent with data from studies of cross-adaptation and cell-cycle delay following ROS treatment, in which there are differences between the way cells respond to the different oxidants.[29,33,37]

This high degree of ROS specificity contrasts with the results obtained from the gene expression studies discussed above, in which there was a degree of similarity between the genes induced by many different stresses. Few of the genes identified by the deletion mutant analysis were represented in the sets identified from the transcription or proteomic analyses, and there was no consistent correlation between the deletion and gene expression data sets in hierarchical clustering. This has been found for DNA damage as well,[66] and reflects the fact that the cell requires many genes to be relatively constitutively expressed to provide the initial resistance to the stress, and that subsequently many genes for repair or detoxification are induced when the damage reaches a critical level that overwhelms these constitutive defences. Clearly about 14% of the genes in yeast that are classified as non-essential have a major role in maintaining the integrity of the cell in the face of an initial ROS challenge. The different genomic approaches therefore provide complementary information and neither on their own gives a complete picture of what is occurring in cells. Moreover, it is our experience that gene over-expression analysis identifies yet another set of genes that are required for response to ROS. One clear case is the *YBP1* gene that encodes a protein required for the transport of activated Yap1 in to the nucleus. This was identified by over-expression analysis; it is only weakly represented in gene expression studies and the deletion mutant has a difficult phenotype to interpret since there is a homologue in the genome.[67]

7. Core Cellular Functions Required to Maintain Resistance

Despite the striking differences between the sensitivities of the deletion strains to the five ROS tested, there were about 30 genes that when deleted led to sensitivity to at least four oxidants.[62] These may identify some core functions that are required for more general tolerance of oxidative damage. These included genes involved in protein synthesis, particularly those encoding the oxidative stress transcription factors Yap1 and Skn7. Other functions in this category included transcriptional coactivators, chromatin and nucleosome remodelling complexes and translation initiation. Protein sorting and vacuolar functions were also highly represented, as was ergosterol metabolism. Several genes involved in cell wall and membrane maintenance were also important.

It is interesting that neither of the genomic approaches (transcriptomics or genome deletion studies) has identified many genes associated with repair of DNA damage as being critical in the response of cells to oxidants,[22,62,66,68] except for those genes involved with maintaining the integrity of the mitochondrial genome. This does not imply that ROS do not damage DNA, nor that some DNA damage systems are involved in the cell cycle delay caused by oxidants (see below), nor even that DNA damage is not critical for mutagenesis and carcinogenesis following ROS treatment. However, for yeast at least, it would appear that DNA damage is not the major cause of cell death, and since protein metabolism and membrane functions were the core ones needed for the survival of all ROS, protein and membrane damage may be the main reasons for the loss of cell viability.

8. Functions Required to Maintain Cellular Resistance to Specific ROS

Hydrogen peroxide. The greatest difference between the deletant strains was seen with H_2O_2 (see Fig. 5), with more than half of the sensitive mutants affected in the function of the respiratory chain (mitochondrial maintenance, mitochondrial genome integrity and respiratory chain components). This contrasted sharply with all of the other ROS tested for which mitochondrial functions were represented to a much lesser extent. It has been speculated that this may represent the fact that damage to the respiratory chain leads to production of superoxide radical, which in combination with the presence of added H_2O_2 catalyzes production of the hydroxy radical via Fenton reaction. The superoxide would reduce the Fe(III) generated in the Fenton reaction back to Fe(II) to promote formation of the very reactive hydroxy radical. This highlights that the effects of H_2O_2 and superoxide on the cell are fundamentally very different, despite the fact that superoxide is converted to H_2O_2 in the cell by SOD.[69]

Superoxide. This ROS gave the fewest sensitive strains, and many of the most sensitive were affected in the pentose phosphate pathway, indicating that NADPH generation in the cytoplasm and antioxidant enzymes using NADPH have a major role in defence against the superoxide anion.

LoaOOH. A range of functions were represented in the mutants that were sensitive only to this compound, including the ones associated with ergosterol metabolism, sterol uptake, peroxisome function, and vacuolar lipid degradation. The peroxisome may be the site of detoxification of the lipid hydroperoxide, and it is known that the peroxisomal biogenesis gene *PEX17* is needed for cell cycle delay in response to LoaOOH.[38] For resistance to this oxidant the control of balance between glycolysis and gluconeogenesis seems to be very critical, although the pentose phosphate pathway is also needed for resistance to the other physiologically significant ROS (H_2O_2 and superoxide). There was also a requirement for mitochondrial respiration, but unlike the situation with H_2O_2, this seemed more directed towards ATP generation.

9. Cell Division Cycle Delay

Prokaryotes and eukaryotes have been known for some time to respond to the inhibition of replication or induction of DNA damage by delaying cell cycle progression until the damage has been repaired.[70,71] This type of checkpoint control has been studied in some detail for cells exposed to DNA-damaging agents[72] but has also been found to occur when cells have been exposed to ROS. Mutants lacking the main cytosolic superoxide dismutase grow slowly due to an increased time spent in the G1 phase of the cell cycle, and in the presence of excess oxygen they arrest in G1 due to inhibition of transcription of the *CLN1* and *CLN2* genes encoding the auto-regulated cyclins involved in progression to S phase.[35] The superoxide generators paraquat and menadione cause a pronounced G1 arrest that is independent of the *RAD9* gene needed for arrest following DNA damage.[36,37] H_2O_2 leads to a subtle arrest at G2/M in a *RAD9*-dependent manner,[37] which would implicate DNA-damage in this delay, although others report that the arrest may be more in the S phase.[73,74] Lipid hydroperoxides and the breakdown product of multiply unsaturated lipid oxidation, 4-hydroxynonenal, also cause G1 arrest.[38,75]

From a secondary screening of all of the LoaOOH-sensitive deletant strains our laboratory has now identified about 45 genes that are implicated in the cell cycle delay caused by LoaOOH treatment (Foong, Moritz and Temple, personal communication). These genes encoded several transcription factors including the S-phase cell-cycle specific Swi6, the oxidative stress responsive Yap1, and various components of the Kornberg mediator complex, and work is underway to identify the mechanisms whereby the stress signal is transduced to control cell cycle progression. Three homologous genes, represented by *OCA1* and *SIW14*, encode putative protein phosphatases that may be involved in such a pathway.[38]

In yeast, there is a program of cell-cycle related gene expression involving several hundred genes. This is sustained by the sequential activation of a small set of transcription regulatory complexes.[73,76] Analyses of cell-cycle progression and genome-wide transcriptional responses caused by menadione and H_2O_2 have indicated that two small co-expressed groups of genes regulated by the Mcm1-Fkh2-Ndd1 transcription complex account for the observed differences in the effects of menadione and H_2O_2 on cell cycle progression discussed above.[73] Deletion of both *FKH1* and *FKH2* led to loss of the difference in expression pattern between menadione and H_2O_2-treated cells. This is very interesting in the light of the facts that the forkhead transcription factors are highly conserved across evolution, the human *FOXO* homologues are involved in cell cycle regulation,[77–79] they respond to oxidative stress and are critical for protection against oxidative stress.[80,81] Moreover, the *Caenorhabditis elegans* homologue Daf-16 is a transcription factor involved in aging,[82] and the human *FOXO* factors that regulate the insulin signaling pathway and act as regulators of organismal longevity are regulated by the SIRT1 deacetylase that is the human homologue of the yeast *SIR2* aging gene.[83] This may be one of the links between oxidative stress and cell aging from yeast to man.

10. The Link Between Apoptosis, Aging and ROS in Yeast

At relatively high doses of oxidants and ROS yeast cells can undergo a form of programmed cell death that resembles apoptosis seen in higher eukaryotes (reviewed in Madeo *et al.*[84]). This involves the flipping of phosphatidylserine from the inner to outer layer of the cell membrane, chromatin condensation, accumulation of DNA strand breaks, nuclear fragmentation and formation of apoptotic bodies. This was first observed in the cells of a *cdc48* mutant at the restrictive temperature,[39] and subsequently was shown to occur in *gsh1* mutants lacking the ability to synthesize glutathione, cells exposed to H_2O_2, other ROS including superoxide,[85] acetic acid[86] sugar or salt stress or antifungal peptides[84] and in cells facing certain forms of starvation. Similar processes have been found in other eukaryotic microorganisms including *Candida albicans*[87] and *Schizosaccharomyces pombe*.[88] In *S. cerevisiae* and *Sch. pombe*, DNA damage and mutations affecting cell cycle progression lead to the generation of ROS and the cells undergo apoptosis.[89]

The apoptotic response to many of these stresses depends on the activity of a caspase-like protein encoded by the *YCA1* gene, and a caspase-regulating serine protease.[40] There is also a yeast homologue Aif1 of the human apoptosis-inducing factor. Aif1 controls yeast apoptosis — it is located in the mitochondrion, but is translocated to the nucleus in response to apoptotic stimuli.[90] Disruption of the gene rescues cells from oxygen stress and delays age-induced apoptosis, while over-expression stimulates apoptotic cell death induced by H_2O_2. While there are no obvious yeast homologues of many apoptotic regulatory proteins such as Bcl and Bax, when these are expressed in yeast they show the appropriate pro-apoptotic or anti-apoptotic activity.[91–93]

Clearly ROS are important, and there are many indications that mitochondrial functions are as relevant to apoptosis in yeast as they are in some forms of apoptosis in higher eukaryotes[94] and there may be a link via the *UTH1* gene (which is involved in cell aging and resistance to H_2O_2) between mitochondrial autophagy and apoptosis.[95] From the genome-wide screen of deletion strains for sensitivity to various ROS described above, the one oxidant that was most deleterious to mitochondrial mutants was H_2O_2. This was proposed to be due to the generation of the very reactive and damaging hydroxyl radical if the mitochondrial mutation affected free radical production (presumed to be superoxide) from the respiratory chain in the presence of H_2O_2, and this may be the mechanism that sets in train, or augments, an initial apoptotic signal in the yeast cells. In this regard Singh[96] has indicated that mitochondria play a role in maintaining genomic stability, and has proposed that there is a "mitochondria damage checkpoint" that co-ordinates the balance between apoptotic and anti-apoptotic signals.

Apoptosis in yeast does occur not just as a response to environmental insults, but also as a natural response to both replicative and chronological cell aging and during mating.[84,97,98] Of these, mother-specific cell aging has been most widely studied. In *S. cerevisiae* (and other yeast species including *S. pombe*), it is possible to distinguish mother and daughter cells after division, and an individual mother cell can undergo a finite number of divisions before enlarging, becoming sterile and ceasing to divide.[99,100] This aging process has many parallels with aging of higher organisms, and shares many features including the involvement of ROS. While there are several tenable theories of aging, each of which has relevance to the processes occurring in most organisms, it has long been known that there is a link between respiratory oxygen metabolism and aging as proposed by Harman[101] and reviewed in Breitenbach *et al.*[98] Senescent cells have been shown to accumulate ROS detectable by dihydrorhodamine (which is relatively indiscriminate in the species detected) and the staining indicates that these are mainly located in the mitochondrion and are not detectable in young cells.[102] Moreover, these aged cells also showed phosphatidylserine flipping in the membrane, diffuse nuclear chromatin and accumulation of DNA strand breaks indicative of apoptosis. One interesting aspect of mother-cell specific aging is that mother cells, but not their daughters, show staining with antibodies to carbonylated proteins, and that this difference is not maintained in a *sir2* mutant which lacks the NAD-dependent histone deacetylase activity that is known to play a role in aging.[11] These results highlight the link between mitochondrial functions, oxidative stress, apoptosis and aging, but much remains to be done to identify the mechanisms that underlie these processes.

In summary, cellular responses to ROS are complex, involving many processes within the cell. The ready availability of genomic techniques in yeast has enabled rapid progress in determining some of the mechanisms that are responsible for these responses. From this several general principles have emerged that are relevant for all organisms. These include the fact that every different reactive oxygen species generates its own unique set of damage, and that the functions in the cell that are required to maintain a constitutive resistance to ROS are very dependent on the ROS involved. This means that it is not really very informative to use one compound like H_2O_2 and make claims that the results of such a study are representative of "oxidative stress." Oxidative stress has been considered to contribute to many pathological conditions, hence each particular condition requires knowledge of the ROS that are being generated to make sense of how cells respond and how damage to cells can be minimized. Moreover, the concentration of a ROS is also clearly important in determining the pattern and nature as well as the level of the response. Clearly much remains to be determined, but at least there are very powerful techniques now available to help answer important questions about how cells sense oxidative damage and how they cope with it.

Acknowledgments

The author expresses his gratitude to his students and colleagues for their contribution to the research from this laboratory. Particular thanks go to Mark Temple and Gabriel Perrone for their helpful advice and suggestions and assistance in producing the manuscript. Thanks also to Geoffrey Thorpe and Nazif Alic for the figures. This work was supported by Discovery Grants from the Australian Research Council.

References

1. Bouveris A, Cadenas E. Production of superoxide radicals and hydrogen peroxide in mitochondria. In: Oberley LW (ed.) *Superoxide Dismutases*. CRC Press, 1982, Vol. 2, pp. 15–30.
2. Halliwell B. The biological significance of oxygen-derived species. In: Valentine JS, Foote CS, Greenberg A, Liebman JF (eds.) *Active Oxygen in Biochemistry*. Blackie Academic and Professional, 1995, pp. 313–335.
3. Scandalios JG. The antioxidant enzyme genes *Cat* and *Sod* of maize: regulation, functional significance, and molecular biology. *Isozymes: Curr. Top. Biol. Med. Res.* 14: 19–44 (1987).
4. Buettner GR. The pecking order of free radicals and antioxidants: lipid peroxidation, α-tocopherol, and ascorbate. *Arch. Biochem. Biophys.* 300: 535–543 (1993).
5. Buettner GR, Schafer FQ. Free radicals, oxidants, and antioxidants. *Teratology* 62: 234 (2000).
6. Wiseman H, Halliwell B. Damage to DNA by reactive oxygen and nitrogen species: role in inflammatory disease and progression to cancer. *Biochem. J.* 313: 17–29 (1996).
7. Gunstone FD. *Fatty Acid and Lipid Chemistry*. Blackie Academic and Professional, 1996.

8. Evans MV, Turton HE, Grant CM, Dawes IW. Toxicity of linoleic acid hydroperoxide to *Saccharomyces cerevisiae*: involvement of a respiration-related process for maximal sensitivity and adaptive response. *J. Bacteriol.* 180: 483–490 (1998).
9. Levine RL. Carbonyl modified proteins in cellular regulation, aging, and disease. *Free Radic. Biol. Med.* 32: 790–796 (2002).
10. Aguilaniu H, Gustafsson L, Rigoulet M, Nystrom T. Protein oxidation in G(0) cells of *Saccharomyces cerevisiae* depends on the state rather than the rate of respiration and is enhanced in *pos9* but not *yap1* mutants. *J. Biol. Chem.* 276: 35396–35404 (2001).
11. Aguilanu H, Gustaffson L, Rigoulet M, Nystrom T. Asymmetric inheritance of oxidatively damaged proteins during cytokinesis. *Science* 299: 1751–1753 (2003).
12. Stadtman ER. Protein oxidation and aging. *Science* 257: 1220–1224 (1992).
13. Gebicki S, Gill KH, Dean RT, Gebicki JM. Action of peroxidases on protein hydroperoxides. *Redox Rep.* 7: 235–242 (2002).
14. Aeschbach R, Amado R, Neukom H. Formation of dityrosine cross-links in proteins by oxidation of tyrosine residues. *Biochim. Biophys. Acta* 439: 292–301 (1976).
15. Fu S, Gebicki S, Jessup W, Gebicki J, Dean RT. Biological fate of amino acid, peptide and protein hydroperoxides. *Biochem. J.* 311: 821–827 (1995).
16. Ames BN, Gold LS. Endogenous mutagens and the causes of aging and cancer. *Mutat. Res.* 214: 41–46 (1991).
17. Joenje H, Lafleur MVM, Retèl J (eds.) *Biological Consequences of Oxidative DNA Damage.* CRC Press, 1991.
18. Brennan RJ, Swoboda BEP, Schiestl RH. Oxidative mutagens induce intrachromosomal recombination in yeast. *Mutat. Res.* 308: 159–167 (1994).
19. Beckman JS, Chen J, Ischiropolous H, Crow JP. Oxidative chemistry of peroxynitrite. *Methods Enzymol.* 233: 229–240 (1994).
20. Buchczyk DP, Briviba K, Harti FU, Sies H. Responses to peroxynitrite in yeast: glyceraldehyde-3-phosphate dehydrogenase (GAPDH) as a sensitive intracellular target for nitration and enhancement of chaperone expression and ubiquitination. *Biol. Chem.* 381: 121–126 (2000).
21. Lashkari DA, DeRisi J, McCusker JH, Namath AF, Gentile C, Hwang SY, Brown PO, Davis RW. Yeast microarrays for genome wide parallel genetic and gene expression analysis. *Proc. Natl. Acad. Sci. USA* 94: 13057–13062 (1997).

22. Gasch AP, Spellman PT, Kao CM, Carmen-Harel O, Eisen MB, Storz G, Botstein D, Brown PO. Genomic expression programs in the response of yeast cells to environmental changes. *Mol. Biol. Cell* 11: 4241–4257 (2000).
23. Winzeler EA. Functional characterization of the *S. cerevisiae* genome by gene deletion and parallel analysis. *Science* 285: 901–906 (1999).
24. Schwikowski B, Uetz P, Fields S. A network of protein-protein interactions in yeast. *Nature* 18: 1257–1261 (2000).
25. Salwinski L, Miller CS, Smith AJ, Pettit FK, Bowie JU, Eisenberg D. The database of interacting proteins. *Nucleic Acids Res.* 32: D449–451 (2004).
26. Martzen MR, McCrith SM, Dpinelli SL, Torres FM, Fields S, Grayhack EJ, Phizicky EM. A biochemical genomics approach for identifying genes by the activity of their products. *Science* 286: 1153–1155 (1999).
27. Tong AHY, Lesage G, Bader GD, Ding HM, Xu H, Xin XF, Young J, Berriz GF, Brost RL, Chang M, Chen YQ, Cheng X, Chua G, Friesen H, Goldberg DS, Haynes J, Humphries C, He G, Hussein S, Ke LZ, Krogan N, Li ZJ, Levinson JN, Lu H, Menard P, Munyana C, Parsons AB, Ryan O, Tonikian R, Roberts T, Sdicu AM, Shapiro J, Sheikh B, Suter B, Wong SL, Zhang LV, Zhu HW, Burd CG, Munro S, Sander C, Rine J, Greenblatt J, Peter M, Bretscher A, Bell G, Roth FP, Brown GW, Andrews B, Busset H, Boone C. Global mapping of the yeast genetic interaction network. *Science* 303: 808–813 (2004).
28. Ren B, Robert F, Wyrick JJ, Aparicio O, Jennings EG, Simon I, Zeitlinger J, Schreiber J, Hannett N, Kanin E, Volkert TL, Wilson CJ, Bell SP, Young RA. Genome-wide location and function of DNA binding proteins. *Science* 290: 2306–2309 (2000).
29. Dawes IW. Stress responses. In: Dickinson JR, Schweizer M (eds.) *The Metabolism and Molecular Physiology of Saccharomyces cerevisiae.* CRC Press LLC, Boca Raton, 2004, pp. 376–438.
30. Santoro N, Thiele DJ. Oxidative stress responses in the yeast *Saccharomyces cerevisiae*. In: Hohmann S, Mager WH (eds.) *Yeast Stress Responses*. RG Landes Co., 1997, pp. 171–211.
31. Collinson LP, Dawes IW. Inducibility of the response of yeast cells to peroxide stress. *J. Gen. Microbiol.* 138: 329–335 (1992).
32. Jamieson DJ. *Saccharomyces cerevisiae* has distinct adaptive responses to both hydrogen peroxide and menadione. *J. Bacteriol.* 174: 6678–6681 (1992).
33. Flattery-O'Brien J, Collinson LP, Dawes IW. *Saccharomyces cerevisiae* has an inducible response to menadione which differs from that to hydrogen peroxide. *J. Gen. Microbiol.* 139: 501–507 (1993).

34. Turton HE, Dawes IW, Grant CM. *Saccharomyces cerevisiae* exhibits an adaptive response to malondialdehyde, a product formed by oxidative stress, and this response is mediated via the yAP-1 transcriptional regulator. *J. Bacteriol.* 179: 1096–1011 (1997).
35. Lee J, Romeo A, Kosman DJ. Transcriptional remodelling and G_1 arrest in dioxygen stress in *Saccharomyces cerevisiae*. *J. Biol. Chem.* 271: 24885–24893 (1997).
36. Nunes E, Siede W. Hyperthermia and paraquat-induced G1 arrest in the yeast *Saccharomyces cerevisiae* is independent of the *RAD9* gene. *Radiat. Environ. Biophys.* 35: 55–57 (1996).
37. Flattery-O'Brien JA, Dawes IW. Hydrogen peroxide causes *RAD9*-dependent cell cycle arrest in G2 in *Saccharomyces cerevisiae* whereas menadione causes G1 arrest independent of *RAD9* function. *J. Biol. Chem.* 273: 8564–8571 (1998).
38. Alic N, Higgins VJ, Dawes IW. Identification of a *Saccharomyces cerevisiae* gene that is required for G1 arrest in response to the lipid oxidation product linoleic acid hydroperoxide. *Mol. Biol. Cell* 12: 1801–1810 (2001).
39. Madeo F, Fröhlich E, Fröhlich KU. A yeast mutant showing diagnostic markers of early and late apoptosis. *J. Cell Sci.* 139: 729–734 (1997).
40. Madeo F, Herker E, Maldena C, Wissing S, Lächelt S, Herlan M, Fehr M, Lauber K, Sigrist SJ, Wesselborg S, Fröhlich KU. A caspase-related protein regulates apoptosis in yeast. *Mol. Cell* 9: 911–917 (2002).
41. Davies JMS, Lowry CV, Davies KJA. Transient adaptation to oxidative stress in yeast. *Arch. Biochem. Biophys.* 317: 1–6 (1995).
42. Branco MR, Marinho HS, Cyrne L, F, A. Decrease of H_2O_2 plasma membrane permeability during adaptation to H_2O_2 in *Saccharomyces cerevisiae*. *J. Biol. Chem.* 279: 6501–6506 (2004).
43. Moye-Rowley WS, Harshman KD, Parker CS. Yeast *YAP1* encodes a novel form of the jun family of transcriptional activator proteins. *Genes Dev.* 3: 283–292 (1989).
44. Lee J, Godon C, Lagniel G, Spector D, Garin J, Labarre J, Toledano MB. Yap1 and Skn7 control two specialized oxidative stress response regulons in yeast. *J. Biol. Chem.* 274: 16040–16046 (1999).
45. Stephen DWS, Rivers SL, Jamieson DJ. The role of *YAP1* and *YAP2* genes in the regulation of the adaptive stress responses of *Saccharomyces cerevisiae*. *Mol. Microbiol.* 16: 415–423 (1995).
46. Izawa S, Inoue Y, Kimura A. Oxidative stress response in yeast: effect of glutathione on adaptation to hydrogen peroxide stress in *Saccharomyces cerevisiae*. *FEBS Lett.* 368: 73–76 (1995).

47. Stephen DWS, Jamieson DJ. Glutathione is an important antioxidant molecule in the yeast *Saccharomyces cerevisiae. FEMS Microbiol. Lett.* 141: 207–212 (1996).
48. Delaunay A, Pflieger D, Barrault MB, Vinh J, Toledano MB. A thiol peroxidase is an H_2O_2 receptor and redox-transducer in gene activation. *Cell* 111: 471–481 (2002).
49. Delauney A, A-D, I, Toledano MB. H_2O_2 sensing through oxidation of the Yap1 transcription factor. *EMBO J.* 19: 5157–5166 (2000).
50. Avery AM, Avery SV. *Saccharomyces cerevisiae* expresses three phospholipid hydroperoxide glutathione peroxidases. *J. Biol. Chem.* 276: 33730–33735 (2001) .
51. Inoue Y, Matsuda T, Sugiyama K, Izawa S, Kimura A. Genetic analysis of glutathione peroxidase in oxidative stress response of *Saccharomyces cerevisiae. J. Biol. Chem.* 274: 27002–27009 (1999).
52. Flattery-O'Brien JA, Grant CM, Dawes IW. Stationary phase regulation of the *Saccharomyces cerevisiae SOD2* gene is dependent on additive effects of HAP2,3,4,5- and STRE-binding elements. *Mol. Microbiol.* 23: 303–312 (1997).
53. Pinkham JL, Wang Z, Alsina J. Heme regulates *SOD2* transcription by activation and repression in *Saccharomyces cerevisiae. Curr. Genet.* 31: 281–291 (1997).
54. Godon C, Lagniel G, Lee J, Buhler J-M, Kieffer S, Perrot M, Boucherie H, Toledano MB, Labarre J. The H_2O_2 stimulon in *Saccharomyces cerevisiae. J. Biol. Chem.* 273: 22480–22489 (1998).
55. Alic N, Felder T, Temple MD, Gloeckner C, Higgins VJ, Briza P, Dawes IW. Genome-wide transcriptional responses to a lipid hydroperoxide: adaptation occurs without induction of oxidant defenses. *Free Radic. Biol. Med.* 37: 23–35 (2004).
56. Koerkamp MG, Rep M, Bussemaker HJ, Hardy GP, Mul A, Piekarska K, Szigyarto CA, De Mattos JM, Tabak HF. *Mol. Biol. Cell* 13: 2783–2794 (2002).
57. Alic N, Higgins VJ, Pichova A, Breitenbach M, Dawes IW. Lipid hydroperoxides activate the mitogen-activated protein kinase Mpk1p in *Saccharomyces cerevisiae. J. Biol. Chem.* 278: 41849–41855 (2003).
58. Grant CM. Role of the glutathione/glutaredoxin and thioredoxin systems in yeast growth and response to stress conditions. *Mol. Microbiol.* 39: 533–541 (2001).
59. Smith A, Ward MP, Garret S. Yeast PKA represses Msn2p/Msn4p-dependent expression to regulate growth, stress response and glycogen accumulation. *EMBO J.* 17: 3556–3564 (1998).

60. Causton HC, Ren B, Koh SS, Harbison CT, Kanin E, Jennings EG, Lee TI, True HL, Lander ES, Young RA. Remodelling of yeast genome expression in response to environmental change. *Mol. Biol. Cell* 12: 323–337 (2001).
61. Higgins VJ, Alic N, Thorpe GW, Breitenbach M, Larsson V, Dawes IW. Phenotypic analysis of gene deletant strains for sensitivity to oxidative stress. *Yeast* 19: 203–214 (2002).
62. Thorpe GW, Fong CS, Alic N, Higgins VJ, Dawes IW. Cells require distinct molecular mechanisms to maintain protection against different reactive oxygen species: oxidative stress-response genes. *Proc. Natl. Acad. Sci. USA* 101: 6564–6569 (2004).
63. Tucker CL, Fields S. Quantitative genome-wide analysis of yeast deletion sensitivities to oxidative and chemical stress. *Comp. Functional Genomics* 5: 216–224 (2004).
64. Draculic T, Dawes IW, Grant CM. A single glutaredoxin or thioredoxin is essential for viability in the yeast *Saccharomyces cerevisiae*. *Mol. Microbiol.* 36: 1167–1174 (2000).
65. Higgins VJ, Rogers PJ, Dawes IW. Application of genome-wide expression analysis to identify molecular markers useful in monitoring industrial fermentations. *Appl. Environ. Microbiol.* 69: 7535–7540 (2003).
66. Birrell GW, Brown JA, Wu HI, Giaever G, Chu AM, Davis RW, Brown JM. Transcriptional response of *Saccharomyces cerevisiae* to DNA-damaging agents does not identify the genes that protect against these agents. *Proc. Natl. Acad. Sci. USA* 99: 8778–8783 (2002).
67. Veal EA, Ross SJ, Malakasi P, Peacock E, Morgan BA. Ybp1 is required for the hydrogen peroxide-induced oxidation of the Yap1 transcription factor. *J. Biol. Chem.* 278: 30896–30904 (2003).
68. Gasch AP, Huang M, Metzner S, Botstein D, Elledge SJ, Brown PO. Genomic expression responses to DNA-damaging agents and the regulatory role of the yeast ATR homolog Mec1p. *Mol. Biol. Cell* 12: 2987–3003 (2001).
69. Gille G, Sigler K. *Folia Microbiol. (Praha)* 40: 131–152 (1995).
70. Burns VW. X-ray induced division delay of individual yeast cells. *Radiat. Res.* 4: 394–412 (1956).
71. Burnborg G, Williamson DH. The relevance of the nuclear division cycle to radiosensitivity in yeast. *Mol. Gen. Genet.* 162: 277–285 (1978).
72. Hartwell LH, Weinert TA. Checkpoints: controls that ensure the order of cell cycle events. *Science* 246: 629–634 (1989).
73. Shapira M, Segal E, Botstein D. Disruption of yeast forkhead-associated cell cycle transcription by oxidative stress. *Mol. Biol. Cell* 15: 5659–5669 (2004).

74. Leroy C, Mann C, Marsolier MC. Silent repair accounts for cell cycle specificity in the signaling of oxidative DNA lesions. *EMBO J.* 20: 2896–2906 (2001).
75. Wonisch W, Tatzber F, Schaur JR, Larkovic N, Guttenberger H, Esterbauer H. Cell cycle inhibition by the lipid peroxidation product 4-hydroxynonenal in the yeast *Saccharomyces cerevisiae*. *Naunyn-Schmiedebergs Archiv. Pharmacol.* 356(Suppl. 1): 72 (1997).
76. Mendenhall MD, Hodge AE. Regulation of Cdc28 cyclin-dependent protein kinase activity during the cell cycle of the yeast *Saccharomyces cerevisiae*. *Microbiol. Molec. Biol. Rev.* 62: 1191–1243 (1998).
77. Wang X, Kiyokawa H, Dennewitz MB, Costa RH. The Forkhead Box m1b transcription factor is essential for hepatocyte DNA replication and mitosis during mouse liver regeneration. *Proc. Natl. Acad. Sci. USA* 99: 16881–16886 (2002).
78. Medema RH, Kops GJ, Bos JL, Burgering BM. AFX-like forkhead transcription factors mediate cell-cycle regulation by Ras and PKB through p27Kip1. *Nature* 404: 782–787 (2000).
79. Alvarez B, Martinez AC, Burgering BM, Carrera AC. Forkhead transcription factors contribute to the execution of the mitotic programme of mammals. *Nature* 413: 744–747 (2001).
80. Nemeto S, Finkel T. Redox regulation of forkhead proteins through a p66shc-dependent signaling pathway. *Science* 295: 2450–2452 (2002).
81. Kops GJ, Dansen TB, Polderman PE, Saarloos I, Wirtz KW, Coffer PJ, Huang TT, Bos JL, Medema RH, Burgering BM. Forkhead transcription factor FOXO3a protects quiescent cells from oxidative stress. *Nature* 419: 316–321 (2002).
82. Murphy CT, McCarroll SA, Bargmann CI, Fraser A, Kamath RS, Ahringer J, Li H, Kenyon C. Genes that act downstream of DAF-16 to influence the lifespan of *Caenorhabditis elegans*. *Nature* 424: 277–283 (2003).
83. Brunet A, Sweeney LB, Sturgill JF, Chua KF, Greer PL, Lin Y, Tran H, Ross SE, Mostoslavsky R, Cohen HY, Hu LS, Cheng H-L, Jedrychowski MP, Gygi SP, Sinclair DA, Alt FW, Greenberg ME. Stress-dependent regulation of FOXO transcription factors by the SIRT1 deacetylase. *Science* 303: 2011–2015 (2004).
84. Madeo F, Herker E, Wissing S, Jungwirth H, Eisenberg T, Frohlich KU. Apoptosis in yeast. *Curr. Opin. Microbiol.* 7: 655–660 (2004).
85. Fabrizio P, Battistella L, Vardavas R, Gattazzo C, Liou LL, Diaspro A, Dossen JW, Gralla EB, Longo VD. Superoxide is a mediator of an altruistic

aging program in *Saccharomyces cerevisiae*. *J. Cell Biol.* 166: 1055–1067 (2004).
86. Ludivico P. *Saccharomyces cerevisiae* commits to a programmed cell death process in response to acetic acid. *Microbiology* 147: 2409–2415 (2001).
87. Phillips AJ, Sudbery I, Ramsdale M. Apoptosis induced by environmental stresses and amphotericin B in *Candida albicans*. *Proc. Natl. Acad. Sci. USA* 100: 14327–14332 (2003).
88. Rodriguez-Menocal L, D'Urso G. Programmed cell death in fission yeast. *FEMS Yeast Res.* 5: 111–117 (2004).
89. Burhans WC, Weinberger M, Marchetti MA, Ramachandran L, D'Urso G, Huberman JA. Apoptosis-like yeast cell death in response to DNA damage and replication defects. *Mutat. Res.* 532: 227–243 (2003).
90. Wissing S, Ludivico P, Herker E, Buttner S, Engelhardt SM, Decker T, Link A, Proksch A, Corte-Real M, Frohlich KU, Manns J, Cande C, Sigrist SJ, Kroemer G, Madeo, F. An AIF orthologue regulates apoptosis in yeast. *J. Cell Biol.* 166: 969–974 (2004).
91. Trancikova A, Weisova P, Kissova I, Zeman I, Kolarov J. Production of reactive oxygen species and loss of viability in yeast mitochondrial mutants: protective effect of Bcl-x(L). *FEMS Yeast Res.* 5: 149–156 (2004).
92. Kang JJ, Schaber MD, Srinivasula S, Alnmeri ES, Litwak G, Hall DJ, Bjornsti MA. Cascades of mammalian caspase activation in the yeast *Saccharomyces cerevisiae*. *J. Biol. Chem.* 274: 3189–3198 (1999).
93. Greenhalf W, Stephan C, Chaudhuri B. Role of mitochondria and C-terminal membrane anchor of Bcl-2 in Bax induced growth arrest and mortality in *Saccharomyces cerevisiae*. *FEBS Lett.* 380: 169–175 (1996).
94. Fannjiang Y, Cheng WC, Lee SJ, Qi B, Pevsner J, McCaffery JM, Hill RB, Basanez G, Hardwick JM. Mitochondrial fission proteins regulate programmed cell death in yeast. *Genes Dev.* 18: 2785–2797 (2004).
95. Camougrand N, Kissova I, Velours G, Manon S. Uth1p: a yeast mitochondrial protein at the crossroads of stress degradation and cell death. *FEMS Yeast Res.* 5: 133–140 (2004).
96. Singh KK. Mitochondria damage checkpoint in apoptosis and genome stability. *FEMS Yeast Res.* 5: 127–132 (2004).
97. Herker E, Jungwirth H, Lehmann KA, Maldener C, Frohlich KU, Wissing S, Buttner S, Fehr M, Sigrist SJ, Madeo F. Chronological aging leads to apoptosis in yeast. *J. Cell Biol.* 164: 501–507 (2004).
98. Breitenbach M, Laun P, Heeren G, Jarolim S, Pichova A. Mother cell-specific aging. In: Dickinson JR, Schweizer M (eds.) *The Metabolism*

and Molecular Physiology of Saccharomyces cerevisiae. CRC Press, 2004, pp. 20–41.

99. Mortimer RK, Johnston JR. Lifespan of individual yeast cells. *Nature* 183: 1751–1752 (1959).
100. Jazwinski SM. The genetics of aging in the yeast *Saccharomyces cerevisiae*. *Genetica* 91: 35–51 (1993).
101. Harman D. Free radical involvement in aging. *Drugs Aging* 3: 60 (1956).
102. Laun PAP, Madeo F, Fuchs J, Ellinger A, Kohlwein S, Dawes I, Fröhlich K-U, Breitenbach M. Aged mother cells of *Saccharomyces cerevisiae* show markers of oxidative stress and apoptosis. *Mol. Microbiol.* 39: 1166–1173 (2001).

9 Oxidative Stress, Cell Proliferation, and Apoptosis

Jennifer S. Carew, Yan Zhou, and Peng Huang

1. Introduction

Oxidative stress in biological systems is broadly defined as an imbalanced redox state in which the production or accumulation of reactive oxygen species (ROS) overwhelms the capacity of antioxidant defenses. Such redox imbalances can result from an overproduction of endogenous ROS, exposure to an exogenous oxidative stressor, and/or an insufficient antioxidant capacity caused by a disturbance in antioxidant production and distribution. In biological systems, reactive oxygen species represent a class of molecules that are derived from the metabolism of oxygen and exist inherently in all aerobic organisms. The sources of ROS include the mitochondrial respiratory chain, metabolic activities catalyzed by the cytochrome P450 system, NAD(P)H oxoreductases, xanthine oxidase, and other enzymes. In addition, inflammatory stimuli, intake of substances with oxidant properties, and exposure to radiation are important sources of oxidative stress. Owing to their reactive chemical property, ROS are generally considered harmful molecules, which can cause various types of damage to the cells, and contribute to the pathological processes of many common diseases, especially neurodegenerative diseases, inflammation, abnormal aging, and cancer. However, it should be emphasized that ROS also play important roles in the normal physiological functions of the cells, including the maintenance of proper redox states of many regulatory molecules, signal transduction, regulation of enzyme activity, and the control of cell cycle and proliferation. Each of these aspects is discussed in the relevant chapters of this book. This article will mainly focus on the role of ROS in cell proliferation, apoptosis, and the implications in cancer therapeutics.

2. Redox Regulation of Cell Proliferation and Survival

Reactive oxygen species (ROS) are known to act as second messengers in a number of signaling cascades including those directly related to cell proliferation. In this respect, ROS can be thought of as important factors involved in the maintenance of cellular homeostasis. A mild increase in the generation of ROS such as superoxide and hydrogen peroxide has been shown to stimulate cell proliferation in a number of different cell types, and may play a role in the carcinogenic process. These effects are most likely mediated by modulation of redox-sensitive sites of key transcription factors and protein kinases and phosphatases involved in cell cycle regulation, leading to alterations in biochemical activity or binding affinities for other proteins. Additionally, the activation of important redox-regulated survival pathways can indirectly promote cell proliferation via survival in the face of oxidative insult. Several key players in these processes are described below in further detail.

3. Transcription Factors

The activity of many key transcription factors involved in cell cycle regulation can be modulated by ROS. This mainly occurs through oxidative modifications of specific amino acid residues in the DNA-binding motif of the protein or redox-induced changes in phosphorylation status. The thiol-containing cysteine residues of the zinc-finger motif in the DNA-binding domains of many transcription factors are particularly sensitive to oxidative modifications. Depending on the transcription factor in question, redox modifications can serve to either increase or decrease transcriptional activity.[1,2]

3.1. *NF-κB*

The nuclear factor kappa B (NFκB) represents a typical example of a transcription factor whose activity can be significantly altered through redox modulation. While not a direct promoter of cell proliferation, NFκB plays an important role in the regulation of many genes involved in immune, inflammatory, and anti-apoptotic responses. Thus, this molecule functions to promote cell survival in response to oxidative insults. When inactive, NF-κB exists as a dimer (usually a p65/p50 heterodimer) bound to its inhibitor IκB in the cytoplasm. IκB is able to keep NFkB cytoplasmic by masking its nuclear localization signal. Upon stimulation by certain cytokines or under certain oxidative stress, IκB proteins are rapidly phosphorylated at 2 N-terminal serine residues and are subsequently ubiquitinated and proteasomally degraded. This exposes NFκB's nuclear localization signal, allowing it to translocate to the nucleus where it activates the transcription of target genes. Phosphorylation of IκB is generally mediated by IKKs, which in turn are regulated by NIK and MEKK3.[3]

The role of reactive oxygen species (ROS) in the regulation of NFκB is still controversial due to inconsistencies in results obtained in different experimental models, even when similar stimuli were used. It has been shown that NFκB activity can be enhanced by reducing glutathione (GSH) levels with diamide treatment, or diminished by treatment with GSH mimetics such as N-acetyl-cysteine.[4,5] A subsequent investigation provided evidence that cysteine 62 of p50 was sensitive to oxidative modification. That particular residue is critical for DNA binding and is regulated by thioredoxin.[6] Some studies have shown that addition of exogenous H_2O_2 can lead to NFkB activation. However, it seems that H_2O_2-related effects are cell type-dependent and could rely heavily upon the redox background of the cells in question.[7–9] Other studies have focused on the effects of modulating expression levels of enzymes that regulate levels of intracellular ROS on NFκB activity. Overexpression of manganese superoxide dismutase (MnSOD) enhanced TNF-induced NFκB activation likely because MnSOD increases levels of H_2O_2 via conversion of O_2^-. This phenomenon seemed to contribute to the resistance to TNF-induced apoptosis.[5,10,11] As a whole, these observations suggest that ROS play a role in regulating NFκB activity. However, a common redox-sensitive step that is required to activate NFκB in response to various stimuli has not been identified. The collective data suggest that ROS do play a role in NFκB activation, but it is not mediated by a universal mechanism and likely depends on the intrinsic redox status of individual cell types.

3.2. *AP-1*

The AP-1 family of transcription factors is comprised of a dimer of basic region leucine zipper proteins of the Jun, Fos, Maf, and ATF subfamilies. All of these proteins have cAMP responsive elements. The most commonly described forms of AP-1 are Jun-Jun homodimers or Jun-Fos heterodimers.[12] The AP-1 dimer can be activated by H_2O_2, which incites a signaling cascade involving the MAP family of serine/threonine kinases. This can occur through several mechanisms. A common consequence of AP-1 activation is increased cell proliferation, due to the induction of cyclin D1 and repression of the cdk inhibitor p21.[13,14] These effects can be inhibited by JunB, a Jun family member, through the transcriptional activation of p16, an inhibitor of the G1/S transition.[15] AP-1 can also influence apoptosis induction in a positive or negative manner, depending upon the balance of pro- and anti-apoptotic target genes in the cells in question.[16]

3.3. *c-myc*

c-myc is a member of a family of transcription factors that contain basic helix-loop-helix and leucine zipper domains.[17] Myc was first implicated as a cell cycle regulator when it was observed that its expression was rapidly induced by growth-promoting stimuli and was not expressed in quiescent cells. Subsequent studies demonstrated that ectopic expression of c-myc alone was sufficient to induce re-entry into S phase in certain types of quiescent cells, suggesting that myc played an important role in the G1/S transition. It is now known that c-myc is a powerful regulator of cell cycle progression from G1 to S phase.[18] This is primarily due to myc-induced expression of genes such as cdk4, Cdc25A and the activation of cyclin E/cdk2 complexes.[19–21] Because of these properties, myc has been demonstrated to play an important role in oncogenic transformation. Two recent reports demonstrated that c-myc overexpression could induce ROS generation and DNA damage while concomitantly disabling the p53-mediated damage response, allowing cells with faulty DNA to progress through the cell cycle. This represents a clear mechanism by which activation of oncogenes contributes to genetic instability and tumor progression.[22,23] Interestingly, malfunction of the biological clock or circadian activity significantly alters the expression of c-myc, and appears to affect genetic stability *in vivo*.[24]

3.4. *Forkhead (FOXO) transcription factors*

The FOXO family of transcription factors represents an important, evolutionarily conserved group of molecules with over 40 members identified to date in mammalian cells alone. All family members contain a highly conserved DNA binding domain known as the forkhead box, which is characterized by the presence of a 110-amino acid butterfly-shaped structure comprised of 3 N-terminal α-helices, 3 β-sheets, and 2 C-terminal loops. Outside of the forkhead box domain, the FOXO family members do not display high sequence homology. Recently, FOXO transcription factors have been shown to regulate cell proliferation and survival in the response to oxidative stress in mammalian cells. FOXO activity is regulated by its phosphorylation status, which is controlled by kinases such as Akt.[25] In affecting cell proliferation, FOXO factors can exert a strong inhibitory effect on the cell cycle progression, mainly due to upregulation of the cyclin-dependent kinase inhibitor p27 and repression of cyclin D, forcing cells into a quiescent state.[26,27] As for direct protection from oxidative stress, activation of FOXO factors results in transcriptional upregulation of the key antioxidant enzymes MnSOD and catalase to assist in the restoration of redox homeostasis.[28,29] Additionally, FOXO proteins can activate Gadd45, a protein that plays a role in DNA repair, to allow for the repair of any DNA damage that occurs as a consequence of oxidative injury.[30]

4. Signaling Molecules

While much of the studies implicating ROS as stimulus of cell proliferation and survival have focused on the role of specific transcription factors, a number of proteins involved in key signal transduction pathways also play a significant role in these processes. In fact, in many cases, upstream signaling events mediated by these non-transcriptionally active proteins lead to the activation of the transcription factors discussed above. Several important signaling molecules involved in redox regulation are discussed below.

4.1. *Phosphatidylinositol 3-kinase (PI3K)/Akt*

PI3K is a lipid kinase that has been identified as an important signaling molecule in a number of cellular transduction pathways including those involving cell proliferation, motility, and survival. Upon activation, PI3K catalyzes the production of PIP3 and recruits Akt (also known as protein kinase B) to the cell membrane. Once localized to the membrane, Akt can be activated upon phosphorylation by 3-phosphoinositide-dependent kinase-1 (PDK-1). This pathway is negatively regulated by the phosphatase PTEN, which serves to remove the activating phosphorylation from PIP3 and thus, downregulate Akt activity.[25] While the functions of PI3K/Akt with respect to cell survival have been well characterized, a number of studies have now provided evidence that ROS may also play a role in regulating Akt activity. For instance, an increase of ROS such as superoxide and hydrogen peroxide leads to the rapid activation of Akt. Conversely, treatment with antioxidants is able to diminish Akt activation. The ROS-induced activation of Akt appears to be PI3K-dependent since PI3K inhibitors block Akt activation even in the presence of exogenous ROS.[31–34] Further studies are needed to clarify how redox status affects Akt activity. Considering that Akt activity is commonly dysregulated in tumor cells, which are known to be under constitutive oxidative stress, investigation in this area is likely to provide significant new insights into the mechanism by which ROS and the PI3K pathway interact to provide a survival advantage in cancer cells.

4.2. *Mitogen-activated protein kinases (MAPKs)*

The MAPKs are an evolutionarily conserved family of serine/threonine kinases involved in many diverse cellular processes such as cell proliferation, energy metabolism, regulation of gene expression, and programmed cell death. The MAPK signaling cascade involves the sequential activation of a series of kinases by phosphorylation events. The specific kinases involved in specific activation steps of the cascade determine which target is affected.[35] Due to the numerous potential MAPK signaling cascades, it may be difficult to define the effect of a particular stimulus in a distinct linear fashion. This is particularly true with respect to the exact mechanistic role ROS play in the activation of the MAPK pathway. In spite of this, some commonalities in ROS-induced MAPK activation have been characterized in the literature. The phosphorylation and thus, activation of the MAPKs p38 and ERK1/2 are commonly observed in response to oxidative insults. These phosphorylation events seem to be redox-dependent since antioxidant treatments abrogate them. The redox-dependent alterations in MAPK activity have also been linked to changes in the cellular proliferative index, indicating that ROS-induced cell proliferation may be, at least in part, dependent upon activation of MAPKs.[36–39]

4.3. *Ras*

The Ras family members of membrane-associated GTPases were first identified as oncogenes in cancer cells. The three major forms of Ras (H-Ras, N-Ras, and K-Ras) are highly related to each other, displaying high levels of sequence homology. While many studies regarding the Ras proteins have focused on their oncogenic properties, these proteins are also active in normal cells where they play an important role in cell cycle regulation, particularly in the transition from G1 to S phase.[40] Several reports have indicated that Ras activity may be redox-dependent. These studies have mainly focused on the opposing effects of oxidants and antioxidants on Ras activity. In general, oxidants seem to increase Ras activity and thus, cell proliferation, while antioxidants diminish both of these related events.[41–44] These findings are in accordance with the effects of changes in redox status on the activation of MAPKs, especially p38 and ERK1/2. Considering that the MAPK pathway is an important downstream effector target of Ras, it is likely that these events are mechanistically linked, and that the Ras-mediated alterations in the proliferation index are likely the consequence of parallel changes in the activity of various MAPKs. A recent report demonstrated that Ras itself can be glutathionylated, suggesting that the alterations in Ras activity observed in different redox environments could be due to direct modification of the protein.[45] Future studies are warranted to explore this possibility. Furthermore, activation of Ras itself can lead to further increases in cellular ROS, mainly due to generation of superoxide by the NAD(P)H oxidase system, a component of which is the Ras-regulated protein Rac.[46] Due to the high frequency of mutations that render Ras constitutively activated in human tumors, it is also possible that Ras may be a contributing factor in the increased ROS generation that is frequently observed in cancer.

5. Redox Regulation of Apoptosis

The role of ROS in the apoptotic process has been a point of controversy for many years. It has been observed that the treatment of cells with certain oxidants results in apoptosis. An increase in the production of ROS has also been observed in response to many apoptotic stimuli. Conversely, treatment with antioxidants can block apoptosis induction due to exposure to oxidants or certain chemotherapeutic agents in a variety of cancer cell types. These effects are likely due, in part, to alterations in the redox status of the glutathione system, and to the malfunction of the mitochondria that commonly occurs during the execution of apoptosis. The requirement for increased ROS generation in apoptosis remains controversial because this increase has been reported to occur at both early and late points during cell death. Thus, a common redox-dependent step in the apoptotic process has not been definitely identified. Nonetheless, redox alterations seem to play a complex but important role in regulating the triggering and execution of apoptosis.[47] Some of the key proteins involved in this process are discussed in further detail below.

5.1. *Apoptosis signal-regulating kinase/thioredoxin: (ASK-1/Trx)*

ASK-1 is a ubiquitously expressed serine/threonine kinase of the MAPK family. Amongst its many functions, ASK-1 has been shown to activate the c-Jun N-terminal kinase (JNK) and p38 MAPK signaling cascades via phosphorylation.[48] Studies conducted in mice deficient in ASK-1 have demonstrated that this molecule is required for execution of the apoptosis in response to oxidative and endoplasmic reticular stress as well as death receptor ligands such as FasL and tumor necrosis factor-α.[49–51] Two mechanisms of ASK-1 regulation have been identified in recent studies. The first mechanism involves the antioxidant molecule thioredoxin (Trx). When in its reduced form, Trx is able to structurally inhibit the activation of ASK-1 by binding to it and preventing its activation. The association between Trx and ASK-1 is redox-dependent and upon stimulation by ROS stress such as H_2O_2, Trx becomes oxidized and dissociates from ASK-1, allowing it to become activated.[52] A second mechanism for regulation of ASK-1 activity involves inhibitory phosphorylation of ASK-1 at Ser83 by Akt. Phosphorylation of this particular amino acid residue leads to a marked reduction in ASK-1 activity and hence, diminished sensitivity to apoptosis induction.[53] A more recently published study has suggested that p53 status may also play a role in ASK-1 regulation. It was shown that certain mutant forms of p53 can interact with Daxx, a Fas-binding protein involved in stress responses, preventing Daxx from activating stress kinases such as ASK-1 and JNK.[54] Considering the high frequency of p53 mutations in cancer, these findings may have potential therapeutic implications.

5.2. *Bcl-2*

Overexpression of the anti-apoptotic protein bcl-2 is able to inhibit apoptosis by numerous stimuli. One of the proposed mechanisms by which bcl-2 exerts its anti-apoptotic function is by increasing the intracellular levels of glutathione (GSH), which plays a role in the detoxification of a variety of compounds.[55] The first indication that bcl-2 was linked to cellular redox status came from studies conducted in bcl-2 -/- mice. Mice deficient in bcl-2 were afflicted with severe polycystic kidney disease and hair hypopigmentation, both of which seem to be attributed to constitutive oxidative stress.[56] A further study by Hockenbery *et al.* substantiated a role for bcl-2 in cellular redox regulation by demonstrating that bcl-2 localizes to sites of ROS generation including the mitochondrion, endoplasmic reticulum, and nucleus. Overexpression of bcl-2 has been demonstrated to inhibit apoptosis induced by oxidants such as menadione and H_2O_2 and potently suppress lipid peroxidation.[57]

While both of the aforementioned studies provided evidence that expression of bcl-2 alters cellular redox potential, they did not identify a specific biochemical mechanism responsible for this effect. Later studies established that bcl-2 expression increased intracellular GSH levels. Resistance to apoptosis in bcl-2 overexpressing cells could be reversed upon depletion of intracellular thiols, further confirming that bcl-2 mediated alterations in redox status influence apoptotic sensitivity.[58,59] A closer examination of the relationship between bcl-2 expression and GSH was conducted using a conditional bcl-2 expression construct in HeLa cells. It was found that when bcl-2 expression was repressed, GSH was uniformly distributed primarily throughout the cytosol. In contrast, when bcl-2 expression was induced GSH became redistributed to the nucleus. Studies in isolated nuclei demonstrated that the nuclear concentration of GSH was maintained in a manner that correlated with nuclear bcl-2 protein levels. Addition of exogenous GSH blocked caspase activity and other apoptotic changes in isolated nuclei.[60] Taken together, these data support a role for bcl-2 as a death repressor and a regulator of the antioxidant pathway.

Overexpression of bcl-2 and elevated intracellular GSH levels have both been associated with resistance to anticancer agents. In addition to direct antioxidant effects, bcl-2-mediated increases in GSH levels could reduce sensitivity to DNA damaging agents by two possible mechanisms. First, it has been established that glutathione-*S*-transferases can use GSH to modify chemotherapeutic agents such as cisplatin, chlorambucil, and cyclophosphamide, forming inactive conjugates.[61,62] Secondly, bcl-2-directed redistribution of GSH to the nucleus could significantly alter the nuclear redox environment. As discussed earlier, several important transcription factors including p53, NF-κB, and AP-1 are subject to redox regulation at conserved cysteine residues in their DNA-binding domains. As such, a high nuclear concentration of GSH could markedly alter apoptotic potential, especially considering that the important pro-apoptotic molecules such as bax, noxa, and puma are under the transcriptional control of p53.[63] While the mechanisms underlying bcl-2 and GSH-mediated resistance to DNA damaging agents remain to be further elucidated, it is clear that both molecules contribute to a drug-resistant phenotype and are attractive targets for therapeutic intervention.

5.3. *c-Jun N-terminal kinase (JNK)*

The JNK family of serine/threonine kinases is comprised of three members: JNK1, JNK2, and JNK3. All three proteins are capable of phosphorylating and activating c-Jun, a component of the dimeric AP-1 transcription factor. Regulation of JNK activity is extremely complex and involves many of the upstream components of the MAPK signaling pathway. Due to this regulatory complexity, numerous studies have suggested both pro- and anti-apoptotic roles for JNKs in stress responses.[35] The conflicting reports are likely due to the specific stimulus in question, the cellular genetic background, and the upstream signaling events that lead to JNK activation. JNKs can be activated by various cellular stresses, including alterations in redox environment and treatment with anticancer agents. JNKs promote apoptosis in several ways. For example, JNK has been shown to translocate to the mitochondria during apoptosis and enhance the release of the pro-apoptotic molecule Smac/DIABLO, as well as bind to Bcl-X_L, preventing its association with Bax.[64,65] In fact, JNK-mediated Smac release is required for TNF-α induced apoptosis.[66] Studies in fibroblasts deficient in all three JNKs demonstrated resistance to stress-induced apoptosis and a failure to release cytochrome c.[67] JNKs have also been shown to phosphorylate the anti-apoptotic protein Bcl-2 and other related family members.[68,69] Recent studies have revealed that JNK activation also promotes translocation of Bax to the mitochondria through phosphorylation of 14-3-3 proteins and that this can be suppressed by activation of the PI3K/Akt pathway.[70] Taken together, these studies have defined a role for JNKs in the promotion of apoptosis at multiple levels in response to stress stimuli.

5.4. *p53*

The p53 protein is the most well-characterized member of a family of three related proteins: p53, p63, and p73. These three proteins share approximately 60% sequence identity, however they are functionally distinct from one another. Many functions have been ascribed to p53, including regulation of gene transcription, cell cycle progression, senescence, DNA synthesis and repair, and apoptosis. Given the important regulatory roles of p53 in these processes, it is not surprising that p53 is considered a key tumor suppressor gene. The p53 protein can be stabilized by specific phosphorylation events in response to cellular stresses such as UV/ionizing radiation, alterations in redox homeostasis, and various chemotherapeutic agents. While p53 is not universally required for apoptosis, the presence of a functional p53 protein enhances the apoptotic response to many stimuli, particularly DNA-damaging agents. This is likely due to p53-mediated transcriptional activation of pro-apoptotic genes such as bax, puma, noxa, and Fas.[71,72] Induction of p53 itself can also lead to changes in metabolic pathways that culminate in increased ROS generation. One proposed mechanism for the observed p53-induced alterations in cellular redox status involves elevation in ferredoxin reductase (FDXR) levels. This increase in FDXR expression has been observed in response to treatment with the anticancer agent 5-fluorouracil (5-FU) only in cells containing wild-type p53. Furthermore, disruption of FDXR resulted in decreased ROS generation and reduced sensitivity to apoptosis induction following exposure to 5-FU. These findings indicate that p53 activation leads to increased ROS generation, which in turn heightens sensitivity to apoptotic stimuli.[73] The exact mechanisms by which p53 alters redox status have not been fully elucidated. However, recent reports have demonstrated that p53 translocates to the mitochondria during apoptosis where it facilitates the activation of the pro-apoptotic proteins bax and bak.[74–77] Considering that the mitochondrion is the primary site of cellular ROS generation, it would be interesting to determine if mitochondrial localization of p53 contributes in a more direct manner to the rise in intracellular ROS frequently observed during apoptosis. It should also be noted that p53 is also a redox-sensitive molecule, and its function can be significantly altered by redox modification of certain cysteine residues in the p53 polypeptide.[78,79]

5.5. *Caspases*

Caspases are evolutionarily conserved proteases directly involved in the apoptotic process. More than ten different human caspases (caspases 1–10 and caspase 14) have been identified to date. While certain caspases play distinct roles in the apoptotic process, there are several features that are shared by all enzymes of this class. All caspases are synthesized as inactive zymogens. They become enzymatically active following cleavage into proper fragments and removal of the prodomain. Other shared features include the presence of a cysteine residue in the active site and a specificity to cleave substrate proteins directly after aspartic acid residues. Caspases can be classified into two main categories — initiator caspases and executioner caspases. Initiator caspases such as caspases 8 and 9 can be structurally distinguished from executioner caspases based on the extended length of their prodomains. Their prodomains are longer due to the presence of a caspase activation and recruitment domain (CARD) in the case of caspases such as 1, 2, 4, 5, and 9 or death effector domain (DED) in caspases 8 and 10 that facilitate interactions with other apoptosis-related proteins. The initiator caspases are usually responsible for processing and activating executioner caspases such as caspases 3, 6, and 7. While certain instances of caspase-independent cell death have been described in the literature, most occurrences of cell death require the activation of specific initiator and executioner caspases.[80]

One mechanism to regulate caspase activity is redox modification. This involves direct modifications of the cysteine residue contained in the active site of the enzyme. The active cysteine of caspase 3 as well as other caspases has been shown to be nitrosylated and oxidatively modified. Most studies have demonstrated that redox modification of caspase 3 is associated with loss of the enzyme activity.[81–85] The extent to which these modifications occur during the apoptotic process remains uncertain. As mentioned earlier, a rise in the production of ROS frequently occurs in the earlier phases of apoptosis. It seems counterintuitive that ROS production would be a common occurrence during programmed cell death if it were to ultimately result in inactivation of key proteins such as caspases involved in this process. It is possible that caspases may only be redox modified in response to extreme elevations in the production of ROS or reactive nitrogen species like nitric oxide (NO). In these extreme situations, modification of the caspase may not abrogate cell death, but rather may lead the cell death process in the direction of necrosis. Alternatively, a minor but constitutive increase in ROS production as in the case of many human tumors could result in caspase oxidation/nitrosylation and thus, inactivation of the protease activity as a mechanism of suppressing apoptotic cell death. This could be of therapeutic importance and may result in reduced sensitivity to anticancer agents. The complexities involved in redox regulation of caspases should be further investigated to dissect the mechanistic roles in apoptosis.

6. Oxidative Stress in Cancer

It is now recognized that oxidative stress is prevalent in cancer cells of various tissue origins.[86–90] Despite such consistent observations, the cause-effect relationship between ROS stress and cancer development remains to be defined. It is likely that there are complex interactions between ROS generation, ROS signaling, ROS-induced damage, and carcinogenesis. Figure 1 illustrates some important aspects of oxidative stress, cancer development, and potential therapeutic implication. Under the influence of certain oncogenic signals, cells may exhibit increased generation of ROS due in part to active metabolic activity associated with uncontrolled cell growth and proliferation. Mitochondria are major sites of endogenous ROS generation owing to leakage of electrons from the respiratory chain. Exogenous ROS insults such as radiation and certain chemicals can also increase oxidative stress in the cells. Persistent oxidative stress may lead to the

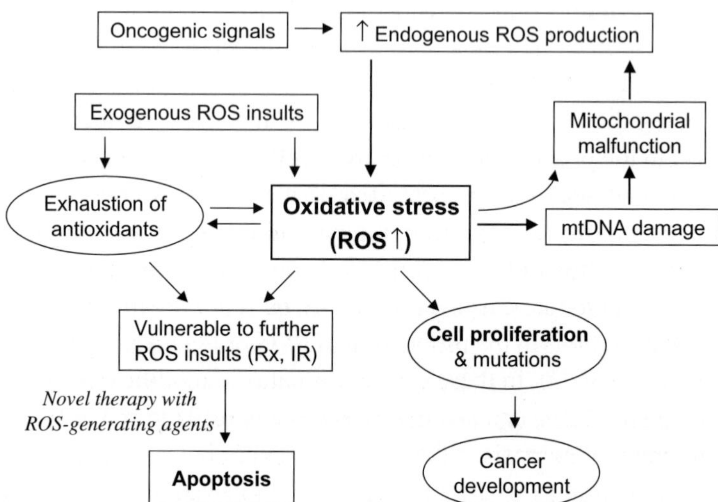

Fig. 1. Schematic illustration of the relationship between ROS stress, cancer development, and therapeutic implication. See text for detail.

consumption of cellular antioxidants and redox imbalance. The increase in cellular ROS can then contribute to cancer initiation, promotion, and progression at multiple levels. For instance, ROS can stimulate cellular proliferation and activate survival pathways by the signaling mechanisms discussed above. ROS may also directly cause damage to DNA leading to mutations. Oxidation of guanine at the C8 position, leading to the formation of 8-hydroxydeoxyguanosine, is probably the most frequent and mutagenic lesion. This oxidative DNA lesion can cause G → T transversions that are often found in mutated oncogenes and tumor suppressor genes.[91–93] These mutational events are known to be involved in cancer development, genetic instability, and disease progression.

As mentioned above, mitochondria constitute the major endogenous source of ROS due to electron bifurcation at complexes I and III of the respiratory chain (for review, see Carew and Huang[94]) Because mitochondrial DNA (mtDNA) encodes for 13 protein components of the respiratory chain, and is physically in close proximity to the site of ROS generation, damage of mtDNA by ROS may cause a malfunction of the respiratory chain, more electron leakage, and a further increase in ROS generation. This will in turn result in additional damage to mtDNA and nuclear DNA. This loop of ROS amplification mechanism may play a significant role in causing endogenous ROS stress, and contribute to genetic instability and cancer progression. The increase in cellular ROS levels and its association with mitochondrial DNA mutation have been observed in primary cancer cells isolated from leukemia patients.[95]

The increase in oxidative stress in cancer cells may have significant therapeutic implications. On one hand, the genetic instability associated with ROS-mediated DNA damage may provide a mechanism for the development of subclones of drug-resistant cancer cells. On the other hand, the increased ROS stress in cancer cells may render them more vulnerable to further oxidative insults by exogenous ROS-generating agents. This may provide a biochemical basis for developing new therapeutic strategies to preferentially kill such cancer cells. It is conceivable that the constant increased ROS stress in cancer cells may largely exhaust the cellular antioxidant capacity, and an additional ROS stress imposed by exogenous anticancer agents is likely to push the ROS stress to a threshold that triggers cell death. Such a threshold hypothesis was proposed by Kong and Lillehei.[96,97]

Indeed, recent studies demonstrated that human leukemia cells and ovarian cancer cells are more sensitive to ROS stress induced by SOD inhibition by 2-methoxyestradiol (2-ME) than normal cells.[89,98] The sensitivity of primary leukemia cells isolated from patients with chronic lymphocytic leukemia (CLL) to 2-ME seems to be positively correlated with the levels of ROS stress in the CLL cells.[88] Thus, the clinical implications of using ROS-generating agents, alone or in combination with other anticancer agents, to kill malignant cells as a therapeutic strategy merit further investigation.

References

1. Marshall HE, Merchant K, Stamler JS. Nitrosation and oxidation in the regulation of gene expression. *FASEB J.* 14: 1889–1900 (2000).
2. Esposito F, Ammendola R, Faraonio R, Russo T, Cimino F. Redox control of signal transduction, gene expression and cellular senescence. *Neurochem. Res.* 29: 617–628 (2004).
3. Li N, Karin M. Is NF-κB the sensor of oxidative stress? *FASEB J.* 13: 1137–1143 (1999).
4. Staal FJ, Roederer M, Hershenberg LA. Intracellular thiols regulate activation of nuclear factor kappa B and transcription of human immunodeficiency virus. *Proc. Natl. Acad. Sci. USA* 87: 9943–9947 (1990).
5. Bowie A, O'Neill LAJ. Oxidative stress and nuclear factor-κB activation: a reassessment of the evidence in light of recent discoveries. *Biochem. Pharmacol.* 59: 13–23 (2000).
6. Matthews JR, Kakasagi N, Vjudsier JL, Yodoi J, Hay RT. Thioredoxin regulates the DNA binding activity of NF-kappa B transcription factor by reduction of a disulphide bind involving cysteine 62. *Nucleic Acids Res.* 20: 3821–3830 (1992).
7. Schreck R, Rieber P, Bauerle PA. Reactive oxygen intermediates as apparently widely used messengers in the activation of the NF-kappa B transcription factor and HIV-1. *EMBO J.* 10: 2247–2258 (1991).
8. Meyer M, Schreck R, Bauerle PA. H_2O_2 and antioxidants have opposite effects on activation of NF-kappa B and AP-1 as a secondary antioxidant-responsive factor. *EMBO J.* 12: 2005–2015 (1993).
9. Bowie AG, Moynagh PN, O'Neill LA. Lipid peroxidation is involved in the activation of NF-kappaB by tumor necrosis factor, but not interleukin-q in the human endothelial cell line ECV304. Lack of involvement of H_2O_2 in

NF-kappaB activation by either cytokine in both primary and transformed endothelial cells. *J. Biol. Chem.* 272: 25941–25950 (1997).

10. Manna SK, Zhang HJ, Yan T, Oberley LW, Aggarwal BB. Overexpression of manganese superoxide dismutase suppresses tumor necrosis factor-induced apoptosis and activation of nuclear transcription factor kappa B and activated protein-1. *J. Biol. Chem.* 273: 13245–13254 (1998).
11. Delhalle S, Deregowski V, Benoit V, Merville MP, Bours V. NF-kappaB-dependent MnSOD expression protects adenocarcinoma cells from TNF-alpha-induced apoptosis. *Oncogene* 21: 3917–3924 (2002).
12. Shaulian E, Karin M. AP-1 in cell proliferation and survival. *Oncogene* 20: 2390–2400 (2001).
13. Brown JR, Nigh E, Lee RJ, Ye H, Thompson MA, Saudon F, Pestell RG, Greenberg ME. Fos family members induce cell cycle entry by activating cyclin D1. *Mol. Cell. Biol.* 18: 5609–5619 (1998).
14. Bakiri LLD, Bossy-Wetzel E, Yaniv M. Cell cycle-dependent variations in c-jun and JunB phosphorylation: a role in the control of cyclin D expression. *EMBO J.* 19: 2969–2979 (2000).
15. Passague E, Wagner EF. JunB suppresses cell proliferation by transcriptional activation of p16(INK4A). *EMBO J.* 19: 2969–2979 (2000).
16. Xia Z, Dickens M, Raingeaud J, Davis RJ, Greenberg ME. Opposing effects of ERK and JNK-p38 kinases on apoptosis. *Science* 270: 1326–1331 (1995).
17. Blackwell TK, Kretzner L, Blackwood EM, Eisenman RN, Weintraub H. Sequence-specific DNA-binding complex with myc. *Science* 250: 1149–1151 (1990).
18. Obaya AJ, Mateyak MK, Sedivy JM. Mysterious liaisons: the relationship between c-myc and the cell cycle. *Oncogene* 18: 2934–2941 (1999).
19. Galaktionov K, Chen X, Beach D. Cdc25 cell-cycle phosphatase as a target of c–myc. *Nature* 382: 511–517 (1996).
20. Leone G, DeGregori J, Sears R, Jakoi L, Nevins JR. Myc and Ras collaborate in inducing accumulation of active cyclin E/cdk2 and E2F. *Nature* 387: 422–426 (1997).
21. Hermeking H, Rago C, Schuhmacher M, Li Q, Barrett JF, Obaya AJ *et al.* Identification of CDK4 as a target of c-MYC. *Proc. Natl. Acad. Sci. USA* 97: 2229–2234 (2000).
22. Vafa O, Wade M, Kern S, Beeche M, Pandita TK, Hampton GM, Wahl GM. c-Myc can induce DNA damage, increase reactive oxygen species, and mitigate p53 function: a mechanism for oncogene-induced genetic instability. *Mol. Cell* 9: 1031–1044 (2002).

23. Tanaka H, Matsumura I, Ezoe S, Satoh Y, Sakamaki T, Albanese C, Machii T, Pestell RG, Kanakura Y. E2F1 and c-Myc potentiate apoptosis through inhibition of NF-kappaB activity that facilitates MnSOD-mediated ROS elimination. *Mol. Cell* 9: 1017–1029 (2002).
24. Fu L, Pelicano H, Liu J, Huang P, Lee C. The circadian gene Period2 plays an important role in tumor suppression and DNA damage response *in vivo. Cell* 111: 41–50 (2002).
25. Burgering BMT, Medema RH. Decisions on life and death: FOXO forkhead transcription factors are in command when PKB/Akt is off duty. *J. Leuk. Bio.* 73: 689–701 (2003).
26. Medema RH, Kops GJ, Bos JL, Burgering BM. AFX-like forkhead transcription factors mediate cell-cycle regulation by Ras and PKB through p27/kip1. *Nature* 404: 782–787 (2000).
27. Schmidt M, de Mattos SF, van der Horst A, Klompmaker R, Kops GJ, Lam EW, Burgering BM, Medema RH. Cell cycle inhibition by foxo forkhead transcription factors involves downregulation of cyclin D. *Mol. Cell. Biol.* 22: 7842–7852 (2002).
28. Kops GJ, Dansen TB, Polderman PB, Saarloos I, Wirtz KW, Coffer PJ, Huang TT, Bos JL, Medema RH, Burgering BM. Forkhead transcription factor FOXO3a protects quiescent cells from oxidative stress. *Nature* 419: 316–321 (2002).
29. Nemoto S, Finkel T. Redox regulation of forkhead proteins through a p66shc-dependent pathway. *Science* 295: 2450–2452 (2002).
30. Tran H, Brunet A, Grenier JM, Datta SR, Fornace Jr. AJ, DiStefano PS, Chiang LW, Greenberg ME. DNA repair pathway stimulated by the forkhead transcription factor FOXO3a through the GADD45 protein. *Science* 296: 530–534 (2002).
31. Nguyen KT, Zong CS, Uttamsingh S, Sachdev P, Bhanot M, Le MT, Chan JL, Wang LH. The role of phosphatidylinositol 3-kinase, rho family GTPases, and STAT3 in Ros-induced cell transformation. *J. Biol. Chem.* 277: 11107–11115 (2002).
32. Liu SL, Lin X, Shi DY, Cheng J, Wu CQ, Zhang YD. Reactive oxygen species stimulated human hepatoma cell proliferation via cross-talk between PI3K/PKB and JNK signaling pathways. *Arch. Biochem. Biophys.* 406: 173–182 (2002).
33. Yacoub A, Mitchell C, Hong V, Gopalkrishnan RV, Su ZZ, Gupta P, Sauane M, Lebedkeva IV, Curiel DT, Mahasreshti PJ, Rosenfeld MR, Broaddus WC, James CD, Grant S, Fisher PB, Dent P. MDA-7 regulates cell growth and radiosensitivity *in vitro* of primary (non-established) human glioma cells. *Cancer Biol. Ther.* 10: Epub ahead of print (2004).

34. Dong-Yun S, Yu-Ru D, Shan-Lin, Ya-Dong Z, Lian W. Redox stress regulates cell proliferation and apoptosis of human hepatoma through Akt protein phosphorylation. *FEBS Lett.* 542: 60–64 (2003).
35. Johnson GL, Lapadat R. Mitogen-activated protein kinase pathways mediated by ERK, JNK, and p38 protein kinases. *Science* 298: 1911–1912 (2002).
36. Preston TJ, Muller WJ, Singh G. Scavenging of extracellular H_2O_2 by catalase inhibits the proliferation of HER-2/Neu-transformed rat-1 fibroblasts through the induction of a stress response. *J. Biol. Chem.* 276: 9558–9564 (2001).
37. Kim BY, Han WJ, Chung AS. Effects of reactive oxygen species on proliferation of Chinese hamster ovary cells. *Free Radic. Biol. Med.* 30: 686–698 (2001).
38. Maeda H, Hori S, Nishitoh H, Ichijo H, Ogawa O, Kakehi Y, Kakizuka A. Tumor growth inhibition by arsenic trioxide (As_2O_3) in the orthotopic metastasis model of androgen-independent prostate cancer. *Cancer Res.* 61: 5432–5440 (2001).
39. Kunduzova OR, Bianchi P, Pizzinat N, Escourrou G, Seguelas MH, Parini A, Cambon C. Regulation of JNK/ERK activation, cell apoptosis, and tissue regeneration by monoamine oxidases after renal ischemia-reperfusion. *FASEB J.* 16: 1129–1131 (2002).
40. Coleman ML, Marshall CJ, Olson MF. Ras and rho GTPases in G1-phasew cell-cycle regulation. *Nat. Rev. Mol. Cell. Biol.* 5: 355–366 (2004).
41. Lion JS, Chen CY, Chen JS, Faller DV. Oncogenic ras mediates spoptosis in response to protein kinase C inhibition through the generation of reactive oxygen species. *J. Biol. Chem.* 275: 39001–39011 (2000).
42. Thannickal VJ, Day RM, Klinz SG, Bastien MC, Larios JM, Fanburg BL. Ras-dependent and -independent regulation of reactive oxygen species generation by mitogenic growth factors and TGF-beta1. *FASEB J.* 14: 1741–1748 (2000).
43. Chuang JL, Chang TY, Lin HS. Glutathione depletion-induced apoptosis of Ha-ras-transformed NIH3T3 cells can be prevented by melatonin. *Oncogene* 23: 1349–1357 (2003).
44. Cullen JJ, Weydert C, Hinkhouse MM, Ritchie J, Domann FE, Spitz D, Oberley LW. The role of manganese superoxide dismutase in the growth of pancreatic adenocarcinoma. *Cancer Res.* 63: 1297–1303 (2003).
45. Adachi T, Pimentel DR, Heibeck T, Hon X, Lee YJ, Jiang B, Ido Y, Cohen RA. S-glutathiolation of Ras mediates redox-sensitive signaling by angiotensin II in vascular smooth muscle cells. *J. Biol. Chem.* Epub ahead of print (2004).
46. Lambeth JD. NOX enzymes and the biology of reactive oxygen. *Nat. Rev. Immunol.* 4: 181–189 (2004).
47. Cai J, Jones DP. Mitochondrial redox signaling during apoptosis. *J. Bioenerg. Biomembr.* 31: 327–334 (1999).

48. Ichijo H, Niishida E, Irie K, ten Dijke P, Saitoh M, Moriguchi T, Takagi M, Matsumoto K, Miyazono K, Gotoh Y. Induction of apoptosis by ASK1, a mammalian MAPKKK that activates SAPK/JNK and p38 signaling pathways. *Science* 275: 90–94 (1997).
49. Nishitoh HS, M, Mochida Y, Takeda K, Nakano H, Rothe M, Miyazono K, Ichijo, H. ASK1 is essential for JNK/SAPK activation by TRAF2. *Mol. Cell.* 2: 389–395 (1998).
50. Tobiume K, Matsuzawa A, Takahashi T, Nishitoh H, Morita K, Takeda K, Minowa O, Miyazono K, Noda T, Ichijo H. ASK1 is required for sustained activation of JNK/p38 MAP kinases and apoptosis. *EMBO Rep.* 2: 222–228 (2001).
51. Nishitoh H, Mastuzawa A, Tobiume K, Saegusa K, Takeda K, Inoue K, Hori S, Kakizuka A, Ichijo H. ASK1 is essential for endoplasmic reticulum stress-induced neuronal cell death triggered by expanded polyglutamine repeats. *Genes Dev.* 16: 1345–1355 (2002).
52. Saitoh M, Nishitoh H, Fujii M, Takeda K, Tobiume K, Sawada Y, Kawabata M, Miyazono K, Ichijo H. Mammalian thioredoxin is a direct inhibitor of apoptosis signal-regulating kinase (ASK) 1. *EMBO J.* 17: 2596–2606 (1998).
53. Kim AH, Khursigara G, Sun X, Franke TF, Chao MV. Akt phosphorylates and negatively regulates apoptosis signal-regulating kinase 1. *Mol. Cell. Biol.* 21: 893–901 (2001).
54. Ohiro Y, Usheva A, Kobayashi S, Duffy SL, Nantz R, Gius D, Horikoshi N. Inihibition of stress-inducible kinase pathways by tumorigenic mutant p53. *Mol. Cell. Biol.* 23: 322–334 (2003).
55. Voehringer DW. Bcl-2 and glutathione: alterations in cellular redox state that regulate apoptotic sensitivity. *Free. Radic. Biol. Med.* 27: 945–950 (1999).
56. Veis DJ, Sorenson CM, Shutter JR, Korsmeyer SJ. Bcl-2-deficient mice demonstrate fulminant lymphoid apoptosis, polycystc kidneys, and hypopigmented hair. *Cell* 75: 229–240 (1993).
57. Hockenbery DM, Ottvai ZN, Yin X-M, Milliman CLl, Korsmeyer SJ. Bcl-2 functions in an antioxidant pathway to prevent apoptosis. *Cell* 75: 241–251 (1993).
58. Meredith MJ, Cusick CL, Soltaninassab S, Sekkar KS, Lu S, Freeman ML. Expression of bcl-2 increases intracellular glutathione by inhibiting methionine-dependent GSH efflux. *Biochem. Biophys. Res. Commun.* 248: 458–463 (1998).
59. Mirkovic N, Voehringer DW, Story MD, McConkey DJ, McDonnell TJ, Meyn RE. Resistance to radiation-induced apoptosis in bcl-2-expressing

cells is reversed by depleting cellular thiols. *Oncogene* 15: 1461–1470 (1997).

60. Voehringer DW, McConkey DJ, McDonnell TJ, Brisbay S, Meyn RE. Bcl-2 expression causes redistribution of glutathione to the nucleus. *Proc. Natl. Acad. Sci. USA* 95: 2956–2960 (1998).
61. Horton JK, Roy G, Piper JT, Van Houten B, Awasthi YC, Mitra S, Alaoui-Jamali MA, Boldogh I, Singhal SS. Characterization of a chlorambucil-resistant human ovarian carcinoma cell line overexpressing glutathione-s-transferase mu. *Biochem. Pharmacol.* 58: 693–702 (1999).
62. Richardson ME, Siemann DW. DNA damage in cyclophosphamide-resistant tumor cells: the role of glutathione. *Cancer Res.* 55: 1691–1695 (1995).
63. Sun Y, Oberley LW. Redox regulation of transcriptional activators. *Free Radic. Biol. Med.* 21: 335–348 (1996).
64. Kharbanda S, Saxena S, Yoshida K, Pandey P, Kaneki M, Wang Q, Cheng K, Chen YN, Campbell A, Sudha T, Yuan ZM, Narula J, Weichselbaum R, Nalin C, Kufe D. Translocation of SAPK/JNK to mitochondria and interaction with Bcl-x(L) in response to DNA damage. *J. Biol. Chem.* 275: 322–327 (2000).
65. Chauhan D, Li G, Hideshima T, Podar K, Mitsiades C, Mitsiades N, Munshi N, Kharbanda S, Anderson KC. JNK-dependent release of mitochondrial protein, Smac, during apoptosis in multiple myeloma (MM) cells. *J. Biol. Chem.* 278: 17593–17596 (2003).
66. Deng Y, Ren X, Yang L, Lin Y, Wu X. A JNK-dependent pathway is required for TNFalpha-induced apoptosis. *Cell* 115: 61–70 (2003).
67. Tournier C, Hess P, Yang DD, Xu J, Turner TK, Nimnual A, Bar-Sagi D, Jones SN, Flavell RA, Davis RJ. Requirement of JNK for stress-induced activation of the cytochrome c-mediated death pathway. *Science* 288: 870–874 (2000).
68. Yamamoto K, Ichijo H, Korsmeyer SJ. Bcl-2 is phosphorylated and inactivated by an ASK1/Jun N-terminal protein kinase pathway normally activated at G(2)/M. *Mol. Cell. Biol.* 19: 8469–8478 (1999).
69. Lei K, Davis RJ. JNK phosphorylation of Bim-related members of the Bcl2 family induces Bax-dependent apoptosis. *Proc. Natl. Acad. Sci. USA* 100: 2432–2437 (2003).
70. Tsuruta F, Sunayama J, Mori Y, Hattori S, Shimizu S, Tsujimoto Y, Yoshioka K, Masuyama N, Gotoh Y. JNK promotes Bax translocation to mitochondria through phosphorylation of 14-3-3 proteins. *EMBO J.* 23: 1889–1899 (2004).

71. Friedman JS, Lowe SW. Control of apoptosis by p53. *Oncogene* 22: 9030–9040 (2003).
72. Slee EA, O'Connor DJ, Lu X. To die or not to die: how does p53 decide? *Oncogene* 23: 2809–2818 (2004).
73. Hwang PM, Bunz F, Yu J, Rago C, Chan TA, Murphy MP, Kelso GF, Smith RA, Kinzler KW, Vogelstein B. Ferredoxin reductase affects p53-dependent, 5-fluorouracil-induced apoptosis in colorectal cancer cells. *Nat. Med.* 7: 1111–1117 (2001).
74. Marchenko ND, Zaika A, Moll U. Death signal-induced localization of p53 protein to mitochondria. A potential role in apoptotic signaling. *J. Biol. Chem.* 275: 16202–16212 (2000).
75. Chipuk JE, Maurer U, Green DR, Schuler M. Pharmacologic activation of p53 elicits BAX-dependent apoptosis in the absence of transcription. *Cancer Cell* 4: 371–381 (2003).
76. Dumont P, Leu JI, Della Pietra III AC, George D, Murphy M. The codon 72 polymorphic variants of p53 have markedly different apoptotic potential. *Nat. Genet.* 33: 357–365 (2003).
77. Mihara M, Erster S, Zaika A, Petrenko O, Chittenden T, Pancoska P, Moll UM. p53 has a direct apoptogenic role at the mitochondria. *Mol. Cell.* 11: 577–590 (2003).
78. Wu HH, Thomas JA, Momand J. p53 protein oxidation in cultured cells in response to pyrrolidine dithiocarbamamte: a novel method for relating the amount of p53 oxidation *in vivo* to the regulation of p53 responsive genes. *Biochem. J.* 351: 87–93 (2000).
79. Sun XZ, Vinci C, Makmura L, Han S, Tran D, Nguyen J, Hamann M, Grazziani S, Sheppard S, Gutova M, Zhou F, Thomas J, Momand J. Formation of disulfide bond in p53 correlates with inhibition of DNA binding and tetramerization. *Antioxid. Redox Signal* 5: 655–665 (2003).
80. Degterev A, Boyce M, Yuan J. A decade of caspases. *Oncogene* 22: 8543–8567 (2003).
81. Melino G, Bernassola F, Knight RA, Corasaniti MT, Nistico G, Finazzi-Agro A. S-nitrosylation regulates caspases. *Nature* 388: 432–433 (1997).
82. Li J, Biliar TR, Talanian RV, Kim YM. Nitric oxide reversibly inhibits seven members of the caspase family via S-nitrosylation. *Biochem. Biophys. Res. Commun.* 240: 419–424 (1997).
83. Mohr S, Zech B, Lapetina EG, Brune B. Inhibition of caspase-3 by S-nitrosation and oxidation caused by nitric oxide. *Biochem. Biophys. Res. Commun.* 238: 387–391 (1997).

84. Hampton MB, Orrenius S. Dual regulation of caspase activity by hydrogen peroxide. *FEBS Lett.* 414: 552–556 (1997).
85. Mannick JB, Schonhoff C, Papeta N, Ghafourifar P, Szibor M, Fang K, Gaston B. S-Nitrosylation of mitochondrial caspases. *J. Cell. Biol.* 154: 1111–1116 (2001).
86. Toyohuni S, Okamoto K, Yodoi J, Hiai H. Persistent oxidative stress in cancer. *FEBS Lett.* 358: 1–3 (1995).
87. Toyohuni S. Oxidative stress and cancer: the role of redox regulation. *Biotherapy* 11: 147–154 (1998).
88. Zhou Y, Hileman EO, Plunkett W, Keating MJ, Huang P. Free radical stress in chronic lymphocytic leukemia cells and its role in cellular sensitivity to ROS-generating anticancer agents. *Blood* 101: 4098–4104 (2003).
89. Hileman EO, Liu J, Albitar M, Keating MJ, Huang P. Intriinsic oxidative stress in cancer cells: a biochemical basis for therapeutic selectivity. *Cancer Chemother. Pharmacol.* 53: 209–219 (2004).
90. Pelicano H, Carney D, Huang P. ROS stress in cancer cells and therapeutic implications. *Drug Resist. Update* 7: 97–110 (2004).
91. Shibutani S, Takeshita M, Grollman AP. Insertion of specific bases during DNA synthesis past the oxidation-damaged base 8-oxo-dG. *Nature* 349: 431–434 (1991).
92. Moriya M. Single-stranded shuttle phagemid for mutagenesis studies in mammalian cells: 8-oxoguanine in DNA induces targeted G:c → T:A transversions in simian kidney cells. *Proc. Natl. Acad. Sci. USA* 90: 1122–1126 (1993).
93. Hussain SP, Harris CC. Molecular epidemiology of human cancer: contribution of mutation spectra studies of tumor suppressor genes. *Cancer Res.* 58: 4023–4037 (1998).
94. Carew JS, Huang P. Mitochondrial defects in cancer. *Mol. Cancer* 1: 9 (2002).
95. Carew JS Zhou Y, Albitar M, Carew JD, Keating MJ, Huang P. Mitochondrial DNA mutations in primary leukemia cells after chemotherapy: clinical significance and therapeutic implications. *Leukemia* 17: 1437–1447 (2003).
96. Kong Q, Lillehei KO. Antioxidant inhibitors for cancer therapy. *Med. Hypotheses* 51: 405–409 (1998).
97. Kong Q, Beel JA, Lillehei KO. A threshold concept for cancer therapy. *Med. Hypotheses* 55: 29–35 (2000).
98. Huang P, Feng L, Oldham EA, Keating MJ, Plunkett W. Superoxide dismutase as a target for the selective killing of cancer cells. *Nature* 407: 390–395 (2000).

10 Oxidative Damage to Carbohydrates and Amino Acids

Marco d'Ischia, Paola Manini, and Alessandra Napolitano

1. Introduction

This chapter attempts to present a conceptual framework for oxidative and nitrosative stress-induced damage to carbohydrates and amino acids. In each section, the effects of exposure of the target molecules to reactive oxygen and nitrogen species will be illustrated, with special emphasis to the highly aggressive OH radical, peroxynitrite ($ONOO^-$), nitrogen dioxide (NO_2), hypochlorous acid (HOCl), and H_2O_2. The pathological implications of oxidative damage as a cause of loss-of-function modifications and/or the generation of geno/cytotoxic breakdown products will then be briefly addressed. Because of space restrictions, coverage of the topic will be illustrative rather than comprehensive, and the essential perspectives to be reviewed are that each class of biomolecules has a range of sites intrinsically more susceptible to free radical attack by oxidizing agents, and that the prevalence of one or the other is determined on a competitive basis by largely chemical factors.

2. Oxidative Damage to Carbohydrates

2.1. *Monosaccharides*

Under oxidative stress conditions, monosaccharides undergo degradation processes leading mainly to fragmentation of the carbon backbone.

Among the various oxygen species, hydroxyl radicals are the most effective in causing oxidative breakdown of carbohydrates. E.s.r. analyses have shown that the Fenton-like system Ti(III)/H_2O_2 or γ-radiolysis induce hydroxyl radical-mediated H-atom abstraction to produce carbon-centered radicals.[1,2] This step is poorly regioselective in the case of pyranoses, leading to the formation of all of the six possible C-radicals, whereas in the case of furanose sugars it takes place preferentially at C-4, the carbon adjacent to the alicyclic oxygen, due to stereoelectronic effects.[3] For D-2-deoxyribose, fragmentation pathways at C-2 are virtually precluded because the lack of the hydroxyl group makes the H-atom abstraction a less favorable process.[4]

Under aerobic conditions, the carbon-centered radicals react with oxygen at diffusion rates to give the corresponding peroxyl radicals[5] to which three different routes are available. The peroxyl radicals can rearrange with loss of $HOO^\bullet$, as shown in Fig. 1 for glucose, to give the corresponding glucosone.[2]

Alternatively, such radicals lead to the formation of the corresponding hydroperoxide via H-atom abstraction from a donor. The resulting hydroperoxides can either undergo Criegee rearrangement with ring expansion followed by hydrolytic cleavage (route A),[6] or can be reduced by Fe^{2+} ions to give an alkoxyl radical which in turn would undergo β-fragmentation (route B), (Fig. 2).[7]

Both mechanistic pathways explain the formation of malondialdehyde from D-2-deoxyribose, a process that represents the basis of a currently used test for evaluating the efficacy of hydroxyl radical scavengers.[8]

A third route would involve dimerization to give tetroxide intermediates, highly reactive species that can decompose either homolytically[9] or heterolytically.[10] However the latter pathways are usually disregarded as being of minor importance.

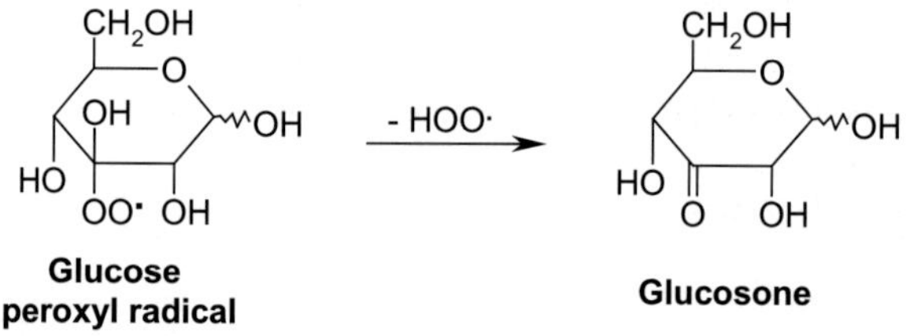

Fig. 1. Formation of glucosone by $HOO^\bullet$ loss from glucose peroxyl radical.

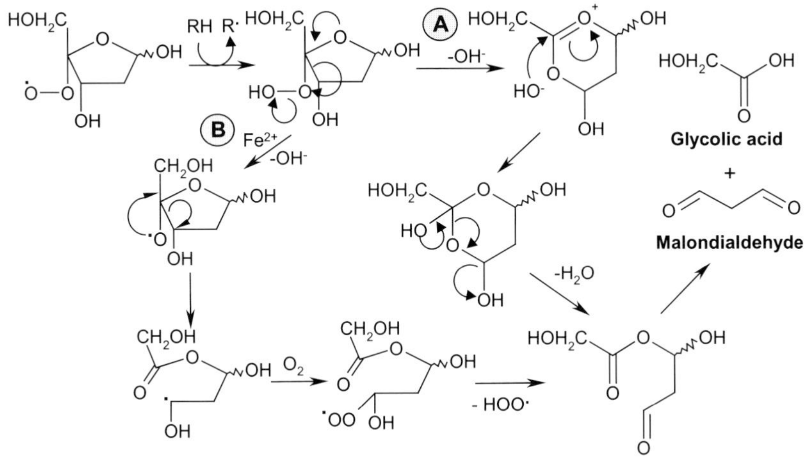

Fig. 2. Mechanisms of the Criegee rearrangement (A) and of the β-fragmentation (B) of monosaccharide hydroperoxide. Highlighted is the formation of malondialdehyde via the hydroxyl radical-induced oxidation of D-2-deoxyribose.

The main products formed by the HO radical-induced oxidation of glucose are reported in Table 1.

In the case of phosphate sugars, the elimination of a phosphate group β to the carbon-centered radical (phosphate release) becomes a competitive pathway with respect to oxygen scavenging.[11] As shown in Fig. 3, phosphate elimination leads to the formation of the radical-cation **1** in which both the charge and the radical are stabilized by the α-oxygen lone pair.

The radical cation **1** can thus rearrange through a ring-opening step followed by hydrogen abstraction from a donor to give the ketoaldehyde **2**, or can suffer hydration with H-atom coupling to give **2** and **3**. Alternative mechanisms of phosphate release have been proposed.[12]

Like most carbohydrates, ascorbic acid can undergo oxidative breakdown following exposure to elevated levels of hydroxyl radicals. Under physiologically relevant conditions, the reaction proceeds with formation of dehydroascorbic acid and diketogulonic acid along with numerous fragmentation products such as threose, glycolaldehyde, glyceraldehyde, dihydroxyacetone, malondialdehyde, glyoxal and formaldehyde (Fig. 4).[13]

Besides hydroxyl radical, other reactive oxygen species that accumulate under oxidative stress conditions can induce the degradation of the carbohydrate backbone.

Table 1. Reaction products formed by the hydroxyl radical-mediated oxidation of D-glucose.[2]

Carbon radical	Oxidation products
C-1	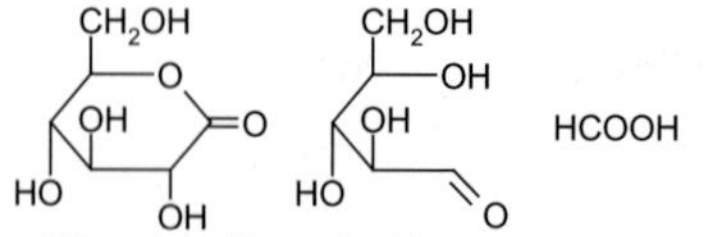 D-Gluconic acid; D-Arabinose; HCOOH Formic acid
C-2	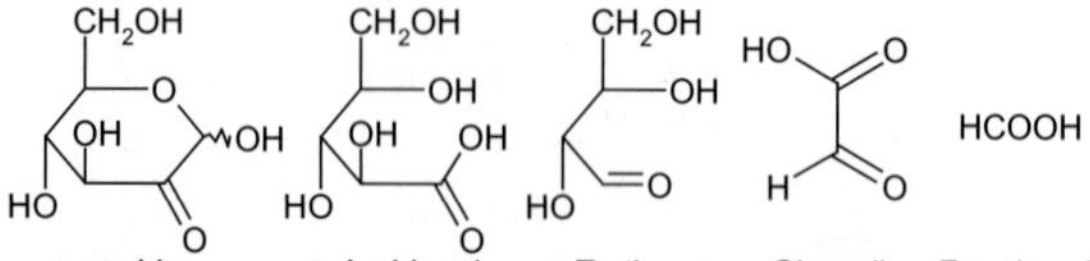 D-*arabino*-Hexosulose; D-Arabinonic acid; D-Erythrose; Glyoxylic acid; HCOOH Formic acid
C-3	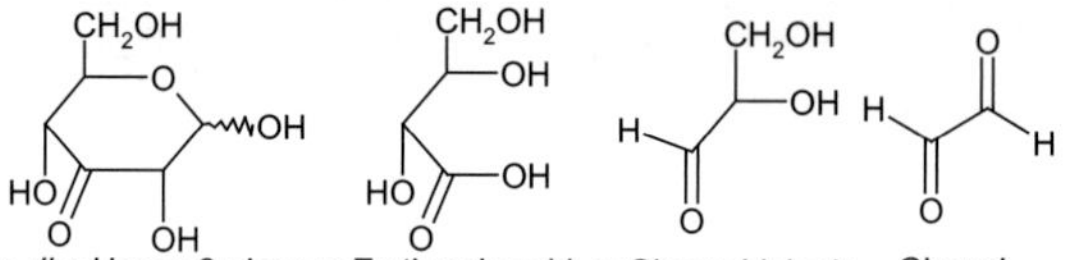 D-*ribo*-Hexos-3-ulose; D-Erythronic acid; D-Glyceraldehyde; Glyoxal
C-4	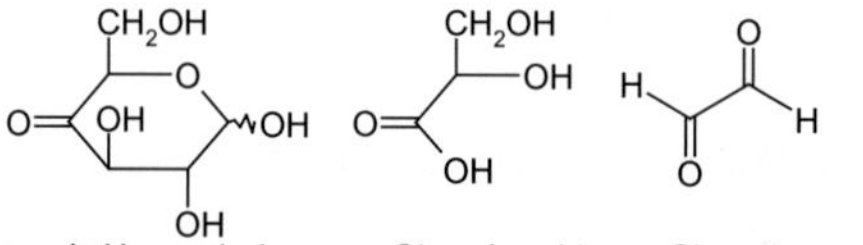 D-*xylo*-Hexos-4-ulose; D-Glyceric acid; Glyoxal
C-5	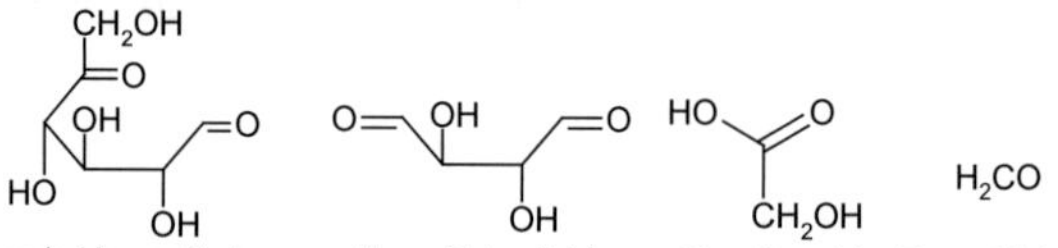 D-*xylo*-Hexos-5-ulose; L-*threo*-Tetrodialdose; Glycolic acid; H_2CO Formaldehyde
C-6	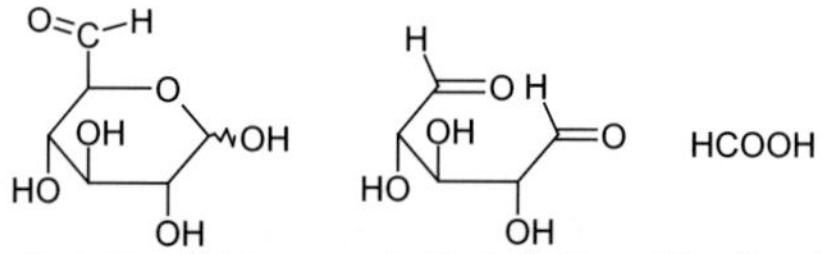 D-*gluco*-Hexodialdose; *xylo*-Pentodialdose; HCOOH Formic acid

One of these is superoxide that oxidizes monosaccharides by a mechanism akin to that of autoxidation, a slow process typically catalyzed by transition metal ions such as Fe^{3+} and Cu^{2+}. This is illustrated in Fig. 5 in the case of glucose. The carbohydrate in its tautomeric enediol form (**4**) can be oxidized by metal ions to the corresponding enediol radical-anion **5**. The

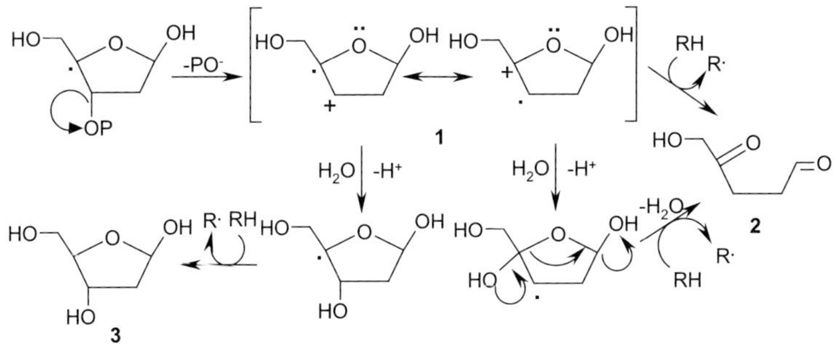

Fig. 3. The phosphate release pathways.

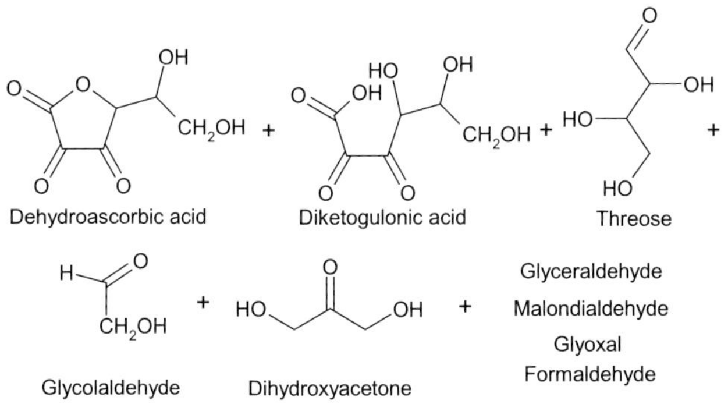

Fig. 4. Main products formed by the hydroxyl radical-induced oxidation of ascorbic acid.

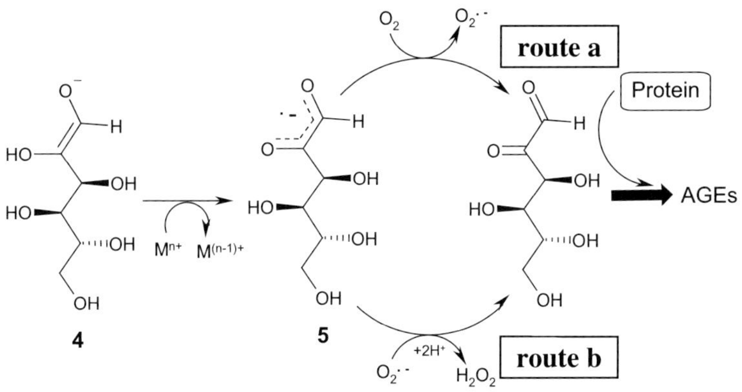

Fig. 5. Mechanisms proposed for the oxygen-promoted (route a) and superoxide radical anion-promoted (route b) oxidation of glucose.

latter is a very reactive specie that reduces molecular oxygen (route a)[14,15] or more rapidly superoxide (route b),[16] to form α-dicarbonyl compounds and superoxide in the former case, or hydrogen peroxide in the latter case.

Overall, these processes can induce cell damage by generating hydroxyl radicals[17] and reactive carbonyl species.[14] These latter can form stable adducts with proteins known as **advanced glycation end-products** (AGEs).[18]

Peroxynitrite ($ONOO^-$) can also cause monosaccharide oxidation.[19] Analysis of the incubation mixtures of glucose with peroxynitrite revealed the formation of 3-deoxyglucosone and glyoxal as main products. This finding underscores the role of nitric oxide in the formation of AGEs and in the pathogenesis of diabetic complications.

Glucose $\xrightarrow{ONOO^-}$ 3-deoxyglucosone + Glyoxal

2.2. *Polysaccharides and nucleic acids*

Polysaccharides are widely distributed in living organisms and subserve both metabolic and structural roles. Hyaluronic acid, heparin, dermatan sulfate, keratan sulfate, and chondroitin sulfate provide the major components of the so-called **ground substance**, a gel-like matrix in which are embedded the collagen and elastin fibers of connective tissues such as cartilage, tendon, skin, and blood vessel walls.

Particular attention has been focused on the oxidative degradation of hyaluronic acid, present at high concentrations in synovial fluid. This process is strictly related to the development of rheumatoid arthritis, a pathology characterized by severe inflammation of the joints.

The alteration of the molecular-weight distribution of synovial fluid in patients with rheumatoid arthritis seems to be a direct consequence of the action of reactive oxygen species on hyaluronic acid.[20] Polymorphonuclear leukocytes invade inflamed joints[21] and, upon stimulation, release myeloperoxidase (MPO), which catalyzes the formation of the oxidant

ClO^- from H_2O_2 and Cl^-;[22] moreover, H_2O_2 produced by stimulated leukocytes may interact with Fe^{2+} to form hydroxyl radicals responsible for the inhibition of chondrocyte proteoglycan synthesis and for inflammatory and degenerative changes.[23]

Degradation of hyaluronic acid with the Fenton reagent or with ClO^- proceeds through cleavage of the glycosidic bond between glucuronic acid and *N*-acetylglucosamine, the two monomers that linearly alternate in the polymeric backbone.[24] The formation of lower molecular weight polysaccharidic units is consistent with the decreased viscosity of the solutions.

Fragmentation of the single monosaccharidic unit could be observed only at high concentrations of the oxidants, leading to *meso*-tartaric acid, arabinaric acid, and glucaric acid as main products. The same products are formed by degradation of glucuronic acid suggesting that the oxidation of hyaluronic acid proceeds preferentially at glucuronic acid residues.

N*-Acetylglucosamine** ***Glucuronic acid

Hyaluronic acid

[O]

***meso*-Tartaric acid** **Arabinaric acid** **Glucaric acid**

It is well recognized that nucleic acids are among the main targets of oxygen radical attack. Besides the bases (as in the case of 8-hydroxydeoxyguanosine formation), also the sugar-phosphate backbone of DNA and RNA is also highly vulnerable to oxidation.[25,26]

As in the case of furanoses, the hydroxyl radical-induced degradation of the 2′-deoxyribose-3′,5′-diphosphate and ribose-3′,5′-diphosphate units in DNA and RNA should proceed via H-atom abstraction to produce carbon-centered radicals preferentially on the C-4′ position.

Nevertheless, due to the complex conformational arrangement of the polymers, particularly DNA, in the solvent, the proneness of each hydrogen on the sugar moiety to be abstracted by $HO^{\bullet}$ depends not only on stereoelectronic factors (the proximity to alicyclic oxygen), but especially on the accessibility of the H-atom to the solvent-borne oxidant. As a matter of fact, both theoretical and experimental studies have demonstrated that hydroxyl radical preference for H-atom abstraction is in the order: H-5′>H-4′>H-2′≈H-3′>H-1′.

As mentioned earlier, the sugar-phosphate carbon-centered radicals can be trapped by molecular oxygen or can release a phosphate group. This latter degradation pathway appears intriguing due to the presence on the ribose/deoxyribose moiety of two different phosphate groups: a primary phosphate on C-5′ and a secondary phosphate on C-3′.

Model studies have shown that the rate of phosphate release from C-5′ ($k \approx 10^3\,s^{-1}$)[27] is three orders of magnitude lower than that from C-3′ ($k \approx 10^6\,s^{-1}$).[28] These data suggest that once the C-4′ radical has formed, the secondary phosphate can be released to form the more stable secondary cation **6**. This latter can undergo hydration to give radicals **7** and **8** as shown in Fig. 6. The former can give the ketoaldehyde **10** by hydrogen abstraction from a donor and base release, whereas the latter can eliminate the

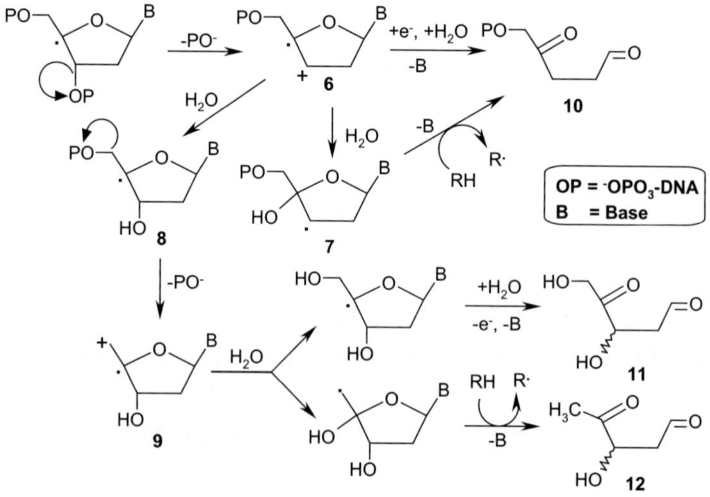

Fig. 6. Proposed mechanisms for hydroxyl radical-mediated degradation of DNA via the phosphate release pathway.

Table 2. Main reaction products formed by the hydroxyl radical-mediated oxidation of the deoxyribose moiety of DNA.

C-radical	Oxidation products	
C-1′	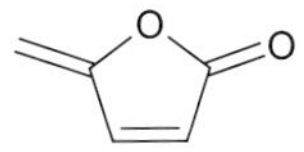 5-Methylene-2-furanone	
C-3′	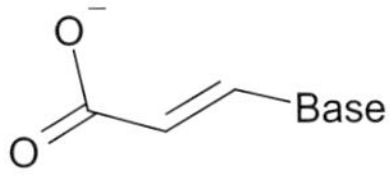 Base propenoate	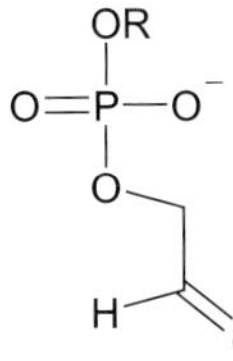 Oligonucleotide 3'-phosphoglycolaldehyde
C-4′	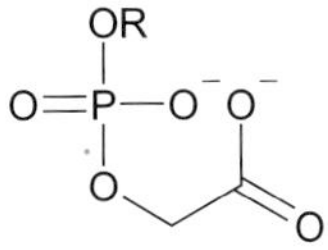 Oligonucleotide 3'-phosphoglycolate	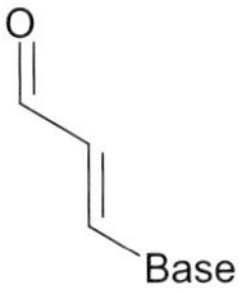 Base propenal
C-5′	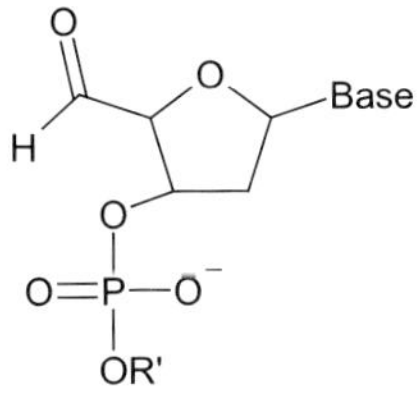 Nucleotide 5'-aldehyde	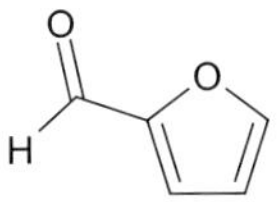 Furfural

phosphate group on C-5′ in the same way as before to give the radical cation **9**. Similarly to **6**, **9** is then converted to hydroxy- and dihydroxyketoaldehydes (**11** and **12**).

On this basis it is possible to account for the formation of the most representative fragments detected in the oxidation mixture of DNA (Table 2).[26]

2.3. *Glycated proteins*

Non-enzymatic glycosylation is an endogenous process, usually slow under physiological conditions, that contributes to the post-translational modification of proteins.[29,30]

Inside the cells, the impact of glycation is counteracted by the high turnover and short half-life of many cellular proteins. Long-lived extracellular proteins, however, accumulate glycation adducts with age. Some of these adducts may be removed by enzymatic repair mechanisms, while others are removed by degradation of the glycated proteins.

Glycation of proteins has been invoked in mechanisms of disease states, particularly the development of chronic clinical complications associated with diabetes mellitus, such as retinopathy, neuropathy, nephropathy, macrovascular disease, Alzheimer's disease, cataract and aging.[30–32]

Studies of protein glycations have focused on the reaction of aldoses and ketoses, particularly glucose, with protein amino acid residues bearing a free amino group, as in the case of lysine and arginine. The reaction proceeds through the condensation of the side chain amino group with the carbonyl functionality of glucose. This leads to the formation of a Schiff base which may undergo Amadori rearrangement to give the corresponding ketoamine, also known as Amadori product or fructosamine.[30]

Following a mechanism analogous to that of monosaccharide autoxidation, fructosamine can undergo glycoxidation, a long term oxidative process triggered by transition metal ions, e.g. Fe^{3+}, Cu^{2+}, and molecular oxygen, to give glyoxal, methylglyoxal and 3-deoxyglucosone.[33]

Also in this case superoxide radical-anion accelerates the glycoxidation process, whereas peroxynitrite induces the accumulation of N^{ε}-(carboxymethyl)lysine, a major antigenic AGE structure, providing the first evidence of protein modification by $ONOO^-$-induced oxidative cleavage of the Amadori product.[19]

Glyoxal
Methylglyoxal
3-Deoxyglucosone
$\xleftarrow{M^{n+}}$ (O_2 or $O_2^{-\cdot}$)
Glycated protein
$\xrightarrow{ONOO^-}$
***N*$^{\varepsilon}$-(carboxymethyl)lysine**

2.4. *Mechanisms of toxicity of carbohydrate breakdown products*

Beside the evident structural modifications and consequential changes in functionality, the oxidative degradation processes of mono/polysaccharides and glycoconjugates cause the overproduction of reactive carbonyl species, mainly α-dicarbonyls. This condition has been referred to as **carbonyl stress** due to the analogy with oxidative and nitrosative stress. Some of the most representative α-dicarbonyl species are glyoxal, methylglyoxal and 3-deoxyglucosone.

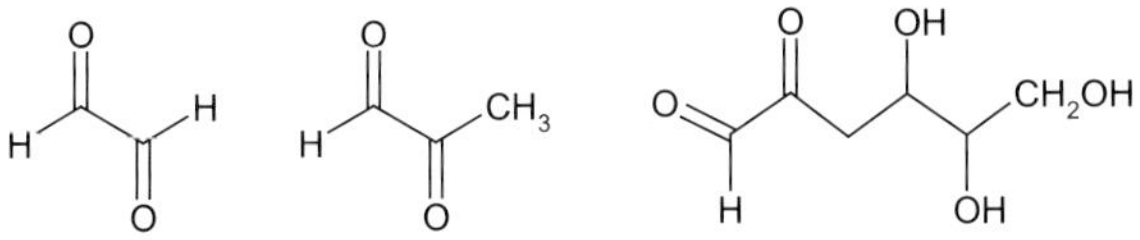

Glyoxal **Methylglyoxal** **3-Deoxyglucosone**

Under physiological conditions, the formation of α-dicarbonyls is counteracted by the action of appropriate enzymes that convert them into non-toxic metabolites. This is the case of the glyoxalase system, constituted by two enzymes, glyoxalase I and glyoxalase II, and a cofactor, reduced glutathione (GSH), that converts glyoxal into glycolate and methylglyoxal into D-lactate.[34] 3-Deoxyglucosone is converted into 3-deoxyfructose by the action of a NADPH-dependent aldehyde reductase.[35]

Under oxidative stress conditions the activity of these enzymatic systems is critically impaired due to the depletion of the cellular levels of GSH and NADPH.[36] This causes the accumulation of high levels of the three α-oxoaldehydes that, because of their electrophilic nature, can form irreversible adducts with proteins, enzymes and nucleic acids, generating the so-called AGEs.

The typical modifications of proteins and enzymes involve the nucleophilic amino groups of lysine and arginine residues. α-Oxoaldehydes can form: a) stable monoadducts with lysine residues, as in the case of carboxymethyllysine, carboxyethyllysine and pyrraline, or with arginine residues, as in the case of hydroimidazolones;[37,38] b) stable biadducts as in the case of argpyrimidine and tetrahydropyrimidine;[39] c) stable crosslinks between two lysine residues, as in the case of bis(lysyl)imidazolium crosslinks GOLD, for glyoxal, and MOLD, for methylglyoxal, and between a lysine and an arginine residue, as in the case of pentosidine crosslinks (Fig. 7).[40]

The typical modifications of nucleic acids involve the nucleophilic sites of the bases, generally guanine, adenine, and cytosine. Glyoxal and methylglyoxal, in particular, can form stable monoadducts as in the case

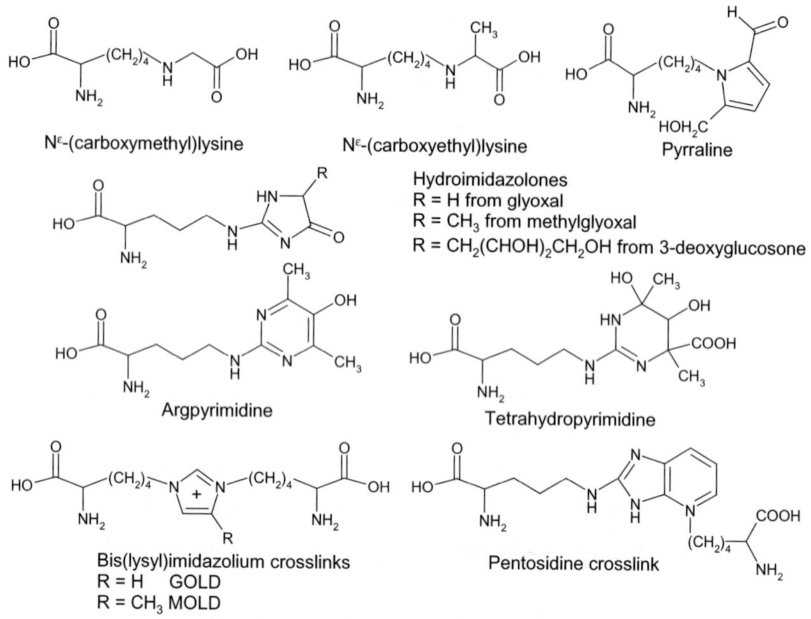

Fig. 7. Some representative examples of amino acid AGEs.

of 6,7-dihydro-6,7-dihydroxyimidazo[2,3-b]-purin-9(8)-ones, and inter- or intra-strands crosslinks mainly between a deoxyguanosine and a deoxycytosine (dG-g-dC) and between a deoxyguanosine and a deoxyadenosine (dG-g-dA).[41,42]

Besides α-oxoaldehydes, other reactive carbonyl species, particularly those generated by the oxidative degradation of the monosaccharidic portion of nucleic acids, can form stable adduct with the nucleophilic sites of bases. This is the case of phosphoglycolaldehyde, base propenal, and *cis*-2-butene-1,4-dial, obtained from the hydroxyl radical-mediated H-atom abstraction from the 3′-, 4′-, and 5′-position of deoxyribose, respectively.[25]

Phosphoglycolaldehyde reacts with 2′-deoxyguanosine to form 6,7-dihydro-6,7-dihydroxyimidazo[2,3-b]-purin-9(8)-one, the same adduct obtained by coupling with glyoxal.[43] Base propenal exhibits a reactivity similar to that of malondialdehyde, a well-recognized genotoxic product of lipid peroxidation, by forming with 2′-deoxyadenosine the pyrimidopurinone adduct,[44] whereas *cis*-2-butene-1,4-dial can form stable oxadiazabicyclooctaimine adducts by coupling with 2′-deoxycytosine residues (Fig. 8).[45]

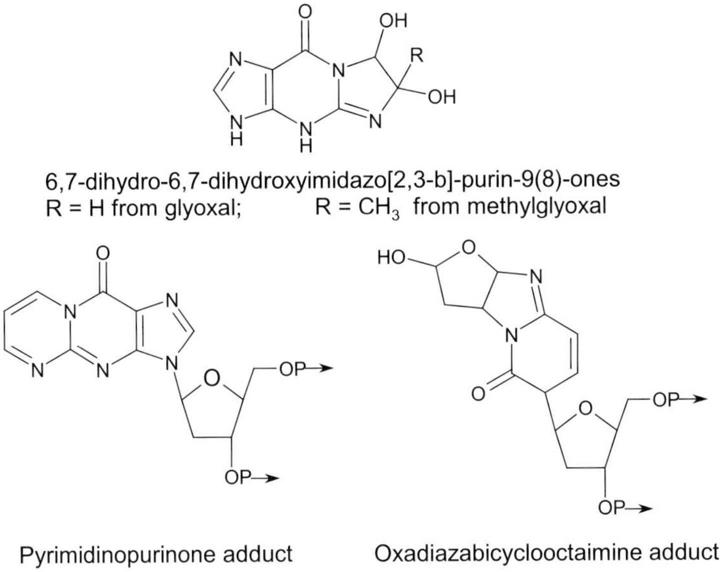

6,7-dihydro-6,7-dihydroxyimidazo[2,3-b]-purin-9(8)-ones
R = H from glyoxal; R = CH_3 from methylglyoxal

Pyrimidinopurinone adduct Oxadiazabicyclooctaimine adduct

Fig. 8. Some representative examples of nucleic acid AGEs.

The formation of AGEs both at protein/enzyme level and at nucleic acid level is the primary cause of α-oxoaldehyde-induced cytotoxicity and genotoxicity, including carcinogenicity. Numerous studies have demonstrated that glyoxal, methylglyoxal and 3-deoxyglucosone can elicit apoptosis and cell growth arrest; moreover, α-oxoaldehyde-modified proteins can undergo receptor-mediated endocytosis and lysosomal degradation in monocytes and macrophages, and can induce adhesion molecule expression, cytokine synthesis and secretion.[46–48]

Excess formation of glyoxal, methylglyoxal and 3-deoxyglucosone has been implicated in the development of diabetic complications, as well as in uremia, atherosclerosis and aging (Table 3).[49,50]

Table 3. Plasma levels of glyoxal, methylglyoxal and 3-deoxyglucosone in some pathologies associated with oxidative stress.[50]

Pathology	Glyoxal (μM)	Methylglyoxal (μM)	3-Deoxyglucosone (μM)
Diabetes	1.34 ± 0.48	2.19 ± 0.64	0.50 ± 0.12
Uremia	3.81 ± 0.48	1.53 ± 0.25	0.36 ± 0.08
Control	1.16 ± 0.35	0.65 ± 0.17	0.16 ± 0.10

3. Amino Acids

Although free amino acids would hardly compete with proteins and other more abundant biomolecules as targets of reactive oxygen species, the cascade of effects of oxidative stress-related processes at various levels makes it possible that changes occur in a myriad of biomolecules that would not normally represent the primary option in terms of accessibility and chemical reactivity. Depending on their structures, amino acids may have a range of reactive sites that can be damaged, but interest has centered mainly on deamination, decarboxylation and side chain modification/breakdown. The degree of α-amino acid oxidation versus side chain modification is determined by the reactivity of the attacking agent (and, hence, its selectivity) and the nature of the side chain. Aliphatic amino acids are more susceptible of being attacked on the amino acid moiety, whereas cysteine, tyrosine, methionine, histidine, tryptophan, lysine can undergo numerous modifications on the side chains following exposure to endogenous oxidants and radicals such as $HO^{\bullet}$, $O_2^{\bullet-}$, HOCl, and $ONOO^-$.

3.1. *The α-amino acid functionality*

One of the major consequences of oxidative free radical damage to amino acids is racemization. The α-hydrogen of an amino acid is readily abstracted by the hydroxyl radical. The free radical thus produced may be quickly repaired by nearby hydrogen donors, e.g. thiols. The repaired product would have a 50% chance of being racemized, a mechanism akin to the formation of amino acid carbanion intermediates and proton re-addition (Fig. 9).[51] D-Amino acids accordingly represent valuable markers of oxidative stress and aging.

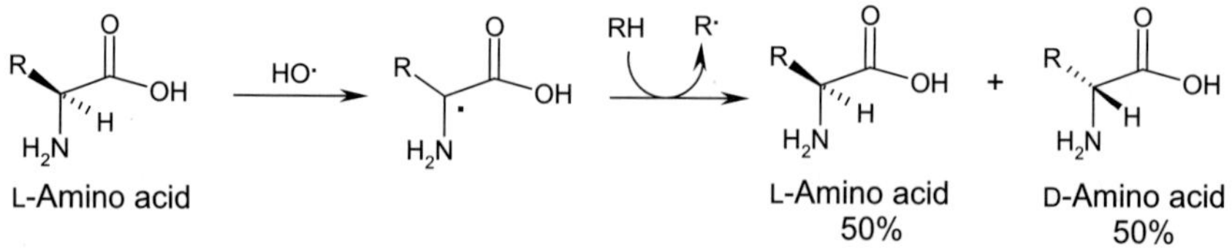

Fig. 9. Hydroxyl radical-induced racemization of L-amino acids.

In addition to racemization, hydroxyl radicals can induce decarboxylation of α-amino acids. This reaction is very effective in basic solutions, i.e. under conditions where the amino group is unprotonated and the lone electron pair at nitrogen is accessible. The decarboxylation mechanism is considered to be initiated by interaction of a hydroxyl radical with the lone electron pair at nitrogen. This hydroxyl radical adduct or a radical cation resulting there from is suggested to decarboxylate spontaneously leaving α-amino radicals.[52]

Almost all free α-amino acids react with hypochlorous acid (HOCl). The reaction proceeds as a rule with the deamination/decarboxylation of the α-amino acidic functionality and the formation of reactive aldehydes bearing the side chain residue.[53,54]

As shown in Fig. 10, the accepted mechanism involves the formation of *N*-chloramines, unstable compounds that spontaneously decompose to give NH_3, CO_2, Cl^-, and the corresponding aldehydes (route A); under forcing conditions, *N*,*N*-dichloramines may also be formed, which decompose to give nitrile species (route B).

Notably, HOCl induces apoptosis on cells in culture media following a process mediated by aminoacyl *N*-chloramines that can be mimicked by the treatment of cells with taurine *N*-chloramine or with long-lived *N*-chloramines generated from modified lysine or arginine.[55]

Moreover, both HOCl and *N*-chloramines can induce thiol oxidation, a process which may be responsible for alterations in regulatory or signaling pathways in cells exposed to neutrophil oxidants.[56]

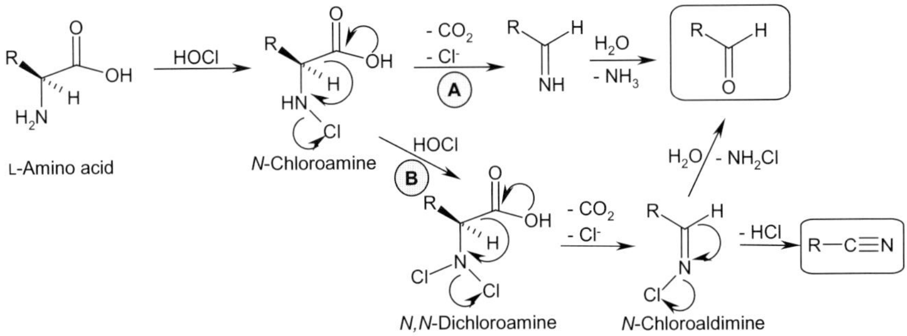

Fig. 10. Mechanisms proposed for the oxidation of L-amino acids with HOCl.

Many of the aldehydes produced by phagocyte-induced amino acid oxidation exert potent biological effects and display signaling properties. L-Alanine yields acetaldehyde, which plays a critical role in the toxic effects of ethanol, whereas glycine generates formaldehyde, a mutagenic agent causing protein crosslinks. L-Serine gives glycolaldehyde, an α-hydroxyaldehyde which mediates protein crosslinking and the formation of N^{ε}-(carboxymethyl)lysine, an advanced glycation end-product.[57] L-Threonine is similarly oxidized to 2-hydroxypropanal and its dehydration product, acrolein, an extremely reactive α,β-unsaturated aldehyde which alkylates proteins and nucleic acids.[57] L-Tyrosine oxidation by the $MPO/H_2O_2/Cl^-$ system yields 4-hydroxyphenylacetaldehyde which can covalently modify ε-amino groups of protein lysine residues in inflammatory tissues; moreover, 4-hydroxyphenylacetaldehyde was found to enhance T-cell proliferation *in vitro* and *in vivo*, suggesting a regulatory role on the immune system.[58]

3.2. *The side chain*

H-Atom abstraction from the carbon skeleton of the amino acids is a typical process brought about by the hydroxyl radical. The relative reaction rates depend on the type of the C-H bonds, on the degree of C-H bond activation by neighboring groups, and on structural effects. The chemical bases of oxidative free radical damage by the Fenton reagent ($Fe^{2+}/EDTA/H_2O_2$) to a variety of amino acids were established as early as 1960.[59] The main oxidation products of some of the most representative α-amino acids are reported in Table 4.

As shown, alanine is hydroxylated to serine which is further oxidized to glycine. Threonine is converted first to hydroxyaspartic acid (**13**), then to serine, and finally to glycine. Reversible oxidation of the sulfhydryl group on cysteine leads to cysteine sulfenic acid (**14**), which can undergo further irreversible oxidation to a sulfinic acid (**15**) and a sulfonic acid (**16**). Upon oxidation, methionine is converted to methionine sulfoxide (**17**) and can be further oxidized to methionine sulfone (**18**). Aspartic acid is decarboxylated, before or after hydroxylation to **13** with the formation of alanine, serine and glycine. Phenylalanine is hydroxylated to *o*-, *m*- and *p*-hydroxyphenylalanines (**19–21**), and tyrosine to 3,4-dihydroxyphenylalanine (**22**).

Table 4. Amino acid oxidation products generated by the Fenton reagent.

Amino acid	Oxidation products
Alanine	Serine, glycine
Serine	Glycine
Threonine	Serine, glycine, 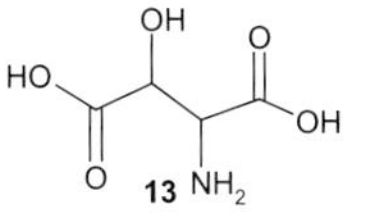 13
Cysteine	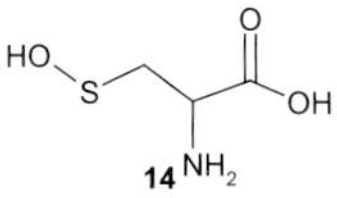 14, 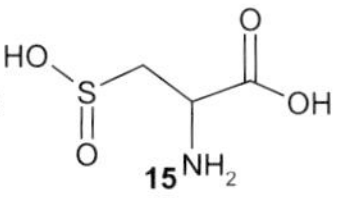 15, 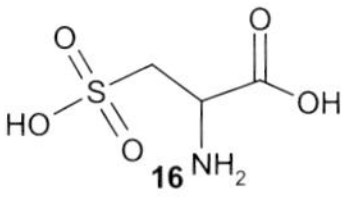 16
Methionine	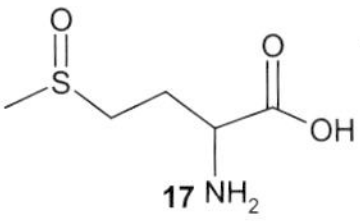 17, 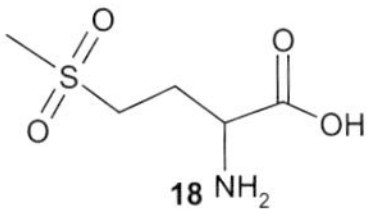 18
Aspartic acid	Alanine, serine, glycine, **13**
Phenylalanine	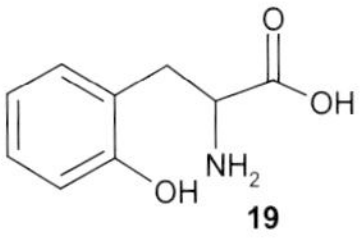 19, 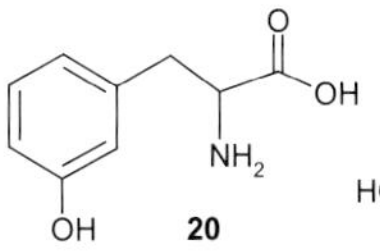 20, 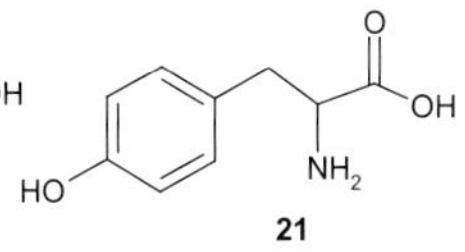 21
Tyrosine	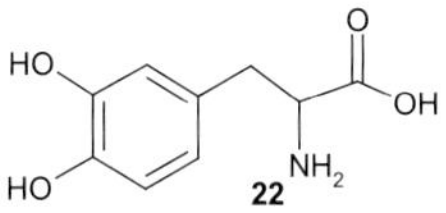 22
Histidine	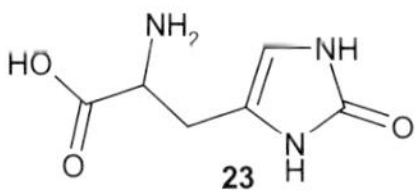 23
Tryptophan	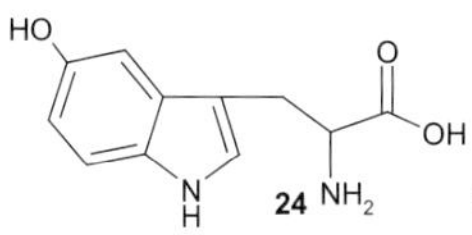 24, 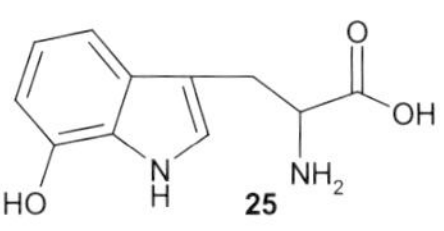 25, 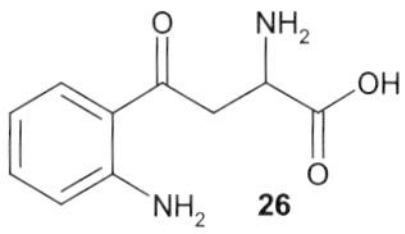 26, 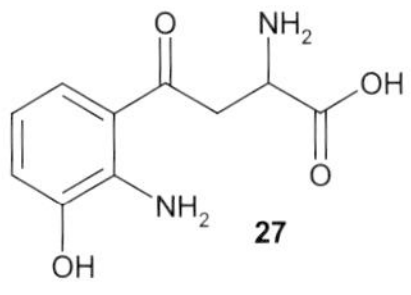 27, 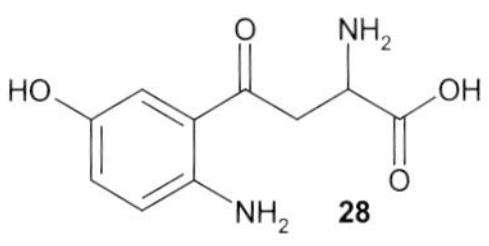 28

Worthy of note is the case of L-histidine, an effective $HO^{\bullet}$ scavenger: it reacts rapidly with hydrogen peroxide to give the 2-imidazolone derivative **23**. Hydroxyl radicals can attack tryptophan inducing the formation of 5- and 7-hydroxytryptophan (**24** and **25**), or can lead to the disruption of the indole nucleus forming kynurenine (**26**) and 3- and 5-hydroxykynurenine (**27** and **28**).

A systematic investigation of the sites of hydroxyl radical reaction with amino acids by ^{2}H NMR detection of induced $^{1}H/^{2}H$ exchange showed that for aliphatic amino acids H-atom abstraction occurs preferentially at the methine and methylene sites, rather than at the methyl ones; moreover, in the case of isoleucine and leucine H-atom abstraction occurs preferentially distal to the α-carbon. Significant $^{1}H/^{2}H$ exchange was observed for the δ positions of proline and arginine and for the ε-methylene of lysine, indicating that a positive charge on a carbon bearing an amino group does not inhibit the $^{1}H/^{2}H$ exchange.

By comparing the ^{2}H NMR integration areas in the amino acid spectra it was possible to establish the relative susceptibility to $HO^{\bullet}$ attack as a measure of $^{1}H/^{2}H$ exchange; this latter, in particular, proceeded according to the following descending order: leucine > isoleucine > valine > arginine > lysine > tyrosine > proline > histidine > phenylalanine > methionine > threonine > alanine > [cysteine, serine, aspartic acid, asparagine, glutamic acid, glutamine, glycine, tryptophan].[60]

Volatile hydrocarbons have been shown to be generated by oxidation of amino acids by a Fe^{2+}/ascorbate/GSH system.[61] Free, but not peptide-bound methionine leads to the generation of ethylene, whereas leucine and isoleucine release small amounts of propane and ethane, respectively. Hydrocarbon generation is inhibited by OH radical scavengers, but catalase and superoxide dismutase are more efficient. Ethane and propane generation is optimal at pH 6.2, suggesting the involvement of protonated superoxide besides OH radicals. These latter would attack the side chains of leucine and isoleucine to produce most likely carbon-centered radicals. H-atom abstraction from the SH group of GSH would account for the formation of saturated hydrocarbons.

The reactions of amino acid side chains with hypochlorous acid have been the subject of considerable interest.[62]

The reaction of HOCl with cysteine and methionine gives oxyacids and cystine, and sulfoxides, respectively, but the same products can be obtained by oxidation with other systems, including hydroxyl and peroxyl radicals.

A more complex situation is observed in the case of tyrosine. Whereas 3-chlorotyrosine formation is an established event in the reaction of HOCl with peptide- or protein-bound tyrosine, the occurrence of similar phenolic ring chlorination on the free amino acid has been a matter of debate. In a systematic assessment of this issue it has been shown that upon exposure to HOCl under physiologic conditions tyrosine is converted to a complex mixture of products including, besides 4-hydroxyphenylacetaldehyde, 3-chlorotyrosine, 3,5-dichlorotyrosine, 3-chloro-4-hydroxyphenylacetaldehyde and 3,5-dichloro-4-hydroxyphenylacetaldehyde.[63] These products are proposed to arise from parallel pathways reflecting sequential competitive attacks of the chlorinating agent(s) on the amino acid and phenol ring moieties. The exact mechanism of phenolic ring chlorination has yet to be defined. It should be noted that HOCl has a pKa of 7.59, therefore at physiologic pH it exists as a mixture of the protonated and unprotonated forms and it has been suggested that several chlorinating agents can concur to product formation, including Cl_2, ClO^- and Cl^+.[64]

The formation of 3-bromotyrosine and 3,5-dibromotyrosine by reaction of tyrosine with brominating agents such as eosinophil peroxidase is also of relevance.[65]

The reaction of L-arginine with HOCl proceeds likewise to give chlorinated products in which the guanidine group is modified.[66]

NO-derived reactive nitrogen species, including nitrogen dioxide (NO_2) and peroxynitrite, the coupling product of NO with superoxide, can target a variety of amino acids, including chiefly tyrosine, cysteine, methionine, tryptophan, phenylalanine and histidine.

Nitration of tyrosine residues is a most typical marker of the contribution of nitric oxide to oxidative damage, and several excellent reviews on protein tyrosine nitration are available.[67–73] The first evidence of tyrosine nitration *in vivo* was obtained by Ohshima *et al.*[74] who reported the occurrence of 3-nitrotyrosine (**29**) and its metabolite 3-nitro-4-hydroxyphenylacetic acid in human urine. Free 3-nitrotyrosine is formed in relatively high levels (1–120 μM) under pathological conditions, e.g. rheumatoid arthritis, liver

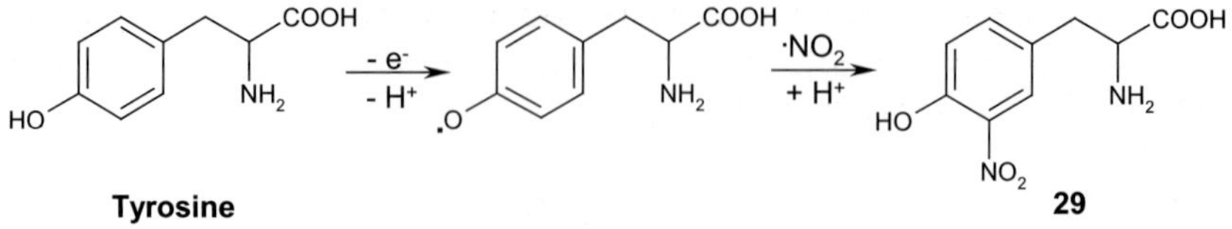

Fig. 11. Mechanism proposed for tyrosine nitration.

transplantation, renal failure, sepsis, atherosclerosis, amyotrophic lateral sclerosis. It may arise either by direct nitration of free tyrosine and/or proteolytic degradation of nitrated proteins. The actual mechanisms of tyrosine nitration have been a controversial issue. Reported systems include nitrite ions at acidic pH,[75] peroxynitrite, peroxidase/H_2O_2, heme/H_2O_2 or the Fenton reagent (chelated Fe^{2+}/H_2O_2) in the presence of nitrite ions,[76,77] and their relative importance *in vivo* is currently under assessment.

Whatever the mechanism, the reaction involves one-electron oxidation of the tyrosine phenol ring to give the phenoxyl radical which couples with NO_2 at the *ortho* position to give **29** (Fig. 11). The tyrosyl radical can also couple with NO to form an unstable nitroso derivative ($k = 2 \times 10^9\,M^{-1}\,s^{-1}$) that can be further oxidized to **29**.

Free 3-nitrotyrosine appears to stimulate superoxide production in the presence of NADH-cytochrome c reductase, and is incorporated into the C-terminus of α-tubulin in mammalian cells[78] and invertebrate nervous tissue.[79] These and other observations suggest that **29** may not be a simple end-product of nitration reactions but rather a species capable of exacerbating the cell's response to injury.

Besides **29**, the peroxynitrite-induced modification of free tyrosine leads to the formation of 3,5-dinitrotyrosine (**30**), 3,3′-dityrosine (**31**) and **22** (Table 5).

Phenylalanine has shown a behavior quite similar to that of tyrosine, leading to the formation, after treatment with peroxynitrite, of **19**, **20**, **21**, nitrophenylalanines (**32–34**), **29** and **31**.

Another target of peroxynitrite is tryptophan, which reacts with a second-order rate constant of 37 $M^{-1}s^{-1}$ at pH 7.4 and 37°C, leading to the formation of 5- and 6-nitrotryptophan (**35** and **36**), *N*-formylkynurenine (**37**), oxindole (**38**), hydropyrroloindole (**39**), **24** and **25**; these latter have been detected *in vitro* in the human Cu,Zn superoxide dismutase after exposure

Table 5. Degradation products obtained by the reaction of amino acids with peroxynitrite.[80]

Amino acid	Oxidation product
Tyrosine	**22, 29**; 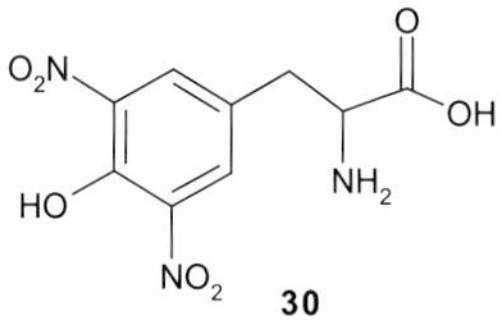 30, 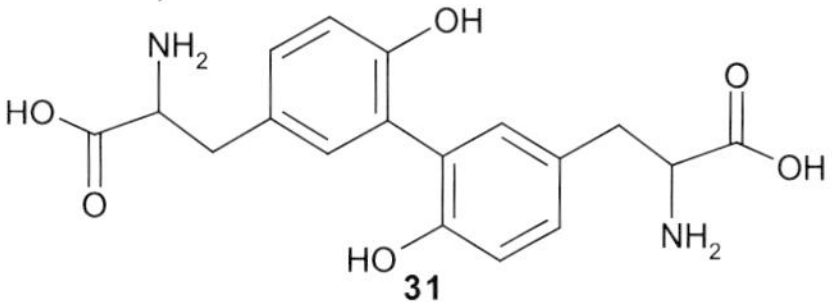 31
Phenylalanine	**19, 20, 21, 29, 31**; 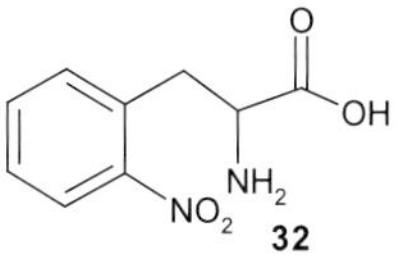 32, 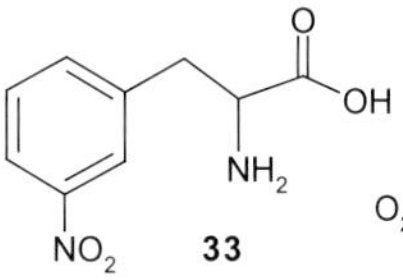 33, 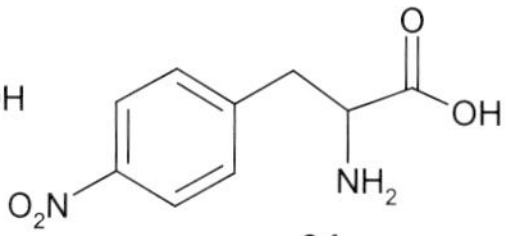 34
Tryptophan	**24, 25**; 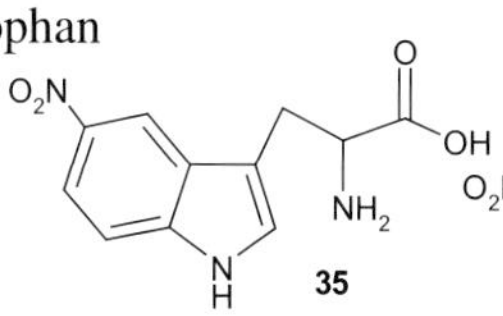 35, 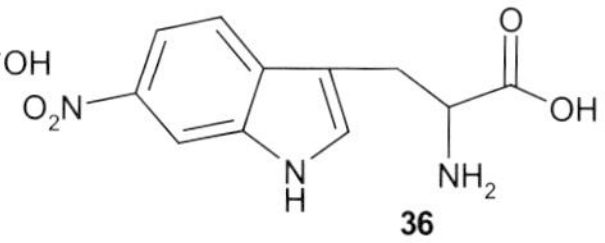 36, 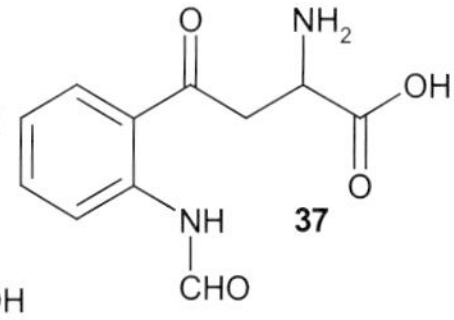 37, 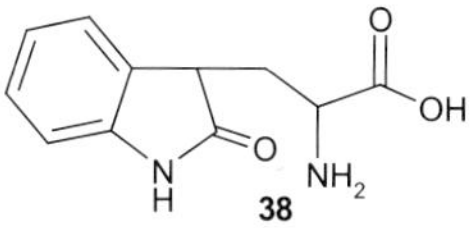 38, 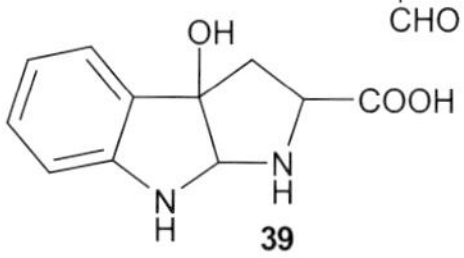 39
Methionine	**17**
Cysteine	**14, 15, 16**; 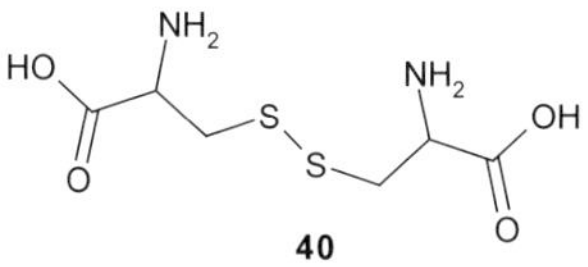 40, 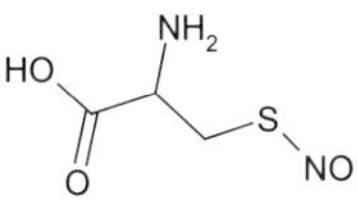 41, 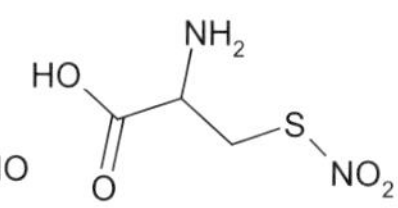 42
Histidine	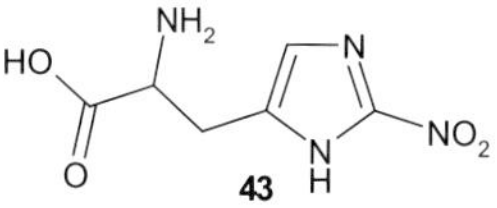 **23**; 43

to peroxynitrite, and are currently recognized as markers of the contribution of nitric oxide pathways to tryptophan damage.

Peroxynitrite can oxidize the sulfur-containing amino acids methionine and cysteine; the first leads to the formation of **17**, whereas the second leads to the formation of **14–16**, of cystine (**40**) and of nitroso- and nitrocysteine (**41** and **42**).

Finally, the exposure of free histidine to peroxynitrite leads to the formation of **23** and nitrohistidine (**43**) via a mechanism that involves the formation of a histidinyl radical which couples with nitrogen dioxide or hydroxyl radical.

References

1. Gilbert BC, King DM, Thomas CB. *J. Chem. Soc. Perkin II* 1186–1199 (1981).
2. Schuchmann MN, von Sonntag C. *J. Chem. Soc. Perkin II* 1958–1963 (1960).
3. Gilbert BC, King DM, Thomas CB. *J. Chem. Soc. Perkin II* 675–683 (1983).
4. Miaskiewicz K, Osman R. *J. Am. Chem. Soc.* 116: 232–238 (1994).
5. Willson RL. *Int. J. Radiat. Biol.* 17: 349–358 (1970).
6. Schreiber SL, Liew W. *Tetrahedron Lett.* 24: 2363–2366 (1983).
7. von Sonntag C *et al. J. Chem. Soc. Perkin II* 171 (1975).
8. Halliwell B, Gutteridge JMC. *FEBS Lett.* 128: 347–352 (1981).
9. von Sonntag C. *The Chemical Basis of Radiation Biology*. Taylor & Francis, London, 1987, pp. 57–93.
10. Russell GA. *J. Am. Chem. Soc.* 79: 3871–3877 (1957).
11. Fitchett M, Gilbert BC, Willson R. *J. Chem. Soc. Perkin II* 673–689 (1988).
12. Koch A *et al. J. Org. Chem.* 58: 1083–1089 (1993).
13. Mlakar A *et al. Free Radic. Res.* 25: 525–539 (1996).
14. Wolff P, Dean T. *Biochem. J.* 245: 243–250 (1987).
15. Hunt JV, Bottoms MA, Mitchinson MJ. *Biochem. J.* 291: 529–535 (1993).
16. Okado-Matsumoto A, Fridovich I. *J. Biol. Chem.* 275: 34853–34857 (2000).
17. Jiang ZY, Woolard ACS, Wolff SP. *FEBS Lett.* 268: 69–71 (1990).
18. Thornalley PJ. *Biochem. J.* 269: 1–11 (1990).
19. Nagai R *et al. Diabetes* 51: 2833–2839 (2002).
20. McCord JM. *Science* 185: 529–531 (1974).
21. Brown KA. *Br. J. Rheumatol.* 27: 150–155 (1988).
22. Albrich JM, McCarthy MC, Hurst JK. *Proc. Natl. Acad. Sci. USA* 78: 210–214 (1981).

23. Schalkwijk J *et al. Arthritis Rheum.* 29: 532–538 (1986).
24. Jahn M, Baynes JW, Spiteller G. *Carbohydr. Res.* 321: 228–234 (1999).
25. Breen AP, Murphy JA. *Free Radic. Biol. Med.* 18: 1033–1077 (1995).
26. Pogozelski WK, Tullius TD. *Chem. Rev.* 98: 1089–1107 (1998).
27. Behrens G *et al. Int. J. Radiat. Biol.* 33: 163–171 (1978).
28. von Sonntag C *et al. Adv. Rad. Biol.* 9: 109–142 (1981).
29. Brownlee M, Vlassara H, Cerami A. *Ann. Intern. Med.* 101: 527–537 (1984).
30. Baynes JW. In: Ikan R (ed.) *The Maillard Reaction: Consequences for the Chemical and Life Sciences*. Wiley, New York, 1996, pp. 55–72.
31. Wolff SP, Jiang ZY, Hunt JV. *Free Radic. Biol. Med.* 10: 339–352 (1991).
32. Thorpe S, Baynes JW. *Drugs Aging* 9: 69–77 (1996).
33. Thornalley PJ, Langborg A, Minhas HS. *Biochem. J.* 344: 109–116 (1999).
34. Thornalley PJ. *Chem. Biol. Interact.* 111–112: 137–151 (1998).
35. Feather MS *et al. Biochim. Biophys. Acta* 1244: 10–16 (1995).
36. Abordo EA, Monhas HS, Thornalley PJ. *Biochem. Pharmacol.* 58: 641–648 (1999).
37. Sady C *et al. Biochim. Biophys. Acta* 1481: 255–264 (2000).
38. Thornalley PJ. *Gen. Pharmacol.* 27: 565–573 (1996).
39. Oya T *et al. J. Biol. Chem.* 274: 18492–18502 (1999).
40. Chellan P, Nagaraj RH. *Arch. Biochem. Biophys.* 368: 98–104 (1999).
41. Shapiro R *et al. Biochemistry* 8: 238–245 (1969).
42. Murata-Kamiya N, Kamiya H, Kaji H, Kasai H. *Nucleic Acids Res.* 25: 1897–1902 (1997).
43. Awada M, Dedon PC. *Chem. Res. Toxicol.* 14: 1247–1253 (2001).
44. Dedon PC, Plastaras JP, Rouzer CA, Marnett LJ. *Proc. Natl. Acad. Sci. USA* 95: 11113–11116 (1998).
45. Gingipalli L, Dedon PC. *J. Am. Chem. Soc.* 123: 2664–2665 (2001).
46. Kalapos MP. *Toxicol. Lett.* 110: 145–175 (1999).
47. Kasper, M *et al. Am. J. Respir. Cell Mol. Biol.* 23: 485–491 (2000).
48. Kikuchi S *et al. J. Neurosci. Res.* 57: 280–289 (1999).
49. Lal S *et al. Arch. Biochem. Biophys.* 342: 254–260 (1997).
50. Odani H *et al. Biochem. Biophys. Res. Commun.* 256: 89–93 (1999).
51. Helfman PM, Bada JL. *Proc. Natl. Acad. Sci. USA* 72: 2891–2894 (1975).
52. Moenig J *et al. J. Phys. Chem.* 89: 3139–3144 (1985).
53. Zgliczynski JM *et al. Biochim. Biophys. Acta* 235: 419–424 (1971).
54. Hazen SL *et al. Biochemistry* 37: 6864–6873 (1998).
55. Englert RP *et al. J. Biol. Chem.* 277: 20518–20526 (2002).
56. Peskin AV, Winterbourn CC. *Free Radic. Biol. Med.* 30: 572–579 (2001).
57. Anderson M *et al. J. Clin. Invest.* 99: 424–432 (1997).

58. Hazen SL *et al. J. Biol. Chem.* 272: 16990–16998 (1997).
59. Nofre C *et al. Compt. Rend.* 251: 811–813 (1960).
60. Nukuna BN *et al. J. Am. Chem. Soc.* 123: 1208–1214 (2001).
61. Kessler W, Remmer H. *Biochem. Pharmacol.* 39: 1347–1351 (1990).
62. Pattison DI, Davies MJ. *Chem. Res. Toxicol.* 14: 1453–1464 (2001).
63. Fu S *et al. J. Biol. Chem.* 275: 10851–10858 (2000).
64. Swain CG, Crist DR. *J. Am. Chem. Soc.* 94: 3195–3200 (1972).
65. Wu W *et al. Biochemistry* 38: 3538–3548 (1999).
66. Zhang C *et al. J. Biol. Chem.* 276: 27159–27165 (2001).
67. Eiserich JP, Patel RP, O'Donnell VB. *Molec. Aspects Med.* 19: 221–357 (1998).
68. Beckman JS. *Chem. Res. Toxicol.* 9: 836–844 (1996).
69. Ischiropulos H. *Arch. Biochem. Biophys.* 356: 1–11 (1998).
70. van der Vliet A *et al. Methods Enzymol.* 269: 175–184 (1996).
71. Alvarez B *et al. J. Biol. Chem.* 274: 842–848 (1999).
72. Ramezanian MS, Padmaja S, Koppenol WH. *Chem. Res. Toxicol.* 9: 232–240 (1996).
73. Zhang H *et al. Nitric Oxide* 1: 301–307 (1997).
74. Ohshima H *et al. Food Chem. Toxicol.* 28: 647–652 (1990).
75. Knowles ME *et al. Nature* 247: 288–289 (1973).
76. Thomas DD *et al. Proc. Natl. Acad. Sci. USA* 99: 12691–12696 (2002).
77. Bian K *et al. Proc. Natl. Acad. Sci. USA* 100: 5712–5717 (2003).
78. Eiserich JP *et al. Proc. Natl. Acad. Sci. USA* 96: 6365–6370 (1999).
79. Palumbo A *et al. Biochem. Biophys. Res. Commun.* 293: 1536–1543 (2002).
80. Alvarez B, Radi R. *Amino Acids* 25: 295–311 (2003).

11 Superoxide Dismutase 2 Deficient Mice: The Role of Increased Reactive Oxygen Species in Genomic Instability

Enrique Samper, Chris Benz, and Simon Melov

1. Sod2, Oxidative Stress, and Genetic Instability

Reactive oxygen species (ROS) are an inevitable by-product of mitochondrial respiration. It has been estimated that between 0.4% to 4% of oxygen used during respiration is converted to superoxide ($O_2^{\bullet -}$).[1,2] The principal defense against superoxide in the mitochondria is the manganese superoxide dismutase (*sod2*) enzyme that catalyzes the conversion of superoxide to hydrogen peroxide (H_2O_2), which may be further metabolized to water by glutathione peroxidase 1, which is a bi-compartmental enzyme located within the mitochondria, as well as the cytosol.

Inactivation of *sod2* by homologous recombination in a CD1 genetic background typically results in neonatal lethality within the first week of life, and the phenotype is characterized by dilated cardiomyopathy and fibrosis, anemia, metabolic acidosis, hepatic lipid accumulation, mitochondrial biochemical abnormalities, and in animals which live longer than two weeks, a spongiform encephalopathy accompanied by profound motor disturbances, and neurodegeneration.[3–6]

Many of these phenotypes can be rescued or modulated via treatment with synthetic catalytic antioxidants that have also been shown to be effective in extending the lifespan of the nematode *Caenorhabditis elegans*.[4,6,7] It is likely that these phenotypes are due to ROS mediated damage, as treatment of these mice with a variety of antioxidants prevents or attenuates many of the disorders, which present during the initial weeks of life. *Sod2* null mice display a marked reduction in the activities of the tricarboxylic acid cycle enzyme aconitase, respiratory chain complexes I and II (NADH dehydrogenase and succinate dehydrogenase respectively),[3,8] although there is tissue-specific variation in the levels of inactivation of mitochondrial enzymes in general.[5,6,8] Like many genetic models, crossing the knockout allele into different genetic backgrounds modulates the severity of the phenotype. In contrast to the *sod2* null phenotype on a CD1 background, inactivation of *sod2* in the C57BL/6 genetic background has been reported to result in a more severe phenotype, with embryonic lethality at around day E15.[9]

Sod2 heterozygous mice on a C57BL/6 background exhibit increased mitochondrial and nuclear DNA oxidation (8-OH-Guanine).[10,11] Indications that the hemizygous loss of *sod2* results in oxidative stress, is shown by a 30–50% reduction of reduced glutathione levels in the lung, brain and muscle.[12] *Sod2* heterozygous animals and cells are hypersensitive to exogenous oxidative stressors such as paraquat, a superoxide generator.[10,13] The consequences of lack of *sod2 in vitro* have been partially analyzed, and it has been reported that primary mouse embryonic fibroblasts (MEFs) from *sod2* null animals show poor cell growth, hypersensitivity to paraquat, increased cell death and chromosomal abnormalities.[14,15] Further, cortical neurons from the *sod2* heterozygous animals are sensitized to glutamate toxicity.[16] *Sod2* heterozygous mice have also been shown to have increased cell turnover and apoptosis through AP-1 and p53 up-regulation, as well as p53 increased mitochondrial localization in the skin after 7,12-dimethylbenz(a)-anthracene (DMBA)/12-O-tetradecanoylphorbol-13-acetate (TPA) treatment.[17] The consequences of the *sod2* deficiency are partially consistent with increased DNA damage as strains of mice deficient for DNA repair show similar phenotypes, particularly embryonic lethality, neuronal apoptosis, neurodegeneration, and cardiomyopathy.[18–24]

2. Antioxidant Interventions and Chronic Mitochondrial Oxidative Stress

Severe phenotypes in the *sod2* null mouse including neuronal cell death, and neonatal lethality can be rescued or attenuated by pharmacological intervention with superoxide dismutase and catalase mimetics such as the synthetic compounds EUK-8, 134 or 189.[5,6] These compounds have been shown to be cyto-protective in this paradigm of oxidative stress, as well as others, both *in vivo* at 1–30 mg/kg and *in vitro* at 100-400 μM concentrations.[5,6,25–27] Long-term consequences of lack of *sod2* are difficult to study due to the severe nature of the insult. However, Friedman and colleagues developed a novel strategy to further understand the consequences of mitochondrial oxidative stress *in vivo* in the hematopoietic system, by using a stem cell transplantation model in myeloablated recipient mice.[26,27]

Sod2 null fetal liver was transplanted into lethally irradiated hosts and the resultant chimeric mice were then able to experience the consequences of long-term lack of *sod2* in the hematopoietic system. These studies showed that deficiency of *sod2* leads to a persistent anemia, with decreased erythrocyte counts and reduced lifespan. In particular the bone marrow reconstituted with the *sod2* null hematopoietic stem cells was reported to contain a marked erythroid hyperplasia with morphological abnormalities in the red cell precursor subpopulation reminiscent of sideroblastic anemia (SA) and a significant reduction in the red cell repopulation ability. This anemia was suggested to be due to increased protein oxidation, altered membrane properties and decreased lifespan of the red cell compartment.[26] Further characterization of the anemia caused in the *sod2* null transplanted animals show that the reticulocytes display an elevated mitochondrial number and membrane thickening.[27] Moreover, peripheral blood smears show a marked increase in iron deposition granules located in the mitochondria of the *sod2* null erythrocytes. Interestingly, a fraction of the *sod2* null splenocytes in the reconstituted animals show nuclear abnormalities, possibly associated with genomic instability *in vivo* due to the lack of *sod2*.[27] Proteomic characterization via 2-D approaches of the *sod2* null cells showed there was a significant reduction in peroxiredoxin 2, a 50-fold increase in the melanotransferin tumor antigen, and an increase in the levels of several subunits of the ATP synthase, and HSP60. The latter suggests a compensatory response to mitochondrial dysfunction and stress.[27]

Recently it was reported that *sod2* null mice have a decreased level of peroxiredoxin 5 (PRDX5) by proteomic analysis.[5] This protein has important functions in oxidative stress and DNA repair[28] implying that a deficiency in *sod2* can lead to decreased levels of other antioxidant enzymes. Peroxiredoxins play a role in DNA damage prevention as overexpression of PRDX 5 in cells results in attenuation of damage to DNA, against the genotoxic insults of H_2O_2 and tert-butylhydroperoxide (tBHP).[28] Further, lack of PRDX-1 (via homologous recombination) in mice leads to increased oxidative stress and a marked propensity to lymphomas, sarcomas and carcinomas, highlighting the role of reactive oxygen species in tumorigenesis.[29]

3. ROS, Genetic Instability, and Cell Fates

Oxidative stress can result in the induction of premature senescence (defined as irreversible growth arrest associated with characteristic morphological cellular changes[30]) apoptosis or transformation (collectively referred to as altered cell fate decisions) in mammalian cells. In fact, oxidative stress from a variety of sources such as oncogene activation (for example, activated *ras*[31] or *c-myc*[32]), culture shock,[33] or exogenous sources such as ionizing radiation[34] can lead to altered cell fates. It appears that oxidative stress is a common denominator in the induction of altered cell fates from a variety of sources as these phenotypes are prevented by treatment with the antioxidant N-acetylcysteine (NAC) or culture under "physiological" (3%) oxygen tension.[31–33,35] Conditions that induce altered cell fate decisions have been associated with genetic instability. For example, cell culture in high serum conditions or oncogene activation promote cellular senescence and are associated with gross chromosomal aneuploidy.[35] Furthermore, the genetic instability caused by oncogene activation is prevented by NAC.[35] Therefore, it is conceivable that many cell fate decisions (e.g. senescence, apoptosis) are determined by the cells' inability to maintain genomic integrity. Further evidence of the relationship between genetic instability and cellular fate comes from studies with Ku86 null mice.[20,23] These mice are severely impaired in their ability to repair double strand breaks[20,36] by non-homologous end joining, and in their telomeric function,[23,37,38] and also show premature senescence *in vivo* and *in vitro*.[20,39]

4. ROS and Cellular Transformation

Evidence for ROS induced transformation comes from studies in which overexpression of a homologous NADPH oxidase to the phagocytic gp91phox, *nox1*, causes increased levels of superoxide and mitogenic signaling as well as cellular transformation of 3T3 mouse cell lines.[40] More recently, it has been shown that the mitogenic signaling and the transformation characteristics of the *nox1* overexpressing cells can be prevented by treatment with catalase, implicating the role of peroxides in the induction of cellular transformation.[41] Interestingly, these studies indicate that the expression of *ras* induces the expression of *nox1* via the MAPK kinase pathway, thus suggesting a mechanism for *ras* induced transformation via the generation of ROS.[42] Further, the downregulation of *nox1* by RNA interference suppresses the transforming ability of oncogenic *ras*, thus directly implicating the generation of ROS in the *ras* induced transformation,[42] confirming and extending previous studies.[31] The exact mechanism by which endogenous ROS mediated stress affects cellular fate is unknown but it may involve the generation of single strand DNA breaks, replication fork stalling, double strand breaks, or the mutation of genes critical for cell cycle checkpoints or DNA repair (reviewed in Lieber and Karanjawala, 2004[43]).

ROS could also induce other types of nuclear defects and affect cell fate decisions in specific genetic backgrounds by mechanisms such as transcriptional interference by inducing DNA lesions which block RNA polymerases,[44] or oxidation of redox sensitive transcription factors such as Sp1 and p53.[45,46] Epigenetic regulation has been shown to impact cell fate and is increasingly recognized as a fundamental mechanism underlying tumor suppression.[47–50]

Further support for the impact of *sod2* deficiency on genetic stability and cell fate comes from previous studies with the *sod2* null MEFs.[15] It was previously shown that *sod2* deficient MEFs display an increased level of chromosomal breaks and fragments, translocations (Fig. 1) as well as poor growth and increased cell death when grown under 20% O_2 tension.

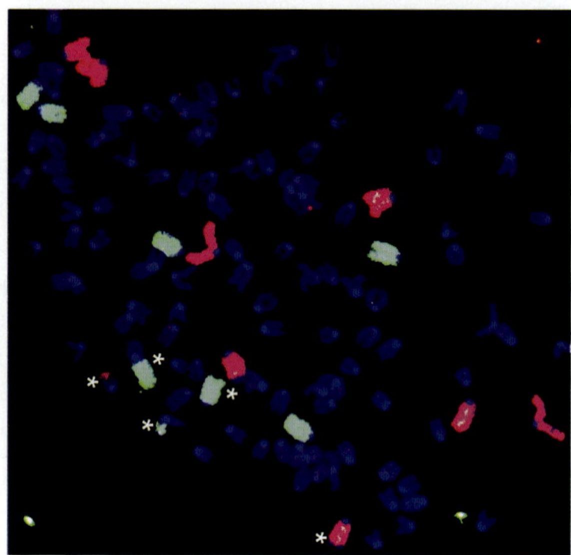

Fig. 1. Genetic instability in *sod2* null MEFs. Cytogenetic analysis of metaphases with chromosome painting probes for chromosome 1 (green) and 2 (red) in an *sod2* null early passage mouse embryonic fibroblast. Chromosomes are counterstained with DAPI. Aneuploidy as well as a dramatic increase in the number of chromosomal translocations (indicated by asterisks) and other structural abnormalities is clearly seen.

5. *Sod2* and DNA Repair

Despite the indications that endogenous oxidative stress may lead to genetic instability *in vitro* we do not yet have a clear mechanistic model of how this occurs. Recently, oxidative stress has been implicated in the activity of the DNA repair enzyme, Endonuclease III (EndoIII). EndoIII is a 4Fe-4S cluster-containing DNA glycosylase with essential repair activity for oxidized pyrimidines in DNA.[51] This enzyme contains an iron-sulfur cluster that appears to play a role in stabilizing the protein folding of the Endo III enzyme.[51] Therefore, it is conceivable that oxidation of this iron-sulfur moiety in the EndoIII protein by ROS can impact the stability of this important DNA repair enzyme and hence promote genetic misrepair. Oxidation of iron-sulfur clusters is a well-known phenomenon[52,53] and is typical of conditions where ROS inactivate Fe-S containing proteins such as aconitase in the *sod2* null mice.[8] Further support for the role of deficiency in DNA repair in mitochondrial dysfunction comes from recent results suggesting that *sod2*$^{+/-}$ and *sod2*$^{-/-}$ cells are increasingly more susceptible to gamma irradiation induced cell death.[13]

6. *Sod2* as a Putative Tumor Suppressor

Increasingly, SOD2 is being recognized as a tumor suppressor protein.[54] Certain polymorphisms in the *sod2* gene have been found to correlate with higher incidence of breast cancer.[55] Importantly, the *sod2* locus at 6q25 in human cells is frequently deleted in a number of lymphomas and other tumors. However, the exact role of *sod2* as a tumor suppressor is still under investigation. Several mechanistic possibilities include the fact that increased steady state level of superoxide may lead to increased mutagenesis and the activation of oncogenes and/or inactivation of other tumor suppressor genes, loss of DNA repair functions, and that ROS is a known second messenger for many types of cell proliferation signals.[56–58] Alternatively, *sod2* mutations may induce tumorigenesis by inactivating mitochondrial complex II (SDH)[59] as mutations in the nuclear encoded genes *sdhb*, *sdhc*, and *sdhc* are known to predispose patients to benign paragangliomas (head and neck tumors of the parasympathetic ganglia), and pheochromocytomas (cathecholamine-producing tumors of the adrenal ganglia).[60–64]

While increased levels of *sod2* have been associated with more aggressive forms of some human cancers, this likely reflects their co-association with pleotropic resistance to chemotherapy,[65,66] as well as the fact that *sod2* is normally upregulated in response to an oxidative environment.[67] *Sod2* gene expression is transcriptionally sensitive to increased ROS since its promoter is regulated by the redox-responsive factors NF-κB, AP-1 and Sp1;[67] and the DNA-binding and transactivating potential of these transcription factors is reported to be dependent on both host age and accumulative oxidative stress in normal and malignant tissues.[68] Additional studies indicate that *sod2* may be justifiably considered a tumor suppressor gene.[67,69,70] Enforced intracellular expression of *sod2* has been shown to inhibit the growth of human cancer cells, prevent malignant transformation by ErbB- and *Ras*-induced mechanisms, and to retard nonmalignant cell senescence.[69,70] Like other tumor suppressor genes, *sod2* can be epigenetically silenced by DNA methylation of a 5′ CpG island within its second intron, potentially accounting for its reduced expression in some malignancies.

Finally, direct support for the role of *sod2* as a novel tumor suppressor comes in recent studies published from the laboratory of Dr. Arlan Richardson indicating that *sod2* hemizygous mice have a 61% incidence of lymphoma at 24–28 months of age (versus an incidence of 22% in controls).[10] It is noteworthy that this increase in lymphomas has been attributed to enhanced initiation or promotion of a malignant cell population as opposed to an increase in the biological aggressiveness (e.g. invasiveness, metastatases) of established malignant cell population.

In summary, there is a large and increasing body of evidence indicating that the *sod2* gene product plays a critical enzymatic role in mitochondrial function and also a protective role in maintaining genomic integrity within mammalian cell nuclei. Future studies are needed to elucidate the pathways and mechanisms by which chronic endogenous mitochondrial oxidative stress results in genetic damage and epigenetic changes promoting the development of such life-threatening diseases as cancer.

References

1. Boveris A. Determination of the production of superoxide radicals and hydrogen peroxide in mitochondria. *Methods Enzymol.* 105: 429–435 (1984).
2. Hansford RG, Hogue BA, Mildaziene V. Dependence of H_2O_2 formation by rat heart mitochondria on substrate availability and donor age. *J. Bioenerg. Biomembr.* 29: 89–95 (1997).
3. Li Y *et al.* Dilated cardiomyopathy and neonatal lethality in mutant mice lacking manganese superoxide dismutase. *Nat. Genet.* 11: 376–381 (1995).
4. Melov S *et al.* A novel neurological phenotype in mice lacking mitochondrial manganese superoxide dismutase. *Nat. Genet.* 18: 159–163 (1998).
5. Hinerfeld D *et al.* Endogenous mitochondrial oxidative stress: neurodegeneration, proteomic analysis, specific respiratory chain defects, and efficacious antioxidant therapy in superoxide dismutase 2 null mice. *J. Neurochem.* 88: 657–667 (2004).
6. Melov S *et al.* Lifespan extension and rescue of spongiform encephalopathy in superoxide dismutase 2 nullizygous mice treated with superoxide dismutase-catalase mimetics. *J. Neurosci.* 21: 8348–8353 (2001).

7. Melov S *et al.* Extension of life-span with superoxide dismutase/catalase mimetics. *Science* 289: 1567–1569 (2000).
8. Melov S *et al.* Mitochondrial disease in superoxide dismutase 2 mutant mice. *Proc. Natl. Acad. Sci. USA* 96: 846–851 (1999).
9. Huang TT *et al.* Genetic modification of prenatal lethality and dilated cardiomyopathy in Mn superoxide dismutase mutant mice. *Free Radic. Biol. Med.* 31: 1101–1110 (2001).
10. Van Remmen H *et al.* Life-long reduction in MnSOD activity results in increased DNA damage and higher incidence of cancer but does not accelerate aging. *Physiol. Genomics* 16: 29–37 (2003).
11. Williams MD *et al.* Increased oxidative damage is correlated to altered mitochondrial function in heterozygous manganese superoxide dismutase knockout mice. *J. Biol. Chem.* 273: 28510–28515 (1998).
12. Van Remmen H *et al.* Characterization of the antioxidant status of the heterozygous manganese superoxide dismutase knockout mouse. *Arch. Biochem. Biophys.* 363: 91–97 (1999).
13. Van Remmen H *et al.* Multiple deficiencies in antioxidant enzymes in mice result in a compound increase in sensitivity to oxidative stress. *Free Radic. Biol. Med.* 36: 1625–1634 (2004).
14. Huang TT *et al.* Superoxide-mediated cytotoxicity in superoxide dismutase-deficient fetal fibroblasts. *Arch. Biochem. Biophys.* 344: 424–432 (1997).
15. Samper E, Nicholls DG, Melov S. Mitochondrial oxidative stress causes chromosomal instability of mouse embryonic fibroblasts. *Aging Cell* 2: 277–285 (2003).
16. Li Y *et al.* Reduced mitochondrial manganese-superoxide dismutase activity exacerbates glutamate toxicity in cultured mouse cortical neurons. *Brain Res.* 814: 164–170 (1998).
17. Zhao Y *et al.* Overexpression of manganese superoxide dismutase suppresses tumor formation by modulation of activator protein-1 signaling in a multistage skin carcinogenesis model. *Cancer Res.* 61: 6082–6088 (2001).
18. Barlow C *et al.* Atm-deficient mice: a paradigm of ataxia telangiectasia. *Cell* 86: 159–171 (1996).
19. Gu Y *et al.* Defective embryonic neurogenesis in Ku-deficient but not DNA-dependent protein kinase catalytic subunit-deficient mice. *Proc. Natl. Acad. Sci. USA* 97: 2668–2673 (2000).
20. Vogel H, Lim DS, Karsenty G, Finegold M, Hasty P. Deletion of Ku86 causes early onset of senescence in mice. *Proc. Natl. Acad. Sci. USA* 96: 10770–10775 (1999).

21. Gao Y *et al.* Interplay of p53 and DNA-repair protein XRCC4 in tumorigenesis, genomic stability and development. *Nature* 404: 897–900 (2000).
22. Karanjawala ZE *et al.* The embryonic lethality in DNA ligase IV-deficient mice is rescued by deletion of Ku: implications for unifying the heterogeneous phenotypes of NHEJ mutants. *DNA Repair (Amst.)* 1: 1017–1026 (2002).
23. Karanjawala ZE, Murphy N, Hinton DR, Hsieh CL, Lieber MR. Oxygen metabolism causes chromosome breaks and is associated with the neuronal apoptosis observed in DNA double-strand break repair mutants. *Curr. Biol.* 12: 397–402 (2002).
24. Leri A *et al.* Ablation of telomerase and telomere loss leads to cardiac dilatation and heart failure associated with p53 upregulation. *EMBO J.* 22: 131–139 (2003).
25. Doctrow SR *et al.* Salen-manganese complexes as catalytic scavengers of hydrogen peroxide and cytoprotective agents: structure-activity relationship studies. *J. Med. Chem.* 45: 4549–4558 (2002).
26. Friedman JS *et al.* Absence of mitochondrial superoxide dismutase results in a murine hemolytic anemia responsive to therapy with a catalytic antioxidant. *J. Exp. Med.* 193: 925–934 (2001).
27. Friedman JS *et al.* SOD2 deficiency anemia: protein oxidation and altered protein expression reveal targets of damage, stress response and anti-oxidant responsiveness. *Blood* (2004).
28. Banmeyer I *et al.* Overexpression of human peroxiredoxin 5 in subcellular compartments of Chinese hamster ovary cells: effects on cytotoxicity and DNA damage caused by peroxides. *Free Radic. Biol. Med.* 36: 65–77 (2004).
29. Neumann CA *et al.* Essential role for the peroxiredoxin Prdx1 in erythrocyte antioxidant defence and tumor suppression. *Nature* 424: 561–565 (2003).
30. Campisi J. The biology of replicative senescence. *Eur. J. Cancer* 33: 703–709 (1997).
31. Lee AC *et al.* *Ras* proteins induce senescence by altering the intracellular levels of reactive oxygen species. *J. Biol. Chem.* 274: 7936–7940 (1999).
32. Vafa O *et al.* *c-myc* can induce DNA damage, increase reactive oxygen species, and mitigate p53 function: a mechanism for oncogene-induced genetic instability. *Mol. Cell* 9: 1031–1044 (2002).
33. Parrinello S *et al.* Oxygen sensitivity severely limits the replicative lifespan of murine fibroblasts. *Nat. Cell Biol.* (2003).
34. Serrano M, Blasco MA. Putting the stress on senescence. *Curr. Opin. Cell Biol.* 13: 748–753 (2001).

35. Woo RA, Poon RY. Activated oncogenes promote and cooperate with chromosomal instability for neoplastic transformation. *Genes Dev.* 18: 1317–1330 (2004).
36. Difilippantonio MJ *et al.* DNA repair protein Ku80 suppresses chromosomal aberrations and malignant transformation. *Nature* 404: 510–514 (2000).
37. Bailey SM *et al.* DNA double-strand break repair proteins are required to cap the ends of mammalian chromosomes. *Proc. Natl. Acad. Sci. USA* 96: 14899–14904 (1999).
38. Samper E, Goytisolo FA, Slijepcevic P, van Buul PP, Blasco MA. Mammalian Ku86 protein prevents telomeric fusions independently of the length of TTAGGG repeats and the G-strand overhang. *EMBO Rep.* 1: 244–252 (2000).
39. Espejel S, Blasco MA. Identification of telomere-dependent "senescence-like" arrest in mouse embryonic fibroblasts. *Exp. Cell Res.* 276: 242–248 (2002).
40. Suh YA *et al.* Cell transformation by the superoxide-generating oxidase Mox1. *Nature* 401: 79–82 (1999).
41. Arnold RS *et al.* Hydrogen peroxide mediates the cell growth and transformation caused by the mitogenic oxidase *Nox1*. *Proc. Natl. Acad. Sci. USA* 98: 5550–5555 (2001).
42. Mitsushita J, Lambeth JD, Kamata T. The superoxide-generating oxidase *Nox1* is functionally required for *Ras* oncogene transformation. *Cancer Res.* 64: 3580–3585 (2004).
43. Lieber MR, Karanjawala ZE. Ageing, repetitive genomes and DNA damage. *Nat. Rev. Mol. Cell Biol.* 5: 69–75 (2004).
44. de Boer J *et al.* Premature aging in mice deficient in DNA repair and transcription. *Science* 296: 1276–1279 (2002).
45. Wu X, Bishopric NH, Discher DJ, Murphy BJ, Webster KA. Physical and functional sensitivity of zinc finger transcription factors to redox change. *Mol. Cell Biol.* 16: 1035–1046 (1996).
46. Cobbs CS *et al.* Inactivation of wild-type p53 protein function by reactive oxygen and nitrogen species in malignant glioma cells. *Cancer Res.* 63: 8670–8673 (2003).
47. Esteller M. Epigenetic lesions causing genetic lesions in human cancer: promoter hypermethylation of DNA repair genes. *Eur. J. Cancer* 36: 2294–2300 (2000).
48. Esteller M, Herman JG. Cancer as an epigenetic disease: DNA methylation and chromatin alterations in human tumors. *J. Pathol.* 196: 1–7 (2002).
49. Gaudet F *et al.* Induction of tumors in mice by genomic hypomethylation. *Science* 300: 489–492 (2003).

50. Neumeister P, Albanese C, Balent B, Greally J, Pestell RG. Senescence and epigenetic dysregulation in cancer. *Int. J. Biochem. Cell Biol.* 34: 1475–1490 (2002).
51. Fromme JC, Verdine GL. Structure of a trapped endonuclease III-DNA covalent intermediate. *EMBO J.* 22: 3461–3471 (2003).
52. Gardner PR, Fridovich I. Inactivation-reactivation of aconitase in *Escherichia coli*. A sensitive measure of superoxide radical. *J. Biol. Chem.* 267: 8757–8563 (1992).
53. Hausladen A, Fridovich I. Superoxide and peroxynitrite inactivate aconitases, but nitric oxide does not. *J. Biol. Chem.* 269: 29405–29408 (1994).
54. Kinnula VL, Crapo JD. Superoxide dismutases in malignant cells and human tumors. *Free Radic. Biol. Med.* 36: 718–744 (2004).
55. Mitrunen K *et al.* Association between manganese superoxide dismutase (MnSOD) gene polymorphism and breast cancer risk. *Carcinogenesis* 22: 827–829 (2001).
56. Finkel T. Oxygen radicals and signaling. *Curr. Opin. Cell Biol.* 10: 248–253 (1998).
57. Irani K *et al.* Mitogenic signaling mediated by oxidants in *Ras*-transformed fibroblasts. *Science* 275: 1649–1652 (1997).
58. Hainaut P, Mann K. Zinc binding and redox control of p53 structure and function. *Antioxid. Redox Signal* 3: 611–623 (2001).
59. Eng C, Kiuru M, Fernandez MJ, Aaltonen LA. A role for mitochondrial enzymes in inherited neoplasia and beyond. *Nat. Rev. Cancer* 3: 193–202 (2003).
60. Astuti D *et al.* Gene mutations in the succinate dehydrogenase subunit SDHB cause susceptibility to familial pheochromocytoma and to familial paraganglioma. *Am. J. Hum. Genet.* 69: 49–54 (2001).
61. Astuti D *et al.* Genetic analysis of mitochondrial complex II subunits SDHD, SDHB and SDHC in paraganglioma and phaeochromocytoma susceptibility. *Clin. Endocrinol. (Oxf.)* 59: 728–733 (2003).
62. Baysal BE *et al.* Mutations in SDHD, a mitochondrial complex II gene, in hereditary paraganglioma. *Science* 287: 848–851 (2000).
63. Gimm O, Armanios M, Dziema H, Neumann HP, Eng C. Somatic and occult germ-line mutations in SDHD, a mitochondrial complex II gene, in nonfamilial pheochromocytoma. *Cancer Res.* 60: 6822–6825 (2000).
64. Niemann S, Muller U. Mutations in SDHC cause autosomal dominant paraganglioma, type 3. *Nat. Genet.* 26: 268–270 (2000).
65. Kong Q, Beel JA, Lillehei KO. A threshold concept for cancer therapy. *Med. Hypotheses* 55: 29–35 (2000).

66. Hur GC *et al.* Manganese superoxide dismutase expression correlates with chemosensitivity in human gastric cancer cell lines. *Clin. Cancer Res.* 9: 5768–5775 (2003).
67. Li Z *et al.* Genes regulated in human breast cancer cells overexpressing manganese-containing superoxide dismutase. *Free Radic. Biol. Med.* 30: 260–267 (2001).
68. Quong J *et al.* Age-dependent changes in breast cancer hormone receptors and oxidant stress markers. *Breast Cancer Res. Treat.* 76: 221–236 (2002).
69. Archibald F. Oxygen toxicity and the health and survival of eukaryote cells: a new piece is added to the puzzle. *Proc. Natl. Acad. Sci. USA* 100: 10141–10143 (2003).
70. Cullen JJ *et al.* The role of manganese superoxide dismutase in the growth of pancreatic adenocarcinoma. *Cancer Res.* 63: 1297–1303 (2003).

12 Oxidative Stress, Genetic Variation, and Disease

Louise Lyrenäs, Elena Zotova, Lena Ekström, and Ralf Morgenstern

1. Introduction

Oxidative stress has been implicated in many disease conditions.[1] It is also becoming evident that the redox state is an important factor in cellular processes such as signal transduction,[2] as well as in controlling cell growth and death.[3] As oxidative stress and redox balance are important in both pathophysiology and physiology, factors that affect this balance may contribute to disease development. Genetic variants in oxidative stress-related genes are attracting considerable interest as tools for understanding oxidative stress-related disease mechanisms.[4] In this overview, we use a broad definition of relevant genes including protective enzymes such as catalase and superoxide dismutase but also 8-OH dG DNA repair, a receptor of advanced glycation end-products (RAGEs) and vitamin uptake/transport proteins. As the information on genetic variants is abundant, the corresponding definition of phenotypic consequences is often lagging. Nevertheless, many, if not a majority of, common genetic variants affecting coding regions or resulting in lack of gene expression due to deletion or splicing defects have been defined. An emerging theme is the discovery and characterization of an increasing number of gene promoter variants that affect expression levels. Here, we give an updated review of the genetic variants in oxidative stress-related genes identifying phenotypically manifested common variants suitable for association studies. A wealth of association studies actually link many of the genetic variants to disease in a predictable fashion; however, conflicting results are common. The strengths and weaknesses of association studies have been discussed[5] and will not be reiterated here. Suffice to say that large well-defined populations are very important and that haplotype analysis can offer additional advantages. Here, a wide selection of association studies relevant to important genes are reviewed. It is also pointed out where studies are lacking.

2. Specific Elimination of Reactive Oxygen Species

2.1. *Superoxide dismutase*

Superoxide dismutases constitute an important antioxidant enzyme defense against reactive oxygen species (ROS) (superoxide anion radicals). At present, three distinct isoforms of superoxide dismutase (SOD) have been identified in mammals, and their genomic structure, cDNA and proteins have been described. Two isoforms of SOD have Cu and Zn in their catalytic center and are localized to either intracellular cytoplasmic compartments (CuZn-SOD or SOD1) or to extracellular elements (EC-SOD or SOD3). A third isoform of SOD has manganese (Mn) as a cofactor and has been localized to the mitochondria of aerobic cells (Mn-SOD or SOD2).[6]

2.2. *Superoxide dismutase 1*

SOD1 is a low molecular weight cytoplasmic protein that catalyzes the disproportionation of superoxide radicals to molecular oxygen and hydrogen peroxide.

The *SOD1* gene contains five exons[7] and is located in a segment enclosing the distal part of chromosome 21q21 and 21q22.1.[8] More than 70 different variations have been described in individuals affected by familial amyotrophic lateral sclerosis (ALS).[7,9–15] Variations in *SOD1* were also identified in sporadic cases of ALS.[16–20]

Using RT-PCR analysis, Hirano *et al.*[21] identified five splice variants of *SOD1*. The variants were expressed in a tissue-specific manner, including expression in brain, a region involved in ALS. Valentine and Hart[22] have reviewed the two hypotheses that had dominated the discussion of the toxicity of ALS mutant SOD1 proteins in the pathogenesis of ALS: the oligomerization and oxidative damage hypotheses (Table 1).

2.3. *Superoxide dismutase 2*

Human mitochondrial SOD2 is a homotetramer located in the mitochondrial matrix, a strategic position since the mitochondrial electron transport chain is believed to be a principal source of endogenous ROS generation.

The *SOD2* gene is located in the region 6q25.3 and consists of five exons.[23] Several genetic variations have been described for the human *SOD2* gene. The substitution of Ala-9Val in the mitochondrial targeting sequence of *SOD2* is associated with an increased risk of sporadic motor neuron disease, especially in females.[24] This polymorphism is associated with non-familial idiopathic cardiomyopathy[25] but has no effect on the occurrence of ALS[26,27] and rheumatoid arthritis (RA) in the US.[28] In Japanese patients an association was shown between the Val allele and Parkinson's disease (PD),[29] but in later studies this association was not confirmed.[30,31]

The alanine variant has been found more frequently in both pre- and post-menopausal breast cancer patients compared with controls in a study in Caucasian women.[32] This finding was replicated in a Finnish case-control study[33] but was not observed in other studies.[34,35] The Ala allele of this polymorphism may be associated with an increased risk of developing colorectal cancer at a young age in Hispanics.[36]

The Val/Val genotype is associated with nephropathy in type 2 diabetes (T2D)[37] and with diabetic polyneuropathy (DPN) in type 1 diabetes (T1D) mellitus.[38]

Another substitution, Ile58Thr, elicits a three-fold decrease in enzymatic activity of SOD2 and reduces the tumor-suppressive effect of the enzyme.[26,39] At least three heterozygous variations in the proximal promoter of human *SOD2* have been identified and linked to reduced transcriptional activity in transient transfection experiments.[40] Recently, a new variation, leucine to phenylalanine, at position 60 in exon 3, was found and suggested to be associated with decreased SOD activity and a malignant phenotype.[41]

Table 1. Genetic variants in oxidative stress-related genes.

Gene	Nucleotide changes	AA change	Effect on enzyme activity/stability	Allele frequency	References
SOD1			81 hits in dbSNP		
SOD2	C>T 47	Ala16Val	Decreased enzyme levels	0.59 T, 0.41 C	
	T>C 339	Ile58Thr	Decreased enzyme activity		489
	C>T −102		Decreased transcriptional activity		463
	Ins A −93				
	C>G −38				
SOD3	C>G 760	Arg213Gly	Increased enzyme levels in plasma	4% G in Swedish population, 3% in Australian population, 6% in Japanese population	45, 46, 48
SOD3	C>G 760	Arg213Gly	Increased enzyme levels in plasma	4% G in Swedish population, 3% in Australian population, 6% in Japanese population	45, 46, 48
	C>T 280				52
	A>G 241	Thr40Ala			52
	C>T 280				52
CAT	G>A 5 intron 4		Abnormal splicing	0.0008	56, 57
	T del 10 exon 4		Frameshift; no activity		58
	G ins 79 exon 2		Frameshift; truncated protein		60, 61
			No activity		
	GA ins 138 exon 2				
	T>G 5 intron 7		Abnormal splicing		
			Decreased activity		

Table 1. (Continued)

Gene	Nucleotide changes	AA change	Effect on enzyme activity/stability	Allele frequency	References
	C>T −262		Altered levels of CAT in erythrocytes	9% homozygotes T in Swedish population	63
				6.6% homozygotes T in Han Chinese	67
	T>C exon 9			0.82 C 0.18 T	
	C>T −844				67
GPX1	C>T 593	Pro197Leu		70% pro, 30% leu	70
	G>C 349	Gly116Arg			151
	C>T 365	Pro121Leu			151
	GCG repeat	Ala*5, Ala*6, Ala*7			70
GPX2	TC repeats				490
	T>A 5′ UTR				491
GPX4			33 hits in dbSNP		81, 82
Prx			309 hits in dbSNP		
GSTA1	G>A −52, −69, −567	GSTA1*A, GSTA1*B	Differential expression and promoter activity		91
GSTM1	G>C 519	Lys173Asn			491
	Del		No protein	From 23 to 62% in different populations	94, 492
GSTO1			66 hits in dbSNP		
GSTP1	A>G 313	Ile105Val		Altered substrate specificity and heat stability	120
	C>T 341	Ala114Val			120
	T>G 103 exon 6	Asp147Tyr			130

(continued)

Table 1. (*Continued*)

Gene	Nucleotide changes	AA change	Effect on enzyme activity/stability	Allele frequency	References
GSTT1	Del		No protein	~38% homozygous deletions	132
	A>C 310	Thr104Pro	Decreased activity	0.65 GSTT1*A allele, 0.01 GSTT1*B in Swedish population	139
GSTZ1	A>G 94	Lys32Glu		0.37 A, 0.63 G	141
GSTZ1	A>G 94	Lys32Glu		0.37 A, 0.63 G	141
	A>G 124	Arg42Gly		0.09 A, 0.91 G	
	C>T 245	Thr82Met	Low activity	0.16 T in Australian population	142
	C>T 245	Thr82Met	Low activity	0.16 T in Australian population	142
MGST1	172 >173 AA del exon 3		Frameshift		151
	4 promoter, 34 intronic, 3 3′UTR, 5 3′flanking				
	T>G pos 598 3′non-coding				
	A>G −314				
	G>C −131			African Zulu	153
	G>C −84				
MGST2			192 hits in dbSNP		
MGST3			193 hits in dbSNP		
FLAP			92 hits in dbSNP		
LTC4S	A>C −444		Increased enzyme levels		169
PON1	G>C −909		Increased concentration and activity		493
	A>G −824		Contribute expression level		
	A>G −162				
	G>C −126				

Table 1. (*Continued*)

Gene	Nucleotide changes	AA change	Effect on enzyme activity/stability	Allele frequency	References
	T>C −108		Contribute activity level 22.8% in expression level		
	A>G 584	Gln192Arg	Decreased enzyme activity	A 0.672, T 0.328	172
	T>A 172	Leu55Met		G 0.55, A 0.45	494
PON2	G>C	Cys311Ser		G 0.77, C 0.23	495
	G>A 475	Ala148Gly			496
NQO1	C>T 609	Pro187Ser	Between 2 and 4% of the activity	0.16 in Caucasians, 0.4 in Native Indians, 0.46 in Inuits and 0.49 in Chinese	497
	C>T 465	Arg139Trp	Increased alternative splicing and decreased expression		193
NQO2			103 hits in dbSNP		
mEH	T>C First nt in	Tyr113His	40–50% decrease in activity	0.28–0.40 His113	207
sEH	G>A pos 860/exon 8	Arg287Gln	Decreased enzyme activity Decreased protein stability	0.4 Gln287 AA 0.7 Gln287 Caucasians	204
	A>G	Lys55Arg	Increased enzyme activity	17% Arg55	
	G>A	Cys154Tyr	Increased enzyme activity		203
	A>G	Glu470Gly	Increased enzyme activity		
	G>A pos 860/exon 8/ C>T	Arg287Gln/ Arg103Cys	Decreased enzyme activity		
	CGT ins pos 1206/exon 13	Arg 402-403	Decreased enzyme activity	4%	202
	C>T 379	Arg127Cys	Decreased activity		265

(*continued*)

Table 1. (*Continued*)

Gene	Nucleotide changes	AA change	Effect on enzyme activity/stability	Allele frequency	References
mEH	T>C First nt in codon 113/exon 3	Tyr113His	40–50% decrease in activity	0.28–0.40 His113	207
	A>G codon 139/exon 4	His139Arg	25% increase in activity	0.15–0.18 Arg139	207
	T>A −4238		53% decrease in promoter activity	0.7% heterozygotes	210
	C>G 2557 intron 1		86% decrease in promoter activity	1.6% homozygotes	
	C>T 14622 exon 2	Arg49Cys		0.67% Caucasian	209
	G>A 31074 exon 9	Arg454Gln		0.73% Caucasian	
	C>T −200			0.88 T mixed population	211
	C>T −259			0.88 T	
	T>G −290			0.88 G	
	A>G −362		Influences transcriptional activity		
	T>C −399			82% C	
	T>C −613		Influences transcriptional activity	68% C	
	T>C −699			68% C	
GLUT1			Xba-RFLP		219
			StuI-RFLP		
	Del	Lys456Ter	Glucose transport defect		
		Tyr449Ter			
		Lys256Val			
		Arg126Leu			

Table 1. (*Continued*)

Gene	Nucleotide changes	AA change	Effect on enzyme activity/stability	Allele frequency	References
		Gly91Asp			
		Arg126His			
	ex10>alter term				
SRB1	G>A 4 exon 1	Gly2Ser			227, 228
	C>T 54 intron 5				
	C>T 1050 exon 8				
TTPA			Several mutations leading to ataxia		222–226
		His101Gln	Associated vitamin E deficiency (AVED)		
	Del T 485				
	Ins TT 513				
		Arg192His			
		Arg134Ter			
	G>A 522				
	Del A 744				
HO-1	(GT)n repeat promoter n = 15–40		Influences transcriptional activity	20% low	236
	A>T −427				242
	T>A −413		Increased promoter activity		174
HO-2			64 hits in dbSNP		
UGT1			56 hits in HGMD		

(*continued*)

Table 1. (*Continued*)

Gene	Nucleotide changes	AA change	Effect on enzyme activity/stability	Allele frequency	References
γ-GCSM	C>T −588		Decreased promoter activity		268
	C>T −23				
	A>C	Glu120Ala			
	A>G	Lys99Glu			
γ-GCSC	C>T −129		Decreased promoter activity		267
	(GAG)n		GSH level		
	CAGCdupl				266
	C>T 256	Ser55Leu		T 0.997, C 0.003	
	A>T 1109	His370Leu	Enzyme deficiency		266
	C>T 473	Pro158Leu			264
	C>T 379	Arg127Cys	Decreased activity		265
GS	A>G 809	Tyr270Cys	Decreased enzyme activity		273
	C>T 847	Arg283Cys	Decreased enzyme activity		
	T>C 808	Tyr270His	Decreased enzyme activity		
	T>C 563	Leu188Pro	Decreased enzyme activity		
	A>G 656 exon 6		Unstable enzyme		274
	Several rare intronic mutations	GS-deficiency			275
GR	Duplication of chrom. 8		Increased activity		279
	G>A −2/54 exon 6	Gly189Ser		0.01	Utah database
	C>T −36/35 exon 4	Arg110Cys		0.03	
	A>G −15 exon 7	Ile218Val		0.01	
TXN			116 hits in dbSNP		

Table 1. (*Continued*)

Gene	Nucleotide changes	AA change	Effect on enzyme activity/stability	Allele frequency	References
TXNRD			554 hits in dbSNP		
GRX			30 hits in dbSNP		
OGG1	G>C 445	Arg46Gln	Four-fold lower activity		498
	C>G 1245	Ser326Cys		C 0.73, G 0.27	326
CYBA	A>G −930		Promoter activity		343
	C>T 242	His72Tyr		C 0.804, T 0.196	344
	A>G 640	3′UTR			362
			Additional 23 hits in dbSNP		
CYBB			267 hits in HGMD		
MPO	G>A −463		Lower expression		378
	G>A −129		Lower levels		385
	T>G 2986 exon 2	Phe53Val		C 0.887, A 0.112	
		Tyr173Cys	MPO deficiency		376
	T>C 4311exon 6	Met251Thr	24% of MPO activity		377
	C>T 569 exon 10	Arg569Trp	Absence of protein		375
	A>G 12684 exon 12	Ile717Val		A 0.991, G 0.003	
	14 bp del		MPO deficiency		377
NOS1	(CA)n repeat exon 29				406
	(AAT)n repeat intron 20	Repeat number: 8–17			406
NOS2	(CCTTT)n promoter				422
	(TAAA)n				421

(*continued*)

Table 1. (*Continued*)

Gene	Nucleotide changes	AA change	Effect on enzyme activity/stability	Allele frequency	References
	G>C −954		Seven-fold higher activity		420
	C>T −1173		Increased fasting urine and plasma NO metabolite concentrations		436
NOS3	C>T −786		Decrease transcription	−786C variant 42.0% in Caucasians, 17.5% in African-Americans or 13.8% Asians	437
	G>T 894	Glu298Asp		G 0.775, T 0.225	439
	27pb ins			4a allele 26.5% in African-Americans, 16.0% in Caucasians or 12.9% Asians	438 454
RAGE	T>A −374		Increased activity	13% A homozygotes	480
	T>C −429		Increased activity	2% C homozygotes	Finnish population
	405>345 del				
	G>A 555 exon 3	Gly82Ser	Ass. to DAMD/MD	92–94% G	480, 482
	G>T 1740 intron 7				
	A>G 2184 intron 8				
	T>A pos 20				480
	G>T −1393				
	G>T −1390				

Table 1. *(Continued)*

Gene	Nucleotide changes	AA change	Effect on enzyme activity/stability	Allele frequency	References
	G>A −1202				
	(GGT)n −1420				
	A>C exon 6	Thr187Pro			
	G>A exon 8	Gly329Arg			
	G>A exon 10	Arg389Gln			
	C>T 540 exon 3	Arg77Cys			
	G>T 718 intron 3				482
	G>T 1704		Loss of Bfa I endonuclease restriction site	5.4% T, 1% TT, 87% GG	
	A ins 1727–1728 intron 7				354
	T>A 1927 exon 8	His305Gln			
	A>T 1931 exon 8	Ser307Cys			
	A>G 2117 intron 8				
	A>G 2184 intron 8		Introducing BsmFI restriction site	16% G	
	G>A 2245 intron 8		Loss of Fau I restriction site		
	AC del 3089 3′UTR				
	C>A −1152			A 0.06	481
	T>A −338			A 0.32	
	A>T exon 1	Arg2Arg		T 0.01	
	Ik	Gly+Arg 196	196 nt after codon stop	A 0.06	

2.4. *Superoxide dismutase 3*

SOD3 is the extracellular equivalent of SOD1. In the vascular system, SOD3 binds on the surface of endothelial cells through the heparan sulfate proteoglycan and can eliminate oxygen radicals formed from the NADPH-dependent oxidative system of neutrophils. In humans, the highest levels of SOD3 are found in lung, pancreas, thyroid, and uterus.[42] Using RNA gel blot analysis, Folz and Crapo[43] determined that the highest expression levels of SOD3 can be found in adult heart, placenta, pancreas, and lung, followed by moderate expression in kidney and skeletal muscle. A low level of SOD3 mRNA was detected in the brain and liver.

The *SOD3* gene is mapped[44] to chromosome 4p15.3-15.1 and contains three exons and two introns.[43]

Substitution of arginine in position 213 to glycine causes an 8- to 15-fold increase in concentration of SOD3 levels in plasma.[45–47] The effect of this *SOD3* polymorphism, which has been found in 4% of Swedish,[48] 3% of Australian,[49] and 6% of Japanese[45] subjects, is not entirely clear, but early studies suggest that this amino acid variation impairs affinity for heparin and endothelial cell surface and may reduce susceptibility to trypsin-like proteases.

The Arg213Gly polymorphism shows association with familial amyloidotic (non-diabetic) polyneuropathy Type I[50] and DPN with T1D,[38] but there was no association with macroangiopathy in patients with T2D mellitus.[51]

Two additional polymorphisms have been identified in the human *SOD3* gene: a transition variation of A>G at position 241 resulting in a Thr40Ala substitution and a silent transition variation of C>T at position 280.[52]

2.5. *Catalase*

Human catalase (CAT) is a heme-containing enzyme that catalyzes the breakdown of hydrogen peroxide to water and oxygen.[53] The gene is located on chromosome 11p13 and contains 13 exons.[54] Catalase can be found in all tissues but is most abundant in liver, kidney, and erythrocytes. Catalase can be upregulated by oxidative stress.[55] Several rare polymorphisms have been found in the *CAT* gene, most of them associated with the catalase deficiency acatalasemia. Acatalasemia is an autosomal recessive trait characterized by erythrocyte CAT levels 0.2–4% of normal levels. Acatalasemia has been found in nine countries but is most common in Japan (91 patients in 46 families) and Switzerland (11 patients in three families). The Japanese type of acatalasemia depends on a G>A substitution in the fifth position in intron 4 leading to abnormal splicing.[56,57] In exon 4 position 10, a T deletion has been found in a Japanese acatalasemia patient, yielding a frameshift variation and introducing a stop codon. The truncated protein that is produced has no catalase activity.[58] The Swiss type of acatalasemia is caused by a point variation leading to an amino acid substitution. The exact type and location of the variation have not been found. This catalase is rapidly degraded and has a unique electrophoretic mobility.[59] In Hungarian acatalasemia, a GA insertion has been located at position 138 in exon 2. This insertion causes a truncated protein with no catalase activity. A frameshift variation is caused by an insertion of G at position 79 in exon 2.[60,61] A G>T substitution at position 5 in intron 7 has been found, leading to abnormal splicing.[62] A common C>T exchange has been found at −262 bp from the transcription start site. This SNP alters the level of catalase in blood and influences transcription factor binding and promoter activity.[63] This polymorphism has shown no association with Alzheimer's disease (AD)[64] but is associated with elevated risks of developing hyperkeratosis[65] and reduced risks of DPN in T1D patients.[66] A promoter polymorphism in a Chinese population (−844C>T) has been associated with blood pressure levels.[67]

3. Elimination of Peroxides and Other Reactive Molecules that Promote Oxidative Stress

3.1. *Glutathione peroxidases*

3.1.1. *Glutathione peroxidase 1*

Glutathione peroxidase (GPX) proteins catalyze the reduction of organic hydroperoxides, lipid peroxides, and hydrogen peroxide, using glutathione as the reducing agent, thereby also protecting cells from oxidative damage resulting from normal oxidative metabolism. There are four known GPXs that contain selenocysteine at the active site.

GPX1 is a homotetramer containing one atom of selenium per subunit that metabolizes hydrogen peroxide and a range of organic peroxides, including cholesterol and long-chain fatty acid peroxides.[68]

The *GPX1* gene is located on chromosome 3p21.3.[69] Two common polymorphisms have been reported in *GPX1*: a proline-to-leucine substitution at codon 198, resulting from a C>T transition at nucleotide 593, and a (GCG)n repeat polymorphism coding for alanine residues in a polyalanine tract.[70]

In a recent study, it was shown that the Pro198Leu polymorphism was significantly associated with the risk of developing lung cancer[71] and breast cancer.[72] The Pro and Leu variants of human GPX1 do not differ in activity and stability of enzyme and are not significantly associated with an increased risk for stroke.[73]

The (GCG)n repeat polymorphism showed significant association with an increased risk of coronary artery disease (CAD) for individuals with at least one ALA6 allele[74,75] but not with prostate cancer.[76]

3.1.2. *Glutathione peroxidase 4*

GPX4 is a monomeric enzyme with mitochondrial and non-mitochondrial forms. GPX4 is highly expressed in the testes and thyroid. This enzyme is capable of reducing peroxidized phospholipids, cholesterol hydroperoxides, and thiamine hydroperoxides. Thus, GPX4 is considered to be an important enzymatic defense against oxidation of biomembranes.[77]

The *GPX4* gene is located[77] on chromosome 19p13.3 and contains seven exons and several hormone-responsive elements in the 5′ untranslated region, which may be related to the function of GPX4 in the testis.[78,79] In testicular tissue, *GPX4* is expressed in three different forms. The full-length cDNA clone of GPX4 has alternative start sites, which can code for proteins of 197 or 170 amino acids. The differences between the two potential forms are 27 amino acids at the N-terminal region. These 27 amino acids constitute a mitochondrial targeting sequence.[80]

A total of 10 variants were found in introns at sites that were not expected to affect splicing.[81]

Recently 23 different variant sites were identified in *GPX4*.[82] Four substitution variants mapped to the promoter region (positions 2221, 2197, 2180, and 2100), and nine mapped to exons, i.e., two in the 5′ untranslated region

(UTR) of the mRNA, four in the coding region, and three in the 3′ UTR of the gene. Only one of the exon variations leads to an Ala93Thr exchange that reduces activity in a porcine GPX4 homolog. Two detected promoter variations were shown by reporter gene constructs to affect transcription in somatic cell lines.

Genetic variants of *GPX2*, *GPX3*, and *GPX5* genes have not been characterized in humans but would certainly be of interest.

3.2. *Peroxiredoxins*

Peroxiredoxins (Prx), also referred to as thioredoxin peroxidases and alkyl-hydroperoxide-reductase-C22 proteins, are proteins capable of directly reducing peroxides.[83,84] Peroxiredoxins have a protective antioxidant role in cells through their peroxidase activity, efficiently detoxifying low levels of hydrogen peroxide, peroxynitrite, and organic hydroperoxides.[85] The enzymes can be upregulated by hydrogen peroxide[86] and are mostly found in the cytosol but can also be found in the mitochondria and peroxisomes (associated with nuclei and membranes) and, in at least one case, exported.[85] There are at least six Prxs (Prx I–VI) identified in mammalian cells.[87] Polymorphisms have been reported for all the six peroxiredoxins in the SNP database. Their functions are however unknown.

3.3. *Glutathione S-transferases*

The glutathione S-transferases (GST) are a family of enzymes responsible for the metabolism of a broad range of xenobiotics and, carcinogens and importantly also function as glutathione peroxidases utilizing lipophilic peroxides.[88] Board[89] showed that the most active GSTs in liver are the products of two autosomal loci, GST1 and GST2, both of which are polymorphic.

Two distinct supergene families encode human proteins with GST activity; firstly at least 16 genes encode proteins expressed in the cytosol, and secondly at least six genes are expressed as membrane proteins. In humans, eight distinct gene families encode the soluble GSTs. The kappa enzymes are expressed in the mitochondria. Polymorphism has been described in many genes in these families, though to date most attention has focused on allelism in the mu, theta, and pi families.[90]

3.3.1. *Glutathione S-transferase A*

The alpha class exhibit glutathione peroxidase activity, thereby protecting the cells from ROS and the products of peroxidation. The *GSTA1* gene is mapped on chromosome 6p12 and contains seven exons.[91]

GSTA1 expression is influenced by a genetic polymorphism that consists of two alleles, GSTA1*A and GSTA1*B, containing three linked base substitutions in the proximal promoter, at positions −567, −69, and −52.[91] A base at position −52 also altered binding of the ubiquitous transcription factor Sp1. Morel *et al.*[91] postulated that *GSTA1* genotyping will be of importance in determining individual susceptibility to certain cancers.

3.3.2. *Glutathione S-transferase M*

The mu class of enzymes are involved in the detoxification of electrophilic compounds, including carcinogens, therapeutic drugs, environmental toxins, and products of oxidative stress.

Five mu class genes are situated in tandem (5′-*GSTM4-GSTM2-GSTM1-GSTM5-GSTM3*-3′) in a 20 kb cluster on chromosome 1p13.3.[92] Polymorphisms have been identified in *GSTM1*, and the clinical consequences of genotypes resulting from combinations of the GSTM1*0, GSTM1*A, and GSTM1*B alleles have been intensively investigated.[90,93] GSTM1*0 is deleted, and homozygotes (GSTM1*0 genotype) express no protein. The frequency of the GSTM1*0 genotype ranges from 23 to 62% in different populations around the world and is approximately 50% in Caucasians, as discussed by Cotton *et al.*[94]

The GSTM1*0 genotype is an independent risk factor for the development of lung cancer,[95–100] thyroid carcinoma,[101] prostate cancer,[102] head/neck cancer,[103] decreased risk for early-onset hepatocellular carcinoma,[104] solar keratoses development;[105] was significantly higher in migraine without aura[106] and in alcoholic chronic pancreatitis patients, especially young female patients.[107] The GSTM1*0 genotype is protective against both CAD and acute myocardial infarction.[108]

There is no evidence of association between GSTM1*0 and glaucoma in the Swedish population;[109] and alcohol withdrawal symptoms[110] and liver status[111] and colon cancer in a United Kingdom population.[112]

Allelism has also been identified in the *GSTM3* gene, with GSTM3*A and GSTM3*B differing in intron 6 by a 3 bp deletion in GSTM3*B. This difference creates a recognition motif for the YY1 transcription factor in GSTM3*B.[113]

Liloglou *et al.*[114] identified a new C>T polymorphism in intron 6 of the *GSTM4* gene (2517 C>T) and termed the allele carrying T at this position allele *A and the allele carrying C, allele *B. The polymorphism did not demonstrate any associations with tumor type.

3.3.3. *Glutathione S-transferase O1*

The *GSTO1* gene is mapped to chromosome 10.[115] Board *et al.*[116] suggested that the wide expression and conserved sequence of *GSTO1* indicate that it may have a significant housekeeping function, such as protection from oxidative stress.

Two functional polymorphisms of *GSTO1* have been identified. One alters a splice junction and causes the deletion of Glu155, and the other results in an Ala140Asp substitution. Deletion of residue Glu155 appears to contribute toward both a loss of heat stability and increased enzymatic activity.[115]

3.3.4. *Glutathione S-transferase P*

The glutathione S-transferase P (GSTP) plays a role in xenobiotic metabolism and may thus play a role in susceptibility to cancer and other diseases. In addition, the protein has been implicated in cellular signalling via protein kinase.[117]

The *GSTP1* gene is mapped to chromosome 11q13 and contains seven exons.[118,119] Three polymorphic *GSTP1* alleles have been described for the human *GSTP1* gene: GSTP1*A, GSTP1*B, and GSTP1*C.[120] The variant cDNAs result from A>G and C>T transitions at nucleotides 313 and 341, respectively. The transitions changed codon 105 from ATC (Ile) in GSTP1*A to GTC (Val) in GSTP1*B and GSTP1*C, and changed codon

114 from GCG (Ala) to GTG (Val) in GSTP1*C. Both amino acid changes are in the electrophile-binding active site of the GSTP polypeptide.

The *GSTP1* Val105 variant is associated with high cancer susceptibility,[121] with familial prostate cancer risk,[122] esophageal adenocarcinoma,[123] lung cancer,[98,124,125] and cervical cancer.[126] The *GSTP1* gene variations are the genetic risk factor for nephrotoxic complications of ifosfamide use.[127]

The gene polymorphism for *GSTP1* was not associated with susceptibility to chronic obstructive pulmonary disease in a Chinese population.[128] Also, no association was found between this genotype and tumor or benign prostatic hyperplasia methylation status.[129]

The *GSTP1* Ile105/Ile105 genotype was associated with an eight-fold increase in the risk of liver disease.[111]

Two new mutant genotypes were discovered recently. A silent A>G substitution at position 99 of exon 6 was found in one healthy child. A T>G bases substitution at position 103 of exon 6 was observed in two children with leukemia, leading to an aspartic acid-to-tyrosine exchange at position 147 in the protein peptide chain (Asp147Tyr).[130]

3.3.5. *Glutathione S-transferase T1*

The *GSTT1* gene is mapped to chromosome 22q11.2.[131] Pemble *et al.*[132] showed that the *GSTT1* gene was absent from 38% of the population. The GSTT1*0 genotype is associated with myelodysplastic syndromes;[133] aplastic anemia;[134] sporadic colorectal adenocarcinoma;[135] and thyroid[136] and lung cancers.[96]

In one study it was suggested that the GSTT1*0 genotype of the *GSTT1* gene is associated with a decreased cancer risk[100] but individuals with the GSTT1*0 genotype were also shown to display an increased risk of Hodgkin's lymphoma.[137] The GSTT1*0 genotype is not associated with colon cancer in the UK population.[112] This genotype might display an interaction with carotid atherosclerosis related to RA in Korean postmenopausal RA women without a history of smoking.[138]

Sequencing of *GSTT1* cDNA revealed a single nucleotide substitution, 310A>C, that altered amino acid residue 104 from threonine to proline (Thr104Pro). Modeling studies of GSTT1 have suggested that residue 104 is located in the middle of alpha-helix 4. Introduction of an alpha-helix-disrupting proline most likely distorts the conformation of the protein. Individuals that lacked GSTT1 activity and carried the variant allele, tentatively denoted GSTT1*B, had no detectable GSTT1 immunoreactive protein. An allele-specific polymerase chain reaction method was developed to determine the frequency of the GSTT1*B allele. In 497 ethnic Swedes, the frequency of the active GSTT1*A allele was 0.65 [95% confidence interval (CI) 0.62–0.68], whereas the frequencies of the non-functional allele GSTT1*O and the novel GSTT1*B allele were 0.34 (CI 0.31–0.37) and 0.01 (CI 0.01–0.02), respectively.[139]

3.3.6. *Glutathione S-transferase Z*

The *GSTZ1* gene contains nine exons and was mapped to chromosome 14q24.3.[140] Three *GSTZ1* alleles resulting from A>G transitions at nucleotides 94 and 124 of the coding region were identified, GSTZ1*A — A94/A124, GSTZ1*B — A94/G124, and GSTZ1*C — G94/G124. These nucleotide substitutions are non-synonymous, with A>G at positions 94 and 124 encoding Lys32Glu and Arg42Gly substitutions, respectively.[141] Additionally a novel allele of the *GSTZ1* gene was identified and termed GSTZ1d. Like GSTZ1b/1b and GSTZ1c/1c, the novel isoform has low activity with dichloroacetic acid compared with GSTZ1a/1a.[142]

3.4. *The MAPEG family*

The membrane-associated proteins in eicosanoid and glutathione metabolism (MAPEG) superfamily consists of structurally and phylogenetically related enzymes, including microsomal glutathione S-transferase 1 (MGST1), microsomal glutathione S-transferase 2 (MGST2), microsomal glutathione S-transferase 3 (MGST3), prostaglandin E synthase (PGES), 5-lipoxygenase activating protein (FLAP), and leukotriene C4 synthase (LTC_4S). Enzymes in this superfamily have distinct or overlapping functions involving detoxification, protection from oxidative stress, glutathione peroxidase activity, or synthesis of prostaglandin E and cysteinyl leukotrienes.[143,144]

3.4.1. *Microsomal glutathione S-transferase 1*

MGST1 is a trimeric, membrane-bound enzyme that catalyzes the conjugation of electrophilic compounds with glutathione and the reduction of lipid hydroperoxides.[145–147] MGST1 has been found in all tissues examined but is most abundant in liver.[148] *MGST1* is 18 kb long and has seven exons: three constitute the coding region and four are alternatively spliced first exons, where one is predominant. The *MGST1* gene has been mapped to chromosome 12p13.3.[148–150] *MGST1* is highly polymorphic: 46 SNPs, four in the promoter region, 34 in introns, three in 3′UTR, and five in the 3′flanking region, and 13 insertion-deletions have been found in a Japanese population. No SNPs were detected in the 5′UTR or coding regions.[151] Forsberg *et al.*[152] report a T>G substitution in the 3′-flanking region, two intronic polymorphisms and an −314A>G promoter polymorphism. The −131G>C and −84G>C polymorphisms have been found in African Zulus but not in northern Europeans.[153] Several polymorphisms have been reported in databases, but as of yet no functional consequences are known.

Using a microarray technique, Chaib *et al.*[154] recently established that expression of *MGST1* in human prostate tumors was twice that of normal tissues.

3.4.2. *MGST2 and MGST3*

Both MGST2 and MGST3 are glutathione-dependent enzymes and catalyze the reduction of 5-hydroperoxyeicosatetraenoic acid and conjugation of leukotrienes (LT)A_4 to form LTC_4. Unlike MGST3, MGST2 shows activity with 1-chloro-2,4-dinitrobenzene (CDNB). MGST2 is found mostly in liver, spleen, skeletal muscle, heart, and pancreas,[155,156] and MGST3 is found in the heart, skeletal muscle, and adrenal cortex.[157] *MGST2* is located on chromosome 4q28.31;[155] *MGST3* is located on chromosome 1q23[157] and has six exons.[158] Iida *et al.*[159] report three SNPs in *MGST2* and Thameem *et al.*[158] report 25 variations, but in the databases over 100 polymorphisms have been reported for both *MGST2* and *MGST3*. *MGST2* has 195 hits in the SNP database (http://www.ncbi.nlm.nih.gov/SNP/). All but 33 are either validated or genotyped or both. Four amino acid exchanges were found. The dbSNP includes 193 reported SNPs for *MGST3*. The majority are either validated or genotyped or both. No association studies have been published for MGST2, whereas an MGST3 variant was reported to have no association with T2D in Pima Indians.[158]

3.4.3. *5-Lipoxygenase activating protein and leukotriene C4 synthase*

The 5-lipoxygenase activating protein (FLAP), 5-lipoxygenase, and leukotriene C_4 synthase (LTC_4S) are required for leukotriene synthesis. Although these enzymes are not antioxidative, they are included as examples of inflammatory modulators. Leukotrienes are arachidonic acid metabolites that have been implicated in various types of inflammatory responses, including asthma, arthritis, and psoriasis. The exact function of the FLAP enzyme remains controversial, but previous studies suggest that it acts as an arachidonic acid transfer protein for 5-lipoxygenase.

The human *FLAP (ALOX5AP)* gene contains four exons within 31 kb located on chromosome 13q12.[160]

A novel G>A substitution at −336 bp and a poly(A) repeat (n = 19 or 23) at positions −169 to −146 bp was identified in the *FLAP* promoter. There was no support for a significant role for these polymorphisms in genetic susceptibility to asthma in the Caucasian population.[161]

A four-SNP marker haplotype in this locus spanning the *FLAP* gene is associated with a two times greater risk of myocardial infarction in Iceland.[162]

The LTC_4S enzyme catalyzes the GSH-dependent conversion of leukotriene A_4 to leukotriene C_4, potent biological compounds derived from arachidonic acid. Leukotrienes have been implicated as mediators of anaphylaxis and inflammatory conditions such as human bronchial asthma. This protein localizes to the nuclear envelope and adjacent endoplasmic reticulum.[163,164]

The human *LTC4S* gene contains four exons and is located on chromosome 5q35.[165] A single nucleotide polymorphism (SNP) consisting of A>C transversion −444 nucleotides upstream of the ATG translation start site in the *LTC4S* gene has been associated with a relative risk for the aspirin-intolerant asthmatic phenotype in Polish patients[166] and in a Japanese population[167] but not in the United States.[168] The −444C allele was associated with higher levels of *LTC4S* mRNA in eosinophils.[169,170]

3.4.4. *Paraoxonase*

Paroxonase (PON) is a high-density lipoprotein (HDL)–associated serum enzyme whose primary physiological role is to protect low-density lipoproteins (LDLs) from oxidative modification. Indeed, the enzyme was initially characterized as an organophosphate hydrolase and is capable of hydrolyzing paroxon to produce *p*-nitrophenol.[171]

The *PON* gene cluster contains at least three members, including *PON1*, *PON2*, and *PON3*, located on chromosome 7q21.3–22.1.[172] PON1 is a calcium-dependent esterase that is known to catalyze hydrolysis of organophosphates and is widely distributed among tissues such as liver, kidney, and intestine.[173]

The *PON1* gene has two common polymorphisms in the coding region, 584A>G and 172T>A, which lead to a glutamine-to-arginine substitution at position 192 (Gln192Arg) and a leucine-to-methionine substitution at position 55 (Leu55Met). The frequencies of the *PON1* alleles vary greatly across human populations.[174–177] Several molecular epidemiological studies have found association with disease as summarized in Ref. 178 and references therein.

PON2 mRNA is ubiquitously expressed in nearly every human tissue, with the highest expression in liver, lung, placenta, testis, and heart.

The human *PON2* gene has two common polymorphisms: the alleles encode either glycine or alanine at codon 148 and either cysteine or serine at codon 311. The polymorphisms are thus designated as 148G>A and Cys311Ser.[179,180] Several reports have showed associations between genetic polymorphisms in *PON2* and different diseases as reviewed in Ref. 178.

3.4.5. *NAD(P)H:quinone oxidoreductase 1*

NAD(P)H:quinone oxidoreductase 1 (NQO1; DT-diaphorase; DTD) is a cytosolic two-electron reductase that detoxifies quinones, is involved in chemoprotection, and can also bioactivate certain antitumor quinones. It is primarily a cytosolic enzyme (~90%) and exists as a homodimer with one molecule of FAD per monomer.[181] NQO1 activity is present in all tissue types.

The *NQO1* is a single copy gene and is located on human chromosome 16q22.1.[182] The *NQO1* gene consists of six exons and five introns for an approximate length of 20 kb.[183]

Currently, there are 22 SNPs reported in the *NQO1* gene. Compared with the human consensus (reference, "wild-type") NQO1*1 allele coding for normal NQO1 enzyme and activity, the NQO1*2 allele encodes a non-synonymous variation, Pro187Ser, that has negligible NQO1 activity. The NQO1*2 allelic frequency ranges between 0.22 (Caucasian) and 0.45 (Asian) in various ethnic populations. A large epidemiologic investigation of a benzene-exposed population has shown that NQO1*2 homozygotes exhibit as much as a seven-fold greater risk of bone marrow toxicity, leading to diseases such as aplastic anemia, leukemia, and some types of cancer.[184–188] The *NQO1*2* allele appears to have little[189] or no [190] association with PD and does not confer increased susceptibility to schizophrenia in Japanese.[191] Ma *et al.*[192] show that *NQO1* 609C>T may be an independent genetic risk factor for sporadic AD in Chinese. A missense variation, Pro187Ser, of the *NQO1* gene showed no significant association with alcohol withdrawal symptoms.[110]

A second polymorphism in *NQO1* (NQO1*3 allele) has also been characterized. This is a 465C>T change coding for an arginine-to-tryptophan substitution at position 139 of the protein.[193,194] The 465C>T SNP disrupts the consensus sequence at the 5′-splice site, which is required for binding by U1 small nuclear RNA (U1 snRNA) in spliceosomes. Thus, alternative splicing of NQO1 at the 5′-splice site of intron 4 increased in cells with NQO1*3 allele. This defective RNA splicing was partially corrected by transfecting HCT-116R30A cells with U1 snRNA constructs, containing base changes to compensate for the 465 SNP. NQO1 protein and enzymatic activity increased with corrected splicing. This SNP was the major cause of increased alternative splicing and decreased expression of NQO1 protein in HCT-116R30A cells.[195]

3.4.6. *NRH:quinone oxidoreductase 2*

NRH:quinone oxidoreductase 2 (NQO2) is a flavoprotein that catalyzes two-electron reduction of various quinones including their derivatives and protect cells from damage associated with redox cycling, oxidative stress, and neoplasia. NQO2 uses dihydronicotinamide riboside (NRH) rather than NAD(P)H as an electron donor.[190]

The human *NQO2* gene is located on chromosome 6p25 and contains seven exons interrupted by six introns. The human *NQO2* gene locus is highly polymorphic.[196,197]

Harada *et al.*[190] identified an insertion/deletion (I/D) of 29 base pairs in the promoter region (652 to 680), 967C>T and 972A>G nucleotide substitutions, and a 13467A>G missense variation, Try76Cys, in exon 4 and show that the I/D polymorphism in the promoter is associated with PD. The frequency of the D allele in the promoter region was found to be significantly higher in patients than in controls. Another association study shows that the D allele is associated with alcohol withdrawal symptoms[110] and schizophrenia.[198]

3.4.7. *Soluble epoxide hydrolase*

Soluble cytoplasmic epoxide hydrolase (sEH, EPXH2) is one of five epoxide hydrolases (the others are hepoxilin EH, leukotriene A_4 hydrolase, cholesterol EH, and microsomal EH) that differ in molecular weight, subcellular localization, pI, and substrate specificity. The enzyme is often involved in the metabolism of endogenous substances, e.g. epoxides of steroids and arachidonic acid derivates, but also participates in xenobiotic metabolism with a preference for *trans*-substituted epoxides. The *sEH* gene is localized on chromosome 8p12-p21.[199] It has 19 exons and encodes 555 amino acids.[200] Several studies have shown high interindividual variation in the *sEH* gene. Thirty-six SNPs were found in a Japanese population: four in the 5′-flanking region, 24 intronic, five exonic, and three in the 3′-flanking region.[201] An arginine insertion was also found in the 5′-flanking region. The arginine insertion leads to a decrease in enzyme activity.[202] In a mixed (Caucasian, Asian, and African-American) population, 44 SNPs were found: 31 intronic and 13 exonic. The arginine insertion was also reported for this population.[203] Six of the exonic SNPs lead to amino acid substitutions. The Arg287Gln substitution is associated with a two-fold increased risk of coronary artery calcification in an African-American population.[204] In cell transfection assays the Arg287Gln single mutant and the Arg287Gln/Arg103Cys double mutant showed statistically significant decreases in enzyme activity when using the exogenous substrates t-SO and t-DPPO. Three single mutants, Lys55Arg, Cys154Tyr, and Glu470Gly, showed statistically significant increases in enzyme activity with the same substrates. Lys55Arg and

Arg287Gln were the most common variants in a mixed population (17 and 14%).[203]

3.4.8. *Microsomal epoxide hydrolase*

Microsomal epoxide hydrolase (mEH, EPHX1) is a phase I metabolic enzyme that catalyzes the hydrolysis of arene, alkene, and aliphatic epoxides from polycyclic aromatic hydrocarbons and aromatic amines. The *mEH* gene is located on chromosome 1q42.1 and has nine exons.[205] mEH is expressed in all tissues and cells but is most abundant in the liver, kidneys, and testis.[206] Within the cell mEH is principally located in the endoplasmic reticulum. In the coding region of the *mEH* gene two relatively common polymorphisms are present in exons 3 and 4.[207] In exon 3 a C is exchanged for a T, leading to a tyrosine-to-histidine exchange at codon 113, resulting in a 40–50% decrease in enzyme activity. In exon 4 a G>A exchange occurs at codon 139. This polymorphism results in a 25% increase in enzyme activity.[207] In Caucasians the allele frequencies in healthy controls vary between 0.28 and 0.40 for the His113 variant and 0.15 and 0.18 for the Arg139 variant.[208] Two missense polymorphisms have also been reported in a French population: a C>T amino acid exchange in exon 2 resulting in an arginine-to-cystein exchange at codon 49; and in exon 9 an arginine-to-glutamine exchange occurs at codon 454. The allele frequencies for the common allele are 0.67 for the exon 2 polymorphism and 0.73 for exon 9.[209] A promoter polymorphism has been reported at −4238T>A that significantly decreases *mEH* promoter activity by 53% in HepG2 cells. This polymorphism also affects binding to a downstream HNF-3β site. HNF-3β could act as a repressor of *mEH*. In intron 1 a 2557C>G substitution significantly suppresses promoter activity by 86% in HepG2 cells. Allele frequencies for these polymorphisms are rather low (−4238T>A heterozygote 0.7% and 2557C>G homozygote 1.6%).[250] Raaka *et al.*[211] report seven promoter polymorphisms, three of them leading to variations in the enzyme activity. Several association studies have been performed by studying the relationship between the exon 3 and 4 polymorphisms and disease, e.g. lung cancer,[208,212] colorectal adenomas,[213] head and neck cancer,[214] Chrons disease,[215] ovarian cancer,[216] and lymphoma,[217] but so far the results are conflicting.

3.5. *Small antioxidant molecule protection*

3.5.1. *Vitamin C transport*

Vitamin C is required for vascular and connective tissue integrity and leukocyte function. Vitamin C also inhibits peroxidation of membrane phospholipids and acts as a scavenger of free radicals.[218] Sodium-dependent vitamin C transporters (SVTC1 and 2) are known to be important proteins for cellular uptake. No polymorphisms have been reported in these genes.

Dehydroascorbic acid (the oxidized form of vitamin C) is transported into the brain through a glucose transporter protein (GLUT1). RFLP analysis with Xba I and Stu I showed the presence of different alleles.[219] The former has been associated with T2D.[220,221] In addition, several variations have been described in patients with defects in glucose transport.

3.5.2. *Vitamin E transport and uptake*

Due to its lipophilicity, vitamin E is transported in the circulation in association with lipoproteins. Several intracellular transport proteins that can bind α-tocopherol with different affinities have been described. Of these, α-tocopherol transfer protein (α-TTP) is the best studied. Many point variations in the α-TTP gene have been described that leed to ataxia-associated vitamin E deficiency (AVED).[222–226]

SRB1 is an essential component in facilitating α-tocopherol uptake into cells. SRB1 is known to play a role in the HDL and LDL metabolism. Five variations have been identified in the *SRB1* gene, whereas three of them are common polymorphisms. They have all been associated with altered lipoprotein metabolism.[227,228]

3.5.3. *CoQ synthesis*

Coenzyme Q (CoQ) or ubiquinone is an endogenously synthesized lipid and exhibits a broad tissue as well as intracellular distribution. Two major functions are attributed to this compound, namely as an electron carrier in the mitochondrial respiratory chain and as a lipid-soluble antioxidant. The CoQ biosynthesis had been investigated in great detail in bacteria and yeast; however, in humans only a few genes have been identified. The synthesis in humans occurs through the mevalonate pathway, where hydroxy-3-methylglutaryl-CoA (HMG-CoA) reductase is the main regulatory enzyme. Three polymorphisms have been identified in this gene.[229–231]

3.5.4. *Heme Oxygenase*

Heme oxygenase-1 (HO-1, HMOX1) is the inducible,[232] rate-limiting enzyme in heme degradation leading to the generation of free iron, biliverdin, and carbon monoxide.[233] It also functions as an antioxidant enzyme since it is induced by various environmental changes and since locally produced biliverdin works as a scavenger of ROS. The *HO-1* gene is located on chromosome 22q12.[234] The human *HO-1* gene has a highly polymorphic $(GT)_n$ promoter region, where n varies between 15 and 40. $(GT)_{22}$ and $(GT)_{27}$ are common in the Japanese population.[235] The GT repeat has been shown to influence transcription.[236] Large repeats give a decrease in HO-1 induction, and short repeats give an increased induction. Large repeats are associated with chronic pulmonary emphysema in Japanese smokers,[236,237] cardiovascular disease (CVD),[16,237] T2D,[238] post-dilation restenosis,[239,240] and decreased longevity[241] but protect against cerebral malaria.[242] A −413T>A substitution in the promoter region has been found to be associated with hypertension in women.[174] In the SNP database 233 possible SNPs are found.

Heme oxygenase-2 (HO-2) has a molecular weight of 38 kDa[243] and is found highly concentrated in the nervous system and testis.[244] HO-2 is constitutively expressed in neurons, and it is also called constitutive or neuronal heme oxygenase. HO-2 acts as a neuroprotective agent in the nervous system. Under normal conditions HO-2 accounts for nearly all of the HO activity in the brain.[245] The *HO-2 (HMOX2)* gene is located on chromosome 16p13.3.[234] In the SNP database 64 SNPs are reported; 33 of these are validated and/or genotyped. There are no amino acid substitutions, and no association studies are reported.

3.5.5. *UDP-glucuronosyltransferase*

UDP-glucuronosyltransferases (UGTs; EC 2.4.1.17) catalyze the addition of the glycosyl group from a nucleotide sugar to a small hydrophobic molecule (aglycone). At least two biological functions are attributed to UGTs: (i) the contribution of UGTs is determinant in the mechanism of protection against some toxic dietary components, tobacco smoke carcinogens, and various environmental pollutants, and (ii) they represent key elements in the homeostasis of a number of endogenous molecules, including bilirubin, steroid and thyroid hormones, and fatty acids as well as biliary acids.[246]

On the basis of the presence of a "signature sequence" a large superfamily of *UGT*s, comprising at least 110 distinct cDNAs/genes.[247] By comparing the cDNA sequences, 33 families have been defined. In mammals, 47 distinct cDNA/genes have been classified into three families, *UGT1*, *UGT2*, and *UGT8*.

The UGT1 family includes isoforms that catalyze the glucuronidation of bilirubin, quinols, and phenols. The *UGT1* gene, which is located on chromosome 2q37, contains at least 12 different promoters/first exons that are spliced to common exons 2 through 5, thus resulting in separate UGT1A forms with unique N-terminals and a conserved 246-amino acid C terminus.[248]

The *UGT2A* subfamily comprises at least one gene with olfactory-specific expression located on chromosome 2q37.[249,250] The *UGT2B* subfamily, located on human chromosome 4, includes phenobarbital-inducible genes, as well as several constitutively expressed genes that are involved in the glucuronidation of endogenous steroids and biogenic amines.[56,251,252] The third family, *UGT8*, is known to have a single member, located on chromosome 4q26, that encodes an enzyme involved in the galactosylation of ceramide.[253]

A number of polymorphisms have been described for both *UGT1* and *UGT2B* genes. Some polymorphic *UGTs* have demonstrated a significant pharmacological impact in addition to being relevant to drug-induced adverse reactions and cancer susceptibility.[254–259]

3.6. *Glutathione synthesis and redox balance*

3.6.1. *γ-Glutamylcysteine synthetase*

γ-Glutamylcysteine synthetase (γ-GCS; also known as glutamate-cysteine ligase, GCL) catalyzes the rate-limiting formation of the amide linkage between cysteine and the γ-carboxyl group of glutamate to form the dipeptide γ-glutamylcysteine. Next, glutathione synthetase catalyzes the addition of glycine to the cysteine carboxyl group of γ-glutamylcysteine to form the tripeptide γ-glutamylcysteinyl-glycine (glutathione, GSH).

γ-GCS is a heterodimer composed of a heavy subunit (γ-GCSH) and a light subunit (γ-GCSL) that associate, through a disulfide bond, to form the holoenzyme. This occurs in response to many cellular insults, particularly oxidative stress.[260] The heavy subunit (73 kDa) governs all the catalytic activity for the enzyme and is also the site of feedback inhibition by GSH. It is encoded by a gene located on chromosome 6p12.[261] The light subunit (31 kDa) serves a modifying function, increasing the affinity of γ-GCS for its substrates, glutamate, and cysteine. It is encoded by a gene on chromosome 1p21.6.[262]

A trinucleotide repeat polymorphism was described in the 5′ UTR of the human γ-*GCSL* gene, which encodes the catalytic subunit of this enzyme and exhibits a range of four to 10 uninterrupted repeats (alleles A1–A5 have nine, eight, seven, 10 and four repeats).[261] In 2001, Walsh *et al.*[263] demonstrated an association between certain alleles and GSH levels and/or drug sensitivity, providing evidence suggesting that polymorphism of the human γ-*GCS* gene is functionally significant.

Several other polymorphisms have been studied in the γ-*GCS* gene, among these a 473C>T variation, predicting a Pro158Leu substitution in the GCSH subunit[264] and a C>T missense variation at nucleotide 379, encoding for a predicted Arg127Cys amino acid change that results in low enzyme activity.[265] A variant A>T at position 1109 produces a deduced amino acid change, His370Leu, of the catalytic subunit that is associated with enzyme deficiency. Additionally, a diallelic polymorphism was found at nt 206 of an intron and additionally a duplication of a CAGC at cDNA nt1972-1975 in the 3′ UTR. These two polymorphisms were found to be only in partial linkage disequilibrium.[266]

The T alleles of two promoter polymorphisms, −588C>T and −129C>T, showed lower promoter activity and were highly frequent in patients with myocardial infarction.[267–269]

3.6.2. *Glutathione synthetase*

Glutathione synthetase (GS) catalyzes the last biosynthetic step in the γ-glutamyl cycle and therefore plays an important role in the synthesis of glutathione. GS is a homodimer of 52 kDa subunits,[270] and the gene is located on chromosome 20q11.2 and has 13 exons.[271,272] Several rare point variations have been reported that lead to GS deficiency.[273] Hereditary GS deficiencies are autosomal recessive and can lead to mental retardation and neuropsychiatric dysfunction in approximately 50% of patients, while this deficiency is routinely accompanied by metabolic acidosis and hemolytic anemia.[274] Among the variations leading to GS deficiency are the amino acid substitutions Tyr270Cys and Tyr270His, which give a 100-fold reduction of GS activity, and the Arg283Cys substitution, which leads to a 10-fold decrease of *in vitro* enzyme activity.[273] A 5G>A exchange in exon 1 leads to the production of two alternative mRNAs. The complete deletion of exon 12 and the insertion of a pseudoexon between exons 2 and 3, a frameshift variation leading to a truncated protein, have also been reported for GS-deficient patients.[275] An Asp219Gly exchange results in an unstable protein.[276]

3.6.3. *Glutathione reductase*

Glutathione reductase (GR, GRS) is a ubiquitous dimeric flavoprotein responsible for maintaining a high ratio of reduced to oxidized glutathione in the cells of most organisms. It is important for protection against oxidative stress and in the production of deoxyribonucleotides.[277] There are two isoenzymes of GR, one cytosolic and one mitochondrial, and the same gene encodes them both. The *GR* gene is located on chromosome 8p21.1.[278] Significantly increased GR activity is found in people with an inverted tandem duplication of chromosome 8, localized to the *GR* gene.[279] This can lead to developmental delay, distinct facial anomalities, and hypotonia in young children. Spastic paraplegia and orthopedic problems frequently occur in adults.[280] Direct duplication of the short arm of chromosome 8 can also occur, leading to mild mental retardation. This is less common than the inverted duplication.[281] Several polymorphisms have been reported in databases (www.genome.utah.edu/genesnps/) (13 SNPs in the 5′flanking region, four in the 5′UTR, and six in the 3′flanking region, and over 100 intronic SNPs); among them are the amino acid substitutions Arg110Cys in exon 4, Gly189Ser in exon 6, and Ile218Val in exon 7. The function of these polymorphisms is unknown.

3.6.4. *Thioredoxin*

The mammalian thioredoxin system consists of thioredoxin (TXN, TRX, Trx), thioredoxin reductase, and NADPH. The thioredoxin system can be found in all organisms. There are several isoforms of TXN; the classical TXN1,[282] mitochondrial TXN2,[283,284] thioredoxin-like protein 1 (Txl-1),[285–288] and Erdj5,[287,288] are all ubiquitously expressed. There are also two testis-specific forms, SpTrx-1[289] and SpTrx-2.[290] TXN1 is a 12 kDa protein,[291] and the gene is located on chromosome 9q31.[292] Mammalian TXN1 is involved in many cellular functions including synthesis of deoxyribonucleotides,[293] redox control of transcription factors,[294] reduction of peroxides,[295] and regulation of apoptosis.[296,297] TXN can be upregulated by several stimuli such as UV irradiation, oxygen, PAH, LPS inflammation and infection.[298–300] The protein is located in the cytoplasm but can relocate to the nucleus, where it acts in transcriptional control.[301] A truncated form of the protein (Trx80) has been found on the surface of monocytic cell lines.[302] Several polymorphisms can be found in the databases, but as of yet no function has been attributed, although TXN has been studied in regard to CVD.[303]

3.6.5. *Thioredoxin reductase*

Thioredoxin reductase (TrxR, TXNRD, TR) isoenzymes are NADPH-dependent homodimer oxidoreductases with one FAD per subunit that reduces the active site disulfide in oxidized thioredoxin.[304] Apart from reducing TXN, the TXNRDs also reduce low molecular weight disulfide and non-disulfide compounds such as lipoic acid,[305] selenite,[306] alloxan,[307] and peroxides.[308] TXNRD can be found in a number of different tissues, e.g. placenta, liver, and kidney. Mammalian TXNRD is about 55 kDa in molecular weight and has broad substrate specificity. There are three TXNRD isoforms found in mammals: the cytosolic TXNRD1, the mitochondrial TXNRD 2,[309–311] and one isoform expressed mainly in testis called thioredoxin and glutathione reductase (TGR).[311] The selenoprotein TXNRD1 has many vital antioxidant and redox regulatory functions. *TXNRD1* spans 100 kb and has 16 exons and can be found on chromosome 12. Mammalian *TXNRD1* and *TXNRD 2* exhibit alternative splicing around the first exon.[312,313] In humans, five different 5′cDNA variants have been reported as well as a variant with an apparent mass of 67 kDa.[313] Twenty-one different exon combinations arise from at least three separate promoters.[313–315] Several polymorphisms have been reported in databases, but their functions are still unknown. TNXRD 1 has also been studied in association with CVD.[303]

3.6.6. *Glutaredoxin*

Glutaredoxin (GRX) is a small (12 kDa) vicinal dithiol protein involved in various cellular functions, including the redox regulation of certain enzyme activities, protection against oxidative stress,[316,317] and apoptosis.[318,319] GRX functions via a disulfide exchange reaction by utilizing the active site Cys-Pro-Tyr-Cys, which specifically and effectively catalyzes the reduction of protein–S–S–glutathione mixed disulfide.[320] GRX is also known as thioltransferase. The *GRX* gene has been mapped to chromosome 5. GRX is generally considered intracellular but has also been found in the human placenta.[321] Human GRX has been shown to rescue cerebellar granule neurons from dopamine (DA)-induced oxidative stress.[319] In the dbSNP there are 35 SNPs reported: 20 of them are validated and four are genotyped. The function of these SNPs is unknown.

4. DNA repair

4.1. *8-Oxoguanine DNA glycosylase*

The 8-oxoguanine DNA glycosylase (OGG1) enzyme is responsible for the excision of 8-oxoguanine, a mutagenic base product that arises as a result of exposure to reactive oxygen. The action of this enzyme includes lyase activity for chain cleavage. The OGG1 is expressed in germinal center B cells, tonsil, and to a lesser extent in other lymphoid cells;[322] in the dark zones of germinal centers and in the nucleus.[323] The function and localization of OGG1 suggest that it may also play a role in somatic hypermutation of immunoglobulin genes.

The human *OGG1* gene is mapped to chromosome 3p25 (3p25.3-p25.2)[324] and consists of seven exons and six introns.[325]

A C>G polymorphism at position 1245 in exon 7 was associated with an exchange of an amino acid, serine to cysteine, in codon 326. A silent polymorphism was found at codon 98 in exon 2, while three others were present in the non-coding region of the *hOGG1* gene. This region shows loss of heterozygosity (LOH) in a variety of human cancers.[326,327] The Ser326Cys polymorphism was not associated with altered OGG1 activity.[328] It was shown that the Cys allele was associated with increased development of different types of cancer,[329–334] but this association was not confirmed in two other studies.[335,336] The mutant forms Arg46Gln (alpha-hOgg1-Gln(46)) and Arg154His (alpha-hOgg1-His(154)) found in human tumors are defective in their catalytic capacities.[337]

4.2. *Generation of reactive oxygen and nitrogen species*

4.2.1. *NADPH oxidase*

The NADPH oxidases are a group of plasma membrane — associated enzymes found in a variety of cells of mesodermal origin. The most thoroughly studied of these is the leukocyte NADPH oxidase, which is found in professional phagocytes and B lymphocytes. It catalyzes the production of superoxide (O_2^-) by the one-electron reduction of oxygen, using NADPH as the electron donor.

The O_2^- generated by this enzyme serves as the starting material for the production of a vast assortment of reactive oxidants, including oxidized halogens, free radicals, and singlet oxygen. The core enzyme comprises five components: p40phox (PHOX for phagocyte oxidase); p47phox and p67phox, existing in the cytosol as a complex; and two components, p22phox and gp91phox, located in the membranes of secretory vesicles and specific granules, where they occur as a heterodimeric flavohemoprotein known as cytochrome b558.[338] Each component is coded by its own gene.

The *CYBA* gene encodes the alpha subunit, also known as the light chain, of cytochrome b558 or p22phox. This gene was mapped to chromosome 16q24 and contains six exons.[339] There are several variations identified in this gene that show association with autosomal recessive cytochrome b-negative chronic granulomatous disease.[340–342] The −930A>G polymorphism in the p22phox promoter may be a novel genetic marker associated with hypertension. It was shown that the G allele had higher promoter activity than did the A allele.[343]

Parkos *et al.*[344] identified a 242C>T polymorphism in the *CYBA* gene that leads to a His72Tyr substitution. This polymorphism affects NAD(P)H oxidase activity and oxidation of lipoproteins by altering the redox state in the vasculature.[345] It also has a major effect on acetylcholine-mediated endothelium-dependent vasodilation and the basal NO-mediated vascular tone of the human forearm circulation in subjects with hypercholesterolemia.[346] Tyr72 is associated with ischemic cerebrovascular disease in Japanese[347–349] and UK populations.[350] The enzyme plays a significant role in atherosclerosis,[351,352] in progression of asymptomatic atherosclerosis,[353] and in development of diabetic nephropathy[354] in subjects with T2D. The polymorphism was not associated with lipid peroxidation and was not a genetic risk marker for several diseases in various populations.[355–361]

A 640A>G polymorphism of the *CYBA* gene is independently associated with the presence and extent of CAD.[362] There is no association between 214C>T, 521C>T, and *24A>G polymorphisms and the occurrence of cerebral aneurysms in Caucasians.[363]

The *CYBB* gene product has also been referred to as gp91phox.[364] The *CYBB* gene was identified at Xp21.[365] In this gene several variations showed an association with chronic granulomatous disease.[364,366–373]

4.2.2. *Myeloperoxidase*

Myeloperoxidase (MPO) is an antimicrobial oxidative enzyme found in phagocytes responsible for the production of hypochlorous acid. MPO catalyzes both one- and two-electron oxidations.

The human *MPO* gene is located on chromosome 17q22-q24.[374] The *MPO* gene has a few common polymorphisms: a C>T transition at codon 569, resulting in an arginine (CGG)-to-tryptophan (TGG) substitution and creating a new *BglII* site,[375] a Tyr173Cys missense variation,[376] a T>C transition causing the non-conservative replacement Met251Thr, and a 14-bp deletion within exon 9.[377] A functional G>A SNP has been identified at position −463, where the A allele is associated with lower MPO expression.[378]

Reynolds *et al.*[379] found that the presence of the *MPO* A allele significantly increased the risk of AD in men in a genetically homogeneous Finnish population, but in Caucasians the *MPO* GG genotype contributes a 1.57-fold increased risk for AD.[380] This association was not confirmed in a Spanish population[381] and in the ApoEurope Study.[382]

This −463G>A promoter polymorphism has been linked with numerous diseases such as acute promyelocytic leukemia,[383] CAD,[378,384–387] aerodigestive tract cancer,[388] hepatoblastoma,[389] and esophageal cancer.[390] London *et al.*[391] were the first to show an association between the *MPO* genotype and lung cancer risk. Subsequently, several studies have been performed and the results concerning the association between lung cancer and this polymorphism are still a matter of debate.[392–400]

A few different variations have been found in the *MPO* gene that are associated with MPO deficiency.[376,377,401]

4.2.3. *Nitric oxide synthase*

Nitric oxide synthases (NOSs) are a group of related proteins that catalyze the five-electron oxidation of the amino acid L-arginine to form L-citrulline and nitric oxide (NO). In mammals, there are three known members of this gene family: neuronal nitric oxide (NO) synthase — nNOS (NOS1), inducible nitric oxide synthase — iNOS (NOS2), and endothelial nitric oxide synthase — eNOS (NOS3).

4.2.4. *Nitric oxide synthase 1*

The neuronal nitric oxide synthase (NOS1; EC 1.14.13.39) is constitutively expressed in a variety of tissues including neurons of the peripheral and central nervous system, skeletal muscle, and airway epithelial cells.[402,403]

The human *NOS1* gene has been mapped to region 12q24.2 on chromosome 12.[404] The gene contains a number of highly polymorphic repeats that are potentially useful in genetic analysis.[405]

Allelic frequencies of a (CA)n dinucleotide repeat in exon 29 and an intronic (AAT)n trinucleotide repeat in *NOS1* vary significantly regarding allele frequency between American-Caucasian and African-American healthy subjects.[406] Recent studies have shown that excessive NO formation from NOS1 in neurological disorders leads to neural injury in the central and peripheral nervous system.[407] *NOS1* may also play a role in Duchenne muscular dystrophy.[408] In genetic studies, the *NOS1* gene has been found to display linkage disequilibrium with infantile pyloric stenosis.[409] Recently an association was observed between a polymorphism in the *NOS1* gene and asthma.[410,411] The number of (AAT)n repeats in intron 20 of the *NOS1* gene may associate with atopy.[412] For an (AAT)n repeat polymorphism in intron 20 of *NOS1* an association with development of cystic fibrosis was observed.[413]

New SNPs have been found in the *NOS1* gene (3391C>T and 5266 C>T) that show association with the development of asthma.[414]

Shinkai *et al.*[415] found genetic association in a novel SNP, a C>T transition located 276 base pairs downstream from the translation termination site of the human *NOS1* gene and schizophrenia, but in another study this association was not confirmed.[416] In a Danish and British case-control study, there was no association between this polymorphism and bipolar disorder.[417]

4.2.5. *Nitric oxide synthase 2*

The *NOS2* gene is mapped to chromosome 17q11.2-q12[418] and contains 27 exons, with translation initiation and termination in exons 2 and 27, respectively.[419]

In the human *NOS2* promoter region three different polymorphisms have been identified: a G>C in position −954 (GenBank accession number: X97821) introducing a restriction enzyme site (*BsaI*)[420] and two microsatellites — a biallelic tetranucleotide repeat sequence, (TAAA)n,[421] and a highly polymorphic (nine alleles) pentanucleotide repeat sequence (CCTTT)n.[422] The G>C exchange has been associated with protection from all forms of severe malaria.[420] *Ex vivo* studies showed that cells isolated from people with this polymorphism have a seven-fold higher baseline NOS activity, compared with the levels detected in cells from subjects with the wild-type gene.[422]

Highly significant differences have been found in the allele frequencies of a (CCTTT)n pentanucleotide repeat in the *NOS2* promoter region between five specific population groups in four continents: Africa, Europe, Asia, and the Caribbean.[424] Allele *14* of (CCTTT)n polymorphic marker correlated with a decreased risk for development of diabetic retinopathy[425] and diabetic nephropathy with T1D.[426] Furthermore, this allele was associated with protection against the development of asthma[427] and essential hypertension.[428] The (CCTTT)n pentanucleotide microsatellite does not play a major role in celiac disease development,[429] RA,[430] brucellosis,[431] and systemic lupus erythematosus,[432] although the −954G>C and CCTTT-8 repeat polymorphisms were in linkage disequilibrium among African-American female systemic lupus erythematosus patients.[433]

The polymorphisms (TAAA)n and (CCTTT)n within the *NOS2* gene promoter did not show a linkage to T1D in a Danish family material.[434]

Johannesen *et al.*[435] performed a scanning of all 27 exons of the human *NOS2* gene and linkage transmission disequilibrium testing of identified *NOS2* polymorphisms in a Danish nationwide T1D family collection. In total, 10 polymorphisms were identified in eight exons, of which four were tested in the family material. A C>T exchange in exon 16 resulting in an amino acid substitution, Ser608Leu, showed linkage to IDDM in humans.

A novel single-nucleotide polymorphism −1173C>T was recently identified in the *NOS2* gene and shows significant association with protection from symptomatic malaria and severe malarial anemia in Tanzania and Kenya.[436] The −1173C>T polymorphism was associated with increased fasting urine and plasma NO metabolite concentrations in Tanzanian children, suggesting that the polymorphism was functional *in vivo*.

4.2.6. *Nitric oxide synthase 3*

The *NOS3* gene is located on chromosome 7q35-q36.[404] Most studies used three polymorphic markers, −786C>T in the promoter region,[437] the 27-bp repeat polymorphism in intron 4 (the larger allele had five tandem 27-bp repeats and the smaller allele had only four repeats — ecNOS4a/4b),[438] and a G>T substitution at position 894 in exon 7, resulting in a change in glutamic acid to aspartic acid at amino acid position 298 (Glu298Asp).[439]

The −786T variant in the promoter region of the *NOS3* reduced transcription of the gene and was strongly associated with coronary spastic angina and myocardial infarction[437] and CAD.[440] The T allele may also reduce vascular invasion in breast cancer and consequently reduce metastatic spread and be a favorable prognostic factor. These results need further validation in larger studies.[441] Allele C of this polymorphism associated with early CAD in Spain[442] and is a risk factor for the development of moderate to severe internal carotid artery stenosis, especially ulcerative lesions.[443] The −786C variant was more common in Caucasians (42.0%) than in African-Americans (17.5%) or Asians (13.8%).

The 4a allele of the ecNOS4a/4b polymorphism of the *NOS3* gene is associated with ischemic heart disease development,[444] diastolic dysfunction in patients with essential hypertension,[445] pre-eclampsia,[446] systolic hypertension,[447] and a risk factor for development of idiopathic recurrent miscarriage.[446] In the same study, allele 4a was also associated with increased development of diabetic nephropathy,[448–450] but not in other studies.[451,452] Moreover, allelic variation within intron 4 of *NOS3* is associated with an advanced tumor stage and positive lymph node involvement in ovarian cancer.[453] The 4a allele in intron 4 was more common in African-Americans (26.5%) than in Caucasians (16.0%) or Asians (12.9%).[454]

The Asp298 variant was more common in Caucasians (34.5%) than in African-Americans (15.5%) or Asians (8.6%). The A allele of the Glu298Asp polymorphism has been linked to an increased risk for stroke,[455,456] myocardial infarction in English, and Japanese subjects,[439,458] hypertension,[459] and hypertension in pregnancy.[460] The Asp298 variant of *NOS3* is associated with poorer event-free survival, particularly in patients with non-ischemic cardiomyopathy,[461] and a risk factor for elevated plasma homocysteine concentrations in healthy non-smoking adults.[462]

In the case of late-onset AD, one study showed a significant association between the Glu allele of *NOS3* and late-onset AD,[463] while other studies showed no association between the missense Glu298Asp variant and AD in different populations.[464–470] There was no association between the missense Glu298Asp variant of *NOS3* and development of idiopathic recurrent miscarriage,[453] familial hypercholestrolemia,[471] and asthma.[472,473]

Derebecka *et al.*[474] studied the distribution of genotypes and frequency of alleles of the 11G>T polymorphism in intron 23 of the *NOS3* gene in patients with hypertension and in a control group of healthy individuals. No major differences in the distribution of the 11G>T polymorphism in the patients and healthy individuals were found.

4.3. *Receptor for advanced glycation end-products*

The receptor for advanced glycation end-products (RAGE) is a 35 kDa polypeptide belonging to the immunoglobin superfamily of receptors. The gene is located on chromosome 6p21.3 in the MHC-region, containing 11 exons and 10 introns.[475] Advanced glycation end-products (AGE) result from non-enzymatic glycation of proteins and lipids.[476,477] Binding of AGEs to RAGE has been shown to induce multiple effects, resulting in oxidative stress, cellular dysfunction, and cellular activation of NF-κB,[478] an oxidative stress marker. RAGE is normally expressed at low levels by the endothelium, smooth muscles, mesangial, and monocytes. High levels are found in the retina, mesangial, and aortic vessels in human diabetic subjects.[479] Several polymorphisms have been found in the 5′regulatory region of *RAGE*. −429 T>C, −374 T>A, and the −407 to −345 deletion, resulting in significantly increased gene transcription in CAT reporter assays.[480] The −374 T>A polymorphism has been associated with diabetic neuropathy in T1D patients with poor metabolic control. The promoter polymorphism −1152C>A is also weakly associated with neuropathy in T1D patients.[481] Three polymorphisms, a common 555G>A in exon 3, 1704G>T intron 7, and 2184A>G intron 8, are together associated with diabetes-associated microvascular dermatoses/microvascular dermatoses (DAMD/MD)).[482,483] The 1704 G>T polymorphism is associated with lower plasma levels of several antioxidants (total carotenoids, lutein, lycopene and tocopherol). The same polymorphism, together with the NADPH oxidase p22 phox 242C>T polymorphism, is significantly associated with an increased risk of diabetic neuropathy in Japanese T2D patients.[354] In the SNP database there are 34 possible SNPs where 17 are verified.

5. Conclusions

In general, it can be stated that lack of expression of protective enzymes only occurs in the large gene family of glutathione transferases. This is perhaps less surprising since humans have more than 20 enzymes displaying overlapping function.[484] What is more remarkable is the rare condition of acatalasemia and the fact that subjects are in general healthy.[485] Most likely, the large number and variety of enzymes (glutathione peroxidases and peroxiredoxins) that can reduce hydrogen peroxide serve as replacements. As many of these enzymes can be upregulated by oxidative stress,[149,486] a compensatory increase could preserve homeostasis. It is remarkable however that overexpression of many of these enzymes confer cellular protection despite the fact that many overlapping protective systems exist. Perhaps, antioxidant enzyme capacity is finely tuned to meet the demands of cellular protection, at the same time allowing redox fluctuations that modulate signal transduction and gene regulatory processes.

Many enzymes, including glutathione transferase, quinone reductase, epoxide hydrolase, superoxide dismutases, and 8-OH dG glycosidase, contain amino acid alterations that affect protein stability, catalytic activity, or subcellular/extracellular distribution and thus are useful tools in association studies. It is interesting that, although diminished/altered function/distribution is tolerated in these enzymes, complete lack of activity does not occur. For some of these enzymes such as mitochondrial superoxide dismutase and phospholipid hydroperoxide glutathione peroxidase, this is consistent with the lethal consequences in mice targeted disruption (knock-outs) experiments.[487,488]

An increasing number of variants in gene regulatory regions are being characterized. The comparative ease and consistent set of experimental tools (gene reporter and gel mobility shift assays) used are an advantage. However, as influences from upstream/downstream, intronic and non-coding-transcribed sequence segments cannot be ruled out, in principle all variants have to be tested. In addition, mRNA stability also needs to be determined. In general, the abundance of genetic variants outside coding and regulatory regions are often more difficult to evaluate functionally. A useful strategy is to study common haplotypes both in functional assays and in association studies. This makes it possible to study the complexity of interacting genetic variants but also potentially adds power to the association analysis. It is known that haplotypes can associate with disease, whereas the individual genetic variants SNPs determining the haplotype do not.[162]

Several new candidate genes that could be used to study oxidative stress related disease are described: examples include the genes involved in vitamin E uptake, peroxiredoxins, and glutaredoxin.

In summary, the molecular genetic tools for studying oxidative stress related disease are becoming more numerous and more well defined, offering the possibility of studying a majority of these genes in association studies.

Acknowledgments

Studies from the authors laboratories were supported by the Swedish Research Council, the Swedish Cancer Society and funds from Karolinska Institutet.

Abbreviations

AD	Alzheimer's disease
AGE	Advanced glycation end-products
α-TTP	α-Tocopherol transfer protein
ALS	Amyotrophic lateral sclerosis
AVED	Ataxia associated vitamin E deficiency
CAD	Coronary artery disease
CAT	Catalase
CoQ	Coenzyme Q
CVD	Cardiovascular disease
DAMD	Diabetes-associated microvascular dermatoses
dbSNP	Database of single nucleotide polymorphisms, small-scale insertions/deletions, polymorphic repetitive elements, and microsatellite variation
DPN	Diabetic polyneuropathy
FAD	Flavin-adenin-dinucleotide
FLAP-5	Lipooxygenase activating enzyme
γ-GCS	γ-Glutamylcysteine synthase
γ-GCSL	Light subunit
γ-GCSH	Heavy subunit
GPX	Glutathione peroxidase
GR	Glutathione reductase
GRX	Glutaredoxin
GS	Glutathione synthetase
GST	Glutathione S-transferase
HDL	High-density lipoprotein
HMG	CoA-hydroxy-3-methylglutaryl
HNF	Hepatic nuclear factor
HO	Heme oxygenase

I/D	Insertion/deletion
LDL	Low-density lipoprotein
LOH	Loss of heterozygosity
LPS	Lipopolysaccharides
LTC_4S	Leukotriene C_4 synthase
MAPEG	Membrane associated proteins in eicosanoid and glutathione metabolism
MD	Microvascular dermatoses
mEH	Microsomal epoxide hydrolase
MGST	Microsomal glutathione S-transferase
MPO	Myeloperoxidase
NADPH	Nicotinamide-adenine-dinucleotide-phosphate
NOS	Nitric oxide synthase
NRH	Dihydronicotinamide riboside
NQO	NAD(P)H:quinone oxidoreductase
OGG1	8-Oxoguanine DNA glycosylase
PAH	Polyaromatic hydrocarbons
PD	Parkinsons disease
PON	Paraoxonase
Prx	Peroxiredoxins
RA	Rhematoid arthritis
RAGE	Receptor for advanced glycation end-products
RFLP	Restriction fragment length polymorphism
ROS	Reactive oxygen species
sEH	Soluble epoxide hydrolase
SNP	Single nucleotide polymorphism
SOD	Superoxide dismutase
Sp1	Specific protein 1
SRB1	Scavenger receptor class B
T1D	Type 1 diabetes
T2D	Type 2 diabetes
TXN	Thioredoxin
TXNRD	Thioredoxin reductase
UGT	UDP-glucuronosyltransferase
UTR	Untranslated region

References

1. Halliwell B, Gutteridge J. *Free Radicals in Biology and Medicine*. Clarendon press, Oxford, 1989.
2. Esposito F, Ammendola R, Faraonio R, Russo T, Cimino F. Redox control of signal transduction, gene expression and cellular senescence. *Neurochem. Res.* 29: 617–628 (2004).
3. Kwon YW, Masutani H, Nakamura H, Ishii Y, Yodoi J. Redox regulation of cell growth and cell death. *Biol. Chem.* 384: 991–996 (2003).
4. Forsberg L, de Faire U, Morgenstern R. Oxidative stress, human genetic variation, and disease [Review]. *Arch. Biochem. Biophys.* 389: 84–93 (2001).
5. Emahazion T, Feuk L, Jobs M, Sawyer SL, Fredman D, St Clair D, Prince JA, Brookes AJ. SNP association studies in Alzheimer's disease highlight problems for complex disease analysis. *Trends Genet.* 17: 407–413 (2001).
6. Zelko IN, Mariani TJ, Folz RJ. Superoxide dismutase multigene family: a comparison of the CuZn-SOD (SOD1), Mn-SOD (SOD2), and EC-SOD (SOD3) gene structures, evolution, and expression. *Free Radic. Biol. Med.* 33: 337–349 (2002).
7. Orrell RW, Marklund SL, deBelleroche JS. Familial ALS is associated with mutations in all exons of SOD1: a novel mutation in exon 3 (Gly72Ser). *J. Neurol. Sci.* 153: 46–49 (1997).
8. Huret JL, Delabar JM, Marlhens F, Aurias A, Nicole A, Berthier M, Tanzer J, Sinet PM. Down syndrome with duplication of a region of chromosome 21 containing the CuZn superoxide dismutase gene without detectable karyotypic abnormality. *Hum. Genet.* 75: 251–257 (1987).
9. Aoki M, Ogasawara M, Matsubara Y, Narisawa K, Nakamura S, Itoyama Y, Abe K. Familial amyotrophic lateral sclerosis (ALS) in Japan associated with H46R mutation in Cu/Zn superoxide dismutase gene: a possible new subtype of familial ALS. *J. Neurol. Sci.* 126: 77–83 (1994).
10. Gaudette M, Hirano M, Siddique T. Current status of SOD1 mutations in familial amyotrophic lateral sclerosis. *Amyotroph. Lateral Scler. Other Motor Neuron Disord.* 1: 83–89 (2000).
11. Hand CK, Mayeux-Portas V, Khoris J, Briolotti V, Clavelou P, Camu W, Rouleau GA. Compound heterozygous D90A and D96N SOD1 mutations in a recessive amyotrophic lateral sclerosis family. *Ann. Neurol.* 49: 267–271 (2001).
12. Lindberg MJ, Tibell L, Oliveberg M. Common denominator of Cu/Zn superoxide dismutase mutants associated with amyotrophic lateral sclerosis: decreased stability of the apo state. *Proc. Natl. Acad. Sci. USA* 99: 16607–16612 (2002).

13. Liu H, Zhu H, Eggers DK, Nersissian AM, Faull KF, Goto JJ, Ai J, Sanders-Loehr J, Gralla EB, Valentine JS. Copper(2+) binding to the surface residue cysteine 111 of His46Arg human copper-zinc superoxide dismutase, a familial amyotrophic lateral sclerosis mutant. *Biochemistry* 39: 8125–8132 (2000).
14. Rosen DR *et al.* Mutations in Cu/Zn superoxide dismutase gene are associated with familial amyotrophic lateral sclerosis. *Nature* 362: 59–62 (1993).
15. Stathopulos PB, Rumfeldt JA, Scholz GA, Irani RA, Frey HE, Hallewell RA, Lepock JR, Meiering EM. Cu/Zn superoxide dismutase mutants associated with amyotrophic lateral sclerosis show enhanced formation of aggregates *in vitro*. *Proc. Natl. Acad. Sci. USA* 100: 7021–7026 (2003).
16. Alexander MD, Traynor BJ, Miller N, Corr B, Frost E, McQuaid S, Brett FM, Green A, Hardiman O. "True" sporadic ALS associated with a novel SOD-1 mutation. *Ann. Neurol.* 52: 680–683 (2002).
17. Gellera C, Castellotti B, Riggio MC, Silani V, Morandi L, Testa D, Casali C, Taroni F, Di Donato S, Zeviani M, Mariotti C. Superoxide dismutase gene mutations in Italian patients with familial and sporadic amyotrophic lateral sclerosis: identification of three novel missense mutations. *Neuromuscul. Disord.* 11: 404–410 (2001).
18. Mancuso M, Filosto M, Naini A, Rocchi A, Del Corona A, Sartucci F, Siciliano G, Murri L. A screening for superoxide dismutase-1 D90A mutation in Italian patients with sporadic amyotrophic lateral sclerosis. *Amyotroph. Lateral Scler. Other Motor Neuron Disord.* 3: 215–218 (2002).
19. Parton MJ, Broom W, Andersen PM, Al-Chalabi A, Nigel Leigh P, Powell JF, Shaw CE. D90A-SOD1 mediated amyotrophic lateral sclerosis: a single founder for all cases with evidence for a Cis-acting disease modifier in the recessive haplotype. *Hum. Mutat.* 20: 473 (2002).
20. Segovia-Silvestre T, Andreu AL, Vives-Bauza C, Garcia-Arumi E, Cervera C, Gamez J. A novel exon 3 mutation (D76V) in the SOD1 gene associated with slowly progressive ALS. *Amyotroph. Lateral Scler. Other Motor Neuron Disord.* 3: 69–74 (2002).
21. Hirano M, Hung WY, Cole N, Azim AC, Deng HX, Siddique T. Multiple transcripts of the human Cu,Zn superoxide dismutase gene. *Biochem. Biophys. Res. Commun.* 276: 52–56 (2000).
22. Valentine JS, Hart PJ. Misfolded CuZnSOD and amyotrophic lateral sclerosis. *Proc. Natl. Acad. Sci. USA* 100: 3617–3622 (2003).
23. Church SL, Grant JW, Meese EU, Trent JM. Sublocalization of the gene encoding manganese superoxide dismutase (MnSOD/SOD2) to 6q25 by

fluorescence in situ hybridization and somatic cell hybrid mapping. *Genomics* 14: 823–825 (1992).

24. Van Landeghem GF, Tabatabaie P, Beckman G, Beckman L, Andersen PM. Manganese-containing superoxide dismutase signal sequence polymorphism associated with sporadic motor neuron disease. *Eur. J. Neurol.* 6: 639–644 (1999).
25. Hiroi S, Harada H, Nishi H, Satoh M, Nagai R, Kimura A. Polymorphisms in the SOD2 and HLA-DRB1 genes are associated with non-familial idiopathic dilated cardiomyopathy in Japanese. *Biochem. Biophys. Res. Commun.* 261: 332–339 (1999).
26. Tomblyn M, Kasarskis EJ, Xu Y, St Clair DK. Distribution of MnSOD polymorphisms in sporadic ALS patients. *J. Mol. Neurosci.* 10: 65–66 (1998).
27. Tomkins J, Banner SJ, McDermott CJ, Shaw PJ. Mutation screening of manganese superoxide dismutase in amyotrophic lateral sclerosis. *Neuroreport* 12: 2319–2322 (2001).
28. Mattey DL, Hassell AB, Dawes PT, Jones PW, Yengi L, Alldersea J, Strange RC, Fryer AA. Influence of polymorphism in the manganese superoxide dismutase locus on disease outcome in rheumatoid arthritis: evidence for interaction with glutathione S-transferase genes. *Arthritis Rheum.* 43: 859–864 (2000).
29. Shimoda-Matsubayashi S, Matsumine H, Kobayashi T, Nakagawa-Hattori Y, Shimizu Y, Mizuno Y. Structural dimorphism in the mitochondrial targeting sequence in the human manganese superoxide dismutase gene. *Biochem. Biophys. Res. Commun.* 226: 561–565 (1996).
30. Farin FM, Hitosis Y, Hallagan SE, Kushleika J, Woods JS, Janssen PS, Smith-Weller T, Franklin GM, Swanson PD, Checkoway H. Genetic polymorphisms of superoxide dismutase in Parkinson's disease. *Mov. Disord.* 16: 705–707 (2001).
31. Grasbon-Frodl EM, Kosel S, Riess O, Muller U, Mehraein P, Graeber MB. Analysis of mitochondrial targeting sequence and coding region polymorphisms of the manganese superoxide dismutase gene in German Parkinson disease patients. *Biochem. Biophys. Res. Commun.* 255: 749–752 (1999).
32. Ambrosone CB, Freudenheim JL, Thompson PA, Bowman E, Vena JE, Marshall JR, Graham S, Laughlin R, Nemoto T, Shields PG. Manganese superoxide dismutase (MnSOD) genetic polymorphisms, dietary antioxidants, and risk of breast cancer. *Cancer Res.* 59: 602–606 (1999).
33. Mitrunen K, Sillanpaa P, Kataja V, Eskelinen M, Kosma VM, Benhamou S, Uusitupa M, Hirvonen A. Association between manganese superoxide

dismutase (MnSOD) gene polymorphism and breast cancer risk. *Carcinogenesis* 22: 827–829 (2001).

34. Knight JA, Onay UV, Wells S, Li H, Shi EJ, Andrulis IL, Ozcelik H. Genetic variants of GPX1 and SOD2 and breast cancer risk at the Ontario site of the Breast Cancer Family Registry. *Cancer Epidemiol. Biomarkers Prev.* 13: 146–149 (2004).
35. Pittman GS, Millikan RC, Bell DA. The SOD2 Val-9Ala polymorphism and its association with breast cancer in a population-based case-control study. *Proc. Am. Assoc. Cancer Res.* 42: 340–341 (2001).
36. Stoehlmacher J, Ingles SA, Park DJ, Zhang W, Lenz HJ. The −9Ala/−9Val polymorphism in the mitochondrial targeting sequence of the manganese superoxide dismutase gene (MnSOD) is associated with age among Hispanics with colorectal carcinoma. *Oncol. Rep.* 9: 235–238 (2002).
37. Nomiyama T, Tanaka Y, Piao L, Nagasaka K, Sakai K, Ogihara T, Nakajima K, Watada H, Kawamori R. The polymorphism of manganese superoxide dismutase is associated with diabetic nephropathy in Japanese type 2 diabetic patients. *J. Hum. Genet.* 48: 138–141 (2003).
38. Zotova EV, Chistiakov DA, Savost'ianov KV, Bursa TR, Galeev IV, Strokov IA, Nosikov VV. Association of the SOD2 Ala(−9)Val and SOD3 Arg213Gly polymorphisms with diabetic polyneuropathy in patients with diabetes mellitus type 1. *Mol. Biol. (Mosk.)* 37: 404–408 (2003).
39. Zhang HJ, Yan T, Oberley TD, Oberley LW. Comparison of effects of two polymorphic variants of manganese superoxide dismutase on human breast MCF-7 cancer cell phenotype. *Cancer Res.* 59: 6276–6283 (1999).
40. Xu Y, Krishnan A, Wan XS, Majima H, Yeh CC, Ludewig G, Kasarskis EJ, St Clair DK. Mutations in the promoter reveal a cause for the reduced expression of the human manganese superoxide dismutase gene in cancer cells. *Oncogene* 18: 93–102 (1999).
41. Hernandez-Saavedra D, McCord JM. Paradoxical effects of thiol reagents on Jurkat cells and a new thiol-sensitive mutant form of human mitochondrial superoxide dismutase. *Cancer Res.* 63: 159–163 (2003).
42. Marklund SL. Extracellular superoxide dismutase in human tissues and human cell lines. *J. Clin. Invest.* 74: 1398–1403 (1984).
43. Folz RJ, Crapo JD. Extracellular superoxide dismutase (SOD3): tissue-specific expression, genomic characterization, and computer-assisted sequence analysis of the human EC SOD gene. *Genomics* 22: 162–171 (1994).
44. Hendrickson DJ, Fisher JH, Jones C, Ho YS. Regional localization of human extracellular superoxide dismutase gene to 4pter-q21. *Genomics* 8: 736–738 (1990).

45. Folz RJ, Peno-Green L, Crapo JD. Identification of a homozygous missense mutation (Arg to Gly) in the critical binding region of the human EC-SOD gene (SOD3) and its association with dramatically increased serum enzyme levels. *Hum. Mol. Genet.* 3: 2251–2254 (1994).
46. Sandstrom J, Nilsson P, Karlsson K, Marklund SL. Ten-fold increase in human plasma extracellular superoxide dismutase content caused by a mutation in heparin-binding domain. *J. Biol. Chem.* 269: 19163–19166 (1994).
47. Yamada H, Yamada Y, Adachi T, Goto H, Ogasawara N, Futenma A, Kitano M, Hirano K, Kato K. Molecular analysis of extracellular-superoxide dismutase gene associated with high level in serum. *Jpn. J. Hum. Genet.* 40: 177–184 (1995).
48. Marklund SL, Nilsson P, Israelsson K, Schampi I, Peltonen M, Asplund K. Two variants of extracellular-superoxide dismutase: relationship to cardiovascular risk factors in an unselected middle-aged population. *J. Intern. Med.* 242: 5–14 (1997).
49. Adachi T, Yamazaki N, Tasaki H, Toyokawa T, Yamashita K, Hirano K. Changes in the heparin affinity of extracellular-superoxide dismutase in patients with coronary artery atherosclerosis. *Biol. Pharm. Bull.* 21: 1090–1093 (1998).
50. Sakashita N, Ando Y, Marklund SL, Nilsson P, Tashima K, Yamashita T, Takahashi K. Familial amyloidotic polyneuropathy type I with extracellular superoxide dismutase mutation: a case report. *Hum. Pathol.* 29: 1169–1172 (1998).
51. Ukkola O, Erkkila PH, Savolainen MJ, Kesaniemi YA. Lack of association between polymorphisms of catalase, copper-zinc superoxide dismutase (SOD), extracellular SOD and endothelial nitric oxide synthase genes and macroangiopathy in patients with type 2 diabetes mellitus. *J. Intern. Med.* 249: 451–459 (2001).
52. Yamada H, Yamada Y, Adachi T, Goto H, Ogasawara N, Futenma A, Kitano M, Miyai H, Fukatsu A, Hirano K, Kakumu S. Polymorphism of extracellular superoxide dismutase (EC-SOD) gene: relation to the mutation responsible for high EC-SOD level in serum. *Jpn. J. Hum. Genet.* 42: 353–356 (1997).
53. Deisseroth A, Dounce AL. Catalase: physical and chemical properties, mechanism of catalysis, and physiological role. *Physiol. Rev.* 50: 319–375 (1970).
54. Quan F, Korneluk R, Tropak M, Gravel R. Isolation and characterization of the human catalse gene. *Nucleic Acids Res.* 14: 5321–5335 (1986).
55. Hunt CR, Sim JE, Sullivan SJ, Featherstone T, Golden W, Von Kapp-Herr C, Hock RA, Gomez RA, Parsian AJ, Spitz DR. Genomic instability and catalase

gene amplification induced by chronic exposure to oxidative stress. *Cancer Res.* 58: 3986–3992 (1998).

56. Chen F, Ritter JK, Wang MG, McBride OW, Lubet RA, Owens IS. Characterization of a cloned human dihydrotestosterone/androstanediol UDP-glucuronosyltransferase and its comparison to other steroid isoforms. *Biochemistry* 32: 10648–10657 (1993).
57. Kishimoto Y, Murakami Y, Hayashi K, Takahara S, Sugimura T, Sekiya T. Detection of a common mutation of the catalase gene in Japanese acatalasemic patients. *Hum. Genet.* 88: 487–490 (1992).
58. Hirono A, Sasaya-Hamada F, Kanno H, Fuji H, Yoshida T, Miwa S. A novel human catalase mutation (358 T-del) causing Japanese type acatalasemia. *Blood Cell. Mol. Dis.* 21: 232–233 (1995).
59. Aebi H, Bossi E, Cantz M, Matsubara S, Suter H. In: Beutler E (ed.) *Hereditary Disorders of Erythrocyte Metabolism*. Grune and Stratton, New York, 1968, pp. 41–83.
60. Goth L, Gorzsas A, Kalmar T. A simple PCR-heteroduplex screening method for detection of a common mutation of the catalase gene in Hungary. *Clin. Chem.* 46: 1199–1200 (2000).
61. Góth L, Shemirani A, Kalmár T. A novel catalase mutation (a GA insertion) causes the Hungarian type of acatalasemia. *Blood Cells Mol. Dis.* 26: 151–154 (2000).
62. Goth L. A new type of inherited catalase deficiencies: its characterization and comparison to the Japanese and Swiss type of acatalasemia. *Blood Cells Mol. Dis.* 27: 512–517 (2001).
63. Forsberg L, Lyrenäs L, de Faire U, Morgenstern R. A common C-T substitution polymorphism in the promoter region of the human catalase gene influences transcription factor binding, reporter gene transcription and is correlated to blood catalase levels. *Free Radic. Biol. Med.* 30: 500–505 (2001).
64. Goulas A, Fidani L, Kotsis A, Mirtsou V, Petersen RC, Tangalos E, Hardy J. An association study of a functional catalase gene polymorphism, $-262C \rightarrow T$, and patients with Alzheimer's disease. *Neurosci. Lett.* 330: 210–213 (2002).
65. Ahsan H, Chen Y, Kibriya MG, Islam MN, Slavkovich VN, Graziano JH, Santella RM. Susceptibility to arsenic-induced hyperkeratosis and oxidative stress genes myeloperoxidase and catalase. *Cancer Lett.* 201: 57–65 (2003).
66. Zotova E, Savost'yanov K, Christyakov D, Bursa T, Galeev I, Strokov I, Nosikov V. Association of polymorphic markers of the antioxidant enzyme genes with diabetic polyneuropathy in type 1 diabetes mellitus. *Mol. Biol.* 38: 244–249 (2004).

67. Jiang Z, Akey JM, Shi J, Xiong M, Chen H, Wu H, Xiao J, Lu D, Huang W, Jin L. A polymorphism in the promoter region of catalase is associated with blood pressure levels. *Hum. Genet.* 109: 95–98 (2001).
68. Arthur JR. The glutathione peroxidases. *Cell. Mol. Life Sci.* 57: 1825–1835 (2000).
69. Kiss CLJ, Szeles A, Gizatullin RZ, Kashuba VI, Lushnikova T, Protopopov AI, Kelve M, Kiss H, Kholodnyuk ID, Imreh S, Klein G, Zabarovsky ER. Assignment of the ARHA and GPX1 genes to human chromosome bands 3p21.3 by *in situ* hybridization and with somatic cell hybrids. *Cytogenet. Cell Genet.* 79: 228–230 (1997).
70. Moscow JA, Schmidt L, Ingram DT, Gnarra J, Johnson B, Cowan KH. Loss of heterozygosity of the human cytosolic glutathione peroxidase I gene in lung cancer. *Carcinogenesis* 15(12): 2769–2773 (1994).
71. Ratnasinghe D, Tangrea JA, Andersen MR, Barrett MJ, Virtamo J, Taylor PR, Albanes D. Glutathione peroxidase codon 198 polymorphism variant increases lung cancer risk. *Cancer Res.* 60(22): 6381–6383 (2000).
72. Hu YJ, Diamond AM. Role of glutathione peroxidase 1 in breast cancer: loss of heterozygosity and allelic differences in the response to selenium. *Cancer Res.* 63(12): 3347–3351 (2003).
73. Forsberg L, de Faire U, Marklund SL, Andersson PM, Stegmayr B, Morgenstern R. Phenotype determination of a common Pro-Leu polymorphism in human glutathione peroxidase 1. *Blood Cells Mol. Dis.* 26(5): 423–426 (2000).
74. Blankenberg S, Rupprecht HJ, Bickel C, Torzewski M, Hafner G, Tiret L, Smieja M, Cambien F, Meyer J, Lackner KJ. Glutathione peroxidase 1 activity and cardiovascular events in patients with coronary artery disease. *N. Engl. J. Med.* 349(17): 1605–1613 (2003).
75. Winter JP, Gongy Y, Grant PJ, Wild CP. Glutathione peroxidase 1 genotype is associated with an increased risk of coronary artery disease. *Coron. Artery Dis.* 14(2): 149–153 (2003).
76. Kote-Jarai Z, Durocha F, Edwards SM, Hamoudi R, Jackson RA, Ardern-Jones A, Murkin A, Dearnaley DP, Kirby R, Houlston R, Easton DF, Eeles R. Association between the GCG polymorphism of the selenium dependent GPX1 gene and the risk of young onset prostate cancer. *Prostate Cancer Prostatic Dis.* 5(3): 189–192 (2002).
77. Kelner MJ, Montoya MA. Structural organization of the human selenium-dependent phospholipid hydroperoxide glutathione peroxidase gene (GPX4): chromosomal localization to 19p13.3. *Biochem. Biophys. Res. Commun.* 249: 53–55 (1998).

78. Brigelius-Flohe R *et al.* Phospholipid-hydroperoxide glutathione peroxidase. Genomic DNA, cDNA, and deduced amino acid sequence. *J. Biol. Chem.* 269: 7342–7348 (1994).
79. Foresta C, Flohe L, Garolla A, Roveri A, Ursini F, Maiorino M. Male fertility is linked to the selenoprotein phospholipid hydroperoxide glutathione peroxidase. *Biol. Reprod.* 67: 967–971 (2002).
80. Pushpa-Rekha TR, Burdsall AL, Oleksa LM, Chisolm GM, Driscoll DM. Rat phospholipid-hydroperoxide glutathione peroxidase. cDNA cloning and identification of multiple transcription and translation start sites. *J. Biol. Chem.* 270: 26993–26999 (1995).
81. Smith CW, Valcarcel J. Alternative pre-mRNA splicing: the logic of combinatorial control. *Trends Biochem. Sci.* 25: 381–388 (2000).
82. Maiorino M, Bosello V, Ursini F, Foresta C, Garolla A, Scapin M, Sztajer H, Flohe L. Genetic variations of gpx-4 and male infertility in humans. *Biol. Reprod.* 68: 1134–1141 (2003).
83. Chae HZ, Chung SJ, Rhee SG. Thioredoxin-dependent peroxide reductase from yeast. *J. Biol. Chem.* 269: 27670–27678 (1994).
84. Chae HZ, Robison K, Poole LB, Church G, Storz G, Rhee SG. Cloning and sequencing of thiol-specific antioxidant from mammalian brain: alkyl hydroperoxide reductase and thiol-specific antioxidant define a large family of antioxidant enzymes. *Proc. Natl. Acad. Sci. USA* 91: 7017–7021 (1994).
85. Hofmann B, Hecht HJ, Flohe L. Peroxiredoxins. *Biol. Chem.* 383: 347–364 (2002).
86. Mitsumoto A, Takanezawa Y, Okawa K, Iwamatsu A, Nakagawa Y. Variants of peroxiredoxins expression in response to hydroperoxide stress. *Free Radic. Biol. Med.* 30: 625–635 (2001).
87. Wood ZA, Schroder E, Robin Harris J, Poole LB. Structure, mechanism and regulation of peroxiredoxins. *Trends Biochem. Sci.* 28: 32–40 (2003).
88. Mannervik B. The isozymes of glutathione transferase. *Adv. Enzym. Relat. Areas Molec. Biol.* 57: 357–417 (1985).
89. Board PG. Biochemical genetics of glutathione-S-transferase in man. *Am. J. Hum. Genet.* 33: 36–43 (1981).
90. Hayes JD, Strange RC. Glutathione S-transferase polymorphisms and their biological consequences. *Pharmacology* 61(3): 154–166 (2000).
91. Morel F, Rauch C, Coles B, Le Ferrec E, Guillouzo A. The human glutathione transferase alpha locus: genomic organization of the gene cluster and functional characterization of the genetic polymorphism in the hGSTA1 promoter. *Pharmacogenetics* 12: 277–286 (2002).

92. Xu S, Wang Y, Roe B, Pearson WR. Characterization of the human class Mu glutathione S-transferase gene cluster and the GSTM1 deletion. *J. Biol. Chem.* 273: 3517–3527 (1998).
93. Rebbeck TR. Molecular epidemiology of the human glutathione S-transferase genotypes GSTM1 and GSTT1 in cancer susceptibility. *Cancer Epidemiol. Biomarkers Prev.* 6: 733–743 (1997).
94. Cotton SC, Sharp L, Little J, Brockton N. Glutathione S-transferase polymorphisms and colorectal cancer: a HuGE review. *Am. J. Epidemiol.* 151: 7–32 (2000).
95. Kiyohara C, Wakai K, Mikami H, Sido K, Ando M, Ohno Y. Risk modification by CYP1A1 and GSTM1 polymorphisms in the association of environmental tobacco smoke and lung cancer: a case-control study in Japanese non-smoking women. *Int. J. Cancer* 107: 139–144 (2003).
96. Kiyohara C, Yamamura KI, Nakanishi Y, Takayama K, Hara N. Polymorphism in GSTM1, GSTT1, and GSTP1 and susceptibility to lung cancer in a Japanese population. *Asian Pac. J. Cancer Prev.* 1: 293–298 (2000).
97. Mohr LC, Rodgers JK, Silvestri GA. Glutathione S-transferase M1 polymorphism and the risk of lung cancer. *Anticancer Res.* 23: 2111–2124 (2003).
98. Perera FP, Mooney LA, Stampfer M, Phillips DH, Bell DA, Rundle A, Cho S, Tsai WY, Ma J, Blackwood A, Tang D. Associations between carcinogen-DNA damage, glutathione S-transferase genotypes, and risk of lung cancer in the prospective Physicians' Health Cohort Study. *Carcinogenesis* 23: 1641–1646 (2002).
99. Pinarbasi H, Silig Y, Cetinkaya O, Seyfikli Z, Pinarbasi E. Strong association between the GSTM1-null genotype and lung cancer in a Turkish population. *Cancer Genet. Cytogenet.* 146: 125–129 (2003).
100. Sgambato A, Campisi B, Zupa A, Bochicchio A, Romano G, Tartarone A, Galasso R, Traficante A, Cittadini A. Glutathione S-transferase (GST) polymorphisms as risk factors for cancer in a highly homogeneous population from southern Italy. *Anticancer Res.* 22: 3647–3652 (2002).
101. Canbay E, Dokmetas S, Canbay EI, Sen M, Bardakci F. Higher glutathione transferase GSTM1 0/0 genotype frequency in young thyroid carcinoma patients. *Curr. Med. Res. Opin.* 19: 102–106 (2003).
102. Acevedo C, Opazo JL, Huidobro C, Cabezas J, Iturrieta J, Quinones Sepulveda L. Positive correlation between single or combined genotypes of CYP1A1 and GSTM1 in relation to prostate cancer in Chilean people. *The Prostate* 57: 111–117 (2003).
103. Lohmueller KE, Pearce CL, Pike M, Lander ES, Hirschhorn JN. Meta-analysis of genetic association studies supports a contribution of common

variants to susceptibility to common disease. *Nat. Genet.* 33: 177–182 (2003).

104. Yu MW, Yang SY, Pan IJ, Lin CL, Liu CJ, Liaw YF, Lin SM, Chen PJ, Lee SD, Chen CJ. Polymorphisms in XRCC1 and glutathione S-transferase genes and hepatitis B-related hepatocellular carcinoma. *J. Natl. Cancer Inst.* 95: 1485–1488 (2003).
105. Carless MA, Lea RA, Curran JE, Appleyard B, Gaffney P, Green A, Griffiths LR. The GSTM1 null genotype confers an increased risk for solar keratosis development in an Australian Caucasian population. *J. Invest. Dermatol.* 119: 1373–1378 (2002).
106. Kusumi M, Ishizaki K, Kowa H, Adachi Y, Takeshima T, Sakai F, Nakashima K. Glutathione S-transferase polymorphisms: susceptibility to migraine without aura. *Eur. Neurol.* 49: 218–222 (2003).
107. Verlaan M, te Morsche RH, Roelofs HM, Laheij RJ, Jansen JB, Peters WH, Drenth JP. Glutathione S-transferase Mu null genotype affords protection against alcohol-induced chronic pancreatitis. *Am. J. Med. Genet.* 120A: 34–39 (2003).
108. Wilson MH, Grant PJ, Kain K, Warner DP, Wild CP. Association between the risk of coronary artery disease in South Asians and a deletion polymorphism in glutathione S-transferase M1. *Biomarkers* 8: 43–50 (2003).
109. Jansson M, Rada A, Tomic L, Larsson LI, Wadelius C. Analysis of the glutathione S-transferase M1 gene using pyrosequencing and multiplex PCR — no evidence of association to glaucoma. *Exp. Eye Res.* 77: 239–243 (2003).
110. Okubo T, Harada S, Higuchi S, Matsushita S. Association analyses between polymorphisms of the phase II detoxification enzymes (GSTM1, NQO1, NQO2) and alcohol withdrawal symptoms. *Alcohol Clin. Exp. Res.* 27: 68S–71S (2003).
111. Henrion-Caude A, Flamant C, Roussey M, Housset C, Flahault A, Fryer AA, Chadelat K, Strange RC, Clement A. Liver disease in pediatric patients with cystic fibrosis is associated with glutathione S-transferase P1 polymorphism. *Hepatology* 36: 913–917 (2002).
112. Ye Z, Parry JM. Genetic polymorphisms in the cytochrome P450 1A1, glutathione S-transferase M1 and T1, and susceptibility to colon cancer. *Teratog. Carcinog. Mutagen* 22: 385–392 (2002).
113. Inskip A *et al.* Identification of polymorphism at the glutathione S-transferase, GSTM3 locus: evidence for linkage with GSTM1*A. *Biochem. J.* 312(Pt 3): 713–716 (1995).
114. Liloglou T, Walters M, Maloney P, Youngson J, Field JK. A T2517C polymorphism in the GSTM4 gene is associated with risk of developing lung cancer. *Lung Cancer* 37: 143–146 (2002).

115. Whitbread AK, Tetlow N, Eyre HJ, Sutherland GR, Board PG. Characterization of the human Omega class glutathione transferase genes and associated polymorphisms. *Pharmacogenetics* 13: 131–144 (2003).
116. Board PG, Coggan M, Chelvanayagam G, Easteal S, Jermiin LS, Schulte GK, Danley DE, Hoth LR, Griffor MC, Kamath AV, Rosner MH, Chrunyk BA, Perregaux DE, Gabel CA, Geoghegan KF, Pandit J. Identification, characterization, and crystal structure of the Omega class glutathione transferases. *J. Biol. Chem.* 275: 24798–24806 (2000).
117. Adler V, Yin ZM, Fuchs SY, Benezra M, Rosario L, Tew KD, Pincus MR, Sardana M, Henderson CJ, Wolf CR, Davis RJ, Ronai Z. Regulation of JNK signaling by GSTp. *EMBO J.* 18: 1321–1334 (1999).
118. Board PG, Webb GC, Coggan M. Isolation of a cDNA clone and localization of the human glutathione S-transferase 3 genes to chromosome bands 11q13 and 12q13-14. *Ann. Hum. Genet.* 53(Pt 3): 205–213 (1989).
119. Moscow JA, Townsend AJ, Goldsmith ME, Whang-Peng J, Vickers PJ, Poisson R, Legault-Poisson S, Myers CE, Cowan KH. Isolation of the human anionic glutathione S-transferase cDNA and the relation of its gene expression to estrogen-receptor content in primary breast cancer. *Proc. Natl. Acad. Sci. USA* 85: 6518–6522 (1988).
120. Ali-Osman F, Akande O, Antoun G, Mao JX, Buolamwini, J. Molecular cloning, characterization, and expression in *Escherichia coli* of full-length cDNAs of three human glutathione S-transferase Pi gene variants. Evidence for differential catalytic activity of the encoded proteins. *J. Biol. Chem.* 272: 10004–10012 (1997).
121. Adams CH, Werely CJ, Victor TC, Hoal EG, Rossouw G, van Helden PD. Allele frequencies for glutathione S-transferase and N-acetyltransferase 2 differ in African population groups and may be associated with oesophageal cancer or tuberculosis incidence. *Clin. Chem. Lab. Med.* 41: 600–605 (2003).
122. Nakazato H, Suzuki K, Matsui H, Koike H, Okugi H, Ohtake N, Takei T, Nakata S, Hasumi M, Ito K, Kurokawa K, Yamanaka H. Association of genetic polymorphisms of glutathione-S-transferase genes (GSTM1, GSTT1 and GSTP1) with familial prostate cancer risk in a Japanese population. *Anticancer Res.* 23: 2897–2902 (2003).
123. Casson AG, Zheng Z, Chiasson D, MacDonald K, Riddell DC, Guernsey JR, Guernsey DL, McLaughlin J. Associations between genetic polymorphisms of Phase I and II metabolizing enzymes, p53 and susceptibility to esophageal adenocarcinoma. *Cancer Detect. Prev.* 27: 139–146 (2003).
124. Miller DP, De Vivo I, Neuberg D, Wain JC, Lynch TJ, Su L, Christiani DC. Association between self-reported environmental tobacco smoke exposure

and lung cancer: modification by GSTP1 polymorphism. *Int. J. Cancer* 104: 758–763 (2003).

125. Wang Y, Spitz MR, Schabath MB, Ali-Osman F, Mata H, Wu X. Association between glutathione S-transferase p1 polymorphisms and lung cancer risk in Caucasians: a case-control study. *Lung Cancer* 40: 25–32 (2003).
126. Jee SH, Lee JE, Kim S, Kim JH, Um SJ, Lee SJ, Namkoong SE, Park JS. GSTP1 polymorphism, cigarette smoking and cervical cancer risk in Korean women. *Yonsei Med. J.* 43: 712–716 (2002).
127. Zielinska E, Zubowska M, Bodalski J. Polymorphism at the glutathione S-transferase pi locus as a risk factor for ifosfamide nephrotoxicity in children. *Pol Merkuriusz Lek* 14: 295–298 (2003).
128. Xiao D, Wang C, Du MJ, Pang BS, Zhang HY, Xiao B, Liu JZ, Weng XZ, Su L, Christiani DC. Association between polymorphisms in the gene coding for glutathione S-transferase P1 and chronic obstructive pulmonary disease. *Zhonghua Jie He He Hu Xi Za Zhi* 26: 555–558 (2003).
129. Jeronimo C, Varzim G, Henrique R, Oliveira J, Bento MJ, Silva C, Lopes C, Sidransky D. I105V polymorphism and promoter methylation of the GSTP1 gene in prostate adenocarcinoma. *Cancer Epidemiol. Biomarkers Prev.* 11: 445–450 (2002).
130. Yuan XJ, Gu LJ, Xue HL, Tang JY, Zhao JC, Chen J, Wang YP, Pan C, Song DL. Analysis on GST-Pi genetic polymorphism in children with acute leukemia. *Zhonghua Yi Xue Za Zhi* 83: 1863–1866 (2003).
131. Webb G, Vaska V, Coggan M, Board P. Chromosomal localization of the gene for the human theta class glutathione transferase (GSTT1). *Genomics* 33: 121–123 (1996).
132. Pemble S, Schroeder KR, Spencer SR, Meyer DJ, Hallier E, Bolt HM, Ketterer B, Taylor JB. Human glutathione S-transferase theta (GSTT1): cDNA cloning and the characterization of a genetic polymorphism. *Biochem. J.* 300(Pt 1). 271–276 (1994).
133. Chen CL, Liu Q, Relling MV. Simultaneous characterization of glutathione S-transferase M1 and T1 polymorphisms by polymerase chain reaction in American whites and blacks. *Pharmacogenetics* 6: 187–191 (1996).
134. Lee KA, Kim SH, Woo HY, Hong YJ, Cho HC. Increased frequencies of glutathione S-transferase (GSTM1 and GSTT1) gene deletions in Korean patients with acquired aplastic anemia. *Blood* 98: 3483–3485 (2001).
135. Zhu Y, Deng C, Zhang Y, Zhou X, He X. The relationship between GSTM1, GSTT1 gene polymorphisms and susceptibility to sporadic colorectal adenocarcinoma. *Zhonghua Nei Ke Za Zhi* 41: 538–540 (2002).

136. Morari EC, Leite JL, Granja F, da Assumpcao LV, Ward LS. The null genotype of glutathione S-transferase M1 and T1 locus increases the risk for thyroid cancer. *Cancer Epidemiol. Biomarkers Prev.* 11: 1485–1488 (2002).
137. Hohaus S, Massini G, D'Alo F, Guidi F, Putzulu R, Scardocci A, Rabi A, Di Febo AL, Voso MT, Leone G. Association between glutathione S-transferase genotypes and Hodgkin's lymphoma risk and prognosis. *Clin. Cancer Res.* 9: 3435–3440 (2003).
138. Park JH, El-Sohemy A, Cornelis MC, Kim HA, Kim SY, Bae SC. Glutathione S-transferase M1, T1, and P1 gene polymorphisms and carotid atherosclerosis in Korean patients with rheumatoid arthritis. *Rheumatol. Int.* 24(3): 157–163 (2003).
139. Alexandrie AK, Rannug A, Juronen E, Tasa G, Warholm M. Detection and characterization of a novel functional polymorphism in the GSTT1 gene. *Pharmacogenetics* 12(8): 613–619 (2002).
140. Blackburn AC, Woollatt E, Sutherland GR, Board PG. Characterization and chromosome location of the gene GSTZ1 encoding the human Zeta class glutathione transferase and maleylacetoacetate isomerase. *Cytogenet. Cell Genet.* 83: 109–114 (1998).
141. Blackburn AC, Tzeng HF, Anders MW, Board PG. Discovery of a functional polymorphism in human glutathione transferase zeta by expressed sequence tag database analysis. *Pharmacogenetics* 10: 49–57 (2000).
142. Blackburn AC, Coggan M, Tzeng HF, Lantum H, Polekhina G, Parker MW, Anders MW, Board PG. GSTZ1d: a new allele of glutathione transferase zeta and maleylacetoacetate isomerase. *Pharmacogenetics* 11: 671–678 (2001).
143. Jakobsson PJ, Morgenstern R, Mancini J, Ford-Hutchinson A, Persson B. Common structural features of MAPEG — a widespread superfamily of membrane associated proteins with highly divergent functions in eicosanoid and glutathione metabolism. *Protein Sci.* 8: 689–692 (1999).
144. Jakobsson PJ, Morgenstern R, Mancini J, Ford-Hutchinson A, Persson B. Membrane-associated proteins in eicosanoid and glutathione metabolism (MAPEG). A widespread protein superfamily. *Am. J. Respir. Crit. Care Med.* 161: S20–S24 (2000).
145. Andersson C, Mosialou E, Weinander R, Morgenstern R. Enzymology of microsomal glutathione S-transferase. *Adv. Pharmacol.* 27: 19–35 (1994).
146. Mosialou E, Ekstrom G, Adang AE, Morgenstern R. Evidence that rat liver microsomal glutathione transferase is responsible for glutathione-dependent protection against lipid peroxidation. *Biochem. Pharmacol.* 45: 1645–1651 (1993).

147. Mosialou E, Piemonte F, Andersson C, Vos RM, van Bladeren PJ, Morgenstern R. Microsomal glutathione transferase: lipid-derived substrates and lipid dependence. *Arch. Biochem. Biophys.* 320: 210–216 (1995).
148. Estonius M, Forsberg L, Danielsson O, Weinander R, Kelner MJ, Morgenstern R. Distribution of microsomal glutathione transferase 1 in mammalian tissues. A predominant alternate first exon in human tissues. *Eur. J. Biochem.* 260: 409–413 (1999).
149. Kelner MJ, Stokely MN, Stovall NE, Montoya MA. Structural organization of the human microsomal glutathione S-transferase gene (GST12). *Genomics* 36: 100–103 (1996).
150. Lee SH, DeJong J. Microsomal GST-I: genomic organization, expression, and alternative splicing of the human gene. *Biochim. Biophys. Acta* 1446: 389–396 (1999).
151. Iida A, Saito S, Sekine A, Harigae S, Osawa S, Mishima C, Kondo K, Kitamura Y, Nakamura Y. Catalog of 46 single-nucleotide polymorphisms (SNPs) in the microsomal glutathione S-transferase 1 (MGST1) gene. *J. Hum. Genet.* 46: 590–594 (2001a).
152. Forsberg L, de Faire U, Morgenstern R. Low yield of polymorphisms from EST blast searching: analysis of genes related to oxidative stress and verification of the P197L polymorphism in GPX1. *Hum. Mutat.* 13: 294–300 (1999).
153. Guy CA, Hoogendoorn B, Smith SK, Coleman S, O'Donovan MC, Buckland PR. Promoter polymorphisms in glutathione-S-transferase genes affect transcription. *Pharmacogenetics* 14: 45–51 (2004).
154. Chaib H, Cockrell EK, Rubin MA, Macoska JA. Profiling and verification of gene expression patterns in normal and malignant human prostate tissues by cDNA microarray analysis. *Neoplasia* 3: 43–52 (2001).
155. Jakobsson PJ, Mancini JA, Ford-Hutchinson AW. Identification and characterization of a novel human microsomal glutathione S-transferase with leukotriene C4 synthase activity and significant sequence identity to 5-lipoxygenase-activating protein and leukotriene C4 synthase. *J. Biol. Chem.* 271: 22203–22210 (1996).
156. Jakobsson PJ, Scoggan KA, Yergey J, Mancini JA, Ford-Hutchinson AW. Characterization of microsomal GST-II by western blot and identification of a novel LTC4 isomer. *J. Lipid. Mediat. Cell Signal.* 17: 15–19 (1997).
157. Jakobsson PJ, Mancini JA, Riendeau D, Ford-Hutchinson AW. Identification and characterization of a novel microsomal enzyme with glutathione-dependent transferase and peroxidase activities, *J. Biol. Chem.* 272: 22934–22939 (1997).

158. Thameem F, Yang X, Permana PA, Wolford JK, Bogardus C, Prochazka M. Evaluation of the microsomal glutathione S-transferase 3 (MGST3) locus on 1q23 as a Type 2 diabetes susceptibility gene in Pima Indians. *Hum. Genet.* 113: 353–358 (2003).
159. Iida A, Saito S, Sekine A, Kitamoto T, Kitamura Y, Mishima C, Osawa S, Kondo K, Harigae S, Nakamura Y. Catalog of 434 single-nucleotide polymorphisms (SNPs) in genes of the alcohol dehydrogenase, glutathione S-transferase, and nicotinamide adenine dinucleotide, reduced (NADH) ubiquinone oxidoreductase families. *J. Hum. Genet.* 46: 385–407 (2001).
160. Yandava CN, Kennedy BP, Pillari A, Duncan AM, Drazen JM. Cytogenetic and radiation hybrid mapping of human arachidonate 5-lipoxygenase-activating protein (ALOX5AP) to chromosome 13q12. *Genomics* 56: 131–133 (1999).
161. Sayers I, Barton S, Rorke S, Sawyer J, Peng Q, Beghe B, Ye S, Keith T, Clough JB, Holloway JW, Sampson AP, Holgate ST. Promoter polymorphism in the 5-lipoxygenase (ALOX5) and 5-lipoxygenase-activating protein (ALOX5AP) genes and asthma susceptibility in a Caucasian population. *Clin. Exp. Allergy* 33: 1103–1110 (2003).
162. Helgadottir A, Manolescu A, Thorleifsson G, Gretarsdottir S, Jonsdottir H, Thorsteinsdottir U, Samani NJ, Gudmundsson G, Grant SF, Thorgeirsson G, Sveinbjornsdottir S, Valdimarsson EM, Matthiasson SE, Johannsson H, Gudmundsdottir O, Gurney ME, Sainz J, Thorhallsdottir M, Andresdottir M, Frigge ML, Topol EJ, Kong A, Gudnason V, Hakonarson H, Gulcher JR, Stefansson K. The gene encoding 5-lipoxygenase activating protein confers risk of myocardial infarction and stroke. *Nat. Genet.* 36: 233–239 (2004).
163. Lam BK, Penrose JF, Freeman GJ, Austen KF. Expression cloning of a cDNA for human leukotriene C4 synthase, an integral membrane protein conjugating reduced glutathione to leukotriene A4. *Proc. Natl. Acad. Sci. USA* 91: 7663–7667 (1994).
164. Welsch DJ, Creely DP, Hauser SD, Mathis KJ, Krivi GG, Isakson PC. Molecular cloning and expression of human leukotriene-C4 synthase. *Proc. Natl. Acad. Sci. USA* 91: 9745–9749 (1994).
165. Penrose JF, Spector J, Baldasaro M, Xu K, Boyce J, Arm JP, Austen KF, Lam BK. Molecular cloning of the gene for human leukotriene C4 synthase. Organization, nucleotide sequence, and chromosomal localization to 5q35. *J. Biol. Chem.* 271: 11356–11361 (1996).
166. Sanak M, Simon HU, Szczeklik A. Leukotriene C4 synthase promoter polymorphism and risk of aspirin-induced asthma. *Lancet* 350: 1599–1600 (1997).

167. Kawagishi Y, Mita H, Taniguchi M, Maruyama M, Oosaki R, Higashi N, Kashii T, Kobayashi M, Akiyama K. Leukotriene C4 synthase promoter polymorphism in Japanese patients with aspirin-induced asthma. *J. Allergy Clin. Immunol.* 109: 936–942 (2002).
168. Van Sambeek R, Stevenson DD, Baldasaro M, Lam BK, Zhao J, Yoshida S, Yandora C, Drazen JM, Penrose JF. 5′ flanking region polymorphism of the gene encoding leukotriene C4 synthase does not correlate with the aspirin-intolerant asthma phenotype in the United States. *J. Allergy Clin. Immunol.* 106: 72–76 (2000).
169. Sampson AP, Siddiqui S, Buchanan D, Howarth PH, Holgate ST, Holloway JW, Sayers I. Variant LTC(4) synthase allele modifies cysteinyl leukotriene synthesis in eosinophils and predicts clinical response to zafirlukast. *Thorax* 55(Suppl 2): S28–S31 (2000).
170. Sanak M, Szczeklik A. Genetics of aspirin-induced asthma. *Thorax* 55(Suppl 2): S45–S47 (2000).
171. Costa LG, Cole TB, Jarvik GP, Furlong CE. Functional genomic of the paraoxonase (PON1) polymorphisms: effects on pesticide sensitivity, cardiovascular disease, drug metabolism. *Annu. Rev. Med.* 54: 371–392 (2003).
172. Humbert R, Adler DA, Disteche CM, Hassett C, Omiecinski CJ, Furlong CE. The molecular basis of the human serum paraoxonase activity polymorphism. *Nat. Genet.* 3: 73–76 (1993).
173. La Du BN. The human serum paraoxonase/arylesterase polymorphism. *Am. J. Hum. Genet.* 43: 227–229 (1988).
174. Ahmed Z, Babaei S, Maguire GF, Draganov D, Kuksis A, La Du BN, Connelly PW. Paraoxonase-1 reduces monocyte chemotaxis and adhesion to endothelial cells due to oxidation of palmitoyl, linoleoyl glycerophosphorylcholine. *Cardiovasc. Res.* 57: 225–231 (2003).
175. Imai Y, Morita H, Kurihara H, Sugiyama T, Kato N, Ebihara A, Hamada C, Kurihara Y, Shindo T, Ohhashi Y, Yazaki Y. Evidence for association between paraoxonase gene polymorphisms and atherosclerotic diseases. *Atherosclerosis* 149: 435–442 (2000).
176. Ko YL, Ko YS, Wang SM, Hsu LA, Chang CJ, Chu PH, Cheng NJ, Chen WJ, Chiang CW, Lee YS. The Gln-Arg 191 polymorphism of the human paraoxonase gene is not associated with the risk of coronary artery disease among Chinese in Taiwan. *Atherosclerosis* 141: 259–264 (1998).
177. Scacchi R, Corbo RM, Rickards O, De Stefano GF. New data on the world distribution of paraoxonase (PON1 Gln 192 $\rightarrow$ Arg) gene frequencies. *Hum. Biol.* 75: 365–373 (2003).

178. Li HL, Liu DP, Liang CC. Paraoxonase gene polymorphisms, oxidative stress, and diseases. *J. Mol. Med.* 81: 766–769 (2003).
179. Mochizuki H, Scherer SW, Xi T, Nickle DC, Majer M, Huizenga JJ, Tsui LC, Prochazka M. Human PON2 gene at 7q21.3: cloning, multiple mRNA forms, and missense polymorphisms in the coding sequence. *Gene* 213: 149–157 (1998).
180. Ng CJ, Wadleigh DJ, Gangopadhyay A, Hama S, Grijalva VR, Navab M, Fogelman AM, Reddy ST. Paraoxonase-2 is a ubiquitously expressed protein with antioxidant properties and is capable of preventing cell-mediated oxidative modification of low density lipoprotein. *J. Biol. Chem.* 276: 44444–44449 (2001).
181. Ross D, Kepa JK, Winski SL, Beall HD, Anwar A, Siegel D. NAD(P)H: quinone oxidoreductase 1 (NQO1): chemoprotection, bioactivation, gene regulation and genetic polymorphisms. *Chem. Biol. Interact.* 129: 77–97 (2000).
182. Chen LZ *et al.* A refined physical map of the long arm of human chromosome 16. *Genomics* 10: 308–312 (1991).
183. Jaiswal AK. Human NAD(P)H: quinone oxidoreductase (NQO1) gene structure and induction by dioxin. *Biochemistry* 30: 10647–10653 (1991).
184. Choi JY, Lee KM, Cho SH, Kim SW, Choi HY, Lee SY, Im HJ, Yoon KJ, Choi H, Choi I, Hirvonen A, Hayes RB, Kang D. CYP2E1 and NQO1 genotypes, smoking and bladder cancer. *Pharmacogenetics* 13: 349–355 (2003).
185. Lin P, Hsueh YM, Ko JL, Liang YF, Tsai KJ, Chen CY. Analysis of NQO1, GSTP1, and MnSOD genetic polymorphisms on lung cancer risk in Taiwan. *Lung Cancer* 40: 123–129 (2003).
186. Nebert DW, Roe AL, Vandale SE, Bingham E, Oakley GG. NAD(P)H: quinone oxidoreductase (NQO1) polymorphism, exposure to benzene, and predisposition to disease: a HuGE review. *Genet. Med.* 4: 62–70 (2002).
187. Park SJ, Zhao H, Spitz MR, Grossman HB, Wu X. An association between NQO1 genetic polymorphism and risk of bladder cancer. *Mutat. Res.* 536: 131–137 (2003).
188. Sarbia M, Bitzer M, Siegel D, Ross D, Schulz WA, Zotz RB, Kiel S, Geddert H, Kandemir Y, Walter A, Willers R, Gabbert HE. Association between NAD(P)H: quinone oxidoreductase 1 (NQ01) inactivating C609T polymorphism and adenocarcinoma of the upper gastrointestinal tract. *Int. J. Cancer* 107: 381–386 (2003).
189. Shao M, Liu Z, Tao E, Chen B. Polymorphism of MAO-B gene and NAD(P)H: quinone oxidoreductase gene in Parkinson's disease. *Zhonghua Yi Xue Yi Chuan Xue Za Zhi* 18: 122–124 (2001).

190. Harada S, Fujii C, Hayashi A, Ohkoshi N. An association between idiopathic Parkinson's disease and polymorphisms of phase II detoxification enzymes: glutathione S-transferase M1 and quinone oxidoreductase 1 and 2. *Biochem. Biophys. Res. Commun.* 288: 887–892 (2001).
191. Hori H, Ohmori O, Matsumoto C, Shinkai T, Nakamura J. NAD(P)H: quinone oxidoreductase (NQO1) gene polymorphism and schizophrenia. *Psychiatry Res.* 118: 235–239 (2003).
192. Ma QL, Yang JF, Shao M, Dong XM, Chen B. Association between NAD(P)H: quinone oxidoreductase and apolipoprotein E gene polymorphisms in Alzheimer's disease. *Zhonghua Yi Xue Za Zhi* 83: 2124–2127 (2003).
193. Hu LT, Stamberg J, Pan S. The NAD(P)H: quinone oxidoreductase locus in human colon carcinoma HCT 116 cells resistant to mitomycin C. *Cancer Res.* 56: 5253–5259 (1996).
194. Pan SS, Forrest GL, Akman SA, Hu LT. NAD(P)H: quinone oxidoreductase expression and mitomycin C resistance developed by human colon cancer HCT 116 cells. *Cancer Res.* 55: 330–335 (1995).
195. Pan SS, Han Y, Farabaugh P, Xia H. Implication of alternative splicing for expression of a variant NAD(P)H: quinone oxidoreductase-1 with a single nucleotide polymorphism at 465C>T. *Pharmacogenetics* 12: 479–488 (2002).
196. Iida A, Saito S, Sekine A, Mishima C, Kondo K, Kitamura Y, Harigae S, Osawa S, Nakamura Y. Catalog of 258 single-nucleotide polymorphisms (SNPs) in genes encoding three organic anion transporters, three organic anion-transporting polypeptides, and three NADH: ubiquinone oxidoreductase flavoproteins. *J. Hum. Genet.* 46: 668–683 (2001).
197. Long DJ II, Jaiswal AK. Mouse NRH: quinone oxidoreductase (NQO2): cloning of cDNA and gene- and tissue-specific expression. *Gene* 252: 107–117 (2000).
198. Harada S, Tachikawa H, Kawanishi Y. A possible association between an insertion/deletion polymorphism of the NQO2 gene and schizophrenia. *Psychiatr. Genet.* 13: 205–209 (2003).
199. Larsson C, White I, Johansson C, Stark A, Meijer J. Localization of the human soluble epoxide hydrolase gene (EPHX2) to chromosomal region 8p21-p12. *Hum. Genet.* 95: 356–358 (1995).
200. Sandberg M, Meijer J. Structural characterization of the human soluble epoxide hydrolase gene (EPHX2). *Biochem. Biophys. Res. Commun.* 221: 333–339 (1996).

201. Saito S, Iida A, Sekine A, Eguchi C, Miura Y, Nakamura Y. Seventy genetic variations in human microsomal and soluble epoxide hydrolase genes (EPHX1 and EPHX2) in the Japanese population. *J. Hum. Genet.* 46: 325–329 (2001).
202. Sandberg M, Hassett C, Adman ET, Meijer J, Omiecinski CJ. Identification and functional characterization of human soluble epoxide hydrolase genetic polymorphisms. *J. Biol. Chem.* 275: 28873–28881 (2000).
203. Przybyla-Zawislak BD, Srivastava PK, Vazquez-Matias J, Mohrenweiser HW, Maxwell JE, Hammock BD, Bradbury JA, Enayetallah AE, Zeldin DC, Grant DF. Polymorphisms in human soluble epoxide hydrolase. *Mol. Pharmacol.* 64: 482–490 (2003).
204. Fornage M, Boerwinkle E, Doris PA, Jacobs D, Liu K, Wong ND. Polymorphism of the soluble epoxide hydrolase is associated with coronary artery calcification in African-American subjects: The Coronary Artery Risk Development in Young Adults (CARDIA) study. *Circulation* 109: 335–339 (2004).
205. Hartsfield JK Jr, Sutcliffe MJ, Everett ET, Hassett C, Omiecinski CJ, Saari JA. Assignment1 of microsomal epoxide hydrolase (EPHX1) to human chromosome 1q42.1 by *in situ* hybridization. *Cytogenet. Cell Genet.* 83: 44–45 (1998).
206. Omiecinski CJ, Aicher L, Holubkov R, Checkoway H. Human peripheral lymphocytes as indicators of microsomal epoxide hydrolase activity in liver and lung. *Pharmacogenetics* 3: 150–158 (1993).
207. Hassett C, Robinson KB, Beck NB, Omiecinski CJ. The human microsomal epoxide hydrolase gene (EPHX1): complete nucleotide sequence and structural characterization. *Genomics* 23: 433–442 (1994).
208. Gsur A, Zidek T, Schnattinger K, Feik E, Haidinger G, Hollaus P, Mohn-Staudner A, Armbruster C, Madersbacher S, Schatzl G, Trieb K, Vutuc C, Micksche M. Association of microsomal epoxide hydrolase polymorphisms and lung cancer risk. *Br. J. Cancer* 89: 702–706 (2003).
209. Belmahdi F, Chevalier D, Lo-Guidice JM, Allorge D, Cauffiez C, Lafitte JJ, Broly F. Identification of six new polymorphisms, g.11177G>A, g.14622C>T (R49C), g.17540T>C, g.17639T>C, g.30929T>C, g.31074G>A (R454Q), in the human microsomal epoxide hydrolase gene (EPHX1) in a French population. *Hum. Mutat.* 16: 450 (2000).
210. Zhu QS, Xing W, Qian B, von Dippe P, Shneider BL, Fox VL, Levy D. Inhibition of human m-epoxide hydrolase gene expression in a case of hypercholanemia. *Biochim. Biophys. Acta.* 1638: 208–216 (2003).

211. Raaka S, Hassett C, Omiencinski CJ. Human microsomal epoxide hydrolase: 5′-flanking region genetic polymorphisms. *Carcinogenesis* 19: 387–393 (1998).
212. Kiyohara C, Otsu A, Shirakawa T, Fukuda S, Hopkin JM. Genetic polymorphisms and lung cancer susceptibility: a review. *Lung Cancer* 37: 241–256 (2002).
213. Harrison DJ, Hubbard AL, MacMillan J, Wyllie AH, Smith CA. Microsomal epoxide hydrolase gene polymorphism and susceptibility to colon cancer. *Br. J. Cancer* 79: 168–171 (1999).
214. Wenghoefer M, Pesch B, Harth V, Broede P, Fronhoffs S, Landt O, Bruning T, Abel J, Bolt HM, Herberhold C, Vetter H, Ko YD. Association between head and neck cancer and microsomal epoxide hydrolase genotypes. *Arch. Toxicol.* 77: 37–41 (2003).
215. de Jong DJ, van der Logt EM, van Schaik A, Roelofs HM, Peters WH, Naber TH. Genetic polymorphisms in biotransformation enzymes in Crohn's disease: association with microsomal epoxide hydrolase. *Gut* 52: 547–551 (2003).
216. Korhonen S, Romppanen EL, Hiltunen M, Helisalmi S, Punnonen K, Hippelainen M, Heinonen S. Two exonic single nucleotide polymorphisms in the microsomal epoxide hydrolase gene are associated with polycystic ovary syndrome. *Fertil. Steril.* 79: 1353–1357 (2003).
217. Soucek P, Sarmanova J, Kristensen VN, Apltauerova M, Gut I. Genetic polymorphisms of biotransformation enzymes in patients with Hodgkin's and non-Hodgkin's lymphomas. *Int. Arch. Occup. Environ. Health* 75(Suppl): S86–S92 (2002).
218. Agus DB, Gambhir SS, Pardridge WM, Spielholz C, Baselga J, Vera JC, Golde DW. Vitamin C crosses the blood-brain barrier in the oxidized form through the glucose transporters. *J. Clin. Invest.* 100: 2842–2848 (1997).
219. Shows TB, Eddy RL, Byers MG, Fukushima Y, Dehaven CR, Murray JC, Bell GI. Polymorphic human glucose transporter gene (GLUT) is on chromosome 1p31.3–p35. *Diabetes* 36: 546–549 (1987).
220. Li SR, Baroni MG, Oelbaum RS, Stock J, Galton DJ. Association of genetic variant of the glucose transporter with non-insulin-dependent diabetes mellitus. *Lancet* 2: 368–370 (1988).
221. Baroni MG, Oelbaum RS, Pozzilli P, Stocks J, Li SR, Fiore V, Galton DJ. Polymorphisms at the GLUT1 (HepG2) and GLUT4 (muscle/adipocyte) glucose transporter genes and non-insulin-dependent diabetes mellitus (NIDDM). *Hum. Genet.* 88: 557–561 (1992).

222. Cavalier L, Ouahchi K, Kayden HJ, Di Donato S, Reutenauer L, Mandel JL, Koenig M. Ataxia with isolated vitamin E deficiency: heterogeneity of mutations and phenotypic variability in a large number of families. *Am. J. Hum. Genet.* 62: 301–310 (1998).
223. Gotoda T, Arita M, Arai H, Inoue K, Yokota T, Fukuo Y, Yazaki Y, Yamada N. Adult-onset spinocerebellar dysfunction caused by a mutation in the gene for the alpha-tocopherol-transfer protein. *N. Engl. J. Med.* 333: 1313–1318 (1995).
224. Hentati A, Deng HX, Hung WY, Nayer M, Ahmed MS, He X, Tim R, Stumpf DA, Siddique T, Ahmed. Human alpha-tocopherol transfer protein: gene structure and mutations in familial vitamin E deficiency. *Ann. Neurol.* 39: 295–300 (1996).
225. Ouahchi K, Arita M, Kayden H, Hentati F, Ben Hamida M, Sokol R, Arai H, Inoue K, Mandel JL, Koenig M. Ataxia with isolated vitamin E deficiency is caused by mutations in the alpha-tocopherol transfer protein. *Nat. Genet.* 9: 141–145 (1995).
226. Schuelke M, Mayatepek E, Inter M, Becker M, Pfeiffer E, Speer A, Hubner C, Finckh B. Treatment of ataxia in isolated vitamin E deficiency caused by alpha-tocopherol transfer protein deficiency. *J. Pediatr.* 134: 240–244 (1999).
227. Tai ES, Adiconis X, Ordovas JM, Carmena-Ramon R, Real J, Corella D, Ascaso J, Carmena R. Polymorphisms at the SRBI locus are associated with lipoprotein levels in subjects with heterozygous familial hypercholesterolemia. *Clin. Genet.* 63: 53–58 (2003).
228. Acton S, Osgood D, Donoghue M, Corella D, Pocovi M, Cenarro A, Mozas P, Keilty J, Squazzo S, Woolf EA, Ordovas JM. Association of polymorphisms at the SR-BI gene locus with plasma lipid levels and body mass index in a white population. *Arterioscler. Thromb. Vasc. Biol.* 19: 1734–1743 (1999).
229. Hubacek JA, Pistulkova H, Valenta Z, Poledne R. (TTA)n repeat polymorphism in the HMG-CoA reductase gene and cholesterolaemia. *Vasa* 28: 169–171 (1999).
230. Leitersdorf E, Hwang M, Luskey KL. ScrFI polymorphism in the 2nd intron of the HMGCR gene. *Nucleic Acids Res.* 18: 5584 (1990).
231. Leitersdorf E, Luskey KL. HgiAI polymorphism near the HMGCR promoter. *Nucleic Acids Res.* 18: 5584 (1990).
232. Otterbein L, Choi A. Heme oxygenase: color of defense against cellular stress. *Am. J. Physiol. Lung Cell. Mol.* 279: L1029–L1037 (2000).
233. Maines M. Heme oxygenase: function, multiplicity, regulatory mechanisms, and clinical applications. *FASEB J.* 2: 2557–2568 (1998).

234. Kutty R, Kutty G, Rodorigues I, Chader G, Wiggert B. Chromosomal localization of the human heme oxygenase genes: heme oxygenase-1 (HMOX1) maps to chromosome 22q12 and heme oxygenase-2 (HMOX2) maps to chromosome 16p13.3. *Genomics* 20: 513–516 (1994).
235. Kimpara T, Takeda A, Watanabe K, Itoyama Y, Ikawa S, Watanabe M, Arai H, Sasaki H, Higuchi S, Okita N, Takase S, Saito H, Takahashi K, Shibahara S. Microsatellite polymorphism in the human heme oxygenase-1 gene promoter and its application in association studies with Alzheimer and Parkinson disease. *Hum. Genet.* 100: 145–147 (1997).
236. Yamada N, Yamaya M, Okinaga S, Nakayama K, Sekizawa K, Shibahara S, Sasaki H. Microsatellite polymorphism in the heme oxygenase-1 gene promoter is associated with susceptibility to emphysema. *Am. J. Hum. Genet.* 66: 187–195 (2000).
237. Kaneda H, Ohno M, Taguchi J, Togo M, Hashimoto H, Ogasawara K, Aizawa T, Ishizaka N, Nagai R. Heme oxygenase-1 gene promoter polymorphism is associated with coronary artery disease in Japanese patients with coronary risk factors. *Arterioscler. Thromb. Vasc. Biol.* 22: 1680–1685 (2002).
238. Chen Y, Lin S, Lin M, Tsa IH, Kuo S, Chen J, Charng M, Wu T, Chen L, Ding Y, Pan W, Jou Y, Chau L. Microsatellite polymorphism in promoter of heme oxygenase-1 gene is associated with susceptibility to coronary artery disease in type 2 diabetic patients, *Hum. Genet.* 111: 1–8 (2002).
239. Chen YH, Chau LY, Lin MW, Chen LC, Yo MH, Chen JW, Lin SJ. Heme oxygenase-1 gene promotor microsatellite polymorphism is associated with angiographic restenosis after coronary stenting. *Eur. Heart J.* 25: 39–47 (2004).
240. Exner M, Schillinger M, Minar E, Mlekusch W, Schlerka G, Haumer M, Mannhalter C, Wagner O. Heme oxygenase-1 gene promoter microsatellite polymorphism is associated with restenosis after percutaneous transluminal angioplasty. *J. Endovasc. Ther.* 8: 433–440 (2001).
241. Yamaya M, Nakayama K, Ebihara S, Hirai H, Higuchi S, Sasaki H. Relationship between microsatellite polymorphism in the haem oxygenase-1 gene promoter and longevity of the normal Japanese population. *J. Med. Genet.* 40: 146–148 (2003).
242. Shibahara S. The heme oxygenase dilemma in cellular homeostasis: new insights for the feedback regulation of heme catabolism. *Tohoku J. Exp. Med.* 200: 167–186 (2003).
243. Maines MD. The heme oxygenase system: a regulator of second messenger gases. *Annu. Rev. Pharmacol. Toxicol.* 37: 517–554 (1997).

244. Verma A, Hirsch DJ, Glatt CE, Ronnett GV, Snyder SH. Carbon monoxide: a putative neural messenger. *Science* 259: 381–384 (1993).
245. McCoubrey WK Jr, Huang TJ, Maines MD. Isolation and characterization of a cDNA from the rat brain that encodes hemoprotein heme oxygenase-3. *Eur. J. Biochem.* 247: 725–732 (1997).
246. Guillemette C. Pharmacogenomics of human UDP-glucuronosyltransferase enzymes. *Pharmacogenomics J.* 3: 136–158 (2003).
247. Mackenzie PI, Owens IS, Burchell B, Bock KW, Bairoch A, Belanger A, Fournel-Gigleux S, Green M, Hum DW, Iyanagi T, Lancet D, Louisot P, Magdalou J, Chowdhury JR, Ritter JK, Schachter H, Tephly TR, Tipton KF, Nebert DW. The UDP glycosyltransferase gene superfamily: recommended nomenclature update based on evolutionary divergence. *Pharmacogenetics* 7: 255–269 (1997).
248. Ritter JK, Yeatman MT, Ferreira P, Owens IS. Identification of a genetic alteration in the code for bilirubin UDP-glucuronosyltransferase in the UGT1 gene complex of a Crigler-Najjar type I patient. *J. Clin. Invest.* 90: 150–155 (1992).
249. Moghrabi N, Sutherland L, Wooster R, Povey S, Boxer M, Burchell B. Chromosomal assignment of human phenol and bilirubin UDP-glucuronosyltransferase genes (UGT1A-subfamily). *Ann. Hum. Genet.* 56(Pt 2): 81–91 (1992).
250. van Es HH, Bout A, Liu J, Anderson L, Duncan AM, Bosma P, Oude Elferink R, Jansen PL, Chowdhury JR, Schurr E. Assignment of the human UDP glucuronosyltransferase gene (UGT1A1) to chromosome region 2q37. *Cytogenet. Cell Genet.* 63: 114–116 (1993).
251. Beaulieu M, Levesque E, Tchernof A, Beatty BG, Belanger A, Hum DW. Chromosomal localization, structure, and regulation of the UGT2B17 gene, encoding a C19 steroid metabolizing enzyme. *DNA Cell Biol.* 16: 1143–1154 (1997).
252. Monaghan G, Clarke DJ, Povey S, See CG, Boxer M, Burchell B. Isolation of a human YAC contig encompassing a cluster of UGT2 genes and its regional localization to chromosome 4q13. *Genomics* 23: 496–499 (1994).
253. Bosio A, Binczek E, Le Beau MM, Fernald AA, Stoffel W. The human gene CGT encoding the UDP-galactose ceramide galactosyl transferase (cerebroside synthase): cloning, characterization, and assignment to human chromosome 4, band q26. *Genomics* 34: 69–75 (1996).
254. Danoff TM, Campbell DA, McCarthy LC, Lewis KF, Repasch MH, Saunders AM, Spurr NK, Purvis IJ, Roses AD, Xu CF. A Gilbert's syndrome UGT1A1

variant confers susceptibility to tranilast-induced hyperbilirubinemia. *Pharmacogenomics J.* 4: 49–53 (2004).

255. Font A, Sanchez JM, Taron M, Martinez-Balibrea E, Sanchez JJ, Manzano JL, Margeli M, Richardet M, Barnadas A, Abad A, Rosell R. Weekly regimen of irinotecan/docetaxel in previously treated non-small cell lung cancer patients and correlation with uridine diphosphate glucuronosyltransferase 1A1 (UGT1A1) polymorphism. *Invest. New Drugs* 21: 435–443 (2003).
256. Kohle C, Mohrle B, Munzel PA, Schwab M, Wernet D, Badary OA, Bock KW. Frequent co-occurrence of the TATA box mutation associated with Gilbert's syndrome (UGT1A1*28) with other polymorphisms of the UDP-glucuronosyltransferase-1 locus (UGT1A6*2 and UGT1A7*3) in Caucasians and Egyptians. *Biochem. Pharmacol.* 65: 1521–1527 (2003).
257. Maruo Y, Serdaroglu E, Iwai M, Takahashi H, Mori A, Bak M, Calkavur S, Sato H, Takeuchi Y. A novel missense mutation of the bilirubin UDP-glucuronosyltransferase gene in a Turkish patient with Crigler-Najjar syndrome type 1. *J. Pediatr. Gastroenterol. Nutr.* 37: 627–630 (2003).
258. Ockenga J, Vogel A, Teich N, Keim V, Manns MP, Strassburg CP. UDP glucuronosyltransferase (UGT1A7) gene polymorphisms increase the risk of chronic pancreatitis and pancreatic cancer. *Gastroenterology* 124: 1802–1808 (2003).
259. Ulgenalp A, Duman N, Schaefer FV, Whetsell L, Bora E, Gulcan H, Kumral A, Oren H, Giray O, Ercal D, Ozkan H. Analyses of polymorphism for UGT1*1 exon 1 promoter in neonates with pathologic and prolonged jaundice. *Biol. Neonate* 83: 258–262 (2003).
260. Wild AC, Mulcahy RT. Regulation of gamma-glutamylcysteine synthetase subunit gene expression: insights into transcriptional control of antioxidant defenses. *Free Radic. Res.* 32: 281–301 (2000).
261. Walsh AC, Li W, Rosen DR, Lawrence DA. Genetic mapping of GLCLC, the human gene encoding the catalytic subunit of gamma-glutamyl-cysteine synthetase, to chromosome band 6p12 and characterization of a polymorphic trinucleotide repeat within its 5′ untranslated region. *Cytogenet. Cell Genet.* 75: 14–16 (1996).
262. Sierra-Rivera E, Dasouki M, Summar ML, Krishnamani MR, Meredith M, Rao PN, Phillips JA III, Freeman ML. Assignment of the human gene (GLCLR) that encodes the regulatory subunit of gamma-glutamylcysteine synthetase to chromosome 1p21. *Cytogenet. Cell Genet.* 72: 252–254 (1996).
263. Walsh AC, Feulner JA, Reilly A. Evidence for functionally significant polymorphism of human glutamate cysteine ligase catalytic subunit: association

with glutathione levels and drug resistance in the National Cancer Institute tumor cell line panel. *Toxicol. Sci.* 61: 218–223 (2001).

264. Ristoff E, Augustson C, Geissler J, de Rijk T, Carlsson K, Luo JL, Andersson K, Weening RS, van Zwieten R, Larsson A, Roos D. A missense mutation in the heavy subunit of gamma-glutamylcysteine synthetase gene causes hemolytic anemia. *Blood* 95: 2193–2196 (2000).
265. Hamilton D, Wu JH, Alaoui-Jamali M, Batist G. A novel missense mutation in the gamma-glutamylcysteine synthetase catalytic subunit gene causes both decreased enzymatic activity and glutathione production. *Blood* 102: 725–730 (2003).
266. Beutler E, Gelbart T, Kondo T, Matsunaga AT. The molecular basis of a case of gamma-glutamylcysteine synthetase deficiency. *Blood* 94: 2890–2894 (1999).
267. Koide S, Kugiyama K, Sugiyama S, Nakamura S, Fukushima H, Honda O, Yoshimura M, Ogawa H. Association of polymorphism in glutamate-cysteine ligase catalytic subunit gene with coronary vasomotor dysfunction and myocardial infarction. *J. Am. Coll. Cardiol.* 41: 539–545 (2003).
268. Nakamura S, Kugiyama K, Sugiyama S, Miyamoto S, Koide S, Fukushima H, Honda O, Yoshimura M, Ogawa H. Polymorphism in the 5′-flanking region of human glutamate-cysteine ligase modifier subunit gene is associated with myocardial infarction. *Circulation* 105: 2968–2973 (2002).
269. Nakamura S, Sugiyama S, Fujioka D, Kawabata K, Ogawa H, Kugiyama K. Polymorphism in glutamate-cysteine ligase modifier subunit gene is associated with impairment of nitric oxide-mediated coronary vasomotor function. *Circulation* 108: 1425–1427 (2003).
270. Gali RR, Board PG. Sequencing and expression of a cDNA for human glutathione synthetase. *Biochem. J.* 310(Pt 1): 353–358 (1995).
271. Webb GC, Vaska VL, Gali RR, Ford JH, Board PG. The gene encoding human glutathione synthetase (GSS) maps to the long arm of chromosome 20 at band 11.2. *Genomics* 30: 617–619 (1995).
272. Whitbread L, Gali RR, Board PG. The structure of the human glutathione synthetase gene. *Chem. Biol. Interact.* 111–112: 35–40 (1998).
273. Dahl N, Pigg M, Ristoff E, Gali R, Carlsson B, Mannervik B, Larsson A, Board P. Missense mutations in the human glutathione synthetase gene result in severe metabolic acidosis, 5-oxoprolinuria, hemolytic anemia and neurological dysfunction. *Hum. Mol. Genet.* 6: 1147–1152 (1997).
274. Corrons JL, Alvarez R, Pujades A, Zarza R, Oliva E, Lasheras G, Callis M, Ribes A, Gelbart T, Beutler E. Hereditary non-spherocytic haemolytic anaemia due to red blood cell glutathione synthetase deficiency in four

unrelated patients from Spain: clinical and molecular studies. *Br. J. Haematol.* 112: 475–482 (2001).

275. Njalsson R, Carlsson K, Winkler A, Larsson A, Norgren S. Diagnostics in patients with glutathione synthetase deficiency but without mutations in the exons of the GSS gene. *Hum. Mutat.* 22: 497 (2003).
276. Shi ZZ, Habib GM, Rhead WJ, Gahl WA, He X, Sazer S, Lieberman MW. Mutations in the glutathione synthetase gene cause 5-oxoprolinuria. *Nat. Genet.* 14: 361–365 (1996).
277. Stoll VS, Simpson SJ, Krauth-Siegel RL, Walsh CT, Pai EF. Glutathione reductase turned into trypanothione reductase: structural analysis of an engineered change in substrate specificity. *Biochemistry* 36: 6437–6447 (1997).
278. Jensen PK, Junien C, Despoisse S, Bernsen A, Thelle T, Friedrich U, de la Chapelle A. Inverted tandem duplication of the short arm of chromosome 8: a non-random *de novo* structural aberration in man. Localization of the gene for glutathione reductase in subband 8p21.1. *Ann. Genet.* 25: 207–211 (1982).
279. Nevin NC, Morrison PJ, Jones J, Reid MM. Inverted tandem duplication of 8p12 — p23.1 in a child with increased activity of glutathione reductase. *J. Med. Genet.* 27: 135–136 (1990).
280. de Die-Smulders CE, Engelen JJ, Schrander-Stumpel CT, Govaerts LC, de Vries B, Vles JS, Wagemans A, Schijns-Fleuren S, Gillessen-Kaesbach G, Fryns JP. Inversion duplication of the short arm of chromosome 8: clinical data on seven patients and review of the literature. *Am. J. Med. Genet.* 59: 369–374 (1995).
281. Moog U, Engelen JJ, Albrechts JC, Baars LG, de Die-Smulders CE. Familial dup(8)(p12p21.1): mild phenotypic effect and review of partial 8p duplications. *Am. J. Med. Genet.* 94: 306–310 (2000).
282. Wollman EE *et al.* Cloning and expression of a cDNA for human thioredoxin. *J. Biol. Chem.* 263: 15506–15512 (1988).
283. Damdimopoulos AE, Miranda-Vizuete A, Pelto-Huikko M, Gustafsson JA, Spyrou G. Human mitochondrial thioredoxin. Involvement in mitochondrial membrane potential and cell death. *J. Biol. Chem.* 277: 33249–33257 (2002).
284. Spyrou G, Enmark E, Miranda-Vizuete A, Gustafsson J. Cloning and expression of a novel mammalian thioredoxin. *J. Biol. Chem.* 272: 2936–2941 (1997).
285. Lee KK, Murakawa M, Takahashi S, Tsubuki S, Kawashima S, Sakamaki K, Yonehara S. Purification, molecular cloning, and characterization of TRP32, a novel thioredoxin-related mammalian protein of 32 kDa. *J. Biol. Chem.* 273: 19160–19166 (1998).

286. Miranda-Vizuete A, Gustafsson JA, Spyrou G. Molecular cloning and expression of a cDNA encoding a human thioredoxin-like protein. *Biochem. Biophys. Res. Commun.* 243: 284–288 (1998).
287. Cunnea PM, Miranda-Vizuete A, Bertoli G, Simmen T, Damdimopoulos AE, Hermann S, Leinonen S, Huikko MP, Gustafsson JA, Sitia R, Spyrou G. ERdj5, an endoplasmic reticulum (ER)-resident protein containing DnaJ and thioredoxin domains, is expressed in secretory cells or following ER stress. *J. Biol. Chem.* 278: 1059–1066 (2003).
288. Hosoda A, Kimata Y, Tsuru A, Kohno K. JPDI, a novel endoplasmic reticulum-resident protein containing both a BiP-interacting J-domain and thioredoxin-like motifs. *J. Biol. Chem.* 278: 2669–2676 (2003).
289. Miranda-Vizuete A, Ljung J, Damdimopoulos AE, Gustafsson JA, Oko R, Pelto-Huikko M, Spyrou G. Characterization of Sptrx, a novel member of the thioredoxin family specifically expressed in human spermatozoa. *J. Biol. Chem.* 276: 31567–31574 (2001).
290. Sadek CM, Damdimopoulos AE, Pelto-Huikko M, Gustafsson JA, Spyrou G, Miranda-Vizuete A. Sptrx-2, a fusion protein composed of one thioredoxin and three tandemly repeated NDP-kinase domains is expressed in human testis germ cells. *Genes Cells* 6: 1077–1090 (2001).
291. Holmgren A. Thioredoxin. 6. The amino acid sequence of the protein from *Escherichia coli* B. *Eur. J. Biochem.* 6: 475–484 (1968).
292. Heppell-Parton A, Cahn A, Bench A, Lowe N, Lehrach H, Zehetner G, Rabbitts P. Thioredoxin, a mediator of growth inhibition, maps to 9q31. *Genomics* 26: 379–381 (1995).
293. Laurent TC, Moore EC, Reichard P. Enzymatic synthesis of deoxyribonucleotides. IV. Isolation and characterization of thioredoxin, the hydrogen donor from *Escherichia coli* B. *J. Biol. Chem.* 239: 3436–3444 (1964).
294. Nakamura H, Nakamura K, Yodoi J. Redox regulation of cellular activation. *Annu. Rev. Immunol.* 15: 351–369 (1997).
295. Chae HZ, Kang SW, Rhee SG. Isoforms of mammalian peroxiredoxin that reduce peroxides in presence of thioredoxin. *Meth. Enzymol.* 300: 219–226 (1999).
296. Saitoh M, Nishitoh H, Fujii M, Takeda K, Tobiume K, Sawada Y, Kawabata M, Miyazono K, Ichijo H. Mammalian thioredoxin is a direct inhibitor of apoptosis signal-regulating kinase (ASK) 1. *EMBO. J.* 17: 2596–2606 (1998).
297. Zhang P, Liu B, Kang SW, Seo MS, Rhee SG, Obeid LM. Thioredoxin peroxidase is a novel inhibitor of apoptosis with a mechanism distinct from that of Bcl-2. *J. Biol. Chem.* 272: 30615–30618 (1997).

298. Higashikubo A, Tanaka N, Noda N, Maeda I, Yagi K, Mizoguchi T, Nanri H. Increase in thioredoxin activity of intestinal epithelial cells mediated by oxidative stress. *Biol. Pharm. Bull.* 22: 900–903 (1999).
299. Nakamura H, Matsuda M, Furuke K, Kitaoka Y, Iwata S, Toda K, Inamoto T, Yamaoka Y, Ozawa K, Yodoi J. Adult T cell leukemia-derived factor/human thioredoxin protects endothelial F-2 cell injury caused by activated neutrophils or hydrogen peroxide. *Immunol. Lett.* 42: 75–80 (1994).
300. Sachi Y, Hirota K, Masutani H, Toda K, Okamoto T, Takigawa M, Yodoi J. Induction of ADF/TRX by oxidative stress in keratinocytes and lymphoid cells. *Immunol. Lett.* 44: 189–193 (1995).
301. Hirota K, Matsui M, Iwata S, Nishiyama A, Mori K, Yodoi J. AP-1 transcriptional activity is regulated by a direct association between thioredoxin and Ref-1. *Proc. Natl. Acad. Sci. USA* 94: 3633–3638 (1997).
302. Sahaf B, Soderberg A, Spyrou G, Barral AM, Pekkari K, Holmgren A, Rosen A. Thioredoxin expression and localization in human cell lines: detection of full-length and truncated species. *Exp. Cell. Res.* 236: 181–192 (1997).
303. Yamawaki H, Haendeler J, Berk BC. Thioredoxin: a key regulator of cardiovascular homeostasis. *Circ. Res.* 93: 1029–1033 (2003).
304. Arner ES, Holmgren A. Physiological functions of thioredoxin and thioredoxin reductase. *Eur. J. Biochem.* 267: 6102–6109 (2000).
305. Arner ES, Nordberg J, Holmgren A. Efficient reduction of lipoamide and lipoic acid by mammalian thioredoxin reductase. *Biochem. Biophys. Res. Commun.* 225: 268–274 (1996).
306. Kumar S, Bjornstedt M, Holmgren A. Selenite is a substrate for calf thymus thioredoxin reductase and thioredoxin and elicits a large non-stoichiometric oxidation of NADPH in the presence of oxygen. *Eur. J. Biochem.* 207: 435–439 (1992).
307. Holmgren A, Lyckeborg C. Enzymatic reduction of alloxan by thioredoxin and NADPH-thioredoxin reductase. *Proc. Natl. Acad. Sci. USA* 77: 5149–5152 (1980).
308. Bjornstedt M, Hamberg M, Kumar S, Xue J, Holmgren A. Human thioredoxin reductase directly reduces lipid hydroperoxides by NADPH and selenocystine strongly stimulates the reaction via catalytically generated selenols. *J. Biol. Chem.* 270: 11761–11764 (1995).
309. Lee SR, Kim JR, Kwon KS, Yoon HW, Levine RL, Ginsburg A, Rhee SG. Molecular cloning and characterization of a mitochondrial selenocysteine-containing thioredoxin reductase from rat liver. *J. Biol. Chem.* 274: 4722–4734 (1999).

310. Miranda-Vizuete A, Damdimopoulos AE, Pedrajas JR, Gustafsson JA, Spyrou G. Human mitochondrial thioredoxin reductase cDNA cloning, expression and genomic organization. *Eur. J. Biochem.* 261: 405–412 (1999).
311. Sun QA, Wu Y, Zappacosta F, Jeang KT, Lee BJ, Hatfield DL, Gladyshev VN. Redox regulation of cell signaling by selenocysteine in mammalian thioredoxin reductases. *J. Biol. Chem.* 274: 24522–24530 (1999).
312. Lescure A, Gautheret D, Carbon P, Krol A. Novel selenoproteins identified *in silico* and *in vivo* by using a conserved RNA structural motif. *J. Biol. Chem.* 274: 38147–38154 (1999).
313. Sun QA, Zappacosta F, Factor VM, Wirth PJ, Hatfield DL, Gladyshev VN. Heterogeneity within animal thioredoxin reductases. Evidence for alternative first exon splicing. *J. Biol. Chem.* 276: 3106–3114 (2001).
314. Osborne SA, Tonissen KF. Genomic organisation and alternative splicing of mouse and human thioredoxin reductase 1 genes. *BMC Genomics* 2: 10 (2001).
315. Rundlof AK, Carlsten M, Giacobini MM, Arner ES. Prominent expression of the selenoprotein thioredoxin reductase in the medullary rays of the rat kidney and thioredoxin reductase mRNA variants differing at the 5′ untranslated region. *Biochem. J.* 347(Pt 3): 661–668 (2000).
316. Luikenhuis S, Perrone G, Dawes IW, Grant CM. The yeast *Saccharomyces cerevisiae* contains two glutaredoxin genes that are required for protection against reactive oxygen species. *Mol. Biol. Cell.* 9: 1081–1091 (1998).
317. Rodriguez-Manzaneque MT, Ros J, Cabiscol E, Sorribas A, Herrero E. Grx5 glutaredoxin plays a central role in protection against protein oxidative damage in *Saccharomyces cerevisiae*. *Mol. Cell. Biol.* 19: 8180–8190 (1999).
318. Chrestensen CA, Starke DW, Mieyal JJ. Acute cadmium exposure inactivates thioltransferase (Glutaredoxin), inhibits intracellular reduction of protein-glutathionyl-mixed disulfides, and initiates apoptosis. *J. Biol. Chem.* 275: 26556–26565 (2000).
319. Daily D, Vlamis-Gardikas A, Offen D, Mittelman L, Melamed E, Holmgren A, Barzilai A. Glutaredoxin protects cerebellar granule neurons from dopamine-induced apoptosis by dual activation of the ras-phosphoinositide 3-kinase and jun n-terminal kinase pathways. *J. Biol. Chem.* 276: 21618–21626 (2001).
320. Gravina SA, Mieyal JJ. Thioltransferase is a specific glutathionyl mixed disulfide oxidoreductase. *Biochemistry* 32: 3368–3376 (1993).
321. Nakamura H, Vaage J, Valen G, Padilla CA, Bjornstedt M, Holmgren A. Measurements of plasma glutaredoxin and thioredoxin in healthy volunteers and during open-heart surgery. *Free Radic. Biol. Med.* 24: 1176–1186 (1998).

322. Kuo FC, Sklar J. Augmented expression of a human gene for 8-oxoguanine DNA glycosylase (MutM) in B lymphocytes of the dark zone in lymph node germinal centers. *J. Exp. Med.* 186: 1547–1556 (1997).
323. Bjoras M, Luna L, Johnsen B, Hoff E, Haug T, Rognes T, Seeberg E. Opposite base-dependent reactions of a human base excision repair enzyme on DNA containing 7,8-dihydro-8-oxoguanine and abasic sites. *EMBO J.* 16: 6314–6322 (1997).
324. Roldan-Arjona T, Wei YF, Carter KC, Klungland A, Anselmino C, Wang RP, Augustus M, Lindahl T. Molecular cloning and functional expression of a human cDNA encoding the antimutator enzyme 8-hydroxyguanine-DNA glycosylase. *Proc. Natl. Acad. Sci. USA* 94: 8016–8020 (1997).
325. Kohno T, Shinmura K, Tosaka M, Tani M, Kim SR, Sugimura H, Nohmi T, Kasai H, Yokota J. Genetic polymorphisms and alternative splicing of the hOGG1 gene, that is involved in the repair of 8-hydroxyguanine in damaged DNA. *Oncogene* 16: 3219–3225 (1998).
326. Shinmura K, Yokota J. The OGG1 gene encodes a repair enzyme for oxidatively damaged DNA and is involved in human carcinogenesis. *Antioxid. Redox. Signal.* 3: 597–609 (2001).
327. Wikman H, Risch A, Klimek F, Schmezer P, Spiegelhalder B, Dienemann H, Kayser K, Schulz V, Drings P, Bartsch H. hOGG1 polymorphism and loss of heterozygosity (LOH): significance for lung cancer susceptibility in a caucasian population. *Int. J. Cancer* 88: 932–937 (2000).
328. Janssen K, Schlink K, Gotte W, Hippler B, Kaina B, Oesch F. DNA repair activity of 8-oxoguanine DNA glycosylase 1 (OGG1) in human lymphocytes is not dependent on genetic polymorphism Ser326/Cys326. *Mutat. Res.* 486: 207–216 (2001).
329. Elahi A, Zheng Z, Park J, Eyring K, McCaffrey T, Lazarus P. The human OGG1 DNA repair enzyme and its association with orolaryngeal cancer risk. *Carcinogenesis* 23: 1229–1234 (2002).
330. He YH, Xu Y, Kobune M, Wu M, Kelley MR, Martin WJ II. *Escherichia coli* FPG and human OGG1 reduce DNA damage and cytotoxicity by BCNU in human lung cells. *Am. J. Physiol. Lung Cell. Mol. Physiol.* 282: L50–L55 (2002).
331. Ito H, Hamajima N, Takezaki T, Matsuo K, Tajima K, Hatooka S, Mitsudomi T, Suyama M, Sato S, Ueda R. A limited association of OGG1 Ser326Cys polymorphism for adenocarcinoma of the lung. *J. Epidemiol.* 12: 258–265 (2002).

332. Le Marchand L, Donlon T, Lum-Jones A, Seifried A, Wilkens LR. Association of the hOGG1 Ser326Cys polymorphism with lung cancer risk. *Cancer Epidemiol. Biomarkers Prev.* 11: 409–412 (2002).
333. Takezaki T, Gao CM, Wu JZ, Li ZY, Wang JD, Ding JH, Liu YT, Hu X, Xu TL, Tajima K, Sugimura H. hOGG1 Ser(326)Cys polymorphism and modification by environmental factors of stomach cancer risk in Chinese. *Int. J. Cancer* 99: 624–627 (2002).
334. Xing DY, Tan W, Song N, Lin DX. Ser326Cys polymorphism in hOGG1 gene and risk of esophageal cancer in a Chinese population. *Int. J. Cancer* 95: 140–143 (2001).
335. Hanaoka T, Yamano Y, Hashimoto H, Kagawa J, Tsugane S. A preliminary evaluation of intra- and interindividual variations of hOGG1 messenger RNA levels in peripheral blood cells as determined by a real-time polymerase chain reaction technique. *Cancer Epidemiol. Biomarkers Prev.* 9: 1255–1258 (2000).
336. Vogel U, Nexo BA, Olsen A, Thomsen B, Jacobsen NR, Wallin H, Overvad K, Tjonneland A. No association between OGG1 Ser326Cys polymorphism and breast cancer risk. *Cancer Epidemiol. Biomarkers Prev.* 12: 170–171 (2003).
337. Audebert M, Radicella JP, Dizdaroglu M. Effect of single mutations in the OGG1 gene found in human tumors on the substrate specificity of the Ogg1 protein. *Nucleic Acids Res.* 28: 2672–2678 (2000).
338. Babior BM. NADPH oxidase: an update. *Blood* 93: 1464–1476 (1999).
339. Dinauer MC, Pierce EA, Bruns GA, Curnutte JT, Orkin SH. Human neutrophil cytochrome b light chain (p22-phox). Gene structure, chromosomal location, and mutations in cytochrome-negative autosomal recessive chronic granulomatous disease. *J. Clin. Invest.* 86: 1729–1737 (1990).
340. de Boer M, de Klein A, Hossle JP, Seger R, Corbeel L, Weening RS, Roos D. Cytochrome b558-negative, autosomal recessive chronic granulomatous disease: two new mutations in the cytochrome b558 light chain of the NADPH oxidase (p22-phox). *Am. J. Hum. Genet.* 51: 1127–1135 (1992).
341. Dinauer MC, Pierce EA, Erickson RW, Muhlebach TJ, Messner H, Orkin SH, Seger RA, Curnutte JT. Point mutation in the cytoplasmic domain of the neutrophil p22-phox cytochrome b subunit is associated with a non-functional NADPH oxidase and chronic granulomatous disease. *Proc. Natl. Acad. Sci. USA* 88: 11231–11235 (1991).
342. Yamada M, Ariga T, Kawamura N, Ohtsu M, Imajoh-Ohmi S, Ohshika E, Tatsuzawa O, Kobayashi K, Sakiyama Y. Genetic studies of three Japanese

patients with p22-phox-deficient chronic granulomatous disease: detection of a possible common mutant CYBA allele in Japan and a genotype-phenotype correlation in these patients. *Br. J. Haematol.* 108: 511–517 (2000).

343. Moreno MU, San Jose G, Orbe J, Paramo JA, Beloqui O, Diez J, Zalba G. Preliminary characterisation of the promoter of the human p22(phox) gene: identification of a new polymorphism associated with hypertension. *FEBS Lett.* 542: 27–31 (2003).
344. Parkos CA, Dinauer MC, Walker LE, Allen RA, Jesaitis AJ, Orkin SH. Primary structure and unique expression of the 22-kilodalton light chain of human neutrophil cytochrome b. *Proc. Natl. Acad. Sci. USA* 85: 3319–3323 (1988).
345. Nakano T, Matsunaga S, Nagata A, Maruyama T. NAD(P)H oxidase p22phox Gene C242T polymorphism and lipoprotein oxidation. *Clin. Chim. Acta* 335: 101–107 (2003).
346. Schneider MP, Hilgers KF, Huang Y, Delles C, John S, Oehmer S, Schmieder RE. The C242T p22phox polymorphism and endothelium-dependent vasodilation in subjects with hypercholesterolaemia. *Clin. Sci. (Lond.)* 105: 97–103 (2003).
347. Inoue N, Kawashima S, Kanazawa K, Yamada S, Akita H, Yokoyama M. Polymorphism of the NADH/NADPH oxidase p22 phox gene in patients with coronary artery disease. *Circulation* 97: 135–137 (1998).
348. Ishii K, Murata M, Oguchi S, Takeshita E, Ito D, Tanahashi N, Fukuuchi Y, Saitou I, Ikeda Y, Watanabe K. Genetic risk factors for ischemic cerebrovascular disease — analysis on fifteen candidate prothrombotic gene polymorphisms in the Japanese population. *Rinsho Byori* 52: 22–27 (2004).
349. Ito D, Murata M, Watanabe K, Yoshida T, Saito I, Tanahashi N, Fukuuchi Y. C242T polymorphism of NADPH oxidase p22 PHOX gene and ischemic cerebrovascular disease in the Japanese population. *Stroke* 31: 936–939 (2000).
350. Spence MS, McGlinchey PG, Patterson CC, Allen AR, Murphy G, Bayraktutan U, Fogarty DG, Evans AE, McKeown PP. Investigation of the C242T polymorphism of NAD(P)H oxidase p22 phox gene and ischaemic heart disease using family-based association methods. *Clin. Sci. (Lond.)* 105: 677–682 (2003).
351. Cahilly C, Ballantyne CM, Lim DS, Gotto A, Marian AJ. A variant of p22(phox), involved in generation of reactive oxygen species in the vessel wall, is associated with progression of coronary atherosclerosis. *Circ. Res.* 86: 391–395 (2000).

352. Guzik TJ, West NE, Black E, McDonald D, Ratnatunga C, Pillai R, Channon KM. Functional effect of the C242T polymorphism in the NAD(P)H oxidase p22phox gene on vascular superoxide production in atherosclerosis. *Circulation* 102: 1744–1747 (2000).
353. Hayaishi-Okano R, Yamasaki Y, Kajimoto Y, Sakamoto K, Ohtoshi K, Katakami N, Kawamori D, Miyatsuka T, Hatazaki M, Hazama Y, Hori M. Association of NAD(P)H oxidase p22 phox gene variation with advanced carotid atherosclerosis in Japanese type 2 diabetes. *Diabetes Care* 26: 458–463 (2003).
354. Matsunaga-Irie S, Maruyama T, Yamamoto Y, Motohashi Y, Hirose H, Shimada A, Murata M, Saruta T. Relation between development of nephropathy and the p22phox C242T and receptor for advanced glycation end-product G1704T gene polymorphisms in type 2 diabetic patients. *Diabetes Care* 27: 303–307 (2004).
355. Cai H, Duarte N, Wilcken DE, Wang XL. NADH/NADPH oxidase p22 phox C242T polymorphism and coronary artery disease in the Australian population. *Eur. J. Clin. Invest.* 29: 744–748 (1999).
356. Stanger O, Renner W, Khoschsorur G, Rigler B, Wascher TC. NADH/NADPH oxidase p22 phox C242T polymorphism and lipid peroxidation in coronary artery disease. *Clin. Physiol.* 21: 718–722 (2001).
357. Li A, Prasad A, Mincemoyer R, Satorius C, Epstein N, Finkel T, Quyyumi AA. Relationship of the C242T p22phox gene polymorphism to angiographic coronary artery disease and endothelial function. *Am. J. Med. Genet.* 86: 57–61 (1999).
358. Wolf G, Panzer U, Harendza S, Wenzel U, Stahl RA. No association between a genetic variant of the p22(phox) component of NAD(P)H oxidase and the incidence and progression of IgA nephropathy. *Nephrol. Dial. Transplant.* 17: 1509–1512 (2002).
359. Renner W, Schallmoser K, Gallippi P, Krauss C, Toplak H, Wascher TC, Pilger E. C242T polymorphism of the p22 phox gene is not associated with peripheral arterial occlusive disease. *Atherosclerosis* 152: 175–179 (2000).
360. Raijmakers MT, Roes EM, Steegers EA, Peters WH. The C242T-polymorphism of the NADPH/NADH oxidase gene p22phox subunit is not associated with pre-eclampsia. *J. Hum. Hypertens.* 16: 423–425 (2002).
361. Matsunaga S, Maruyama T, Yamada S, Motohashi Y, Shigihara T, Shimada A, Saruta T. Nicotinamide adenine dinucleotide phosphate oxidase (NADPH oxidase) P22 Phox C242T gene polymorphism in type 1 diabetes. *Ann. NY Acad. Sci.* 1005: 324–327 (2003).

362. Gardemann A, Mages P, Katz N, Tillmanns H, Haberbosch W. The p22 phox A640G gene polymorphism but not the C242T gene variation is associated with coronary heart disease in younger individuals. *Atherosclerosis* 145: 315–323 (1999).
363. Krex D, Ziegler A, Konig IR, Schackert HK, Schackert G. Polymorphisms of the NADPH oxidase P22PHOX gene in a Caucasian population with intracranial aneurysms. *Cerebrovasc. Dis.* 16: 363–368 (2003).
364. Schapiro BL, Newburger PE, Klempner MS, Dinauer MC. Chronic granulomatous disease presenting in a 69-year-old man. *N. Engl. J. Med.* 325: 1786–1790 (1991).
365. Royer-Pokora B, Kunkel LM, Monaco AP, Goff SC, Newburger PE, Baehner RL, Cole FS, Curnutte JT, Orkin SH. Cloning the gene for an inherited human disorder — chronic granulomatous disease — on the basis of its chromosomal location. *Nature* 322: 32–38 (1986).
366. Bolscher BG, de Boer M, de Klein A, Weening RS, Roos D. Point mutations in the beta-subunit of cytochrome b558 leading to X-linked chronic granulomatous disease. *Blood* 77: 2482–2487 (1991).
367. Brouha B, Meischl C, Ostertag E, de Boer M, Zhang Y, Neijens H, Roos D, Kazazian HH Jr. Evidence consistent with human L1 retrotransposition in maternal meiosis I. *Am. J. Hum. Genet.* 71: 327–336 (2002).
368. Dinauer MC, Curnutte JT, Rosen H, Orkin SH. A missense mutation in the neutrophil cytochrome b heavy chain in cytochrome-positive X-linked chronic granulomatous disease. *J. Clin. Invest.* 84: 2012–2016 (1989).
369. Ishibashi F, Mizukami T, Kanegasaki S, Motoda L, Kakinuma R, Endo F, Nunoi H. Improved superoxide-generating ability by interferon gamma due to splicing pattern change of transcripts in neutrophils from patients with a splice site mutation in CYBB gene. *Blood* 98: 436–441 (2001).
370. Ishibashi F, Nunoi H, Endo F, Matsuda I, Kanegasaki S. Statistical and mutational analysis of chronic granulomatous disease in Japan with special reference to gp91-phox and p22-phox deficiency. *Hum. Genet.* 106: 473–481 (2000).
371. Meischl C, Boer M, Ahlin A, Roos D. A new exon created by intronic insertion of a rearranged LINE-1 element as the cause of chronic granulomatous disease. *Eur. J. Hum. Genet.* 8: 697–703 (2000).
372. Noack D, Heyworth PG, Newburger PE, Cross AR. An unusual intronic mutation in the CYBB gene giving rise to chronic granulomatous disease. *Biochim. Biophys. Acta.* 1537: 125–131 (2001).
373. Stasia MJ, Lardy B, Maturana A, Rousseau P, Martel C, Bordigoni P, Demaurex N, Morel F. Molecular and functional characterization of a new

X-linked chronic granulomatous disease variant (X91+) case with a double missense mutation in the cytosolic gp91phox C-terminal tail. *Biochim. Biophys. Acta* 1586: 316–330 (2002).

374. Miki T, Weil SC, Rosner GL, Reid MS, Kidd KK. An MPO cDNA clone identifies an RFLP with PstI. *Nucleic Acids Res.* 16: 1649 (1988).
375. Kizaki M, Miller CW, Selsted ME, Koeffler HP. Myeloperoxidase (MPO) gene mutation in hereditary MPO deficiency. *Blood* 83: 1935–1940 (1994).
376. DeLeo FR, Goedken M, McCormick SJ, Nauseef WM. A novel form of hereditary myeloperoxidase deficiency linked to endoplasmic reticulum/proteasome degradation. *J. Clin. Invest.* 101: 2900–2909 (1998).
377. Romano M, Dri P, Dadalt L, Patriarca P, Baralle FE. Biochemical and molecular characterization of hereditary myeloperoxidase deficiency. *Blood* 90: 4126–4134 (1997).
378. Pecoits-Filho R, Stenvinkel P, Marchlewska A, Heimburger O, Barany P, Hoff CM, Holmes CJ, Suliman M, Lindholm B, Schalling M, Nordfors L. A functional variant of the myeloperoxidase gene is associated with cardiovascular disease in end-stage renal disease patients. *Kidney Int. Suppl.* 84: S172–S176 (2003).
379. Reynolds WF, Hiltunen M, Pirskanen M, Mannermaa A, Helisalmi S, Lehtovirta M, Alafuzoff I, Soininen H. MPO and APOEepsilon4 polymorphisms interact to increase risk for AD in Finnish males. *Neurology* 55: 1284–1290 (2000).
380. Crawford FC, Freeman MJ, Schinka JA, Morris MD, Abdullah LI, Richards D, Sevush S, Duara R, Mullan MJ. Association between Alzheimer's disease and a functional polymorphism in the Myeloperoxidase gene. *Exp. Neurol.* 167: 456–459 (2001).
381. Combarros O, Infante J, Llorca J, Pena N, Fernandez-Viadero C, Berciano J. The myeloperoxidase gene in Alzheimer's disease: a case-control study and meta-analysis. *Neurosci. Lett.* 326: 33–36 (2002).
382. Leininger-Muller B, Hoy A, Herbeth B, Pfister M, Serot JM, Stavljenic-Rukavina M, Massana L, Passmore P, Siest G, Visvikis S. Myeloperoxidase G-463A polymorphism and Alzheimer's disease in the ApoEurope study. *Neurosci. Lett.* 349: 95–98 (2003).
383. Reynolds WF, Chang E, Douer D, Ball ED, Kanda V. An allelic association implicates myeloperoxidase in the etiology of acute promyelocytic leukemia. *Blood* 90: 2730–2737 (1997).
384. Eiserich JP, Baldus S, Brennan ML, Ma W, Zhang C, Tousson A, Castro L, Lusis AJ, Nauseef WM, White CR, Freeman BA. Myeloperoxidase, a leukocyte-derived vascular NO oxidase. *Science* 296: 2391–2394 (2002).

385. Hoy A, Tregouet D, Leininger-Muller B, Poirier O, Maurice M, Sass C, Siest G, Tiret L, Visvikis S. Serum myeloperoxidase concentration in a healthy population: biological variations, familial resemblance and new genetic polymorphisms. *Eur. J. Hum. Genet.* 9: 780–786 (2001).
386. Nikpoor B, Turecki G, Fournier C, Theroux P, Rouleau GA. A functional myeloperoxidase polymorphic variant is associated with coronary artery disease in French-Canadians. *Am. Heart J.* 142: 336–339 (2001).
387. Zhang R, Brennan ML, Fu X, Aviles RJ, Pearce GL, Penn MS. Topol EJ, Sprecher DL, Hazen SL. Association between myeloperoxidase levels and risk of coronary artery disease. *JAMA* 286: 2136–2142 (2001).
388. Cascorbi I, Henning S, Brockmoller J, Gephart J, Meisel C, Muller JM, Loddenkemper R, Roots I. Substantially reduced risk of cancer of the aerodigestive tract in subjects with variant — 463A of the myeloperoxidase gene. *Cancer Res.* 60: 644–649 (2000).
389. Pakakasama S, Chen TT, Frawley W, Muller C, Douglass EC, Tomlinson GE. Myeloperoxidase promotor polymorphism and risk of hepatoblastoma. *Int. J. Cancer* 106: 205–207 (2003).
390. Matsuo K, Hamajima N, Shinoda M, Hatooka S, Inoue M, Takezaki T, Onda H, Tajima K. Possible risk reduction in esophageal cancer associated with MPO-463 A allele. *J. Epidemiol.* 11: 109–114 (2001).
391. London SJ, Lehman TA, Taylor JA. Myeloperoxidase genetic polymorphism and lung cancer risk. *Cancer Res.* 57: 5001–5003 (1997).
392. Chevrier I, Stucker I, Houllier AM, Cenee S, Beaune P, Laurent-Puig P, Loriot MA. Myeloperoxidase: new polymorphisms and relation with lung cancer risk. *Pharmacogenetics* 13: 729–739 (2003).
393. Dally H, Gassner K, Jager B, Schmezer P, Spiegelhalder B, Edler L, Drings P, Dienemann H, Schulz V, Kayser K, Bartsch H, Risch A. Myeloperoxidase (MPO) genotype and lung cancer histologic types: the MPO-463 A allele is associated with reduced risk for small cell lung cancer in smokers. *Int. J. Cancer* 102: 530–535 (2002).
394. Feyler A, Voho A, Bouchardy C, Kuokkanen K, Dayer P, Hirvonen A, Benhamou S. Point: myeloperoxidase-463G → a polymorphism and lung cancer risk. *Cancer Epidemiol. Biomarkers. Prev.* 11: 1550–1554 (2002).
395. Kantarci OH, Lesnick TG, Yang P, Meyer RL, Hebrink DD, McMurray CT, Weinshenker BG. Myeloperoxidase-463 (G → A) polymorphism associated with lower risk of lung cancer. *Mayo Clin. Proc.* 77: 17–22 (2002).
396. Le Marchand L, Seifried A, Lum A, Wilkens LR. Association of the myeloperoxidase-463G → a polymorphism with lung cancer risk. *Cancer Epidemiol. Biomarkers Prev.* 9: 181–184 (2000).

397. Lu W, Qi J, Xing D, Tan W, Miao X, Su W, Wu M, Lin D. Lung cancer risk associated with genetic polymorphism in myeloperoxidase (−463 G/A) in a Chinese population. *Zhonghua Zhong Liu Za Zhi* 24: 250–253 (2002).
398. Misra RR, Tangrea JA, Virtamo J, Ratnasinghe D, Andersen MR, Barrett M, Taylor PR, Albanes D. Variation in the promoter region of the myeloperoxidase gene is not directly related to lung cancer risk among male smokers in Finland. *Cancer Lett.* 164: 161–167 (2001).
399. Schabath MB, Spitz MR, Hong WK, Delclos GL, Reynolds WF, Gunn GB, Whitehead LW, Wu X. A myeloperoxidase polymorphism associated with reduced risk of lung cancer. *Lung Cancer* 37: 35–40 (2002).
400. Xu LL, Liu G, Miller DP, Zhou W, Lynch TJ, Wain JC, Su L, Christiani DC. Counterpoint: the myeloperoxidase-463G → a polymorphism does not decrease lung cancer susceptibility in Caucasians. *Cancer Epidemiol. Biomarkers Prev.* 11: 1555–1559 (2002).
401. Nauseef WM, Brigham S, Cogley M. Hereditary myeloperoxidase deficiency due to a missense mutation of arginine 569 to tryptophan. *J. Biol. Chem.* 269: 1212–1216 (1994).
402. Asano K, Chee CB, Gaston B, Lilly CM, Gerard C, Drazen JM, Stamler JS. Constitutive and inducible nitric oxide synthase gene expression, regulation, and activity in human lung epithelial cells. *Proc. Natl. Acad. Sci. USA* 91: 10089–10093 (1994).
403. Forstermann U, Boissel JP, Kleinert H. Expressional control of the "constitutive" isoforms of nitric oxide synthase (NOS I and NOS III). *FASEB J.* 12: 773–790 (1998).
404. Marsden PA, Heng HH, Scherer SW, Stewart RJ, Hall AV, Shi XM, Tsui LC, Schappert KT. Structure and chromosomal localization of the human constitutive endothelial nitric oxide synthase gene. *J. Biol. Chem.* 268: 17478–17488 (1993).
405. Hall AV, Antoniou H, Wang Y, Cheung AH, Arbus AM, Olson SL, Lu WC, Kau CL, Marsden PA. Structural organization of the human neuronal nitric oxide synthase gene (NOS1). *J. Biol. Chem.* 269: 33082–33090 (1994).
406. Grasemann H, Drazen JM, Yandava CN. Protein sequence of the human neuronal nitric oxide synthase (Type I NOS): an error in the sequence database. *Nitric Oxide* 1: 441 (1997).
407. Yun HY, Dawson VL, Dawson TM. Nitric oxide in health and disease of the nervous system. *Mol. Psychiatry* 2: 300–310 (1997).
408. Brenman JE, Chao DS, Xia H, Aldape K, Bredt DS. Nitric oxide synthase complexed with dystrophin and absent from skeletal muscle sarcolemma in Duchenne muscular dystrophy. *Cell* 82: 743–752 (1995).

409. Chung E, Curtis D, Chen G, Marsden PA, Twells R, Xu W, Gardiner M. Genetic evidence for the neuronal nitric oxide synthase gene (NOS1) as a susceptibility locus for infantile pyloric stenosis. *Am. J. Hum. Genet.* 58: 363–370 (1996).
410. Gao PS, Kawada H, Kasamatsu T, Mao XQ, Roberts MH, Miyamoto Y, Yoshimura M, Saitoh Y, Yasue H, Nakao K, Adra CN, Kun JF, Morooka S, Inoko H, Ho LP, Shirakawa T, Hopkin JM. Variants of NOS1, NOS2, and NOS3 genes in asthmatics. *Biochem. Biophys. Res. Commun.* 267: 761–763 (2000).
411. Grasemann H, Knauer N, Buscher R, Hubner K, Drazen JM, Ratjen F. Airway nitric oxide levels in cystic fibrosis patients are related to a polymorphism in the neuronal nitric oxide synthase gene. *Am. J. Respir. Crit. Care Med.* 162: 2172–2176 (2000).
412. Ali M, Khoo SK, Turner S, Stick S, Le Souef P, Franklin P. NOS1 polymorphism is associated with atopy but not exhaled nitric oxide levels in healthy children. *Pediatr. Allergy Immunol.* 14: 261–265 (2003).
413. Grasemann H, Storm van's Gravesande K, Gartig S, Kirsch M, Buscher R, Drazen JM, Ratjen F. Nasal nitric oxide levels in cystic fibrosis patients are associated with a neuronal NO synthase (NOS1) gene polymorphism. *Nitric Oxide* 6: 236–241 (2002).
414. Immervoll T, Loesgen S, Dutsch G, Gohlke H, Herbon N, Klugbauer S, Dempfle A, Bickeboller H, Becker-Follmann J, Ruschendorf F, Saar K, Reis A, Wichmann HE, Wjst M. Fine mapping and single nucleotide polymorphism association results of candidate genes for asthma and related phenotypes. *Hum. Mutat.* 18: 327–336 (2001).
415. Shinkai T, Ohmori O, Hori H, Nakamura J. Allelic association of the neuronal nitric oxide synthase (NOS1) gene with schizophrenia. *Mol. Psychiatry* 7: 560–563 (2002).
416. Liou YJ, Tsai SJ, Hong CJ, Liao DL. Association analysis for the CA repeat polymorphism of the neuronal nitric oxide synthase (NOS1) gene and schizophrenia. *Schizophr. Res.* 65: 57–59 (2003).
417. Buttenschon HN, Mors O, Ewald H, McQuillin A, Kalsi G, Lawrence J, Gurling H, Kruse TA. No association between a neuronal nitric oxide synthase (NOS1) gene polymorphism on chromosome 12q24 and bipolar disorder. *Am. J. Med. Genet.* 124B: 73–75 (2004).
418. Marsden PA, Heng HH, Duff CL, Shi XM, Tsui LC, Hall AV. Localization of the human gene for inducible nitric oxide synthase (NOS2) to chromosome 17q11.2-q12. *Genomics* 19: 183–185 (1994).

419. Xu W, Charles IG, Liu L, Moncada S, Emson P. Molecular cloning and structural organization of the human inducible nitric oxide synthase gene (NOS2). *Biochem. Biophys. Res. Commun.* 219: 784–788 (1996).
420. Kun JF, Mordmuller B, Lell B, Lehman LG, Luckner D, Kremsner PG. Polymorphism in promoter region of inducible nitric oxide synthase gene and protection against malaria. *Lancet* 351: 265–266 (1998).
421. Bellamy R, Hill AV. A bi-allelic tetranucleotide repeat in the promoter of the human inducible nitric oxide synthase gene. *Clin. Genet.* 52: 192–193 (1997).
422. Xu W, Liu L, Emson PC, Harrington CR, Charles IG. Evolution of a homopurine-homopyrimidine pentanucleotide repeat sequence upstream of the human inducible nitric oxide synthase gene. *Gene* 204: 165–170 (1997).
423. Kun JF, Mordmuller B, Perkins DJ, May J, Mercereau-Puijalon O, Alpers M, Weinberg JB, Kremsner PG. Nitric oxide synthase 2(Lambarene) (G-954C), increased nitric oxide production, and protection against malaria. *J. Infect. Dis.* 184: 330–336 (2001).
424. Xu W, Humphries S, Tomita M, Okuyama T, Matsuki M, Burgner D, Kwiatkowski D, Liu L, Charles IG. Survey of the allelic frequency of a NOS2A promoter microsatellite in human populations: assessment of the NOS2A gene and predisposition to infectious disease. *Nitric Oxide* 4: 379–383 (2000).
425. Warpeha KM, Xu W, Liu L, Charles IG, Patterson CC, Ah-Fat F, Harding S, Hart PM, Chakravarthy U, Hughes AE. Genotyping and functional analysis of a polymorphic (CCTTT)(n) repeat of NOS2A in diabetic retinopathy. *FASEB J.* 13: 1825–1832 (1999).
426. Johannesen J, Tarnow L, Parving HH, Nerup J, Pociot F. CCTTT-repeat polymorphism in the human NOS2-promoter confers low risk of diabetic nephropathy in type 1 diabetic patients. *Diabetes Care* 23: 560–562 (2000).
427. Konno S, Hizawa N, Yamaguchi E, Jinushi E, Nishimura M. (CCTTT)n repeat polymorphism in the NOS2 gene promoter is associated with atopy. *J. Allergy. Clin. Immunol.* 108: 810–814 (2001).
428. Rutherford S, Johnson MP, Curtain RP, Griffiths LR. Chromosome 17 and the inducible nitric oxide synthase gene in human essential hypertension. *Hum. Genet.* 109: 408–415 (2001).
429. Rueda B, Lopez-Nevot MA, Pascual M, Ortega E, Maldonado J, Lopez ML, Koeleman BP, Martin J. Polymorphism of the inducible nitric oxide synthase gene in celiac disease. *Hum. Immunol.* 63: 1062–1065 (2002).

430. Pascual M, Lopez-Nevot MA, Caliz R, Koeleman BP, Balsa A, Pascual-Salcedo D, Martin J. Genetic determinants of rheumatoid arthritis: the inducible nitric oxide synthase (NOS2) gene promoter polymorphism. *Genes. Immun.* 3: 299–301 (2002).
431. Orozco G, Sanchez E, Lopez-Nevot MA, Caballero A, Bravo MJ, Morata P, de Dios Colmenero J, Alonso A, Martin J. Inducible nitric oxide synthase promoter polymorphism in human brucellosis. *Microbes Infect.* 5: 1165–1169 (2003).
432. Lopez-Nevot MA, Ramal L, Jimenez-Alonso J, Martin J. The inducible nitric oxide synthase promoter polymorphism does not confer susceptibility to systemic lupus erythematosus. *Rheumatology (Oxford)* 42: 113–116 (2003).
433. Oates JC, Levesque MC, Hobbs MR, Smith EG, Molano ID, Page GP, Hill BS, Weinberg JB, Cooper GS, Gilkeson GS. Nitric oxide synthase 2 promoter polymorphisms and systemic lupus erythematosus in African-Americans. *J. Rheumatol.* 30: 60–67 (2003).
434. Johannesen J, Pociot F, Kristiansen OP, Karlsen AE, Nerup J. No evidence for linkage in the promoter region of the inducible nitric oxide synthase gene (NOS2) in a Danish type 1 diabetes population. *Genes. Immun.* 1: 362–366 (2000).
435. Johannesen J, Pie A, Pociot F, Kristiansen OP, Karlsen AE, Nerup J. Linkage of the human inducible nitric oxide synthase gene to type 1 diabetes. *J. Clin. Endocrinol. Metab.* 86: 2792–2796 (2001).
436. Hobbs MR, Udhayakumar V, Levesque MC, Booth J, Roberts JM, Tkachuk AN, Pole A, Coon H, Kariuki S, Nahlen BL, Mwaikambo ED, Lal AL, Granger DL, Anstey NM, Weinberg JB. A new NOS2 promoter polymorphism associated with increased nitric oxide production and protection from severe malaria in Tanzanian and Kenyan children. *Lancet* 360: 1468–1475 (2002).
437. Nakayama M, Yasue H, Yoshimura M, Shimasaki Y, Kugiyama K, Ogawa H, Motoyama T, Saito Y, Ogawa Y, Miyamoto Y, Nakao K. T-786 → C mutation in the 5′-flanking region of the endothelial nitric oxide synthase gene is associated with coronary spasm. *Circulation* 99: 2864–2870 (1999).
438. Miyahara K *et al.* Cloning and structural characterization of the human endothelial nitric-oxide-synthase gene. *Eur. J. Biochem.* 223: 719–726 (1994).
439. Shimasaki Y, Yasue H, Yoshimura M, Nakayama M, Kugiyama K, Ogawa H, Harada E, Masuda T, Koyama W, Saito Y, Miyamoto Y, Ogawa Y, Nakao K. Association of the missense Glu298Asp variant of the endothelial nitric oxide synthase gene with myocardial infarction. *J. Am. Coll. Cardiol.* 31: 1506–1510 (1998).

440. Miyamoto Y, Saito Y, Nakayama M, Shimasaki Y, Yoshimura T, Yoshimura M, Harada M, Kajiyama N, Kishimoto I, Kuwahara K, Hino J, Ogawa E, Hamanaka I, Kamitani S, Takahashi N, Kawakami R, Kangawa K, Yasue H, Nakao K. Replication protein A1 reduces transcription of the endothelial nitric oxide synthase gene containing a $-786 \rightarrow$ C mutation associated with coronary spastic angina. *Hum. Mol. Genet.* 9: 2629–2637 (2000).
441. Ghilardi G, Biondi ML, Cecchini F, DeMonti M, Guagnellini E, Scorza R. Vascular invasion in human breast cancer is correlated to T $\rightarrow$ 786C polymorphism of NOS3 gene. *Nitric Oxide* 9: 118–122 (2003).
442. Alvarez R, Gonzalez P, Batalla A, Reguero JR, Iglesias-Cubero G, Hevia S, Cortina A, Merino E, Gonzalez I, Alvarez V, Coto E. Association between the NOS3 (−786 T/C) and the ACE (I/D) DNA genotypes and early coronary artery disease. *Nitric Oxide* 5: 343–348 (2001).
443. Ghilardi G, Biondi ML, DeMonti M, Bernini M, Turri O, Massaro F, Guagnellini E, Scorza R. Independent risk factor for moderate to severe internal carotid artery stenosis: T786C mutation of the endothelial nitric oxide synthase gene. *Clin. Chem.* 48: 989–993 (2002).
444. Chistiakov DA, Voron'ko OE, Savost'ianov KV, Minushkina LO. Polymorphic markers of endothelial NO-synthase and angiotensin II vascular receptor genes and predisposition to ischemic heart disease. *Genetika* 36: 1707–1711 (2000).
445. Minushkina LO, Zateishchikov DA, Zateishchikova AA, Zotova IV, Kudriashova OY, Nosikov VV, Sidorenko BA. NOS3 gene polymorphism and left ventricular hypertrophy in patients with essential hypertension. *Kardiologiia* 42: 30–34 (2002).
446. Tempfer C, Unfried G, Zeillinger R, Hefler L, Nagele F, Huber JC. Endothelial nitric oxide synthase gene polymorphism in women with idiopathic recurrent miscarriage. *Hum. Reprod.* 16: 1644–1647 (2001).
447. Kimura T, Yokoyama T, Matsumura Y, Yoshiike N, Date C, Muramatsu M, Tanaka H. NOS3 genotype-dependent correlation between blood pressure and physical activity. *Hypertension* 41: 355–360 (2003).
448. Neugebauer S, Baba T, Watanabe T. Association of the nitric oxide synthase gene polymorphism with an increased risk for progression to diabetic nephropathy in type 2 diabetes. *Diabetes* 49: 500–503 (2000).
449. Voron'ko OE, Chistiakov DA, Kobalava Zh D, Tereshchenko SN, Moiseev SV, Nosikov VV. Polymorphic minisatellite of ecNOS4a/4b in the endothelial NO-synthase gene amd cardiovascular diseases. *Mol. Biol. (Mosk.)* 34: 875–878 (2000).
450. Zanchi A, Moczulski DK, Hanna LS, Wantman M, Warram JH, Krolewski AS. Risk of advanced diabetic nephropathy in type 1 diabetes is associated

with endothelial nitric oxide synthase gene polymorphism. *Kidney Int.* 57: 405–413 (2000).

451. Fujita H, Narita T, Meguro H, Ishii T, Hanyu O, Suzuki K, Kamoi K, Ito S. Lack of association between an ecNOS gene polymorphism and diabetic nephropathy in type 2 diabetic patients with proliferative diabetic retinopathy. *Horm. Metab. Res.* 32: 80–83 (2000).
452. Rippin JD, Patel A, Belyaev ND, Gill GV, Barnett AH, Bain SC. Nitric oxide synthase gene polymorphisms and diabetic nephropathy. *Diabetologia* 46: 426–428 (2003).
453. Hefler LA, Ludwig E, Lampe D, Zeillinger R, Leodolter S, Gitsch G, Koelbl H, Tempfer CB. Polymorphisms of the endothelial nitric oxide synthase gene in ovarian cancer. *Gynecol. Oncol.* 86: 134–137 (2002).
454. Tanus-Santos JE, Desai M, Flockhart DA. Effects of ethnicity on the distribution of clinically relevant endothelial nitric oxide variants. *Pharmacogenetics* 11: 719–725 (2001).
455. Elbaz A, Poirier O, Moulin T, Chedru F, Cambien F, Amarenco P. Association between the Glu298Asp polymorphism in the endothelial constitutive nitric oxide synthase gene and brain infarction. The GENIC Investigators. *Stroke* 31: 1634–1639 (2000).
456. MacLeod MJ, Dahiyat MT, Cumming A, Meiklejohn D, Shaw D, St Clair D. No association between Glu/Asp polymorphism of NOS3 gene and ischemic stroke. *Neurology* 53: 418–420 (1999).
457. Hingorani AD, Liang CF, Fatibene J, Lyon A, Monteith S, Parsons A, Haydock S, Hopper RV, Stephens NG, O'Shaughnessy KM, Brown MJ. A common variant of the endothelial nitric oxide synthase (Glu298 → Asp) is a major risk factor for coronary artery disease in the UK. *Circulation* 100: 1515–1520 (1999).
458. Hibi K, Ishigami T, Tamura K, Mizushima S, Nyui N, Fujita T, Ochiai H, Kosuge M, Watanabe Y, Yoshii Y, Kihara M, Kimura K, Ishii M, Umemura S. Endothelial nitric oxide synthase gene polymorphism and acute myocardial infarction. *Hypertension* 32: 521–526 (1998).
459. Jachymova M, Horky K, Bultas J, Kozich V, Jindra A, Peleska J, Martasek P. Association of the Glu298Asp polymorphism in the endothelial nitric oxide synthase gene with essential hypertension resistant to conventional therapy. *Biochem. Biophys. Res. Commun.* 284: 426–430 (2001).
460. Kobashi G, Yamada H, Ohta K, Kato E, Ebina Y, Fujimoto S. Endothelial nitric oxide synthase gene (NOS3) variant and hypertension in pregnancy. *Am. J. Med. Genet.* 103: 241–244 (2001).

461. McNamara DM, Holubkov R, Postava L, Ramani R, Janosko K, Mathier M, MacGowan GA, Murali S, Feldman AM, London B. Effect of the Asp298 variant of endothelial nitric oxide synthase on survival for patients with congestive heart failure. *Circulation* 107: 1598–1602 (2003).
462. Brown KS, Kluijtmans LA, Young IS, Woodside J, Yarnell JW, McMaster D, Murray L, Evans AE, Boreham CA, McNulty H, Strain JJ, Mitchell LE, Whitehead AS. Genetic evidence that nitric oxide modulates homocysteine: the NOS3 894TT genotype is a risk factor for hyperhomocystenemia. *Arterioscler. Thromb. Vasc. Biol.* 23: 1014–1020 (2003).
463. Dahiyat M, Cumming A, Harrington C, Wischik C, Xuereb J, Corrigan F, Breen G, Shaw D, St Clair D. Association between Alzheimer's disease and the NOS3 gene. *Ann. Neurol.* 46: 664–667 (1999).
464. Crawford F, Freeman M, Abdullah L, Schinka J, Gold M, Duara R, Mullan M. No association between the NOS3 codon 298 polymorphism and Alzheimer's disease in a sample from the United States. *Ann. Neurol.* 47: 687 (2000).
465. Higuchi S, Ohta S, Matsushita S, Matsui T, Yuzuriha T, Urakami K, Arai H. NOS3 polymorphism not associated with Alzheimer's disease in Japanese. *Ann. Neurol.* 48: 685 (2000).
466. Kalman J, Juhasz A, Rimanoczy A, Palotas A, Palotas M, Boda K, Marki-Zay J, Csibri E, Janka Z. The nitric oxide synthase-3 codon 298 polymorphism is not associated with late-onset sporadic Alzheimer's dementia and Lewy body disease in a sample from Hungary. *Psychiatr. Genet.* 13: 201–204 (2003).
467. Kunugi H, Akahane A, Ueki A, Otsuka M, Isse K, Hirasawa H, Kato N, Nabika T, Kobayashi S, Nanko S. No evidence for an association between the Glu298Asp polymorphism of the NOS3 gene and Alzheimer's disease. *J. Neural. Trans.* 107: 1081–1084 (2000).
468. Monastero R, Cefalu AB, Camarda C, Buglino CM, Mannino M, Barbagallo CM, Lopez G, Camarda LK, Travali S, Camarda R, Averna MR. No association between Glu298Asp endothelial nitric oxide synthase polymorphism and Italian sporadic Alzheimer's disease. *Neurosci. Lett.* 341: 229–232 (2003).
469. Tedde A, Nacmias B, Cellini E, Bagnoli S, Sorbi S. Lack of association between NOS3 poly morphism and Italian sporadic and familial Alzheimer's disease. *J. Neurol.* 249: 110–111 (2002).
470. Via M, Gonzalez-Perez E, Esteban E, Lopez-Alomar A, Vacca L, Vona G, Dugoujon JM, Harich N, Moral P. Molecular variation in endothelial nitric oxide synthase gene (eNOS) in western Mediterranean populations. *Coll. Antropol.* 27: 117–124 (2003).

471. Hirata RD, Salaza LA, Cavalli SA, Yoshioka KK, Matsumoto LO, Santos ST, Giannini SD, Forti N, Diament J, Doi SQ, Hirata MH. A method to detect the G894T polymorphism of the NOS3 gene. Clinical validation in familial hypercholesterolemia. *Clin. Chem. Lab. Med.* 40: 436–440 (2002).
472. Holla LI, Buckova D, Kuhrova V, Stejskalova A, Francova H, Znojil V, Vacha J. Prevalence of endothelial nitric oxide synthase gene polymorphisms in patients with atopic asthma. *Clin. Exp. Allergy* 32: 1193–1198 (2002).
473. van's Gravesande KS, Wechsler ME, Grasemann H, Silverman ES, Le L, Palmer LJ, Drazen JM. Association of a missense mutation in the NOS3 gene with exhaled nitric oxide levels. *Am. J. Respir. Crit. Care Med.* 168: 228–231 (2003).
474. Derebecka N, Holysz M, Dankowski R, Wierzchowiecki M, Trzeciak WH. Polymorphism in intron 23 of the endothelial nitric oxide synthase gene (NOS3) is not associated with hypertension. *Acta Biochim. Pol.* 49: 263–268 (2002).
475. Sugaya K, Fukagawa T, Matsumoto K, Mita K, Takahashi E, Ando A, Inoko H, Ikemura T. Three genes in the human MHC class III region near the junction with the class II: gene for receptor of advanced glycosylation end-products, PBX2 homeobox gene and a notch homolog, human counterpart of mouse mammary tumor gene int-3. *Genomics* 23: 408–419 (1994).
476. Brownlee M. Lilly Lecture 1993. Glycation and diabetic complications. *Diabetes* 43: 836–841 (1994).
477. Vlassara H, Bucala R, Striker L. Pathogenic effects of advanced glycosylation: biochemical, biologic, and clinical implications for diabetes and aging. *Lab. Invest.* 70: 138–151 (1994).
478. Schmidt AM, Hori O, Brett J, Yan SD, Wautier JL, Stern D. Cellular receptors for advanced glycation end-products. Implications for induction of oxidant stress and cellular dysfunction in the pathogenesis of vascular lesions. *Arterioscler. Thromb.* 14: 1521–1528 (1994).
479. Soulis T, Thallas V, Youssef S, Gilbert RE, McWilliam BG, Murray-McIntosh RP, Cooper ME. Advanced glycation end-products and their receptors co-localise in rat organs susceptible to diabetic microvascular injury. *Diabetologia* 40: 619–628 (1997).
480. Hudson BI, Stickland MH, Grant PJ. Identification of polymorphisms in the receptor for advanced glycation end-products (RAGE) gene: prevalence in type 2 diabetes and ethnic groups. *Diabetes* 47: 1155–1157 (1998).
481. Poirier O, Nicaud V, Vionnet N, Raoux S, Tarnow L, Vlassara H, Parving HH, Cambien F. Polymorphism screening of four genes encoding advanced glycation end-product putative receptors. Association study with nephropathy in type 1 diabetic patients. *Diabetes* 50: 1214–1218 (2001).

482. Kankova K, Marova I, Zahejsky J, Muzik J, Stejskalova A, Znojil V, Vacha J. Polymorphisms 1704G/T and 2184A/G in the RAGE gene are associated with antioxidant status. *Metabolism* 50: 1152–1160 (2001).
483. Kankova K, Zahejsky J, Marova I, Muzik J, Kuhrova V, Blazkova M, Znojil V, Beranek M, Vacha J. Polymorphisms in the RAGE gene influence susceptibility to diabetes-associated microvascular dermatoses in NIDDM. *J. Diabetes Complications* 15: 185–192 (2001b).
484. Strange RC, Spiteri MA, Ramachandran S, Fryer AA. Glutathione-S-transferase family of enzymes. *Mutat. Res.* 482: 21–26 (2001).
485. Ogata M. Acatalasemia. *Hum. Genet.* 86: 331–340 (1991).
486. Kelner MJ, Bagnell RD, Montoya MA, Lanham KA. Structural organization of the human gastrointestinal glutathione peroxidase (GPX2) promoter and 3′-non-transcribed region: transcriptional response to exogenous redox agents. *Gene* 248: 109–116 (2000).
487. Huang TT, Carlson EJ, Raineri I, Gillespie AM, Kozy H, Epstein CJ. The use of transgenic and mutant mice to study oxygen free radical metabolism. *Ann. NY Acad. Sci.* 893: 95–112 (1999).
488. Yant LJ, Ran Q, Rao L, Van Remmen H, Shibatani T, Belter JG, Motta L, Richardson A, Prolla TA. The selenoprotein GPX4 is essential for mouse development and protects from radiation and oxidative damage insults. *Free Radic. Biol. Med.* 34: 496–502 (2003).
489. Ho YS, Crapo JD. Isolation and characterization of complementary DNAs encoding human manganese-containing superoxide dismutase. *FEBS Lett.* 229: 256–260 (1988).
490. Chua FF, Rotan de Silva HA, Esworthy RS, Boteva KK, Walters CE, Roses A, Raod PN, Pettenati MJ. Polymorphism and chromosomal localization of the GI-form of human glutathione peroxidase (GPX2) on 14q24.1 by *in situ* hybridization. *Genomics* 32(2): 272–276 (1996).
491. Widersten M, Pearson WR, Engstrom A, Mannervik B. Heterologous expression of the allelic variant mu-class glutathione transferases mu and psi. *Biochem. J.* 276(Pt 2): 519–524 (1991).
492. Seidegard J, Vorachek WR, Pero RW, Pearson WR. Hereditary differences in the expression of the human glutathione transferase active on trans-stilbene oxide are due to a gene deletion. *Proc. Natl. Acad. Sci. USA* 85: 7293–7297 (1988).
493. Brophy VH, Jampsa RL, Clendenning JB, McKinstry LA, Jarvik GP, Furlong CE. Effects of 5′ regulatory-region polymorphisms on paraoxonase-gene (PON1) expression. *Am. J. Hum. Genet.* 68: 1428–1436 (2001).
494. Garin MC, James RW, Dussoix P, Blanche H, Passa P, Froguel P, Ruiz J. Paraoxonase polymorphism Met-Leu54 is associated with modified serum

concentrations of the enzyme. A possible link between the paraoxonase gene and increased risk of cardiovascular disease in diabetes. *J. Clin. Invest.* 99: 62–66 (1997).

495. Sanghera DK, Aston CE, Saha N, Kamboh MI. DNA polymorphisms in two paraoxonase genes (PON1 and PON2) are associated with the risk of coronary heart disease. *Am. J. Hum. Genet.* 62: 36–44 (1998).
496. Hegele RA, Connelly PW, Scherer SW, Hanley AJ, Harris SB, Tsui LC, Zinman B. Paraoxonase-2 gene (PON2) G148 variant associated with elevated fasting plasma glucose in non-insulin-dependent diabetes mellitus. *J. Clin. Endocrinol. Metab.* 82: 3373–3377 (1997).
497. Traver RD, Horikoshi T, Danenberg KD, Stadlbauer TH, Danenberg PV, Ross D, Gibson NW. NAD(P)H: quinone oxidoreductase gene expression in human colon carcinoma cells: characterization of a mutation which modulates DT-diaphorase activity and mitomycin sensitivity. *Cancer Res.* 52: 797–802 (1992).
498. Audebert M, Chevillard S, Levalois C, Gyapay G, Vieillefond A, Klijanienko J, Vielh P, El Naggar AK, Oudard S, Boiteux S, Radicella JP. Alterations of the DNA repair gene OGG1 in human clear cell carcinomas of the kidney. *Cancer Res.* 60: 4740–4744 (2000).

13 Oxidative Stress and Autoimmune Diseases

Jun Saegusa, Seiji Kawano and Shunichi Kumagai

1. Introduction

Autoimmune diseases develop on complex backgrounds, in which both genetic and environmental factors are involved. For example, the frequency of systemic lupus erythematosus (SLE) concordance in identical twins is about 25%, compared with 1–2% among fraternal twins.[1] The frequency of rheumatoid arthritis (RA) concordance in identical twins is 15–34%.[2,3] Although this suggests a strong role of genetic factors in SLE and RA, this also tells that genetics cannot explain the whole scenario of the development of these diseases. The etiology of autoimmune diseases can thus be viewed as a multideterminant process involving one or more environmental stimuli, which acts on a genetically susceptible host, probably in conjunction with some element of chance.

Infections, ultraviolet (UV) irradiation, coldness and emotional stress have been clinically well known as triggering and exacerbating factors for autoimmune diseases. All these environmental factors have the potential to induce some degree of oxidative stress. At an individual level, various types of stresses affect the immune system through neuro-endocrine-immune network. In particular, oxidative stress directly affects the immune cells. Infection or inflammation activates monocytes and neutrophils, which generate a large amount of reactive oxygen species (ROS), resulting in the breakdown of the homeostasis of the immune system. Oxidative stress also acts as an apoptosis effector upon UV irradiation, TNF-α stimuli or viral infections.

Intracellularly, oxidative stress acts on both protein and deoxyribonucleic acid (DNA) levels. Oxidative stress induces a large number of proteins (e.g. heat shock protein), phosphorylates certain types of proteins, and activates some transcription factors such as NF-κB and AP-1.[4,5] Upon oxidative stress, DNA receives multiple types of damages such as oxidation of the pyrimidine or purine bases in the nucleoside, and the oxidation of the sugar moieties.

The maintenance of an appropriate intracellular reduction/oxidation (redox) balance is of crucial importance for normal cellular functioning that involves cell viability, signaling, activation and proliferation. The deleterious effects of oxidative stress are counterbalanced by a complex antioxidant system consisting of both low molecular weight antioxidants, such as glutathione (GSH), thioredoxin (TRX), ascorbic acid and tocopherols, and enzymes such as catalase, superoxide dismutase and glutathione peroxidase.

As shown in Fig. 1, excessive oxidative stress or an ineffective antioxidant system is thought to have an important role in the pathogenesis of autoimmune diseases by exacerbating the inflammatory process, inducing apoptotic cell death, modifying autoantigens, and breaking down the immunological tolerance.[6,7]

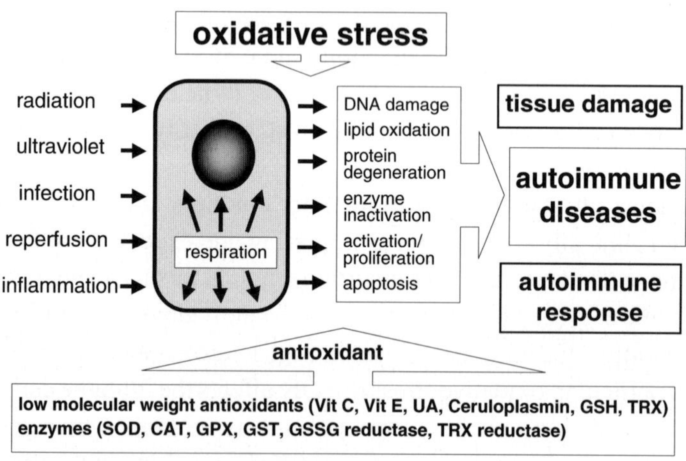

Fig. 1. Oxidative stress and autoimmune reaction.

1.1. *Breakdown of immunological tolerance by oxidative stress*

One of the recent prodigious advances in the research of autoimmune diseases is the clarification of the mechanism of tolerance, and the demonstration of the fact that the breakdown of tolerance induces autoimmune responses.[8,9] Autoantibody-producing B lymphocytes and/or autoreactive T lymphocytes play important roles in the pathogenesis of autoimmune diseases. Under normal conditions, these autoreactive lymphocytes are in immunological tolerance by clonal deletion, clonal anergy or active suppression. Apoptosis is regarded as the surest way to carry out clonal deletion. It has been demonstrated that defects in the apoptotic pathway could induce autoimmune diseases through the breakdown of tolerance in animal model experiments.[10]

In fact, some human cases of autoimmune lymphoproliferative syndrome (ALPS) with a deleterious *Fas* gene mutation and SLE patients with a deletion of *Fas-L* gene have been reported.[11,12] However, genetic defects of Fas or Fas-L, in which autoreactive lymphocytes may survive, are rarely seen in human autoimmune diseases. Rather, increased apoptosis could be demonstrated in patients with SLE.[13] Increased apoptosis might provide abundant autoantigens to the immune system, leading to induced autoimmune reaction. Reports have shown that oxidative stress induces apoptosis by stimulating the release of cytochrome c from mitochondria or by activating apoptosis-stimulating kinase 1 (ASK-1).[14] Thus, oxidative stress is one of the most important environmental factors that could induce autoimmune reaction through releasing autoantigen by apoptosis.

1.2. *Thioredoxin and 8-hydroxy-2′-deoxyguanosine as a biomarker for oxidative stress in patients with autoimmune diseases*

In order to investigate the involvement of oxidative stress in the pathogenesis of autoimmune diseases, it is very important to detect the state of oxidative stress and to quantify it at an individual level. There may be two ways to quantify the state of oxidative stress and antioxidants: one is to measure the amount of chemical compound modified by oxidative stress, and another is to measure the amount of low molecular weight antioxidant or enzyme which can remove ROS. As an example of the former, it has been reported that plasma malondialdehyde and 4-hydroxynonenal levels of children with active SLE were significantly higher than those of healthy children.[15] In nuclear and mitochondrial DNA, 8-hydroxydeoxyguanosine (8-OHdG), an oxidized nucleoside of DNA, is the most frequently detected and studied DNA-associated product. Upon DNA repair, 8-OHdG is excreted into urine. Numerous evidences have indicated that urinary 8-OHdG is a biomarker of generalized cellular oxidative stress.[16] Recently, urinary 8-OHdG has been reported to be significantly increased in RA patients than in healthy subjects.[17]

Measurement of substance that plays a role in antioxidant system has also been investigated. TRX is a multifunctional and ubiquitous protein that has a redox-active disulfide/dithiol bond within the conserved active site. TRX has been reported to possess multiple biological functions and to regulate various cellular functions via thiol redox control.[18] TRX can be induced not merely by viral infection but also by a variety of cellular stress. TRX gene has a novel *cis*-regulatory element responsible for oxidative stress in its promoter region, and can be strongly induced by oxidative stress such as various oxidative agents, ultraviolet irradiation, and ischemic reperfusion. Upon oxidative stress, TRX expression is induced in lymphocytes and keratinocytes and is also secreted extracellularly. Recently, increased TRX production in synovial tissue from RA patients has been reported.[19] Therefore, plasma TRX level could be a good indicator of oxidative stress in patients with autoimmune diseases.

1.3. *High levels of TRX and 8-OHdG in patients with autoimmune diseases*

As shown in Fig. 2, the TRX levels in peripheral blood were significantly higher in patients with SLE, RA, and polymyositis (PM)/dermatomyositis (DM) than in healthy subjects.[19] Urinary excretion of 8-OHdG was also significantly increased in patients with SLE, Sjögren's syndrome (SS), RA, and mixed connective tissue disease (MCTD) compared with healthy subjects. In RA patients, significant positive correlation was found between plasma TRX levels and urinary excretion of 8-OHdG. Furthermore, these values were correlated with disease activity.[19] Taken together, patients with

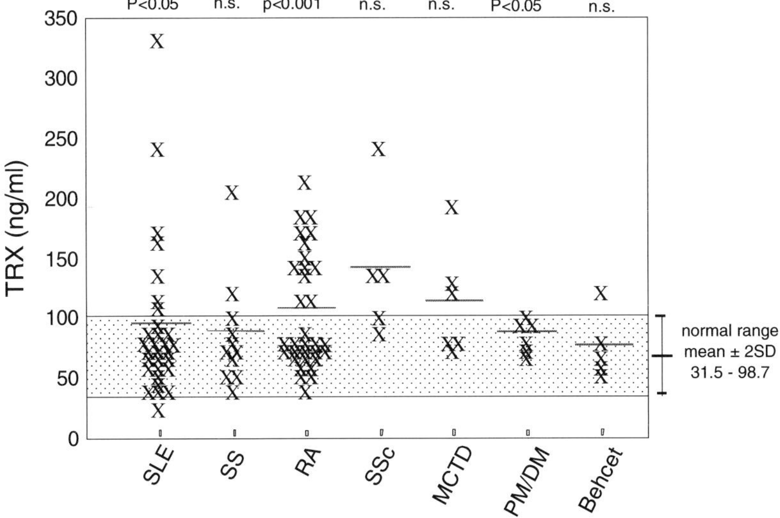

Fig. 2. Plasma TRX levels in patients with autoimmune diseases.

autoimmune diseases have higher levels of oxidative stress than healthy individuals.

2. Pathological Roles of Oxidative Stress in Autoimmune Diseases

If patients with autoimmune diseases are exposed to higher levels of oxidative stress than healthy individuals, it is important next to clarify how oxidative stress is implicated in the pathophysiology of each autoimmune disease.

2.1. *Oxidative stress and rheumatoid arthritis*

RA is a chronic inflammatory joint disease characterized by the proliferation of synovial cells and by the influx of a variety of inflammatory cells with rich blood vessels into synovial tissue. Infiltration of T cells, B cells, macrophages, and polymorphonuclear cells is observed in the joints. These cells and cell-derived factors such as cytokines and proteolytic enzymes are thought to have important roles in the joint destruction. ROS is also produced at the site of synovitis by macrophages and polymorphonuclear cells or by mechanical reperfusion, and may contribute to the maintenance of chronic inflammation through the activation of pro-inflammatory molecules, leading to the destruction of cartilage and bone.[20]

There are several lines of evidences indicating the involvement of increased oxidative stress on RA. It has been demonstrated that the levels of GSH, the most abundant cellular thiol, are significantly lower in patients with RA than in controls, and that the plasma activity of GSH peroxidase is significantly lower in RA.[21,22] Impaired GSH reductase activity in synovial fluid (SF) in RA has also been reported.[23] The presence of catalytic iron was shown in SF from RA patients, and increased concentration of nitrate in SF and serum samples from RA patients were reported.[24,25] Changes in a variety of markers for oxidative stress such as decreased sulphydryl, increased mitochondrial radical production, and increased pentosidine, an advanced glycation end-product, in the blood or SF from RA patients have also been reported.[26–28] In a Finnish cohort study, elevated risks of RA were observed when the antioxidant such as α-tocopherol, β-carotene and selenium remained at low levels.[29]

As mentioned above, plasma TRX levels and urinary excretion of 8-OHdG in RA patients were higher than those in healthy subjects. As shown in Fig. 3, the TRX concentration in SF from RA patients was significantly higher than that in SF from osteoarthritis (OA) patients.[19] As SF from RA patients contained significantly higher concentration of TRX than their plasma, TRX might have originated from the SF in RA patients. The histological examination of synovial tissue from RA patients showed that TRX was present on the surface of the synovial lining layer as well as in some leukocytes.[19] These results suggest that TRX may protect synovial tissues and joints from oxidative damage by scavenging the hydrogen peroxide and hydroxyl radical, or regenerating the proteins deactivated by oxidative stress.

2.2. *Oxidative stress and Sjögren's syndrome*

Sjögren's syndrome (SS) is an immune-mediated disorder in which both T cells and B cells infiltrate and progressively destroy the salivary and lacrimal glands, resulting in dry mouth and dry eyes. Previous report has

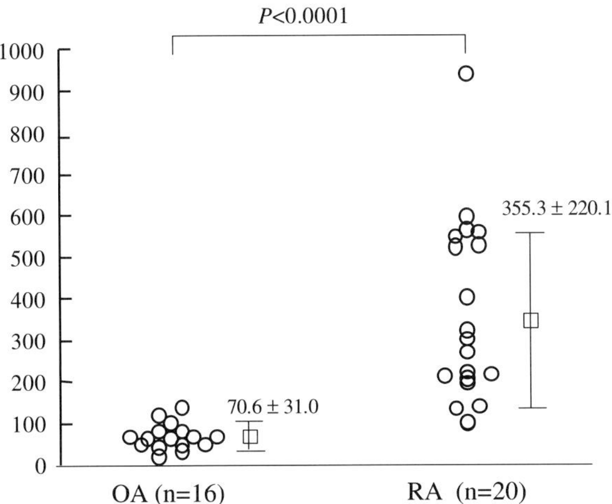

Fig. 3. The TRX concentrations of SF of RA patients.

shown an increased expression of human TRX in salivary gland tissue from patients with SS, suggesting that oxidative stress may play a role in the destruction of salivary glands in patients with SS.[30]

The glutathione S-transferase (GST) superfamily of enzymes plays an important role in the detoxification or inactivation of various drugs and xenobiotics, and in the limitation of toxic effects of ROS. Among the four classes of GST, GST-θ (GSTT) and GST-μ (GSTM) contain members that exhibit a genetic polymorphism, and a large percentage of individuals display a homozygous deletion in the GSTT1 and GSTM1 gene loci. The GST null genotype has been shown to be associated with various malignancies, including smoking-related cancer, stomach cancer, bladder cancer, squamous cell carcinoma, pituitary adenoma, astrocytoma, myelodysplastic syndrome, and acute lymphoblastic leukemia.[31] Interestingly, an association between the GST null genotype and inflammatory bowel disorders such as ulcerative colitis and Crohn's disease has also been reported.[32] As shown in Table 1, frequency of the GSTM1 homozygous null genotype was significantly increased in SS and SLE patients compared with controls. Moreover, a significantly higher frequency of anti-SS-A/Ro antibodies was found among SS patients with the GSTM1 null genotype than among those with the GSTM1 non-null genotype.[31] These data suggest that GST null

Table 1. Frequency of the GSTM1 and/or GSTT1 null homozygotes in autoimmune diseases.

Subjects	n	GSTM1 null % (n)	GSTT1 null % (n)	Double null % (n)
Healthy	143	44.1 (63)	43.4 (62)	15.4 (22)
Sjögren	106	57.5 (61)*	44.3 (47)	24.5 (26)
SLE	185	57.8 (107)*	51.9 (96)	31.4 (58)**
RA	123	52.0 (64)	43.9 (54)	22.0 (27)

*$p < 0.05$ versus controls, **$p < 0.001$ versus controls.

genotype would degrade the antioxidant capacity of the body, leading to autoimmune responses.

2.3. *UV-B-induced oxidative stress and cutaneous manifestations*

Cutaneous manifestations are common in autoimmune diseases, and are often used as one of the classification criteria for autoimmune diseases. Since the skin is always in contact with atmospheric oxygen and is occasionally exposed to UV light, skin is one of the best target organs of environmental photo-oxidative stress.

UV irradiation is regarded as one of the major environmental factors in autoimmune diseases, since UV exposure is known not only to aggravate the skin lesions but also to exacerbate the systemic disease activity.[33] It is, however, not clear how UV irradiation induces biological reactions and affects a living body. There is now a growing body of evidence that increased levels of ROS are observed after UV exposure. A photon of UV-B has enough energy to elevate oxygen to the singlet state. Furthermore, not only singlet oxygen but also other species of oxygen intermediates are generated in the epidermis by UV irradiation. There are many reports supporting the free radical hypothesis for UV-induced cutaneous damage.[34] Sunburn cell formation, a hallmark of UV-B-damaged epidermis, can be moderated by free radical scavengers. The contact photosensitization process may be partly attributed to UV-derived oxidants. Products of lipid peroxidation, lipid radicals and other free radicals are also noted in UV irradiated skin. While short-lived, these ROS can reversibly or irreversibly damage nucleic acids, proteins, free amino acids, lipids, lipoproteins, and connective tissue macromolecules.[34] These reports demonstrate that the damage caused by ROS and other oxidants after UV irradiation. Therefore, ROS and other oxidants are thought to be responsible for some, if not all, of the biological and pathological effects of UV.

2.4. *UV-B-induced oxidative stress and SS-A/Ro antigen*

Autoimmune diseases are characterized by various circulating autoantibodies. Autoantibodies may be related to the pathogenesis of cutaneous lesions of autoimmune diseases since deposits of immunoglobulin and complement occur at the dermal-epidermal junction in sun-exposed skin. Of these autoantibodies, anti-SS-A/Ro antibody is known to be closely associated with the development of skin lesions of autoimmune diseases. Anti-SS-A/Ro autoantibodies are commonly found in the sera of patients with SS, SLE and subacute cutaneous lupus erythematosus (SCLE). SS-A/Ro antigen, the target antigen of anti-SS-A/Ro autoantibody, is a ribonucleoprotein consisting of at least two proteins, 52 (Ro52) and 60 kDa (Ro60). Both proteins contain zinc finger motifs, while Ro52 was shown to also contain a leucine zipper motif in its hydrophilic domain, which was found to be the main epitope recognized by anti-SS-A/Ro autoantibodies. Although it is not known how antibodies to these sequestered intracellular proteins arise, the strong association of anti-SS-A/Ro antibodies with cutaneous lesions suggests that these antibodies may participate in the development of skin lesions in autoimmune diseases. SS-A/Ro antigens are usually present in the nucleus and cytoplasm, but interestingly, clinical and experimental observations have demonstrated that exposure to UV-B induces SS-A/Ro antigen expression on the surface of keratinocytes.[35,36] Thus, anti-SS-A/Ro antibodies in the sera can bind to the relevant antigens expressed on the surface of UVB-irradiated keratinocytes. This phenomenon is now considered to answer two long-standing questions in the field of autoimmune diseases, namely how autoantibodies interact with self-antigens, which are located in the nucleus or cytoplasm of the cell, and why the anti-SS-A/Ro antibody is closely associated with the development of skin lesions in autoimmune diseases.

Recently, the mechanism that induces SS-A/Ro antigen on the cell surface by UV-B has been identified.[37] The exclusive induction by UV-B

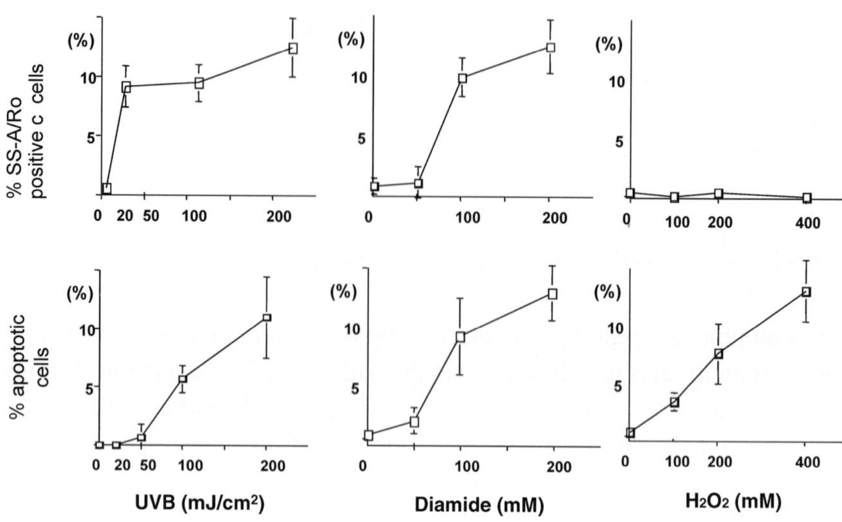

Fig. 4. Diamide induced surface expression of Ro52.

irradiation of the Ro52 but not of Ro60 was demonstrated by means of indirect immunofluorescence. The surface expression of Ro52 induced by UV-B irradiation was concentration-dependently inhibited by *N*-acetyl-L-cysteine, an antioxidant. Furthermore, surface expression of Ro52 was similarly induced by diamide, a chemical oxidant (Fig. 4).[37] Previous report has shown that autoantigens including the SS-A/Ro antigen are clustered in the surface blebs of UV-B-induced apoptotic keratinocytes.[38] As numerous autoantigens are cleaved during apoptosis, this redistribution could potentially expose modified autoantigens to autoantibodies and trigger a proinflammatory phagocytosis. In contrast, UV-B-induced oxidative stress is able to induce cell surface expression of Ro52, independent of the apoptotic pathway as shown in Fig. 4.[37] These findings led to the conclusion that oxidative stress induces the cell surface expression of Ro52 on keratinocytes and that UV-B-induced oxidative stress is capable of inducing cell surface expression of Ro52, either dependent on or independent of the apoptotic pathway.

It is known that congenital heart block (CHB) in neonatal lupus erythematosus (NLE) is strongly associated with maternal anti-SS-A/Ro antibody.[39] It has been found that the 52β isoform, an alternative transcript of Ro52, is expressed on the fetal heart, and that 87% of sera from mothers whose children were NLE immunoprecipitated the 52β form.[40] It

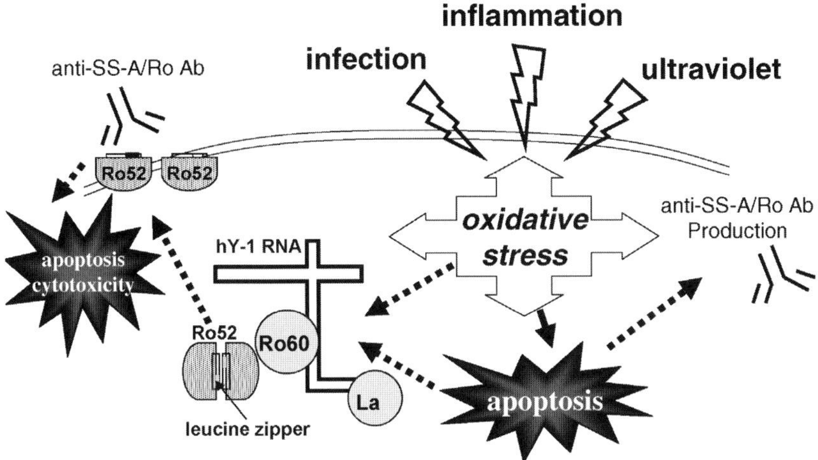

Fig. 5. Oxidative stress and pathophysiology of Sjögren's syndrome.

can be hypothesized that some oxidative stresses (e.g. hypoxia) may induce surface expression of 52β on the fetal heart, which would make it recognizable by means of maternal anti-SS-A/Ro antibody. In addition to UV-B and diamide, estrogen, viral infection, and heat shock have been reported to induce the surface expression of SS-A/Ro antigen on keratinocytes.[41–43] All these stimuli have the potential to induce some degree of oxidative stress. Oxidative stress may therefore be a key to understanding the SS-A/Ro antigen expression induced by these stimuli.

Figure 5 shows the hypothetical scheme of pathophysiology of SS.[7] Not only UV irradiation but inflammation or infection also acts as oxidative stress and induces apoptosis on various cells. Increased apoptosis might provide autoantigen to the immune system, leading to induce autoimmune reaction. On the other hand, these oxidative stresses may induce surface expression of SS-A/Ro52 on cells, leading to anti-SS-A/Ro antibody-dependent cellular cytotoxicity or, through antigen presentation to T cells, T cell mediated cytotoxicity or anti-SS-A/Ro antibody production.

3. Concluding Remarks

Infections, UV irradiation, coldness, and emotional stress have been clinically well known as developing and exacerbating factors for autoimmune diseases. These environmental factors are closely related to oxidative stress, which induces inflammatory and autoimmune biological responses. The form and function of oxidative stress are extremely varied, and the same is true of antioxidant system. Therefore, elucidating the mechanism of oxidative stress or antioxidant system may lead us to understand the pathogenesis of autoimmune diseases, or to the discovery of novel therapeutic strategy in the near future.

References

1. Cooper GS, Dooley MA, Treadwell EL, St Clair EW, Parks CG, Gilkeson GS. Hormonal, environmental, and infectious risk factors for developing systemic lupus erythematosus. *Arthritis Rheum.* 41: 1714–1724 (1998).
2. Lawrence JS. Heberden Oration, 1969. Rheumatoid arthritis — nature or nurture? *Ann. Rheum. Dis.* 29: 357–379 (1970).
3. Jarvinen P, Aho K. Twin studies in rheumatic diseases. *Semin. Arthritis Rheum.* 24: 19–28 (1994).
4. Saliou C, Kitazawa M, McLaughlin L, Yang JP, Lodge JK, Tetsuka T, Iwasaki K, Cillard J, Okamoto T, Packer L. Antioxidants modulate acute solar ultraviolet radiation-induced NF-kappa-B activation in a human keratinocyte cell line. *Free Radic. Biol. Med.* 26: 174–183 (1999).
5. Isoherranen K, Westermarck J, Kahari VM, Jansen C, Punnonen K. Differential regulation of the AP-1 family members by UV irradiation *in vitro* and *in vivo*. *Cell Signal.* 10: 191–195 (1998).
6. Kumagai S, Jikimoto T, Saegusa J. Pathological roles of oxidative stress in autoimmune diseases. *Rinsho Byori* 52: 126–132 (2003) (in Japanese).
7. Kumagai S, Nobuhara Y, Saegusa J. Oxidative stress and autoimmune diseases. *Nippon Naika Gakkai Zasshi* 92: 1096–1103 (2003) (in Japanese).
8. Herrmann M, Voll RE, Kalden JR. Etiopathogenesis of systemic lupus erythematosus. *Immunol. Today* 21: 424–426 (2000).
9. Utz PJ, Anderson P. Post-translational protein modifications, apoptosis, and the bypass of tolerance to autoantigens. *Arthritis Rheum.* 41: 1152–1160 (1998).
10. Nagata S, Suda T. Fas and Fas ligand: lpr and gld mutations. *Immunol. Today* 16: 39–43 (1995).
11. Fisher GH, Rosenberg FJ, Straus SE, Dale JK, Middleton LA, Lin AY, Strober W, Lenardo MJ, Puck JM. Dominant interfering Fas gene mutations

impair apoptosis in a human autoimmune lymphoproliferative syndrome. *Cell* 81: 935–946 (1995).

12. Wu J, Wilson J, He J, Xiang L, Schur PH, Mountz JD. Fas ligand mutation in a patient with systemic lupus erythematosus and lymphoproliferative disease. *J. Clin. Invest.* 98: 1107–1113 (1996).
13. Mevorach D. Systemic lupus erythematosus and apoptosis: a question of balance. *Clin. Rev. Allergy Immunol.* 25: 49–60 (2003).
14. Tobiume K, Matsuzawa A, Takahashi T, Nishitoh H, Morita K, Takeda K, Minowa O, Miyazono K, Noda T, Ichijo H. ASK1 is required for sustained activations of JNK/p38 MAP kinases and apoptosis. *EMBO Rep.* 2: 222–228 (2001).
15. Grune T, Michel P, Sitte N, Eggert W, Albrecht-Nebe H, Esterbauer H, Siems WG. Increased levels of 4-hydroxynonenalmodified proteins in plasma of children with autoimmune diseases. *Free Radic. Biol. Med.* 23: 357–360 (1997).
16. Toyokuni S. Reactive oxygen species-induced molecular damage and its application in pathology. *Pathol. Int.* 49: 91–102 (1999).
17. Rall LC, Roubenoff R, Meydani SN, Han SN, Meydani M. Urinary 8-hydroxy-2-deoxyguanosine (8-OHdG) as a marker of oxidative stress in rheumatoid arthritis and aging: effect of progressive resistance training. *J. Nutr. Biochem.* 11: 581–584 (2000).
18. Nakamura H, Nakamura K, Yodoi J. Redox regulation of cellular activation. *Annu. Rev. Immunol.* 15: 351–369 (1997).
19. Jikimoto T, Nishikubo Y, Koshiba M, Kanagawa S, Morinobu S, Morinobu A, Saura R, Mizuno K, Kondo S, Toyokuni S, Nakamura H, Yodoi J, Kumagai S. Thioredoxin as a biomarker for oxidative stress in patients with rheumatoid arthritis. *Mol. Immunol.* 38: 765–772 (2002).
20. Mapp PI, Grootveld MC, Blake DR. Hypoxia, oxidative stress and rheumatoid arthritis. *Br. Med. Bull.* 51: 419–436 (1995).
21. Hassan MQ, Hadi RA, Al-Rawi ZS, Padron VA, Stohs SJ. The glutathione defense system in the pathogenesis of rheumatoid arthritis. *J. Appl. Toxicol.* 21: 69–73 (2001).
22. Karatas F, Ozates I, Canatan H, Halifeoglu I, Karatepe M, Colakt R. Antioxidant status and lipid peroxidation in patients with rheumatoid arthritis. *Indian J. Med. Res.* 118: 178–181 (2003).
23. Bazzichi L, Ciompi ML, Betti L, Rossi A, Melchiorre D, Fiorini M, Giannaccini G, Lucacchini A. Impaired glutathione reductase activity and levels of collagenase and elastase in synovial fluid in rheumatoid arthritis. *Clin. Exp. Rheumatol.* 20: 761–766 (2002).

24. Rowley D, Gutteridge JM, Blake D, Farr M, Halliwell B. Lipid peroxidation in rheumatoid arthritis: thiobarbituric acid-reactive material and catalytic iron salts in synovial fluid from rheumatoid patients. *Clin. Sci. (Lond.)* 66: 691–695 (1984).
25. Hilliquin P, Borderie D, Hernvann A, Menkes CJ, Ekindjian OG. Nitric oxide as S-nitrosoproteins in rheumatoid arthritis. *Arthritis Rheum.* 40: 1512–1517 (1997).
26. Halliwell B. Oxygen radicals, nitric oxide and human inflammatory joint disease. *Ann. Rheum. Dis.* 54: 505–510 (1995).
27. Miesel R, Murphy MP, Kroger H. Enhanced mitochondrial radical production in patients which rheumatoid arthritis correlates with elevated levels of tumor necrosis factor alpha in plasma. *Free Radic. Res.* 25: 161–169 (1996).
28. Miyata T, Ishiguro N, Yasuda Y, Ito T, Nangaku M, Iwata H, Kurokawa K. Increased pentosidine, an advanced glycation end-product, in plasma and synovial fluid from patients with rheumatoid athritis and its relation with inflammatory markers. *Biochem. Biophys. Res. Commun.* 244: 45–49 (1998).
29. Heliovaara M, Knekt P, Aho K, Aaran RK, Alfthan G, Aromaa A. Serum antioxidants and risk of rheumatoid arthritis. *Ann. Rheum. Dis.* 53: 51–53 (1994).
30. Saito I, Shimuta M, Terauchi K, Tsubota K, Yodoi J, Miyasaka N. Increased expression of human thioredoxin/adult T cell leukemia-derived factor in Sjogren's syndrome. *Arthritis Rheum.* 39: 773–782 (1996).
31. Morinobu A, Kanagawa S, Koshiba M, Sugai S, Kumagai S. Association of the glutathione S-transferase M1 homozygous null genotype with susceptibility to Sjogren's syndrome in Japanese individuals. *Arthritis Rheum.* 42: 2612–2615 (1999).
32. Duncan H, Swan C, Green J, Jones P, Brannigan K, Alldersea J, Fryer AA, Strange RC. Susceptibility to ulcerative colitis and Crohn's disease: interactions between glutathione S-transferase GSTM1 and GSTT1 genotypes. *Clin. Chim. Acta* 249: 53–61 (1995).
33. Zamansky GB. Sunlight-induced pathogenesis in systemic lupus erythematosus. *J. Invest. Dermatol.* 85: 179–180 (1985).
34. Miyachi Y. Photoaging from an oxidative standpoint. *J. Dermatol. Sci.* 9: 79–86 (1995).
35. LeFeber WP, Norris DA, Ryan SR, Huff JC, Lee LA, Kubo M, Boyce ST, Kotzin BL, Weston WL. Ultraviolet light induces binding of antibodies to selected nuclear antigens on cultured human keratinocytes. *J. Clin. Invest.* 74: 1545–1551 (1984).

36. Furukawa F, Kashihara-Sawami M, Lyons MB, Norris DA. Binding of antibodies to the extractable nuclear antigens SS-A/Ro and SS-B/La is induced on the surface of human keratinocytes by ultraviolet light (UVL): implications for the pathogenesis of photosensitive cutaneous lupus. *J. Invest. Dermatol.* 94: 77–85 (1990).
37. Saegusa J, Kawano S, Koshiba M, Hayashi N, Kosaka H, Funasaka Y, Kumagai S. Oxidative stress mediates cell surface expression of SS-A/Ro antigen on keratinocytes. *Free Radic. Biol. Med.* 32: 1006–1016 (2002).
38. Casciola-Rosen LA, Anhalt G, Rosen A. Autoantigens targeted in systemic lupus erythematosus are clustered in two populations of surface structures on apoptotic keratinocytes. *J. Exp. Med.* 179: 1317–1330 (1994).
39. Buyon JP, Slade SG, Reveille JD, Hamel JC, Chan EK. Autoantibody responses to the "native" 52-kDa SS-A/Ro protein in neonatal lupus syndromes, systemic lupus erythematosus, and Sjogren's syndrome. *J. Immunol.* 152: 3675–3684 (1994).
40. Buyon JP, Tseng CE, DiDonato F, Rashbaum W, Morris A, Chan EK. Cardiac expression of 52beta, an alternative transcript of the congenital heart block associated 52-kd SS-A/Ro autoantigen, is maximal during fetal development. *Arthritis Rheum.* 40: 655–660 (1997).
41. Furukawa F, Lyons MB, Lee LA, Coulter SN, Norris DA. Estradiol enhances binding to cultured human keratinocytes of antibodies specific for SS-A/Ro and SS-B/La. Another possible mechanism for estradiol influence of lupus erythematosus. *J. Immunol.* 141: 1480–1488 (1998).
42. Zhu J. Ultraviolet B irradiation and cytomegalovirus infection synergize to induce the cell surface expression of 52-kD/Ro antigen. *Clin. Exp. Immunol.* 103: 47–53 (1996).
43. Igarashi T, Itoh Y, Fukunaga Y, Yamamoto M. Stress-induced cell surface expression and antigenic alteration of the Ro/SSA autoantigen. *Autoimmunity* 22: 33–42 (1995).

14 Does Oxidative Stress Determine Lifespan?

Florian L. Muller and Holly Van Remmen

1. Introduction

The origins of the free radical theory of aging go back to the mid-20th century when it was discovered that oxygen free radicals, normally only associated with radiation biochemistry, are formed *in situ* and are responsible for the toxic effects of hyperbaric oxygen.[1] Noting the close parallels between histological effects of radiation damage and aging, Denham Harman proposed that oxygen free radicals play an important role in the aging process. In the last 50 years of research, this simple hypothesis has been refined, encompassing not just free radicals *per se* but also other forms of activated oxygen. Special attention has focused on the mitochondria, since these organelles generate the majority of reactive oxygen species (ROS) in cells.[2] However, it is still unclear at present whether the hypothesis that ROS contribute to aging is correct or not. In a recent review, Beckman and Ames[3] made a useful addition to the debate by dividing the hypothesis into "strong" and "weak" versions of the theory. The strong version of the oxidative theory of aging states that oxidative damage determines lifespan, while the weaker version postulates that oxidative damage is most strongly associated with age-related disease.

Obviously there also exists a continuum between these two extreme hypotheses. We suggest that the weak version of the oxidative theory of aging is already well established, namely that there are multiple studies showing an association between elevated oxidative damage and age and age-related disorders.[3] However, in this chapter we will review and evaluate the evidence for and against the "strongest" version of the oxidative stress hypothesis of aging. We will place special emphasis on genetic modifications leading to elevated or reduced oxidative stress, and the resulting effect on lifespan.

2. Oxidative Stress as a Lifespan-Determining Factor in *Drosophila melanogaster*

The oldest method of modulating *in situ* oxidative damage is through the manipulation of oxygen tension. Indeed, the oxygen "poisoning" experiments of Gerschman *et al.*[1] were an important foundation to Harman's free radical theory of aging. The zest of these experiments is that *in situ* oxidative damage can be elevated by increasing oxygen tension, which we now know to be due to increased (mitochondrial) ROS formation.[4,5] Indeed, there is a quasi-linear, inverse relationship between lifespan and oxygen tension in *Drosophila*.[6,7] Thus, if oxygen tension is increased above 21%, lifespan is correspondingly shortened. At 40% oxygen, lifespan is reduced by over 30%. Interestingly, however, reducing oxygen tension below 21% does not increase lifespan, but this is readily explained by the fact that hypoxia can (paradoxially) lead to an increase in ROS formation and oxidative stress.[8] It is difficult to say whether the decrease in lifespan in these experiments is due to "oxygen poisoning" or true accelerated aging. In a recent microarray study comparing gene expression patterns in old flies, young flies, and young flies treated with 100% oxygen, it was discovered that young flies treated with 100% oxygen exhibit many of the gene expression changes seen in old untreated flies.[9] The same microarray experiment could theoretically be employed to determine whether flies treated with 40% O_2 exhibit true accelerated aging. On the whole, these experiments certainly indicate that oxidative damage *can* be a lifespan limiting factor, but do not truly answer whether it actually *is* at normal atmospheric O_2 tension.

3. Genetic Manipulations Aimed at Modulating Oxidative Stress in *Drosophila*

In *Drosophila*, superoxide dismutase (SOD), which scavenges superoxide anion, occurs in both cytoplasmic and mitochondrial isoforms (encoded by two different genes, *Sod1* and *Sod2*, respectively). Assuming an inverse linear relationship between $O_2^{\bullet -}$ levels and SOD, increasing the levels of SOD would be predicted to decrease oxidative damage (which is still a contentious point),[10] providing a good model to test the oxidative stress theory of aging. The first such experiments were conducted in the early 1990s.[11–13] Generally, a constitutive promoter (such as β-actin) was used to overexpress *Sod1*. The results were contradictory: some studies reported an increase in average lifespan,[13] some found no effect, and some others found a decrease in lifespan.[11] A study in 1995 by Orr and Sohal found that while overexpression of either *Sod1* or *catalase* alone led to no extension of lifespan, the concomitant overexpression of both genes resulted in an increase in average and maximum lifespan.[14] However, transgenic studies in *Drosophila* using P-element mediated transformation are problematic due to the fact that the control and experimental lines have different genetic backgrounds, a factor that has been shown to alter lifespan independently from any transgenetic manipulation.[15] To minimize these background issues, Parkes *et al.*[16] targeted the overexpression of CuZnSOD in *Drosophila* to motorneurons using a yeast UAS element that was regulated by a GAL4 activator and found that overexpression of CuZnSOD in motorneurons resulted in an increase in lifespan (40%), as well as an increase in resistance to paraquat and γ-irradiation. The Philips group also reported that MnSOD overexpression increased lifespan, albeit to a somewhat smaller extent.[17] Although this seems unlikely, there still remains a small chance that genetic background might have played a role in lifespan extension independently of the SOD1 transgene. To address this issue, the UAS-SOD1 transgene and the GAL4 activator were crossed into different strains of *Drosophila*. The SOD1 transgene did increase lifespan in some, but not all *Drosophila* strains.[18] To settle the genetic background question once and for all, Tower's group used a conditional promoter to overexpress SOD1 (as well as SOD2), allowing for isogeny in both the experimental and control groups.[19–21] Using this approach, a statistically significant extension of mean lifespan was obtained, but maximum lifespan remained essentially unchanged. Although the magnitude of the lifespan increase is relatively low, this work remains the best evidence that superoxide, and by extension, oxidative damage, is a lifespan-limiting factor in *Drosophila*. While the results of Phillip's and Tower's lab are supportive of the oxidative theory, Sohal's group has recently published that constitutive (as opposed to inducible in the studies above) overexpression of catalase, MnSOD, and thioredoxin reductase had no effect on lifespan,[22–24] despite the fact that some of these transgenic interventions actually increased acute-oxidative stress resistance. However, no actual oxidative damage measurements, under basal conditions, were reported. Thus, while these results do not support the oxidative theory, they cannot be used to disprove it either.

While ablation of SOD1 was already known for some years,[25] only very recently were the phenotypical results of an ablation of SOD2 published. Phillips *et al.* used an RNAi knock down strategy to repress expression of the *Drosophila* SOD2 gene.[26,27] This resulted in postnatal lethality (about 10 days after birth), somewhat similar to what was observed in the SOD1 m/m.[28] Duttaroy *et al.*[29] used the excision of a P-insertional element proximal to the SOD2 locus to delete this gene. They thus generated a true knockout, whose phenotype was even more deleterious than that observed by Phillip's group using RNAi. Duttaroy's SOD2 knockout was found do be post-natal lethal, dying around 36 h after birth (hatching). While this result confirms the toxicity of mitochondria superoxide, it does not *per se* prove that it causes aging: to complement Tower's studies of SOD2 overexpression, the lifespan of the heterozygous knockout SOD2 needs to be determined. If the lifespan of the heterozygote is intermediate between wildtype and SOD2 null, the oxidative stress theory will have survived an important challenge.

Very recent transgenic studies provide more evidence for the oxidative stress theory in *Drosophila*. Overexpression of the protein oxidative damage repair enzyme, peptide-S-methionine sulfoxide reductase (MsrA), was found to increase average lifespan up to 85%.[30] Maximum lifespan was also increased. This study took great pains to establish that the changes in lifespan were not due to genetic background issues as previously discussed. As things stand, the validity of this result has not been questioned and this experiment remains a very convincing piece of evidence in favor of the oxidative stress theory.

As the data now stand, the preponderance of evidence suggests that oxidative stress is indeed a lifespan-limiting factor in *Drosophila*. We would argue that a better understanding of the *in vivo* oxidative chemistry will, in the future, explain the previous contradictory results.

4. Oxidative Stress as a Lifespan-Determining Factor in *Caenorhabditis elegans*

Caenorhabditis elegans is an invertebrate model system much used in developmental biology. The study of aging in this organism has centered around the *dauer* mutants,[31] which are thought to be similar in mechanism to lifespan-extending Ames-dwarf mutation previously identified in mice,[32] in that insulin-like growth factor signaling is ablated. The *dauer* mutants are generally consistent with the oxidative hypothesis and point mutations in the mitochondrial electron transfer chain, which lead to increased superoxide production and have been shown to reduce lifespan;[33,34] however, recent work by two independent groups has shown that knockdown of the mitochondrial electron transport chain leads to a greatly extended lifespan, which is additive with the *dauer* mutants.[35,36] Interestingly, partial inhibition of Complex III with antimycin A also extended lifespan.[35] This would seem to go against the oxidative hypothesis, since antimycin A treatment drastically increases superoxide production. However, it has been observed that near complete inhibition of Complex III must be attained before antimycin A stimulates superoxide production.[37] The findings by Ruvkun and Kenyon are highly intriguing, considering that in mammals partial inhibition of the mitochondrial electron transport chain leads to Parkinsonism,[38–40] and a host of severe disease such as mitochondrial myopathies and encephalomyopathies.[41] Thus, there is a fundamental difference in energy metabolism (and its potential relationship to aging) between *C. elegans* and mammals. Indeed, while mammals rely overwhelmingly on aerobic metabolism to remain alive, *C. elegans* can survive for extended periods of time (~48 h for wild type, considerably longer for *dauer* mutants[42] in complete anaerobiosis.[43] This tolerance is due to an anaerobic energy generating pathway, not found in mammals, involving a fumarate reductase and malate dismutation.[31,44] Indeed, the long-lived *dauer* larva's metabolism is shifted even more toward anaerobiosis.[44] The reliance on non-mitochondrial anaerobic metabolism may also explain *C. elegan*'s extreme tolerance to hyperoxia: it is quite distinct from higher metazoans by its ability to grow, live, and reproduce at 100% O_2.[45] Johnson has presented a detailed hypothesis integrating the above findings, arguing that upregulation of the malate dismutation pathway and the ensuing decrease in mitochondrial superoxide production is responsible for the extended lifespan observed in the electron transport chain complex knockdowns.[31]

5. Oxidative Stress as a Lifespan-Determining Factor in Mice

Since the oxidative stress hypothesis, in its strongest version, broadly predicts that modulations in oxidative stress and damage should alter lifespan, the phenotype of mice enhanced or deficient in antioxidant protection is of great interest. In the past two decades, several mouse models that overexpress or lack primary components of the antioxidant defense system have been generated and characterized. We will summarize the effects of these with respect to oxidative damage and alteration in lifespan.

5.1. *Manganese superoxide dismutase*

MnSOD is the only scavenger of superoxide in the mitochondrial matrix.[46] Genetic ablation of this enzyme in mice ($Sod2^{-/-}$) results in neonatal lethality between 1 and 24 days after birth, depending on genetic background.[47–49] These mice have approximately fourfold increase in oxidative damage as measured by 8-OH-guanine, 8-OH-adenine, and 5-OH-cytosine, and severe enzymatic deficits strongly consistent with massively elevated oxidative stress.[50] $Sod2^{-/-}$ mice are extremely sensitive to hyperoxia.[51,52] The cause of death in the longest-lived genetic background (dead by ~24 days after birth) is neurodegeneration.[47] Although the neonatal lethality of $Sod2^{-/-}$ does indicate that maintaining superoxide levels low is necessary for life, i.e., that elevated superoxide is toxic, these do not prove (although clearly fail to disprove) that mitochondrial superoxide (and by extension oxidative stress) causes aging. However, if increased superoxide levels were responsible for accelerated aging and if there exists a linear correlation between the concentration of superoxide and superoxide dismutase, one would expect that a modest decrease (rather than an outright elimination) of *Sod2* should lead to an increase in endogenous oxidative damage, and a diminution of lifespan. To address this question, we have measured oxidative damage and lifespan in *Sod2*$^{+/-}$ mice, i.e., mice possessing one wildtype and one deleted allele for *Sod2*. The activity of MnSOD is decreased on average by 50% as one would expect and there was no compensatory increase in activity of glutathione peroxidase 1 or CuZnSOD.[53–55] Oxidative damage to both nuclear and mitochondrial DNA was increased as measured by 8-oxo-dG.[53–56] However, mtDNA deletions were not significantly elevated in *Sod2*$^{+/-}$ mice compared to wildtype.[57] Interestingly, *Sod2*$^{+/-}$ mice were no more sensitive to hyperoxia than wildtype littermates.[51,52] Sensitivity to 10 Gy of γ-irradiation was also not significantly different from wildtype.[58] The natural lifespan of the *Sod2*$^{+/-}$ mice was statistically indistinguishable from that of wildtype. Various aging biomarkers also failed to show any differences between *Sod2*$^{+/-}$ mice and wildtype mice. Intriguingly, the tumor burden at 26 months of age was significantly higher in *Sod2*$^{+/-}$ mice, but this did not result in a difference in survival.[56]

5.2. *Glutathione peroxidase 1 (Gpx1)*

Glutathione peroxidase 1 is located in both the mitochondrial and cytosolic compartments of the cell, and together with catalase is a primary cellular scavenger of H_2O_2. Knockout mice completely lacking catalase develop normally and show no overt phenotype, even in response to hyperoxia-induced lung injury.[59] Likewise, a knockout of Gpx1 fails to generate a dramatic phenotype.[60,61] Mice lacking Gpx1 are sensitive to severe oxidative stress induced by paraquat/diquat toxicity; however, they are not more sensitive to less severe stress such as that induced by hyperoxia.[60–63] The only pathological finding to date is that *Gpx1*$^{-/-}$ mice develop cataracts at a considerably younger age than wildtype.[64] Although no detailed lifespan studies have been published, in our laboratory we have found that there is no difference in mortality curves between *Gpx1*$^{-/-}$ and wildtype to at least 30 months (Van Remmen *et al.*, unpublished results). In other words, lifespan is almost certainly unaltered by a complete deficiency of this antioxidant enzyme. This leads to the question of whether a lack of Gpx1 results in an increase in oxidative stress or damage. Measures of DNA oxidative damage (8-oxo-dG) suggest a modest (between 10 and 35%) increase in oxidative stress (Van Remmen, unpublished data). In preliminary measurements of F_2-isoprostanes, perhaps currently the most robust marker of *in situ* oxidative damage,[65] we did not observe elevation in the *Gpx1*$^{-/-}$ as compared to wildtype. Finally, H_2O_2 release, as measured with the Amplex Red method,[66,67] is not increased in skeletal muscle mitochondria from *Gpx1*$^{-/-}$ mice (Muller, unpublished). To summarize, there are some serious doubts as to whether *Gpx1*$^{-/-}$ mice are in fact under oxidative stress. Obviously, if there is no significant increase in oxidative stress, the normal lifespan of *Gpx1*$^{-/-}$ does not disprove the strong version of the oxidative theory.

5.3. *CuZn superoxide dismutase*

CuZnSOD is the major cytoplasmic superoxide scavenger.[46] Recent studies also place this enzyme in the mitochondrial intermembrane space,[68] where it may play an important role in detoxifying superoxide released by from Complex III.[69,70] At first glance, *Sod1*$^{-/-}$ knockout mice appear surprisingly normal. However, on closer inspection, there are some strong deleterious phenotypes. Fibroblasts form *Sod1*$^{-/-}$ mice do not grow in culture (cells from *Sod2*$^{-/-}$, *Sod2*$^{+/-}$, and *Gpx1*$^{-/-}$ grow just fine).[71] *Sod1*$^{-/-}$ females have very low fertility due to ovarian dysfunction.[72,73] *Sod1*$^{-/-}$ mice are sucescptible to age-related hearing loss.[74–76] and there are considerable age-dependent neuromuscular abnormalities.[77–79] We have confirmed in a cohort of *Sod1*$^{-/-}$ mice that the ratio of skeletal muscle to body mass is considerably lower in *Sod1*$^{-/-}$ than in age-matched wildtype mice, an effect exaggerated as the mice age (Van Remmen *et al.*, unpublished data). In our preliminary work with these animals, we have found liver 8-oxo-dG and plasma F_2-isoprostanes to be considerably elevated (approximately two- to threefold) as compared to wildtype, indicating a profound level of oxidative stress.

5.4. *Combination of primary antioxidant knockouts*

The question of redundancy and complementarity in the antioxidant system is often raised. For example, crossing *Gpx1*$^{-/-}$ and *Gpx2*$^{-/-}$ (neither of which has a particularly strong deleterious phenotype on their own) results in a lethal intestinal inflammation.[80] We decided to explore this issue by crossing *Sod2*$^{+/-}$, *Sod1*$^{-/-}$, and *Gpx1*$^{-/-}$. *Sod2*$^{+/-}$ *Gpx1*$^{-/-}$ mice are normal with respect to gross physiology but we found that the *Gpx1*$^{-/-}$ *Sod2*$^{+/-}$ double knockout mice are more sensitive to exogenous oxidative stress (paraquat, diquat) than either knockout alone.[58] Further, the double knockout strain becomes sensitive to exogenous oxidative stressors to which the single knockouts are not sensitive alone (γ-irradiation). Although the lifespan experiments are not fully complete, there is at present no difference in survival and mortality up to 37 months of age, between *Gpx1*$^{-/-}$ *Sod2*$^{+/-}$ and wildtype mice (Van Remmen *et al.*, unpublished data). Quite surprisingly, *Sod1*$^{-/-}$ *Gpx1*$^{-/-}$ and *Sod1*$^{-/-}$ *Sod2*$^{+/-}$ *Gpx1*$^{-/-}$ knockout mice are viable. No formal survival experiments have been conducted but the oldest *Sod1*$^{-/-}$ *Sod2*$^{+/-}$mouse in our colony lived to 27 months, and the oldest *Sod1*$^{-/-}$ *Gpx1*$^{-/-}$ mouse to 25 months. This is about the same as *Sod1*$^{-/-}$ mice alone. The oldest living *Sod1*$^{-/-}$ *Sod2*$^{+/-}$*Gpx1*$^{-/-}$ mouse is currently 16 months old.

5.5. *Peroxiredoxins*

While most experimental attention has focused on antioxidant enzymes, there is now increasing evidence that these enzymes are only a part of a larger redox-balance maintenance system. Among the more recently discovered members of the antioxidant family are the peroxiredoxins, most of which are thioredoxin peroxidases.[81] Their substrates include (but are not limited to) hydrogen peroxide, organic peroxides, and peroxynitrite.[81,82] Six peroxiredoxins have been identified in the mammalian genome.[81] Knockouts of peroxiredoxin 1, 2, and 6 have been generated (unfortunately, knockouts of peroxiredoin 3, located in mitochondria, have not yet been reported) and their phenotypes are of considerable interest to the oxidative theory of aging.[83–85] Peroxiredoxin 1 is thioredoxin peroxidase found in the cytoplasm of most tissues. Knockout of peroxiredoxin 1 (*Prxd1*$^{-/-}$)

causes hemolytic anemia, and increased cancer, culminating in decreased lifespan.[84] Oxidative damage as measured by protein carbonyls was also increased.[84] Interestingly, just as in our *Sod2*$^{+/-}$ study,[56] *Prxd1*$^{+/-}$ mice exhibited increased tumor burden, but no decrease in lifespan, as compared to wildtype.[84] Just as peroxiredoxin 1, peroxiredoxin 2 is found in most tissue but is especially abundant in the erythrocyte.[36,83] A knockout of *Prxd2* causes a hemolytic anemia,[83] but apparently in a milder form than that observed in the *Prxd1*$^{-/-}$ mice.[84] The *Prxd2*$^{-/-}$ mice also show decreased circulating half-life of their erythrocytes. No data on lifespan are yet available for *Prxd2*$^{-/-}$ mice.[83] It is interesting to note that neither *Gpx1*$^{-/-}$ nor hypocatalasemic mice develop anemia, which leads to the conclusion that peroxiredoxins are apparently much more important in antioxidant protection than previously thought.[83] This is all the more puzzling considering that the rate constant of Gpx1 reacting with H_2O_2 is higher than the rate of reaction of H_2O_2 with peroxiredoxins.[81] Localization and the high abundance of peroxiredoxins might explain why their ablation is so deleterious, while removal of Gpx1 is not.

5.6. *Methionine sulfoxide reductase*

Another component of the antioxidant system that has received recent experimental attention is methionine sulfoxide reductase. This enzyme selectively reduces (using thioredoxin as an electron source) the sulfoxide of methionine back to its thioether; it is found in the cytoplasm as well as in mitochondria.[86] As discussed in Sec. 2, overexpression of one isoform of this enzyme (methionine-S-sulfoxide reductase, MsrA) leads to lifespan increase in flies[30] and yeast.[87] Thus, it is interesting to note that a knockout of MsrA actually shortens lifespan in mice.[88] The cause of death was not analyzed, nor was the general pathology reported. However, the heterozygous knockout (*MsrA*$^{+/-}$) did not have a changed lifespan.

6. Overexpression of Antioxidant Enzymes

While the study of antioxidant knockouts can be used to attempt to disprove the strong oxidative hypothesis, the more powerful experiment (but also the more potentially confounding) is to overexpress antioxidant enzymes with the intention of reducing *in vivo* oxidative stress. As discussed above, this approach has provided some positive results (but also its fair share of controversy) in *D. melanogaster*. Only a handful of studies examining lifespan in antioxidant overexpressing mice have been published. As we discussed previously,[70] the studies so far indicate that neither overexpression of *Sod1* nor *Sod2* actually increase lifespan. The big problem with overexpression of antioxidant enzymes is that it is not always clear this actually reduces endogenous oxidative stress.[10,89,90] While by the virtue of their name antioxidant enzymes ought to be purely beneficial, it is worth remembering that the active centers of CuZnSOD and MnSOD house some of the strongest oxidants in the cell. Indeed, high overexpression of both *Sod1* and *Sod2* leads to very deleterious phenotypes.[10,89–91] Cross-species comparisons reveal that although lifespan negatively correlates with oxidative damage (as the oxidative theory would predict), the levels of antioxidant enzymes are consistently lower in longer lived ones.[92,93]

The only published study to have demonstrated an increase in lifespan by overexpression of a specific gene was that of Yodoi's group. These investigators reported that overexpressing thioredoxin 1 (a substrate for the peroxiredoxins and MsrA) results in an increase in both average and maximum lifespan.[94] Unfortunately, the sample size used was limited. Clearly, if this study were confirmed using a larger sample size, the significance for the strong oxidative theory would be considerable.

7. Conclusions and Future Directions

If we only consider the experiments that are directly relevant to aging, we are left with the results of *Sod2*$^{+/-}$ and *Prxd1*$^{+/-}$ mice with the startling result that although antioxidant enzyme deficiency causes elevated tumor burden, this does not actually decrease survival (lifespan). On the other hand, *Sod2*$^{+/-}$ seems to have a profound negative effect on several mouse models of age-related diseases.[95–99] Obviously, such results are in great accordance with the weak version of the oxidative hypothesis of aging, i.e., (mitochondrial) oxidative damage seems to play an important pathogenic role in several age-related disorders. It also leads to some very important questions on the role of oxidative damage in tumor initiation and progression. But what does it mean for the strong version? If we make no additional assumptions and we take the data showing an elevation of oxidative damage in the *Sod2*$^{+/-}$ to be correct, the simplest explanation is that the strong version of the oxidative stress theory is wrong, i.e., oxidative damage does not determine lifespan. How confident can we be in this conclusion? There are at least four lines of argumentation to defend the strong version of the oxidative theory against these results: (1) the underlying *in vitro* data do not reflect the *in vivo* situation (oxidative damage is not increased *in vivo*); (2) some types of oxidative damage are elevated while others are unchanged (e.g., mtDNA deletions in the *Sod2*$^{+/-}$), the types that remain unchanged are the ones relevant to aging;[100] (3) oxidative damage is increased across the board, but there is a compensatory, hormesis-type response; (4) lifespan is unchanged because *Sod2*$^{+/-}$ restricts tumor progression. It is too early to say whether the results of the *Sod2*$^{+/-}$ are a "bump in the road" or are actually the beginning of the end for the strong version of the oxidative stress theory of aging. Only time and additional research will tell.

References

1. Gerschman R, Gilbert DL, Nye SW, Dwyer P, Fenn WO. Oxygen poisoning and x-irradiation: a mechanism in common. *Science* 119: 623–626 (1954).
2. Chance B, Sies H, Boveris A. Hydroperoxide metabolism in mammalian organs. *Physiol. Rev.* 59: 527–605 (1979).
3. Beckman KB, Ames BN. The free radical theory of aging matures. *Physiol. Rev.* 78: 547–581 (1998).
4. Boveris A, Chance B. The mitochondrial generation of hydrogen peroxide. General properties and effect of hyperbaric oxygen. *Biochem. J.* 134: 707–716 (1973).
5. Li J, Gao X, Qian M, Eaton JW. Mitochondrial metabolism underlies hyperoxic cell damage. *Free Radic. Biol. Med.* 36: 1460–1470 (2004).
6. Miquel J, Lundgren PR, Bensch KG. Effects of exygen-nitrogen (1:1) at 760 Torr on the life span and fine structure of *Drosophila melanogaster*. *Mech. Ageing Dev.* 4: 41–57 (1975).
7. Baret P, Fouarge A, Bullens P, Lints FA. Life-span of *Drosophila melanogaster* in highly oxygenated atmospheres. *Mech. Ageing Dev.* 76: 25–31 (1994).

8. Mansfield KD, Simon MC, Keith B. Hypoxic reduction in cellular glutathione levels requires mitochondrial reactive oxygen species (mtROS). *J. Appl. Physiol.* 97: 1358–1366 (2004).
9. Landis GN, Abdueva D, Skvortsov D, Yang J, Rabin BE, Carrick J, Tavare S, Tower J. Similar gene expression patterns characterize aging and oxidative stress in *Drosophila melanogaster*. *Proc. Natl. Acad. Sci. USA* 101: 7663–7668 (2004).
10. Rando TA, Epstein CJ. Copper/zinc superoxide dismutase: more is not necessarily better! *Ann. Neurol.* 46: 135–136 (1999).
11. Seto NO, Hayashi S, Tener GM. Overexpression of Cu–Zn superoxide dismutase in *Drosophila* does not affect life-span. *Proc. Natl. Acad. Sci. USA* 87: 4270–4274 (1990).
12. Staveley BE, Phillips JP, Hilliker AJ. Phenotypic consequences of copper–zinc superoxide dismutase overexpression in *Drosophila melanogaster*. *Genome* 33: 867–872 (1990).
13. Reveillaud I, Niedzwiecki A, Bensch KG, Fleming JE. Expression of bovine superoxide dismutase in *Drosophila melanogaster* augments resistance of oxidative stress. *Mol. Cell Biol.* 11: 632–640 (1991).
14. Sohal RS, Agarwal A, Agarwal S, Orr WC. Simultaneous overexpression of copper- and zinc-containing superoxide dismutase and catalase retards age-related oxidative damage and increases metabolic potential in *Drosophila melanogaster*. *J. Biol. Chem.* 270: 15671–15674 (1995).
15. Kaiser M, Gasser M, Ackermann R, Stearns SC. P-element inserts in transgenic flies: a cautionary tale. *Heredity* 78: 1–11 (1996).
16. Parkes TL, Elia AJ, Dickinson D, Hilliker AJ, Phillips JP, Boulianne GL. Extension of *Drosophila* lifespan by overexpression of human SOD1 in motorneurons. *Nat. Genet.* 19: 171–174 (1998).
17. Phillips JP, Parkes TL, Hilliker AJ. Targeted neuronal gene expression and longevity in *Drosophila*. *Exp. Gerontol.* 35: 1157–1164 (2000).
18. Spencer CC, Howell CE, Wright AR, Promislow DE. Testing an "aging gene" in long-lived Drosophila strains: increased longevity depends on sex and genetic background. *Aging Cell* 2: 123–130 (2003).
19. Sun J, Molitor J, Tower J. Effects of simultaneous over-expression of Cu/ZnSOD and MnSOD on *Drosophila melanogaster* life span. *Mech. Ageing Dev.* 125: 341–349 (2004).
20. Sun J, Tower J. FLP recombinase-mediated induction of Cu/Zn-superoxide dismutase transgene expression can extend the life span of adult *Drosophila melanogaster* flies. *Mol. Cell Biol.* 19: 216–228 (1999).

21. Sun J, Folk D, Bradley TJ, Tower J. Induced overexpression of mitochondrial Mn-superoxide dismutase extends the life span of adult *Drosophila melanogaster. Genetics* 161: 661–672 (2002).
22. Mockett RJ, Bayne AC, Kwong LK, Orr WC, Sohal RS. Ectopic expression of catalase in *Drosophila* mitochondria increases stress resistance but not longevity. *Free Radic. Biol. Med.* 34: 207–217 (2003).
23. Mockett RJ, Sohal RS, Orr WC. Overexpression of glutathione reductase extends survival in transgenic *Drosophila melanogaster* under hyperoxia but not normoxia. *FASEB J.* 13: 1733–1742 (1999).
24. Mockett RJ, Orr WC, Rahmandar JJ, Benes JJ, Radyuk SN, Klichko VI, Sohal RS. Overexpression of Mn-containing superoxide dismutase in transgenic *Drosophila melanogaster. Arch. Biochem. Biophys.* 371: 260–269 (1999).
25. Reveillaud I, Phillips J, Duyf B, Hilliker A, Kongpachith A, Fleming JE. Phenotypic rescue by a bovine transgene in a Cu/Zn superoxide dismutase-null mutant of *Drosophila melanogaster. Mol. Cell Biol.* 14: 1302–1307 (1994).
26. Kirby K, Hu J, Hilliker AJ, Phillips JP. RNA interference-mediated silencing of Sod2 in *Drosophila* leads to early adult-onset mortality and elevated endogenous oxidative stress. *Proc. Natl. Acad. Sci. USA* 99: 16162–16167 (2002).
27. Missirlis F, Hu J, Kirby K, Hilliker AJ, Rouault TA, Phillips JP. Compartment-specific protection of iron-sulfur proteins by superoxide dismutase. *J. Biol. Chem.* 278: 47365–47369 (2003).
28. Mockett RJ, Radyuk SN, Benes JJ, Orr WC, Sohal RS. Phenotypic effects of familial amyotrophic lateral sclerosis mutant Sod alleles in transgenic *Drosophila. Proc. Natl. Acad. Sci. USA*100: 301–306 (2003).
29. Duttaroy A, Paul A, Kundu M, Belton A. A Sod2 null mutation confers severely reduced adult life span in *Drosophila. Genetics* 165: 2295–2299 (2003).
30. Ruan H, Tang XD, Chen ML, Joiner ML, Sun G, Brot N, Weissbach H, Heinemann SH, Iverson L, Wu CF, Hoshi T, Chen ML, Joiner MA. High-quality life extension by the enzyme peptide methionine sulfoxide reductase. *Proc. Natl. Acad. Sci. USA* 99: 2748–2753 (2002).
31. Rea S, Johnson TE. A metabolic model for life span determination in *Caenorhabditis elegans. Dev. Cell* 5: 197–203 (2003).
32. Brown-Borg HM, Borg KE, Meliska CJ, Bartke A. Dwarf mice and the ageing process. *Nature* 384: 33 (1996).
33. Hartman PS, Ishii N, Kayser EB, Morgan PG, Sedensky MM. Mitochondrial mutations differentially affect aging, mutability and anesthetic sensitivity in *Caenorhabditis elegans. Mech. Ageing Dev.* 122: 1187–1201 (2001).

34. Ishii N, Fujii M, Hartman PS, Tsuda M, Yasuda K, Senoo-Matsuda N, Yanase S, Ayusawa D, Suzuki K. A mutation in succinate dehydrogenase cytochrome b causes oxidative stress and ageing in nematodes. *Nature* 394: 694–697 (1998).
35. Dillin A, Hsu AL, Arantes-Oliveira N, Lehrer-Graiwer J, Hsin H, Fraser AG, Kamath RS, Ahringer J, Kenyon C. Rates of behavior and aging specified by mitochondrial function during development. *Science* 298: 2398–2401 (2002).
36. Lee SS, Lee RY, Fraser AG, Kamath RS, Ahringer J, Ruvkun G. A systematic RNAi screen identifies a critical role for mitochondria in *C. elegans* longevity. *Nat. Genet.* 33: 40–48 (2003).
37. Sipos I, Tretter L, Adam-Vizi V. Quantitative relationship between inhibition of respiratory complexes and formation of reactive oxygen species in isolated nerve terminals. *J. Neurochem.* 84: 112–118 (2003).
38. Betarbet R, Sherer TB, MacKenzie G, Garcia-Osuna M, Panov AV, Greenamyre JT. Chronic systemic pesticide exposure reproduces features of Parkinson's disease. *Nat. Neurosci.* 3: 1301–1306 (2000).
39. Panov AV, Gutekunst CA, Leavitt BR, Hayden MR, Burke JR, Strittmatter WJ, Greenamyre JT. Early mitochondrial calcium defects in Huntington's disease are a direct effect of polyglutamines. *Nat. Neurosci.* 5: 731–736 (2002).
40. Sherer TB, Betarbet R, Stout AK, Lund S, Baptista M, Panov AV, Cookson MR, Greenamyre JT. An *in vitro* model of Parkinson's disease: linking mitochondrial impairment to altered alpha-synuclein metabolism and oxidative damage. *J. Neurosci.* 22: 7006–7015 (2002).
41. Wallace DC. Mitochondrial defects in neurodegenerative disease. *Ment. Retard. Dev. Disabil. Res. Rev.* 7: 158–166 (2001).
42. Scott BA, Avidan MS, Crowder CM. Regulation of hypoxic death in *C. elegans* by the insulin/IGF receptor homolog DAF-2. *Science* 296: 2388–2391 (2002).
43. Foll RL, Pleyers A, Lewandovski GJ, Wermter C, Hegemann V, Paul RJ. Anaerobiosis in the nematode *Caenorhabditis elegans*. *Comp Biochem. Physiol B Biochem. Mol. Biol.* 124: 269–280 (1999).
44. Holt SJ, Riddle DL. SAGE surveys *C. elegans* carbohydrate metabolism: evidence for an anaerobic shift in the long-lived dauer larva. *Mech. Ageing Dev.* 124: 779–800 (2003).
45. van Voorhies WA, Ward S. Broad oxygen tolerance in the nematode *Caenorhabditis elegans*. *J. Exp. Biol.* 203 (Pt 16): 2467–2478 (2000).
46. Fridovich I. Fundamental aspects of reactive oxygen species, or what's the matter with oxygen? *Ann. NY Acad. Sci.* 893: 13–18 (1999).

47. Huang T-T, Carlson EJ, Gillespie AM, Epstein CJ. Genetic modification of the dilated cardiomyopathy and neonatal lethality phenotype of mice lacking mangnese superoxide dismutase. *Age* 21: 83–84 (1998).
48. Lebovitz RM, Zhang H, Vogel H, Cartwright J, Dionne L, Lu N, Huang S, Matzuk MM. Neurodegeneration, myocardial injury, and perinatal death in mitochondrial superoxide dismutase-deficient mice. *Proc. Natl. Acad. Sci. USA* 93: 9782–9787 (1996).
49. Li Y, Huang T-T, Carlson EJ, Melov S, Ursell PC, Olson JL, Noble LJ, Yoshimura MP, Berger C, Chan PH, Wallace DC, Epstein CJ. Dilated cardiomyopathy and neonatal lethality in mutant mice lacking manganese superoxide dismutase. *Nat. Genet.* 11: 376–381 (1995).
50. Melov S, Coskun P, Patel M, Tuinstra R, Cottrell B, Jun AS, Zastawny TH, Dizdaroglu M, Goodman SI, Huang T-T, Miziorko H, Epstein CJ, Wallace DC. Mitochondrial disease in superoxide dismutase 2 mutant mice. *Biochemistry* 96: 846–851 (1999).
51. Tsan M-F, White JE, Caska B, Epstein CJ, Lee CY. Susceptibility of heterozygous MnSOD gene-knockout mice to oxygen toxicity. *Am. J. Respir. Cell Mol. Biol.* 19: 114–120 (1998).
52. Asikainen TM, Huang TT, Taskinen E, Levonen AL, Carlson E, Lapatto R, Epstein CJ, Raivio KO. Increased sensitivity of homozygous Sod2 mutant mice to oxygen toxicity. *Free Radic. Biol. Med.* 32: 175–186 (2002).
53. Van Remmen H, Salvador C, Epstein CJ, Richardson A. Characterization of the antioxidant status of the heterozygous manganese superoxide dismutase knockout mouse. *Arch. Biochem. Biophys.* 363: 91–97 (1999).
54. Van Remmen H, Williams MD, Guo Z, Estlack L, Yang H, Carlson EJ, Epstein CJ, Huang TT, Richardson A. Knockout mice heterozygous for Sod2 show alterations in cardiac mitochondrial function and apoptosis. *Am. J. Physiol. Heart Circ. Physiol.* 281: H1422–H1432 (2001).
55. Williams MD, Van Remmen H, Conrad CC, Huang T-T, Epstein CJ, Richardson A. Increased oxidative damage is correlated to altered mitochondrial function in heterozygous manganese superoxide dismutase knockout mice. *J. Biol. Chem.* 273: 28510–28515 (1998).
56. Van Remmen H, Ikeno Y, Hamilton M, Pahlavani M, Wolf N, Thorpe SR, Alderson NL, Baynes JW, Epstein CJ, Huang TT, Nelson J, Strong R, Richardson A. Life-long reduction in MnSOD activity results in increased DNA damage and higher incidence of cancer but does not accelerate aging. *Physiol. Genomics* 16: 29–37 (2003).

57. Lynn S, Van Remmen H, Epstein CJ, Huang T-T. Investigation of mitochondrial DNA deltions in post-mitotic tissues of teh heterozygous superoxide dismutase 2 knockout mouse: effect of aging and genotype on the tissue-specific accumulation. *Free Radic. Biol. Med.* 31: S58 (2001).
58. Van Remmen H, Qi W, Sabia M, Freeman G, Estlack L, Yang H, Mao GZ, Huang TT, Strong R, Lee S, Epstein CJ, Richardson A. Multiple deficiencies in antioxidant enzymes in mice result in a compound increase in sensitivity to oxidative stress. *Free Radic. Biol. Med.* 36: 1625–1634 (2004).
59. Ho YS, Xiong Y, Ma W, Spector A, Ho DS. Mice lacking catalase develop normally but show differential sensitivity to oxidant tissue injury. *J. Biol. Chem.* 279: 32804–32812 (2004).
60. De Haan JB, Bladier C, Griffiths P, Kelner M, O'Shea RD, Cheung NS, Bronson RT, Silvestro MJ, Wild S, Zheng SS, Beart PM, Hertzog PJ, Kola I. Mice with a homozygous null mutation for the most abundant glutathione peroxidase, Gpx1, show increased susceptibility to the oxidative stress-inducting agents paraquat and hydrogen peroxide. *J. Biol. Chem.* 273: 22528–22536 (1998).
61. Ho Y-S, Magnenat JL, Bronson RT, Cao J, Gargano M, Sugawara M, Funk CD. Mice deficient in cellular glutathione peroxidase develop normally and show no increased sensitivity to hyperoxia. *J. Biol. Chem.* 272: 16644–16651 (1997).
62. Cheng W, Fu YX, Porres JM, Ross DA, Lei XG. Selenium-dependent cellular glutathione peroxidase protects mice against a pro-oxidant-induced oxidation of NADPH, NADH, lipids, and protein. *FASEB J.* 13: 1467–1475 (1999).
63. Cheng WH, Ho YS, Valentine BA, Ross DA, Combs GF, Jr, Lei XG. Cellular glutathione peroxidase is the mediator of body selenium to protect against paraquat lethality in transgenic mice. *J. Nutr.* 128: 1070–1076 (1998).
64. Reddy VN, Giblin FJ, Lin LR, Dang L, Unakar NJ, Musch DC, Boyle DL, Takemoto LJ, Ho YS, Knoernschild T, Juenemann A, Lutjen-Drecoll E. Glutathione peroxidase-1 deficiency leads to increased nuclear light scattering, membrane damage, and cataract formation in gene-knockout mice. *Invest Ophthalmol. Vis. Sci.* 42: 3247–3255 (2001).
65. Morrow JD, Roberts LJ. Mass spectrometric quantification of F2-isoprostanes in biological fluids and tissues as measure of oxidant stress. *Methods Enzymol.* 300: 3–12 (1999).
66. Zhou Z, Kang YJ. Cellular and subcellular localization of catalase in the heart of transgenic mice. *J. Histochem. Cytochem.* 48: 585–594 (2000).

67. Zhou M, Diwu Z, Panchuk-Voloshina N, Haugland RP. A stable nonfluorescent derivative of resorufin for the fluorometric determination of trace hydrogen peroxide: applications in detecting the activity of phagocyte NADPH oxidase and other oxidases. *Anal. Biochem.* 253: 162–168 (1997).
68. Okado-Matsumoto A, Fridovich I. Subcellular distribution of superoxide dismutases (SOD) in rat liver: Cu,Zn-SOD in mitochondria. *J. Biol. Chem.* 276: 38388–38393 (2001).
69. Han D, Williams E, Cadenas E. Mitochondrial respiratory chain-dependent generation of superoxide anion and its release into the intermembrane space. *Biochem. J.* 353: 411–416 (2001).
70. Muller F, Mele J, Van Remmen H, Richardson A. Probing the *in vivo* relevance of oxidative stress in aging using knockout and transgenic mice. In: Von Zglinicki T (ed.) *Aging at the Molecular Level.* Kluwer Academic Publishers, Dordrecht, 2003, pp. 131–144.
71. Huang T-T, Yasunami M, Carlson EJ, Gillespie AM, Reaume AG, Hoffman EK, Chan PH, Scott RW, Epstein CJ. Superoxide-mediated cytotoxicity in superoxide dismutase-deficient fetal fibroblasts. *Arch. Biochem. Biophys.* 344: 424–432 (1997).
72. Ho Y-S, Gargano M, Cao J, Bronson RT, Heimler I, Hutz RJ. Reduced fertility in female mice lacking CuZn superoxide dismutase. *J. Biol. Chem.* 273: 7765–7769 (1998).
73. Matzuk MM, Dionne L, Guo Q, Kumar TR, Lebovitz RM. Ovarian function in superoxide dismutase 1 and 2 knockout mice. *Endocrinology* 139: 4008–4011 (1998).
74. McFadden SL, Ding D, Burkard RF, Jiang H, Reaume AG, Flood DG, Salvi RJ. Cu/Zn SOD deficiency potentiates hearing loss and cochlear pathology in aged 129,CD-1 mice. *J. Comp. Neurol.* 413: 101–112 (1999).
75. McFadden SL, Ding D, Reaume AG, Flood DG, Salvi RJ. Age-related cochlear hair cell loss is enhanced in mice lacking copper/zinc superoxide dismutase. *Neurobiol. Aging* 20: 1–8 (1999).
76. Ohlemiller KK, McFadden SL, Ding DL, Flood DG, Reaume AG, Hoffman EK, Scott RW, Wright JS, Putcha GV, Salvi RJ. Targeted deletion of the cytosolic Cu/Zn-superoxide dismutase gene (Sod1) increases susceptibility to noise-induced hearing loss. *Audiol. Neurootol.* 4: 237–246 (1999).
77. Flood DG, Reaume AG, Gruner JA, Hoffman EK, Hirsch JD, Lin YG, Dorfman KS, Scott RW. Hindlimb motor neurons require Cu/Zn superoxide dismutase for maintenance of neuromuscular junctions. *Am. J. Pathol.* 155: 663–672 (1999).

78. Reaume AG, Elliott JL, Hoffman EK, Kowall NW, Ferrante RJ, Siwek DF, Wilcox HM, Flood DG, Beal MF, Brown RH, Jr, Scott RW, Snider WD. Motor neurons in Cu/Zn superoxide dismutase-deficient mice develop normally but exhibit enhanced cell death after axonal injury. *Nat. Genet.* 13: 43–47 (1996).
79. Shefner JM, Reaume AG, Flood DG, Scott RW, Kowall NW, Ferrante RJ, Siwek DF, Upton-Rice M, Brown RH, Jr. Mice lacking cytosolic copper/zinc superoxide dismutase display a distinctive motor axonopathy. *Neurology* 53: 1239–1246 (1999).
80. Esworthy RS, Aranda R, Martin MG, Doroshow JH, Binder SW, Chu FF. Mice with combined disruption of Gpx1 and Gpx2 genes have colitis. *Am. J. Physiol Gastrointest. Liver Physiol.* 281: G848–G855(2001).
81. Wood ZA, Schroder E, Robin HJ, Poole LB. Structure, mechanism and regulation of peroxiredoxins. *Trends Biochem. Sci.* 28: 32–40 (2003).
82. Dubuisson M, Vander SD, Clippe A, Etienne F, Nauser T, Kissner R, Koppenol WH, Rees JF, Knoops B. Human peroxiredoxin 5 is a peroxynitrite reductase. *FEBS Lett.* 571: 161–165 (2004).
83. Lee TH, Kim SU, Yu SL, Kim SH, Park DS, Moon HB, Dho SH, Kwon KS, Kwon HJ, Han YH, Jeong S, Kang SW, Shin HS, Lee KK, Rhee SG, Yu DY. Peroxiredoxin II is essential for sustaining life span of erythrocytes in mice. *Blood* 101: 5033–5038 (2003).
84. Neumann CA, Krause DS, Carman CV, Das S, Dubey DP, Abraham JL, Bronson RT, Fujiwara Y, Orkin SH, Van Etten RA. Essential role for the peroxiredoxin Prdx1 in erythrocyte antioxidant defence and tumour suppression. *Nature* 424: 561–565 (2003).
85. Wang X, Phelan SA, Forsman-Semb K, Taylor EF, Petros C, Brown A, Lerner CP, Paigen B. Mice with targeted mutation of peroxiredoxin 6 develop normally but are susceptible to oxidative stress. *J. Biol. Chem.* 278: 25179–25190 (2003).
86. Hansel A, Kuschel L, Hehl S, Lemke C, Agricola HJ, Hoshi T, Heinemann SH. Mitochondrial targeting of the human peptide methionine sulfoxide reductase (MSRA), an enzyme involved in the repair of oxidized proteins. *FASEB J.* 16: 911–913 (2002).
87. Koc A, Gasch AP, Rutherford JC, Kim HY, Gladyshev VN. Methionine sulfoxide reductase regulation of yeast lifespan reveals reactive oxygen species-dependent and -independent components of aging. *Proc. Natl. Acad. Sci. USA* 101: 7999–8004 (2004).
88. Moskovitz J, Bar-Noy S, Williams WM, Requena J, Berlett BS, Stadtman ER. Methionine sulfoxide reductase (MsrA) is a regulator of antioxidant defense

and lifespan in mammals. *Proc. Natl. Acad. Sci. USA* 98: 12920–12925 (2001).

89. Jaarsma D, Haasdijk ED, Grashorn JA, Hawkins R, van Duijn W, Verspaget HW, London J, Holstege JC. Human Cu/Zn superoxide dismutase (SOD1) overexpression in mice causes mitochondrial vacuolization, axonal degeneration, premature motoneuron death and accelerates motoneuron disease in mice expressing a familial amyotrophic lateral sclerosis mutant SOD1. *Neurobiol. Dis.* 7: 623–643 (2000).
90. Rando TA, Crowley RS, Carlson EJ, Epstein CJ, Mohapatra PK. Overexpression of copper/zinc superoxide dismutase: a novel cause of murine muscular dystrophy. *Ann. Neurol.* 44: 381–386 (1998).
91. Raineri I, Carlson EJ, Gacayan R, Carra S, Oberley TD, Huang TT, Epstein CJ. Strain-dependent high-level expression of a transgene for manganese superoxide dismutase is associated with growth retardation and decreased fertility. *Free Radic. Biol. Med.* 31: 1018–1030 (2001).
92. Barja G. Rate of generation of oxidative stress-related damage and animal longevity. *Free Radic. Biol. Med.* 33: 1167–1172 (2002).
93. Muller F. The nature and mechanism of superoxide production by the electron transport chain: its relevance to aging. *J. Am. Aging Assoc.* 23: 227–253 (2000).
94. Mitsui A, Hamuro J, Nakamura H, Kondo N, Hirabayashi Y, Ishizaki-Koizumi S, Hirakawa T, Inoue T, Yodoi J. Overexpression of human thioredoxin in transgenic mice controls oxidative stress and life span. *Antioxid. Redox Signal.* 4: 693–696 (2002).
95. Li F, Calingasan NY, Yu F, Mauck WM, Toidze M, Almeida CG, Takahashi RH, Carlson GA, Flint BM, Lin MT, Gouras GK. Increased plaque burden in brains of APP mutant MnSOD heterozygous knockout mice. *J. Neurochem.* 89: 1308–1312 (2004).
96. Ballinger SW, Patterson C, Knight-Lozano CA, Burow DL, Conklin CA, Hu Z, Reuf J, Horaist C, Lebovitz R, Hunter GC, McIntyre K, Runge MS. Mitochondrial integrity and function in atherogenesis. *Circulation* 106: 544–549 (2002).
97. Asimakis GK, Lick S, Patterson C. Postischemic recovery of contractile function is impaired in SOD2(+/−) but not SOD1(+/−) mouse hearts. *Circulation* 105: 981–986 (2002).
98. Andreassen OA, Ferrante RJ, Klivenyi P, Klein AM, Shinobu LA, Epstein CJ, Beal MF. Partial deficiency of manganese superoxide dismutase exacerbates a transgenic mouse model of amyotrophic lateral sclerosis. *Ann. Neurol.* 47: 447–455 (2000).

99. Andreassen OA, Ferrante RJ, Dedeoglu A, Albers DW, Klivenyi P, Carlson EJ, Epstein CJ, Beal MF. Mice with a partial deficiency of manganese superoxide dismutase show increased vulnerability to the mitochondrial toxins malonate, 3-nitropropionic acid, and MPTP. *Exp. Neurol.* 167: 189–195 (2001).
100. de Grey AD. The reductive hotspot hypothesis of mammalian aging: membrane metabolism magnifies mutant mitochondrial mischief. *Eur. J. Biochem.* 269: 2003–2009 (2002).

15 Oxidative Stress and Ataxia–Telangiectasia

Emily M. Dunner and Dianne J. Watters

1. Introduction — The Ataxia–Telangiectasia Disease

Ataxia–telangiectasia (A–T) is a debilitating childhood disease with a frequency in the United States and British populations of between 1:40,000 and 1:100,000 live births, respectively.[1] The cause of the disease is the functional loss of the ataxia–telangiectasia-mutated (ATM) protein due to mutations in the *ATM* gene.[2,3] Clinical features of A–T present within the first few years of life and progress to severe neurological abnormalities and immunodeficiencies, rendering A–T patients immobile and predisposing them to recurrent sinopulmonary infections.[4] Due to severe neurological deterioration and a predisposition to malignancies, predominantly lymphomas, individuals homozygous for A–T mutations generally do not live longer than the second decade of life. Heterozygotes, estimated to be 0.5–1.0% of the general population, have no clinical disease but do have a predisposition to malignancies,[5] and heart disease[6] and intermediate radiosensitivity at the cellular level.[7]

The initial symptom of A–T, ataxia or gaited walk, is observed when the child begins to walk. This progresses into general neuromotor dysfunction, the signs of which include involuntary eye movements and dysarthric (uncoordinated or inarticulated) speech and leads to immobilization by about age 10 years. The cause of the neuromotor deterioration, identified at autopsy in A–T patients, is continual neuronal degeneration of the central nervous system.[8] The regions of the brain affected are the cortical layers of the cerebellum, owing initially to the loss of the Purkinje cells. Additionally, the granule and basket cells deteriorate.[9–11] Subsequently, it has been detected in a substantial number of cases that neuronal loss has occurred outside the cerebellum, in the substantia nigra and the ocular motor neurones.[8] Degenerative changes in the peripheral nervous system have also been evident in the spinal motor neurones, dorsal root, and sympathetic motor neurones.[8] This indicates that the relentless advancement of ataxia in A–T patients results from cumulative loss of neurones, extending from the Purkinje cells of the cerebellum to neurones of the peripheral nervous system.

The second hallmark of A–T is the onset of telangiectases. Typically appearing between the ages of two and eight years, these capillary dilations occur primarily in the eyes.[4,8] Hair-like telangiectases may also be observed on the butterfly area of the face and neck, resembling that found in aged individuals, perhaps indicating premature aging in A–T patients.[4] Moreover, the appearance of telangiectases in A–T patients is most probably due to the radiation hypersensitivity, as they are commonly observed in radiotherapy patients.[4,12] At the cellular level, fibroblasts from A–T patients fail to undergo cell cycle arrest in response to DNA damage from ionizing radiation.[13,14] The residual double-strand break repair defect underlies a significant component of radiosensitivity of A–T cells.[15] Also A–T patients fail to respond to ultraviolet light type C,[16] but exhibit a normal response to ultraviolet light type A.[17] In addition, the radiation sensitivity in A–T is dependent on the specific cell type. ATM-deficient fibroblasts are radiosensitive whereas ATM-deficient neurones are radioresistant[18] but astrocytes lacking ATM are indistinguishable from wild type and yet require ATM for growth.[19]

In addition to the neuromotor and radiosensitive signs, there are many other cellular features that assist in the diagnosis of A–T. Growth retardation is another defining feature, that is, A–T patients are short in stature relative to their age while they also appear to prematurely age.[4,8] Cells from A–T patients, such as fibroblast and lymphoblastoid cells, exhibit a range of anomalies in culture including higher serum requirements, slow growth rate, and a reduced lifespan such that senescent-like growth arrest is observed after very few passages.[20] More specifically, premature senescence and accelerated aging has been linked to telomere dysfunction.[21] In addition, defects in meiosis cause gonadal abnormalities characteristic of

A–T. Infertility occurs in homozygote A–T patients due to a reduced number of germ cells[8] such that females have hypoplastic ovaries lacking mature follicles, while males display abnormalities in the testes with incomplete spermatogenesis.[4] Further diagnosing features of A–T include immune system defects. A–T patients display selective deficiency of immunoglobulin isotypes IgA, IgE, and IgG.[22] While the total circulating B-cell population could be either normal or slightly increased, responses to bacterial or viral antigens are greatly reduced in A–T patients.[4] Furthermore, the thymus is hypoplastic and dysfunctional and this was initially predicted to be the result of chromosomal rearrangement.[23] However, chromosomal V(D)J recombinations are normal.[24] The T- and B-cell repertoires have been shown to be highly skewed and restricted in A–T, with patients' T-cells predominantly being represented by terminally differentiated effector memory cells.[24,25] Giovannetti *et al.*[26] suggest that T-cell immunity in A–T is more likely to depend on a developmental defect rather than defects in T-cell activation since these memory cells have undergone terminal differentiation. On the other hand, there are several reports of defective signal transduction in T-lymphocytes of A–T patients.[25,26] The more variable features between A–T patients include a rare type of diabetes mellitus, involving marked hyperinsulinemia with peripheral insulin resistance.[27,28] This indicates possible abnormalities in the number, affinity, or response of the receptor.[28] Hence, growth retardation, infertility, immunodeficiencies, and a predisposition to malignancies are all characteristic features of A–T.[4,8]

1.1. *ATM gene and protein*

Initial characterization of the genetic heterogeneity in A–T patients revealed at least four complementation groups based on the rate of inhibition of DNA synthesis by X-rays,[29,30] indicating the possibility that the disease could have been determined by mutations in four genes. However, linkage analysis of two of these groups located the A–T locus to chomosome 11, region q22–23[31,32] and subsequent positional cloning found a mutation common to all groups, identifying a single gene, *ATM*, as responsible for the disorder.[2,3] *ATM* is a large gene consisting of 66 exons that span a region approximately 150 kb in length.[2,3,33] The transcript of *ATM* is 12 kb in length, including a 9.2 kb open reading frame.[2]

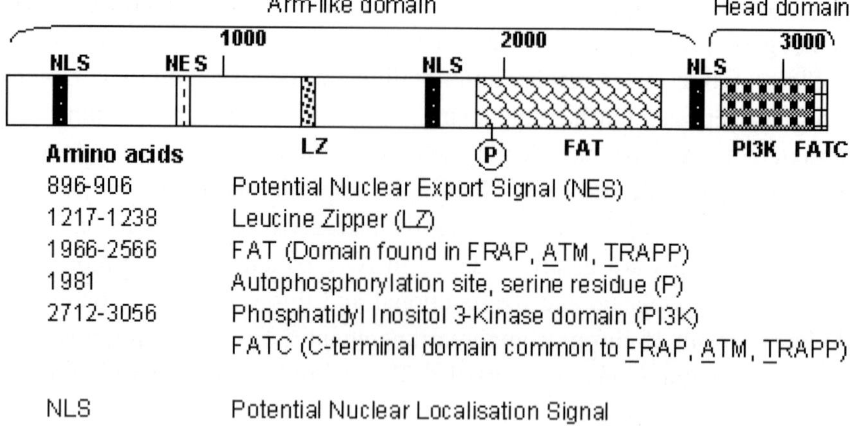

Fig. 1. Schematic diagram of the ATM protein.

The gene product, the ATM protein kinase, is predicted to contain 3056 amino acid residues with a mass of 350–370 kDa.[3,34] The ATM protein (Fig. 1) is identified by the small catalytic domain at the C-terminal region in the head of the protein,[35] which is highly homologous to the phosphatidyl inositol 3-kinase (PI3 kinase) family. The PI3 kinase region is common to a variety of lipid and protein related kinases, found in various organisms, most of which are involved in cell cycle control, responses to DNA damage, and maintenance of genome stability.[36] However, the high homology between members of the PI3 kinase family and ATM does not extend further than the sharing of this common domain.[2] Indeed, the highest homology exists between *S. cerevisiae* TEL1 with only 45% of amino acids of the carboxy terminus shared with ATM.[3] Furthermore, the existence of highly conserved residues that occurs in two domains within the core of the PI3 kinase domain are predicted to be involved in the binding of ATP and phosphotransferase activity.[2,37] The remainder of the protein is dominated by N-terminal HEAT repeats (a sequence element found in huntingtin, elongation factor 3, protein phosphatase 2A and TOR1).[38] A HEAT repeat is a pair of antiparallel helices linked by a flexible loop and when in a series, adjacent HEAT repeats interlock forming a superhelical matrix that provides a scaffold to allow interaction of proteins.[39] Hence, a major part of this large protein is believed to interact with downstream targets. The ATM protein also contains other known protein interaction domains such as a potential leucine zipper,[40] a proline rich region,[41] and several motifs encoding potential nuclear localization signals.[42]

1.2. *Mouse models*

Following the cloning of the human *ATM* gene, the mouse homolog was characterized.[43] The encoding sequence of the mouse *atm* gene has 84% homology to the human form,[43] so a mammalian model was created in the mouse,[18,36,44–47] based on the theory that with an expected high degree of similarity of phenotype between species, the model would provide further clues to understanding the roles of the ATM protein.

As most mutations in human A–T patients result in a truncated gene product,[48] the models were created by gene targeting techniques to develop a mouse strain that failed to express a functional Atm protein. In general, mice lacking the Atm protein display a series of pleiotropic abnormalities that closely resemble the human phenotype.[36,44–46] Features of the *atm* knock-out (Atm deficient) mice include growth abnormalities, such that A–T mice weigh 10–25% less than their sex-matched wild-type or heterozygous littermates, and infertility, as a result of meiotic arrest owing to chromosomal fragmentation. Furthermore, these mice display immunodeficiencies, such as a reduction in the number of T-cells and thymic lymphomas, which develop by the expansions of T-cells bearing chromosomal translocations.[44–46]

In addition, a knock-in mouse was developed by the deletion of three amino acids leading to the expression of a non-functional near-full-length protein product.[49] A number of differences in the A–T phenotype were displayed in the knock-in mouse, including a longer lifespan and variety of tumors not seen in the *atm* knock-out mouse. Borghesani and colleagues[50] have developed an *atm* mutant model whereby the exons comprising the catalytic kinase domain have been replaced with a neomycin-resistance gene in a reverse orientation such that no atm protein is detected by using N-terminal or C-terminal antibodies. The mutant mice from this model display reduced incidence of thymic tumors, motor defects, and abnormally differentiated Purkinje cells in mice of all ages.[50]

Despite some evidence of *atm* mutant mice presenting neuropathological abnormalities,[50] mice from almost all other A–T mouse models present less severe behavioral ataxia compared to the human A–T phenotype or no gross cerebellar degeneration.[44–46] The brain histology of the mutant mice at 1–3 months of age showed normal architecture with no neuronal degeneration in the brain, spinal cord, dorsal root ganglia, or peripheral nerves by hematoxylin and eosin staining,[44,46] although a significant increase in lysosomes has been detected in 4-month-old *atm*-deficient mice.[51] Also, there is evidence of selective loss of dopaminergic neurones in the substantia nigra,[52] to some extent supporting findings of structural abnormalities seen in the human central nervous system. However these mice appear to have negligible degeneration of the Purkinje cell region. Recent studies on the Atm-deficient mice during development suggest neurodegeneration may be instigated by defective Purkinje cell maturation during mid-gestation[53] and that the presence of early predegenerative lesions is indicated by decreased sodium currents.[47]

Studies in mice doubly null for *atm* and telomerase RNA component (*Terc*) revealed no cerebellar ataxia suggesting that the cerebellar defects in A–T might be independent of the role of atm in telomere dynamics[21] however, neural stem cells from these mice did show diminished ability to proliferate and differentiate into viable neurons and there were fewer dopamine-containing neurons in the substantia nigra. Interestingly, the presence of telomere dysfunction was associated with a near complete suppression of thymic lymphomas in fourth generation *Terc−/− atm−/−* mice. Therefore, creating models of A–T by disruption of the *atm* gene in mice provides a means for understanding the cellular processes involved in the phenotypical features of the disease and the roles of the protein product; however, the mice do not display the characteristic neurological degeneration seen in human patients for reasons that are presently unclear.

1.3. *Localization of ATM*

Various techniques have been employed in the detection of the ATM protein. Based on the results from Northern blotting, the human ATM major transcript is present in relatively uniform expression in the pancreas, kidney, liver, skeletal muscle, brain, thymus, prostrate, testes, ovary, colon, small intestine, and placenta, with higher levels expected in the heart, spleen, and leukocytes[2,54] Furthermore, western blotting has revealed that ATM protein is present within the cerebellar cortex but not the cerebral cortex, in developing human brains.[55] In comparison, the distribution of the ATM transcript in mice, reveals a different pattern. High levels of expression were detected in the skeletal muscle, brain, and testes, with barely detectable expression in the heart, spleen, lung, and kidney.[43]

The localization of ATM has also been investigated on the cellular level. The ATM protein is reduced or absent in A–T homozygote cells.[56–58] In control fibroblasts[58] and lymphoblasts,[57] the ATM protein is predominantly present in the nucleus. Detectable levels of microsome-associated ATM are observed in lymphoblasts and peripheral lymphocytes from A–T patients.[57] In fibroblasts, approximately 80% of ATM is nuclear and the remainder is cytoplasmic.[58] In the A–T cells that do express low levels of the mutant ATM protein, a similar cellular distribution was detected.[56,58] In a study using a subcellular fractionation method, a significant proportion of ATM of the post-mitochondrial fraction was shown to be localized to an organelle responsible for oxidative metabolism, the peroxisome.[59] Thus, a role for ATM in redox balance is indicated. In contrast, in immunocytochemistry of Purkinje cells from human cerebellum, the cells most affected by neurodegeneration, the ATM protein was detected in the cytoplasm but not within the nuclei.[55] Similarly, Atm is predominantly expressed in the nucleus of undifferentiated neural progenitor cells in wild-type mice[60] but has predominant extranuclear expression in differentiated mouse Purkinje cells.[51] The Atm protein has also been located in mouse neuronal endosomes.[61] The expression of Atm in the adult rat cerebellum neuronal cells was predominantly nuclear; however, in Purkinje cells, cells of the cerebellar nuclei, and spinal cord ventral horn neurones, ATM was found in the cytoplasm.[62] Thus, ATM is located in both the nuclear and cytoplasmic fractions of cells. This implicates ATM could have important roles in nuclear functions, such as cell cycle progression, and extranuclear mechanisms, for example, signal transduction from the cell surface, particularly in cells of neuronal origin.

1.4. *ATM activation*

ATM is the key molecule in orchestrating cellular responses to DNA damage. Upon induction of DNA double-strand breaks by exogenous chemical agents or ionizing radiation, endogenous oxidative stresses, or

DNA recombinational processing errors, a portion of nuclear ATM rapidly migrates to the site of damage and is activated upon binding to the DNA break where it serves in a signal transducer role for other reactions that take place at the site.[63] In addition to activated ATM bound to the DNA breaks, it is thought that a free floating portion of ATM exists in the nucleus which becomes active in response to alterations to chromatin structure rather than direct contact between ATM and the DNA lesion.[64] Regardless, a dramatic increase in ATM kinase activity immediately follows, and this involves an autophosphorylation mechanism as demonstrated by specific activation of ATM by ATP.[37] Inactive ATM exists as a dimer in uncompromised cells, with the kinase (head) domain (see Fig. 1) of one ATM molecule bound to the FAT domain containing a serine residue at amino acid position 1981, within the arm-like region[35] of the adjoining ATM.[64] Following DNA damage, the kinase domain of each ATM molecule phosphorylates serine 1981 of the adjoining molecule.[64] This causes a large conformational change in the position of the arm-like domains,[35] releasing two individual proteins. Each active ATM monomer serves as a platform for many cellular substrates, conveying the damage signal simultaneously to multiple effector pathways. The arm-like region is specifically capable of binding around the DNA double helix.[35] The leucine zipper domain and adjacent sequences, in particular, have been shown to be essential for regulating the cell survival response following DNA damage.[40] The exact mechanism by which double strand breaks are recognized and the activation of ATM has been the subject of intense investigation. The presently available evidence indicates that the MRN complex (consisting of the proteins MRE11, RAD50 and NBS1) binds directly to DNA and senses DSBs. It unwinds the ends, and recruits ATM leading to dissociation of the ATM dimer and activation of ATM by autophosphorylation.[65] Additional proteins are recruited to the DSBs, including H2AX, MDC1/NFBD1, 53BP1, BRCA1, and SMC1 and these accumulate at distinct foci.[66] These proteins are also substrates of ATM (see Sec. 1.5). No other mechanism for sensing the DNA damage in A–T has been suggested in the literature to date. A schematic summary of the activation of ATM in response to DNA double-strand breaks is shown in Fig. 2.

There are also a number of other activators of ATM. One such activator is the nucleotide, ATP, which has been shown to activate ATM in a time- and concentration-dependent manner in unirradiated cells without the

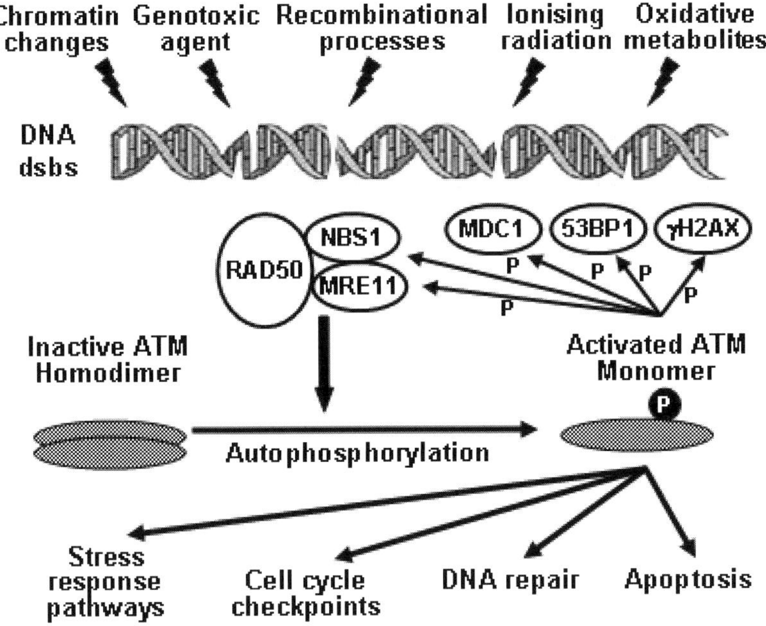

Fig. 2. ATM activation is central to the cellular response to DNA double-strand breaks (dsbs).

requirement of DNA.[37] Insulin exposure also leads to ATM activation and initiation of protein synthesis via the phosphorylation of the binding protein 4E-BP1 and release of the translation initiation factor, EIF-4E.[67] It is noteworthy that 4E-BP1 has an entirely cytoplasmic localization. A recent paper has shown that ATM is activated by polyglutamine protein expression in response to DNA damage from the resulting accumulation of reactive oxygen species in cells.[68] In addition, ATM-deficient cells are in a constant state of oxidative stress[59] and are sensitive to hydrogen peroxide.[69] ATM is activated in response to reactive oxygen species during re-oxygenation after hypoxia.[70] ATM is also activated in response to oxygen-glucose deprivation,[71] whereby an AMP-activated protein kinase, ARK5, activates ATM in an Akt-dependent manner, promoting cell survival.[72] Furthermore, ultraviolet A irradiation triggers ATM kinase activity and induces apoptotic signalling.[17] In this case, ATM is activated in response to ultraviolet A induced generation of reactive oxygen species.[17] Evidence also suggests ATM is activated in response to DNA alkylation, but this response could be caused by DNA scission associated with DNA repair endonuclease activity.[73] Thus, ATM activity is regulated by various stimuli and depends on the redox state of the cell.

1.5. *ATM substrates and functions*

The many substrates of ATM have complex roles in maintaining cellular homeostasis. ATM phosphorylates all substrates on a general consensus motif, either a serine or threonine residue that is followed by a glutamine.[74,75] ATM has a central role in orchestrating the arrest of cell cycle progression in response to cellular stresses, by activating or inhibiting substrates that control specific check points of the cell cycle, to allow homologous recombinational repair and cell survival. Substrates of ATM that are involved in cell cycle control and DNA damage response include p53,[76–78] MDM2,[79] CHK1,[80] CHK2,[81] NBS1 of the MRN complex (see Sec. 1.4),[82] BRCA1,[83] CtIP,[84] FANCD2,[85] BLM,[86] RAD9,[87] and RAD17.[88] In addition, some substrates of ATM are involved in chromosome and telomere maintenance. These include H2AX,[89] SMC1,[90] and PIN2.[91] Stress response substrates include IκBα[92] and c-Abl.[41,93] Transcription factor E2F1 is a known substrate of ATM, resulting in accumulation of E2F1 after DNA damage.[94] ATM can also phosphorylate 4E-BP1 after insulin treatment, allowing the initiation of translation.[67] Hence, ATM has a critical role, linking many of the signaling pathways in the cell. Full activation of Akt (protein kinase B) in response to ionizing radiation or insulin is mediated through ATM.[95]

1.6. *Gene expression in A–T*

From the above discussion, it is clear that ATM has a wide role in cellular homeostasis. A comprehensive analysis of gene expression patterns using oligonucleotide microarrays was undertaken in control and ATM−/− cells as well as NBS−/− cells.[96] ATM up- and downregulated genes fall into six broad groups — cell cycle/DNA replication, apoptosis, signal transduction, cell–cell adhesion, growth and differentiation, and metabolism. In addition, heterozygotes for ATM mutations, although showing no clinical disease, also have altered gene expression patterns.[97]

2. Evidence of Oxidative Stress in A–T

There is extensive evidence of oxidative stress in A–T. Elevated levels of lipid hydroperoxides have been detected in fibroblasts from A–T patients indicating that cells lacking functional ATM protein are in a chronic state of oxidative stress.[59] In addition to lipid peroxidation, Reichenbach and colleagues[98] found that oxidative damage to DNA was markedly increased in ten A–T patients compared to controls. A–T cells are also hypersensitive to nitric oxide, superoxide anion, and hydrogen peroxide,[69,99] implicating a role for ATM in redox balance. The preferential loss of neurons and T-lymphocytes could be in part due to chronic oxidative damage.[99,100] Indeed, Kamsler and colleagues[101] have reported increased activity of the redox regulatory enzyme, thioredoxin, and the reactive oxygen species detoxifier, superoxide dismutase, in the cerebellum of *atm*-deficient mice, reflecting an altered redox state in the region of the brain that is most affected by the neuronal degeneration. Significantly reduced catalase activity is also reported for the cerebellum of *atm*-deficient mice[101] and in human A–T cells,[59,69] reflecting overall alterations in reactive oxygen species. However, it is thought that a reduction of the intracellular catalase enzyme cofactor, NADPH, is attributed to the reduced enzymatic activity, as a consequence of accumulated DNA strand breaks.[102]

2.1. *Signal transduction*

Oxidative stress can lead to activations and alterations in signal transduction in A–T cells. Hydrogen peroxide treatment of endothelial cells activates p53 via the transactivation of platelet-derived growth factor-β and subsequent activation of ATM kinase.[103] Thus, oxidative stress affects signal transduction from growth factor receptors in A–T. Moreover, the coordinated degradation of regulatory proteins via the ubiquitin pathway and subsequent apoptosis is modulated by redox status in A–T cells. The research indicates that A–T cells have higher levels of ubiquitin conjugates relative to controls, and a milder response to induced stress,[104] consistent with A–T cells being chronically under oxidative stress. There is also evidence that suggests oxidative stress affects cell cycle signaling. A–T fibroblasts exposed to *t*-butyl-hydroperoxide were unable to induce normal G1 and

G2 cell cycle checkpoint stress responses.[105] Hence, oxidative stress can induce defective signaling responses in A–T.

2.2. *Gene regulation*

Chronic oxidative damage leads to a critical disturbance of cell homeostasis. In the cerebella of *atm*-deficient mice where elevated oxidative stress levels are exhibited, the transcription factor AP-1 remains continuously activated.[106] Eventually, effective AP-1 activated DNA-binding activity in response to ionizing radiation is lost in these mice. A recent report links ATM and DNA turnover to redox balance. ATM regulates redox-sensitive cell cycle checkpoints reducing DNA turnover and determining the cell fate of developing lymphocytes.[107] Cell fate is further determined by the activation of transcription factors. Exposure of control and A–T fibroblasts to *t*-butyl-hydroperoxide has shown the involvement of ATM in the regulation of the transcription factors, AP1, SP1, and MTF1.[108] So, ATM could regulate gene expression via redox signaling pathways. However, there is no apparent link between oxidative stress and loss of gene regulation leading to cancer. A murine model deficient for *atm* and overexpressing the human Cu/Zn superoxide dismutase (*SAT*) displayed moderate levels of oxidative stress relative to the *atm*+/+ mice.[109] Growth retardation, defective maturation of T-cells, and radiosensitivity similar to the A–T phenotype were augmented, although there was no enhancement of thymic lymphomas indicating oxidative stress did not contribute to tumorigenesis in A–T.[109] The evidence suggests that ATM has a role in redox balance and in the regulation of gene expression.

2.3. *Neurodegeneration*

The A–T murine model provides evidence of oxidative damage in important neurons. While no gross neuronal abnormalities are displayed in most of the *atm*−/− and *SAT* mice,[52,109,110] oxidative damage has been identified in the *atm*−/− mouse Purkinje cells.[101,111,112] Reduced dendritic arborization of *atm*−/− mouse Purkinje cells could be attributable to continuous oxidative stress.[113] Furthermore, *atm*−/− mice have altered activities of thioredoxin, catalase, and superoxide dismutase[101,112] as well as increased hem-oxygenase-1 and 3-nitrotyrosine[111] in the affected neuronal populations. Hence, ATM could modulate redox balance in the neuronal populations affected in A–T. Additionally, genotoxic stress during development may affect neuronal survival. Evidence indicates ATM could act in neuronal development to activate apoptosis and eliminate DNA damaged cells early in neurogenesis.[114] In theory, ATM acts at a checkpoint in early development such that DNA damage left unrepaired in ATM deficient cells consolidates during development and is critical to progressive degeneration.[114] Dopaminergic neurons in the substantia nigra pars compacta form normally but progressively degenerate over time in *atm−/−* mice.[110] Evidence shows that neural progenitor cells from wild-type mice differentiate along a neuronal linage but neuronal survival of neural progenitor cells from *atm−/−* mice is reduced after an environmental stimulus.[60] Also, the defective c-Abl signaling in A–T after genotoxic stress could contribute to the defective development of the nervous system.[115] Interestingly, α-synuclein bodies, which are shown to exacerbate oxidative stress levels in Parkinson's disease,[116] are found in *atm−/−* mice[110] and in A–T patients.[117] Thus, neurodegeneration in A–T may be a result of unrepaired damage during development; however, it is likely that there is a significant contribution from oxidative stress.

2.4. *Immunodeficiencies*

Oxidative stress also contributes to defective immunoresponses in A–T. There is evidence indicating that naive T-cells are particularly sensitive to oxidative stress compared to memory T-cells.[118] It has been shown that oxidative stress induces increased apoptosis and cell death of naive T-cells in blood plasma from A–T patients.[100] This is supported by findings in *atm−/−* mice, which have elevated oxidative stress levels and display premature loss of lymphocytes.[44,107] So thymic dysfunction[24] could in part result from chronic oxidative stress. Hence, redox imbalance in A–T may contribute to immune signaling defects.

2.5. *Aging*

The aging process has been linked to cumulative oxidative stress[119] and this is accelerated in A–T patients. Critically shortened telomeres are a defining feature of A–T cells.[120,121] Recent results indicate telomere dysfunction leads to accelerated aging and premature cell death in A–T and potentially compromises whole organ systems.[21] There is evidence to suggest that telomere shortening and premature senescence in A–T is induced by cellular oxidative damage.[122,123] Chronic hydrogen peroxide induced oxidative stress increased the telomere shortening rate in both control and A–T cells,[123] despite higher than normal telomerase activity[124] precluding defective enzymatic activity and indicating elevated oxidative stress responses observed in untreated A–T cells[59,69] as the likely cause of premature senescence. Further, it is proposed that ATM could have a maintenance role in sensing oxidative damage to telomere function[125] as a significant increase in extra-chromosomal fragments of telomeric DNA were detected in A–T cells under oxidative stress compared to control cells.[123,126] Therefore, ATM is an important redox sensor involved in telomere maintenance.

2.6. *Heterozygotes*

Although A–T heterozygotes display no clinical signs of A–T, they do have some cellular features of the disease. Apart from a predisposition to malignancies[5] and heart disease,[6] and intermediate radiosensitivity at the cellular level,[7] cells from A–T heterozygotes also show signs of oxidative stress. A study on red blood cells from A–T homozygotes and heterozygotes showed the cell membranes had increased fluidity, decreased microviscosity, and decreased sulfyldryl group content due to increased lipid oxidation and elevated oxidative stress levels.[127] In addition, telomere shortening due to oxidative damage has been detected in A–T heterozygote cells.[123]

3. Therapy

To date, there is no effective therapy to halt the progression of A–T symptoms. However, there are some treatments that relieve some aspects of the A–T phenotype examined in culture and by the use of mouse models. Several reports investigate expression of various genes to restore cellular homeostasis in A–T. The expression of full length ATM cDNA reprieves A–T cells of the cellular features of A–T[128] and antisense expression results in the A–T phenotype in normal cells.[129] Consistently, the expression of recombinant ATM in a viral vector in A–T cells showed the survival of A–T cells expressing the recombinant ATM was far greater than non-transduced A–T cells after hydrogen peroxide treatment.[62] Additionally, A–T and normal cells stably transfected with hTERT, an expression vector for the catalytic subunit of human telomerase, resulted in telomere elongation and prevented premature senescence in A–T cells.[122] Unfortunately, the hypersensitivity to ionizing radiation and the defect in G1 checkpoint activation were not corrected in A–T fibroblasts expressing hTERT.[122] Hence, the expression hTERT in A–T could be useful in treating A–T patients, if used in combination with, for example, an antioxidant.

It is indicated that A–T patients have reduced endogenous antioxidant capacity, mainly reduced vitamin A and vitamin E, due to elevated cellular levels of reactive oxygen species.[130] Apart from reactive oxygen species scavaging, vitamins are implicated as having other important stimulatory roles in immune response, aging, and neuropathology.[131,132] A recent study has shown the use of an antioxidant, isoindoline nitroxide, prevented cell death and promoted dendritogenesis to wild-type levels in *atm*-deficient mice Purkinje cells in culture.[113] It has been shown that the use of the antioxidant, α-lipoic acid, reduces the chronic oxidative stress-induced activation of p53 and p21 in A–T cells.[133] The iron chelators, desferrioxamine, apoferritin and quercetin increase the resistance of A–T but not normal cells to oxidative stress.[134] Furthermore labile iron was found to be elevated in the sera of Atm-deficient mice.[135,136] Intracellular labile iron is an oxidant that can cause hydroxyl radical generation and oxidative damage. These findings suggest that iron chelators may slow Purkinje cell death in A–T. The use of antioxidant phenyl-butyl-nitrone in A–T and control cells decreased the rate of telomere shortening when exposed to hydrogen peroxide.[123] Hence, antioxidants can also decrease premature aging defects in A–T cells.

Treatment of atm−/− mice with the catalytic antioxidant EUK189 (a catalase/superoxide dismutase mimetic) which is known to cross the blood brain barrier, improved their performance on the rotarod, increased their lifespan and retarded the development of thymomas.[137] Treatment of Atm-deficient mice with the antioxidant N-acetylcysteine (NAC) counteracted the oxidative damage.[138] The self-renewal capacity of hematopoietic stem cells is reduced in Atm-deficient mice and this was shown to be recovered by treatment with NAC indicating that oxidative stress may be responsible and that A–T patients might benefit from antioxidant treatment.[139]

In conclusion, oxidative stress appears to play a significant role in the pathophysiology of ataxia–telangiectasia. The source of the oxidative stress is not yet clear: ATM could directly sense ROS and prevent DSBs or the excess ROS may arise from unrepaired DSBs via elevation of poly (ADP ribose) polymerase (PARP) activity and the resulting depletion of NAD^+ pools.[140] A clinical trial is currently underway at the A–T Clinical Center, Johns Hopkins Hospital, using nicotinamide (an inhibitor of PARP) in conjunction with an antioxidant, α-lipoic acid. It is hoped that antioxidant treatment will slow or halt the progessive neuronal loss of this disease.

References

1. Taylor AM, Metcalfe JA, Thick J, Mak YF. *Blood* 87: 423–438 (1996).
2. Savitsky K *et al. Science* 268: 1749–1753 (1995a).
3. Savitsky K *et al. Hum. Mol. Genet.* 4: 2025–2032 (1995b).
4. Lavin MF, Shiloh Y. *Annu. Rev. Immunol.* 15: 177–202 (1997).
5. Easton DF. *Int. J. Radiat. Biol.* 66: S177–S182 (1994).
6. Su Y, Swift M. *Ann. Intern. Med.* 133: 770–778 (2000).
7. Pernin D, Bay J-O, Uhrhammer N, Bignon Y-J. *Eur. J. Cancer* 35: 1130–1135 (1999).
8. Sedgwick RP, Boder E. In: Vianney De Jong JMV (ed.) *Hereditary Neuropathies and Spinocerebellar Atrophies*. Elsevier, Amsterdam, 1991, pp. 347–423.
9. Farina L *et al. J. Comput. Assist. Tomogr.* 18: 724–727 (1994).
10. Paula-Barbosa MM *et al. Ann. Neurol.* 13: 297–302 (1983).
11. Sardanelli F *et al. Neuroradiology* 37: 77–82 (1995).
12. Scott D. *Strahlenther. Onkol.* 176: 229–234 (2000).
13. Ford MD, Martin L, Lavin MF. *Mutat. Res.* 125: 115–122 (1984).
14. Beamish H *et al. Oncogene* 13: 963–970 (1996).
15. Kuhne M *et al. Cancer Res.* 64: 500–508 (2004).
16. Shafman TD *et al. Cancer Res.* 55: 3242–3245 (1995).
17. Zhang Y *et al. J. Biol. Chem.* 277: 3124–3131 (2002).
18. Herzog KH *et al. Science* 280: 1089–1091 (1998).
19. Gosink EC, Chong MJ, McKinnon PJ *Cancer Res.* 59: 5294–5298 (1999).
20. Shiloh Y. *Eur. J. Hum. Genet.* 3: 116–138 (1995).

21. Wong KK *et al. Nature* 421: 643–648 (2003).
22. Strober W *et al. J. Clin. Invest.* 47: 1905–1915 (1968).
23. Kojis TL, Gatti RA, Sparkes RS. *Cancer Genet. Cytogenet.* 56: 143–156 (1991).
24. Giovannetti A *et al. Blood* 100: 4082–4089 (2002).
25. Schubert R, Reichenbach J, Zielen S. *Clin. Exp. Immunol.* 129: 125–132 (2002).
26. Kondo N *et al. Scand. J. Immunol.* 38: 45–48 (1993).
27. Schalch DS, McFarlin DE, Barlow MH. *N. Engl. J. Med.* 282: 1396–1402 (1970).
28. Bar RS *et al. N. Engl. J. Med.* 298: 1164–1171 (1978).
29. Murnane JP, Painter RB. *Proc. Natl. Acad. Sci. USA* 79: 1960–1963 (1982).
30. Jaspers NG *et al. Cytogenet. Cell Genet.* 49: 259–263 (1988).
31. Gatti RA *et al. Nature* 336: 577–580 (1988).
32. Ziv Y *et al. Genomics* 9: 373–375 (1991).
33. Uziel T *et al. Genomics* 33: 317–320 (1996).
34. Chen G, Lee E. *J. Biol. Chem.* 271: 33693–33697 (1996).
35. Llorca O, Rivera-Calzada A, Grantham J, Willison KR. *Oncogene* 22: 3867–3874 (2003).
36. Abraham RT. *DNA Repair* 3: 883–887 (2004).
37. Kozlov S *et al. J. Biol. Chem.* 278: 9309–9317 (2003).
38. Perry J, Kleckner N. *Cell* 112: 151–155 (2003).
39. Groves MR, Barford D. *Curr. Opin. Struct. Biol.* 9: 383–389 (1999).
40. Chen S, Paul P, Price BD. *Oncogene* 22: 6332–6339 (2003).
41. Shafman T *et al. Nature* 387: 520–523 (1997).
42. Shiloh Y, Kastan MB. *Adv. Cancer Res.* 83: 209–254 (2001).
43. Pecker I *et al. Genomics* 35: 39–45 (1996).
44. Barlow C *et al. Cell* 86: 159–171 (1996).
45. Elson A *et al. Proc. Natl. Acad. Sci. USA* 93: 13084–13089 (1996).
46. Xu Y *et al. Genes Dev.* 10: 2411–2422 (1996).
47. Chiesa N *et al. Neuroscience* 96: 575–583 (2000).
48. Gilad S *et al. Hum. Mol. Genet.* 5: 433–439 (1996).
49. Spring K *et al. Cancer Res.* 61: 4561–4568 (2001).
50. Borghesani PR *et al. Proc. Natl. Acad. Sci. USA* 97: 3336–3341 (2000).
51. Barlow C *et al. Proc. Natl. Acad. Sci. USA* 97: 871–876 (2000).
52. Eilam R *et al. Proc. Natl. Acad. Sci. USA* 95: 12653–12656 (1998).
53. Soares HD, Morgan JI, McKinnon PJ. *Neuroscience* 86: 1045–1054 (1998).
54. Chan DW *et al. J. Biol. Chem.* 275: 7803–7810 (2000).
55. Oka A, Takashima S. *Neurosci. Lett.* 252: 195–198 (1998).

56. Lakin ND *et al. Oncogene* 13: 2707–2716 (1996).
57. Brown KD *et al. Proc. Natl. Acad. Sci. USA* 94: 1840–1845 (1997).
58. Watters D *et al. Oncogene* 14: 1911–1921 (1997).
59. Watters D *et al. J. Biol. Chem.* 274: 34277–34282 (1999).
60. Allen DM *et al. Genes Dev.* 15: 554–566 (2001).
61. Kuljis RO *et al. Brain Res.* 842: 351–358 (1999).
62. Qi J *et al. Gene Ther.* 11: 25–33 (2004).
63. Andegeko Y *et al. J. Biol. Chem.* 276: 38224–38230 (2001).
64. Bakkenist CJ, Kastan MB. *Nature* 421: 499–506 (2003).
65. Lee J-H, Pauli T. *Science* 308: 551–554 (2005).
66. Löbrich M, Jeggo P. *DNA Repair* 4: 749–759 (2005).
67. Yang DQ, Kastan MB. *Nat. Cell. Biol.* 2: 893–898 (2000).
68. Giuliano P *et al. Hum. Mol. Genet.* 12: 2301–2309 (2003).
69. Takao N, Li Y, Yamamoto K-I. *FEBS Lett.* 472: 133–136 (2000).
70. Hammond EM, Dorie MJ, Giaccia AJ. *J. Biol. Chem.* 278: 12207–12213 (2003).
71. Yin KJ *et al. Stroke* 33: 2471–2477 (2002).
72. Suzuki A *et al. J. Biol. Chem.* 278: 48–53 (2003).
73. Adamson AW *et al. J. Biol. Chem.* 277: 38222–38229 (2002).
74. Kim S-T, Lim D-S, Canman CE, Kastan MB. *J. Biol. Chem.* 274: 37538–37543 (1999).
75. O'Neill T *et al. J. Biol. Chem.* 275: 22719–22727 (2000).
76. Siliciano JD *et al. Genes Dev.* 11: 3471–3481 (1997).
77. Banin S *et al. Science* 281: 1674–1677 (1998).
78. Canman CE *et al. Science* 281: 1677–1679 (1998).
79. Maya R *et al. Genes Dev.* 15: 1067–1077 (2001).
80. Gatei M *et al. J. Biol. Chem.* 278: 14806–14811 (2003).
81. Falck J *et al. Nature* 410: 842–847 (2001).
82. Zhao S *et al. Nature* 405: 473–477 (2000).
83. Cortez D, Wang Y, Qin J, Elledge SJ. *Science* 286: 1162–1166 (1999).
84. Li S *et al. Nature* 406: 210–215 (2000).
85. Taniguchi T *et al. Cell* 109: 459–472 (2002).
86. Beamish H *et al. J. Biol. Chem.* 28: 28 (2002).
87. Chen MJ *et al. J. Biol. Chem.* 276: 16580–16586 (2001).
88. Bao S *et al. Nature* 411: 969–974 (2001).
89. Burma S *et al. J. Biol. Chem.* 276: 42462–42467 (2001).
90. Yazdi PT *et al. Genes Dev.* 16: 571–582 (2002).
91. Kishi S *et al. J. Biol. Chem.* 276: 29282–29291 (2001).
92. Jung M *et al. Cancer Res.* 57: 24–27 (1997).

93. Baskaran R *et al. Nature* 387: 516–519 (1997).
94. Lin WC, Lin FT, Nevins JR. *Genes Dev.* 15: 1833–1844 (2001).
95. Viniegra JG *et al. J. Biol. Chem.* 280: 4029–4036 (2005).
96. Jang ER, Lee JH, Lim DS, Lee JS. *J. Cancer Res. Clin. Oncol.* 130: 225–234 (2004).
97. Watts JA *et al. Am. J. Hum. Genet.* 71: 791–800 (2002).
98. Reichenbach J *et al. Antioxid. Redox Signal.* 4: 465–469 (2002).
99. Rotman G, Shiloh Y. *Cancer Surv.* 29: 285–304 (1997).
100. Schubert R *et al. Clin. Exp. Immunol.* 119: 140–147 (2000).
101. Kamsler A *et al. Cancer Res.* 61: 1849–1854 (2001).
102. Hoffschir F *et al. Free Radic. Biol. Med.* 24: 809–816 (1998).
103. Chen K, Albano A, Ho A, Keaney JF Jr. *J. Biol. Chem.* 278: 39527–39533 (2003).
104. Taylor A *et al. Oncogene* 21: 4363–4373 (2002).
105. Shackelford RE *et al. J. Biol. Chem.* 276: 21951–21959 (2001).
106. Weizman N, Shiloh Y, Barzilai A. *J. Biol. Chem.* 278: 6741–6747 (2003).
107. Yan M *et al. FASEB J.* 15: 1132–1138 (2001).
108. Heinloth AN *et al. Radiat. Res.* 160: 273–290 (2003).
109. Peter Y *et al. EMBO J.* 20: 1538–1546 (2001).
110. Eilam R, Peter Y, Groner Y, Segal M. *Neuroscience* 121: 83–98 (2003).
111. Barlow C *et al. Proc. Natl. Acad. Sci. USA* 96: 9915–9919 (1999).
112. Quick KL, Dugan LL. *Ann. Neurol.* 49: 627–635 (2001).
113. Chen P *et al. J. Neurosci.* 23: 11453–11460 (2003).
114. Lee Y, Chong MJ, McKinnon PJ. *J. Neurosci.* 21: 6687–6693 (2001).
115. Miller HL *et al. Brain Res. Dev. Brain Res.* 145: 31–38 (2003).
116. Junn E, Mouradian MM. *Neurosci. Lett.* 320: 146–150 (2002).
117. Agamanolis DP, Greenstein JI. *J. Neuropathol. Exp. Neurol.* 38: 475–489 (1979).
118. Lahdenpohja N, Hurme M. *Cell. Immunol.* 173: 282–286 (1996).
119. Finkel T, Holbrook NJ. *Nature* 408: 239–247 (2000).
120. Harley CB, Vaziri H, Counter CM, Allsopp RC. *Exp. Gerontol.* 27: 375–382 (1992).
121. Xia SJ, Shammas MA, Shmookler Reis RJ. *Mutat. Res.* 364: 1–11 (1996).
122. Naka K, Tachibana A, Ikeda K, Motoyama N. *J. Biol. Chem.* 279: 2030–2037 (2004).
123. Tchirkov A, Lansdorp PM. *Hum. Mol. Genet.* 12: 227–232 (2003).
124. Pandita TK, Pathak S, Geard CR. *Cytogenet. Cell Genet.* 71: 86–93 (1995).
125. Pandita TK. *Oncogene* 21: 611–618 (2002).
126. Hande MP *et al. Hum. Mol. Genet.* 10: 519–528 (2001).

127. Rybczynska M, Pawlak AL, Sikorska E, Ignatowicz R. *Biochim. Biophys. Acta* 1302: 231–235 (1996).
128. Zhang N *et al. Proc. Natl. Acad. Sci. USA* 94: 8021–8026 (1997).
129. Zhang N *et al. Oncogene* 17: 811–818 (1998).
130. Reichenbach J *et al. Clin. Exp. Immunol.* 117: 535–539 (1999).
131. Harding AE, Muller DP, Thomas PK, Willison HJ. *Ann. Neurol.* 12: 419–424 (1982).
132. Meydani SN, Hayek MG. *Clin. Geriatr. Med.* 11: 567–576 (1995).
133. Gatei M *et al. J. Biol. Chem.* 276: 17276–17280 (2001).
134. Shackelford RE *et al. DNA Repair (Amst.)* 2: 971–981 (2003).
135. Barbouti A *et al. Free Radic. Biol. Med.* 31: 490–498 (2001).
136. Shackelford RE *et al. DNA Repair* 3: 1263–1272 (2004).
137. Browne SE *et al. Free Radic. Biol. Med.* 36: 934–942 (2004).
138. Reliene R *et al. Cancer Res.* 64: 5148–5153 (2004).
139. Ito K *et al. Nature* 431: 997–1002 (2004).
140. Barzilai A *et al. DNA Repair* (*Amst.*) 1: 3–25 (2002).

16 Oxidative Stress and Cardiovascular Disease

Sofian Johar, Philip A. MacCarthy, and Ajay M. Shah

1. Introduction

Oxidative stress can be defined as a pathological imbalance between production of reactive oxygen species (ROS) and antioxidant defenses. Thus it can result from either excess production of ROS or deficiencies in antioxidant systems. Historically, oxidative stress has been thought to exert its deleterious effects via free radical-induced oxidation and damage to DNA, proteins, and other macromolecules. High levels can also trigger apoptosis and necrosis. The direct toxic effects can be illustrated using the example of the neutrophil, which produces ROS in large quantities to facilitate microbial killing. A second mechanism for pathophysiological effects of increased ROS production involves inactivation of the signaling molecule nitric oxide (NO), leading to the development of endothelial dysfunction, which is now recognized as important in the pathophysiology of several cardiovascular disorders and a predictor of future adverse cardiovascular events. Recently, the view that ROS are implicated mainly in causing damage or endothelial dysfunction has been challenged by the appreciation that virtually all cells produce small amounts of ROS, both as a by-product of cellular metabolism and in a tightly controlled manner to modulate many cellular processes. Many experimental studies have shown that small amounts of ROS influence cell signaling pathways including the MAPK family of kinases[1] and the transcription factors NF-κB[2] and AP-1,[3] a process generally termed "redox signaling."

ROS are highly reactive molecules that include not only free radicals such as superoxide ($O_2^{\bullet -}$) and the hydroxyl radical ($OH^{\bullet -}$) but other non-radical derivatives of superoxide such as hydrogen peroxide (H_2O_2) and hypochlorous acid (HOCl). Other ROS are generated by the reaction of radicals with other molecules, e.g. superoxide and nitric oxide ($NO^{\bullet}$) to form peroxynitrite ($ONOO^-$). Living organisms have developed a variety of antioxidant defenses to minimize potential damage from ROS in both extracellular and intracellular compartments. Important enzymes include superoxide dismutase (SOD), catalase, and glutathione peroxidase. SOD catalyzes the dismutation of superoxide into hydrogen peroxide and oxygen. The hydrogen peroxide is hydrolyzed by catalase and by glutathione peroxidase. Other endogenous antioxidants include vitamins C and E. Thus the overall level of ROS within a cell reflects the balance between production of ROS and the levels of antioxidant systems. However, this is complicated by evidence that suggests that production of a particular species of ROS may be localized to specific subcellular compartments.[4]

A large body of evidence has implicated oxidative stress in pathologies such as atherosclerosis, hypertension, heart failure, myocardial infarction, and cardiac hypertrophy. Potential sources of ROS include mitochondria, cytochrome P450-based enzymes, NADPH oxidases, dysfunctional NO synthases, and xanthine oxidase.

1.1. *Xanthine oxidase*

Xanthine oxidase is a member of the molybdoenzyme family, which metabolizes hypoxanthine and xanthine to uric acid with the formation of superoxide. Xanthine oxidase-derived ROS are known to be important in ischemia–reperfusion injury and play a role in endothelial dysfunction. For example, in rat hearts subjected to ischemia–reperfusion injury, elevated levels of H_2O_2 and ventricular dysfunction can be partially attenuated by free radical scavengers or allopurinol (a xanthine oxidase inhibitor).[5] In a rabbit model of cardiac ischemia, allopurinol attenuates left ventricular dysfunction on reperfusion.[6] Attenuation of endothelial dysfunction with enhancement of endothelial-dependent vasodilatation has been demonstrated with clinical trials of allopurinol in human heart failure.[7]

1.2. *Dysfunctional nitric oxide synthase*

NO is generated by NO synthases (NOS) through the oxidation of L-arginine. It is an important signaling molecule with particular relevance for normal endothelial functions. Interestingly, under conditions where there is a deficiency of the NOS cofactor tetrahydrobiopterin (BH_4), the enzyme can become uncoupled and generate superoxide rather than NO. Furthermore, BH_4 itself is highly sensitive to degradation by oxidation so that in settings where ROS are generated by other sources, subsequent degradation of BH_4 may result in amplification of ROS production due to NOS uncoupling. This mechanism has been shown to be operative in experimental hypertension[8] and diabetes.[9]

1.3. *NADPH oxidases*

A major source of ROS that are involved specifically in redox signaling is a family of complex enzymes termed NADPH oxidases (or Noxes). The classical NADPH oxidase is a complex multi-subunit enzyme originally described in phagocytes that produces a burst of superoxide on stimulation.[10] However, its existence has been now described in virtually all cardiovascular cells, where it differs from its phagocyte counterpart in that there is continuous low level production of superoxide.[11–13]

NADPH oxidase consists of several subunits: $p22^{phox}$ and $gp91^{phox}$ (= Nox2), which are cell membrane associated, and $p47^{phox}$, $p67^{phox}$, and rac1, which are the cytosolic subunits.[14] The main catalytic subunit is $gp91^{phox}$, which catalyzes the formation of superoxide from the one-electron reduction of molecular oxygen using NADPH as the electron donor. Several homologues of $gp91^{phox}$ have been described, such as Nox1[15] and Nox4,[16] which are expressed in the cardiovascular system and may have roles distinct from those of Nox2 (Table 1).

2. ROS and Endothelial Dysfunction

The normal endothelium is the major regulator of vascular homeostasis with effects on vascular tone, smooth muscle proliferation and migration,

Table 1. Expression of Nox mRNAs in the cardiovasculature.[17]

	Nox1	Nox2	Nox3	Nox4	Nox5	Duox1
Cardiac myocytes	ND	++	ND	+	ND	ND
Cardiac fibroblasts	+	+	ND	+++	ND	ND
Endothelial cells	+	+	ND	++++	+[a]	ND
VSMCs from conduit vessels	+			+++	+	+
VSMCs from resistance vessels		+		+++	+[a]	+

[a]Human only.
VSMC, vascular smooth muscle cells; ND, not detected.

thrombogenesis, and fibrinolysis. Endothelial dysfunction occurs when the balance between these various processes are disturbed. It has been implicated in different forms of cardiovascular disease such as hypertension,[18] atherosclerosis,[19] chronic heart failure,[20] and diabetes.[21]

The major regulator of vasodilatory tone is NO, and decreased production or bio-availability of NO is considered to be the hallmark of endothelial dysfunction. Inactivation of NO can occur by rapid diffusion-limited reaction with superoxide to form peroxynitrite. In fact the rate constant for this reaction exceeds that of the dismutation of superoxide by SOD. As previously discussed, ROS can also oxidize BH_4, uncoupling eNOS and further increasing superoxide production. Peroxynitrite itself causes cellular damage. There is thus significant evidence implicating ROS in the pathogenesis of endothelial dysfunction.

The major sources of superoxide in the vasculature include xanthine oxidase, uncoupled eNOS, and NADPH oxidase. Many experiments have highlighted their role in endothelial superoxide production. Increasing evidence suggests that NADPH oxidase is the major contributor, but in conditions resulting in endothelial dysfunction, uncoupled eNOS also plays a major role. In many cases multiple sources are involved and may act synergistically.[22]

3. ROS and Hypertension

In both experimental and genetic hypertension vascular oxidative stress has been observed. In the spontaneously hypertensive rat (SHR) and stroke-prone spontaneously hypertensive rat (SP-SHR) models of spontaneous hypertension, both resistance vessels and conduit vessels exhibit increased NADPH oxidase activity,[23,24] which appears to be at least partly due to increased expression of several component subunits.[25] Interestingly there have been several polymorphisms of the $p22^{phox}$ promoter that have been identified in these models,[26] which in essential hypertension in humans is associated with increased atherosclerosis and endothelial dysfunction.[27]

Treatment with antioxidant vitamins and NADPH oxidase inhibitors and supplementation with the eNOS cofactor tetrahydrobiopterin (BH_4) and SOD mimetics have all been shown to reduce vascular superoxide production and attenuate the development of hypertension in some of these models.[28] This provides further evidence for the role of increased superoxide production in the development of hypertension.

Increased superoxide production has also been demonstrated in other models of hypertension such as angiotensin II-driven hypertension, mineralocorticoid-induced hypertension, obesity-induced hypertension, and hypertension in the Dahl salt-sensitive rat. In these models decreased superoxide production has been observed with apocynin, an NADPH oxidase inhibitor, free radical scavengers, or antioxidant vitamins, with a con sequent attenuation of the hypertensive response.[28]

In humans, essential hypertension is usually associated with increased levels of superoxide and hydrogen peroxide. However in "never treated" mild-to-moderate essential hypertensives, markers of lipid peroxidation and oxidative stress are not increased, suggesting that ROS may be more important in the later stages of hypertension.[29] Interestingly, the levels of free radical scavengers such as vitamin E, SOD, and GSH have also been reported to be depressed in this situation.[30] Other forms of hypertension including pre-eclampsia, renovascular hypertension, and malignant hypertension also have increased superoxide levels. In most of these studies measurements of plasma thiobarbituric acid-reactive substances (TBARS), isoprostanes, and markers of lipid peroxidation have been used as markers of oxidative stress.

The renin–angiotensin system is an important pathway involved in many types of hypertension and may be the main pathway through which the NADPH oxidase enzyme is activated. Consonant with this, ACE inhibitors and AT1 receptor antagonists have been shown to decrease NADPH oxidase activity[31] and superoxide production.[32]

4. ROS and Atherosclerosis

Abundant experimental evidence suggests that oxidative stress is important in atherogenesis. All components of the atherosclerotic plaque have been shown to produce ROS. In cholesterol-fed rabbits, increased levels of superoxide production and attenuated NO-mediated responses have been demonstrated.[33] In these animals treatment with SOD was able to partially restore endothelial function.[34] Supplementation with L-arginine was also able to reduce superoxide production and restore NO production.[35] Increased NADPH activity has also been described and may in part be responsible for increased superoxide levels.[36] In Watanabe heritable hyperlipidemic rabbits (WHHL), superoxide levels are also raised.[37]

In apoE and LDL receptor knockout mice exhibiting atherosclerosis there are increased levels of isoprostanes, which are markers of oxidative stress.[38,39] Uncoupling of eNOS may be a potential source of superoxide in this model. Macrophage-derived ROS may also be an important initiator of atherogenesis. In CD36 (a receptor for oxidized LDL) or 12/15 lipooxygenase (important in lipid peroxidation)-deficient mice crossed with apoE$^{-/-}$ mice there is a significant reduction in atherosclerotic lesion size.[40,41] This suggests that macrophage-derived ROS are important in atherogenesis. However, p47phox or gp91phox-deficient mice show no attenuation of lesion size when crossed with apoE$^{-/-}$ mice in the ascending aorta.[42,43] In contrast, another study demonstrated decreased lesion formation in the descending aorta of p47phox/apoE double knockout mice.[44] The different results suggest that further experiments are required in order to resolve these discrepancies.

The renin–angiotensin system may also be important in mediating the production of ROS in atherosclerosis. In the hypercholesterolemic rabbit model, both endothelial function and lesion formation are favorably influenced by treatment with an angiotensin II receptor antagonist.[36] In apoE$^{-/-}$ mice, angiotensin II can also accelerate lesion formation.[45] Angiotensin II can also upregulate expression of adhesion molecules in the endothelium, thus potentially encouraging adhesion of macrophages. Vascular smooth muscle can also be induced to hypertrophy by angiotensin II, which may potentially be important in arterial remodeling.

A prominent feature of the mature atherosclerotic plaque is the presence of fibrous tissue. ROS have been shown to modulate matrix-metalloproteinase (MMP) activity. MMP-2 and MMP-9 have been shown to be expressed in the shoulder area of atherosclerotic plaques.[46,47]

In humans, hypercholesterolemia is associated with increases in markers of oxidative stress such as isoprostanes and antibodies to oxidized LDL.[48,49] However, drugs such as statins are also capable of effecting a decrease in oxidase stress independent of changes in cholesterol levels. One possible mechanism by which this may occur is by interfering with the geranylgeranylation of rac, a component of NADPH oxidase.[50]

Other vascular risk factors are also associated with oxidative stress. Cigarette smoking is associated with a dose-dependent increase in serum isoprostanes that is reduced on quitting.[51] Endothelial function is also impaired by cigarette smoking. Other risk factors such as diabetes and hyperhomocystinemia are also associated with increased levels of isoprostanes.

5. ROS and Heart Failure

The mechanisms underlying the clinical syndrome of heart failure are incompletely understood. However, a significant body of clinical and experimental evidence suggests a role for oxidative stress in the pathophysiology of heart failure. It is also recognized that many of the antecedent conditions that lead to heart failure, such as cardiac hypertrophy and myocardial infarction, are themselves linked with oxidative stress.

5.1. *ROS and hypertrophy*

Cardiac hypertrophy *in vivo* occurs in response to increased load. This process is initially adaptive and minimizes wall stress but eventually becomes maladaptive and ultimately leads to cardiac failure. Experiments have indicated that cells undergo hypertrophy in response to a wide variety of stimuli including mechanical stretch and hormones such as endothelin-1, noradrenaline, and angiotensin II. In vascular smooth muscle cells (VSMCs), at least part of the response is in fact ROS dependent. The role of the $p22^{phox}$

subunit of NADPH oxidase has also been demonstrated in the hypertrophic response.

In cultured cardiac myocytes angiotensin II and TNF-α induce hypertrophy. This effect is inhibited by vitamin E and catalase.[52] Mechanical stretching also causes increases in ROS production, and this effect is inhibited by free radical scavengers such as *N*-acetylcysteine and *N*-2-mercaptoproprionyl-glycine.[53] *In vivo* development of pressure-overload hypertrophy may also involve free radicals. During the transition from hypertrophy to heart failure, increased oxidative stress was evident. Treatment with vitamin E delayed the development of heart failure.[54]

Recent studies from our laboratory have demonstrated an important role for a phagocyte-type NADPH oxidase.[55] Mice infused with a subpressor dose of angiotensin II demonstrated cardiac hypertrophy and increased NADPH oxidase activity. Interestingly, angiotensin II infusion in $gp91^{phox-/-}$ mice failed to induce hypertrophy and was not associated with any changes in NADPH oxidase activity. In experimental pressure-overload in a guinea pig model, left ventricular hypertrophy was accompanied by increased NADPH oxidase activity and increases in expression of the subunits $p22^{phox}$, $gp91^{phox}$, $p67^{phox}$, and $p47^{phox}$ in the transition to heart failure. Further work has also demonstrated inactivation of NO and diastolic dysfunction in this model.[56] In a model of cardiac hypertrophy induced by aldosterone infusion, apocynin, an NADPH oxidase inhibitor, was able to block this response and was associated with decreased expression of $p22^{phox}$.[57] Interestingly we have also shown that different NADPH oxidases may mediate different responses to hypertrophic stimuli such as pressure-overload and angiotensin II infusion.[58]

Pathological hypertrophy is also associated with excess interstitial fibrosis, which has deleterious effects on cardiac function. ROS can regulate fibroblast collagen synthesis and increase MMP activity, thus causing unfavorable remodeling.[59] Further evidence of the importance of ROS in fibrosis is suggested by the absence of excess fibrosis in $gp91^{phox}$ knockout mice infused with angiotensin II, implicating a role for NADPH oxidase-derived superoxide in the profibrotic effects of angiotensin II.[55] We have recently also reported evidence of increased NADPH oxidase activity in failing human hearts.[60]

5.2. *ROS and myocardial infarction*

Myocardial infarction (MI) is the leading cause of heart failure. It can result in either acute failure or more chronic heart failure via a process known as cardiac remodeling that is characterized by a series of changes in cardiac structure, volume, and geometry that ultimately have an adverse effect on cardiac function.

Reperfusion of ischemic myocardium is associated with the production of large amounts of ROS and is associated with deleterious effects on cardiac function. Cardiac dysfunction is also correlated with decreases in antioxidant defense mechanisms and an increase in lipid peroxidation.[61] Increases in levels of MDA and decreases in SOD and catalase are evident in hearts exposed to 30 minutes of ischemia.[62] SOD and catalase treatment was able to reduce infarct size and improve cardiac function in MI.[63,64] Overexpression of Mn-SOD in mice also decreased ischemia–reperfusion injury.[65] Conversely, disruption of Cu/Zn-SOD resulted in an increase in infarct size and impaired recovery of contractile function after repeated periods of ischemia.[66] In a rat model of MI, treatment with vitamin E reduced the size of the infarct and attenuated markers of oxidative stress.[67]

Oxidative stress has also been implicated in remodeling following MI. Dimethylthiourea (DMTU) attenuated LV dilatation and contractile impairment in a mouse model of MI.[68] Another antioxidant, probucol, also favorably influenced remodeling in a rat model of MI.[69]

Remodeling is also associated with excess extracellular matrix deposition in non-infarcted areas. Activity of MMPs has also been shown to be influenced by ROS in MI.[70] Interestingly, cardiac inhibitor of metalloproteinase (CIMP) was able to reduce NADPH oxidase activity, decrease MMP activity, and attenuate LV dilatation.[71]

6. Clinical Trials to Reduce Oxidative Stress

As is evident from the above discussion, there is a wealth of experimental evidence implicating oxidative stress in cardiovascular disease states. A greater intake of antioxidant vitamins such as vitamin E, vitamin C, and beta carotene is associated with a reduced risk of cardiovascular disease.[72] Other animal studies also support this hypothesis.[73,74] In humans, vitamin E has been shown to decrease LDL oxidation[75] and improve endothelial function.[76] Vitamin C also improves endothelium-mediated vasodilatation.[77]

However, larger prospective randomized trials in humans have had contrasting results. The Cambridge Heart Anti-oxidant Study suggested that vitamin E was capable of reducing the incidence of cardiovascular death and non-fatal MI.[78] The Anti-oxidant Supplementation in Atherosclerosis Prevention Study showed that vitamins A and E retarded the progression of carotid atherosclerosis at six years.[79] However, in other studies such as Heart Outcomes Prevention Evaluation and the Heart Protection Study, antioxidants failed to have any benefit on cardiovascular outcomes. In fact, the majority of studies have been negative with regard to the primary endpoint of cardiovascular events.[75]

These results may be explained by the possibility that the role of oxidative stress in the endpoints usually measured in trials such as myocardial infarction, stroke, and vascular death may be overestimated. Also, no biochemical evidence for increased ROS production was obtained in these trials. Thus the patients selected in these studies may not have been expected to benefit from therapy. Another possible reason is that the antioxidants used in clinical practice may be relatively ineffective. Future studies are likely to include novel antioxidants with the capacity to scavenge ROS, target specific sources of ROS, and gain access to intracellular compartments.

7. Conclusion

Current evidence supports a pathophysiological role for oxidative stress in diverse cardiovascular diseases. Levels of ROS are elevated in virtually all pathophysiological states and have been shown to affect cellular signaling, gene transcription, and cell growth/differentiation. Low-level production may be important in cell signaling, while higher levels are associated with cell apoptosis and necrosis. Whilst antioxidant therapy offers a potential mechanism for favorably influencing a wide variety of cardiovascular diseases, disappointing results in human studies suggest that our understanding of the processes involved in oxidative stress is incomplete. Further studies into the basic mechanisms underlying oxidative stress are essential for developing a rational strategy for the development of future therapies.

Acknowledgment

We acknowledge support by the British Heart Foundation.

References

1. Das DK, Maulik N, Engelman RM. Redox regulation of angiotensin II signaling in the heart. *J. Cell. Mol. Med.* 8: 144–152 (2004).
2. Li N, Karin M. Is NF-kappaB the sensor of oxidative stress? *FASEB J.* 13: 1137–1143 (1999).
3. Karin M, Shaulian E. AP-1: linking hydrogen peroxide and oxidative stress to the control of cell proliferation and death. *IUBMB Life* 52: 17–24 (2001).
4. Hilenski LL, Clempus RE, Quinn MT, Lambeth JD, Griendling KK. Distinct subcellular localizations of Nox1 and Nox4 in vascular smooth muscle cells. *Arterioscler. Thromb. Vasc. Biol.* 24(4): 677–683 (2003).
5. Brown JM, Terada LS, Grosso MA, Whitmann GJ, Velasco SE, Patt A, Harken AH, Repine JE. Xanthine oxidase produces hydrogen peroxide which contributes to reperfusion injury of ischemic, isolated, perfused rat hearts. *J. Clin. Invest.* 81: 1297–1301 (1988).
6. Terada LS, Rubinstein JD, Lesnefsky EJ, Horwitz LD, Leff JA, Repine JE. Existence and participation of xanthine oxidase in reperfusion injury of ischemic rabbit myocardium. *Am. J. Physiol.* 260: H805–H810 (1991).
7. Doehner W, Schoene N, Rauchhaus M, Leyva-Leon F, Pavitt DV, Reaveley DA, Schuler G, Coats AJS, Anker SD, Hambrecht R. Effects of xanthine oxidase inhibition with allopurinol on endothelial function and peripheral blood flow in hyperuricemic patients with chronic heart failure: results from 2 placebo-controlled studies. *Circulation* 105: 2619–2624 (2002).
8. Landmesser U, Dikalov S, Price SR, McCann L, Fukai T, Holland SM, Mitch WE, Harrison DG. Oxidation of tetrahydrobiopterin leads to uncoupling of endothelial cell nitric oxide synthase in hypertension. *J. Clin. Invest.* 111: 1201–1209 (2003).
9. Alp NJ, Mussa S, Khoo J, Cai S, Guzik T, Jefferson A, Goh N, Rockett KA, Channon KM. Tetrahydrobiopterin-dependent preservation of nitric oxide-mediated endothelial function in diabetes by targeted transgenic GTP-cyclohydrolase I overexpression. *J. Clin. Invest.* 112: 725–735 (2003).

10. Sbarra AJ, Karnovsky ML. The biochemical basis of phagocytosis. I. Metabolic changes during the ingestion of particles by polymorphonuclear leukocytes. *J. Biol. Chem.* 234: 1355–1362 (1959).
11. Pagano PJ, Clark JK, Cifuentes-Pagano ME, Clark SM, Callis GM, Quinn MT. Localization of a constitutively active, phagocyte-like NADPH oxidase in rabbit aortic adventitia: enhancement by angiotensin II. *Proc. Natl. Acad. Sci. USA* 94: 14483–14488 (1997).
12. Griendling KK, Sorescu D, Ushio-Fukai M. NAD(P)H oxidase: role in cardiovascular biology and disease. *Circ. Res.* 86: 494–501 (2000).
13. Lambeth JD. NOX enzymes and the biology of reactive oxygen. *Nat. Rev. Immunol.* 4: 181–189 (2004).
14. Babior BM. NADPH oxidase: an update. *Blood* 93: 1464 (1999).
15. Lassegue B, Sorescu D, Szocs K, Yin Q, Akers M, Zhang Y, Grant SL, Lambeth JD, Griendling KK. Novel gp91phox homologues in vascular smooth muscle cells: nox1 mediates angiotensin II-induced superoxide formation and fedox-sensitive signaling pathways. *Circ. Res.* 88: 888–894 (2001).
16. Lassegue B, Clempus RE. Vascular NAD(P)H oxidases: specific features, expression, and regulation. *Am. J. Physiol. Regul. Integr. Comp. Physiol.* 285: R277–R297 (2003).
17. Griendling KK. Novel NAD(P)H oxidases in the cardiovascular system. *Heart* 90: 491–493 (2004).
18. Park JB, Schiffrin EL. Small artery remodeling is the most prevalent (earliest?) form of target organ damage in mild essential hypertension. *J. Hypertens.* 19: 921–930 (2001).
19. Luscher TF, Barton M. Biology of the endothelium. *Clin. Cardiol.* 20: II-3–II-10 (1997).
20. Landmesser U, Spiekermann S, Dikalov S, Tatge H, Wilke R, Kohler C, Harrison DG, Hornig B, Drexler H. Vascular oxidative stress and endothelial dysfunction in patients with chronic heart failure: role of xanthine-oxidase and extracellular superoxide dismutase. *Circulation* 106: 3073–3078 (2002).
21. Rizzoni D, Porteri E, Guelfi D, Muiesan ML, Valentini U, Cimino A, Girelli A, Rodella L, Bianchi R, Sleiman I, Rosei EA. Structural alterations in subcutaneous small arteries of normotensive and hypertensive patients with non-insulin-dependent diabetes mellitus. *Circulation* 103: 1238–1244 (2001).
22. Li JM, Shah AM. Endothelial cell superoxide generation: regulation and relevance for cardiovascular physiology. *Am. J. Physiol. Regul. Integr. Comp. Physiol.* 287: R1014–R1030 (2004).

23. Shokoji T, Nishiyama A, Fujisawa Y, Hitomi H, Kiyomoto H, Takahashi N, Kimura S, Kohno M, Abe Y. Renal sympathetic nerve responses to tempol in spontaneously hypertensive rats. *Hypertension* 41: 266–273 (2003).
24. Park JB, Touyz RM, Chen X, Schiffrin EL. Chronic treatment with a superoxide dismutase mimetic prevents vascular remodeling and progression of hypertension in salt-loaded stroke-prone spontaneously hypertensive rats. *Am. J. Hypertens.* 15: 78–84 (2002).
25. Paravicini TM, Chrissobolis S, Drummond GR, Sobey CG. Increased NADPH-oxidase activity and Nox4 expression during chronic hypertension is associated with enhanced cerebral vasodilatation to NADPH *in vivo*. *Stroke* 35: 584–589 (2004).
26. Zalba G, Jose GS, Beaumont FJ, Fortuno MA, Fortuno A, Diez J. Polymorphisms and promoter overactivity of the p22phox gene in vascular smooth muscle cells from spontaneously hypertensive rats. *Circ. Res.* 88: 217–222 (2001).
27. Schachinger V, Britten MB, Dimmeler S, Zeiher AM. NADH/NADPH oxidase p22 phox gene polymorphism is associated with improved coronary endothelial vasodilator function. *Eur. Heart J.* 22: 96–101 (2001).
28. Touyz RM. Reactive oxygen species, vascular oxidative stress, and redox signaling in hypertension: what is the clinical significance? *Hypertension* 44: 248–252 (2004).
29. Ormezzano O, Cracowski JL, Baguet JP, Francois P, Bessard J, Bessard G, Mallion JM. Oxidative stress and baroreflex sensitivity in healthy subjects and patients with mild-to-moderate hypertension. *J. Hum. Hypertens.* 18: 517–521 (2004).
30. Sagar S, Kallo IJ, Kaul N, Ganguly NK, Sharma BK. Oxygen free radicals in essential hypertension. *Mol. Cell. Biochem.* 111: 103–108 (1992).
31. Rueckschloss U, Quinn MT, Holtz J, Morawietz H. Dose-dependent regulation of NAD(P)H oxidase expression by angiotensin II in human endothelial cells: protective effect of angiotensin II type 1 receptor blockade in patients with coronary artery disease. *Arterioscler. Thromb. Vasc. Biol.* 22: 1845–1851 (2002).
32. Berry C, Anderson N, Kirk AJ, Dominiczak AF, McMurray JJ. Renin angiotensin system inhibition is associated with reduced free radical concentrations in arteries of patients with coronary heart disease. *Heart* 86: 217–220 (2001).
33. Ohara Y, Peterson TE, Harrison DG. Hypercholesterolemia increases endothelial superoxide anion production. *J. Clin. Invest.* 91: 2546–2551 (1993).

34. Mugge A, Elwell JH, Peterson TE, Hofmeyer TG, Heistad DD, Harrison DG. Chronic treatment with polyethylene-glycolated superoxide dismutase partially restores endothelium-dependent vascular relaxations in cholesterol-fed rabbits. *Circ. Res.* 69: 1293–1300 (1991).
35. Boger RH, Bode-Boger SM, Mugge A, Kienke S, Brandes R, Dwenger A, Frolich JC. Supplementation of hypercholesterolaemic rabbits with L-arginine reduces the vascular release of superoxide anions and restores NO production. *Atherosclerosis* 117: 273–284 (1995).
36. Warnholtz A, Nickenig G, Schulz E, Macharzina R, Brasen JH, Skatchkov M, Heitzer T, Stasch JP, Griendling KK, Harrison DG, Bohm M, Meinertz T, Munzel T. Increased NADH-oxidase mediated superoxide production in the early stages of atherosclerosis: evidence for involvement of the renin–angiotensin system. *Circulation* 99: 2027–2033 (1999).
37. Miller FJ, Gutterman DD, Rios CD, Heistad DD, Davidson BL. Superoxide production in vascular smooth muscle contributes to oxidative stress and impaired relaxation in atherosclerosis. *Circ. Res.* 82: 1298–1305 (1998).
38. Pratico D, Tangirala RK, Rader DJ, Rokach J, FitzGerald GA. Vitamin E suppresses isoprostane generation *in vivo* and reduces atherosclerosis in ApoE-deficient mice. *Nat. Med.* 4: 1189–1192 (1998).
39. Tangirala RK, Pratico D, FitzGerald GA, Chun S, Tsukamoto K, Maugeais C, Usher DC, Pure E, Rader DJ. Reduction of isoprostanes and regression of advanced atherosclerosis by apolipoprotein E. *J. Biol. Chem.* 276: 261–266 (2001).
40. Febbraio M, Podrez EA, Smith JD, Hajjar DP, Hazen SL, Hoff HF, Sharma K, Silverstein RL. Targeted disruption of the class B scavenger receptor CD36 protects against atherosclerotic lesion development in mice. *J. Clin. Invest.* 105: 1049–1056 (2000).
41. Cyrus T, Witztum JL, Rader DJ, Tangirala R, Fazio S, Linton MF, Funk CD. Disruption of the 12/15-lipoxygenase gene diminishes atherosclerosis in apo E-deficient mice. *J. Clin. Invest.* 103: 1597–1604 (1999).
42. Hsich E, Segal BH, Pagano PJ, Rey FE, Paigen B, Deleonardis J, Hoyt RF, Holland SM, Finkel T. Vascular effects following homozygous disruption of p47phox: an essential component of NADPH oxidase. *Circulation* 101: 1234–1236 (2000).
43. Kirk EA, Dinauer MC, Rosen H, Chait A, Heinecke JW, LeBoeuf RC. Impaired superoxide production due to a deficiency in phagocyte NADPH oxidase fails to inhibit atherosclerosis in mice. *Arterioscler. Thromb. Vasc. Biol.* 20: 1529–1535 (2000).

44. Barry-Lane PA, Patterson C, van der Merwe M, Hu Z, Holland SM, Yeh ET, Runge MS. p47phox is required for atherosclerotic lesion progression in ApoE(−/−) mice. *J. Clin. Invest.* 108: 1513–1522 (2001).
45. Weiss D, Kools JJ, Taylor WR. Angiotensin II-induced hypertension accelerates the development of atherosclerosis in ApoE-deficient mice. *Circulation* 103: 448–454 (2001).
46. Galis ZS, Sukhova GK, Lark MW, Libby P. Increased expression of matrix metalloproteinases and matrix degrading activity in vulnerable regions of human atherosclerotic plaques. *J. Clin. Invest.* 94: 2493–2503 (1994).
47. Faia KL, Davis WP, Marone AJ, Foxall TL. Matrix metalloproteinases and tissue inhibitors of metalloproteinases in hamster aortic atherosclerosis: correlation with *in situ* zymography. *Atherosclerosis* 160: 325–337 (2002).
48. Reilly MP, Pratico D, Delanty N, DiMinno G, Tremoli E, Rader D, Kapoor S, Rokach J, Lawson J, FitzGerald GA. Increased formation of distinct F2 isoprostanes in hypercholesterolemia. *Circulation* 98: 2822–2828 (1998).
49. Yamaguchi Y, Kunitomo M, Haginaka J. Assay methods of modified lipoproteins in plasma. *J. Chromatogr. B Analyt. Technol. Biomed. Life Sci.* 781: 313–330 (2002).
50. Delbosc S, Morena M, Djouad F, Ledoucen C, Descomps B, Cristol JP. Statins, 3-hydroxy-3-methylglutaryl coenzyme A reductase inhibitors, are able to reduce superoxide anion production by NADPH oxidase in THP-1-derived monocytes. *J. Cardiovasc. Pharmacol.* 40: 611–617 (2002).
51. Morrow JD, Frei B, Longmire AW, Gaziano JM, Lynch SM, Shyr Y, Strauss WE, Oates JA, Roberts LJ. Increase in circulating products of lipid peroxidation (F2-isoprostanes) in smokers. Smoking as a cause of oxidative damage. *N. Engl. J. Med.* 332: 1198–1203 (1995).
52. Nakamura K, Fushimi K, Kouchi H, Mihara K, Miyazaki M, Ohe T, Namba M. Inhibitory effects of antioxidants on neonatal rat cardiac myocyte hypertrophy induced by tumor necrosis factor-{alpha} and angiotensin II. *Circulation* 98: 794–799 (1998).
53. Aikawa R, Nagai T, Tanaka M, Zou Y, Ishihara T, Takano H, Hasegawa H, Akazawa H, Mizukami M, Nagai R, Komuro I. Reactive oxygen species in mechanical stress-induced cardiac hypertrophy. *Biochem. Biophys. Res. Commun.* 289: 901–907 (2001).
54. Dhalla AK, Hill MF, Singal PK. Role of oxidative stress in transition of hypertrophy to heart failure. *J. Am. Coll. Cardiol.* 28: 506–514 (1996).
55. Bendall JK, Cave AC, Heymes C, Gall N, Shah AM. Pivotal role of a gp91phox-containing NADPH oxidase in angiotensin II-induced cardiac hypertrophy in mice. *Circulation* 105: 293–296 (2002).

56. MacCarthy PA, Grieve DJ, Li JM, Dunster C, Kelly FJ, Shah AM. Impaired endothelial regulation of ventricular relaxation in cardiac hypertrophy: role of reactive oxygen species and NADPH oxidase. *Circulation* 104: 2967–2974 (2001).
57. Park YM, Park MY, Suh YL, Park JB. NAD(P)H oxidase inhibitor prevents blood pressure elevation and cardiovascular hypertrophy in aldosterone-infused rats. *Biochem. Biophys. Res. Commun.* 313: 812–817 (2004).
58. Byrne JA, Grieve DJ, Bendall JK, Li JM, Gove C, Lambeth JD, Cave AC, Shah AM. Contrasting roles of NADPH oxidase isoforms in pressure-overload versus angiotensin II-induced cardiac hypertrophy. *Circ. Res.* 93: 802–805 (2003).
59. Siwik DA, Pagano PJ, Colucci WS. Oxidative stress regulates collagen synthesis and matrix metalloproteinase activity in cardiac fibroblasts. *Am. J. Physiol. Cell Physiol.* 280: C53–C60 (2001).
60. Heymes C, Bendall JK, Ratajczak P, Cave AC, Samuel JL, Hasenfuss G, Shah AM. Increased myocardial NADPH oxidase activity in human heart failure. *J. Am. Coll. Cardiol.* 41: 2164–2171 (2003).
61. Palace V, Kumar D, Hill MF, Khaper N, Singal PK. Regional differences in non-enzymatic antioxidants in the heart under control and oxidative stress conditions. *J. Mol. Cell. Cardiol.* 31: 193–202 (1999).
62. Prasad K, Lee P, Mantha SV, Kalra J, Prasad M, Gupta JB. Detection of ischemia–reperfusion cardiac injury by cardiac muscle chemiluminescence. *Mol. Cell. Biochem.* 115: 49–58 (1992).
63. Jolly SR, Kane WJ, Bailie MB, Abrams GD, Lucchesi BR. Canine myocardial reperfusion injury. Its reduction by the combined administration of superoxide dismutase and catalase. *Circ. Res.* 54: 277–285 (1984).
64. Temsah RM, Netticadan T, Chapman D, Takeda S, Mochizuki S, Dhalla NS. Alterations in sarcoplasmic reticulum function and gene expression in ischemic–reperfused rat heart. *Am. J. Physiol.* 277: H584–H594 (1999).
65. Chen EP, Bittner HB, Davis RD, Van Trigt P, Folz RJ. Physiologic effects of extracellular superoxide dismutase transgene overexpression on myocardial function after ischemia and reperfusion injury. *J. Thorac. Cardiovasc. Surg.* 115: 450–458 (1998).
66. Yoshida T, Maulik N, Engelman RM, Ho YS, Das DK. Targeted disruption of the mouse Sod I gene makes the hearts vulnerable to ischemic reperfusion injury. *Circ. Res.* 86: 264–269 (2000).
67. Sethi R, Takeda N, Nagano M, Dhalla NS. Beneficial effects of vitamin E treatment in acute myocardial infarction. *J. Cardiovasc. Pharmacol. Ther.* 5: 51–58 (2000).

68. Kinugawa S, Tsutsui H, Hayashidani S, Ide T, Suematsu N, Satoh S, Utsumi H, Takeshita A. Treatment with dimethylthiourea prevents left ventricular remodeling and failure after experimental myocardial infarction in mice: role of oxidative stress. *Circ. Res.* 87: 392–398 (2000).
69. Sia YT, Lapointe N, Parker TG, Tsoporis JN, Deschepper CF, Calderone A, Pourdjabbar A, Jasmin JF, Sarrazin JF, Liu P, Adam A, Butany J, Rouleau JL. Beneficial effects of long-term use of the antioxidant probucol in heart failure in the rat. *Circulation* 105: 2549–2555 (2002).
70. Spinale FG. Matrix metalloproteinases: regulation and dysregulation in the failing heart. *Circ. Res.* 90: 520–530 (2002).
71. Cox MJ, Hawkins UA, Hoit BD, Tyagi SC. Attenuation of oxidative stress and remodeling by cardiac inhibitor of metalloproteinase protein transfer. *Circulation* 109: 2123–2128 (2004).
72. Rimm EB, Stampfer MJ. Antioxidants for vascular disease. *Med. Clin. North Am.* 84: 239–249 (2000).
73. Crawford RS, Kirk EA, Rosenfeld ME, LeBoeuf RC, Chait A. Dietary antioxidants inhibit development of fatty streak lesions in the LDL receptor deficient mouse. *Arterioscler. Thromb. Vasc. Biol.* 18: 1506–1513 (1998).
74. Davidge ST, Ojimba J, McLaughlin MK. Vascular function in the vitamin E deprived rat: an interaction between nitric oxide and superoxide anions. *Hypertension* 31: 830–835 (1998).
75. Jialal I, Devaraj S. Antioxidants and atherosclerosis: don't throw out the baby with the bath water. *Circulation* 107: 926–928 (2003).
76. Heitzer T, Herttuala SY, Wild E, Luoma J, Drexler H. Effect of vitamin E on endothelial vasodilator function in patients with hypercholesterolemia, chronic smoking or both. *J. Am. Coll. Cardiol.* 33: 499–505 (1999).
77. Gokce N, Keaney JF Jr, Frei B, Holbrook M, Olesiak M, Zachariah BJ, Leeuwenburgh C, Heinecke JW, Vita JA. Long-term ascorbic acid administration reverses endothelial vasomotor dysfunction in patients with coronary artery disease. *Circulation* 99: 3234–3240 (1999).
78. Stephens NG, Parsons A, Schofield PM, Kelly F, Cheeseman K, Mitchinson MJ. Randomised controlled trial of vitamin E in patients with coronary disease: Cambridge Heart Antioxidant Study (CHAOS). *Lancet* 347: 781–786 (1996).
79. Salonen RM, Nyyssonen K, Kaikkonen J, Porkkala-Sarataho E, Voutilainen S, Rissanen TH, Tuomainen TP, Valkonen VP, Ristonmaa U, Lakka HM, Vanharanta M, Salonen JT, Poulsen HE. Six-year effect of combined vitamin C and E supplementation on atherosclerotic progression: the Antioxidant Supplementation in Atherosclerosis Prevention (ASAP) Study. *Circulation* 107: 947–953 (2003).

17 Oxidative Stress, Insulin Resistance, and Cardiovascular Disease

Antonio Ceriello

1. Introduction

In the last few decades, type 2 diabetes mellitus (T2DM) has rapidly increased worldwide world and it has been estimated that the number of diabetic patients will more than double within 15 years.[1] Moreover, while T2DM was previously considered a slow-onset disease of middle-aged and older subjects, an emerging issue is the recent increase in diagnoses of T2DM and prediabetic conditions in children.[2]

As T2DM is mainly characterized by the development of increased morbidity and mortality for cardiovascular disease (CVD),[3] it has been suggested that diabetes may be considered a cardiovascular disease.[4] However, CVD risk is elevated long before the development of diabetes.[5] The close relationship between T2DM and CVD has led to the "common-soil" hypothesis,[6] which postulates that T2DM and CVD share common genetic and environmental antecedents. One of the most important of these possible antecedents is considered insulin resistance. In genetically predisposed subjects the combination of excess caloric intake and relatively scarce physical activity, with the likely consequence of obesity, can induce a state of resistance to the action of insulin.[7] Insulin resistance is an important component of the metabolic syndrome, first described as a clinical syndrome in which the clustering of factors such as obesity, dyslipidemia, and hypertension leads to a substantial increase in CVD risk.[8] Insulin resistance is also a crucially important metabolic abnormality in T2DM and overt diabetes is thought to be preceded by a long period of insulin resistance, during which blood glucose is maintained near normal levels by compensatory hyperinsulinemia.[7] When β-cells are no more able to compensate for insulin resistance by adequately increasing insulin production, impaired glucose tolerance (IGT) appears.[7] This condition is characterized by an excessive blood glucose concentration in the postprandial phase, fasting glucose being in the normal range.[7] Persistence of imbalance between caloric intake and expenditure eventually leads to overt diabetes, characterized by high glycemia in any condition, whether fasting or postprandial.[7] It is worth noting that studies currently carried out in children point out the coexistence of obesity, insulin resistance, and β-cell dysfunction, as occurs in classic older T2DM-prone subjects.[9] The mix of overfeeding and sedentary habits has extended to children.

All of these three conditions, i.e., insulin resistance, IGT, and overt diabetes, appear to be associated, although to a variable degree, with an increased risk of CVD.[10,11] Recent trials have confirmed the hypothesis that lifestyle modifications, in terms of reduced caloric intake and increased physical activity, can reduce the incidence of new cases of diabetes.[12,13] In other intervention trials the same goal has been attained by means of several drugs.

There have been studies specifically aimed to demonstrate the ability of known antidiabetic drugs, i.e., metformin,[12] troglitazone,[14] and acarbose,[15] to hamper the evolution from IGT to diabetes. Each of the three drugs was successful in that regard. Interestingly, while metformin and troglitazone were expected to act by abating insulin resistance, and secondarily hyperglycemia, acarbose lowers postprandial hyperglycemia by impairing carbohydrate absorption from the intestinal lumen, without any direct effect on insulin resistance. It appears, then, that prevention of the development of diabetes is obtainable by simply lowering postprandial glycemic peaks. But the picture is more intricate: in studies aimed to reduce the incidence of cardiovascular disease in high-risk populations by means of calcium channel blockers (CCBs), angiotensin-converting enzyme (ACE) inhibitors, angiotensin-1 (AT-1) receptor antagonists, and statins, all of which are devoid of any effect on glycemia, a significant reduction of new cases of diabetes has been incidentally discovered.[16–20] It appears that in the prevention of diabetes a direct action on insulin resistance is not a requisite, nor is the reduction of postprandial hyperglycemia. Now the question is: what sort of effect of CCBs, ACE inhibitors, AT-1 receptor antagonists, and statins is responsible for the prevention of diabetes? Do these compounds share any mechanism of action with the aforementioned antidiabetic drugs? It has been shown that CCBs,[21] statins,[22] ACE inhibitors,[23] and AT-1 receptor antagonists[24] have a strong intracellular "preventive" antioxidant activity, and it has been suggested that many of their beneficial ancillary effects, such as a decrease in cardiovascular mortality not fully accounted for by hypotensive or lipid-lowering effects, may be due to this property.[21–24] If we consider that glitazones are intracellular antioxidants too,[25] and that postprandial hyperglycemia itself produces an oxidative stress,[26] so that acarbose (an inhibitor of intestinal glucose absorption) and glinides (i.e., repaglinide, nateglinide, and metiglinide which restore the first phase of insulin secretion) may be expected to reduce oxidative stress by specifically lowering postprandial hyperglycemia, the antioxidant effect is the only known property that all of these drugs have in common.

Since evidence suggests that overnutrition, insulin resistance, IGT, diabetes, and CVD share in common the presence of an oxidative stress,[27–29] in this chapter oxidative stress generation is proposed as the common, persistent pathogenic factor mediating the appearance of insulin resistance as well as the passage from insulin resistance to overt diabetes, via IGT, while producing the increased cardiovascular risk condition typical of prediabetic and diabetic subjects by favoring atherosclerotic complications. This hypothesis may help us understand why diverse therapeutic interventions, which have in common the ability to reduce oxidative stress, can impede or delay the onset of diabetes and CVD.

2. From Overfeeding to Insulin Resistance: The Role of Oxidative Stress

The most important tissues involved in the pathogenesis of insulin resistance are muscle and adipose tissue.

When caloric intake exceeds the energy expenditure, the substrate-induced increase in citric acid cycle activity generates an excess of mitochondrial NADH (mNADH) and reactive oxygen species (ROS).[30] To protect themselves against harmful effects of ROS, cells may reduce the formation of ROS and/or enhance ROS removal. Prevention of ROS formation is accomplished by preventing the build-up of mNADH by inhibiting insulin-stimulated nutrient uptake and preventing the entrance of energetic substrates (pyruvate, fatty acids) into the mitochondria.

Controversy exists as to whether FFA or glucose is the primary fuel source in the overnourished muscle and adipose tissue. In either case, an influx of substrates into the citric acid cycle generates mitochondrial acetyl CoA and NADH.[30] Acetyl CoA, either derived from glucose through pyruvate, or from beta-oxidation of FFA, combines with oxaloacetate to form citrate which enters the citric acid cycle and is converted to isocitrate. NAD+-dependent isocitrate dehydrogenase generates NADH. When excessive NADH cannot be dissipated by oxidative phosphorylation (or other mechanisms) the mitochondrial proton gradient increases and single electrons are transferred to oxygen leading to the formation of free radicals, particularly superoxide anion[31] (Fig. 1). The generation

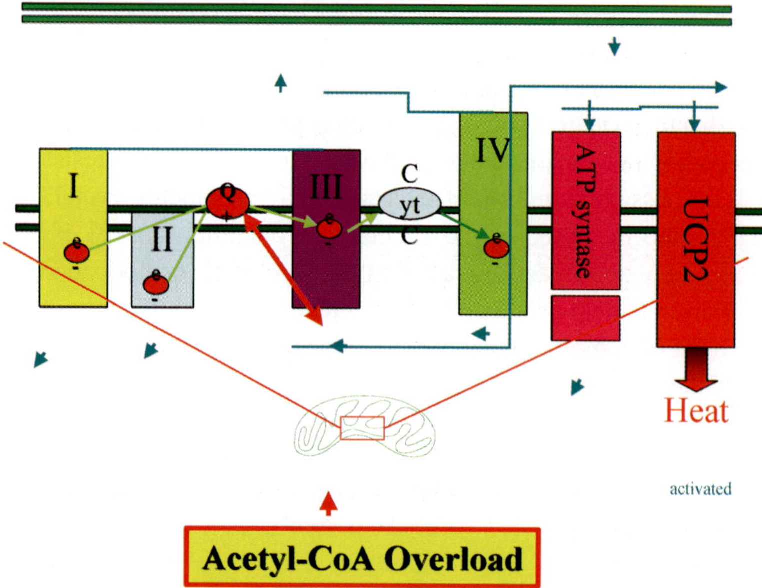

Fig. 1. Possible mechanism of increased superoxide generation on mitochondrial electron-transport chain during FFA and glucose overload. FFA and glucose overload increases the generation of acetyl CoA, which, in turn, increases the production of electron donors from the tricarboxylic acid cycle (NADH). This increases the membrane potential ($\Delta\mu$H+), because protons are pumped across the mitochondrial inner membrane in proportion to electron flux through the electron-transport chain. Inhibition of electron transport at Complex III by increased $\Delta\mu$H+ increases the half-life of free radical intermediates of coenzyme Q, which reduce O_2 to superoxide. Uncoupling protein 2 modulates this phenomenon producing heat. Pi, inorganic phosphorus.

of excessive NADH may be prevented in several ways, one of which is the inhibition of FFA oxidation.[32] An increase in intracellular FFA, in turn, leads to reduced GLUT4 translocation to the plasma membrane, resulting in resistance to insulin-stimulated glucose uptake in both muscle and adipose tissue.[33–35] In this setting, insulin resistance may be considered a compensatory mechanism that protects the cells against further insulin-stimulated glucose and fatty acid uptake and therefore oxidative damage.

Many studies support this hypothesis: in *in vitro* studies and in animal models antioxidants have been shown to improve insulin sensitivity.[36] Several clinical trials have demonstrated that treatment with vitamin E, vitamin C, or glutathione improves insulin sensitivity in insulin-resistant individuals,[36,37] while there is evidence from molecular biology studies to support the possibility that oxidative stress alters the intracellular signaling pathway inducing insulin resistance.[28] The recent finding that insulin resistance is associated in humans with reduced intracellular antioxidant defense also support this hypothesis.[38]

3. Oxidative Stress as a Common Pathogenic Factor for the Dysfunction of β and Endothelial Cells

It is a reasonable hypothesis that what happens in muscle and fat cells may also occur in other cells, particularly in β-cells and endothelial cells. Moreover, these cell types may be particularly affected by overfeeding. These cells are notably not dependent on insulin for glucose uptake, which is here via facilitative diffusion instead of insulin-regulated glucose transporters. Therefore, if overfed, they cannot downregulate the influx of nutrients by means of insulin resistance, and must allow intracellular concentrations to rise further.

Many studies have suggested that β-cell dysfunction results from prolonged exposure to high glucose, elevated FFA levels, or a combination of the two.[28]

β-cells are particularly sensitive to ROS because they are low in free-radical quenching (antioxidant) enzymes such as catalase, glutathione peroxidase, and superoxide dismutase.[39] Therefore, the ability of oxidative stress to damage mitochondria and markedly blunt insulin secretion is not surprising:[40] for example, it has been demonstrated that oxidative stress generated by short exposure of β-cell preparations to H_2O_2 increases production of p21, decreases insulin mRNA, cytosolic ATP, and calcium flux in cytosol and mitochondria.[41] The key role of increased glucose metabolism in producing impaired β-cell function, through oxidative stress, has recently been confirmed. Intracellular ROS increased 15 min after exposure to high glucose and this effect was blunted by inhibitors of the mitochondrial function.[42] Glucose-induced insulin secretion was also suppressed by H_2O_2, a chemical substitute for ROS.[42] Interestingly, the first phase of glucose-induced insulin secretion could be suppressed by 50 μM H_2O_2. H_2O_2 or high glucose suppressed the activity of glyceraldehyde 3-phosphate dehydrogenase (GAPDH), a glycolytic enzyme, and inhibitors of the mitochondrial function abolished the latter effects. These data suggest that high glucose concentrations induce mitochondrial ROS, which suppress the first phase of glucose-induced insulin secretion, at least in part, through the suppression of GAPDH activity.[42]

These results have been confirmed *in vivo*. In subjects with normal glucose tolerance, glutathione infusion failed to affect β-cell response to glucose.[43] In contrast, glutathione significantly potentiated glucose-induced insulin secretion in patients with IGT.[43] Furthermore, in the latter group studied in the condition of hyperglycemic clamp, glutathione infusion significantly potentiated the β-cell response to glucose when plasma glucose levels varied between 10 and 15 mM.[43]

Impaired insulin secretion has been associated with an FFA-induced increase in ROS, both *in vitro*[44,45] and *in vivo*.[46] Interestingly, it has been reported that both FFA and glucose may impair insulin secretion in β-cells by activating uncoupling protein 2.[45,47] In the case of hyperglycemia, it has been shown that such activation is accomplished by hyperglycemia-induced superoxide formation in mitochondria.[47] Therefore, as glucose as well as FFA overload is present during increased caloric disposal, it is possible that the combination with high glucose will maximize β-cell toxicity. This hypothesis is supported by recent studies showing that when either isolated islets or HIT cells were exposed to chronically elevated glucose and FFA levels, there was a distinct decrease in insulin mRNA and the activation of an insulin–gene reporter construct.[48] In other studies, coculture of islets with high levels of glucose and palmitate resulted in almost complete impairment of glucose-stimulated insulin secretion, despite partially sustained stored insulin.[45] Recent studies have suggested that β-cell lipotoxicity is enhanced by concurrent hyperglycemia and that oxidative stress may be the mediator.[49,50]

The response-to-injury hypothesis of atherosclerosis states that the initial damage affects the arterial endothelium, in terms of endothelial dysfunction.[51] Notably, today's evidence confirms that endothelial dysfunction, associated to oxidative stress, predicts cardiovascular disease[52,53] Insulin resistance is associated with impaired endothelial function.[54]

Glucose and FFA overload may be supposed to influence endothelial cells, as well as β-cells, producing an endothelial dysfunction through an oxidative stress. Indeed, many studies show that high glucose concentrations induce endothelial dysfunction. *In vitro*, the direct role of hyperglycemia has been suggested by evidence that arteries isolated from normal animals and subsequently exposed to exogenous hyperglycemia exhibit attenuated endothelium-dependent relaxation.[55] Consistently, *in vivo* studies have also shown that hyperglycemia directly induces, in diabetic as well as normal subjects, endothelial dysfunction.[56,57]

The role of free radical generation in producing the hyperglycemia-dependent endothelial dysfunction is suggested by studies showing that, both *in vitro*[58] and *in vivo*,[59,60] the acute effects of hyperglycemia are counterbalanced by antioxidants.

Recent studies demonstrate that a single hyperglycemia-induced process of overproduction of superoxide by the mitochondrial electron-transport chain seems to be the first and key event in the activation of all other pathways involved in the pathogenesis of endothelial dysfunction in the case of hyperglycemia.[61,62] Superoxide overproduction is accompanied by increased nitric oxide generation, due to eNOS and iNOS uncoupled state,[63] a phenomenon favoring the formation of the strong oxidant peroxynitrite, which in turn damages DNA.[62] DNA damage is an obligatory stimulus for the activation of the nuclear enzyme poly(ADP-ribose) polymerase.[62] Poly(ADP-ribose) polymerase activation in turn depletes the intracellular concentration of its substrate NAD+, slowing the rate of glycolysis, electron transport, and ATP formation and produces an ADP-ribosylation of the GAPDH.[62] These processes result in acute endothelial dysfunction. Convincingly, FFA may work through the same way[28]: FFAs increase oxidative stress generation in humans,[47] and induce endothelial dysfunction, which can be reversed by antioxidants.[64]

4. From Insulin Resistance to Impaired Glucose Tolerance: The Role of Oxidative Stress

Initially, insulin resistance is compensated by hyperinsulinemia, through which a normal glucose tolerance is preserved. Deterioration to impaired glucose tolerance occurs when insulin resistance increases further, and/or the compensatory insulin secretory response decreases. An increase in insulin, FFA, and/or glucose levels can increase ROS production and oxidative stress as well as activate stress-sensitive pathways.[28] This, in turn, can worsen both insulin action and secretion, thereby accelerating the progression to overt type 2 diabetes.

IGT, i.e., postprandial hyperglycemia with fasting glycemia in the normal range, is a risk factor for increased cardiovascular mortality.[65] Many studies show that postprandial hyperglycemia is associated with oxidative stress generation.[65]

A loss of early-phase insulin response is a common event in subjects with impaired glucose metabolism.[66] This alteration may not simply be a marker of the risk of developing diabetes, but rather an important pathogenic mechanism causing excessive postprandial hyperglycemia.[66]

In response to intravenous glucose, insulin secretion is biphasic. The first phase is a rapid release of insulin into the bloodstream in response to the ingestion of carbohydrates or a mixed meal.[7] The rapid increase in portal blood insulin concentration and the avid binding of the hormone to its receptors on liver cell membranes account for a prompt suppression of endogenous glucose production and a reduced rate of increase in plasma glucose concentrations.[66] In experiments carried out in animals and humans the selective abolition of early insulin secretion in healthy subjects resulted in IGT, excessive glycemic excursions, and possible hampering of the thermic effects of ingested carbohydrates.[7,66] In non-diabetic subjects, the loss of early insulin secretion is a determinant for the subsequent development of diabetes.[66] The critical role of the early-phase insulin response in determining postprandial hyperglycemia is supported by the demonstration that glucose tolerance is improved by restoring the acute rise in plasma insulin concentrations after the ingestion of both glucose and a mixed meal.[66] This amelioration of the glycemic profile can prevent late hyperglycemia and hyperinsulinemia. Oxidative stress contributes, *in vivo*, to specifically alter the early phase of insulin secretion since the latter can be restored by antioxidants.[36] Moreover, it has been proposed that mitochondrial overproduction of free radicals is a potential mechanism causing impaired first phase of glucose-induced insulin secretion.[42]

Evidence indicates that postprandial hyperglycemia is directly implicated in the development of cardiovascular disease, while evidence linking fasting glycemia to diabetic complications is inconclusive as yet.[65] Moreover, in many studies postprandial glycemia is a better predictor of the cardiovascular risk than HbA_{1c}, which reflects both fasting and postprandial blood glucose levels.[65] Postprandial glucose may be directly involved in cardiovascular complications through a toxic effect on the vascular endothelium, mediated by oxidative stress.[26] This atherogenic effect appears to be independent of other cardiovascular risk factors such as hyperlipidemia.[67]

5. From IGT to Diabetes and Endothelial Dysfunction

Repeated exposure to hyperglycemia and increased levels of FFA can lead to β-cell dysfunction that may become irreversible over time.[68]

In its initial stages, this damage is characterized by a reversible defective insulin gene expression.[38] Glucose and lipid toxicity induce the gradual, time-dependent establishment of irreversible damage to cellular components of insulin production, and, therefore, to insulin content and secretion.[66] Oxidative stress is convincingly the mediator of such damage.[28]

Recent studies in type 2 diabetic animal models report that the progressive reduction of islet β-cells is associated with excessive oxidative stress.[69] In these animal models, when hyperglycemia is allowed to continue, a so-called "glucotoxicity" to β-cells impairs insulin secretion and eventually causes fatal islet cell injury, accelerating β-cell loss.[69] Consistently, Japanese type 2 diabetic patients show a reduction of β-cell mass and evidence of increased oxidative stress-related tissue damage that is correlated with the extent of the β-cell lesions.[70]

Vascular function in diabetes mellitus has been studied extensively in both animal models and humans. Impaired endothelium-dependent vasodilation has been a consistent finding in animal models of diabetes induced by alloxan or streptozotocin.[71,72] Similarly, studies in humans with insulin-dependent and noninsulin-dependent diabetes have found endothelial dysfunction when compared to vascular function in non-diabetic subjects.[73,74] Strong evidences suggest that oxidative stress is the mediator of impaired endothelial function in diabetes.[75]

6. The Possible Link Between Oxidative Stress and Inflammation in Insulin Resistance, Diabetes, and CVD

While the concept of atherosclerosis as an inflammatory disease is now well established, line of evidence suggests that chronic inflammation may be involved in the pathogenesis of insulin resistance and T2DM.[76] This led to the hypothesis that inflammatory changes may be considered a common pathogenic step in all of these conditions.[76]

The concept that oxidative stress is the common factor underlying insulin resistance, T2DM, and CVD may explain the presence of inflammation in all these conditions. Indeed, it is well recognized that inflammation is one manifestation of oxidative stress,[77] and the pathways that generate the mediators of inflammation, such as adhesion molecules and interleukins, are all induced by oxidative stress.[77]

Interestingly, it has recently been proposed that the subclinical proinflammatory state observable in many conditions including atherosclerosis, cancer, and aging is due to a mitochondrial overgeneration of free radicals.[78] Moreover, the hypothesis is supported by *in vivo* studies, showing that FFA and glucose induce inflammation through oxidative stress, having a cumulative and independent effect, and that antioxidants reverse the phenomenon.[79–82]

7. Oxidative Stress as the Connection Between Nutrition Overload and Diabetes and Related Cardiovascular Complications: Therapeutic Implications

Available evidence, as presented above, lead to the hypothesis, summarized in Fig. 2, that oxidative stress can be considered the clue to the association

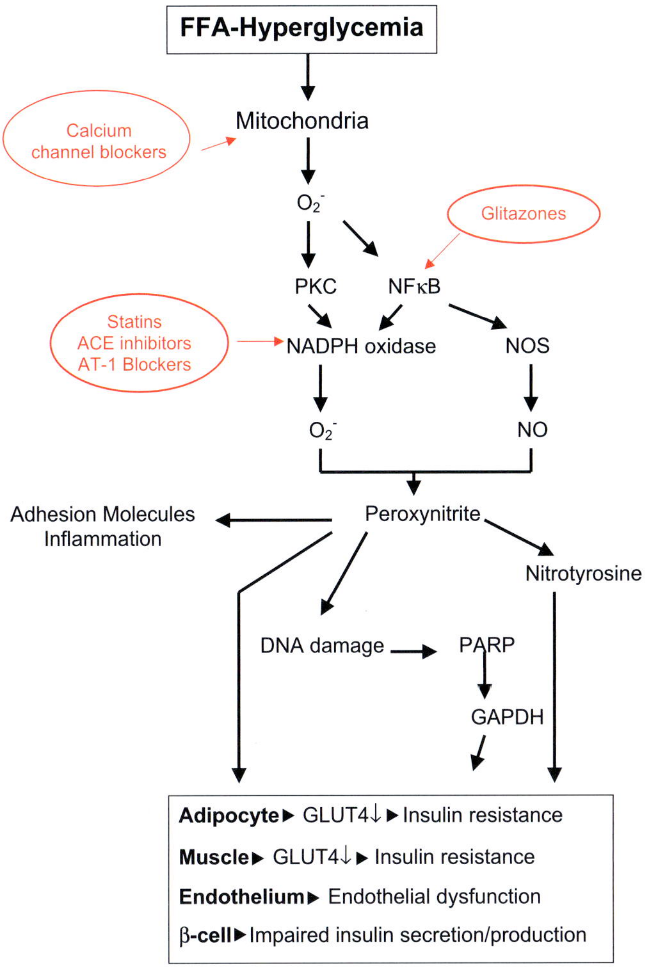

Fig. 2. In the cells, hyperglycemia and free fatty acids induce overproduction of superoxide at the mitochondrial level, and nitric oxide overproduction through NOS, while also PKC and NF-κB are activated and favor an overexpression of the enzyme NADPH. NADPH generates a great amount of superoxide. Superoxide overproduction, accompanied by increased nitric oxide generation, favors the formation of the strong oxidant peroxynitrite, which, in turn, damages DNA. DNA damage is an obligatory stimulus for the activation of the nuclear enzyme poly(ADP-ribose) polymerase. Poly(ADP-ribose) polymerase activation, in turn, reduces the GAPDH activity. This process results in the adipocyte and muscle in reduced GLUT4 expression and the subsequent insulin resistance, in endothelial cell in endothelial dysfunction, while in β-cells in decreased insulin secretion/production. Calcium channel blockers, statins, ACE inhibitors, ATI inhibitors, and glitazones may intervene, at different levels, in preventing this phenomenon.

of overnutrition with the development of overt diabetes. It may also link the progressive β-cell failure to an increased cardiovascular risk, a prominent association in the clinical setting.

However, this hypothesis can also contribute to understand why different therapeutic strategies, apparently having in common only the ability to reduce oxidative stress, appear to simultaneously decrease cardiovascular mortality and lower incidence of diabetes. If oxidative stress is the pathogenic mechanism leading from insulin resistance to overt diabetes, the ability of a drug to prevent or reverse oxidant stress can account for its clinical usefulness.[21–25] Furthermore, the beneficial effect of controlling postprandial hyperglycemia on both the development of diabetes[15] and the prevention of cardiovascular disease[83] also supports this hypothesis, since it has been shown that in the postprandial state there is an oxidative stress generation that is strictly dependent on the level of glycemia reached.[84]

However, even convincing evidence is now available supporting the hypothesis that oxidative stress may play a key role on the development of both diabetes and CVD, clinical trials with antioxidants, in particular with vitamin E, have failed to demonstrate any beneficial effect.[85]

On this matter, it has recently been suggested that antioxidant therapy with vitamin E or other antioxidants is limited to scavenging already formed oxidants and may, therefore, be considered a more "symptomatic" rather than a causal treatment for oxidative stress.[86]

According to the evidence discussed in this chapter, it is suggested that interrupting the overproduction of superoxide by the mitochondrial electron-transport chain would normalize the pathways involved in the development of the oxidative stress.[87] It might, however, be difficult to accomplish this using conventional antioxidants, as these scavenge RDS in a stoichiometric manner. However, while waiting for more focused tools,[88] CCBs,[21] statins,[22] ACE inhibitors,[23] and ATI receptor antagonists[24] and glitazones,[25] which have a strong ability to prevent intracellular oxidant activity,[87] seem to be valid options already available. For an extensive review on this topic see Refs. 21, 86, 87, while this concept is summarized in Fig. 2.

In conclusion, a puzzle of many pieces of evidence suggests that free radical overgeneration may be considered the key and continuous lifestyle-dependent event that has a pivotal role in the development of overt diabetes, on the one hand, and of the associated cardiovascular complications on the other. This approach is of particular interest because, even if a change in lifestyle remains the best preventive and therapeutic approach, many new "specific and causal" antioxidants are being developed[86,87] and may become important tools to oppose the rising epidemic of diabetes, a real emergency in our future. Moreover, this concept can explain why treating cardiovascular risk with drugs such as CCBs, ACE inhibitors, AT-1 receptor antagonists, and statins may also prevent diabetes. Last but not least, since it has been demonstrated that insulin resistance is associated in humans with reduced intracellular antioxidant defense[38] and that diabetic subjects prone to complications may have a defective intracellular antioxidant response,[89,90] even what we call genetic predisposition to diabetes, as well as liability to its late complications, might be based on a deficient ROS scavenging ability in β-cells and/or in target tissues such as endothelium.

References

1. Amos A, McCarthy D, Zimmet P. The rising global burden of diabetes and its complications: estimates and projections to the year 2010. *Diabet. Med.* 14 (Suppl 5): S1–S85 (1997).
2. Rosembloom AL, Joe JR, Young RS, Winter WE. Emerging epidemic of type 2 diabetes in youth. *Diabetes Care* 22: 345–354 (1999).
3. Kannel WB, McGee DL. Diabetes and cardiovascular diseases. The Framingham Study. *JAMA* 241: 2035–2038 (1979).
4. Expert Panel on Detection, Evaluation, and Treatment of High Blood Cholesterol in Adults. Executive Summary of the Third Report of the National Cholesterol Education Program (NCEP) (Adult Treatment Panel III). *JAMA* 285: 2486–2497 (2001).
5. Hu FB, Stampfer MJ, Haffner SM, Solomon CG, Willett WC, Manson JE. Elevated risk of cardiovascular disease prior to clinical diagnosis of type 2 diabetes. *Diabetes Care* 25: 1129–1134 (2002).
6. Stern MP. Diabetes and cardiovascular disease. The "common soil" hypothesis. *Diabetes* 44: 369–374 (1995).
7. Kahan SE. The relative contributions of insulin resistance and beta-cell dysfunction to the pathophysiology of type 2 diabetes. *Diabetologia* 46: 3–19 (2003).
8. Haffner SM, Stern MP, Hazuda HP, Mitchell BD, Patterson JK. Cardiovascular risk factors in confirmed prediabetic individuals. Does the clock for coronary

heart disease start ticking before the onset of clinical diabetes? *JAMA* 263: 2893–2898 (1990).

9. Sinha R, Fisch G, Teague B, Tamborlane WV, Banyas B, Allen K, Savoye M, Rieger V, Taksali S, Barbetta G, Sherwin RS, Caprio S. Prevalence of impaired glucose tolerance among children and adolescents with marked obesity. *N. Engl. J. Med.* 346: 802–810 (2002).
10. Lakka HM, Laaksonen DE, Lakka TA, Niskanen LK, Kumpusalo E, Tuomilehto J, Salonen JT. The metabolic syndrome and total and cardiovascular disease mortality in middle-aged men. *JAMA* 288: 2709–2716 (2002).
11. Balkau B, Bertrais S, Ducimetiere P, Eschwege E. Is there a glycaemic threshold for mortality risk? *Diabetes Care* 22: 696–699 (1999).
12. Knowler WC, Barrett-Connor E, Fowler SE, Hamman RF, Lachin JM, Walker EA, Nathan DM, Diabetes Prevention Program Research Group. Reduction in the incidence of type 2 diabetes with lifestyle intervention or metformin. *N. Engl. J. Med.* 346: 393–403 (2002).
13. Tuomilehto J, Lindstrom J, Eriksson JG, Valle TT, Hamalainen H, Ilanne-Parikka P, Keinanen-Kiukaanniemi S, Laakso M, Louheranta A, Rastas M, Salminen V, Uusitupa M, Finnish Diabetes Prevention Study Group. Prevention of type 2 diabetes mellitus by changes in lifestyle among subjects with impaired glucose tolerance. *N. Engl. J. Med.* 344: 1343–1350 (2001).
14. Buchanan TA, Xiang AH, Peters RK, Kjos SL, Marroquin A, Goico J, Ochoa C, Tan S, Berkowitz K, Hodis HN, Azen SP. Preservation of pancreatic beta-cell function and prevention of type 2 diabetes by pharmacological treatment of insulin resistance in high-risk hispanic women. *Diabetes* 51: 2796–2803 (2002).
15. Chiasson JL, Josse RG, Gomis R, Hanefeld M, Karasik A, Laakso M, STOP-NIDDM Trail Research Group. Acarbose for prevention of type 2 diabetes mellitus: the STOP-NIDDM randomised trial. *Lancet* 359: 2072–2077 (2002).
16. Brown MJ, Palmer CR, Castaigne A, de Leeuw PW, Mancia G, Rosenthal T, Ruilope LM. Morbidity and mortality in patients randomised to double-blind treatment with a long-acting calcium-channel blocker or diuretic in the International Nifedipine GITS study: intervention as a goal in hypertension treatment (INSIGHT). *Lancet* 356: 366–372 (2000).
17. Yusuf S, Gerstein H, Hoogwerf B, Pogue J, Bosch J, Wolffenbuttel BH, Zinman B. HOPE Study Investigators: ramipril and the development of diabetes. *JAMA* 286: 1882–1885 (2001).
18. Freeman DJ, Norrie J, Sattar N, Neely RD, Cobbe SM, Ford I, Isles C, Lorimer AR, Macfarlane PW, McKillop JH, Packard CJ, Shepherd J, Gaw A.

Pravastatin and the development of diabetes mellitus: evidence for a protective treatment effect in the West of Scotland Coronary Prevention Study. *Circulation* 103: 357–362 (2001).

19. Dahlof B, Devereux RB, Kjeldsen SE, Julius S, Beevers G, Faire U, Fyhrquist F, Ibsen H, Kristiansson K, Lederballe-Pedersen O, Lindholm LH, Nieminen MS, Omvik P, Oparil S, Wedel H, LIFE Study Group. Cardiovascular morbidity and mortality in the Losartan Intervention For Endpoint reduction in hypertension study (LIFE): a randomised trial against atenolol. *Lancet* 359: 995–1003 (2002).
20. Vermes E, Ducharme A, Bourassa MG, Lessard M, White M, Tardif JC, Studies of Left Ventricular Dysfunction. Enalapril reduces the incidence of diabetes in patients with chronic heart failure: insight from the Studies Of Left Ventricular Dysfunction (SOLVD). *Circulation* 107: 1291–1296 (2003).
21. Mason RP, Marche P, Hintze TH. Novel vascular biology of third-generation L-type calcium channel antagonists: ancillary actions of amlodipine. *Arterioscler. Thromb. Vasc. Biol.* 23: 2155–2163 (2003).
22. Takemoto M, Liao JK. Pleiotropic effects of 3-hydroxy-3-methylglutaryl coenzyme A reductase inhibitors. *Arterioscler. Thromb. Vasc. Biol.* 21: 1712–1719 (2001).
23. Münzel T, Keaney JF Jr. Are ACE inhibitors a "magic bullet" against oxidative stress? *Circulation* 104: 1571–1579 (2001).
24. Ceriello A, Motz E. Angiotensin-receptor blockers, type 2 diabetes, and renoprotection. *N. Engl. J. Med.* 346: 705–707 (2002).
25. Da Ros R, Assaloni R, Ceriello A. The preventive antioxidant action of thiazolinediones: a new therapeutic prospect in diabetes and insulin resistance. *Diabet. Med.* 21(11): 1249–1252 (2004).
26. Ceriello A. Acute hyperglycaemia and oxidative stress generation. *Diabet. Med.* 14 (Suppl 3): S45–S49 (1997).
27. Heilbronn LK, Ravussin E. Calorie restriction and aging: review of the literature and implications for studies in humans. *Am. J. Clin. Nutr.* 78: 361–369 (2003).
28. Evans JL, Goldfine ID, Maddux BA, Grodsky GM. Are oxidative stress-activated signaling pathways mediators of insulin resistance and β-cell dysfunction? *Diabetes* 52: 1–8 (2003).
29. Griendling KK, FitzGerald GA. Oxidative stress and cardiovascular injury: Part I: basic mechanisms and *in vivo* monitoring of ROS. *Circulation* 108: 1912–1916 (2003).
30. Maddux BA, See W, Lawrence JC Jr, Goldfine AL, Goldfine ID, Evans JL. Protection against oxidative stress-induced insulin resistance in rat L6 muscle

cells by micromolar concentrations of α-lipoic acid. *Diabetes* 50: 404–410 (2001).

31. Maechler P, Jornot L, Wolheim CB. Hydrogen peroxide alters mitochondrial activation and insulin secretion in pancreatic beta cells. *J. Biol. Chem.* 274: 27905–27913 (1999).
32. Williamson JR, Cooper RH. Regulation of the citric acid cycle in mammalian systems. *FEBS Lett.* 117 (Suppl): K73–K85 (1980).
33. Tretter L, Adam-Vizi V. Inhibition of Krebs cycle enzymes by hydrogen peroxide: a key role of alpha-ketoglutarate dehydrogenase in limiting NADH production under oxidative stress. *J. Neurosci.* 20: 8972–8979 (2000).
34. Rudich A, Tirosh A, Potashnik R, Hemi R, Kanety H, Bashan N. Prolonged oxidative stress impairs insulin-induced GLUT4 translocation in 3T3-L1 adipocytes. *Diabetes* 47: 1562–1569 (1998).
35. Talior I, Yarkoni M, Bashan N, Eldar-Fielman H. Increased glucose uptake promotes oxidative stress and PKC delta activation in adipocytes of obese, insulin-resistant mice. *Am. J. Physiol.* 285: E295–E302 (2003).
36. Paolisso G, Giugliano D. Oxidative stress and insulin action. Is there a relationship? *Diabetologia* 39: 357–363 (1996).
37. Ceriello A. Oxidative stress and glycemic regulation. *Metabolism* 49: 27–29 (2000).
38. Bruce CR, Carey AL, Hawley JA, Febbraio MA. Intramuscular heat shock protein 72 and heme oxygenase-1 mRNA are reduced in patients with type 2 diabetes: evidence that insulin resistance is associated with a disturbed antioxidant defence mechanism. *Diabetes* 52: 2338–2345 (2003).
39. Tiedge M, Lortz S, Drinkgern J, Lenzen S. Relation between antioxidant enzyme gene expression and antioxidative defense status of insulin producing cells. *Diabetes* 46: 1733–1742 (1997).
40. Robertson RP, Harmon J, Tran PO, Tanaka Y, Takahashi H. Glucose toxicity in β-cells: type 2 diabetes, good radicals gone bad, and the glutathione connection. *Diabetes* 52: 581–587 (2003).
41. Maechler P, Jornot L, Wollheim CB. Hydrogen peroxide alters mitochondrial activation and insulin secretion in pancreatic beta cells. *J. Biol. Chem.* 274: 27905–27913 (1999).
42. Sakai K, Matsumoto K, Nishikawa T, Suefuji M, Nakamaru K, Hirashima Y, Kawashima J, Shirotani T, Ichinose K, Brownlee M, Araki E. Mitochondrial reactive oxygen species reduce insulin secretion by pancreatic beta-cells. *Biochem. Biophys. Res. Commun.* 300: 216–222 (2003).
43. Paolisso G, Giugliano D, Pizza G, Gambardella A, Tesauro P, Varricchio M, D'Onofrio F. Glutathione infusion potentiates glucose-induced insulin

secretion in aged patients with impaired glucose tolerance. *Diabetes Care* 15: 1–7 (1992).

44. Carlsson C, Borg LA, Welsh N. Sodium palmitate induces partial mitochondrial uncoupling and reactive oxygen species in rat pancreatic islets *in vitro*. *Endocrinology* 140: 3422–3428 (1999).
45. Lameloise N, Muzzin P, Prentki M, Assimacopoulos-Jeannet F. Uncoupling protein 2: a possible link between fatty acid excess and impaired glucose-induced insulin secretion? *Diabetes* 50: 803–809 (2001).
46. Paolisso G, Gambardella A, Tagliamonte MR, Saccomanno F, Salvatore T, Gualdiero P, D'Onofrio F, Howard B. Does free fatty acid infusion impair insulin action also though an increase in oxidative stress? *J. Clin. Endocrinol. Metab.* 81: 4244–4248 (1996).
47. Krauss S, Zhang CY, Scorrano L, Dalgaard LT, St-Pierre J, Grey ST, Lowell BB. Superoxide-mediated activation of uncoupling protein 2 causes pancreatic beta cell dysfunction. *J. Clin. Invest.* 112: 1831–1842 (2003).
48. Jacqueminet S, Briaud I, Rouault C, Reach G, Poitout V. Inhibition of insulin gene expression by long-term exposure of pancreatic beta cells to palmitate is dependent on the presence of a stimulatory glucose concentration. *Metabolism* 49: 532–536 (2002).
49. El-Assad W *et al.* Saturated fatty acids synerize with elevated glucose to cause pancreatic beta-cell death. *Endocrinology* 144: 4154–4163 (2003).
50. Piro S, Anello M, Di Pietro C, Lizzio MN, Patane G, Rabuazzo AM, Vigneri R, Purrello M, Purrello F. Chronic exposure to free fatty acids or high glucose induces apoptosis in rat pancreatic islets: possible role of oxidative stress. *Metabolism* 51: 1340–1347 (2002).
51. Ross R. The pathogenesis of atherosclerosis: a perspective for 1990s. *Nature* 326: 801–809 (1993).
52. Perticone F, Ceravolo R, Pujia A, Ventura G, Iacopino S, Scozzafava A, Ferraro A, Chello M, Mastroroberto P, Verdecchia P, Schillaci G. Prognostic significance of endothelial dysfunction in hypertensive patients. *Circulation* 104: 191–196 (2001).
53. Heitzer T, Schlinzig T, Krohn K, Meinertz T, Munzel T. Endothelial dysfunction, oxidative stress, and risk of cardiovascular events in patients with coronary artery disease. *Circulation* 104: 2673–2678 (2001).
54. Baron AD. Insulin resistance and vascular function. *J. Diabetes. Complicat.* 16: 92–102 (2002).
55. Bohlen HG, Lash JM. Topical Hyperglycemia rapidly suppresses EDRF-mediated vasodilatation of normal rat arterioles. *Am. J. Physiol.* 265: H219–H225 (1993).

56. Giugliano D, Marfella R, Coppola L, Verrazzo G, Acampora R, Giunta R, Nappo F, Lucarelli C, D'Onofrio F. Vascular effects of acute hyperglycemia in humans are reversed by L-arginine. Evidence for reduced availability of nitric oxide during hyperglycemia. *Circulation* 95: 1783–1790 (1997).
57. Kawano H, Motoyama T, Hirashima O, Hirai N, Miyao Y, Sakamoto T, Kugiyama K, Ogawa H, Yasue H. Hyperglycemia rapidly suppresses flow-mediated endothelium-dependent vasodilation of brachial artery. *J. Am. Coll. Cardiol.* 34: 146–154 (1999).
58. Tesfamariam B, Cohen RA. Free radicals mediate endothelial cell dysfunction caused by elevated glucose. *Am. J. Physiol.* 263: H321–H326 (1992).
59. Marfella R, Verrazzo G, Acampora R, La Marca C, Giunta R, Lucarelli C, Paolisso G, Ceriello A, Giugliano D. Glutathione reverses systemic hemodynamic changes by acute hyperglycemia in healthy subjects. *Am. J. Physiol.* 268: E1167–E1173 (1995).
60. Ting HH, Timimi FK, Boles KS, Creager SJ, Ganz P, Creager MA. Vitamin C improves endothelium-dependent vasodilation in patients with non-insulin-dependent diabetes mellitus. *J. Clin. Invest.* 97: 22–28 (1996).
61. Nishikawa T, Edelstein D, Du X-L, Yamagishi S, Matsumura T, Kaneda Y, Yorek M, Beebe D, Oates P, Hammes HP, Giardino I, Brownlee M. Normalizing mitochondrial superoxide production blocks three pathways of hyperglycaemic damage. *Nature* 404: 787–790 (2000).
62. Garcia Soriano F, Virag L, Jagtap P, Szabo E, Mabley JG, Liaudet L, Marton A, Hoyt DG, Murthy KG, Salzman AL, Southan GJ, Szabo C. Diabetic endothelial dysfunction: the role of poly(ADP-ribose) polymerase activation. *Nat. Med.* 7: 108–113 (2001).
63. Hink U, Li H, Mollnau H, Oelze M, Matheis E, Hartmann M, Skatchkov M, Thaiss F, Stahl RAK, Warnholtz A, Meinertz T, Griendling K, Harrison DG, Forstermann U, Munzel T. Mechanisms underlying endothelial dysfunction in diabetes mellitus. *Circ. Res.* 88: 14–22 (2001).
64. Pleiner J, Schaller G, Mittermayer F, Bayerle-Eder M, Roden M, Woltz M. FFA-induced endothelial dysfunction can be corrected by vitamin C. *J. Clin. Endocrinol. Metab.* 87: 2913–2917 (2002).
65. Ceriello A. The possible role of postprandial hyperglycaemia in the pathogenesis of diabetic complications. *Diabetologia* 46 (Suppl 1): M9–M16 (2003).
66. Del Prato S. Loss of early insulin secretion leads to postprandial hyperglycaemia. *Diabetologia* 46 (Suppl 1): M2–M8 (2003).
67. Ceriello A, Taboga C, Tonutti L, Quagliaro L, Piconi L, Bais B, Da Ros R, Motz E. Evidence for an independent and cumulative effect of postprandial hypertriglyceridemia and hyperglycemia on endothelial dysfunction and

oxidative stress generation. Effects of short- and long-term simvastatin treatment. *Circulation* 106: 1211–1218 (2002).
68. Poitout V, Robertson RP. Minireview: secondary beta-cell failure in type 2 diabetes — a convergence of glucotoxicity and lipotoxicity. *Endocrinology* 143: 339–342 (2002).
69. Bast A, Wolf G, Oberbaumer I, Walther R. Oxidative and nitrosative stress induces peroxiredoxins in pancreatic beta cells. *Diabetologia* 45: 867–876 (2002).
70. Sakuraba H, Mizukami H, Yagihashi N, Wada R, Hanyu C, Yagihashi S. Reduced beta-cell mass and expression of oxidative stress-related DNA damage in the islet of Japanese Type II diabetic patients. *Diabetologia* 45: 85–96 (2002).
71. Meraji S, Jayakody L, Senaratne PJ, Thomson ABR, Kappagoda T. Endothelium-dependent relaxation in aorta of BB rat. *Diabetes* 36: 978–981 (1987).
72. Mayhan WG. Impairment of endothelium-dependent dilatation of cerebral arterioles during diabetes mellitus. *Am. J. Physiol.* 256: H621–H625 (1989).
73. Johnstone MT, Creager SJ, Scales KM, Cusco JA, Lee BK, Creager MA. Impaired endothelium-dependent vasodilation in patients with insulin-dependent diabetes mellitus. *Circulation* 88: 2510–2516 (1993).
74. McVeigh GE, Brennan GM, Johnston GD, McDermott BJ, McGrath LT, Henry WR, Andrews JW, Hayes JR. Impaired endothelium-dependent and independent vasodilation in patients with type 2 (non-insulin dependent) diabetes mellitus. *Diabetologia* 35: 771–776 (1992).
75. Giugliano D, Ceriello A, Paolisso G. Oxidative stress and diabetic vascular complications. *Diabetes Care* 19: 257–267 (1996).
76. Hu FB, Stampfer MJ. Is type 2 diabetes mellitus a vascular condition? *Arterioscler. Thromb. Vasc. Biol.* 23: 1715–1716 (2003).
77. Roebuck KA. Oxidant stress regulation of IL-8 and ICAM-1 gene expression: differential activation and binding of the transcription factors AP-1 and NF-kappaB. *Int. J. Mol. Med.* 4: 223–230 (1999).
78. Lane N. A unifying view of ageing and disease: the double-agent theory. *J. Theor. Biol.* 225: 531–540 (2003).
79. Tripathy D, Mohanty P, Dhindsa S, Syed T, Ghanim H, Aljada A, Dandona P. Elevation of free fatty acids induces inflammation and impairs vascular reactivity in healthy subjects. *Diabetes* 52: 2882–2887 (2003).
80. Esposito K, Nappo F, Marfella R, Giugliano G, Giugliano F, Ciotola M, Quagliaro L, Ceriello A, Giugliano D. Inflammatory cytokine concentrations

are acutely increased by hyperglycemia in humans: role of oxidative stress. *Circulation* 106: 2067–2072 (2002).

81. Nappo F, Esposito K, Cioffi M, Giugliano G, Molinari AM, Paolisso G, Marfella R, Giugliano D. Postprandial endothelial activation in healthy subjects and in type 2 diabetic patients: role of fat and carbohydrate meals. *J. Am. Coll. Cardiol.* 39: 1145–1150 (2002).
82. Ceriello A, Quagliaro L, Piconi L, Assaloni R, Da Ros R, Maier A, Esposito K, Giugliano D. Effect of postprandial hypertriglyceridemia and hyperglycemia on circulating adhesion molecules and oxidative stress generation and the possible role of simvastatin treatment. *Diabetes* 53: 701–710 (2004).
83. Chiasson JL, Josse RG, Gomis R, Hanefeld M, Karasik A, Laakso M, STOP-NIDDM Trial Research Group. Acarbose treatment and the risk of cardiovascular disease and hypertension in patients with impaired glucose tolerance: the STOP-NIDDM trial. *JAMA* 290: 486–494 (2003).
84. Ceriello A, Quagliaro L, Catone B, Pascon R, Piazzola M, Bais B, Marra G, Tonutti L, Taboga C, Motz E. The role of hyperglycemia in nitrotyrosine postprandial generation. *Diabetes Care* 25: 1439–1443 (2002).
85. Marchioli R, Schweiger C, Levantesi G, Gavazzi L, Valagussa F. Antioxidant vitamins and prevention of cardiovascular disease: epidemiological and clinical trial data. *Lipids* 36: S53–S63 (2001).
86. Cuzzocrea S, Riley DP, Caputi AP, Salvemini D. Antioxidant therapy: a new pharmacological approach in shock, inflammation, and ischemia/reperfusion injury. *Pharmacol. Rev.* 53: 135–159 (2001).
87. Ceriello A. New insights on oxidative stress and diabetic complications may lead to a "causal" antioxidant therapy. *Diabetes Care* 26: 1589–1596 (2003).
88. Smith RA, Porteous CM, Gane AM, Murphy MP. Delivery of bioactive molecules to mitochondria *in vivo*. *Proc. Natl. Acad. Sci. USA* 100: 5407–5412 (2003).
89. Ceriello A, Morocutti A, Mercuri F, Quagliaro L, Moro M, Damante G, Viberti GC. Defective intracellular antioxidant enzyme production in type 1 diabetic patients with nephropathy. *Diabetes* 49: 2170–2177 (2000).
90. Hodgkinson AD, Bartlett T, Oates PJ, Millward BA, Demaine AG. The response of antioxidant genes to hyperglycemia is abnormal in patients with type 1 diabetes and diabetic nephropathy. *Diabetes* 52: 846–851 (2003).

18 Pathogenesis and Etiology of Down's Syndrome in Relation to Oxidative Stress

Svetlana Arbuzova and Howard Cuckle

1. Introduction

Down's syndrome (DS) is the most common cause of mental retardation, with a prevalence in the absence of prenatal diagnosis of 1–2 per 1000 births. In 95% of cases there is non-disjunction of chromosome 21, in 4% there is a Robertsonian translocation, mostly t(14;21) or t(21;21), and 1% are mosaic.[1]

Advanced maternal age is by far the strongest epidemiological variable, with birth prevalence increasing from 0.6 per 1000 at age 15 to 4.1 per 1000 by age 45.[2] There is familial aggregation: having had a previous DS pregnancy confers a 5.4 per 1000 higher risk than the age-specific prevalence, other types of aneuploidy are also more frequent, and there is an excess of double aneuploidies including trisomy 21.[3] Other risk factors, such as a family history of Alzheimer's disease (AD), diabetes, and hypothyroidism, are weaker.[4,5] Recently a familial association with neural tube defects has been reported, but this remains to be confirmed.[6]

Genetic mapping shows that in about 90% of non-disjunction trisomy 21 the extra chromosome is maternal in origin and that certain types of crossover at maternal meiosis I confer a substantial susceptibility.[6] Parental DNA studies have reported an altered distribution of polymorphisms in the genes for apolipoprotein E[7] and presenilin-1[8] and those involved in folate metabolism, but the effects are not great and the results inconsistent between studies.[9–14] Despite considerable research over many decades the principle cause of DS is unclear.

Also, the mechanisms by which aneuploidy produces the clinical features of DS are still uncertain. In addition to severe learning difficulties, the typical appearance, and cardiac and digestive tract abnormalities, DS is associated with a general acceleration in the aging process. In particular, affected individuals develop changes in the brain by about age 30 similar to those of AD, and there is a substantial early onset of autoimmune diseases and cataracts.

Numerous attempts have been made to ascertain whether it is the consequence of given segments of chromosome 21 being triplicated. The chromosome has now been completely sequenced, and it includes a number of important genes, such as those for Cu, Zn-superoxide dismutase (SOD-1) and the amyloid precursor protein (AβPP). There is no evidence, however, that any individual loci are by themselves responsible for specific anatomical, physiological, and functional features of the syndrome.[15] In addition, the wide variation in onset and severity of dementia in those affected suggests that factors other than direct changes to chromosome 21 genes are involved in the pathogenesis.

2. Oxidative Stress

There are convincing data, epidemiological, *in vitro*, and *in vivo*, of oxidative stress in DS. The process is evident during fetal and postnatal development and critically influences subsequent neuronal death in the older DS individuals.[16–23]

The level of intracellular reactive oxygen species (ROS) is increased three- to fourfold in fetal DS neurons, with substantially elevated levels of lipid peroxidation that precede neuronal death.[18] The level of malondialdehyde (MDA), a biomarker of lipid peroxidation, is elevated by 30–60% in the brain, erythrocytes, fibroblasts, and urine.[16,18,24,25] There is also a disturbance in lipid metabolism and lipid composition.[19]

There is evidence that accelerated brain glycoxidation occurs very early in DS. A study of 18–20 week gestation fetuses found elevated levels of thiobarbituric acid reactive substances, 4-hydroxynonenal, a strong toxic aldehyde resulting from lipoperoxidation, and two end-products of advanced glycation involved in the process of cellular oxidation, pyrraline and pentosidine.[26] The same study also showed a high level of protein carbonyl groups, confirming direct injury by oxidation.

The level of 8-hydroxy-2′-deoxyguanosine, a biomarker of oxidative damage to DNA, is increased by 70%.[17] In a study of cerebral neurons from DS individuals of various ages, ranging from 4 months to 65 years, there was a parallel increase of 8-hydroxyguanosine (8OHG), an oxidized nucleoside, and nitrotyrosine, an oxidation product of protein.[27] The study concluded that nucleic acid and protein oxidation are prominent features of cerebral neurons in DS.

Another indication of oxidative stress is the elevation of plasma or serum uric acid, an efficient antioxidant, and allantoin, a product of uric acid oxidation,[20–22] and glutathione deficiency.[23,28]

Neuropathologic stigmata of AD in DS individuals are also consistent with the role of chronic oxidative injury in the age-related changes in the DS brain. All individuals with DS by the fourth decade of life develop senile plaques, neurofibrillary tangles, and granulovacuolar bodies, which is virtually identical with the AD pathology, as well as a similar neurochemical deficit pattern.[29,30] Increased lipid, protein, and DNA oxidation was demonstrated in the brain of subjects with AD, and the contribution of oxidative stress in the progression of AD is well documented (for a review see Ref. 31). High expression of excision repair-cross-complementing proteins 80 and 89, encoded for on genes ERCC2 and ERCC3, which are responsible for repairing DNA lesions from oxidative stress, was found in brain samples from AD subjects and adults with DS with a mean age of 54 years.[32] This confirms increased oxidative DNA damage *in vivo* for both disorders and the role of chronic oxidative injury in subsequent neuronal death. Negative effects of oxidative stress on neuronal function in DS are also supported by studies on DS mouse models, trisomy 16 (Tr16), and mice transgenic for, and overexpressing, SOD-1 (TgSOD).[28,33,34]

There is general agreement that a disturbance in the balance of reactive oxygen species may be a key point in the DS pathogenesis, but there are too many contradictions to favor a dosage effect of the genes located on chromosome 21 as the reason for the oxidative damage in DS.

3. Genes Connected to Oxidative Stress

The imbalance of ROS homeostasis is generally considered to be mainly the consequence of the overexpression of SOD-1 and AβPP genes.[35]

3.1. *Superoxide dismutase*

It is widely believed that the oxidative stress in DS is due to a direct gene dosage effect resulting from a 50% increase in the activity of SOD-1, which is encoded for at 21q22.1.[36] However, examination of the available evidence reveals many contradictions to this proposal.

Changes in SOD-1 activity cannot be solely due to a direct gene dosage effect; in fact it varies according to cell or tissue type, and genotype. In blood cells and fibroblasts with complete trisomy 21, activity is increased by 30–90% on average; whilst about one-fifth have normal activity and plasma SOD-1, activity is markedly decreased.[24,37–40] SOD-1 activity was found to be increased in fetal brain in some studies but not in others.[16,41] There are DS patients with partial trisomy 21, translocations or mosaicism, and no excess of SOD-1, and in contrast, there are documented cases of partial trisomy 21 with increased SOD-1 but without any of the usual symptoms.[15,38] No significant correlation was found between levels of SOD-1 and percentage of trisomic cells in erythrocytes and fibroblasts of children with mosaic trisomy 21.[42] Similar discrepancies, as well as an extremely wide range of values, were found in studies which analyzed the concentration of SOD-1.[43,44]

Despite numerous studies, there is no clear evidence that the elevated lipid peroxidation seen in DS is a consequence of increased SOD-1 activity. This suggestion was generally considered to be plausible, but even early investigators failed to confirm that increased SOD-1 activity was developmentally deleterious or necessarily increased lipid peroxidation.[24]

One study group, using cultured cells overexpressing a transfected SOD-1 gene and transgenic mice harbouring the h-CuZnSOD gene, claimed that increased SOD-1 activity resulted in enhanced lipid peroxidation.[45] However, extrapolating from their results, the SOD-1 increase in DS would only be expected to enhance lipid peroxidation by about 10%. In addition, the results do not support the authors' claim that elevated SOD-1 activity did not protect the cells from the damage caused by a paraquat-generator of superoxide radicals. The same group also reported that kainic acid neurotoxicity, mediated by oxidative stress, is exacerbated in cultures of neurons derived from TgSOD mice that are transgenic for, and overexpressing, SOD-1.[46] However, other groups have shown that mixed neuro and glial cultures derived from Tri16 and TgSOD mice are less vulnerable to N-methyl-4-phenyl-1,2,3,6-tetrahydropyridine-induced neurotoxicity as well as to direct oxidative injury.[47–50] Elroy-Stein and Groner[51] have indicated that overexpression of SOD-1 leads to deficits in peripheral markers of neurochemical function. To test this the concentrations of amino acids and biogenic amines, and activities of synthetic enzymes, were measured in both control mice and TgSOD mice that overexpressed SOD-1 by two- to fivefold compared with control values.[52] The results indicated that overexpression of SOD-1 by itself, even higher than expected by gene dosage effect, was not sufficient to cause the synaptic neurochemical deficits reported in DS. The same conclusion was reached by other scientists who investigated the relationship between excess gene dosage and neurophysiological abnormalities, having compared dorsal root ganglion neurons from Tr16 mice with normal neurons.[53] No electrophysiological differences were found between the two groups of neurons, indicating that increased dosage of the SOD-1 gene alone is not sufficient to cause potential dysfunction found in trisomy 21 and trisomy 16 neurons.

In general, despite the ability of SOD-1 to have peroxidative activity,[54] a 1.5-fold increase alone is insufficient for an enzyme to bring this about, and a similar elevation or greater in SOD-1 is known in response to increased ROS for diseases that have nothing to do with gene dosage effect. For example, Bloom syndrome cells exhibit elevated levels of superoxide dismutase activity due to increased concentration of $O_2^{\bullet-}$, which leads to elevated sister chromatid exchanges — the major cytological characteristic of this disorder[55] or AD, where elevated SOD-1 activity has also been reported in first-degree relatives.[56,57]

Having analyzed the SOD-1 activity and the level of lipid peroxidation in DS individuals of different ages, we have found that SOD-1 activity decreases, whereas MDA increases with age.[58,59] Thus the enhanced lipid peroxidation in DS is unlikely to be a consequence of a direct SOD-1 gene dosage effect.

It has also been suggested that the ability of increased SOD-1 to lead to oxidative stress is enhanced by an imbalance of other antioxidants such as glutathione peroxidase (GSH-Px) and catalase, as well as the trace elements copper, zinc, and selenium. However, there is an even greater discrepancy between published studies than for SOD-1 itself, including a significant increase, a null effect, and a significant decrease.[16,24,40,60–62]

3.2. *Amyloid precursor protein*

The gene for AβPP maps to q21.3-22.05 and codes for a transmembrane protein expressed in neurons and astrocytes. It was proposed that amyloid-β (Aβ) is the source of oxidative stress in DS,[63,64] and some studies have shown that Aβ peptide is capable of generating free radical damage, is involved in membrane lipid peroxidation, and induces apoptosis.[64–67]

Since the AβPP gene is located on chromosome 21, it was hypothesized that the increased gene dosage of AβPP leads to an increase in soluble Aβ in the DS brain[68] with consequent Aβ40 and/or Aβ42 deposition[69,70] and development of AD-type brain pathology.[71] Indeed abnormal AβPP metabolism in DS has been demonstrated in brain, platelets, and fibroblasts.[72–74] A systemic abnormality was suggested mainly by elevated plasma concentrations of Aβ40 and Aβ42, but these forms were found to be increased by two- to threefold in DS plasma,[75] which is not consistent with a gene dosage effect, suggesting that other factors determine Aβ production.

It was shown that the level of soluble Aβ in DS brain structures increases exponentially with age and soluble Aβ is present during the first decade of life, clearly preceding plaque formation.[68] However, there is a lack of correlation between the Aβ plaque load and the levels of either soluble or insoluble Aβ.[76]

Some studies indicate that glutamate transport (GT) may be impaired by Aβ, and GT activity correlates with AβPP level.[77–79] However, decreased GT in DS brain does not correlate with the number of AD-like plaques and tangles or the severity of dementia.[80]

Finally, if Aβ is the source of oxidative stress, as was suggested,[64] then oxidative damage should positively correlate with Aβ deposition. However, marked paralleling accumulation of oxidized nucleic acid, 8OHG, and oxidized protein, nitrotyrosine, found in the cytoplasm of cerebral neurons in DS preceded Aβ deposition.[27] These findings mean that in brains of patients with DS, increased levels of oxidative damage occur prior to the onset of plaque formation. Moreover, deposition of Aβ, particularly Aβ42, was associated with a decrease in the level of neuronal oxidative stress.

4. SOD-1 and AβPP — Gene Dosage Effects or Protective Response?

An alternative and compelling interpretation of the data on elevated SOD-1 activity is that it has a protective, rather than harmful, effect in DS individuals and that the increase of this scavenger is of benefit for the homeostasis between generated reactive oxygen metabolites and their propagation.

It is known that SOD-1 plays an important role in the protection of cells from oxidative damage and decreased SOD-1 expression in a variety of species increases their vulnerability to oxidative stress.[81,82]

In one study, SOD-1 activity in red cells was increased among DS individuals without AD manifestations, whereas those with symptoms had lower SOD-1 levels than did matched controls.[60]

Strong evidence for the protective effect of increased SOD-1 activity in DS individuals can be found in the study of *M. pneumoniae* injury to trisomy 21 and control cells.[83] Following infection, the level of MDA was raised in trisomy 21 fibroblasts by only 10–32%, whereas, in normal cells, MDA was increased by 140–870%. Supplementation of SOD-1 to the control cells following infection reduced the extent of lipid peroxidation. The inactivation of the cellular antioxidative defence mechanism results in progressive oxidative damage. The protective effect of increased SOD-1 activity has also been repeatedly shown in a number of experimental studies with transgenic mice overexpressing CuZn superoxide dismutase.[47–50,84,85]

We believe that the reason for increased SOD-1 activity in DS is chronic overproduction of the superoxide radical anion. In cases where the 21q22.1 region is triplicated, SOD-1 activity has more potential to increase in response to overproduction of $O_2^{\bullet -}$ and can exceed a theoretically expected 50% increase, depending on the level of $O_2^{\bullet -}$ in various cells and tissues, since SOD-1 activity reflects the intracellular superoxide contents. The consequence of high $O_2^{\bullet -}$ levels concomitant with induced SOD activity is the formation of large amounts of H_2O_2, which can apparently inactivate the enzyme responsible for its elimination.[54]

As SOD-1 activity decreases with age, spontaneous dismutation of $O_2^{\bullet -}$ becomes more prevalent. Changes in SOD-1 activity appear to be the consequence, rather than the cause, of oxidative stress in DS.

Likewise, the overexpression of AβPP may also be a neuronal protective response rather than a consequence of the direct gene dosage effect. Neuronal oxidative damage has been shown to be reduced as senile plaques increase, suggesting that increased AβPP production is a protective response.[27] Indeed, Busciglio and coworkers demonstrated the neuroprotective effect of secreted AβPP on astrocytes.[86] The authors also found reduced AβPP in DS astrocytes and cortex throughout life. The same conclusion was reached by another group, who showed that the extent of deposition of Aβ, particularly Aβ42, was associated with a reduction in the level of neuronal oxidative stress.[27] The negative correlation between Aβ and the extent of oxidative damage in these studies is in contrast with *in vitro* toxicity studies or studies with transgenic mice overexpressing AβPP, where Aβ precipitated oxidative damage.[64,87,88] It may be related to an extremely high level of AβPP expression (about 6 times higher) in the AβPP transgenic mice[89] or to the much higher concentrations of H_2O_2 used *in vitro* compared with those found physiologically *in vivo*, used in both experimental AβPP and SOD-1 studies. For example, cultures were treated with at least 50 μM and much higher doses of H_2O_2. In comparison, 75 μM H_2O_2 induces death of more than 90% of neurons, in a one-hour exposure, and 50 μM results in death of about 70% of neurons.[90]

Despite numerous attempts to connect the genes for SOD-1 and AβPP to oxidative stress, it must be concluded that there is no consistent evidence to support this. Moreover, molecular investigation of some DS individuals with partial trisomy 21 shows that the DS region may include parts of bands 21q22.2 and 21q22.3, but it must exclude bands encoding SOD-1 and AβPP.[91,92] Hence, these two genes could not be responsible for the phenotypic and neurobiological abnormalities in DS. Interestingly, Ets-2, a transcription factor located on the distal part of chromosome 21 at 21q22.3 and considered to be linked to apoptosis, is overexpressed in DS cells and tissues by five- to sevenfold. Such an increase in Ets-2 expression cannot be explained by the gene dosage alone and was shown to be induced by oxidative stress.[93]

5. MtDNA Mutations

Rather than a gene-dosage effect related to the oxidative stress in trisomy 21, a more compelling explanation is that mitochondrial (mt) DNA mutations are involved. The mitochondrial respiratory system is the most important intracellular source of ROS and free radicals, and mitochondria have a central role in different types of apoptosis.

We have suggested that mtDNA mutations have a role in the pathogenesis of DS.[49–59] Apart from helping to explain free radical damage and development of AD, the presence of mtDNA mutations could explain the association of DS with premature ageing and diabetes, which can result from mtDNA mutations.[94] Our data on mtDNA sequencing of three DS individuals are consistent with this concept as a high incidence of mtDNA base changes was found, including those not previously described.[95] These variations may lead to a decreased mitochondrial function with a consequent defect in AβPP processing or, alternatively, leave the cells more vulnerable to neurotoxic insults.

Numerous studies have demonstrated that the accumulation of mtDNA mutations is a major contributor to degenerative diseases and ageing. A specific heteroplasmic point mutation in the mtDNA D-loop region, T414G, has been found[96] in individuals aged over 65, and the same mutation with a different level of heteroplasmy was found in DS individuals aged 45 and older,[97] indicating mitochondrial signs of premature ageing.

A significant reduction in the activities of the mitochondrial enzymes, monoamine oxidase, cytochrome oxidase, and isocitrate dehydrogenase, in platelets from DS individuals has been found, suggesting that these reductions are a consequence of a generalized mitochondrial disturbance.[98] It is known that mtDNA is much more vulnerable to oxidative damage than is nuclear DNA. Defective repair of oxidative damage in mtDNA was shown in DS fibroblasts.[99]

Oxidative stress in fetal DS was suggested to be linked to decreased expression of peroxiredoxin (Prx) proteins, a newly characterized family of highly conserved antioxidant enzymes.[100] It is notable that among the subtypes which have been studied, only Prx III, mainly found in the mitochondria, was significantly decreased.

Direct evidence for increased mitochondrial superoxide production in DS was demonstrated using a lucigenen-derived chemiluminescence (LDCL) assay. DS individuals had significantly elevated LDCL signal compared with control subjects, providing support for the mitochondria being a major source of superoxide radicals in this condition.[101] Increased mitochondrial superoxide generation was also shown in neurons from Ts16 mice.[102]

In DS astrocytes, impaired mitochondrial function, indicated by reduced mitochondrial redox activity and membrane potential, has been demonstrated.[86] The same group also showed a defect in AβPP processing in DS astrocytes that might either be the cause or effect of the observed mitochondrial dysfunction. However, inhibition of mitochondrial function in normal cells induced similar abnormalities of AβPP processing, implying that mitochondrial dysfunction in DS cells is a cause of the AβPP processing defect.

The authors concluded that mitochondrial dysfunction in the DS brain may contribute to the pathogenesis of AD by inducing oxidative stress and interfering with AβPP processing. They also observed a similar impairment of mitochondrial function in primary cultures of DS fibroblasts, suggesting that mitochondrial dysfunction is widespread in DS.

As with DS pathogenesis, there are many unanswered questions about the non-disjunction leading to trisomy 21,[103] and it has been hypothesized that mtDNA mutations may play a role.[6,58,59,104,105] Mutations in mtDNA may bring about an increase in the generation of free radicals and reduce ATP levels. This, in turn, could affect the synaptonemal complex, chromosome segregation and division spindle, alter recombination (the enzymes participating in recombination and DNA repair are ATP-dependent),[106,107] and so lead to aneuploidy.

There is a congruity between the salient facts of mtDNA mutation and the epidemiology of DS. The number of mtDNA mutations increases with age in different cells, particularly in oocytes,[108] and mtDNA is almost entirely of maternal origin.[109] There are proven associations between mtDNA mutations and AD, diabetes, and hypothyroidism.[110]

Impaired function of the oxidant–antioxidant system has been found in mothers of infants with DS, and entire mtDNA sequencing in one donor of the extra chromosome 21 identified four mutations, not previously described, all causing amino acid changes.[59]

Moreover, experimental work with animals supports the idea. The Dip 1 mutation in mice, which produces a high incidence of ovulated diploid oocytes, is carried by the mitochondria.[111]

The evidence for mtDNA involvement in DS etiology is particularly strong when there is a family history of DS recurrence or the occurrence of both DS and one or more other types of aneuploidy.[112–116]

6. Down's Syndrome Inheritance

DS recurrence is a relatively rare but well-documented event in liveborn children, spontaneous abortions, and prenatally diagnosed cases.[113–115,117–121] In a meta-analysis of four second-trimester amniocentesis series totalling 4953 pregnancies to women having the procedure because of a previous affected pregnancy, the DS incidence was 5.4 per 1000 higher than that expected from the maternal-age distribution.[3] In an unpublished study of more than 2500 women who had first-trimester invasive prenatal diagnosis for the same reason, the excess risk was 7.5 per 1000 (Kypros Nicolaides, personal communication). A meta-analysis of 433 livebirths had 5 recurrences, an excess risk of 5.2 per 1000.[112]

There are many reports of families in which both DS and another autosomal trisomy or a sex chromosome abnormality occur.[113–115,117,121–125] There are families that include both DS and two other types of aneuploidy, for example Edwards' syndrome and Patau's syndrome.[126] As with the DS recurrences, this association is not attributable to chance alone. The above meta-analysis also documented aneuploidies other than DS among women having an amniocentesis because of a previous trisomy 21 pregnancy, and there was an excess of 2.4 per 1000.[3] The phenomenon of double aneuploidy involving DS is well known.[1,118–120,127–133] This can be due to chance in some cases, but an analysis of data from a large national DS register found a highly statistically significant excess of 2.1 per 1000.[3]

In an attempt to explain DS recurrences, researchers have invoked either parental mosaicism or inheritance of genes that favor nondisjunction.[113–126,134] Mosaicism is rarely found in families with one affected child — under 5% of published cases[134] and although the incidence is higher in families with DS recurrence, it is still under 25%.[118] Mosaicism in gonads has also been considered to be an important etiological factor;[119,135] however, it was acknowledged that even a high percentage of trisomic cells in a mother's ovaries cannot be a complete explanation for the multiple DS recurrences.[119] Even if all the germ cells were trisomic, half of the gametes would have a normal chromosome complement. Besides, studies on preimplantation genetic diagnosis have shown that aneuploidy in oocytes and embryos is not a rare event and it increases markedly with maternal age, being the consequence of both a trisomic germ line and further disruption in meiotic division.[136] Furthermore, the occurrence of more than one type of aneuploidy in a family and double aneuploidy are unlikely to be explained by mosaicism.

Mosaicism was put forward as an alternative explanation to genetic predisposition, but they are not necessarily alternatives. The possible involvement of genetic factors has also been raised to explain the extremely high DS recurrence in women with gonadal mosaicism.[119] The fact that mosaicism can occur in successive generations[137,138] suggests a familial tendency toward mitotic non-disjunction that can reflect general abnormalities in the genetic control of non-disjunction. Moreover, mosaicism itself requires explanation: we believe that it is not the initial cause but rather the consequence of the same factors that can lead to non-disjunction of chromosomes in meiosis. Taking all these considerations together, genetic predisposition to both events cannot be excluded.

The possibility of genes predisposing to non-disjunction in humans was suggested in numerous studies (for a review see reference 139). The finding of increased DS incidence in highly inbred populations has led to the hypothesis that autosomal recessive genes are involved in the genetic control of non-disjunction.[140] However, there is no evidence for this or for any other form of nuclear inheritance. Nevertheless, the fact that there is familial aggregation that cannot be accounted for by chance strongly favors some form of inheritance.

Studies of families with either two DS cases with regular trisomy 21 or one DS and another aneuploidy in which there were different reproductive partners in the parental or grand-parental generation suggests the inheritance of a cytoplasmic factor. Seven pedigrees were analyzed from such families referred to two regional genetics centers.[3] Four families had recurrences of trisomy 21, and three had combinations of more than one type of aneuploidy, including Edwards' and Turner's syndromes, and in every pedigree the recurrence was on the maternal side. In the literature there are six case reports of half-siblings born to the same mother but different fathers where one has DS and the other either has DS or a different aneuploidy and only one report of affected half-siblings to the same father and different mothers, but this was in a highly inbred population (see citations in Ref. 3).

There are three reports of familial DS where the origin of the additional chromosome 21 can be traced between generations, and they too support inheritance of a cytoplasmic factor. In one family the father of a child with DS had twin siblings with DS.[118] He was the source (meiosis II) of the extra chromosome in his child, and it was identical to that in his mother, which was duplicated (meiosis I) in the twins. In a similar study the mother of the child with DS had a sister with DS, and the extra chromosome 21 (meiosis I) that she passed to her child was identical to that in her mother which was duplicated in her affected sister.[116] In the third family a brother and sister both had children with DS; they were each the origin of the extra chromosome (paternal meiosis II and maternal meiosis I), and they had inherited it from their mother.[118] Thus the pattern of inheritance in all these families with DS recurrence or concurrence of more one type of aneuploidy fits a cytoplasmic inheritance.

An intriguing aspect of DS, which although obvious has not been emphasised in the literature, is that there are features in common between the pathogenesis and etiology of the disorder. The effect of age is present both in the DS individuals and in maternal meiotic non-disjunction. Similarly, diseases associated with DS, such as AD, diabetes, and autoimmune disease, are relatively common in affected families. The involvement of mtDNA mutations in both the etiology and pathogenesis of the syndrome can explain the similarities between the origin and manifestation including oxidative stress in DS.

7. Conclusions

Although oxidative damage is a well described and established phenomenon in DS individuals, it is unlikely to be explained by chromosome 21 gene-dosage effects, and there are convincing data of mitochondrial dysfunction being the cause of oxidative stress. It is likely that mtDNA mutations are involved in both the etiology of non-disjunction and the pathogenesis of DS. This concept opens up a new area of research into aneuploidy.

References

1. Mutton D, Alberman E, Hook EB. *J. Med. Genet.* 33: 387–394 (1996).
2. Cuckle HS, Wald NJ, Thompson SG. *Br. J. Obstet. Gynaecol.* 94: 387–402 (1987).
3. Arbuzova S, Cuckle H, Mueller R, Sehmi I. *Clin. Genet.* 60: 456–462 (2001).
4. Schupf N, Kapell D, Lee JH, Ottman R, Mayeux R. *Lancet* 344: 353–356 (1994).
5. Narchi H, Kulaylat N. *Arch. Dis. Child.* 77: 242–244 (1997).
6. Hassold T, Sherman S. *Clin. Genet.* 57: 95–100 (2000).
7. Avramopoulos D, Mikkelsen M, Vassilopoulos D, Grigoriadou M, Petersen MB. *Lancet* 347: 862–865 (1996).
8. Petersen MB, Karadima G, Samaritaki M, Avramopoulos D, Vassilopoulos D, Mikkelsen M. *Am. J. Med. Genet.* 93(5): 366–372 (2000).
9. James SJ, Pogribna M, Pogribny IP, Melnyk S, Hine RJ, Gibson JB, Yi P, Tafoya DL, Swenson DH, Wilson VL, Gaylor DW. *Am. J. Clin. Nutr.* 70(4): 495–501 (1999).
10. Hobbs CA, Sherman SL, Yi P, Hopkins SE, Torfs CP, Hine RJ, Pogribna M, Rozen R, James SJ. *Am. J. Hum. Genet.* 67(3): 623–630 (2000).
11. Petersen MB, Grigoriadou M, Mikkelsen M. *Am. J. Hum. Genet.* 69(Suppl) 323 (2001).
12. Chadefaux-Vekemans B, Coude M, Muller F, Oury JF, Chabli A, Jais J, Kamoun P. *Pediatr. Res.* 51(6): 766–767 (2002).
13. O'Leary VB, Parle-McDermott A, Molloy AM, Kirke PN, Johnson Z, Conley M, Scott JM, Mills JL. *Am. J. Med. Genet.* 107(2): 151–155 (2002).
14. Stuppia L, Gatta V, Gaspari AR, Antonucci I, Morizio E, Calabrese G, Palka G. *Eur. J. Hum. Genet.* 10(6): 388–390 (2002).
15. Shapiro BL. *J. Neural. Transm. Suppl.* 57: 41–60 (1999).
16. Brooksbank BW, Balazs R. *Brain Res.* 318(1): 37–44 (1984).
17. Jovanovic SV, Clements D, MacLeod K. *Free Radic. Biol. Med.* 25(9): 1044–1048 (1998).
18. Busciglio J, Yankner BA. *Nature* 378(6559) 776–779 (1995).
19. Pueschel SM, Craig WY, Haddow JE. *J. Intellect. Disabil. Res.* 36: 365–369 (1992).
20. Zitnanova I, Korytar P, Aruoma OI, Sustrova M, Garaiova I, Muchova J, Kalnovicova T, Pueschel S, Durackova Z. *Clin. Chim Acta.* 341(1–2): 139–146 (2004).
21. Nagyova A, Sustrova M, Raslova K. *Physiol. Res.* 49(2): 227–231 (2000).

22. Pueschel SM, Pueschel JK. (eds.) *Biomedical Concerns in Persons with Down Syndrome.* Paul H Brookers Publishing Co., Baltimore, 1992, pp. 159–259.
23. Pastore A, Tozzi G, Gaeta LM, Giannotti A, Bertini E, Federici G, Digilio MC, Piemonte F, *J. Pediatr.* 142(5): 583–585 (2003).
24. Anneren KG, Epstein CJ. *Pediatr. Res.* 21(1): 88–92 (1987).
25. Bras A, Monteiro C, Rueff J. *Ophthalmic Paediatr. Genet.* 10(4): 271–277 (1989).
26. Odetti P, Angelini G, Dapino D, Zaccheo D, Garibaldi S, Dagna-Bricarelli F, Piombo G, Perry G, Smith M, Traverso N, Tabaton M. *Biochem. Biophys. Res. Commun.* 243(3): 849–851 (1998).
27. Nunomura A, Perry G, Pappolla MA, Friedland RP, Hirai K, Chiba S, Smith MA. *J. Neuropathol. Exp. Neurol.* 59(11): 1011–1017 (2000).
28. Behar TN, Colton CA. *Free Radic. Biol. Med.* 35(6): 566–575 (2003).
29. Yates CM, Simpson J, Gordon A, Maloney AF, Allison Y, Ritchie IM, Urquhart A. *Brain Res.* 280(1): 119–126 (1983).
30. Godridge H, Reynolds GP, Czudek C, Calcutt NA, Benton M. *J. Neurol. Neurosurg. Psychiatr.* 50(6): 775–778 (1987).
31. Capone GT. *J. Dev. Behav. Pediatr.* 22(1): 40–59 (2001).
32. Hermon M, Cairns N, Egly JM, Fery A, Labudova O, Lubec G, *Neurosci. Lett.* 251(1): 45–48 (1998).
33. Colton CA, Yao JB, Gilbert D, Oster-Granite ML. *Brain Res.* 519(1–2): 236–242 (1990).
34. Stabel-Burow J, Kleu A, Schuchmann S, Heinemann U. *Brain Res.* 765(2): 313–318 (1997).
35. Iannello RC, Crack PJ, de Haan JB, Kola I. *J. Neural. Transm. Suppl.* 57: 257–267 (1999).
36. Sinet PM. *Ann. NY Acad. Sci.* 396: 83–94 (1982).
37. Feaster WW, Kwok LW, Epstein CJ. *Am. J. Hum. Genet.* 29: 563–570 (1977).
38. De La Torre R, Casado A, Lopez-Fernandez E, Carrascosa D, Ramires V, Saez J. *Experientia* 52(9): 871–873 (1996).
39. Jeziorowska A, Jakubowski L, Lach J, Kaluzewski B. *Clin. Genet.* 33(1): 11–19 (1988).
40. Teksen F, Sayli BS, Aydin A, Sayal A, Isimer A. *Biol. Trace Elem. Res.* 63(2): 123–127 (1998).
41. Gulesserian T, Engidawork E, Fountoulakis M, Lubec G. *J. Neural Transm.* 61(Suppl): 71–84 (2001).
42. Baeteman MA, Mattei MG, Baret A, Mattei JF. *Acta. Paediatr. Scand.* 73(3): 341–344 (1984).

43. Kimura H, Nakano M. *FEBS Lett.* 239(2): 347–350 (1988).
44. Porstmann T, Wietschke R, Schmechta H, Grunow R, Porstmann B, Bleiber R, Pergande M, Stachat S, von Baehr R. *Clin. Chim. Acta.* 171(1): 1–10 (1988).
45. Elroy-Stein O, Bernstein Y, Groner Y. *EMBO J.* 5: 615–622 (1986).
46. Bar-Peled O, Korkotian E, Segal M, Groner Y. *Proc. Natl. Acad. Sci. USA* 93: 8530–8535 (1996).
47. Chan PH. *J. Neurotrauma.* 9: 417–423 (1992).
48. Chan PH, Chu L, Chen SF, Carlson EJ, Epstein CJ. *Stroke* 21: 80–82 (1990).
49. Schwartz PJ, Coyle JT. *Synapse* 29(3): 206–212 (1998).
50. Przedborski S, Kostic V, Jackson-Lewis V, Naini AB, Simonetti S, Fahn S, Carlson E, Epstein CJ, Cadet JL. *J. Neurosci.* 12(5): 1658–1667 (1992).
51. Elroy-Stein O, Groner Y. *Cell* 52: 259–267 (1988).
52. Schwartz PJ, Berger UV, Coyle JT. *J. Neurochem.* 65(2): 660–669 (1995).
53. Ault B, Caviedes P, Hidalgo J, Epstein CJ, Rapoport SI. *Brain Res.* 497(1): 191–194 (1989).
54. Fridovich I. *Adv. Enzymol. Relat. Areas Mol. Biol.* 58: 61–97 (1986).
55. Nicotera TM, Notaro J, Notaro S, Schumer J, Sandberg AA. *Cancer Res.* 49(19): 5239–5243 (1989).
56. Zemlan FP, Thienhaus OJ, Bosmann HB. *Brain Res.* 476(1): 160–162 (1989).
57. Serra JA, Famulari AL, Kohan S, Marschoff ER, Dominguez RO, de Lustig ES. *J. Neurol. Sci.* 122(2): 179–188 (1994).
58. Arbuzova S. *Cytol. Genet.* 30(B2): 25–34 (1996) (in Russian).
59. Arbuzova S. *Down's Syndr. Res. Pract.* 5(3): 26–29 (1998).
60. Percy ME, Dalton AJ, Markovic VD, McLachlan DR, Hammel JT, Rusk AC, Andrews DF. *Am. J. Med. Genet.* 35(4): 459–467 (1990).
61. Neve J, Sinet PM, Molle L, Nicole A. *Clin. Chim. Acta.* 133(2): 209–214 (1983).
62. Kadrabova J, Madaric A, Sustrova M, Ginter E. *Biol. Trace Elem. Res.* 54(3): 201–206 (1996).
63. Behl C, Davis JB, Lesley R, Schubert D. *Cell* 77: 817–827 (1994).
64. Hensley K, Carney JM, Mattson MP, Aksenova M, Harris M, Wu JF, Floyd RA, Butterfield DA. *Proc. Natl. Acad. Sci. USA* 91(8): 3270–3274 (1994).
65. Mattson MP, Cheng B, Davis D, Bryant K, Lieberburg I, Rydel RE. *J. Neurosci.* 12(2): 376–389 (1992).
66. Loo DT, Copani A, Pike CJ, Whittemore ER, Walencewicz AJ, Cotman CW. *Proc. Natl. Acad. Sci. USA* 90(17): 7951–7955 (1993).

67. Mark RJ, Pang Z, Geddes JW, Uchida K, Mattson MP. *J. Neurosci.* 17(3): 1046–1054 (1997).
68. Teller JK, Russo C, DeBusk LM, Angelini G, Zaccheo D, Dagna-Bricarelli F, Scartezzini P, Bertolini S, Mann DM, Tabaton M, Gambetti P. *Nat. Med.* 2(1): 93–95 (1996).
69. Iwatsubo T, Mann DMA, Odaka A, Suzuki N, Ihara Y. *Ann. Neurol.* 37: 294–299 (1995).
70. Lemere CA, Blusztajn JK, Yamaguchi H, Wisniewski T, Saido TC, Selkoe DJ. *Neurobiol. Dis.* 3(1): 16–32 (1996).
71. Mann DMA. *Mech. Ageing Dev.* 43: 99–136 (1988).
72. Di Luca M, Pastorino L, Cattabeni F, Zanardi R, Scarone S, Racagni G, Smeraldi E, Perez J. *Arch. Neurol.* 53(11): 1162–1166 (1996).
73. Govoni S, Bergamaschi S, Gasparini L, Quaglia S, Racchi M, Cattaneo E, Binetti G, Bianchetti A, Giovetti F, Battaini F, Trabucchi M. *Neurology* 47(4): 1069–1075 (1996).
74. Urakami K, Kataoka J, Okade A, Isoe K, Wakutani Y, Ji Y, Adach Y, Ohno K, Takahashi K. *Dementia* 7(2): 82–85 (1996).
75. Tokuda T, Fukushima T, Ikeda S, Sekijima Y, Shoji S, Yanagisawa N, Tamaoka A. *Ann. Neurol.* 41(2): 271–273 (1997).
76. McLean CA, Cherny RA, Fraser FW, Fuller SJ, Smith MJ, Beyreuther K, Bush AI, Masters CL. *Ann. Neurol.* 46(6): 860–866 (1999).
77. Lauderback M, Hackett JM, Huang FF, Keller JN, Szwerda LI, Markesbery WR, Butterfield DA. *J. Neurochem.* 78(2): 413–416 (2001).
78. Li S, Mallory M, Alford M, Tanaka S, Masliah E. *J. Neuropathol. Exp. Neurol.* 56(8): 901–911 (1997).
79. Masliah E, Alford M, Mallory M, Roskenstein E, Moechars D, Van Leuven F. *Exp. Neurol.* 163(2): 381–387 (2000).
80. Simpson MD, Slater P, Cross AJ, Mann DM, Royston MC, Deakin JF, Reynolds GP. *Brain Res.* 484(1–2): 273–278 (1989).
81. Warner HR. *Free Radic. Biol. Med.* 17(3): 249–258 (1994).
82. Fridovich I. *Ann. NY Acad. Sci.* 893: 13–18 (1999).
83. Almagor M, Kahane I, Yatziv S. *J. Clin. Invest.* 73(3): 842–847 (1984).
84. Kinouchi H, Epstein CJ, Mizui T, Carlson E, Chen SF, Chan PH. *Proc. Natl. Acad. Sci. USA* 88: 11158–11162 (1991).
85. Huang T, Carlson EJ, Leadon SA, Epstein CJ. *FASEB J.* 6: 903–910 (1992).
86. Busciglio J, Pelsman A, Wong C, Pigina G, Yuan M, Mori H, Yanker BA. *Neuron* 33: 677–688 (2002).
87. Pappolla MA, Chyan YJ, Omar RA, Hsiao K, Perry G, Smith MA, Bozner P. *Am. J. Pathol.* 152(4): 871–877 (1998).

88. Smith MA, Hirai K, Hsiao K, Pappolla MA, Harris PL, Siedlak SL, Tabaton M, Perry G. *J. Neurochem.* 70(5): 2212–2215 (1998).
89. Hsiao K, Chapman P, Nilsen S, Eckman C, Harigaya Y, Younkin S, Yang F, Cole G. *Science* 274(5284): 99–102 (1996).
90. Pelsman A, Hoyo-Vadillo C, Gudasheva TA, Seredenin SB, Ostrovskaya RU, Busciglio J. *Int. J. Dev. Neurosci.* 21(3): 117–124 (2003).
91. Korenberg JR, Kawashima H, Pulst SM, Ikeuchi T, Ogasawara N, Yamamoto K, Schonberg SA, West R, Allen L, Magenis E *et al. Am. J. Hum. Genet.* 47(2): 236–246 (1990).
92. Pellissier MC, Laffage M, Philip N, Passage E, Mattei MG, Mattei JF. *Hum. Genet.* 80(3): 277–281 (1988).
93. Sanij E, Hatzistavrou T, Hertzog P, Kola I, Wolvetang EJ. *Biochem. Biophys. Res. Commun.* 287: 1003–1008 (2001).
94. Wallace DC. *Science* 283(5407): 1482–1488 (1999).
95. Arbuzova S, Hutchin T, Cuckle H. *DSNews* 7(2): 27 (2000).
96. Michikawa Y, Mazzucchelli F, Bresolin N, Scarlato G, Attardi G. *Science* 286(5440): 774–779 (1999).
97. Del Bo R, Comi GP, Perini MP, Strazzer S, Bresolin N, Scarlato G. *Ann. Neurol.* 49(1): 137–138 (2001).
98. Prince J, Jia S, Bave U, Anneren G, Oreland L. *J. Neural. Transm. Park. Dis. Dement. Sect.* 8(3): 171–181 (1994).
99. Druzhyna N, Nair RG, LeDoux SP, Wilson GL. *Mutat. Res.* 409(2): 81–89 (1998).
100. Krapfenbauer K, Engidawork E, Cairns N, Fountoulakis M, Lubec G. *Brain Res.* 967: 152–160 (2003).
101. Capone G, Kim P, Jovanovich S, Payne L, Freund L, Welch K, Miller E, Trush M. *Life Sci.* 70: 2885–2895 (2002).
102. Schuchmann S, Heinemann U. *Free Radic. Biol. Med.* 28(2): 235–250 (2000).
103. Gaulden ME. *Mutat. Res.* 296(1–2): 69–88 (1992).
104. Arbuzova S. *Cytol. Genet.* 29(B3): 77–80 (1995). (In Russian.)
105. Schon EA, Kim SH, Ferriera JC, Magalhaes P, Grace M, Warburton D, Gross SJ. *Hum. Redrod.* 15(Suppl.): 160–172 (2000).
106. Strick TR, Croquette V, Bensimon D. *Nature* 404(6780): 901–904 (2000).
107. Schar P, Herrman G, Daly G, Lindahl T. *Genes Dev.* 11(15): 1912–1924 (1997).
108. Keefe DL, Niven-Fairchild T, Powell S, Buradagunta S. *Fertil. Steril.* 64(B3): 577–583 (1995).
109. Marchington DR, Scott Brown MS, Lamb VK, van Golde RJ, Kremer JA, Tuerlings JH, Mariman EC, Balen AH, Poulton J. *Mol. Hum. Reprod.* 8(11): 1046–1049 (2002).

110. Wallace DC. *J. Bioenerg. Biomembr.* 26: 241–250 (1994).
111. Beerman F, Hummler E, Franke U, Hansmann I. *Hum. Genet.* 79(4): 338–340 (1988).
112. Hook EB. Chromosomal abnormalities: prevalence risks and recurrence. In: Brock DJH, Rodeck CH, Ferguson-Smith MA (eds). *Prenatal Diagnosis and Screening*. Churchill Livingstone, Edinburgh, 1992, pp. 351–392.
113. Mikkelsen M, Stene J. Previous child with Down syndrome and other chromosome aberration. In: Murken J, Stengel-Rutkowski S, Schwinger EW (eds.). *Prenatal Diagnosis. Proceedings of the Third European Conference on Prenatal Diagnosis of Genetic Disorders.* Enke, Stuttgart, 1979, pp. 22–29.
114. Stene J, Stene E, Mikkelsen M. *Prenat. Diagn.* 4: 81–95 (1984).
115. Uehara S, Yaegashi N, Maeda T, Hoshi N, Fujimoto S, Fujimori K, Yanagida K, Yamanaka M, Hirahara F, Yajima A. *J. Obstet. Gynaecol. Res.* 25(6): 373–379 (1999).
116. Stinissen P, Van Roy B, Van Camp G, Backhovens H, Partoens P, Wehnert A, Verniers H, Dumon J, Vandenberghe A, Van Broeckhoven C. *Am. J. Med. Genet. Suppl.* 7: 133–136 (1990).
117. Krishna Murthy DS, Farag TI. *Ann Genet.* 38(4): 217–224 (1995).
118. Pangalos CG, Conover Talbot C, Lewis JG, Adelsberger PA, Petersen MB, Serre J-L, Rethore M-O, de Blois M-C, Parent P, Schinzel AA, Binkert F, Boue J, Corbin E, Croquette MF, Gilgenkrantz S, de Grouchy J, Bertheas MF, Prieur M, Raoul O, Serville F, Siffroi JP, Thepot F, Lejeune J, Antonarakis SE. *Am. J. Hum. Genet.* 51: 1015–1027 (1992).
119. Nielsen KG, Poulsen H, Mikkelsen M, Steuber E. *Hum. Genet.* 78: 103–105 (1988).
120. James RS, Ellis K, Pettay D, Jacobs PA. *Eur. J. Hum. Genet.* 6(3): 207–212 (1998).
121. Medical Research Council of Canada. *Diagnosis of Genetic Disease by Amniocentesis during the Second Trimester of Pregnancy. A Canadian Study.* Report No. 5, Supply Services, Ottawa, 1977.
122. Hecht F, Bryant JS, Gruber D, Townes PL. *New Engl. J. Med.* 271: 1081–1086 (1964).
123. Wright SW, Day RW, Mosier HD, Koons A, Mueller H. *J. Pediatr*. 62: 217–224 (1963).
124. Benirschke K, Brownhill L, Hoefnagel D, Allen FH. *Cytogenetics* 1: 75–89 (1962).
125. David TJ, Jones AJ. *Humangenetik* 27: 351–352 (1975).
126. FitzPatrick DR, Boyd E. *Hum. Genet.* 82: 301 (1989).
127. Wilson MG, Fujimoto A, Alfi OS. *J. Med. Genet.* 11(1): 96–101 (1974).
128. Reddy KS. *Hum. Genet.* 101: 339–345 (1997).

129. Van Buggenhout GJCM, Hamel BCJ, Trommelen JCM, Mieloo H, Smeets DFCM. *J. Med. Genet.* 31: 807–810 (1994).
130. Park VM, Bravo RR, Shulman LP. *J. Med. Genet.* 32(8): 650–653 (1995).
131. Ikonen RS, Lindlof M, Janas MO, Simola KO, Millington-Ward A, de la Chapelle A. *Hum. Genet.* 83(3): 235–238 (1989).
132. Chen CP, Chern SR, Yeh LF, Chen WL, Chen LF, Wang W. *Prenat. Diagn.* 20(9): 750–753 (2000).
133. Lorda-Sanchez I, Petersen MB, Binkert F, Maechler M, Schmid W, Adelsberger PA, Antonarakis SE, Schinzel AA. *Hum. Genet.* 87(1): 54–56 (1991).
134. Uchida IA, Freeman VC. *Hum. Genet.* 70(3): 246–248: (1985).
135. Tseng L-H, Huang S-M, Lee T-Y, Ko T-M. *Arch. Gynecol. Obstet.* 255: 213–216 (1994).
136. Munne S, Cohen J. *Hum. Reprod.* 4(6): 842–855 (1998).
137. Parke JC, Grass FS, Pixley R, Deal J. *J. Med. Genet.* 17: 48–49 (1980).
138. Werner W, Herrmann FH, John B. *Hum. Genet.* 60: 202–204 (1982).
139. Hook EB. In: de la Cruz FF, Gerald PS (eds.). *Trisomy 21 (Down Syndrome) Research Perspectives*, NICHD Mental Retardation Research Centres Series. University Park Press, Baltimore, 1981, pp. 3–69.
140. Alfi OS, Chang R, Azen SP. *Am. J. Hum. Genet.* 32: 477–483 (1980).

19 Oxidative Stress and Ulcerative Colitis: Experimental Evidence and Implications for Treatment

Darren N. Seril, Jie Liao, Guang-Yu Yang, and Chung S. Yang

1. Approaches to Studying Oxidative Stress in Ulcerative Colitis

Much of the evidence implicating oxidative stress in the pathogenesis of Ulcerative Colitis (UC) has come from studies on biopsy and colectomy samples obtained from UC patients. A combination of endoscopic, histologic, biochemical, and immunochemical approaches have revealed correlations between reactive oxygen species (ROS) and reactive nitrogen species (RNS) production by human tissue samples and clinical and histological parameters of disease activity. In addition, experimental models of colon inflammation, in which colitis arises spontaneously or by treatment with cytotoxic chemicals in animals, have provided invaluable insights into the role of oxidative stress and oxidant-producing cells in the pathogenesis of UC, as well as the potential usefulness of treatments targeting oxidative stress.

The most relevant animal model of UC is that of spontaneous colitis in monkeys, which resembles human UC endoscopically and histologically, responds to clinical treatments, and exhibits similar complications and systemic manifestations.[1] However, the use of primates in the study of UC is limited by animal availability and the long time-course of disease progression. The genetic and chemically induced models of intestinal inflammation in rodents have become the systems of choice, despite their own limitations, because of their ready availability, rapid disease development, and potential for genetic manipulation.[1] Among the genetic models, the interleukin (Il)-2-deficient mouse develops colitis that most closely resembles human UC,[2] whereas the Il-10 knockout mouse develops colitis manifesting a mixture of the qualities of UC and Crohn's disease.[3] Transgenic rats bearing the human major histocompatibility complex antigen, HLA-B27, develop colitis spontaneously.[4] The chemically induced models are the most widely used, and the most common of these is trinitrobenzene sulfonic acid (TNBS)-induced colitis in rodents. TNBS forms hapten/protein complexes, leading to a T-cell or macrophage response and histology similar to inflammatory bowel disease (IBD). In contrast, the acetic acid model is based on direct irritation of the colonic epithelium, leading to short-lived ulceration and inflammation.[5] Colitis induced by sulfated polysaccharides bears many histological similarities to human IBD, although the mechanism of action is unclear. Dextran sulfate sodium (DSS), a synthetic, sulfated polysaccharide, induces colitis in rodents, which is clinically and histologically reminiscent of human UC, possibly due to altered colonic microflora or macrophage activity, or direct toxicity to crypt cells.[6–8] DSS is administered orally, and so can be conveniently used to study acute and chronic UC.[8,9] Like human UC, DSS-induced colitis is strongly influenced by background genetics.[10] These genetic and chemically induced models, studied in combination with specific genetic deficiencies, antioxidants, and pharmacological enzyme inhibitors, have proved useful in studying the mechanisms and treatment of UC.

2. UC and Oxidative Stress

2.1. *Mucosal inflammation: the role of lamina propria leukocytes*

UC is characterized by large infiltrates of inflammatory cells into the colonic mucosa: the lamina propria of UC patients is populated by a mixture of neutrophils, eosinophils, mast cells, macrophages, and lymphocytes. B lymphocyte and T lymphocyte (CD4+ and CD8+) activities are increased in UC patients.[11] Indeed, T-cell dysfunction and an abnormal cell-mediated immune response may drive the persistent colonic inflammation seen in UC patients.[12–14] Cell mediators of innate immunity are involved as well. Myeloperoxidase (MPO) is a lysosomal enzyme present predominately in the azurophilic granules of neutrophils, and, to a lesser extent, in eosinophils and monocytes. MPO activity, which is used as an index of neutrophil infiltration, is elevated in mucosal samples from UC patients and correlates with disease activity.[15] Isolated circulating neutrophils from active UC patients have been reported to exhibit increased oxidant production compared to those from non-UC individuals, with further elevations during disease flare-ups.[16] However, others have shown that circulating neutrophils from UC patients actually have decreased oxidative burst activity in response to triggers *in vitro* as compared to healthy individuals.[17,18] In addition to neutrophils, monocyte activity is increased in UC patients.[17,18] Mucosal mononuclear cells from IBD patients exhibit a significantly higher respiratory burst activity compared to those of normal controls with or without activation by triggers, including interferon (IFN)-γ and lipopolysaccharide (LPS). This activity was shown to increase from non-inflamed IBD samples to "minimally" inflamed samples, and the percentage of cells with elevated respiratory burst activity increased in response to cytokines and other triggers as well.[19]

Phagocytic leukocytes carry out the destruction of foreign organisms through the release of cytotoxic oxygen metabolites and lysosomal enzymes.[20–22] Activated neutrophils and macrophages reduce oxygen to the superoxide anion via the oxidization of nicotinamide-adenine dinucleotide phosphate (NADPH) by the NADPH oxidase complex. The spontaneous or enzyme-catalyzed dismutation of superoxide yields hydrogen peroxide (H_2O_2), which may result in the generation of highly reactive molecules. MPO catalyzes the conversion of H_2O_2 to hypochlorous acid, which takes part in halogenation and oxidation reactions. The reduction of H_2O_2 via the iron-catalyzed fenton reaction yields the hydroxyl radical. Both cell types, especially macrophages, also express inducible nitric oxide synthase (iNOS), a cytokine inducible enzyme that catalyzes the reduction of L-arginine to L-citrulline, with the release of nitric oxide (NO). NO is a free radical gas and signal transduction second messenger, and participates in the anti-microbial actions of leukocytes as well. The product of the reaction of NO with the superoxide anion is peroxynitrite, a stable molecule with reactivity similar to the hydroxyl radical.[23]

Regardless of their relative activity levels, activated neutrophils and macrophages are present in large numbers in the inflamed UC mucosa, closely apposed to the colonic glands and within the crypts themselves. As will be discussed in the next two sections, ROS and RNS overproduction in the colonic mucosa is characteristic of UC. A large proportion of these reactive molecules are likely derived from activated mucosal leukocytes.

2.2. *UC and the production of reactive oxygen species*

The results of several studies on tissue samples from UC patients have indicated that the overproduction of ROS is a hallmark of UC. Measuring oxidant production by luminol-amplified chemiluminescence, Simmonds *et al.* detected significantly increased oxidant levels in UC biopsies as compared to samples from normal patients. Chemiluminescence was correlated with endoscopic and microscopic grades of UC, as well as with MPO activity, implicating neutrophil-generated oxidants. Indeed, the MPO inhibitor sodium azide significantly reduced chemiluminescence produced by UC biopsies in this study; catalase and dimethylsulfoxide (DMSO, a hydroxyl radical scavenger) had smaller but significant effects.[24] Lih-Brody *et al.* detected a 20-fold increase in chemiluminescence in UC mucosal biopsies from areas of active inflammation, but not in non-inflamed UC biopsies, suggesting an association between the level of oxidant production and disease activity.[25]

Studying mucosal biopsies from UC patients, Kruidenier *et al.* found that the levels of malondialdehyde (MDA), a lipid peroxidation product, are elevated in the inflamed mucosa of UC patients. Schiff staining for lipid peroxides was present in luminal epithelial cells in inflamed mucosa, but absent in the lamina propria and in the morphologically normal mucosa of normal control patients. Bivariate and multiple linear regression analysis showed that the increased MDA levels were associated with catalase levels and MPO activity, suggesting that this membrane damage is mediated by ROS elaborated by infiltrating neutrophils.[26] Inflamed biopsies from UC patients also exhibit increases in markers of protein oxidation (protein carbonyls) and oxidative DNA modification (8-hydroxydeoxyguanosine, 8-OHdG).[27] The mucosal levels of 8-OHdG were more than two-fold higher in UC patients than in normal controls.[28] The levels of 8-OHdG were elevated in peripheral blood leukocytes from UC patients versus controls, suggestive of increased oxidative burst activity. 8-OHdG levels in this study were dependent on treatment, being lower in patients treated with a combination of 5-aminosalicylic acid (5-ASA) plus a corticosteroid versus those treated with 5-ASA alone. However, there was no difference in the levels of this DNA oxidation marker between active UC patients and patients in remission.[27] The colons of UC patients have also shown a two-fold increase in mucosal iron,[25] possibly due to local hemorrhaging, hemolysis, and breakdown of iron-containing proteins.[29] Iron catalyzes the production of the highly reactive hydroxyl radical, which reacts with DNA to form 8-OHdG residues *in vitro*.

Excessive ROS production is also a feature of the animal models of colitis. DSS-induced colitis is associated with increases in mucosal MDA[30] and DSS-dose dependent increases in 8-OHdG levels.[31] Urinary output of 8-OHdG was increased four- to five-fold after DSS treatment in rats, and approximately 3.5-fold after TNBS treatment. Urinary 8-OHdG levels correlated with MPO activity and neutrophil recruitment in both models, and were significantly diminished by inhibition of neutrophil recruitment using an anti-PMN antibody.[32] DSS treatment in mice had no effect on protein carbonyl levels in the colon, but increased the carbonyl content of specific proteins, as assayed by Western blot detection of dinitrophenyl hydrazine-modified proteins.[33] Loguercio *et al.* observed large increases in colonic mucosal lipoperoxide (~40-fold) and MDA (greater than 100-fold) just 1 h after TNBS treatment in rats. The increase in lipid peroxidation products preceded the peak of histological severity, which occurred at week 1.[34] Numerous studies have also been performed in animal models assessing the effectiveness of radical scavengers, antioxidant enzymes, and pro-oxidant enzyme inhibitors on the severity of colitis (see the sections on colitis treatments targeting oxidative stress and colitis pathogenesis for a discussion of these studies).

2.3. *The role of nitric oxide in UC*

Nitric oxide (NO), a free radical gas, serves as a cell signaling molecule but can also give rise to reactive species that can damage cellular constituents. The cytochrome P450-like enzyme nitric oxide synthase (NOS) catalyzes the seven electron reduction of L-arginine that yields NO and L-citrulline. Three isoforms of NOS have been characterized to date. The neuronal and endothelial enzymes (nNOS and eNOS, respectively) are calcium-dependent, producing low levels of NO that appear to serve signal transduction functions. The third isoform (iNOS), in contrast, is calcium-independent and cytokine inducible. Inducible NOS was first detected in macrophages, where it serves an anti-microbial role by the production of cytotoxic levels of NO.[35]

NO was increased 100-fold in colonic luminal gas from UC patients compared to controls, and was increased in inflamed and uninflamed areas. Treatment with salicylates, or salicylates plus corticosteroids, had no impact on luminal NO levels.[36] Herulf *et al.* measured NO levels in rectal gas samples obtained with a balloon catheter. Chemiluminescence of NO was increased greater than 10-fold in samples from patients with active UC versus inactive UC patients and controls.[37] Rachmilewitz *et al.*, using an NO electrode method, detected a more modest two-fold increase in colonic levels of the NO end-products nitrite and nitrate (NO_x) in active UC patients versus patients in remission or normal controls. NO_x levels correlated with NOS activity in mucosal biopsies, as well as with indices of clinical and endoscopic disease activity.[38] In a study by Kimura *et al.*, the plasma levels of NO_x were increased two-fold in patients with active UC versus those with UC in remission or normal controls.[39] In another study, the serum levels of NO_x were significantly elevated in UC patients with active inflammation versus inactive UC, independent of the proximal extension of the disease (e.g., total versus left-sided disease). The nitrate levels were positively correlated with indices of active inflammation, including leukocyte count.[40] Mucosal NO_x levels have been found to increase from control samples to samples from UC patients with inactive disease, to those with active disease of mild, moderate, and severe intensity.[41] Rachmilewitz *et al.*, using organ explant cultures of colonic mucosa from biopsy specimens, reported a four-fold increase in nitrate levels in samples from UC patients compared to normal controls. Nitrate generation was inhibited by the L-arginine analog, N^{ω}-nitro-L-arginine. Mucosal NOS activity, which was nearly undetectable in normal mucosa, was greatly elevated in explants from UC biopsies.[42]

NOS activity, measured by the conversion of radiolabeled L-arginine to L-citrulline, has been shown to be elevated in mucosal biopsy specimens from UC patients.[39,43,44] The NOS activity in UC mucosa was increased eight-fold compared to normal control mucosa in a study by Boughton-Smith *et al.* Incubation with the NOS inhibitor N^{ω}-monomethyl-L-arginine (L-NMMA) *in vitro* eliminated NOS activity. The NOS activity in the mucosa of UC biopsies was only partially decreased by the calcium chelator EGTA, indicating that the enzyme activity was largely attributable to the calcium-independent, inducible NOS isoform.[43] Godkin *et al.* reported a 50-fold increase in calcium-independent citrulline formation in UC biopsies, indicative of iNOS activity.[44] Colonic mucosa NOS activity increased in samples from patients in remission to those with active disease, as well as from morphologically normal mucosa to inflamed mucosa. NOS activity correlated positively with serum NO_x levels and with endoscopic and histological grades of UC.[39]

Immunohistochemical staining using an antibody specific for the inducible isoform showed that iNOS is expressed in lamina propria inflammatory cells and colonic epithelial cells.[44] Immunohistochemistry of colectomy samples showed iNOS staining in mononuclear cells at the base of ulcers in regions of active inflammation. Inducible NOS was also localized in epithelial cells and fibroblasts in ulcerated regions. Few iNOS-positive cells were present in normal mucosa. The number of iNOS-expressing mucosal cells increased from inactive to active UC, and fewer positive cells were observed in infectious and ischemic forms of colitis.[45] Dijkstra *et al.* detected increased immunohistochemical expression of iNOS in UC biopsies, predominately in epithelial cells in inflamed mucosa with fewer lamina propria cells staining positive. In contrast, eNOS staining was only observed in vascular endothelial cells.[45,46] In IBD patients, unstimulated monocytes express iNOS, and the percentage of iNOS-positive monocytes detected by flow cytometry was significantly increased (but there was no correlation with disease activity, and no difference in monocyte activation observed between normal controls and IBD patients).[46] Immunostaining for nitrotyrosine, a marker of NO-mediated protein modification, was observed in lamina propria inflammatory cells and occasionally surface epithelia in inflamed mucosa, and increased with disease activity.[47] Dijksta *et al.* detected nitrotyrosine in CD15-positive monocytes but not in epithelial cells.[48] Keshavarzian *et al.* reported that protein nitration, detected by anti-nitrotyrosine slot blotting, correlated with NO_x levels, and increased in mucosal samples from control patients to UC patients with inactive disease, to patients with active disease. Interestingly, this study also found correlations among protein carbonylation, NO_x levels, and protein nitration.[41]

The studies on NO using tissue samples from UC patients have been complemented by numerous studies in animal models. For example, like human UC, colitis in the rhesus macaque is associated with induction of iNOS and increased plasma NO_x levels.[49] The chemically induced and genetic rodent models also exhibit increases in iNOS expression in the colonic mucosa. Further mechanistic studies of the role of NO in rodent colitis have employed pharmacological NOS inhibitors, NO-generating agents, and mice genetically deficient in NOS isoforms. Depending on the study, the NOS inhibitors have been shown to improve, worsen, or have no effect on colitis in these models (see the next section on colitis treatments targeting oxidative stress for a fuller discussion of the NOS inhibitors). Increasing NO levels through the use of NO-generating compounds seems to have an ameliorative effect. Surprisingly, as with the NOS inhibitors, the studies examining the susceptibility of iNOS knockout (iNOS −/−) mice to experimental colitis have yielded mixed results as well.

The administration of L-arginine in the drinking fluid two days before TNBS in rats significantly increased macroscopic damage nearly two-fold, concomitant with increases in plasma NO_x (1.5-fold), TBARS (1.4-fold), and GSH content (1.6-fold). Administration of the NOS inhibitor, N-ω-nitro-L-arginine methyl ester (L-NAME) in the drinking water reversed the effects of L-arginine.[50] In the TNBS model, iNOS (−/−) mice lack expression of the iNOS protein in surface epithelial cells or lamina propria inflammatory cells.[51,52] The iNOS knockout mouse has also shown a four-fold decrease in plasma NO_x, and a two- to three-fold reduction in nitrotyrosine staining in apical epithelia, damaged epithelia, and inflammatory cells in this model. In the study by Zingarelli *et al.*, TNBS-treated iNOS (−/−) mice showed improved 7-day survival, decreased microscopic colonic damage, and two-fold lower mucosal MDA levels as compared to wild-type mice.[52] In another study, iNOS (−/−) mice were more susceptible to colonic damage at early time-points, showing significantly elevated macroscopic damage and MPO activity 1–3 days after TNBS, but no difference from controls after 7 days.[51] In the acetic acid-induced model, iNOS mRNA levels were elevated 1–3 days after colitis induction. However, iNOS (–/–) mice showed significantly increased macroscopic and microscopic colonic damage and delayed mucosal healing 7 days after acetic acid treatment.[53] In the Il-10 gene knockout mouse, iNOS mRNA and protein expression are increased compared to wild-type mice, and plasma NO_x levels are persistently elevated three- to nine-fold.[54] Double gene knockout mice lacking both Il-10 and the iNOS gene showed a six- to nine-fold decrease in macroscopic colonic damage and plasma NO_x compared to mice lacking Il-10 only. However, iNOS gene deficiency had no effect on histological colitis grade or MPO activity.[54]

DSS-treated mice have shown increased immunohistochemical expression of iNOS in surface epithelia and lamina propria inflammatory cells, as well as elevated serum NO_x and mucosal nitrotyrosine staining.[55,56] Lack of iNOS expression ameliorated colitis in studies using the DSS model, decreasing disease severity and increasing survival concomitant with decreases in MPO activity, serum NO_x, and nitrotyrosine staining.[55–57] We have observed that the administration of two-fold iron-supplemented diet can affect the susceptibility of iNOS knockout mice to DSS-induced colitis. In our study, consistent with the results of other investigators, iNOS-deficient mice administered DSS and a control diet containing the normal level of iron exhibited decreased histological inflammation scores as compared to wild-type mice. However, iNOS knockout mice fed two-fold iron-enriched diet showed no difference in DSS-induced colitis compared to wild-type mice given the same diet (unpublished data). Thus, the enhancement of ROS production in the presence of iron may compensate for the lack of iNOS gene expression.

The continuous intracolonic infusion of 1 mg/kg/day sodium nitroprusside (SNP), an NO donor, decreased TNBS-induced macroscopic mucosal damage and MPO activity by greater than 50%, while increasing NO levels in colonic luminal contents by greater than two-fold.[58] The effects of SNP were partially reversed by treatment with hemoglobin, which binds NO with high affinity. Similarly, the daily subcutaneous administration of DETA/NO (1 mg/kg), another NO donor, to DSS-treated mice increased plasma NO_x levels but decreased colitis-associated weight loss, colon weight, and MPO activity. These effects may have been mediated by inhibition of inflammatory cell infiltration or activity: DETA/NO significantly reduced vascular adhesion molecule expression and leukocyte rolling and adhesion by 50%, and decreased pro-inflammatory cytokine mRNA levels as well.[59] In contrast to the effects of NO donors, the intrarectal administration of peroxynitrite (the stable product of the reaction of NO with the superoxide anion) induced acute injury and inflammation in rats in a dose-dependent manner. Peroxynitrite-induced colitis is associated with increases in mucosal NOS activity, NO_x production, and MPO activity.[60]

The conflicting reports on the effects of iNOS deficiency on TNBS-induced colitis[51,52] may reflect on the complex roles of NO in inflammation and the maintenance of gut integrity. NO produced by phagocytic leukocytes is cytotoxic. However, iNOS activity may also take part in the resolution of inflammation by inhibiting inflammatory cell infiltration and fostering wound healing.[61,62] Indeed, the ameliorative effects of the NO donors, SNP and NO-DETA, in the TNBS and DSS models may be examples of the ulcer healing and anti-inflammatory effects of NO.[58] Thus, depending on the time point after the induction of TNBS colitis that is assessed, iNOS deficiency may appear to have differing effects. The presence or absence of luminal pathogens, affected by the conditions under which the experimental animals are housed, has also been suggested to influence the outcome in the iNOS knockout mouse.[57] Our results indicate that the presence or absence of iron can also impact the susceptibility of iNOS-deficient mice to chemically induced colitis.

2.4. *Antioxidant capacity*

Cells utilize several enzymatic and non-enzymatic activities to control potentially cytotoxic reactive side-products of respiration. These include antioxidant vitamins, and enzymes such as superoxide dismutase, catalase, and glutathione peroxidase. Based on the data from UC tissue samples, many of these antioxidant defenses are upregulated in UC patients, or reduced (presumably due to the presence of increased amounts of ROS and RNS) compared to individuals without UC. Plasma levels of lipid-soluble antioxidants, including retinol, α-tocopherol, and β-carotene, and total carotenoids, are frequently decreased in UC patients. Many of these nutrients showed a decrease during the transition from disease remission to active disease.[27] These depletions are likely a result of a combination of increased oxidant formation, malabsorption, and loss, and decreased intake.[63] Buffinton *et al.* measured total aqueous radical scavenging capacity in inflamed and non-inflamed biopsies from UC patients by the inhibition of peroxyl radical-mediated phycoerythrin damage. Radical scavenging capacity was significantly decreased in inflamed versus non-inflamed samples, and was increased in samples from healed mucosa. Mucosal levels of urate and ubiquinol-10 were significantly depleted in inflamed UC mucosa, but α-tocopherol was unchanged in the study by Buffinton *et al.*[64]

Decreased levels of GSH and total glutathione in UC biopsies versus normal controls have been observed and associated with UC disease activity.[64,65] Oxidized glutathione (GSSG) levels were increased in actively inflamed UC samples compared to inactive UC and normal controls, and GSSG levels in active UC were positively correlated with the UC disease activity index, composed of both sigmoidoscopy and histology scores. The GSH/GSSG ratio was decreased in actively inflamed UC, and inversely correlated with the disease index. Importantly, the positive correlation between disease activity and mucosal GSSG content was maintained in a longitudinal study: GSSG levels were decreased during inactive disease periods, but increased during active disease flare-ups (the GSH/GSSG ratio exhibited the opposite trend). GSSG levels also correlated with the extent of neutrophil infiltration.[65] In a study using biopsies from 24 UC patients before and after treatment with a steroid and an aminosalicylate, mucosal levels of reduced glutathione were increased and oxidized glutathione decreased at follow-up.[66] In patients undergoing colectomy, the plasma levels of cysteine and total thiols were significantly decreased prior to surgery as compared to normal individuals, and the levels were inversely correlated with UC disease activity. In contrast, the glutathione precursors, glutamate and glycine, were significantly increased prior to surgery. All of these parameters returned to control levels after surgery.[67] McKenzie *et al.* isolated colonic epithelial crypts from inflamed UC biopsies and found that reduced thiols were depleted as compared to normal controls. The thiols of the enzyme glyceraldehyde-3-phosphate dehydrogenase (GAPDH) were consistently oxidized in these samples, and correlated with decreased GAPDH activity. Further, *in vitro* studies on normal isolated colonic crypt epithelial cells showed that among oxidants formed in the inflamed colon, the hypochlorite ion was the most potent *in vitro* thiol oxidizer, followed by chloramines T, hydrogen peroxide, and nitric oxide.[68]

In the colons of rats treated with TNBS, mucosal GSH levels increased to a maximum value 14 days after colitis induction (greater than 10-fold increase), then decreased to values below that of controls after 4 weeks,[34] suggestive of an initial response to increased ROS and RNS production followed by depletion. Nieto *et al.* described a significant decrease (25–50%) in the levels of reduced glutathione in the colonic mucosa of TNBS-treated rats.[69] Togashi *et al.* used the spin clearance rate of a stable nitroxide radical as a measure of the levels of thiol compounds, in the colons of TNBS-treated mice. The reduction in spin clearance mirrored the reduction in GSH levels (−75% versus non-TNBS controls) and macroscopic damage scores.[70] Increasing concentrations of DNBS administration in rats increased colonic damage and decreased GSH levels (−30 to 80%) dose-dependently. DNBS also decreased the content of low molecular weight antioxidants in the colonic mucosa (25–70%) in a dose-dependent manner.[71] A study using the DSS model in mice showed a non-significant decrease in mucosal total thiols (−13%) compared to non-treated mice.[33]

Among the antioxidant enzymes, catalase activity was found to be increased in the inflamed mucosa of UC patients, more so than in non-inflamed UC mucosa. Catalase expression was increased in non-inflamed and inflamed epithelium and in the lamina propria.[72] Glutathione peroxidase (GPx) activity was increased in UC mucosa as well, as were total glutathione levels. However, the numbers of GPx-positive cells in inflamed epithelium were decreased compared to non-inflamed epithelium and normal control tissue. Similarly, the antioxidant enzyme metallothionein was decreased in inflamed epithelium.[72] In a study by Krudenier *et al.*, manganese (Mn)-SOD protein levels were increased in epithelia and inflammatory cells in non-inflamed (two-fold) and inflamed (2.5-fold) mucosa from UC patients, but there was no change in Mn-SOD activity, as compared to normal controls. Copper/zinc (Cu/Zn)-SOD levels were increased 25% in non-inflamed mucosa, but unchanged in inflamed mucosa. Extracellular (EC)-SOD was decreased in inflamed mucosa.[73] Deficiencies for selenium and zinc may compromise the functions of antioxidant enzymes like Cu/Zn-SOD and GPx. In a study of 24 UC patients, plasma selenium was reduced by 33% in patients with disease of moderate severity; GPx activity was decreased as well. In the inflamed mucosa, zinc levels were decreased compared to controls, as were metallothionein levels, but GPx was increased.[74] However, Rannem *et al.*, in a study of 40 UC patients, reported that decreased plasma or erythrocyte levels of selenium and GPx were rare, and likely due to malabsorption and malnutrition.[75]

In TNBS-treated rats, studies have shown both decreased and increased SOD activity following the induction of colitis.[34,69,76] In a study by Seo *et al.*, SOD activity was decreased more than 50%, and the protein levels of Mn-SOD and Cu/Zn-SOD were decreased about 70%.[76] In contrast, the mucosal SOD activity increased to a peak 1 week after TNBS, and then declined to control values.[34] The mucosal levels of SOD were increased greater than two-fold as compared to control rats after 2 weeks in the study by Nieto *et al.* Enzymes of the glutathione antioxidant system (γ-glutamyltranspeptidase, GPx, glutathione reductase, glutathione transferase) and catalase were also elevated.[69] Similar to UC patients, colon levels of zinc and selenium are decreased compared in the acetic acid and TNBS models.[77] The activity of the inducible form of heme oxygenase, expressed by epithelia, endothelia, and inflammatory cells, is significantly increased in TNBS-treated rats. Inhibition of heme oxygenase by tin mesoporphyrin (s.c. 3 h before TNBS) increased mucosal lesion area and luminol-amplified chemiluminescence.[78]

In the DSS model in mice, the colonic activities of Mn-SOD, catalase, and GPx were elevated.[79] SOD activity was increased 50% after one DSS cycle, and 80% after two cycles.[30] The 5- to 10-fold overexpression of human Cu/Zn-SOD in hSOD1-Tg transgenic mice had no effect on DSS-induced disease activity, although it did increase survival in one study.[79] Conversely, the three-fold overexpression of Cu/Zn-SOD in a study by Krieglstein *et al.* was associated with increased disease activity indices (1.5-fold) in DSS-treated mice, as well as increased histological damage (1.33-fold) and MPO activity (1.7-fold).[57] DSS-treated mice showed 50% increases in plasma GPx activity and extracellular GPx protein levels after 7 days of treatment. In contrast, colonic E-GPx protein decreased about 30%, and cytoplasmic GPx increased 40%, by day 7.[80] Interestingly, mice lacking both the Gpx1 gene and the gastrointestinal epithelium-specific GPx (Gpx2) gene develop colitis spontaneously, whereas mice lacking either gene alone do not.[81]

3. Targeting Oxidative Stress in the Study and Treatment of UC

The clinical management of UC currently utilizes a combination of aminosalicylates (sulfasalazine and related drugs), corticosteroids, and immunosuppressive agents (e.g., cyclosporine). Typically, depending on the severity of acute UC flare-ups, one or a combination of the above therapies is used to induce disease remission. The maintenance of remission requires long-term treatment, most commonly with the active moiety of sulfasalazine, 5-ASA. However, non-responsiveness to treatment, toxicity, and opportunistic infection can make the use of these drugs problematic. Many newer therapies are being explored in the treatment of UC, including anti-tumor necrosis factor antibodies (e.g., Infliximab), nicotine, heparin, and probiotics, as well as antibiotics.[82] All of these approaches have shown only modest benefits to UC patients, however, and are usually no more effective than the current mainstays of therapy. The inhibition of oxidative stress via radical scavenging actions or inhibition of ROS generation may be effective strategies for treating UC. Indeed, the aminosalicylates are thought to function, at least, in part, via anti-oxidative mechanisms. Natural compounds with antioxidant actions and specific enzyme inhibitors may be useful either alone or in combination with established therapies for the amelioration of UC. The therapeutic efficacies of several such agents have been assessed, predominately in rodent model systems (see Table 1). At the same time, these agents have served as tools for further assessing the role of oxidative stress in UC.

3.1. *Antioxidant activity of aminosalicylates*

The aminosalicylate sulfasalazine, 5-ASA, and sulfapyridine react with the superoxide radical, the hydroxyl radical, and the hypochlorite anion. All of these agents provide protection from oxidant-induced deoxyribose degradation at physiological concentrations *in vitro*, but this effect appears to be due to scavenging of HOCl rather than the hydroxyl radical.[83] In UC patients, the therapeutic effect of sulfasalazine correlates with reduced MDA levels in colonic mucosal biopsies.[84] Sulfasalazine also inhibited NO_x formation by a macrophage cell line, possibly by reducing the expression

Table 1. Effects of agents targeting oxidative stress on UC and experimental colitis.

Agent	System/dose/route	Effects	Ref.
Vitamin E	Clinical; 480 IU, p.o.	↑ Serum α-tocopherol (three-fold), no effect on disease activity	93
	TNBS, rats; 0.025% (~25 mg/kg), p.o.	↓ Macro damage (40%), MPO activity	91
	DSS, rats 49 mg/kg, p.o.	↓ Inflammation score w/iron (35%), crypt scores (25%), plasma 8-isoprostane (30%), no effect on lipid peroxides	92
Vitamin E + selenium	TNBS, rats; 30 mg/kg, i.p.	α-Tocopherol: ↓ MDA, protein carbonyls; Combo: ↓ macro damage, MDA, protein carbonyls	90
Retinol	TNBS, rats; ~1.5 mg/kg, p.o.	↓ Inflammation and fibrosis, MDA (45%)	94
NAC	Acetic acid, rats; 40,100 mg/ml (~4, 10 g/kg), p.o.	↓ Macro damage (45–85%), MPO (70–85%), vascular permeability (55%)	95
	TNBS, rats; 40 mM (~650 mg/kg), p.o.	↓ Macro damage (50%) ↑ GSH (>two-fold), γGCS (four-fold)	97
	DSS, mice 200 mg/kg, p.o.	↓ Chronic inflammation area (17%), N-Tyr and iNOS-positive cell number (50% and 33%)	98
WR-2721	Acetic acid, rats 200 mg/kg, i.p. 100–300 mg/kg, i.r.	i.p.: ↓ Inflammation score (~45%), chemiluminescence (50%); i.r.: no effect	99
Mesna	TNBS, rats 360 mg/kg, i.r.	↓ Chronic macro and micro damage (75%), acute MPO (80%); ↑ iNOS mRNA (60%)	100
Tea catechins	TNBS, rats 0.5% catechin mix (~3250 mg/kg), p.o.	↓ Macro damage (60%), MPO (55%); TBARS no change; ↑ colonic α-tocopherol (40%)	91
Green tea polyphenols	Il-2 (−/−) mouse 5 g/L (~500 mg/kg), p.o.	↓ Micro damage (40%), colon wt (40%), serum amyloid A (75%)	102
Thearubigens	TNBS, mice 40–100 mg/kg, i.g.	↓ Macro damage (50–60%), colon wt (50%), NO_x (60%), superoxide (50%), MDA(60%)	103
Curcumin	TNBS, mice ~2000–5000 mg/kg, p.o.	↓ Histological alteration, weight loss, NFκB activation	106

Table 1. (*Continued*).

Agent	System/dose/route	Effects	Ref.
	TNBS, mice 50–300 mg/kg, i.g.	↓ Macro (40%) and micro damage (40–50%), NO_x (50%), superoxide (50%), MDA (50–60%), iNOS mRNA (45%), NFκB activation	107
	DNBS, mice ∼250 mg/kg, p.o.	↓ Macro (40%) and micro (40–50%) damage, MPO (80%), NFκB activation	108
Paepalantine	TNBS, rats 5–25 mg/kg, i.g.	↓ Acute (12%) and chronic (50–66%) macro damage, NOS activity (40%); ↑ GSH (1.4-fold)	109
Ellagic acid	DSS, rats 10,100 mg/kg, p.o.	↓ Macro damage (80–85%), MPO (non-sig), TBARS (50%); ↑ colon length (1.3–1.5-fold)	115
Resveratrol	TNBS, rats 10 mg/kg, i.g.	↓ Macro damage (55%), MPO (30%) ↑ epithelial apoptosis (1.5-fold)	112
Lycopene	TNBS, rats ∼1.5 mg/kg, p.o.	↓ Area of inflammation (70%), MPO (65%)	113
β-Carotene	TNBS, rats ∼1.5 mg/kg, p.o.	↓ Area of inflammation (non-significant)	113
Zerumbone	DSS, mice 0.1% (∼1000 mg/kg), p.o.	↓ Inflammation score (45%), ulceration (33%), edema (60%); ↑ regenerative change (three-fold)	114
Quercetin	TNBS, rats 1 or 5 mg/kg, p.o.	No effect on macro damage; ↓ MDA (50%), NOS activity (25%); ↑ water absorption capacity	116
Baicalein	DSS, mice 20 mg/kg, p.o.	↓ Macro damage (50%), IFNγ (25%)	117
Morin	TNBS, rats 2 mg/kg, p.o.	↓ Macro (12–20%), micro (20–75%) damage, MPO (20–40%), iNOS act (50%), MDA (25%)	118
Rutoside	TNBS, rats 10–25 mg/kg, i.g.	↓ Acute (15–20%) and chronic (40–50%) macro damage, MPO (30%); ↑ GSH (30–66%)	119
DA-6034	Acetic acid, rats 2–6 mg/kg, p.o.	↓ Lesion area (50–70%)	153
	TNBS, rats 1–3 mg/kg, p.o.	↓ Acute, chronic lesion score (33–50%)	
	HLA-B27 rat 6 mg/kg, p.o.	↓ Micro lesion (60%)	

Table 1. (*Continued*).

Agent	System/dose/route	Effects	Ref.
Compound A	TNBS, rats 0.6 mmol/kg (∼140 mg/kg), i.v.	↓ Extent of damage (80%), serum TNFα (80%)	120
Trimetazidine	Acetic acid, rats 5 mg/kg, i.p. or i.r.	↓ Macro damage (40%, i.p.), MPO (85%, i.p. and i.r.), NO_x (non-sig); SOD act (60%, i.r.)	121
	TNBS, rats ∼150 mg/kg, i.p. or i.r.	No effect on macro, micro damage, MPO, GSH (i.p. and i.r.); ↓ MDA (66%, i.p.); ↑ MDA (2x, i.r.)	122
Zolimid	Acetic acid, rats 200–400 mg/kg, i.g. or i.r.	i.r.: ↓ Macro (40–60%), micro (40%) damage, MPO i.g.: ↓ macro (40%), micro (40%) damage, MPO	123
AEOL11201	Acetic acid, rats 5 mg/kg, i.p.	↓ Macro (80%), micro (50%) damage, MPO (90%)	123
Rebamipide	TNBS, rats 50 mg/kg, i.p. +50 mg/kg, i.r.	↓ Macro, micro damage (50%), Gpx activity (25%), MPO; ↑ GST, Cu/Zn-SOD act (1.3-fold)	126
	Acetic acid, rats 30 mg/kg, p.o.	↓ Lesion score (60%), TBARS (25%); no effect on MPO; ↑ GSH (1.5-fold), SOD act	125
Stobadine	TNBS, rats 10 or 20 mg/kg, intracolonic	↓ Macro damage (50–70%), MPO (40–75%), vascular permeability (45–66%); ↑ GSH (1.5-fold)	127
TEMPOL	TNBS, rats 500 mg/kg, i.g, i.r.	↓ Lesion area (70%), MPO (70%), no effect on colon weight, LTB_4, LTC_4	129
	Acetic acid, rats 0.1–0.75 g/kg, i.g.	↓ Lesion area (60–85%), MPO (70%); no effect on colon weight, LTB_4, LTC_4	129
Deferoxamine	Acetic acid, rats 50 mg/kg, i.m.	↑ Inflammation (non-sig)	131
SOD	Acetic acid, rats 15,000 U/kg, i.p.	↓ Inflammation score (50%)	131
	TNBS, rats 30,000 U/kg, s.c.	↓ Acute and chronic macro damage (33, 75%), chemi-luminescence (non-significant)	132
	DSS, mice 30,000 U/kg, i.r.	↓ Macro damage (60%); ↑ colon length (40%)	115
M40403	TNBS, rats 5 mg/kg, i.p.	↓ Macro damage (50%), MDA (50%), MPO (45%), TNF-α, N-tyr	133

Table 1. (*Continued*).

Agent	System/dose/route	Effects	Ref.
PEG: catalase/bovine catalase	Acetic acid, rats 100,000 U/kg PEG: catalase + 300 mg/kg bovine catalase, i.p.	↓ Inflammation score (33%), chemiluminescence (70%)	99
Catalase	TNBS, rats 400,000 U/kg, s.c.	↓ Acute and chronic macro damage (50, 80%), micro damage (50%), chemiluminescence (non-significant)	132
CuDIPS	Acetic acid, rats 80 mg/kg, p.o.	↓ Micro inflammation score (25%), chemiluminescence (75%)	99
Allopurinol + sulfasalazine	Clinical 200 mg/day, p.o.	↓ WBC count, erythrocyte sedimentation rate, relapse rate	134
Allopurinol + 5-ASA	Clinical 200 mg/day, p.o.	↓ Relapse rate	135
Allopurinol	Acetic acid, rats oral	↓ Inflammation score (40%), XO activity (98%)	131
Oxypurinol	TNBS, rats 25 mg/kg, p.o.	↓ Inflammation (non-quantitative), TBARS (30%)	136
Aminoguanidine	TNBS, rats 1.5 μmol/kg (~0.2 mg/kg), p.o.	↓ Macro, micro damage (33%), ulcera area (60%), MPO, NO_x (20%); no effect on iNOS activity	139
	TNBS, rats 500, 2500 mg/l (~50, 250 mg/kg), p.o.	No effect on macro damage; ↑ weight loss (1.4-fold); ↓ citrulline levels (50–75%)	140
	TNBS, rats ~200 mg/kg, p.o.	↑ Acute macro damage (1.3–1.8-fold), acute MPO (1.7-fold); ↓ serum NO_x (70%)	141
	HLA-B27 rats 52 μmol/kg (~6 mg/kg), p.o.	↓ Mucosal permeability (50%) and thickness (33%), crypt depth (33%), MPO (50–60%), NO_x (33%)	142
L-NAME	Acetic acid + capsaicin, rats 0.1 mg/ml (~10 mg/kg), p.o.	↓ Lesion area (60%), LTB_4 (33%), LTC_4 (60%), colonic NO_x (>95%), NOS activity (60%)	143
	TNBS, rats 30 mg/kg, p.o.	↓ Lesion area (30–55%), MPO (30–70%), NOS activity (15–50%)	143
	TNBS, rats 40 mg/kg, s.c. inject or minipump	Inject: ↑ acute lesion area (1.7–2.5-fold); ↓ MPO pump: ↓ lesion area, ulcer (20–30%, low dose); ↑ lesion area, ulcer (1.2–2-fold, high dose)	144

Table 1. (*Continued*).

Agent	System/dose/route	Effects	Ref.
	TNBS, rats 100 μg/ml (~10 mg/kg, p.o (before TNBS) or p.o. + i.g. (after TNBS)	Before TNBS: ↑ macro damage (25–33%), iNOS activity (two-fold); after TNBS: ↓ macro damage (25–45%), lesion area (25–50%), iNOS activity (50–60%), MPO	145
L-NAME	TNBS, rats 500 mg/l (~50 mg/kg), p.o.	No effect on macro damage; ↑ weight loss (two-fold) ↓ citrulline levels (75%)	140
	TNBS, rats 500 mg/l (~50 mg/kg), p.o.	No effect on macro damage ↓ NO_x (40%), TBARS (30%)	50
	TNBS, rats 35 mg/kg, s.c.	No effect on damage area ratio, distal colon weight, MPO	146
	HLA-B27 rats 45 μmol/kg (~12 mg/kg), p.o.	↑ Mucosal permeability (two-fold); crypt depth (33%); ↓ MPO (50–60%), serum NO_x (50%)	142
L-NMMA	TNBS, rats 50 mg/kg, i.p.	Early: ↑ chronic macro damage (1.3-fold), late: no effect on macro damage	147
1400W	TNBS, rats 5 or 10 mg/kg, s.c.	↓ Damage area ratio (33%), distal colon weight (33–60%), MPO (60%)	146
	TNBS, rats 2 mg/kg, i.p.	↓ Chronic macro damage (40–50%), acute MPO (50%), acute iNOS activity (50–66%), mucosal NO_x (33–50%)	148
	DSS, mice 10 mg/kg/h, s.c.	↓ Disease activity index (40–66%), microscopic damage (45%), MPO activity (50%)	157
L-NIL	TNBS, rats 10 mg/kg, i.p.	↓ MPO (50%), iNOS activity (90%), N-Tyr cell no. (80%), apoptotic cell no. (80%), apoptotic/N-tyr cell no. (90%)	150
MEG	TNBS, rats 20 mg/kg, i.v.	↓ Macro damage (60%), MPO (33%), iNOS and N-Tyr IHC	151
ONO-1714	DSS, mice 0.03–3 mg/kg, i.p.	↑ Weight gain, colon length; ↓ MPO (70–80%), TBARS (40–50%), serum (40%) and luminal (80–90%) NO_x, iNOS mRNA, epithelial N-Tyr IHC	152

Abbreviations: i.g., intragastric; i.v., intravenous; p.o., per os (oral); s.c., subcutaneous; U, units; IHC, immunohistochemistry; IU, international units; macro or micro damage, macroscopic or microscopic (histologic) mucosal damage score; MDA, malondialdehyde; MPO, myeloperoxidase activity; N-Tyr, nitrotyrosine; TBARS, thiobarbituric acid reactive substance. Estimates of doses are given as ~mg/kg for comparison purposes. Estimates were for a 200 g rat consuming 20 g diet/day or 20 ml drinking fluid/day, or a 20 g mouse consuming 2 g diet/day or 2 ml drinking fluid/day.

of iNOS. 5-ASA and sulfapyridine are much less potent suppressors of NO_x levels.[85] Other studies indicate that 5-ASA is the active antioxidant moiety of sulfasalazine. 5-ASA has been shown to rapidly reduce the free radical 1,1-diphenyl-2,2-picryhydrazyl (DPPHL) *in vitro*, and is a more potent DPPHL scavenger than α-tocopherol and ascorbate. However, sulfasalazine and sulfapyridine, as well as acetylated 5-ASA, do not reduce DPPHL.[86] 5-ASA has been shown to inhibit superoxide radical production, and scavenges the hydroxyl radical and hypochlorite anion.[87] 5-ASA dose-dependently inhibits neutrophil-mediated cell lysis and HOCl production,[88] and has been shown to inhibit nitrite formation from SNP.[89] Exposure of 5-ASA to ROS *in vitro* yields 5-ASA oxidation products, many of which are also detectable in fecal extracts from UC patients treated with sulfasalazine, but are absent in extracts from rheumatoid arthritis patients treated with sulfasalazine.[84]

3.2. *Antioxidant vitamins*

Antioxidant vitamins are deficient in UC patients, and supplementation of these agents has shown potential applicability in the management of UC based on results in animal models. The lipid-soluble vitamin α-tocopherol, administered by intraperitoneal injection (30 mg/kg) decreased MDA levels and protein carbonyl content in the colons of TNBS-treated rats.[90] Selenium, which has been found to be deficient in UC patients and is required for the activity of Gpx, was ineffective in the same study when administered alone via the drinking water, but the combination of α-tocopherol and selenium significantly decreased lipid and protein oxidation, as well colonic mucosal XO activity and macroscopic damage.[90] Dietary supplementation of 0.025% (~25 mg/kg) α-tocopherol (five times the basal level) decreased TNBS-induced macroscopic damage by 40%, as well as mucosal MPO activity, in the study by Sato *et al.*[91] In the DSS model in rats, feeding with a diet supplemented with α-tocopherol (49 mg/kg) partially reversed increases in crypt inflammation and plasma 8-isoprostane levels induced by dietary iron supplementation, but had no effect on increases in lipid peroxides.[92] However, the oral administration of α-tocopherol (480 international units per day) for 14 days was minimally effective in decreasing clinical and endoscopic disease activity in UC patients, despite a three-fold rise in serum α-tocopherol levels.[93] Reifen *et al.* examined the effect of retinol (vitamin A)-deficient diet, as well as retinol supplementation, on TNBS colitis in rats. Rats fed retinol-deficient diet for 7 weeks exhibited significantly reduced serum, colon, and liver retinol levels. Colonic NF-κB activation was increased and MDA levels were elevated two-fold following TNBS treatment compared to animals fed the retinol-sufficient diet. Conversely, retinol supplementation (~1.5 mg/kg) decreased TNBS-induced inflammation and fibrosis, as well as MDA levels (45%).[94]

3.3. *Thiol compounds*

The water-soluble antioxidant, *N*-acetyl L-cysteine (NAC), attenuated acetic acid-induced acute colitis in rats, with inhibitory effects on MPO activity, vascular permeability, and severity of colonic damage.[95] NAC is a GSH precursor, and has also shown direct radical scavenging activity.[96] Similar to the observations in UC patients, acetic acid-induced colitis is associated with a reduction in GSH levels, which is remedied by NAC treatment.[95] The administration of 40 mM (~650 mg/kg) NAC in the drinking water 4 h after TNBS reduced microscopic mucosa damage approximately 50%, and mucosal increased GSH (two-fold) and γ-GCS levels (four-fold).[97] In our study, dietary administration of 200 mg/kg NAC had a mild inhibitory effect on chronic colitis induced by long-term, cyclic DSS administration (15 DSS cycles) and enhanced by dietary iron supplementation. Interestingly, NAC significantly decreased colitis-associated colorectal carcinoma development in this model, and also decreased the numbers of lamina propria nitrotyrosine and iNOS immunostain-positive cells (~50%).[98] The thiol agent *S*-2-(3-aminopropylamino)ethylphosphorothiotic acid (WR-2721) administered by intraperitoneal injection or intrarectally had no effect on acetic acid-induced colitis, despite a 50% reduction in luminol-enhanced chemiluminescence *in vitro*.[99] Intrarectal administration of mesna (2-mercaptoethane sulfonate, 360 mg/kg), decreased iNOS message levels (60%), but increased MPO activity by 80% at early time-points after TNBS administration. However, mesna reduced macroscopic damage by 75% as compared to controls 14 days after TNBS.[100]

3.4. *Plant-derived compounds*

Many naturally occurring compounds, including food and plant components, exhibit antioxidant activities and may be useful non-toxic alternatives or supplements to UC therapy. The components of tea (*Camellia sinensis*) have received much attention as potential cancer chemopreventive agents based on epidemiological data and anti-cancer effects in animal models. Tea is rich in polyphenolic compounds (catechins) and flavonols, which are *in vitro* scavengers of ROS and RNS, including the superoxide anion, the hydroxyl radical, the peroxyl radical, nitric oxide, and peroxynitrite.[101] A mixture of tea catechins (including 46% epigallocatechin 3-gallate by weight) has been shown to ameliorate TNBS-induced colitis in rats. Dietary administration of the catechin mixture reduced colonic MPO activity and decreased TNBS-induced macroscopic damage by 60% after 7 days.[91] Varilek *et al.* reported that an extract of green tea polyphenols reduced clinical and histological parameters of colitis in the Il-2 knockout mouse model. Consumption of the polyphenol extract in the drinking water for 6 weeks significantly decreased the levels of serum amyloid A, which correlates with the severity of colitis in that model. These disease-inhibitory effects were also associated with reduced production of pro-inflammatory cytokines by colon tissue explant cultures and isolated lamina propria lymphocytes, but no parameters of oxidative stress were measured.[102] Thearubigens, accounting for approximately 20% of the dry weight of black tea extract, have shown an inhibitory effect on TNBS-induced colitis in mice. Daily intragastric administration of 40–100 mg/kg thearubigens starting 10 days before and continuing 8 days after TNBS treatment reduced colonic macroscopic damage, decreased spleen and liver weight, and reduced colitis-associated weight loss. Thearubigens also reduced MPO activity, reduced colonic NO_x (50–60%) and superoxide anion production (50%), and decreased colonic MDA levels (60%).[103]

Another natural compound that has been widely studied in the chemoprevention field is curcumin (diferuloyl methane), a component of the spice turmeric (derived from the root, *Curcuma longa*) that gives curry its characteristic yellow color. Curcumin is an *in vitro* inhibitor of iNOS and cyclooxygenase-2 expression,[104,105] and has radical scavenging capacity most likely due to its β-diketone structure and phenolic groups.

Diet containing 2–5% curcumin (~2000–5000 mg/kg) was effective in inhibiting weight loss, histological alteration, and pro-inflammatory transcription factor NF-κB activation in mice when given before or after TNBS administration.[106] Ukil *et al.*, also studying TNBS colitis in mice, observed significant decreases in macroscopic and microscopic colonic mucosal damage and colon weight with curcumin administered intragastrically (50–300 mg/kg). Curcumin also reduced tissue NO_x (50%) and iNOS mRNA levels, superoxide anion levels (50%) in isolated neutrophils, and tissue MDA levels (50–60%). As in the study by Sugimoto *et al.*, pro-inflammatory cytokine expression and NF-κB activation were suppressed.[107] Similar results were obtained with dinitrobenzene sulfonic acid (DNB)-induced colitis in mice: treatment with 0.25% curcumin (~250 mg/kg) in the diet for 5 days prior to intrarectal DNB instillation decreased macroscopic and microscopic colonic damage by 40–50%, and decreased MPO activity by 80%.[108]

Paepalantine, an isocoumarin (polphenolic) derived from the plant *Paepalanthus bromelioides*, is an *in vitro* DPPH radical scavenger. Administration of paepalantine by oral gavage (5–10 mg/kg) decreased chronic macroscopic colonic damage 50–66% and increased GSH content by 40% three weeks after TNBS treatment, but had little effect at earlier time points and at higher doses.[109] Resveratrol, or 3,5,4′-trihydroxy-trans-stilbene, is found in the skin of grapes and in red wines and has been shown to be an inhibitor of lipid peroxidation, as well as iNOS expression and NO production.[110,111] In the TNBS model in rats, resveratrol administered by oral gavage (10 mg/kg) before and after TNBS treatment decreased macroscopic damage by 55% and colonic MPO activity by 30%. Resveratrol also induced epithelial cell apoptosis (1.5-fold).[112] Lycopene is a carotenoid found in tomatoes that reacts with singlet oxygen, H_2O_2, and nitrogen dioxide, and suppresses lipid peroxidation. The oral administration of lycopene (300 μg/rat/day; ~1.5 mg/kg) decreased the mucosal area of inflammatory involvement (70%) and MPO activity by about 60% in the TNBS rat model.[113] Another carotenoid, β-carotene (a pro-retinol compound with radical scavenging activity), also decreased inflammatory area and MPO in the same study, but the effects did not reach statistical significance.[113]

In a study by Murakami *et al.*, zerumbone (a sesquiterpenoid found in rhizomes) decreased ulceration (33%) and edema, as well as pro-inflammatory cytokine levels, in mice subjected to short-term DSS treatment.[114] The plant phenol ellagic acid has shown anti-inflammatory and antioxidant effects in the DSS model. Oral administration of plain ellagic acid significantly reduced macroscopic damage (80–85%) and colonic MPO activity. The use of microspheres to increase colonic delivery markedly enhanced the potency of ellagic acid, with significant inhibitory effects on DSS-induced lesion area and thiobarbituric acid reactive substance (TBARS) levels (50%), a marker of lipid peroxidation.[115] Oral administration of quercitin, an antioxidant flavonoid (1 or 5 mg/kg), decreased epithelial permeability and improved water absorption capacity when administered starting 2 h before TNBS treatment. Quercetin also reduced colonic iNOS activity (25%) detected in explant culture, and MDA levels (−50%). However, quercetin had no affect on macroscopic damage scores.[116] Baicalein (a flavonoid from the root of the plant *Scutellaria baicalensis*) significantly decreased macroscopic damage 50% when administered orally (20 mg/kg) for 10 days with DSS. Two other related flavonoids, baicalin and wogonin, were ineffective in the same study.[117] Morin, a flavonoid found in figs with antioxidant and radical scavenging capabilities, showed an inhibitory effect on TNBS-induced chronic colitis. Rats given morin after TNBS administration (2 mg/kg) showed decreased macroscopic (12–20%) and microscopic damage (20–75%) after 1–4 weeks, together with decreases in MPO activity, iNOS activity (40–50%), and acute MDA levels (25%).[118]

3.5. *Synthetic antioxidants, antioxidant derivatives, and iron chelators*

Synthetic antioxidants and derivatives of natural antioxidant compounds have also shown therapeutic potential in colitis models. Rutoside, a flavonoid glycosidic derivative of quercetin, inhibits acute and chronic colitis induced by TNBS in rats. Administered via an esophageal catheter (25 mg/kg), rutoside significantly decreased macroscopic damage and MPO activity, and significantly increased GSH levels, compared to TNBS-treated controls.[119] Compound A (5-[2-hydroxy-ethylamino]-1-cyclohexyl-2-pentanone), a hydroxyl radical scavenger, attenuates TNBS-induced colitis in rats when administered intravenously at a concentration of 0.6 mmol/kg (~140 mg/kg).[120] Trimetazidine (TMZ), an anti-anginal drug that reportedly exerts its effects by inhibiting ROS-mediated membrane damage, showed inhibitory actions in the acetic acid model but was ineffective against TNBS-induced colitis. Administration of 50 mg/kg TMZ via intraperitoneal or intrarectal injection attenuated MPO activity, acute macroscopic damage (50%), and microscopic mucosal damage in acetic acid-treated rats.[121] In a study by Girgin *et al.*, intraperitoneal and intrarectal administration of TMZ (~150 mg/kg) had no effects on TNBS-induced macroscopic or microscopic colonic damage, or MPO activity, despite increased (intrarectal) or decreased (intraperitoneal) MDA levels compared to controls.[122] Choudhary *et al.* assessed the effects of zolimid (an L-histidine analog and antioxidant) and AEOL11201 (a manganese porphyrin and catalytic antioxidant) on acetic acid-induced injury in rats. Zolimid (enema and gavage) and AEOL11201 (i.p.) significantly decreased colonic MPO activity as well as macroscopic and histological disease severity.[123] Rebamipide (2-(4-chlorobenzoyl-amino)-3-[2-(1H)-quinolinon-4-yl]-propionic acid), a quinolone derivative, has been shown to significantly inhibit the respiratory burst of activated polymorphonuclear cells,[124] scavenge hydroxyl radicals, and inhibit lipid peroxidation *in vitro*. Rebamipide administered by intraperitoneal injection (50 mg/kg) and enema (50 mg/kg) 3 days before and 13 days after TNBS decreased macroscopic and microscopic indices of mucosal damage by about 50%. The oral administration of rebamipide (30 mg/kg) significantly ameliorated lesion severity (60%) and TBARS levels (25%) associated with acetic acid treatment. Rebamipide treatment was also associated with restoration of depleted GSH and α-tocopherol levels and SOD activity, in colon homogenates or isolates colonocytes.[125,126] Stobadine is a pyridoindole similar to melatonin that is known to scavenge the hydroxyl and peroxyl radicals, peroxynitrite and hypochlorite anions, and singlet oxygen. In the acetic acid model in rats, stobadine (10–20 mg/kg, i.r.) reduced macroscopic damage 50–70%, decreased MPO activity, and increased colonic GSH levels 1.5- to 1.8-fold.[127] Melatonin, itself a pyridoindole with similar scavenging activities to stobadine, has been reported to be ameliorative in the DSS murine model.[128] Treatment with TEMPOL (4-hydroxy-2,2,6,6-tetramethyl-piperidine-*N*-oxyl), a stable nitroxide radical with radical scavenging activity, has been shown to decrease colonic lesion area in rats when administered intragastrically after TNBS treatment or intrarectally with TNBS (500 mg/kg). Intragastric TEMPOL (100–750 mg/kg) has also shown an ameliorative effect on macroscopic lesion area (60–85%) when administered before acetic acid treatment.[129] Oral administration of the iron chelator, deferiprone, significantly decreased macroscopic mucosal damage, as well as MPO and NOS activities, in the acetic acid model in rats.[130] However, deferoxamine, another iron chelator, had no significant effect on inflammation in the same model when administered intramuscularly 7 days before acetic acid treatment.[131]

3.6. *Antioxidant enzymes and related compounds*

The enzymes SOD and catalase play vital roles in controlling oxidant production by cellular respiration. Together, these enzymes catalyze the disproportionation of the partially reduced oxygen species, superoxide anion, to oxygen and water. In the TNBS rat model, subcutaneous SOD injection (30,000 U/kg) prior to TNBS decreased acute macroscopic damage (24 h after TNBS) by about 33%, and decreased damage 75% after 6 days. SOD also decreased luminol-enhanced chemiluminescence in the acute and chronic stages, although not significantly.[132] Intraperitoneal injection of SOD (15,000 U/kg) decreased acetic acid-induced inflammation by 50%.[131] SOD given intrarectally (30,000 U/kg) during DSS administration reduced macroscopic damage 60%.[115] An SOD mimetic (M40403) administered by intraperitoneal injection (5 mg/kg) to rats decreased mortality by 60% and macroscopic mucosal damage by 50% when given 2 days after TNBS treatment. M40403 treatment was associated with a 50% decrease in MDA levels, as well as a marked reduction in nitrotyrosine expression by epithelial cells and inflammatory cells.[133] In a study by Keshavarzian *et al.*, a combination of PEG:catalase (100,000 U/kg, i.p.) and bovine catalase (300 mg/kg, i.p.) decreased acetic acid-induced inflammation 33%, and decreased luminol-enhanced chemiluminescence 70% *in vitro*.[99] Catalase was also effective in the TNBS model in the study by Yavuz *et al*. Catalase administered subcutaneously (400,000 U/kg) reduced acute and chronic macroscopic damage by 50 and 80%, respectively.[132] Oral copper $(II)_2(3,5\text{-}DIPS)_4$ (CuDIPS) at 40 mg/kg showed similar efficacy in the same study (25% decrease in inflammation and 75% reduction in chemiluminescence *in vitro*). CuDIPS is a lipophilic compound that may function to deliver copper to cells that can be utilized by enzymes such as Cu/Zn-SOD.[99]

3.7. *Inhibitors of pro-oxidative enzymes*

The addition of the xanthine oxidase (XO) inhibitor, allopurinol (200 mg/day orally), to a maintenance regimen of 2 g/day sulfasalazine improved the control of symptoms in patients with recurrent procto-sigmoidal UC, and also reduced the frequency of 12-month relapse (5% with allopurinol versus 25% without).[134] In a study of 199 UC patients in remission, the addition of allopurinol (200 mg/day) to 5-ASA maintenance therapy was associated with 23% relapse at 6 months versus 41% relapse in the placebo-plus-5-ASA group. Relapse at 12 months was 38% and 47%, respectively, but the difference did not reach statistical significance.[135] The administration of allopurinol (100 μg/ml) in the drinking water 7 days before acetic acid administration in rats decreased inflammation about 40% and reduced XO activity 98% *in vitro*. Two other XO inhibitors, tungsten and pterin aldehyde, had no effect on acetic acid-induced colitis, despite inhibition of XO activity by greater than 50%.[131] Oxypurinol (an oxidation product of allopurinol) administered orally (~25 mg/kg) after TNBS treatment significantly reduced colonic lipid peroxidation products by 30%.[136] Oxypurinol, like allopurinol, most likely acts via XO inhibition.

Aminoguanidine, L-NAME, and L-NMMA are considered non-selective nitric oxide synthase inhibitors.[137,138] Nakamura *et al.* assessed the effect of aminoguanidine on TNBS-induced colitis in rats. Starting 7 days after TNBS treatment and continuing for 1 week (1.5 μmol/kg, ~0.1 mg/kg) aminoguanidine decreased macroscopic and microscopic mucosal damage by one-third compared to controls, and reduced serum NO_x levels by 20%. However, aminoguanidine had no effect on colonic iNOS activity in this study.[139] In another study using the same model, aminoguanidine (500–2500 mg/l, ~50–250 mg/kg) administered in the drinking water starting 1 day before TNBS significantly reduced tissue citrulline levels (50–75%), but had no effect on macroscopic colonic damage.[140] In a study by Dikopoulos *et al.*, rats given aminoguanidine (200 mg/kg) in the drinking fluid starting 3 days before TNBS instillation showed reduced acute serum NO_x as much as 70%. However, MPO and macroscopic damage were increased by 1.3- to 1.8-fold by this relatively non-specific NOS inhibitor.[141] Three weeks treatment with 52 μmol/kg/day aminoguanidine (∼4 mg/kg) decreased plasma NO_x by 33%, mucosal thickness by 33%, colonic MPO activity by 50–60% in HLA-B27 transgenic rats.[142]

L-NAME had differing effects in the TNBS rat model depending on the time of administration and dose. Rachmilewitz *et al.* reported inhibition of TNBS-induced lesion area by L-NAME (30 mg/kg) together with a 50% reduction in NOS activity.[143] Delivery of 0.042–1.667 mg/kg/h L-NAME via subcutaneous osmotic pump for 5 days prior to TNBS instillation significantly decreased MPO activity but increased lesion area at high doses (1.2- to 2-fold). Subcutaneous administration of L-NAME in the same study also increased lesion area. However, at lower doses, pre-administration of L-NAME decreased lesion area and ulcer index (20–30%).[144] Given 48 h before TNBS, 100 μg/ml (∼10 mg/kg) L-NAME in the drinking fluid significantly increased macroscopic damage 25–33%, and increased iNOS activity two-fold. When administered 6 h after TNBS, L-NAME decreased macroscopic damage 25–45%, as well as iNOS and MPO activities.[145] In other studies, L-NAME had no effect on TNBS colitis in rats when administered subcutaneously just prior to TNBS at a concentration of 35 mg/kg,[146] at 500 mg/l (∼50 mg/kg) in the drinking water starting 1 day before TNBS,[140] or at ∼50 mg/kg in the drinking water after TNBS treatment.[50] In the latter study, L-NAME was ineffective in attenuating TNBS-induced colitis despite reducing NO_x levels 40% and TBARS levels 30%. However, similar to the results for aminoguanidine, L-NAME (∼3 mg/kg) was effective in attenuating spontaneous colitis in the HLA-B27 transgenic rat.[142] L-NAME (0.1 mg/ml, p.o.) was also inhibitory when administered for 7 days before treatment with acetic acid plus capsaicin in rats, with significant reductions in lesion area (60%), NO_x (>95%), and NOS activity (60%).[143] L-NMMA administered by intraperitoneal injection (50 mg/kg) significantly increased TNBS-induced colitis (1.3-fold) in rats in the chronic stage (day 14) when administered immediately after TNBS (days 0–4). However, L-NMMA had no effect when administered after day 4. The authors indicated that L-NMMA may have delayed the resolution of inflammation.[147] It is interesting that the effect of the non-selective NOS inhibitors, especially in the TNBS model, tended to vary based on the time of administration. Inducible NOS activity has been reported to be maximal between 1 and 7 days after the instillation of the chemical.[51] Drug administration before TNBS may have detrimental effects by inhibiting constitutive NOS isoforms, while later administration may be beneficial by inhibiting iNOS activity.

The partially iNOS-selective and iNOS-specific inhibitors[137,138] have been shown to be more effective in ameliorating experimental colitis. The potent iNOS inhibitor, *N*-[3-(aminomethyl)benzyl]acetamidine (1400W), significantly decreased MPO activity (60%) and reduced colon weight loss, as well as the area of mucosal damage (33%), when administered subcutaneously (5 or 10 mg/kg).[146] In a study by Menchen *et al.*, intraperitoneal injection of 1400W (2 mg/kg) from day 5 to day 10 after TNBS treatment reduced macroscopic mucosal damage by 40–50% in rats. In the same study, 1400W decreased tissue iNOS activity (50–66%) and mucosal NO_x (33–50%) levels at earlier time points.[148] In mucosal samples obtained from proctocolectomy samples from active UC patients, 1400W significantly reduced the production of pro-inflammatory cytokines.[149] DSS-induced colitis is also effectively inhibited by 1400W. Krieglstein *et al.* reported that the subcutaneous administration of 1400W (10 mg/kg/h) via miniosmotic pump during DSS treatment reduced the disease activity (40–66%) and histological colonic damage (45%), MPO activity (50%), and serum NO_x levels (55%).[57] The iNOS-selective inhibitor, L-N^G-(1-iminoethyl) lysine (L-NIL), decreased MPO (50%) and iNOS activities (90%) in the colon when administered by intraperitoneal injection after TNBS. Interestingly, L-NIL also reduced the number of apoptotic epithelial cells and the number of such cells co-expressing nitrotyrosine in this model.[150] Zingarelli *et al.* showed that mercaptoethylguanidine (MEG, 20 mg/kg, i.v.) inhibited TNBS-induced macroscopic damage by 60%, concomitant with decreases in the numbers of iNOS and nitrotyrosine immunostain-positive cells in the colonic mucosa.[151] In the DSS model in mice, the iNOS inhibitor (1*S*,5*S*,6*R*,7*R*)-7-chloro-3-imino-5-methyl-2-azabicyclo-[4.1.0.]heptane hydrochloride (ONO-1714, 3 mg/kg, i.p.) reduced lipid peroxidation (TBARS levels, 40–50%), iNOS mRNA levels, luminal and serum NO_x (40–90%), and nitrotyrosine immunostaining in the colonic mucosa.[152] In contrast to the non-selective NOS inhibitors, the iNOS-specific agents have consistently proved effective in treating experimental colitis independent of the timing of administration. This is presumably due to a minimization of constitutive NOS inhibition.

4. The Role of Oxidative Stress in UC Pathogenesis

As indicated by the results discussed above, oxidative stress is a prominent feature of UC. However, the manner in which oxidative stress contributes to the pathogenesis of UC is still in question. ROS and RNS have been shown to directly mediate cell damage. Highly reactive molecules like the hydroxyl radical, HOCL, and peroxynitrite can react with most cellular constituents, including lipids, carbohydrates, proteins, and nucleic acids.[29,154,155] Lipid peroxidation, or alteration of membrane proteins, can adversely modify the regulatory properties of cell membranes, leading to epithelial cell death. Lipid peroxides thus formed can themselves react with other molecules. Oxidation of essential cellular enzymes, signaling proteins, and the cell support proteins can all lead to loss of cell viability.[154,156] DNA oxidation can lead to altered gene expression, and initiate programmed cell death cascades.

At the same time, ROS and RNS may act indirectly to facilitate mucosal ulceration and perpetuate the inflammatory response. ROS have been shown to inactivate protease inhibitors, leaving the interstitial cells of the colonic mucosa open to degradation by leukocyte-derived proteases. ROS can also activate matrix metalloproteinases, leading to the destruction of the tissue stroma.[21] The hydroxyl radical has been shown to react with mucin glycoproteins, and the negatively charged glycoproteins may bind luminal iron, leading to oxidative degradation of the mucus barrier and enhanced infiltration of luminal antigens into the epithelium.[29,157]

The reactions of molecules such as the hydroxyl radical require their production in very close proximity to the cellular structures. Babbs has noted that the activity of adherent neutrophils can theoretically generate very high local concentrations of superoxide in the colonic mucosa. Combined with adequate sources of iron, such as those present in the feces due to iron supplementation and within the mucosa due to local hemorrhaging and hemolysis, the environment is ideal for hydroxyl radical formation.[29] This hypothesis is supported by observations in animal models, which have shown that elevated iron levels exacerbate experimental colitis. The central role of iron in the generation of oxidants via Fenton chemistry, *in vitro* as well as *in vivo*, is well established.[158,159] Iron deficiency is a common complication in UC patients. Iron losses in these patients are due to persistent colonic mucosal injury and bleeding. Dietary iron supplementation to treat anemia and consumption of an iron-rich diet, combined with local hemolysis, exposes the colonic mucosa to large amounts of iron.[29] In addition, oxidation of storage proteins like ferritin releases iron, adding to the free iron pool. We and others have demonstrated in rodent models that iron supplementation through the diet increases colitis-associated mucosal damage, as well as parameters of oxidative stress. In a study by Reifen *et al.*, looking at iodoacetamide-induced colitis, rats fed a diet containing four times the normal iron level showed a 20% increase in colon thickness, and 10% increases in colon weight and inflammation area compared to controls. Colonic MDA levels were increased by 80% with iron supplementation.[160] Carrier *et al.*, reporting on the DSS model in rats, found that 3000 or 30,000 mg iron/kg diet increased inflammation scores (two-fold), colonic lipid peroxides (six-fold), and reduced α-tocopherol levels.[161] Excessive body iron stores also increased colitis severity. The creation of iron overload by intraperitoneal injection of iron-dextran (1000 mg/kg b.w.) increased crypt and inflammation scores 1.8- to 2-fold versus DSS-treated control rats. Colonic lipid peroxides were increased nearly two-fold, and plasma α-tocopherol levels were reduced by 30%.[162] Using the DSS model in mice, we observed that feeding with two- to five-fold iron supplemented diet significantly increased mucosal inflammation and damage by 2- to 2.5-fold. Iron supplementation was associated with increases in mucosal iNOS and nitrotyrosine-positive cell numbers, including lamina propria inflammatory cells and adjacent epithelial cells.[163] Dietary iron supplementation was associated with increased prussian blue staining of ferric iron at the mucosal surface and in areas of ulceration.[161,163] Interestingly, consumption of two-fold iron diet in our study increased colorectal carcinoma development in association with cyclic, long-term DSS treatment by approximately four-fold.[163] The effects of iron supplementation on acute colitis and chronic colitis-associated carcinogenesis are likely related. The cytotoxic effects of oxidative stress, which are enhanced by iron, may lead to increased mutagenesis as well as cell death and ulceration.[9] Indeed, the antioxidant NAC (200 mg/kg, p.o.) decreased iron-enhanced colorectal tumor incidence by 25% in the DSS model.[98] The role of iron in UC is also indicated by the inhibitory effect of the iron chelator, deferipone, on acetic acid-induced colitis. Thus, increased luminal iron in UC patients, brought into close proximity to oxidants produced by the surface mucosa and adherent phagocytic leukocytes, may combine to promote cellular injury and mucosal ulceration.

What insights into the mechanistic roles of ROS and RNS can be gained from the studies on the effects of antioxidants on experimental colitis (see Table 1)? There is certainly abundant data indicating that compounds with antioxidant activities have ameliorative effects in animal models of colitis. The effective natural compounds, such as the tea components and curcumin, are particularly interesting because of their relatively low toxicity. Many of the agents have been shown to target multiple ROS and RNS, as well as pro-inflammatory enzymes. In addition, in many of the studies no correlations were made between inhibitory effects on clinical and histological aspects of colitis and parameters of oxidative stress, making it difficult to draw mechanistic conclusions. The antioxidant enzymes and pro-oxidant enzyme inhibitors are more specific, and so perhaps more informative. In the study by Keshavarzian *et al.*, administration of SOD and inhibition of XO by allopurinol had ameliorative effects on acetic acid-induced colitis.[131] Thus, the superoxide radical, generated either by phagocytic leukocytes or by epithelial cells, appears to play an important role in that model. The role of the hydroxyl radical in the acetic acid model is uncertain. DMSO and deferoxamine were ineffective in the study by Keshavarzian *et al.*, but another iron chelator, deferiprone, had an inhibitory effect on macroscopic injury in the same model,[130] as did catalase.[99] Thus, the involvement of H_2O_2 and the hydroxyl radical in the pathogenesis of the acetic acid model cannot be excluded. Perhaps peroxynitrite, formed by the reaction of superoxide with equimolar amounts of NO, is a mediator of acetic acid-induced inflammation. A NOS inhibitor was ameliorative in this model,[143] but the iNOS knockout mouse shows increased sensitivity to acetic acid.[53] Both SOD and catalase treatments show clear inhibitory effects on macroscopic injury in the TNBS model, together with antioxidant effects *in vitro*.[99,132] SOD also reduced colitis in the DSS model.[115] But the overexpression of Cu/Zn-SOD in the hSOD1-Tg transgenic mouse did not affect DSS-induced mucosal injury,[79] and actually exacerbated colitis in another study.[57]

As mentioned above, the mixed effects of the NOS inhibitors (aminoguanidine, L-NAME, and L-NMMA) on TNBS-induced colitis may be due to their relative non-selectivity for specific NOS isoforms, and their timing of administration.[50,139–141,143–146] NOS inhibition after colitis induction appears to ameliorate colitis in this model, possibly by suppressing iNOS activity when it is at its highest levels. In contrast, NOS inhibition prior to TNBS treatment may adversely affect colitis by inhibiting the constitutive NOS isoforms as well as iNOS. The more specific iNOS inhibitors (1400W, L-NIL, MEG, ONO-1714) are more consistent: all have been demonstrated to decrease TNBS or DSS-associated colonic injury, while at the same time decreasing parameters of NO production and NO-associated protein modification.[57,146,148,150,151] The studies using iNOS gene knockout mice have indicated that NO plays a role in colitis-associated injury.[53,55–57] However, the contradictory results obtained using the TNBS model,[51,52] and the results of the NO-donor studies[58,59] reinforce the idea that NO has multiple roles in inflammation and wound healing.[61,62] In light of the differing roles of NO in inflammation, more experimental studies are needed to assess the applicability of iNOS-specific inhibitors for use in UC patients. The toxicity of compounds such as 1400W with prolonged use is also a concern.[137]

For the most part, the animal data strongly suggest that ROS and RNS are involved in the mediation of colonic mucosal injury, but it is difficult to implicate specific molecules and cell types, and to determine whether the involvement is direct or indirect. Multiple cell types, and their associated ROS and RNS, may contribute in redundant or overlapping fashions to produce mucosal ulceration (e.g., macrophages are capable of producing many of the same inflammatory mediators as neutrophils, and epithelial cells produce superoxide and NO). The results of Krieglstein *et al.* indicate that ROS and RNS have complex, somewhat compensatory roles in the pathogenesis of colitis, at least in the DSS model. Using mice genetically deficient in the p47 subunit of the NADPH oxidase complex (p47*phox* [-/-] mice), it was found that the lack of superoxide production by phagocytic leukocytes had no effect on disease activity or histological grades of DSS-induced colitis. But when p47*phox* (−/−) mice were also administered the iNOS-specific inhibitor, 1400W, colonic injury was nearly completely ablated (−90% compared to DSS controls), with histological scores significantly lower than wild-type mice administered 1400W.[57] Thus, NO may completely compensate for the absence of leukocyte superoxide production in the DSS model. Conversely, it appears that superoxide can compensate for NO, but only partially. The finding that intrarectal administration of the superoxide and NO reaction product, peroxynitrite, can induce colonic injury and inflammation in rodents also provides support for the joint role of ROS and RNS in the production of mucosal injury.[60] Such redundancy in the pathogenic roles of ROS and RNS may explain the observation that colonic injury in the chemically induced rodent models is unaffected by neutropenia produced by anti-neutrophil antibodies.[32,164,165] Still, the studies in neutropenic animals could also indicate that neutrophils are not involved in the production of colitis-associated mucosal injury, or serve to highlight a limitation of chemically induced colitis. Cellular injury in these models may be initiated by the cytotoxicity of the chemicals themselves, and not by infiltrating inflammatory cells. Thus, the possibility remains that genetic manipulations or pharmacological interventions exert their effects in these models by impacting the initial reactions of the inducing chemicals. More studies are needed to differentiate among these possibilities and to help clarify the applicability of the current model systems.

5. Conclusions

Studies in tissue samples from UC patients have shown that ROS and RNS production in the colonic mucosa is a prominent feature of that disease. The likely sources of ROS and RNS in this setting are the large numbers of activated lamina propria phagocytic leukocytes that are characteristic of UC. UC patients also present with antioxidant deficiencies over the long term, which combined with ROS and RNS overproduction, results in an oxidative stress environment. While the overabundance of ROS and RNS is consistently observed in the colons of UC patients, and often correlated with indices of disease severity, it is impossible to discern a cause and effect relationship between the presence of the reactive molecules and mucosal injury from such studies. Several animal models of UC are available that have the potential to provide information on the mechanistic role of oxidative stress in the initiation and propagation of UC, as well as the usefulness of therapies targeting oxidative stress. The chemically induced animal models have been the most widely used, and a combination of pharmacological and gene-targeting approaches have suggested that ROS and RNS have definitive roles in the pathogenesis of these models. They also suggest that a mixture of reactive species is involved with overlapping cytotoxic effects. The most compelling evidence supporting a role for oxidative stress has come from studies utilizing the administration of antioxidant enzymes and mice genetically deficient in iNOS. Still, it is difficult to conclude from these studies if the targeted reactive molecules have direct or indirect effects on mucosal ulceration. The chemically induced and genetic colitis models are useful screening tools for potential therapies for UC. Given the experimental evidence for the role of oxidative stress in UC pathogenesis, natural or synthetic compounds that have demonstrated antioxidant activities could be helpful to UC patients, most likely in combination with current therapeutic mainstays. Several promising, non-toxic compounds have been identified in experimental systems. However, the relevance of the animal models to the human situation must be considered. Many of these potential therapies need to be tested in multiple animal models before considering translation to clinical studies.

References

1. Warren BF, Watkins PE. Animal models of inflammatory bowel disease. *J. Pathol.* 172: 313–316 (1994).
2. Sadlack B, Merz H, Schorle H, Schimpl A, Feller AC, Horak I. Ulcerative colitis-like disease in mice with a disrupted interleukin-2 gene. *Cell* 75: 253–261 (1993).
3. Kuhn R, Lohler J, Rennick D, Rajewsky K, Muller W. Interleukin-10-deficient mice develop chronic enterocolitis. *Cell* 75: 263–274 (1993).
4. Taurog JD, Maika SD, Simmons WA, Breban M, Hammer RE. Susceptibility to inflammatory disease in HLA-B27 transgenic rat lines correlates with the level of B27 expression. *J. Immunol.* 150: 4168–4178 (1993).
5. MacPherson B, Pfeiffer CJ. Experimental colitis. *Digestion* 14: 424–452 (1976).
6. Cooper HS, Murthy SN, Shah RS, Sedergran DJ. Clinicopathologic study of dextran sulfate sodium experimental murine colitis. *Lab. Invest.* 69: 238–249 (1993).
7. Ohkusa T, Okayasu I, Tokoi S, Araki A, Ozaki Y. Changes in bacterial phagocytosis of macrophages in experimental ulcerative colitis. *Digestion* 56: 159–164 (1995).

8. Okayasu I, Hatakeyama S, Yamada M, Ohkusa T, Inagaki Y, Nakaya R. A novel method in the induction of reliable experimental acute and chronic ulcerative colitis in mice. *Gastroenterology* 98: 694–702 (1990).
9. Seril DN, Liao J, Yang GY, Yang CS. Oxidative stress and ulcerative colitis-associated carcinogenesis: studies in humans and animal models. *Carcinogenesis* 24: 353–362 (2003).
10. Mahler M, Bristol IJ, Leiter EH, Workman AE, Birkenmeier EH, Elson CO, Sundberg JP. Differential susceptibility of inbred mouse strains to dextran sulfate sodium-induced colitis. *Am. J. Physiol.* 274: G544–G551 (1998).
11. Schreiber S, MacDermott RP, Raedler A, Pinnau R, Bertovich MJ, Nash GS. Increased activation of isolated intestinal lamina propria mononuclear cells in inflammatory bowel disease. *Gastroenterology* 101: 1020–1030 (1991).
12. Farrell RJ, Peppercorn MA. Ulcerative colitis. *Lancet* 359: 331–340 (2002).
13. Fiocchi C. Inflammatory bowel disease: etiology and pathogenesis. *Gastroenterology* 115: 182–205 (1998).
14. Podolsky DK. Inflammatory bowel disease. *N. Engl. J. Med.* 347: 417–429 (2002).
15. Sedghi S, Fields JZ, Klamut M, Urban G, Durkin M, Winship D, Fretland D, Olyaee M, Keshavarzian A. Increased production of luminol enhanced chemiluminescence by the inflamed colonic mucosa in patients with ulcerative colitis. *Gut* 34: 1191–1197 (1993).
16. Shiratora Y, Aoki S, Takada H, Kiriyama H, Ohto K, Hai K, Teraoka H, Matano S, Matsumoto K, Kamii K. Oxygen-derived free radical generating capacity of polymorphonuclear cells in patients with ulcerative colitis. *Digestion* 44: 163–171 (1989).
17. Verspaget HW, Pena AS, Weterman IT, Lamers CB. Diminished neutrophil function in Crohn's disease and ulcerative colitis identified by decreased oxidative metabolism and low superoxide dismutase content. *Gut* 29: 223–228 (1988).
18. Williams A. Macrophage activity in inflammatory bowel disease. *Gut* 31: 481 (1990).
19. Mahida YR, Wu KC, Jewell DP. Respiratory burst activity of intestinal macrophages in normal and inflammatory bowel disease. *Gut* 30: 1362–1370 (1989).
20. Bogdan C, Rollinghoff M, Diefenbach A. Reactive oxygen and reactive nitrogen intermediates in innate and specific immunity. *Curr. Opin. Immunol.* 12: 64–76 (2000a).
21. Grisham MB, Granger DN. Neutrophil-mediated mucosal injury. Role of reactive oxygen metabolites. *Dig. Dis. Sci.* 33: 6S–15S (1988).

22. Grisham MB. Oxidants and free radicals in inflammatory bowel disease. *Lancet* 344: 859–861 (1994).
23. Jaiswal M, LaRusso NF, Gores GJ. Nitric oxide in gastrointestinal epithelial cell carcinogenesis: linking inflammation to oncogenesis. *Am. J. Physiol. Gastrointest. Liver Physiol.* 281: G626–G634 (2001).
24. Simmonds NJ, Allen RE, Stevens TR, Van Someren RN, Blake DR, Rampton DS. Chemiluminescence assay of mucosal reactive oxygen metabolites in inflammatory bowel disease. *Gastroenterology* 103: 186–196 (1992).
25. Lih-Brody L, Powell SR, Collier KP, Reddy GM, Cerchia R, Kahn E, Weissman GS, Katz S, Floyd RA, McKinley MJ, Fisher SE, Mullin GE. Increased oxidative stress and decreased antioxidant defenses in mucosa of inflammatory bowel disease. *Dig. Dis. Sci.* 41: 2078–2086 (1996).
26. Kruidenier L, Kuiper I, Lamers CB, Verspaget HW. Intestinal oxidative damage in inflammatory bowel disease: semi-quantification, localization, and association with mucosal antioxidants. *J. Pathol.* 201: 28–36 (2003a).
27. D'Odorico A, Bortolan S, Cardin R, D'Inca R, Martines D, Ferronato A, Sturniolo GC. Reduced plasma antioxidant concentrations and increased oxidative DNA damage in inflammatory bowel disease. *Scand. J. Gastroenterol.* 36: 1289–1294 (2001).
28. D'Inca R, Cardin R, Benazzato L, Angriman I, Martines D, Sturniolo GC. Oxidative DNA damage in the mucosa of ulcerative colitis increases with disease duration and dysplasia. *Inflamm. Bowel. Dis.* 10: 23–27 (2004).
29. Babbs CF. Oxygen radicals in ulcerative colitis. *Free Radic. Biol. Med.* 13: 169–181 (1992).
30. Korenaga D, Takesue F, Kido K, Yasuda M, Inutsuka S, Honda M, Nagahama S. Impaired antioxidant defense system of colonic tissue and cancer development in dextran sulfate sodium-induced colitis in mice. *J. Surg. Res.* 102: 144–149 (2002).
31. Tardieu D, Jaeg JP, Cadet J, Embvani E, Corpet DE, Petit, C. Dextran sulfate enhances the level of an oxidative DNA damage biomarker, 8-oxo-7,8-dihydro-2′-deoxyguanosine, in rat colonic mucosa. *Cancer Lett.* 134: 1–5 (1998).
32. Dykens JA, Baginski TJ. Urinary 8-hydroxydeoxyguanosine excretion as a non-invasive marker of neutrophil activation in animal models of inflammatory bowel disease. *Scand. J. Gastroenterol.* 33: 628–636 (1998).
33. Blackburn AC, Doe WF, Buffinton GD. Protein carbonyl formation on mucosal proteins *in vitro* and in dextran sulfate-induced colitis. *Free Radic. Biol. Med.* 27: 262–270 (1999).

34. Loguercio C, D'Argenio G, Delle Cave M, Cosenza V, Della Valle N, Mazzacca G, del Vecchio Blanco C. Direct evidence of oxidative damage in acute and chronic phases of experimental colitis in rats. *Dig. Dis. Sci.* 41: 1204–1211 (1996).
35. Bogdan C, Rollinghoff M, Diefenbach A. The role of nitric oxide in innate immunity. *Immunol. Rev.* 173: 17–26 (2000b).
36. Lundberg JO, Hellstrom PM, Lundberg JM, Alving K. Greatly increased luminal nitric oxide in ulcerative colitis. *Lancet* 344: 1673–1674 (1994).
37. Herulf M, Ljung T, Hellstrom PM, Weitzberg E, Lundberg JO. Increased luminal nitric oxide in inflammatory bowel disease as shown with a novel minimally invasive method. *Scand. J. Gastroenterol.* 33: 164–169 (1998).
38. Rachmilewitz D, Eliakim R, Ackerman Z, Karmeli F. Direct determination of colonic nitric oxide level — a sensitive marker of disease activity in ulcerative colitis. *Am. J. Gastroenterol.* 93: 409–412 (1998).
39. Kimura H, Miura S, Shigematsu T, Ohkubo N, Tsuzuki Y, Kurose I, Higuchi H, Akiba Y, Hokari R, Hirokawa M, Serizawa H, Ishii H. Increased nitric oxide production and inducible nitric oxide synthase activity in colonic mucosa of patients with active ulcerative colitis and Crohn's disease. *Dig. Dis. Sci.* 42: 1047–1054 (1997).
40. Oudkerk Pool M, Bouma G, Visser JJ, Kolkman JJ, Tran DD, Meuwissen SG, Pena AS. Serum nitrate levels in ulcerative colitis and Crohn's disease. *Scand. J. Gastroenterol.* 30: 784–788 (1995).
41. Keshavarzian A, Banan A, Farhadi A, Komanduri S, Mutlu E, Zhang Y, Fields JZ. Increases in free radicals and cytoskeletal protein oxidation and nitration in the colon of patients with inflammatory bowel disease. *Gut* 52: 720–728 (2003).
42. Rachmilewitz D, Stamler JS, Bachwich D, Karmeli F, Ackerman Z, Podolsky DK. Enhanced colonic nitric oxide generation and nitric oxide synthase activity in ulcerative colitis and Crohn's disease. *Gut* 36: 718–723 (1995).
43. Boughton-Smith NK, Evans SM, Hawkey CJ, Cole AT, Balsitis M, Whittle BJ, Moncada S. Nitric oxide synthase activity in ulcerative colitis and Crohn's disease. *Lancet* 342: 338–340 (1993).
44. Godkin AJ, De Belder AJ, Villa L, Wong A, Beesley JE, Kane SP, Martin JF. Expression of nitric oxide synthase in ulcerative colitis. *Eur. J. Clin. Invest.* 26: 867–872 (1996).
45. Ikeda I, Kasajima T, Ishiyama S, Shimojo T, Takeo Y, Nishikawa T, Kameoka S, Hiroe M, Mitsunaga A. Distribution of inducible nitric oxide synthase in ulcerative colitis. *Am. J. Gastroenterol.* 92: 1339–1341 (1997).

46. Dijkstra G, Zandvoort AJ, Kobold AC, de Jager-Krikken A, Heeringa P, van Goor H, van Dullemen HM, Tervaert JW, van de Loosdrecht A, Moshage H, Jansen PL. Increased expression of inducible nitric oxide synthase in circulating monocytes from patients with active inflammatory bowel disease. *Scand. J. Gastroenterol.* 37: 546–554 (2002).
47. Kimura H, Hokari R, Miura S, Shigematsu T, Hirokawa M, Akiba Y, Kurose I, Higuchi H, Fujimori H, Tsuzuki Y, Serizawa H, Ishii H. Increased expression of an inducible isoform of nitric oxide synthase and the formation of peroxynitrite in colonic mucosa of patients with active ulcerative colitis. *Gut* 42: 180–187 (1998).
48. Dijkstra G, Moshage H, van Dullemen HM, de Jager-Krikken A, Tiebosch AT, Kleibeuker JH, Jansen PL, van Goor H. Expression of nitric oxide synthases and formation of nitrotyrosine and reactive oxygen species in inflammatory bowel disease. *J. Pathol.* 186: 416–421 (1998).
49. Ribbons KA *et al.* Potential role of nitric oxide in a model of chronic colitis in rhesus macaques. *Gastroenterology* 108: 705–711 (1995).
50. Seven A, Seymen O, Inci F, Oz B, Yigit G, Burcak G. Evaluation of oxidative stress in experimental colitis: effects of L-arginine-nitric oxide pathway manipulation. *J. Toxicol. Environ. Health A* 61: 167–176 (2000).
51. McCafferty DM, Miampamba M, Sihota E, Sharkey KA, Kubes P. Role of inducible nitric oxide synthase in trinitrobenzene sulphonic acid induced colitis in mice. *Gut* 45: 864–873 (1999).
52. Zingarelli B, Szabo C, Salzman AL. Reduced oxidative and nitrosative damage in murine experimental colitis in the absence of inducible nitric oxide synthase. *Gut* 45: 199–209 (1999).
53. McCafferty DM, Mudgett JS, Swain MG, Kubes P. Inducible nitric oxide synthase plays a critical role in resolving intestinal inflammation. *Gastroenterology* 112: 1022–1027 (1997).
54. McCafferty DM, Sihota E, Muscara M, Wallace JL, Sharkey KA, Kubes P. Spontaneously developing chronic colitis in IL-10/iNOS double-deficient mice. *Am. J. Physiol. Gastrointest Liver Physiol.* 279: G90–G99 (2000).
55. Beck PL, Xavier R, Wong J, Ezedi I, Mashimo H, Mizoguchi A, Mizoguchi E, Bhan AK, Podolsky DK. Paradoxical roles of different nitric oxide synthase isoforms in colonic injury. *Am. J. Physiol. Gastrointest. Liver Physiol.* 286: G137–G147 (2004).
56. Hokari R, Kato S, Matsuzaki K, Kuroki M, Iwai A, Kawaguchi A, Nagao S, Miyahara T, Itoh K, Sekizuka E, Nagata H, Ishii H, Miura S. Reduced sensitivity of inducible nitric oxide synthase-deficient mice to chronic colitis. *Free Radic. Biol. Med.* 31: 153–163 (2001).

57. Krieglstein CF, Cerwinka WH, Laroux FS, Salter JW, Russell JM, Schuermann G, Grisham MB, Ross CR, Granger DN. Regulation of murine intestinal inflammation by reactive metabolites of oxygen and nitrogen: divergent roles of superoxide and nitric oxide. *J. Exp. Med.* 194: 1207–1218 (2001).
58. Lamine F, Fioramonti J, Bueno L, Nepveu F, Cauquil E, Lobysheva I, Eutamene H, Theodorou V. Nitric oxide released by *Lactobacillus farciminis* improves TNBS-induced colitis in rats. *Scand. J. Gastroenterol.* 39: 37–45 (2004).
59. Salas A, Gironella M, Soriano A, Sans M, Iovanna J, Pique JM, Panes J. Nitric oxide supplementation ameliorates dextran sulfate sodium-induced colitis in mice. *Lab. Invest.* 82: 597–607 (2002).
60. Rachmilewitz D, Stamler JS, Karmeli F, Mullins ME, Singel DJ, Loscalzo J, Xavier RJ, Podolsky DK. Peroxynitrite-induced rat colitis — a new model of colonic inflammation. *Gastroenterology* 105: 1681–1688 (1993).
61. Calatayud S, Barrachina D, Esplugues JV. Nitric oxide: relation to integrity, injury, and healing of the gastric mucosa. *Microsc. Res. Tech.* 53: 325–335 (2001).
62. Witte MB, Barbul A. Role of nitric oxide in wound repair. *Am. J. Surg.* 183: 406–412 (2002).
63. Geerling BJ, Stockbrugger RW, Brummer RJ. Nutrition and inflammatory bowel disease: an update. *Scand. J. Gastroenterol. Suppl.* 230: 95–105 (1999).
64. Buffinton GD, Doe WF. Depleted mucosal antioxidant defences in inflammatory bowel disease. *Free Radic. Biol. Med.* 19: 911–918 (1995).
65. Holmes EW, Yong SL, Eiznhamer D, Keshavarzian A. Glutathione content of colonic mucosa: evidence for oxidative damage in active ulcerative colitis. *Dig. Dis. Sci.* 43: 1088–1095 (1998).
66. Tsunada S, Iwakiri R, Ootani H, Aw TY, Fujimoto K. Redox imbalance in the colonic mucosa of ulcerative colitis. *Scand. J. Gastroenterol.* 38: 1002–1003 (2003).
67. Sido B, Hack V, Hochlehnert A, Lipps H, Herfarth C, Droge W. Impairment of intestinal glutathione synthesis in patients with inflammatory bowel disease. *Gut* 42: 485–492 (1998).
68. McKenzie SJ, Baker MS, Buffinton GD, Doe WF. Evidence of oxidant-induced injury to epithelial cells during inflammatory bowel disease. *J. Clin. Invest.* 98: 136–141 (1996).
69. Nieto N, Torres MI, Fernandez MI, Giron MD, Rios A, Suarez MD, Gil A. Experimental ulcerative colitis impairs antioxidant defense system in rat intestine. *Dig. Dis. Sci.* 45: 1820–1827 (2000).

70. Togashi H, Oikawa K, Adachi T, Sugahara K, Ito J, Takeda T, Watanabe H, Saito K, Saito T, Fukui T, Takeda H, Ohya H, Kawata S. Mucosal sulfhydryl compounds evaluation by *in vivo* electron spin resonance spectroscopy in mice with experimental colitis. *Gut* 52: 1291–1296 (2003).
71. Blau S, Kohen R, Bass P, Rubinstein A. Relation between colonic inflammation severity and total low-molecular-weight antioxidant profiles in experimental colitis. *Dig. Dis. Sci.* 45: 1180–1187 (2000).
72. Kruidenier L, Kuiper I, Van Duijn W, Mieremet-Ooms MA, van Hogezand RA, Lamers CB, Verspaget HW. Imbalanced secondary mucosal antioxidant response in inflammatory bowel disease. *J. Pathol.* 201: 17–27 (2003c).
73. Kruidenier L, Kuiper I, van Duijn W, Marklund SL, van Hogezand RA, Lamers CB, Verspaget HW. Differential mucosal expression of three superoxide dismutase isoforms in inflammatory bowel disease. *J. Pathol.* 201: 7–16 (2003b).
74. Sturniolo GC, Mestriner C, Lecis PE, D'Odorico A, Venturi C, Irato P, Cecchetto A, Tropea A, Longo G, D'Inca R. Altered plasma and mucosal concentrations of trace elements and antioxidants in active ulcerative colitis. *Scand. J. Gastroenterol.* 33: 644–649 (1998).
75. Rannem T, Ladefoged K, Hylander E, Hegnhoj J, Staun M. Selenium depletion in patients with gastrointestinal diseases: are there any predictive factors? *Scand. J. Gastroenterol.* 33: 1057–1061 (1998).
76. Seo HG, Takata I, Nakamura M, Tatsumi H, Suzuki K, Fujii J, Taniguchi N. Induction of nitric oxide synthase and concomitant suppression of superoxide dismutases in experimental colitis in rats. *Arch. Biochem. Biophys.* 324: 41–47 (1995).
77. Al-Awadi FM, Khan I, Dashti HM, Srikumar TS. Colitis-induced changes in the level of trace elements in rat colon and other tissues. *Ann. Nutr. Metab.* 42: 304–310 (1998).
78. Wang WP, Guo X, Koo MW, Wong BC, Lam SK, Ye YN, Cho CH. Protective role of heme oxygenase-1 on trinitrobenzene sulfonic acid-induced colitis in rats. *Am. J. Physiol. Gastrointest. Liver Physiol.* 281: G586–G594 (2001).
79. Kruidenier L, van Meeteren ME, Kuiper I, Jaarsma D, Lamers CB, Zijlstra FJ, Verspaget HW. Attenuated mild colonic inflammation and improved survival from severe DSS-colitis of transgenic Cu/Zn-SOD mice. *Free Radic. Biol. Med.* 34: 753–765 (2003d).
80. Tham DM, Whitin JC, Cohen HJ. Increased expression of extracellular glutathione peroxidase in mice with dextran sodium sulfate-induced experimental colitis. *Pediatr. Res.* 51: 641–646 (2002).

81. Esworthy RS, Aranda R, Martin MG, Doroshow JH, Binder SW, Chu FF. Mice with combined disruption of Gpx1 and Gpx2 genes have colitis. *Am. J. Physiol. Gastrointest. Liver Physiol.* 281: G848–G855 (2001).
82. Rutgeerts P. Modern therapy for inflammatory bowel disease. *Scand. J. Gastroenterol. Suppl.* 237: 30–33 (2003).
83. Aruoma OI, Wasil M, Halliwell B, Hoey BM, Butler J. The scavenging of oxidants by sulphasalazine and its metabolites. A possible contribution to their anti-inflammatory effects? *Biochem. Pharmacol.* 36: 3739–3742 (1987).
84. Ahnfelt-Ronne I, Nielsen OH, Christensen A, Langholz E, Binder V, Riis P. Clinical evidence supporting the radical scavenger mechanism of 5-aminosalicylic acid. *Gastroenterology* 98: 1162–1169 (1990).
85. Hasko G, Szabo C, Nemeth ZH, Deitch EA. Sulphasalazine inhibits macrophage activation: inhibitory effects on inducible nitric oxide synthase expression, interleukin-12 production and major histocompatibility complex II expression. *Immunology* 103: 473–478 (2001).
86. Ahnfelt-Ronne I, Nielsen OH. The antiinflammatory moiety of sulfasalazine, 5-aminosalicylic acid, is a radical scavenger. *Agents Actions* 21: 191–194 (1987).
87. Kimura I, Kumamoto T, Matsuda A, Kataoka M, Kokuba Y. Effects of BX661A, a new therapeutic agent for ulcerative colitis, on reactive oxygen species in comparison with salazosulfapyridine and its metabolite sulfapyridine. *Arzneimittelforschung* 48: 1007–1011 (1998).
88. Dallegri F, Ottonello L, Ballestrero A, Bogliolo F, Ferrando F, Patrone F. Cytoprotection against neutrophil derived hypochlorous acid: a potential mechanism for the therapeutic action of 5-aminosalicylic acid in ulcerative colitis. *Gut* 31: 184–186 (1990).
89. Reynolds PD, Middleton SJ, Shorthouse M, Hunter JO. The effects of aminosalicylic acid derivatives on nitric oxide in a cell-free system. *Aliment. Pharmacol. Ther.* 9: 491–495 (1995).
90. Ademoglu E, Erbil Y, Tam B, Barbaros U, Ilhan E, Olgac V, Mutlu-Turkoglu U. Do vitamin E and selenium have beneficial effects on trinitrobenzenesulfonic acid-induced experimental colitis. *Dig. Dis. Sci.* 49: 102–108 (2004).
91. Sato K, Kanazawa A, Ota N, Nakamura T, Fujimoto K. Dietary supplementation of catechins and alpha-tocopherol accelerates the healing of trinitrobenzene sulfonic acid-induced ulcerative colitis in rats. *J. Nutr. Sci. Vitaminol. (Tokyo)* 44: 769–778 (1998).
92. Carrier J, Aghdassi E, Cullen J, Allard JP. Iron supplementation increases disease activity and vitamin E ameliorates the effect in rats with dextran sulfate sodium-induced colitis. *J. Nutr.* 132: 3146–3150 (2002).

93. Lauritsen K, Laursen LS, Bukhave K, Rask-Madsen J. Does vitamin E supplementation modulate *in vivo* arachidonate metabolism in human inflammation? *Pharmacol. Toxicol.* 61: 246–249 (1987).
94. Reifen R, Nur T, Ghebermeskel K, Zaiger G, Urizky R, Pines M. Vitamin A deficiency exacerbates inflammation in a rat model of colitis through activation of nuclear factor-kappaB and collagen formation. *J. Nutr.* 132: 2743–2747 (2002).
95. Nosal'ova V, Cerna S, Bauer V. Effect of N-acetylcysteine on colitis induced by acetic acid in rats. *Gen. Pharmacol.* 35: 77–81 (2000).
96. Cotgreave IA. N-acetylcysteine: pharmacological considerations and experimental and clinical applications. *Adv. Pharmacol.* 38: 205–227 (1997).
97. Ardite E, Sans M, Panes J, Romero FJ, Pique JM, Fernandez-Checa JC. Replenishment of glutathione levels improves mucosal function in experimental acute colitis. *Lab. Invest.* 80: 735–744 (2000).
98. Seril DN, Liao J, Ho KL, Yang CS, Yang GY. Inhibition of chronic ulcerative colitis-associated colorectal adenocarcinoma development in a murine model by N-acetylcysteine. *Carcinogenesis* 23: 993–1001 (2002b).
99. Keshavarzian A, Haydek J, Zabihi R, Doria M, D'Astice M, Sorenson JR. Agents capable of eliminating reactive oxygen species. Catalase, WR-2721, or Cu(II)2(3,5-DIPS)4 decrease experimental colitis. *Dig. Dis. Sci.* 37: 1866–1873 (1992).
100. Shusterman T, Sela S, Cohen H, Kristal B, Sbeit W, Reshef R. Effect of the antioxidant Mesna (2-mercaptoethane sulfonate) on experimental colitis. *Dig. Dis. Sci.* 48: 1177–1185 (2003).
101. Yang CS, Maliakal P, Meng X. Inhibition of carcinogenesis by tea. *Annu. Rev. Pharmacol. Toxicol.* 42: 25–54 (2002).
102. Varilek GW, Yang F, Lee EY, deVilliers WJ, Zhong J, Oz HS, Westberry KF, McClain CJ. Green tea polyphenol extract attenuates inflammation in interleukin-2-deficient mice, a model of autoimmunity. *J. Nutr.* 131: 2034–2039 (2001).
103. Maity S, Ukil A, Karmakar S, Datta N, Chaudhuri T, Vedasiromoni JR, Ganguly DK, Das PK. Thearubigin, the major polyphenol of black tea, ameliorates mucosal injury in trinitrobenzene sulfonic acid-induced colitis. *Eur. J. Pharmacol.* 470: 103–112 (2003).
104. Hong J, Bose M, Ju J, Ryu JH, Chen X, Sang S, Lee MJ, Yang CS. Modulation of arachidonic acid metabolism by curcumin and related {beta}-diketone derivatives: effects on cytosolic phospholipase A2, cyclooxygenases, and 5-lipoxygenase. *Carcinogenesis* 25(9): 1671–1679 (2004).
105. Surh YJ, Chun KS, Cha HH, Han SS, Keum YS, Park KK, Lee SS. Molecular mechanisms underlying chemopreventive activities of anti-inflammatory

phytochemicals: down-regulation of COX-2 and iNOS through suppression of NF-kappa B activation. *Mutat. Res.* 480–481: 243–268 (2001).

106. Sugimoto K, Hanai H, Tozawa K, Aoshi T, Uchijima M, Nagata T, Koide Y. Curcumin prevents and ameliorates trinitrobenzene sulfonic acid-induced colitis in mice. *Gastroenterology* 123: 1912–1922 (2002).

107. Ukil A, Maity S, Karmakar S, Datta N, Vedasiromoni JR, Das PK. Curcumin, the major component of food flavour turmeric, reduces mucosal injury in trinitrobenzene sulphonic acid-induced colitis. *Br. J. Pharmacol.* 139: 209–218 (2003).

108. Salh B, Assi K, Templeman V, Parhar K, Owen D, Gomez-Munoz A, Jacobson K. Curcumin attenuates DNB-induced murine colitis. *Am. J. Physiol. Gastrointest. Liver Physiol.* 285: G235–G243 (2003).

109. Di Stasi LC, Camuesco D, Nieto A, Vilegas W, Zarzuelo A, Galvez J. Intestinal anti-inflammatory activity of paepalantine, an isocoumarin isolated from the capitula of *Paepalanthus bromelioides*, in the trinitrobenzenesulphonic acid model of rat colitis. *Planta Med.* 70: 315–320 (2004).

110. Chan MM, Mattiacci JA, Hwang HS, Shah A, Fong D. Synergy between ethanol and grape polyphenols, quercetin, and resveratrol, in the inhibition of the inducible nitric oxide synthase pathway. *Biochem. Pharmacol.* 60: 1539–1548 (2000).

111. Martinez J, Moreno JJ. Effect of resveratrol, a natural polyphenolic compound, on reactive oxygen species and prostaglandin production. *Biochem. Pharmacol.* 59: 865–870 (2000).

112. Martin AR, Villegas I, La Casa C, de la Lastra CA. Resveratrol, a polyphenol found in grapes, suppresses oxidative damage and stimulates apoptosis during early colonic inflammation in rats. *Biochem. Pharmacol.* 67: 1399–1410 (2004).

113. Reifen R, Nur T, Matas Z, Halpern Z. Lycopene supplementation attenuates the inflammatory status of colitis in a rat model. *Int. J. Vitam. Nutr. Res.* 71: 347–351 (2001).

114. Murakami A, Hayashi R, Tanaka T, Kwon KH, Ohigashi H, Safitri R, Takana T. Suppression of dextran sodium sulfate-induced colitis in mice by zerumbone, a subtropical ginger sesquiterpene, and nimesulide: separately and in combination. *Biochem. Pharmacol.* 66: 1253–1261 (2003).

115. Ogawa Y, Kanatsu K, Iino T, Kato S, Jeong YI, Shibata N, Takada K, Takeuchi K. Protection against dextran sulfate sodium-induced colitis by microspheres of ellagic acid in rats. *Life Sci.* 71: 827–839 (2002).

116. Sanchez de Medina F, Vera B, Galvez J, Zarzuelo A. Effect of quercitrin on the early stages of hapten induced colonic inflammation in the rat. *Life Sci.* 70: 3097–3108 (2002).
117. Hong T, Jin GB, Cho S, Cyong JC. Evaluation of the anti-inflammatory effect of baicalein on dextran sulfate sodium-induced colitis in mice. *Planta Med.* 68: 268–271 (2002).
118. Galvez J, Coelho G, Crespo ME, Cruz T, Rodriguez-Cabezas ME, Concha A, Gonzalez M, Zarzuelo A, Intestinal anti-inflammatory activity of morin on chronic experimental colitis in the rat. *Aliment. Pharmacol. Ther.* 15: 2027–2039 (2001).
119. Cruz T, Galvez J, Ocete MA, Crespo ME, Sanchez de Medina LHF, Zarzuelo A. Oral administration of rutoside can ameliorate inflammatory bowel disease in rats. *Life Sci.* 62: 687–695 (1998).
120. Andreadou I, Papalois A, Triantafillidis JK, Demonakou M, Govosdis V, Vidali M, Anagnostakis E, Kourounakis PN. Beneficial effect of a novel non-steroidal anti-inflammatory agent with basic character and antioxidant properties on experimental colitis in rats. *Eur. J. Pharmacol.* 441: 209–214 (2002).
121. Kuralay F, Yildiz C, Ozutemiz O, Islekel H, Caliskan S, Bingol B, Ozkal S. Effects of trimetazidine on acetic acid-induced colitis in female Swiss rats. *J. Toxicol. Environ. Health A* 66: 169–179 (2003).
122. Girgin F, Karaoglu O, Erkus M, Tuzun S, Ozutemiz O, Dincer C, Batur Y, Tanyalcin T. Effects of trimetazidine on oxidant/antioxidant status in trinitrobenzenesulfonic acid-induced chronic colitis. *J. Toxicol. Environ. Health A* 59: 641–652 (2000).
123. Choudhary S, Keshavarzian A, Yong S, Wade M, Bocckino S, Day BJ, Banan A. Novel antioxidants zolimid and AEOL11201 ameliorate colitis in rats. *Dig. Dis. Sci.* 46: 2222–2230 (2001).
124. Farhadi A, Keshavarzian A, Fitzpatrick LR, Mutlu E, Zhang Y, Banan A. Modulatory effects of plasma and colonic milieu of patients with ulcerative colitis on neutrophil reactive oxygen species production in presence of a novel antioxidant, rebamipide. *Dig. Dis. Sci.* 47: 1342–1348 (2002).
125. Sakurai K, Osaka T, Yamasaki K. Protection by rebamipide against acetic acid-induced colitis in rats: relationship with its antioxidative activity. *Dig. Dis. Sci.* 43: 125S–133S (1998).
126. Zea-Iriarte WL, Makiyama K, Goto S, Murase K, Urata Y, Sekine I, Hara K, Kondo T. Impairment of antioxidants in colonic epithelial cells isolated

from trinitrobenzene sulphonic acid-induced colitis rats. Protective effect of rebamipide. *Scand. J. Gastroenterol.* 31: 985–992 (1996).

127. Nosal'ova V, Bauer V. Protective effect of stobadine in experimental colitis. *Life Sci.* 65: 1919–1921 (1999).
128. Pentney PT, Bubenik GA. Melatonin reduces the severity of dextran-induced colitis in mice. *J. Pineal Res.* 19: 31–39 (1995).
129. Karmeli F, Eliakim R, Okon E, Samuni A, Rachmilewitz D. A stable nitroxide radical effectively decreases mucosal damage in experimental colitis. *Gut* 37: 386–393 (1995).
130. Ablin J, Shalev O, Okon E, Karmeli F, Rachmilewitz D. Deferiprone, an oral iron chelator, ameliorates experimental colitis and gastric ulceration in rats. *Inflamm. Bowel. Dis.* 5: 253–261 (1999).
131. Keshavarzian A, Morgan G, Sedghi S, Gordon JH, Doria M. Role of reactive oxygen metabolites in experimental colitis. *Gut* 31: 786–790 (1990).
132. Yavuz Y, Yuksel M, Yegen BC, Alican I. The effect of antioxidant therapy on colonic inflammation in the rat. *Res. Exp. Med. (Berl.)* 199: 101–110 (1999).
133. Cuzzocrea S, Mazzon E, Dugo L, Caputi AP, Riley DP, Salvemini D. Protective effects of M40403, a superoxide dismutase mimetic, in a rodent model of colitis. *Eur J. Pharmacol.* 432: 79–89 (2001).
134. Salim AS. Role of oxygen-derived free radical scavengers in the management of recurrent attacks of ulcerative colitis: a new approach. *J. Lab. Clin. Med.* 119: 710–717 (1992).
135. Jarnerot G, Strom M, Danielsson A, Kilander A, Loof L, Hultcrantz R, Lofberg R, Floren C, Nilsson A, Brostrom O. Allopurinol in addition to 5-aminosalicylic acid based drugs for the maintenance treatment of ulcerative colitis. *Aliment. Pharmacol. Ther.* 14: 1159–1162 (2000).
136. Siems WG, Grune T, Werner A, Gerber G, Buntrock P, Schneider W. Protective influence of oxypurinol on the trinitrobenzene sulfonic acid (TNB) model of inflammatory bowel disease in rats. *Cell. Mol. Biol.* 38: 189–199 (1992).
137. Crowell JA, Steele VE, Sigman CC, Fay JR, Is inducible nitric oxide synthase a target for chemoprevention? *Mol. Cancer Ther.* 2: 815–823 (2003).
138. Vallance P, Leiper J. Blocking NO synthesis: how, where and why? *Nat. Rev. Drug. Discov.* 1: 939–950 (2002).
139. Nakamura H, Tsukada H, Oya M, Onomura M, Saito T, Fukuda K, Kodama M, Taniguchi T, Tominaga M, Hosokawa M, Seino Y. Aminoguanidine has both an anti-inflammatory effect on experimental colitis and a proliferative effect on colonic mucosal cells. *Scand. J. Gastroenterol.* 34: 1117–1122 (1999).

140. Armstrong AM, Campbell GR, Gannon C, Kirk SJ, Gardiner KR. Oral administration of inducible nitric oxide synthase inhibitors reduces nitric oxide synthesis but has no effect on the severity of experimental colitis. *Scand. J. Gastroenterol.* 35: 832–838 (2000).
141. Dikopoulos N, Nussler AK, Liptay S, Bachem M, Reinshagen M, Stiegler M, Schmid RM, Adler G, Weidenbach H. Inhibition of nitric oxide synthesis by aminoguanidine increases intestinal damage in the acute phase of rat TNB-colitis. *Eur. J. Clin. Invest.* 31: 234–239 (2001).
142. Aiko S, Fuseler J, Grisham MB. Effects of nitric oxide synthase inhibition or sulfasalazine on the spontaneous colitis observed in HLA-B27 transgenic rats. *J. Pharmacol. Exp. Ther.* 284: 722–727 (1998).
143. Rachmilewitz D, Karmeli F, Okon E, Bursztyn M. Experimental colitis is ameliorated by inhibition of nitric oxide synthase activity. *Gut* 37: 247–255 (1995).
144. Pfeiffer CJ, Qiu BS. Effects of chronic nitric oxide synthase inhibition on TNB-induced colitis in rats. *J. Pharm. Pharmacol.* 47: 827–832 (1995).
145. Kiss J, Lamarque D, Delchier JC, Whittle BJ. Time-dependent actions of nitric oxide synthase inhibition on colonic inflammation induced by trinitrobenzene sulphonic acid in rats. *Eur. J. Pharmacol.* 336: 219–224 (1997).
146. Kankuri E, Vaali K, Knowles RG, Lahde M, Korpela R, Vapaatalo H, Moilanen E. Suppression of acute experimental colitis by a highly selective inducible nitric-oxide synthase inhibitor. N-[3-(aminomethyl)benzyl]acetamidine. *J. Pharmacol. Exp. Ther.* 298: 1128–1132 (2001).
147. Hosoi T, Goto H, Arisawa T, Niwa Y, Okada N, Ohmiya N, Hayakawa T. Role of nitric oxide synthase inhibitor in experimental colitis induced by 2,4,6-trinitrobenzene sulphonic acid in rats. *Clin. Exp. Pharmacol. Physiol.* 28: 9–12 (2001).
148. Menchen LA, Colon AL, Moro MA, Leza JC, Lizasoain I, Menchen P, Alvarez E, Lorenzo P. N-(3-(aminomethyl)benzyl)acetamidine, an inducible nitric oxide synthase inhibitor, decreases colonic inflammation induced by trinitrobenzene sulphonic acid in rats. *Life Sci.* 69: 479–491 (2001).
149. Kankuri E, Hamalainen M, Hukkanen M, Salmenpera P, Kivilaakso E, Vapaatalo H, Moilanen E. Suppression of pro-inflammatory cytokine release by selective inhibition of inducible nitric oxide synthase in mucosal explants from patients with ulcerative colitis. *Scand. J. Gastroenterol.* 38: 186–192 (2003).
150. Yue G, Lai PS, Yin K, Sun FF, Nagele RG, Liu X, Linask KK, Wang C, Lin KT, Wong PY. Colon epithelial cell death in 2,4,6-trinitrobenzenesulfonic acid-induced colitis is associated with increased inducible

nitric-oxide synthase expression and peroxynitrite production. *J. Pharmacol. Exp. Ther.* 297: 915–925 (2001).

151. Zingarelli B, Cuzzocrea S, Szabo C, Salzman AL. Mercaptoethylguanidine, a combined inhibitor of nitric oxide synthase and peroxynitrite scavenger, reduces trinitrobenzene sulfonic acid-induced colonic damage in rats. *J. Pharmacol. Exp. Ther.* 287: 1048–1055 (1998).
152. Naito Y, Takagi T, Ishikawa T, Handa O, Matsumoto N, Yagi N, Matsuyama K, Yoshida N, Yoshikawa T. The inducible nitric oxide synthase inhibitor ONO-1714 blunts dextran sulfate sodium colitis in mice. *Eur. J. Pharmacol.* 412: 91–99 (2001).
153. Kim YS, Son M, Ko JI, Cho H, Yoo M, Kim WB, Song IS, Kim CY. Effect of DA-6034, a derivative of flavonoid, on experimental animal models of inflammatory bowel disease. *Arch. Pharm. Res.* 22: 354–360 (1999).
154. Kehrer JP. Free radicals as mediators of tissue injury and disease. *Crit. Rev. Toxicol.* 23: 21–48 (1993).
155. Marnett LJ. Oxyradicals and DNA damage. *Carcinogenesis* 21: 361–370 (2000).
156. Banan A, Zhang Y, Losurdo J, Keshavarzian A. Carbonylation and disassembly of the F-actin cytoskeleton in oxidant induced barrier dysfunction and its prevention by epidermal growth factor and transforming growth factor alpha in a human colonic cell line. *Gut* 46: 830–837 (2000).
157. Grisham MB, Von Ritter C, Smith BF, Lamont JT, Granger DN. Interaction between oxygen radicals and gastric mucin. *Am. J. Physiol.* 253: G93–G96 (1987).
158. Herbert V, Shaw S, Jayatilleke E, Stopler-Kasdan T. Most free-radical injury is iron-related: it is promoted by iron, hemin, holoferritin and vitamin C, and inhibited by desferoxamine and apoferritin. *Stem Cells* 12: 289–303 (1994).
159. Kadiiska MB, Burkitt MJ, Xiang QH, Mason RP. Iron supplementation generates hydroxyl radical *in vivo*. An ESR spin-trapping investigation. *J. Clin. Invest.* 96: 1653–1657 (1995).
160. Reifen R, Matas Z, Zeidel L, Berkovitch Z, Bujanover Y. Iron supplementation may aggravate inflammatory status of colitis in a rat model. *Dig. Dis. Sci.* 45: 394–397 (2000).
161. Carrier J, Aghdassi E, Platt I, Cullen J, Allard JP. Effect of oral iron supplementation on oxidative stress and colonic inflammation in rats with induced colitis. *Aliment. Pharmacol. Ther.* 15: 1989–1999 (2001).
162. Aghdassi E, Carrier J, Cullen J, Tischler M, Allard JP. Effect of iron supplementation on oxidative stress and intestinal inflammation in rats with acute colitis. *Dig. Dis. Sci.* 46: 1088–1094 (2001).

163. Seril DN, Liao J, Ho KL, Warsi A, Yang CS, Yang GY. Dietary iron supplementation enhances DSS-induced colitis and associated colorectal carcinoma development in mice. *Dig. Dis. Sci.* 47: 1266–1278 (2002a).
164. Buell MG, Berin MC. Neutrophil-independence of the initiation of colonic injury. Comparison of results from three models of experimental colitis in the rat. *Dig. Dis. Sci.* 39: 2575–2588 (1994).
165. Yamada T, Zimmerman BJ, Specian RD, Grisham MB. Role of neutrophils in acetic acid-induced colitis in rats. *Inflammation* 15: 399–411 (1991).

20 Oxidative Stress and Neurodegenerative Disease

Katrin Schüssel, Uta Keil and Anne Eckert

1. Introduction

The brain is considered to be especially vulnerable toward oxidative stress due to high levels of prooxidant factors and relatively low antioxidant defence. Putative prooxidant factors consist of a high metabolic rate, high levels of unsaturated fatty acids that readily undergo lipid peroxidation reactions, and relatively high levels of iron in some brain regions that facilitate hydroxyl radical formation from Fenton reactions.[1] Furthermore, neuronal activity results in high levels of intracellular calcium ions after depolarization, which are linked to activation of phospholipase A2, release of arachidonic acid, and subsequent formation of reactive oxygen species (ROS) from cyclooxygenase and lipoxygenase reactions. Calcium ions also facilitate mitochondrial depolarization with release of mitochondrial factors that promote ROS formation. Furthermore, calcium ions are required for nitric oxide synthesis from endothelial and neuronal nitric oxide synthases (eNOS and nNOS). The brain contains relatively high levels of nitric oxide that can give rise to formation of highly reactive peroxynitrite. Also, catecholamine metabolism involves increased ROS formation: superoxide can be generated from semiquinone formation, and hydrogen peroxide is released as by-product of catecholamine synthesis by tyrosine hydroxylase and degradation by monoamonoxidases.

Despite these prooxidant factors, the brain possesses only relatively low levels of antioxidant defenses. Catalase activity is extremely low in

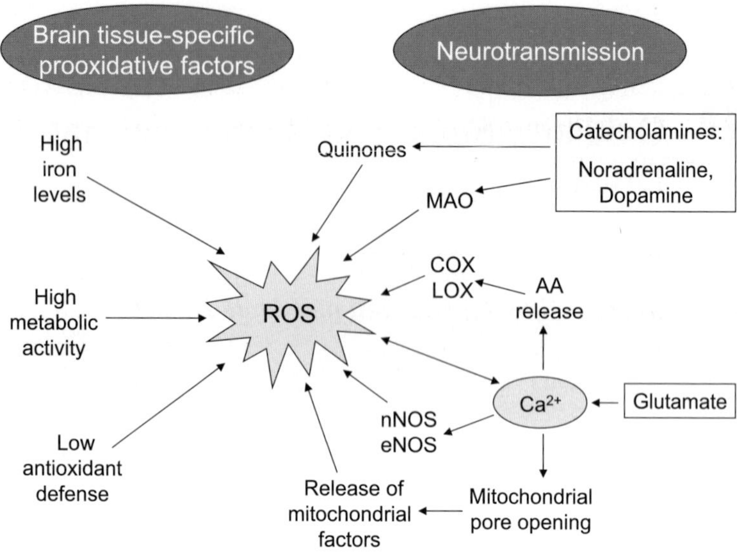

Fig. 1. Factors contributing to accumulation of reactive oxygen species (ROS) in brain tissue. See text for details. MAO, monoamine oxidase; COX, cyclooxygenase; LOX, lipoxygenase; AA, arachidonic acid; eNOS/nNOS, endothelial/neuronal nitric oxide synthase.

brain tissue, and glutathione peroxidase and superoxide dismutase show low activity compared with other organs like liver, heart, and kidney.[2] As a consequence, increased levels of ROS can be especially detrimental to brain tissue (Fig. 1).

Oxidative stress has accordingly been suggested to be a primary factor in the pathogenesis of several chronic neurodegenerative disorders, most prominently Alzheimer's disease (AD), Parkinson's disease (PD), amyotrophic lateral sclerosis (ALS), and Huntington's disease (HD).

2. Evidence for a Pathological Role for Oxidative Stress in Alzheimer's Disease

AD is a neurodegenerative brain disease and the most common form of dementia among the elderly. It is characterized by clinical symptoms of severe and progressive loss of memory, language skills as well as spatial and temporal orientation. Neuropathological hallmarks found in the brains of AD patients are extracellular senile plaques, composed of aggregated amyloid beta peptide (Aβ), and intracellular neurofibrillary tangles, consisting of hyperphosphorylated tau protein. The pathogenic events that lead to the neurodegeneration observed in the brains of AD patients are not understood in detail.

Identification of factors that contribute to the pathology of AD comes from epidemiological as well as genetic studies: AD can be classified into two different forms, rare familial forms (fAD) where the disease onset is at an age younger than 60 years, and the vast majority of sporadic AD (sAD) cases where onset occurs at an age over 60 years. Both forms of AD show the same clinical symptoms and neuropathology. Genetic studies in familial AD patients have identified mutations in the genes encoding for the amyloid precursor protein APP and for the presenilins PS1 and PS2 that cause an autosomal inherited form of AD with 100% penetrance. These fAD mutations consistently lead to increased production of Aβ from its precursor protein APP, which prompted Hardy and Higgins to suggest a direct and pathological role for Aβ accumulation in the development of AD.[3] In the sporadic form of the disease, several risk factors have been found that increase the risk to develop the disease, but — unlike fAD mutations — do not necessarily lead to development of AD. Aging is by far the most important risk factor for AD, but also the apolipoprotein E4 allele and female gender predispose to the development of AD.

Immunohistochemical studies of postmortem AD brains have established that neurons undergo apoptotic cell death. Since reactive oxygen species can elicit apoptotic signaling, the hypothesis that oxidative stress is involved in the pathogenic steps that lead to the development of AD has been proposed in the 1990s by several groups.[4–7] There is a large body of evidence in support of this hypothesis: oxidative stress has been repeatedly shown to be associated with Aβ toxicity and with risk factors for sporadic AD — mostly aging and the apolipoprotein E4 genotype.

2.1. *Evidence for a role for oxidative stress in sporadic AD*

Oxidative stress has been associated with the risk factors for sporadic AD, most prominently with aging,[8] suggesting that an age-associated rise in accumulation of ROS can render the brain more vulnerable toward the development of AD. Consequently, increased markers of oxidative stress have been found in AD patients: several studies have reported elevated levels of lipid peroxidation products, oxidatively modified proteins, and oxidized DNA and RNA bases in brains and cerebrospinal fluid from AD patients compared to age-matched non-demented controls.[9–11] Furthermore, tissue samples from AD brains display a higher susceptibility toward *in vitro* oxidation,[12] suggesting an impairment of antioxidant defense in AD patients. Reports on antioxidant parameters in AD brains have however been contradictory so far. Several antioxidant enzymes have been studied in AD brains with inconsistent results, but the majority of reports found elevations in antioxidant enzymes suggesting an upregulation of antioxidant defense in response to increased ROS levels.[13] Interestingly, upregulation of antioxidant defense was more pronounced in female patients and levels of 4-hydroxynonenal (HNE), a neurotoxic aldehyde derived from lipid peroxidation reactions, were elevated in female compared to male patients. These findings suggest that brains from female AD patients are under higher oxidative pressure,[13] consistent with epidemiological findings that AD is more frequent in women compared to age-matched men. Potential sources of ROS in AD brains include ROS derived from impaired mitochondrial function[14] and secondary ROS formation due to inflammatory reactions. Furthermore, increased monoamine oxidase B activity and increased levels of potentially prooxidative heavy metals like iron have been identified in AD brains.[15,16]

Apart from aging, the apolipoprotein E4 allele is the second most important risk factor for the development of AD. Apolipoprotein E seems to play a role in brain lipid metabolism and neuronal and glial development. It can exist in three different alleles: E2, E3, or E4, which differ in only two amino acids: the E2 isoform contains two and the E3 isoform one cysteine residue, while the E4 isoform contains none. Carriers of the apolipoprotein E4 are at increased risk to develop sporadic AD, especially when they are homozygous carriers. The apolipoprotein E4 allele has been associated with increased oxidative damage in AD brains depending on the numbers of E4 alleles present: oxidative damage was highest in homozygous carriers.[17] *In vitro* studies have evidenced that apolipoprotein E4 is least efficient in binding HNE, a cytotoxic lipid peroxidation product. These findings suggest that the Apo E4 isoform increases susceptibility to oxidative damage thereby possibly predisposing to the development of AD.

2.2. *Oxidative stress and toxicity of mutant APP and presenilins*

Since the proposal of the amyloid hypothesis of AD, toxic mechanisms caused by mutant APP and presenilins related to increased production of Aβ have been extensively studied. Cells exposed to Aβ undergo apoptotic cell death, and the toxicity of Aβ has been shown to be related to production of ROS.[18] Furthermore, toxicity of Aβ depends on its aggregation state, which can be influenced by oxidation. Thus, oxidative stress can cause formation of toxic Aβ species, which in turn can further exacerbate accumulation of ROS in a vicious cycle. This could also explain why the prevalence of AD increases with advancing age — due to rising oxidative stress levels with aging favoring Aβ toxicity.

Toxicity of Aβ is also evident in APP-transfected cells. PC12 cells transfected with mutant APP show higher sensitivity to ROS-induced cell death and increased mitochondrial impairment after challenge with hydrogen peroxide.[19] Toxicity of Aβ has also been evidenced in animal models of the disease. Mice transgenic for mutant APP have high levels of Aβ in their brains and show an age-dependent formation of Aβ plaques similar to the plaques found in AD patients. Increased markers of oxidative stress have been detected in brains of transgenic mice transgenic for mutant APP, accompanied by markers for mitochondrial damage.[20] Furthermore, mutant APP transgenic mice show reduced levels of the antioxidant enzyme copper/zinc superoxide dismutase.[21] Of note, this deficit could be reversed by dietary copper supplementation, which also had an impact on the formation of amyloid plaques in the brains of these mice. These results suggest that augmentation of antioxidant defense by copper supplementation might help to slow the disease progress. Similar observations supporting a role of oxidative stress — partially accounted for by impaired antioxidant defense — in fAD cases in humans has been provided by a study on postmortem brain tissue from patients bearing a familial APP mutation. Increased markers of oxidative stress and reduced antioxidant defense by catalase as well as a trend toward reduced activity of SOD were found in these patients.[22] The results provide an important link of studies on toxicity of mutant APP in cell culture and animal models with the pathogenesis of the disease in fAD patients.

Mutations in the presenilins PS1 and PS2 account for the majority of fAD cases and have similarly been linked with oxidative stress. Oxidative toxicity of mutant presenilins can be either (i) due to increased formation of toxic Aβ, especially the Aβ_{1-42} isoform, or (ii) due to direct toxic effects of mutant presenilins. Several mutations in the presenilins have been found that consistently lead to increased production of Aβ from its precursor protein APP,[23] resulting in increased Aβ levels and toxicity via the above-mentioned mechanisms. However, direct toxic effects of mutant presenilins cannot be ruled out. Expression of mutant presenilins in cell culture and transgenic mice sensitizes cells to apoptotic stimuli by increasing ROS production and mitochondrial damage.[24,25] Furthermore, brains from PS1 mutant transgenic mice display reduced activities of antioxidant enzymes,[26] and lymphocytes from these mice display increased sensitivity to apoptosis accompanied by high intracellular ROS and calcium levels.[14] Interestingly, increased ROS accumulation, disturbed calcium homeostasis, and diminished levels of antioxidants have also been identified in peripheral cells from fAD patients bearing APP or PS mutations as well as in cells from sporadic AD patients.[27] These results suggest that oxidative toxicity observed in transgenic animal models of the disease can indeed play an important role to the pathogenesis of sporadic as well as familial AD in man.

2.3. *Is oxidative stress an early event in the pathogenesis of AD?*

From the above evidence it can be concluded that oxidative stress is a feature of sporadic as well as familial forms of AD. However, it remains to be elucidated whether oxidative stress is a primary factor in the pathogenesis of the disease or only a secondary contributing mechanism. The fact that oxidative damage and mitochondrial dysfunction can be detected at early stages in animal models[20] — even before the presence of Aβ plaques[28] — and that oxidative stress parameters have been detected at highest levels in the early stages of the disease in AD patients[29] suggest that oxidative stress is a primary event in the course of the disease. This is supported by a recent study that reported a reduced risk of AD in users of antioxidant vitamin supplements.[30] Although further clinical trials are needed, antioxidant therapeutic approaches are probably most effective at very early stages of AD or are even better utilized for prevention of the disease.

3. Evidence for an Involvement of Oxidative Stress in Parkinson's Disease

PD is a progressive neurodegenerative disorder that is characterized by impairment in motor function such as bradykinesia, rest tremor, and rigidity. The mean age at onset is 55 and the incidence increases with age. The pathological hallmark of the disease is the selective loss of dopaminergic neurons in the substantia nigra pars compacta (SNPC) accompanied by the formation of intracellular fibrillar α-synuclein and ubiquitin, two protein components of the Lewy bodies.

3.1. *Evidence for oxidative stress in familial PD*

Most PD cases are sporadic, but there are a few rare cases in which PD is inherited (fPD). Mutations in fPD have been found in the genes encoding α-synuclein and parkin. The normal physiological role of α-synuclein seems to be the modulation of synaptic vesicle function.[31] Mutations in α-synuclein may lead to the formation of highly toxic protein aggregates or fibrils that ultimately lead to neuronal cell death.[32] Importantly, expression of mutant α-synuclein was also shown to increase cellular oxidative stress, as determined through the oxidation of DNA, proteins, and lipids.[33] Oxidative damage to α-synuclein can augment its ability to misfold and to aggregate.[34] Accumulation of misfolded proteins is also associated with parkin mutations. Parkin is an E3 ubiquitin ligase,[35] a component of the ubiquitin–proteasome system that identifies and targets misfolded proteins to the proteasome for degradation.[36] Parkin mutations are found in fPD patients with onset before an age of 30.[37] Many parkin mutations abolish this E3 ligase activity, suggesting that accumulation of misfolded parkin substrates could be responsible for the cell death of SNPC dopaminergic neurons in PD. Furthermore, mutations in parkin cause oxidative stress (increased protein oxidation and lipid peroxidation) and sensitize neurons against cell death processes.[38] In addition, parkin knockout mice show decreased serum antioxidant capacity and increased protein and lipid peroxidation levels.[39] From these findings it can be established that oxidative stress seems to be involved in the pathogenesis of fPD.

3.2. *Mitochondrial dysfunction and oxidative stress in sporadic PD*

PD is characterized by a selective loss of dopaminergic neurons in the SNPC. A reason for this selective vulnerability of dopaminergic neurons could be oxidative damage since the biosynthesis and metabolism of dopamine produces hydrogen peroxide and superoxide radicals.[40] Thus, the metabolism of dopamine might be responsible for the high basal levels of oxidative stress found in the substantia nigra. Oxidative stress-induced mitochondrial damage and energy failure may disrupt the vesicular storage of dopamine causing a rise in free cytosolic concentration of dopamine and allowing harmful dopamine-mediated reactions. Thus, dopaminergic neurons seem to be especially susceptible to oxidative attack.

Twenty years ago it was discovered that 1-methyl-4-phenyl-1,2,3,6-tetrahydro-pyridine (MPTP) causes parkinsonism in humans and in laboratory animals.[41] MPTP is known to inhibit complex I of the mitochondrial respiratory chain,[42] but only indirectly, as it is the MPTP metabolite *N*-methyl-4-phenylpyridinium ion (MPP^+) produced by the mitochondrial outer membrane protein monoamine oxidase B (MAO-B) that causes mitochondrial damage. Impairment of the mitochondrial respiratory chain through the attack of MPP^+ might exacerbate superoxide formation that can then initiate apoptotic cell death signaling. Subsequent studies identified abnormalities in complex I activity in PD[43] mostly in the SNPC of PD patients. But the complex I deficiency is not confined to the brain,[44] as reduced complex I activity was also found in platelets from PD patients.[45] Interestingly, cybrid cell lines containing mtDNA derived from PD platelets also show a deficiency of complex I activity and increased ROS levels.[46] Similarly, defiency of complex I activity could lead to increased DNA damage and lipid peroxidation found in PD brains.[47] One target of ROS may be the mitochondrial respiratory chain itself, leading to mitochondrial damage and further production of ROS in a vicious cycle. Thus, several biological markers of oxidative damage are elevated in the SNPC of PD brains,[48] which may be causally related to increased levels of iron in the substantia nigra in PD.[49–51] Increased levels of 4-hydroxynonenal HNE,[52,53] oxidatively modified proteins,[54–56] and DNA bases[55–57] have been identified in vulnerable brain regions from PD patients. In addition, the antioxidative defense system seems to be impaired in PD. Studies show that GSH levels in the SNPC of PD brains are reduced resulting in increased ROS accumulation in this brain region.[58]

Additionally, there is increasing evidence that oxidative damage also results from nitric oxide. Nitric oxide might react with superoxide to form peroxynitrite. In the SNPC of PD patients there is increased immunoreactivity for inducible NO synthase.[59] Thus, mitochondrial respiratory chain complexes might be damaged by sustained exposure to NO.[60] NO itself also may affect GSH levels by inhibition of GSH reductase[61] leading to a reduced antioxidant capacity.

An apoptotic type of cell death that might be related to mitochondrial dysfunction has been suggested to occur in PD. The demonstration of increased numbers of TUNEL-positive dopaminergic neurons and increased caspase-3 and -9 activity in the brains of PD patients supports the occurrence of apoptosis in this disease.[62–64] Additionally, the neuronal expression of the proapoptotic molecule Bax is increased in PD[65] and immunolocalization of Bax shows that a greater percentage of dopaminergic neurons in the SNPC were positive in brains of patients with PD.[63] Moreover Bax content seems to be higher in the remaining dopaminergic neurons.[66] Taken together, these findings suggest that the intrinsic pathway of apoptosis via mitochondria is involved in neuronal cell loss in PD patients.

A number of therapies targeting oxidative stress and mitochondrial dysfunction, e.g., iron chelators, radical scavenger antioxidants, MAO-B inhibitors, glutamate antagonists, and nitric oxide synthase inhibitors, are efficacious in the MPTP model of PD. Coenzyme Q(10), an essential electron carrier and an important antioxidant in the mitochondrial inner membrane, appears to be particularly promising based on the results of a recent phase 2 clinical trial in which it significantly slowed the progression of PD.[67]

4. Evidence for an Involvement of Oxidative Stress in Amyotrophic Lateral Sclerosis ALS

ALS is a disorder with onset in mid-life, which is characterized by a selective and progressive degeneration of lower and upper motor neurons in spinal cord and cerebral cortex. Clinical symptoms are progressive muscle weakness leading in later stages to paralysis and death due to respiratory failure. The disease can occur as a sporadic form (sALS) with no clear genetic influence or in a familial form (fALS), which is genetically inherited. In a subset of patients suffering from familial forms of ALS (fALS), rare mutations in the genes encoding copper/zinc-superoxide dismutase (Cu/Zn-SOD) and ALS-2 have been identified. The toxic properties of mutant of Cu/Zn-SODs are still a matter of debate and the function of ALS-2 is unknown — it is a putative guanine exchange factor for a yet unidentified G protein.

Direct evidence for an involvement of oxidative stress in ALS comes from studies on postmortem spinal cord and motor cortex tissue and analysis of cerebrospinal fluid from sALS and fALS patients. Oxidatively modified proteins and DNA bases as well as 4-hydroxynonenal (HNE), a marker for lipid peroxidation, were increased in ALS patients.[68–70] Furthermore, 3-nitrotyrosine, a marker for peroxynitrite formation, was elevated in tissue from sporadic and familial ALS patients and also in a transgenic animal model of ALS overexpressing mutant Cu/Zn-SOD.[71,72]

4.1. *Oxidative toxicity of fALS mutant Cu/Zn-SOD*

Under physiological conditions, Cu/Zn-SOD plays an important role in detoxification of superoxide radical anions. Transgenic mouse models overexpressing fALS mutant Cu/Zn-SOD display progressive motor neuron disease similar to ALS in humans[73] suggesting a direct pathological role for mutant Cu/Zn-SOD in the pathogenesis of the disease. For some ALS mutations, reduced enzymatic activity has been shown, thought to be associated with increased accumulation of superoxide radicals and thus probably causally detrimental to neurons. However, reduced Cu/Zn-SOD activity was neither found in other familial forms of ALS nor in sporadic ALS patients. Furthermore, a knockout of the Cu/Zn-SOD does not lead to ALS symptoms in mice. Therefore, rather a toxic gain-of-function mechanism has been associated with fALS mutant Cu/Zn-SOD. Enhanced formation of superoxide radicals, increased peroxidase activity, and superoxide reductase activity have been implicated as toxic mechanisms of mutated Cu/Zn-SODs.[74] This toxic function of mutant Cu/Zn-SOD is probably related to altered metal-binding properties of the protein resulting in increased peroxidative ability and increased levels of free copper and/or zinc ions. Copper ions can mediate one-electron oxidation and reduction reactions and thus propagate formation of highly reactive hydroxyl radicals from hydrogen peroxide via Fenton chemistry. Alternatively, altered protein conformation and copper binding could facilitate access of peroxynitrite — a highly reactive ROS derived from nitric oxide and superoxide radical anions — to the active site of the enzyme, thus facilitating nitration of tyrosine residues. Increased levels of nitrotyrosine have been found in sALS as well as fALS patients and moreover in fALS mutant Cu/Zn-SOD transgenic mice. Furthermore, immunohistochemical studies have shown that nitrotyrosine immunoreactivity was predominantly found in degenerating neurons suggesting a pathogenic role for peroxynitrite in motor neurodegeneration in ALS.

4.2. *Oxidative toxicity due to AMPA/kainate receptor overstimulation*

Other sources of ROS in the disease could be attributed to a rise in intracellular calcium levels caused by overstimulation of AMPA/kainate receptors.[75] Large numbers of a subset of AMPA/kainate receptors that are calcium-permeable have been identified in motor neurons which could explain the selective vulnerability of these neurons in ALS. Increased intracellular calcium levels have been shown to elicit mitochondrial calcium overload and dysfunction accompanied by increased ROS formation. Oxidative damage to glutamate transporters GLT-1 on astrocytes could subsequently lead to accumulation of extracellular glutamate and further stimulation of AMPA/kainate receptors on motor neurons in a vicious cycle. Impaired activity of GLT-1 was detected in ALS patients[76] and mutant Cu/Zn-SOD transgenic mice. In accordance with these observations, elevated levels of CSF glutamate have been found in a subset of patients. Of note, the only drug approved for the treatment of ALS, riluzole, can reduce excitotoxic signaling by glutamate. However, clinical efficacy of riluzole is rather limited, which necessitates the search for new therapeutic approaches. Although vitamin E was efficient in an ALS mouse model, it has shown only a marginal benefit in ALS patients.[77] Recent studies on animal models support the idea that combinations of several therapeutic approaches — e.g., inhibition of microglial activation, blockade of glutamate signaling, and calcium antagonists — can have additive effects, an approach that might be valuable for further studies of neuroprotective therapies in ALS patients.

5. Evidence for a Pathological Role for Oxidative Stress in Huntington's Disease

HD is an autosomal dominant neurodegenerative disorder characterized by chronic involuntary movements. Pathologically there is a selective neuronal loss in the striatum and cerebral cortex. HD is a trinucleotide repeat disorder, with expansions of a CAG repeat in the gene that encodes for huntingtin, a cytoplasmic protein of unknown function. The CAG triplet codes for glutamine. When mutated, the protein contains a polyglutamine tract at the N-terminus. Polyglutamine fragments are able to accumulate as aggregates in the cytoplasm or in the nucleus in striatum and cortex. Intraneuronal and cytoplasmic aggregates of mutant huntingtin have been identified in both human HD brains and in transgenic animal models of HD.[78,79] The role of these inclusions in the pathogenesis remains unclear. Probably, the accumulation of mutant huntingtin may induce neuronal cell death. In postmortem tissue from patients with HD, TUNEL-positive cells have been detected in the neostriatum.[80,81] In addition, caspases-1 and -8 are activated in the brain of HD patients. Although these findings indicate that caspases might be valuable targets for therapeutic intervention in HD, how mutant huntingtin triggers neuronal cell death remains unclear.

5.1. *Mitochondrial dysfunction and oxidative stress in HD*

Defects in mitochondrial complex II and III activity and in aconitase have been found in postmortem HD brains.[82] Moreover, mitochondrial respiratory chain inhibitors such as 3-nitropropionic acid and malonate induce brain lesions in animals that mimic the pathology of HD. Occipital cortex and basal ganglia of HD patients show elevated lactate levels,[83] suggesting an increase in anerobic energy metabolism. In addition, lymphoblasts from HD patients show increased cyanide-induced depolarization of mitochondria. Recently, it was demonstrated that lymphoblast mitochondria from patients with HD have a lower mitochondrial membrane potential than control mitochondria. In brain mitochondria from transgenic mice expressing mutant huntingtin, similar mitochondrial defects can be observed.[84]

Oxidative damage is one of the major consequences of defects in energy metabolism. Bogdanov and coworkers could show that oxidative damage to DNA in the striatum of a transgenic mouse model of Huntington's disease is elevated,[85] suggesting increased oxidative stress in the brains of these mice. In accordance with this finding, other studies have shown that lipid peroxidation is increased in these transgenic mice.[86] Moreover, there is a significant increase of DNA damage in HD caudate and in mitochondrial DNA from parietal cortex of HD patients.[87] Moreover, DNA strand breaks could be found in HD postmortem tissue, which might be a consequence of oxidative damage.[81] The activity of glutamine synthetase, an enzyme that is especially susceptible to oxidative damage, is significantly reduced in HD postmortem tissue[88] suggesting that oxidative stress is involved in the pathogenesis of HD.

A defect in energy metabolism leading to increased susceptibility to excitotoxic injury has also been proposed as a potential pathogenic mechanism underlying HD.[89] Increasing evidence suggests that glutamate mediated excitotoxicity via NMDA receptors may be involved in the neurodegeneration of HD. Neurons bearing NMDA receptors appear to be relatively lost in HD. Moreover, intrastriatal lesions of NMDA receptor agonists mimic the lesions seen in HD.

6. Concluding Remarks

From the above evidence it can be concluded that oxidative stress is a feature of several neurodegenerative disorders. However, it has to be carefully considered whether oxidative stress is a primary factor in the pathogenesis of the disease or only a secondary contributing mechanism. The mere presence of oxidative stress markers in tissues from patients is not sufficient to decide on this matter. Rather prospective studies of different disease stages in humans or studies on different mouse models mimicking the respective disease pathology will be helpful to determine at which stages oxidative damage occurs — and if it is causally related to functional deficits. As a consequence, therapeutic approaches utilizing antioxidants will probably be effective only under neurodegenerative disease conditions where oxidative stress is an early and causal trigger of the disease process, and these approaches are best taken advantage of in very early stages of the disease.

References

1. Halliwell B. Reactive oxygen species and the central nervous system. *J. Neurochem.* 59: 1609–1623 (1992).
2. Marklund SL, Westman NG, Lundgren E, Roos G. Copper- and zinc-containing superoxide dismutase, manganese-containing superoxide dismutase, catalase, and glutathione peroxidase in normal and neoplastic human cell lines and normal human tissues. *Cancer Res.* 42: 1955–1961 (1982).
3. Hardy JA, Higgins GA. Alzheimer's disease: the amyloid cascade hypothesis. *Science* 256: 184–185 (1992).
4. Blass JP, Gibson GE. The role of oxidative abnormalities in Alzheimer's disease. *Rev. Neurol. (Paris)* 147: 513–525 (1991).
5. Benzi G, Moretti A. Are reactive oxygen species involved in Alzheimer's disease? *Neurobiol. Aging* 16: 661–674 (1995).
6. Markesbery WR. Oxidative stress hypothesis in Alzheimer's disease. *Free Radic. Biol. Med.* 23: 134–147 (1997).
7. Smith MA, Sayre LM, Monnier VM, Perry G. Radical ageing in Alzheimer's disease. *Trends Neurosci.* 18: 172–176 (1995).
8. Leutner S, Eckert A, Muller WE. ROS generation, lipid peroxidation and antioxidant enzyme activities in the aging brain. *J. Neural Transm.* 108: 955–967 (2001).
9. Lovell MA, Ehmann WD, Butler SM, Markesbery WR. Elevated thiobarbituric acid-reactive substances and antioxidant enzyme activity in the brain in Alzheimer's disease. *Neurology* 45: 1594–1601 (1995).
10. Smith CD, Carney JM, Starke-Reed PE, Oliver CN, Stadtman ER, Floyd RA, Markesbery WR. Excess brain protein oxidation and enzyme dysfunction in normal aging and in Alzheimer disease. *Proc. Natl. Acad. Sci. USA* 88: 10540–10543 (1991).

11. Lyras L, Cairns NJ, Jenner A, Jenner P, Halliwell B. An assessment of oxidative damage to proteins, lipids, and DNA in brain from patients with Alzheimer's disease. *J. Neurochem.* 68: 2061–2069 (1997).
12. Subbarao KV, Richardson JS, Ang LC. Autopsy samples of Alzheimer's cortex show increased peroxidation *in vitro*. *J. Neurochem.* 55: 342–345 (1990).
13. Schuessel K, Leutner S, Cairns NJ, Müller WE, Eckert A. Impact of gender on upregulation of antioxidant defence mechanisms in Alzheimer's disease brain. *J. Neural. Transm.*, in press (2004).
14. Eckert A, Schindowski K, Leutner S, Luckhaus C, Touchet N, Czech C, Muller WE. Alzheimer's disease-like alterations in peripheral cells from presenilin-1 transgenic mice. *Neurobiol. Dis.* 8: 331–342 (2001).
15. Deibel MA, Ehmann WD, Markesbery WR. Copper, iron, and zinc imbalances in severely degenerated brain regions in Alzheimer's disease: possible relation to oxidative stress. *J. Neurol. Sci.* 143: 137–142 (1996).
16. Cornett CR, Markesbery WR, Ehmann WD. Imbalances of trace elements related to oxidative damage in Alzheimer's disease brain. *Neurotoxicology* 19: 339–345 (1998).
17. Ramassamy C, Averill D, Beffert U, Bastianetto S, Theroux L, Lussier-Cacan S, Cohn JS, Christen Y, Davignon J, Quirion R, Poirier J. *Free. Radic. Biol. Med.* 27: 544–553 (1999).
18. Butterfield DA, Drake J, Pocernich C, Castegna A. Evidence of oxidative damage in Alzheimer's disease brain: central role for amyloid beta-peptide. *Trends Mol. Med.* 7: 548–554 (2001).
19. Marques CA, Keil U, Bonert A, Steiner B, Haass C, Muller WE, Eckert A. Neurotoxic mechanisms caused by the Alzheimer's disease-linked Swedish amyloid precursor protein mutation: oxidative stress, caspases, and the JNK pathway. *J. Biol. Chem.* 278: 28294–28302 (2003).
20. Blanchard V, Moussaoui S, Czech C, Touchet N, Bonici B, Planche M, Canton T, Jedidi I, Gohin M, Wirths O, Bayer TA, Langui D, Duyckaerts C, Tremp G, Pradier L. Time sequence of maturation of dystrophic neurites associated with Abeta deposits in APP/PS1 transgenic mice. *Exp. Neurol.* 184: 247–263 (2003).
21. Bayer TA, Schafer S, Simons A, Kemmling A, Kamer T, Tepest R, Eckert A, Schuessel K, Eikenberg O, Sturchler-Pierrat C, Abramowski D, Staufenbiel M, Multhaup G. Dietary Cu stabilizes brain superoxide dismutase 1 activity and reduces amyloid Abeta production in APP23 transgenic mice. *Proc. Natl. Acad. Sci. USA* 100: 14187–14192 (2003).
22. Bogdanovic N, Zilmer M, Zilmer K, Rehema A, Karelson E. The Swedish APP670/671 Alzheimer's disease mutation: the first evidence for strikingly

increased oxidative injury in the temporal inferior cortex. *Dement. Geriatr. Cogn. Disord.* 12: 364–370 (2001).

23. Duff K, Eckman C, Zehr C, Yu X, Prada CM, Perez-tur J, Hutton M, Buee L, Harigaya Y, Yager D, Morgan D, Gordon MN, Holcomb L, Refolo L, Zenk B, Hardy J, Younkin S. Increased amyloid-beta42(43) in brains of mice expressing mutant presenilin 1. *Nature* 383: 710–713 (1996).
24. Guo Q, Furukawa K, Sopher BL, Pham DG, Xie J, Robinson N, Martin GM, Mattson MP. Alzheimer's PS-1 mutation perturbs calcium homeostasis and sensitizes PC12 cells to death induced by amyloid beta-peptide. *Neuroreport* 8: 379–383 (1996).
25. Guo Q, Sebastian L, Sopher BL, Miller MW, Ware CB, Martin GM, Mattson MP. Increased vulnerability of hippocampal neurons from presenilin-1 mutant knock-in mice to amyloid beta-peptide toxicity: central roles of superoxide production and caspase activation. *J. Neurochem.* 72: 1019–1029 (1999).
26. Leutner S, Czech C, Schindowski K, Touchet N, Eckert A, Muller WE. Reduced antioxidant enzyme activity in brains of mice transgenic for human presenilin-1 with single or multiple mutations. *Neurosci. Lett.* 292: 87–90 (2000).
27. Schindowski K, Kratzsch T, Peters J, Steiner B, Leutner S, Touchet N, Maurer K, Czech C, Pradier L, Frolich L, Muller WE, Eckert A. Impact of aging: sporadic, and genetic risk factors on vulnerability to apoptosis in Alzheimer's disease. *Neuromol. Med.* 4: 161–178 (2003).
28. Pratico D, Uryu K, Leight S, Trojanoswki JQ, Lee VM. Increased lipid peroxidation precedes amyloid plaque formation in an animal model of Alzheimer amyloidosis. *J. Neurosci.* 21: 4183–4187 (2001).
29. Nunomura A, Perry G, Aliev G, Hirai K, Takeda A, Balraj EK, Jones PK, Ghanbari H, Wataya T, Shimohama S, Chiba S, Atwood CS, Petersen RB, Smith MA. Oxidative damage is the earliest event in Alzheimer disease. *J. Neuropathol. Exp. Neurol.* 60: 759–767 (2001).
30. Zandi PP, Anthony JC, Khachaturian AS, Stone SV, Gustafson D, Tschanz JT, Norton MC, Welsh-Bohmer KA, Breitner JC. Reduced risk of Alzheimer disease in users of antioxidant vitamin supplements: the Cache County Study. *Arch. Neurol.* 61: 82–88 (2004).
31. Kahle PJ, Haass C, Kretzschmar HA, Neumann M. Structure/function of alpha-synuclein in health and disease: rational development of animal models for Parkinson's disease and related diseases. *J. Neurochem.* 82: 449–457 (2002).

32. Dawson TM, Mandir AS, Lee MK. Animal models of PD: pieces of the same puzzle? *Neuron* 35: 219–222 (2002).
33. Lee M, Hyun D, Halliwell B, Jenner P. Effect of the overexpression of wild-type or mutant alpha-synuclein on cell susceptibility to insult. *J. Neurochem.* 76: 998–1009 (2001).
34. Giasson BI, Duda JE, Murray IV, Chen Q, Souza JM, Hurtig HI, Ischiropoulos H, Trojanowski JQ, Lee VM. Oxidative damage linked to neurodegeneration by selective alpha-synuclein nitration in synucleinopathy lesions. *Science* 290: 985–989 (2000).
35. Zhang Y, Gao J, Chung KK, Huang H, Dawson VL, Dawson TM. Parkin functiond as an E2-dependent ubiquitin-protein ligase and promotes the degradation of the synaptic vesicle-associated protein, CDCrel-1. *Proc. Natl. Acad. Sci.* 97: 13354–13359 (2000).
36. Sherman MY, Goldberg AL, Cellular defenses against unfolded proteins: a cell biologist thinks about neurodegenerative diseases. *Neuron* 29: 15–32 (2001).
37. Mizuno Y, Hattori N, Mori H, Suzuki T, Tanaka K. Parkin and Parkinson's disease. *Curr. Opin. Neurol.* 14: 477–482 (2001).
38. Hyun DH, Lee M, Hattori N, Kubo S, Mizuno Y, Halliwell B, Jenner P. Effect of wild-type or mutant Parkin on oxidative damage, nitric oxide, antioxidant defenses, and the proteasome. *J. Biol. Chem.* 277: 28572–28577 (2002).
39. Palacino JJ, Sagi D, Goldberg MS, Krauss S, Motz C, Klose J, Shen J. Mitochondrial dysfunction and oxidative damage in Parkin-deficient mice. *J. Biol. Chem.* 279: 18614–18622 (2004).
40. Graham DG. Oxidative pathways for catecholamines in the genesis of neuromelanin and cytotoxic quinines. *Mol. Pharmacol.* 14: 633–643 (1978).
41. Langston JW, Ballard P, Tetrud JW, Irwin I. Chronic Parkinsonism in humans due to a product of meperidine-analog synthesis. *Science* 219: 979–980 (1983).
42. Nicklas WJ, Youngster SK, Kindt MV, Heikkila RE. MPTP, MPP+ and mitochondrial function. *Life Sci.* 40: 721–729 (1987).
43. Greenamyre JT, Sherer TB, Betarbet R, Panov AV. Complex I and Parkinson's disease. *IUBMB Life* 52: 135–141 (2001).
44. Schapira AH, Cooper JM, Dexter D, Clark JB, Jenner P, Marsden CD. Mitochondrial complex I deficiency in Parkinson's disease. *J. Neurochem.* 54: 823–827 (1990).
45. Parker WD Jr, Boyson SJ, Parks JK. Abnormalities of the electron transport chain in idiopathic Parkinson's disease. *Ann. Neurol.* 26: 719–723 (1989).
46. Swerdlow RH, Parks JK, Miller SW, Tuttle JB, Trimmer PA, Sheehan JP, Bennett JP Jr., Davis RE, Parker WD Jr. Origin and functional consequences

of the complex I defect in Parkinson's disease. *Ann. Neurol.* 40: 663–671 (1996).
47. Dexter DT, Holley AE, Flitter WD, Slater TF, Wells FR, Daniel SE, Lees AJ, Jenner P, Marsden CD. Increased levels of hydroperoxides in the Parkinsonian substantia nigra: an HPLC and ESR study. *Mov. Disord.* 9: 92–97 (1994).
48. Przedborski S, Jacksin-Lewis V. ROS and Parkinson's disease: a view to a kill. In: Poli G, Cadenas E, Packer L (eds.) Free Radicals in Brain Pathophysiology. Marcel Dekker, New York, 2000, pp. 273–290.
49. Dexter DT, Carter CJ, Wells FR, Javoy-Agid F, Agid Y, Lees A, Jenner P, Marsden CD. Basal lipid peroxidation in substantia nigra is increased in Parkinson's disease. *J. Neurochem.* 52: 381–389 (1989).
50. Sofic E, Riederer P, Heinsen H, Beckmann H, Reynolds GP, Hebenstreit G, Youdim MB. Increased iron (III) and total iron content in post mortem substantia nigra of Parkinsonian brain. *J. Neural. Transm.* 74: 199–205 (1988).
51. Hirsch EC, Brandel JP, Galle P, Javoy-Agid F, Agid Y. Iron and aluminium increase in the the substantia nigra of patients with Parkinson's disease: an X-ray microanalysis. *J. Neurochem.* 56: 446–451 (1991).
52. Yoritaka A, Hattori N, Uchida K, Tanaka M, Stadtman ER, Mizuno Y. Immunohistochemical detection of 4-hydroxynonenam protein adducts in Parkinson disease. *Proc. Natl. Acad. Sci. USA* 93: 2696–2701 (1996).
53. Picklo MJ, Amarnath V, McIntyre JO, Graham DG, Montine TJ. 4-Hydroxy-2(E)-nonenal inhibits CNS mitochondrial respiration at multiple sites. *J. Neurochem.* 72: 1617–1624 (1999).
54. Floor E, Wetzel MG. Increased protein oxidation in human substantia nigra pars compacta in comparison with basal ganglia and prefrontal cortex measured with an improved dinitrophenylhydrazine assay. *J. Neurochem.* 70: 268–275 (1998).
55. Alam ZI, Daniel SE, Lees AJ, Marsden DC, Jenner P, Halliwell B. A generalised increase in protein carbonyls in the brain in Parkinson's but not incidental Lewy body disease. *J. Neurochem.* 69: 1326–1329 (1997).
56. Alam ZI, Jenner A, Daniel SE, Lees AJ, Cairns N, Marsden CD, Jenner P, Halliwell B. Oxidative DNA damage in the Parkinsonian brain: an apparent selective increase in 8-hydroxyguanine levels in substantia nigra. *J. Neurochem.* 69: 1196–1203 (1997).
57. Zhang Y, Gao J, Chung KK, Huang H, Dawson VL, Dawson TM. Parkin function as an E2-dependent ubiquitin-protein ligase and promotes the degradation of the synaptic vesicle-associated protein, CDCrel-1. *Proc. Natl. Acad. Sci. USA* 97: 13354–13359 (2000).

58. Sian J, Dexter DT, Lees AJ, Daniel S, Jenner P, Marsden CD. Glutathione-related enzymes in brain in Parkinson's disease. *Ann. Neurol.* 36: 356–361 (1994).
59. Hunot S, Boissiere F, Faucheux B, Brugg B, Mouatt-Prigent A, Agid Y, Hirsch EC. Nitric oxide synthase and neuronal vulnerability in Parkinson's disease. *Neuroscience* 72: 355–363 (1996).
60. Clementi E, Brown GC, Feelisch M, Moncada S. Persistent inhibition of cell respiration by nitric oxide: crucial role of S-nitrosylation of mitochondrial complex I and protective action of glutathione. *Proc. Natl. Acad. Sci. USA* 95: 7631–7636 (1998).
61. Barker JE, Heales SJ, Cassidy A, Bolanos JP, Land JM, Clark JB. Depletion of brain glutathione results in a decrease of glutathione reductase activity; an enzyme susceptible to oxidative damage. *Brain Res.* 716: 118–122 (1996).
62. Mochizuki H, Goto K, Mori H, Mizuno Y. Histochemical detection of apoptosis in Parkinson's disease. *J. Neurol. Sci.* 137: 120–123 (1996).
63. Hartmann A, Troadec JD, Hunot S, Kikly K, Faucheux BA, Mouatt-Prigent A, Ruberg M, Agid Y, Hirsch EC. Caspase-8 is an effector in apoptotic death of dopaminergic neurons in Parkinson's disease, but pathway inhibition results in neuronal necrosis. *J. Neurosci.* 21: 2247–2255 (2001).
64. Viswanath V, Wu Y, Boonplueang R, Chen S, Stevenson FF, Yantiri F, Yang L, Beal MF, Andersen JK. Caspase-9 activation results in downstream caspase-8 activation and bid cleavage in 1-methyl-4-phenyl-1,2,3,6-tetrahydropyridine-induced Parkinson's disease, *J. Neurosci.* 21: 9519–9528 (2001).
65. Hartmann A, Michel PP, Troadec JD, Mouatt-Prigent A, Faucheux BA, Ruberg M, Agid Y, Hirsch EC. Is Bax a mitochondrial mediator in apoptotic death of dopaminergic neurons in Parkinson's disease? *J. Neurochem.* 76: 1785–1793 (2001).
66. Tatton NA. Increased caspase 3 and Bax immunoreactivity accompany nuclear GAPDH translocation and neuronal apoptosis in Parkinson's disease. *Exp. Neurol.* 166: 29–43 (2000).
67. Beal MF. Mitochondria, oxidative damage, and inflammation in Parkinson's disease. *Ann. N. Y. Acad. Sci.* 991: 120–131 (2003).
68. Ferrante RJ, Browne SE, Shinobu LA, Bowling AC, Baik MJ, MacGarvey U, Kowall NW, Brown RH Jr., Beal MF. Evidence of increased oxidative damage in both sporadic and familial amyotrophic lateral sclerosis. *J. Neurochem.* 69: 2064–2074 (1997).
69. Smith RG, Henry YK, Mattson MP, Appel SH. Presence of 4-hydroxynonenal in cerebrospinal fluid of patients with sporadic amyotrophic lateral sclerosis. *Ann. Neurol.* 44: 696–699 (1998).

70. Pedersen WA, Fu W, Keller JN, Markesbery WR, Appel S, Smith RG, Kasarskis E, Mattson MP. Protein modification by the lipid peroxidation product 4-hydroxynonenal in the spinal cords of amyotrophic lateral sclerosis patients. *Ann. Neurol.* 44: 819–824 (1998).
71. Beal MF, Ferrante RJ, Browne SE, Matthews RT, Kowall NW, Brown RH Jr. Increased 3-nitrotyrosine in both sporadic and familial amyotrophic lateral sclerosis. *Ann. Neurol.* 42: 644–654 (1997).
72. Bruijn LI, Beal MF, Becher MW, Schulz JB, Wong PC, Price DL, Cleveland DW. Elevated free nitrotyrosine levels, but not protein-bound nitrotyrosine or hydroxyl radicals, throughout amyotrophic lateral sclerosis (ALS)-like disease implicate tyrosine nitration as an aberrant *in vivo* property of one familial ALS-linked superoxide dismutase 1 mutant. *Proc. Natl. Acad. Sci. USA* 94: 7606–7611 (1997).
73. Gurney ME, Pu H, Chiu AY, Dal Canto MC, Polchow CY, Alexander DD, Caliendo J, Hentati A, Kwon YW, Deng HX, Chen W, Zhai P, Sufit RL, Siddique T. Motor neuron degeneration in mice that express a human Cu,Zn superoxide dismutase mutation. *Science* 264: 1772–1775 (1994).
74. Liochev SI, Fridovich I. Mutant Cu,Zn superoxide dismutases and familial amyotrophic lateral sclerosis: evaluation of oxidative hypotheses. *Free Radic. Biol. Med.* 34: 1383–1389 (2003).
75. Rao SD, Weiss JH. Excitotoxic and oxidative cross-talk between motor neurons and glia in ALS pathogenesis. *Trends Neurosci.* 27: 17–23 (2004).
76. Rothstein JD, Van Kammen M, Levey AI, Martin LJ, Kuncl RW. Selective loss of glial glutamate transporter GLT-1 in amyotrophic lateral sclerosis. *Ann. Neurol.* 38: 73–84 (1995).
77. Desnuelle C, Dib M, Garrel C, Favier AA. A double-blind, placebo-controlled randomized clinical trial of alpha-tocopherol (vitamin E) in the treatment of amyotrophic lateral sclerosis. ALS riluzole-tocopherol Study Group. *Amyotroph. Lateral. Scler. Other Motor Neuron Disord.* 2: 9–18 (2001).
78. Davies SW, Turmaine M, Cozens BA, DiFiglia M, Sharp AH, Ross CA, Scherzinger E, Wanker EE, Mangiarini L, Bates GP. Formation of neuronal intranuclear inclusions underlies the neurological dysfunction in mice transgenic for the HD mutation. *Cell* 90: 537–548 (1997).
79. DiFiglia M, Sapp E, Chase KO, Davies SW, Bates GP, Vonsattel JP, Aronin N. Aggregation of huntingtin in neuronal intranuclear inclusions and dystrophic neuritis in brain. *Science* 277: 1990–1993 (1997).
80. Thomas LB, Gates DJ, Richfield EK, O'Brien TF, Schweitzer JB, Steindler DA. DNA end labeling (TUNEL) in Huntington's disease and other neuropathological conditions. *Exp. Neurol.* 133: 265–272 (1995).

81. Portera-Cailliau C, Hedreen JC, Price DL, Koliatsos VE. Evidence for apoptotic cell death in Huntington disease and excitotoxic animal models. *J. Neurosci.* 15: 3775–3787 (1995).
82. Brennan W, Bird E, Aprille J. Regional mitochondrial respiratory activity in Huntington's disease brain. *J. Neurochem.* 44: 1948–1950 (1985).
83. Jenkins JG, Koroshetz WJ, Beal MF, Rosen BR. Evidence for impairment of energy metabolism *in vivo* in Huntington's disease using localized 1H NMR spectroscopy. *Neurology* 43: 2689–2695 (1993).
84. Panov AV, Gutekunst CA, Leavitt BR, Hayden MR, Burke JR, Strittmatter WJ, Greenamyre JT. Early mitochondrial calcium defects in Huntington's disease are a direct effct of polyglutamines. *Nat. Neurosci.* 5: 731–736 (2002).
85. Bogdanov MB, Andreassen OA, Dedeoglu A, Ferrante RJ, Beal MF. Increased oxidative damage to DNA in atransgenic mouse model of Huntington's disease. *J. Neurochem.* 79: 1246–1249 (2001).
86. Perez-Severiano F, Rios C, Segovia, J. Striatal oxidative damage parallels the expression of a neurological phenotype in mice transgenic for the mutation of Huntington's disease. *Brain Res.* 862: 234–237 (2000).
87. Browne SE, Bowling AC, MacGarvey U, Baik MJ, Berger SC, Muquit MM, Bird ED, Beal MF. Oxidative damage and metabolic dysfunction in Huntington's disease: selective vulnerability of the basal ganglia. *Ann. Neurol.* 41: 646–653 (1997).
88. Butterworth J, Yates CM, Reynolds GP. Distribution of phosphate-activated glutaminase, succinic dehydrogenase, pyruvate dehydrogenase and γ-glutamyl transpeptidase in post-mortem brain from Huntington's disease and agonal cases. *J. Neurol. Sci.* 67: 161–171 (1985).
89. Beal MF. Does impairment of energy metabolism result in excitotoxic neuronal cell death in neurodegenerative illnesses? *Ann. Neurol.* 31: 119–130 (1992).

21 Oxidative Stress and Mitochondrial Disease

Ching-You Lu, Cheng-Feng Lee, Yi-Shing Ma, Chun-Yi Liu, Chia-Yu Wei, Yin-Chiu Chen, Shi-Bei Wu, and Yau-Huei Wei

1. Introduction

Generation of energy in the form of ATP from fuel molecules in foodstuff by biological oxidation in human cells is not a perfect metabolic process. Reactive oxygen species (ROS) including superoxide anions ($\bullet O_2^-$), hydrogen peroxide (H_2O_2), and hydroxyl radicals (•OH) are continually produced in tissue cells as byproducts of aerobic metabolism.[1] Although ROS at low concentrations can serve as physiological signals in the regulation of cell proliferation and other cellular functions,[2,3] they may damage nucleic acids,[4] proteins,[5] lipids,[6] and other cellular components at high concentrations.

To cope with the oxidative stress elicited by aerobic metabolism, human cells have developed an antioxidant defense system.[7,8] Superoxide dismutase (SOD), catalase (CAT), glutathione peroxidase (GPx), and glutathione reductase (GR) together with low-molecular-weight antioxidants such as ascorbic acid, α-tocopherol, retinal, and glutathione constitute the antioxidant defense system to dispose of ROS and free radicals to minimize their damaging effects. However, this antioxidant defense system may be altered by various intrinsic and extrinsic factors such that a fraction of the ROS may escape destruction and get transformed to the far more reactive hydroxyl radicals.[7–10] It has been reported that the expression profile of free radical scavenging enzymes is altered and oxidative damage to DNA and lipids are increased in skin fibroblasts or leukocytes of patients with CPEO and mitochondrial respiratory chain deficiency cause by deletions and point mutations of mitochondrial DNA (mtDNA).[11,12] Based on these reports and recent work, we have proposed that oxidative stress plays a role in the pathophysiology of mitochondrial diseases.

2. Mitochondria are the Major Producer and Target of ROS in Mammalian Cells

It is established that intracellular ROS production is directly proportional to the rate of mitochondrial oxygen consumption of human and animal cells.[13] Most of the tissue oxygen (more than 90%) is consumed by mitochondria in human cells and about 1–5% of the O_2 is transformed to $\bullet O_2^-$ by electron leakage from Complex I (NADH: ubiquinone oxidoreductase) and the protonmotive Q cycle of the respiratory chain.[1,8,10] In mitochondria, most of the $\bullet O_2^-$ is rapidly metabolized to H_2O_2 by manganese-dependent superoxide dismutase (Mn-SOD).[7] However, if H_2O_2 is not efficiently removed, highly reactive hydroxyl radicals may be produced in mitochondria via Fenton reaction in the presence of Fe^{2+} or Cu^+.[1]

It has been established that due to its continual exposure to ROS and lack of histones protection, mtDNA is inflicted with more oxidative damage compared with nuclear DNA in mammalian cells.[14] The mutation rate of human and bovine mtDNA has been estimated to be about 20 times higher than that of nuclear DNA.[15] Moreover, mitochondrial membrane phospholipids are extremely susceptible to lipid peroxidation due to high contents of unsaturated fatty acids and proximity to the sites of ROS generation.[8,10]

3. Mitochondrial Diseases

Mitochondrial diseases are a heterogeneous group of metabolic diseases mostly caused by inborn errors of enzymes or proteins involved in cellular respiration and oxidative phosphorylation.[16] Most of the mitochondrial diseases documented so far are maternally inherited, but some are sporadic or transmitted as Mendelian traits. They may arise from mutations in either nuclear DNA or the mitochondrial genome. Mutations in nuclear DNA may affect structures and/or functions of the structural proteins or enzymes in mitochondria at the levels of transcription, translation, protein import, or inter-genomic signaling. Examples of the mitochondrial diseases caused by nuclear DNA defects include Leigh syndrome, autosomal dominant progressive external ophthalmoplegia, Friedreich ataxia, Wilson disease, and spastic paraplegia.[17] Otherwise, more than 150 pathogenic mutations, including point mutations in tRNA or protein-coding genes and deletion and duplication of mtDNA have been reported to associate with a wide spectrum of mitochondrial diseases. These include mitochondrial encephalopathy, lactic acidosis and stroke-like episodes (MELAS), myoclonic epilepsy with ragged-red fibers (MERRF), Leigh syndrome, neurogenic muscle weakness, ataxia, and retinitis pigmentosa (NARP), Leber's hereditary optic neuropathy (LHON), chronic progressive external ophthalmoplegia (CPEO), Kearns–Sayre syndrome (KSS), maternally inherited diabetes mellitus and deafness, hypertrophic cardiomyopathy and dilated cardiomyopathy.[18–20] However, the correlation between phenotype and genotype is poor for most of the mitochondrial diseases.[20] The molecular mechanisms underlying the great diversity of clinical phenotype and complexity of the pathophysiology of these overt diseases have remained unclear. This implies that the etiology of mitochondrial diseases may involve other unidentified etiology factors that affect mitochondrial structure or function,[19–21] which exacerbates bioenergetic dysfunction of mitochondria caused by mtDNA mutation. It has been demonstrated that defects in the respiratory chain can lead to an increase of electron leakage and overproduction of ROS.[9–12] In light of these observations, we have hypothesized that an increase of oxidative stress and oxidative damage is involved in the age-related deterioration of bioenergetic function of patients with mitochondrial diseases. To test this hypothesis, we have investigated the production of ROS and alterations in gene expression of free radical scavenging enzymes at the levels of mRNA, protein, and enzyme activities in muscle and skin fibroblasts of a dozen patients with mitochondrial diseases. The results from this and other laboratories[11,18,22,23] have provided compelling evidence to support the notion that oxidative stress elicited by impairment of the respiratory chain in the affected tissues of the patients plays an important role in the pathogenesis and progression of mitochondrial diseases.

4. Role of Free Radicals in the Pathogenesis of Mitochondrial Diseases

Excess production of ROS and free radicals in defective mitochondria has been recognized more than three decades ago and is thought to be one of the pathological factors of mitochondrial diseases.[11,12,18] An elevated level of ROS in the affected tissues of patients with mitochondrial diseases may cause oxidative damage to nucleic acids, proteins, lipids, and other biomolecules.[8,10,11] It was reported that there were excess amounts of hydroxyl radicals and aldehydic lipid peroxidation products in cultured skin fibroblasts from patients with Complex I deficiency.[24] Decreased levels of small-molecular-weight antioxidants were also noted in serum of the patients with mitochondrial encephalomyopathies.[25] Barrientos and Moraes[26] also reported that human xenomitochondrial cybrids with 40% deficiency in Complex I and rotenone-treated human osteosarcoma 143B cells exhibited retarded growth, declined respiratory function, and lower mitochondrial membrane potential accompanied by enhanced ROS production and lipid peroxidation. Interestingly, they showed that cell death was quantitatively associated with free radical production rather than with a decrease in respiratory chain function. Piccolo *et al.*[27] found that lipid peroxides and fluorescent adducts of organic aldehyde with plasma proteins were elevated in blood cells of the patients with CPEO syndrome. Moreover, it was reported that the skeletal muscle with a significant increase of 8-OHdG content and higher intensity of immunohistochemical staining for Mn-SOD displayed remarkable bounty of ragged-red fibers (RRFs) in the patients with KSS or CPEO syndrome.[28]

5. Alteration of Antioxidant Enzymes in Mitochondrial Diseases

There is abundant evidence to show that alterations of the activities of free radical scavenging enzymes were found in the affected tissues of patients with mitochondrial diseases. The skeletal muscle with RRFs in patients with CPEO syndrome showed increased expression of Mn-SOD but not of Cu,Zn-SOD.[29–31] In patients with CPEO syndrome, Mn-SOD-positive fibers were found to display decreased activity of cytochrome *c* oxidase (COX). Mitsui *et al.*[32] reported that COX-negative muscle with RRFs showed strong immunohistochemical staining with anti-Mn-SOD and anti-Cu,Zn-SOD antibodies in several patients with KSS and CPEO syndromes, respectively. Recently, Filosto *et al.*[33] detected very strong expression of Mn-SOD and GSH, but very weak expression of Cu,Zn-SOD in the muscle with COX-negative RRFs of patients with CPEO or MELAS syndrome. By immunohistochemical staining, Kunishige *et al.*[34] also demonstrated that the protein level of Mn-SOD was dramatically increased in COX-deficient RRFs, and that the expression levels of Cu,Zn-SOD, CAT, and GPx were only slightly increased. In this laboratory, we have cultured skin and muscle fibroblasts from patients with CPEO and MERRF syndromes, respectively, for study of alterations in the expression of free radical scavenging enzymes. We found that skin and muscle fibroblasts from the CPEO patients all had significantly higher enzyme activity and mRNA levels of Mn-SOD but those of CAT and GPx were not increased or even decreased in some cases.[11] Furthermore, we showed that the expression of these antioxidant enzymes is also imbalanced in skin fibroblasts of three patients with MERRF syndrome (Fig. 1).

It is not clear as to what causes the antioxidant enzymes induction and whether this bears any relationship with the severity of the mitochondrial disease in the patient. To investigate the biochemical responses associated with the respiratory-deficient phenotype, U937 cells were cultured in the presence of either ethidium bromide (EtBr) or chloramphenicol (CP). Brambilla and coworkers found that U937 cells grown in the medium containing EtBr or CP were rapidly led to respiratory deficiency and the activities and mRNA levels of Se-dependent and Se-independent GPx were increased but not those of CAT.[30] An increase in the gene expression of heme oxygenase 1 (HO-1) was also found in EtBr-treated cells. This response is commonly considered to be an indicator of oxidative stress. On the other hand, the severity of the enzyme deficiency in Complex I was found to correlate with the increase of production of $\bullet O_2^-$ and induction of mRNA of the Mn-SOD gene.[28] Notably, it was observed that the rate of $\bullet O_2^-$ production was decreased, but H_2O_2 was increased, by the induction of Mn-SOD gene expression in cultured cells with Complex I deficiency. These findings

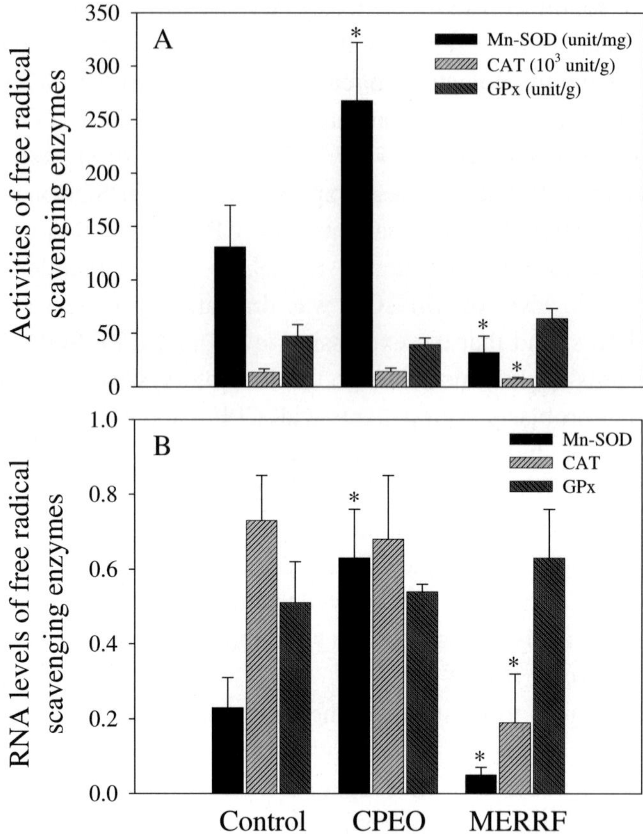

Fig. 1. Comparison of the activities (A) and RNA levels of free radical scavenging enzymes (B) in skin fibroblasts from CPEO and MERRF patients with those of the age-matched healthy subjects. The data for the enzyme activities were obtained from three independent experiments and are expressed as mean ± SD. The asterisks indicate significant differences ($p < 0.01$) in the free radical scavenging enzyme activities and RNA levels of skin fibroblasts between the patients and healthy subjects. Values for the mRNAs of free radical scavenging enzymes, manganese superoxide dismutase (Mn-SOD), catalase (CAT), and glutathione peroxidase (GPx), were normalized with the level of β-actin RNA. Control data were obtained from the skin fibroblasts of 18 healthy subjects aged between 25 and 70 years. The skin fibroblasts examined were primary cultures between three and six population doublings. The fibroblasts were established from the skin biopsies of eight CPEO patients, three MERRF patients, and 18 healthy subjects who had been ruled out to have any of the known mitochondrial diseases.

have been confirmed by our recent work on the muscle fibroblasts of CPEO patients.[11]

Taken together, these observations suggest that there must be a redox-sensitive factor that is able to sense oxidative stress and induce antioxidant gene expression. The alteration in the expression pattern of free radical scavenging enzymes can be considered as the adaptive response of human cells to the deleterious effects of ROS produced in the defective respiratory chain of affected tissues in patients with mitochondrial diseases.

6. Consequences of Imbalanced Expression of Free Radical Scavenging Enzymes

A delicate balance exists between the expression of both types of SOD and CAT plus GPx or thioredoxin reductase to confer the ability to cope with oxidative stress and live longer in animals.[35] Therefore, a low activity level of SOD relative to GPx or CAT could lead to the accumulation of ROS such as superoxide anions in affected cells. Superoxide anions, acting alone or by reacting with nitric oxide, may damage proteins containing iron–sulfur centers such as aconitase, succinate dehydrogenase and mitochondrial NADH-ubiquinone reductase and impair the normal function of the TCA cycle and electron transport chain. On the other hand, a high activity level of SOD relative to GPx or CAT may lead to an increase in the production of H_2O_2 (Fig. 2), which was indeed observed in skin and muscle fibroblasts of the CPEO patients that we examined in a recent study.[11] Chen and Ames[36] demonstrated that H_2O_2 induces senescence-like growth arrest in human diploid fibroblasts. Therefore, a significant increase in the activity of SOD must be accompanied by a comparable increase in CAT and/or GPx activity to prevent excessive buildup of H_2O_2 in the cell. As mentioned in the previous sections, we found that skin and muscle fibroblasts from patients with CPEO syndrome had significantly higher enzyme activity and mRNA levels of Mn-SOD, but those of CAT and GPx were not increased or even decreased.[11] These results suggest that there must be an imbalance between the generation and disposal systems of H_2O_2 in skin fibroblasts from the patients with CPEO syndrome. It is worthy of mentioning that this imbalance was much more pronounced in the fibroblasts

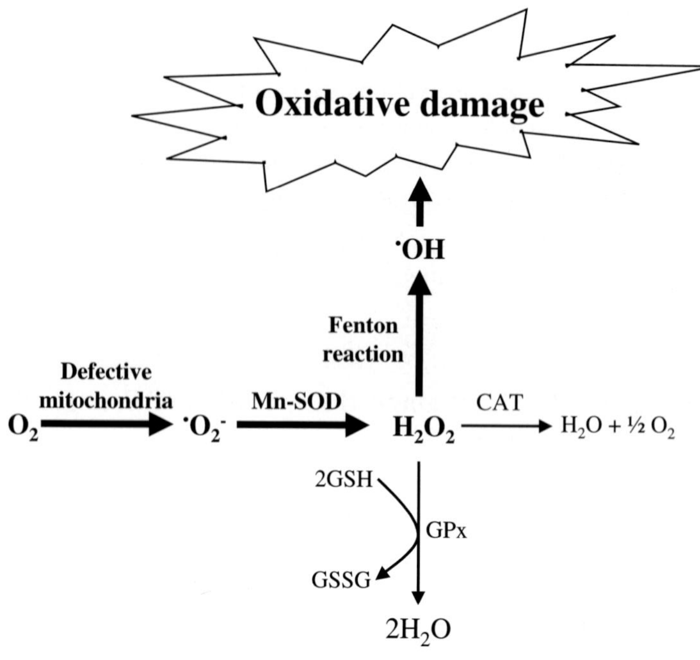

Fig. 2. Overexpression of Mn-SOD in mitochondria induces an imbalance of free radical scavenging enzymes and leads to accumulation of H_2O_2 in the mitochondria and the cell as a whole. When Mn-SOD is overexpressed in the human cell without concurrent increase in the expression of catalase (CAT) or glutathione peroxidase (GPx), the H_2O_2 thus generated will be accumulated in mitochondria or cytoplasm and can be converted to the far more reactive and damaging •OH radicals via Fenton reaction. Under such kind of "oxidative stress" condition, the cellular components of the affected cells may be subjected to a wide spectrum of oxidative damage.

from muscle (target tissue) than in those from skin biopsies. It might lead to higher oxidative stress in muscle because the average protein level of CAT of muscle fibroblasts was only about half that of the skin fibroblasts from patients (Table 1). Most importantly, we noted that the oxidative damage to DNA in muscle of CPEO patients is much more extensive than that in muscle of patients with other types of diseases that are not associated with any of the pathogenic mtDNA mutations.

To investigate the consequences of the imbalance in free radical scavenging enzymes, the effects of overexpression of SOD have been measured in several cell types including mouse L cells, neuroblastoma cells,

Table 1. Comparison of the activities and mRNA levels of free radical scavenging enzymes in muscle and skin fibroblasts from the patients with CPEO syndrome with those of age-matched controls.

Subject	Original tissue	No.	MnSOD		CAT		GPx	
			Activity (unit/mg)	RNA	Activity (10^3 unit/g)	RNA	Activity (unit/g)	RNA
CPEO	M	8	260 ± 24*	0.68 ± 0.17*	6.2 ± 1.3	0.34 ± 0.07*	56.0 ± 15.0	0.69 ± 0.20
	S	8	268 ± 54*	0.54 ± 0.25*	13.5 ± 3.3	0.73 ± 0.12	39.6 ± 6.2	0.54 ± 0.02
Control	M	5	116 ± 34	0.22 ± 0.06	6.6 ± 1.6	0.16 ± 0.04	65.9 ± 6.7	0.72 ± 0.09
	S	23	123 ± 33	0.26 ± 0.06	13.5 ± 3.2	0.68 ± 0.17	47.3 ± 10.8	0.52 ± 0.11

Values for mRNAs of free radical scavenging enzymes Mn-SOD, catalase, and GPx were normalized with the level of β-actin RNA. The data are presented as mean ± SD.

*Significantly ($p < 0.001$) different from skin or muscle fibroblasts of control subjects using the Student t-test. The ages of controls were between 25 and 70 years. The skin and muscle fibroblasts examined were the primary cultures established between three and six passages.

murine fibroblasts, mouse epidermal cells, and NIH/3T3 fibroblasts transfected with the cDNA of human Cu,Zn-SOD.[37–39] It is worth noting that the clones overexpressing Cu,Zn-SOD alone were much more susceptible to DNA strand breaks, growth retardation, easy killing by an extracellular burst of $\bullet O_2^-$ and H_2O_2, and showed the phenotypes of cell senescence.[39] Some clones showed adaptation to Cu,Zn-SOD overproduction by an increase in GPx or CAT activity, and the double transfectants of Cu,Zn-SOD and CAT or GPx were better protected from H_2O_2-induced oxidative damage. Recently, Li *et al.*[40] obtained two stable Mn-SOD-overexpressed clones by transfection of NIH/3T3 mouse fibroblasts with the Mn-SOD cDNA. The two clones showed different sensitivities to H_2O_2 and menadione and altered cell cycle progression, which was accompanied by the accumulation of cells in G_2/M phase and decrease in mitosis. Furthermore, a higher intracellular level of H_2O_2 was found in the Mn-SOD-overexpressed cells and resulted in a 9.5-fold induction of mRNA level of matrix-degrading metalloprotease-1 (MMP-1), which has been shown to play a major role in the process of cytoskeleton remodeling and tumor metastasis.[41]

The most striking consequences of defects in free radical scavenging enzymes were observed in gene-knock-out animals.[21,42–45] Li *et al.*[42] were the first to establish homozygous mutant mice by target disruption of the Mn-SOD gene, which resulted in dilated cardiomyopathy and neonatal lethality. Cytochemical analysis of the mutant mice revealed a severe reduction in succinate dehydrogenase and aconitase activities in the heart and, to a lesser extent, in other organs. Williams *et al.*[43] demonstrated that increased oxidative damage to mitochondria result in decreased activities of the enzymes containing iron–sulfur clusters (aconitase and NADH: coenzyme Q oxidoreductase), increased carbonyl groups in proteins, and increased contents of 8-OHdG in mitochondria of heterozygous *Sod2′* mice. Melvo *et al.*[21,44] first demonstrated that mice lacking Mn-SOD develop neurological disorders similar to those found in patients with mitochondrial encephalomyopathies. The *Sod2* mutant mice exhibit a tissue-specific impairment of electron transport activities of Complexes I and II, inactivation of aconitase, development of urine organic aciduria in conjunction with a partial defect in 3-hydroxy-3-methylglutaryl-CoA lyase, and accumulation of oxidative damage to DNA. Furthermore, the initial results showed that homozygous mutant *Gpx1* mice display normal development, but no histopathologies or mitochondrial abnormalities were observed in mutant mice that had been exposed to oxidative stress.[45,46] However, controversial results have been reported in other laboratories. Mice with a homozygous null mutation for *Gpx1* gene have shown increased susceptibility to oxidative stress-inducing agents such as paraquat and H_2O_2.[47] This group of investigators found that $Gpx1^{-/-}$ fibroblasts were more susceptible to H_2O_2-induced apoptosis and showed senescence-like morphological changes, increased NF-κB activation, elevated levels of Cip1, and reduced activity of cell proliferation and DNA synthesis, and poor responses to EGF and serum.[48] Moreover, Esposito *et al.*[49] showed that mice lacking *Gpx1* display a growth deficiency at 8 months of age. Livers from $Gpx1tm1Mgr^{(-/-)}$ mice showed increased levels of lipid peroxides. Liver mitochondria isolated from the $Gpx1tm1Mgr^{(-/-)}$ mice displayed an increased rate of H_2O_2 production, reduced mitochondrial respiratory control, and decreased mitochondrial power output.

By using cDNA microarray and RT-PCR, we discovered that alteration in the expression pattern of free radical scavenging enzymes in fibroblasts of patients with mitochondrial encephalomyopathies such as MERRF is frequently associated with a dramatic increase in the expression of several matrix metalloproteinases (MMPs) such as MMP-1 and MMP-3. The upregulation of these genes was apparently induced by an increase in the production of ROS in affected cells, because the same change could be brought about by treatment of the fibroblasts with 100–300 μM H_2O_2. One of the most conspicuous features of the mitochondria in these disease cells was the striking derangement of the mitochondrial network, which normally serves as a dynamic vehicle for transmission of energy through the cytoskeleton in normal cells. We believe that the gross morphological change of mitochondria in the affected tissues from the patients with mitochondrial disease is a result of activation of MMPs by elevated oxidative stress (Fig. 3). This notion is supported by a recent report that MMP-1 gene expression is highly induced in human fibroblasts upon treatment with H_2O_2.[50] Taken together, these results suggest that oxidative stress elicits the degradation and deterioration of the structural proteins of skeletal muscle in the patients with mitochondrial encephalomyopathies such as MERRF and MELAS syndromes. These observations and other lines of evidence have been accumulated to support the notion that overproduction of ROS

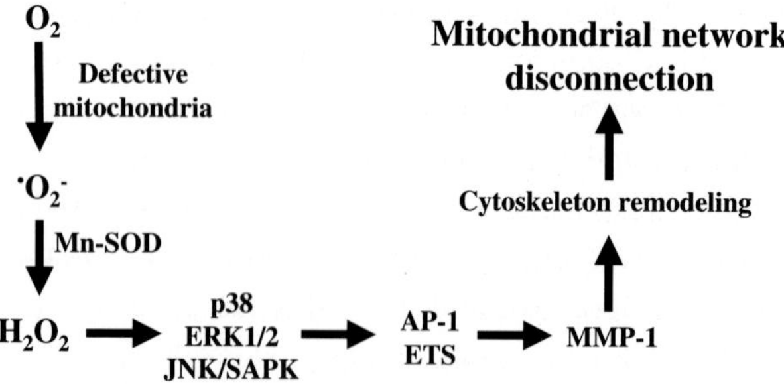

Fig. 3. Upregulation of the gene expression of MMP-1 in skin fibroblasts of patients with mitochondrial diseases under oxidative stress. In skin fibroblasts of the patients with mitochondrial diseases such as MERRF syndrome, MMP-1 gene expression may be increased by H_2O_2 through the signaling pathway involving p38, Erk1/2, and JNK/SAPK. The activated transcription factors (AP-1, ETS) then trans-activate the MMP-1 gene expression, which results in cytoskeleton remodeling of the fibroblasts and other types of cells of patients. These molecular and cellular events may be involved in the pathological manifestation (e.g., muscle weakness and muscle wasting) and clinical progression of mitochondrial diseases.

and defects in the free radical scavenging enzyme system are important contributory factor to the pathogenesis and progression of mitochondrial diseases.[18,51]

7. Oxidative DNA Damage and DNA Repair in Mitochondria

Oxidative damage to DNA may occur at nucleobases, sugar-phosphates, and the DNA backbones leading to single- and double-strand breaks in DNA.[52] During DNA replication, the adjacent single-strand breaks in the opposite strands may be converted to double-strand breaks. Unless these damages are repaired, both single- and double-strand breaks will result in defects in the DNA template, and accumulated damages may inhibit the DNA replication.[52] When this occurs in mitochondria that are continually exposed to oxidative stress, it may result in mtDNA depletion in the affected tissues of patients with mitochondrial diseases.

Base excision repair (BER) is an important mechanism for the removal of oxidative DNA damage. Extensive studies in the past decade have revealed that mitochondria contain the BER system including uracil- or 8-OHdG DNA glycosylase,[53,54] apurinic/apyrimidinic (AP) endonucleases.[55–57] and

8-OHdGTPase.[58] The first line of repair system for oxidative DNA damage in human cells is the removal of 8-oxodGTP from the nucleotide pool by nucleotidyl hydrolase hMTH1 (human MutT homolog 1), which can efficiently degrade 8-oxodGTP (as well as 8-oxodATP and 2-hydroxy-dATP) to their respective nucleoside monophosphates.[52] The hMTH1 is located in the nucleus, cytosol, and mitochondria of the human cell.[58] The physiological importance of hMTH1 in mitochondria remains obscure. It was reported that the level of hMTH1 in mitochondria of mice was increased in myocardial infarction, which suggests an important role of the enzyme in protection of cells against oxidative damage to mitochondria.[59] However, some 8-oxodGTP molecules may escape sanitation by hMTH1 and get incorporated into DNA opposite to either dA or dC. Human 8-oxoguanine DNA glycosylase 1 (hOGG1) is responsible for efficient removal of 8-oxodG from DNA. The hOGG1 gene encodes two major isoforms of the enzyme, α-hOGG1 and β-hOGG1, which are made by alterative mRNA splicing.[54,60,61] Mitochondria-targeting signals are present in the N-terminus of both isoforms of hOGG1, while only α-hOGG1 contains a nuclear localization signal in its C-terminus,[61] and only β-hOGG1 appears to be translocated into mitochondria. In the execution of DNA repair by BER, DNA glycosylase recognizes a damaged nucleobase and cleaves the N-glycosidic bond between the sugar and nucleobase to generate an apurinic (AP) site in DNA. Some glycosylases have AP lyase activity that cleaves the phosphate backbone of DNA, whereas others rely on AP endonucleases to cleave the DNA strands being repaired. A phosphodiesterase then excises the unsaturated sugar derivatives at the 3′-end of the DNA, and the gap of one nucleotide thus generated is then bridged by a DNA polymerase and the ends are sealed by a DNA ligase.[52] When the repair of 8-oxodG:C lesions is not completed before the next round of DNA replication, dATP could be incorporated instead of dCTP and thereby leads to GC $\rightarrow$ TA transversion. Human MutY homolog (hMYH) has a function of removing A, which is misincorporated at the nucleotide positions opposite to 8-oxodG. It has been shown that different isoforms of hMYH are translocated, respectively, to the nuclei and mitochondria in human cells.[62,63] Together with mitochondrial hMTH1 and hOGG1 isoforms, hMYH constitutes a DNA repair system to protect human cells against the accumulation of 8-oxodG in mtDNA. In addition, recombinational DNA repair has also been reported to be present in mammalian mitochondria.[64,65] However, UV-induced pyrimidine dimers cannot be repaired in mitochondria, because the nucleotide excision repair (NER) system exists only in the nucleus and is absent in mitochondria.[66–68] Moreover, hOGG1 function may be compromised by defects in the translocation of the enzyme to mitochondria. In a recent study, we found that the 8-OHdG levels in leukocyte DNA of LHON patients are significantly higher than those of controls.[12] By using a PCR-based technique,[14] we demonstrated that 8-OHdG contents in cellular DNA of primary cultures of skin fibroblasts of MERRF patients were significantly higher than those of skin fibroblasts from age-matched healthy subjects (data not shown). The incomplete and inefficient DNA repair system in mitochondria is one of the major factors contributing to the accumulation of oxidative damage and mutation to mtDNA in somatic tissues during human aging and in the affected tissues of patients with mitochondrial diseases.[10–12]

8. Antioxidant Therapy for Mitochondrial Disease

As extensively discussed above, endogenous oxidative stress plays a key role in the onset and progression of mitochondrial diseases. To counteract the deleterious effect of oxidative stress, several synthetic catalytic antioxidants have been developed for alleviation of oxidative stress in animal models for neurodegenerative diseases. Melov *et al.*[44] treated *sod2* nullizygous mice (*sod2*$^{\mathrm{tm1Cje}}$) with the catalytic antioxidant manganese 5,10,15,20-tetrakis (4-benzoic acid) porphyrin (MnTBAP). The *Sod2* nullizygous mice died within the first week of life and showed dilated cardiomyopathy, hepatic lipid accumulation, metabolic defects, mitochondrial enzyme defects, oxidative DNA damage, and organic aciduria.[21] Treatment of the mutant mice with MnTBAP significantly increased the mean lifespan of the mice and ameliorated dilated cardiomyopathy and hepatic lipid accumulation. However, MnTBAP was not able to cross the blood–brain barrier and the MnTBAP-treated *sod2* nullizygous mice had a severe disturbance in motor control and spongiform changes within the frontal cortex and focally in brainstem nuclei.[44] They also treated the *sod2* nullizygous mice with synthetic mimetics of SOD and CAT. The results showed that *sod2* nullizygous mice that had been treated with SOD/CAT mimetics extended their lifespan, the spongiform encephalopathy was cured, and mitochondrial defects were attenuated.[69] In addition, these compounds showed therapeutic effects in a variety of oxidative stress paradigms, including animal models for stroke, Parkinson's disease, autoimmune disease, excitotoxic neuronal death, and familial ALS.[70–73]

Moreover, several oxygen radical scavengers including CoQ_{10} and its analogs (i.e., idebenone, decylubiquinone, CoQ_2) have been utilized in the treatment of mitochondrial diseases. CoQ_{10} is an endogenously synthesized provitamin, which is mainly located in the inner membrane of mitochondria. It seems to have membrane-stabilizing properties and is an efficient free radical scavenger.[74] We and other investigators reported significant clinical and biochemical improvements in patients with mitochondrial diseases after treatment with CoQ_{10}.[75–77] CoQ_{10} improved lactate/pyruvate ratio in some patients with mitochondrial diseases and increased pancreatic function in a patient with diabetes mellitus and MELAS syndrome.[75,76] Furthermore, the ROS-triggered cell death has been hypothesized to contribute to optic nerve degeneration in LHON patients. Treatment of some patients with LHON with CoQ_{10} and idebenone together with vitamin E were found to have therapeutic effects.[77] Furthermore, idebenone was found to be effective in the treatment of mitochondrial cardiomyopathy in patients with Friedreich's ataxia (FRDA). FRDA is the hereditary ataxia caused by a GAA expansion in the first intron of the gene coding for frataxin, a mitochondrial protein which is most probably involved in the biosynthesis or maintenance of iron–sulfur clusters.[78,79] Patients suffering from FRDA are caused by the loss of activities of mitochondrial enzymes containing iron–sulfur clusters,[78] perturbation of antioxidant reserves,[80] and an increase in the urine level of DNA with oxidative modification.[81] In a recent clinical study, 40 FRDA patients received idebenone, a short-chain quinone-containing antioxidant, for more than 6 months, and a significant decrease of heart hypertrophy (>20%) was observed in about 50% of the patients.[82]

9. Concluding Remarks

Mitochondrial diseases may be caused by mutations in mtDNA and/or nuclear DNA. Although more than 150 mtDNA mutations have been detected in the affected tissues of patients, the molecular mechanisms underlying the pathogenesis of mitochondrial diseases are still poorly understood. It remains a mystery as to how and why mutations in different genes lead to similar clinical features and symptoms, and how the same mtDNA mutation leads to widely varied clinical phenotypes. We believe that the formation and accumulation of noxious metabolic intermediates in the affected tissues of patients with mitochondrial disease may be involved in the onset and progression of this prominent group of metabolic disorders.[18] While the classical role of mitochondria in generation of ATP by aerobic metabolism has been established for more than half a century, the other faces of mitochondria in producing excess ROS and leading to apoptosis have just been recognized in recent years. We have proposed that defective mitochondria not only produce less ATP but also generate more ROS and free radicals via electron leakage from the respiratory chain. As a result, enhanced oxidative stress and oxidative damage are most frequently manifest in the affected tissues,[24] and less often in peripheral blood cells of the patients with mitochondrial diseases.[12] Due to inefficient disposal of ROS in mitochondria[8,10,11] and shortage of energy supply for repair and elimination of the oxidative damage to cellular components, various damages to lipids, proteins, and DNA are accumulated with time in the affected tissues of these patients. Although most of the mtDNA damages can be repaired by an array of repair enzymes in mitochondria, some forms of damage (e.g., pyrimidine dimers) are not removed due to the lack of some DNA repair enzymes in the organelle. Once the damage persists too long or gets too extensive to be repaired, the mitochondria could sense and integrate the extra-mitochondrial stress and signals to drive the affected cell into an irreversible death process.[18,83] This scenario may explain, at least, in part, the age-dependent progression (e.g., neuronal cell death and muscle wasting) and worsening of most, if not all, mitochondrial diseases.

It has been increasingly appreciated that enhanced oxidative stress plays an important role in the pathophysiology of mitochondrial diseases. Many clinical phenotypes of this overt group of human diseases are associated with a gradual accumulation of oxidative damage in the affected tissues, which may explain the clinical features that are somewhat similar to those observed in degenerative diseases. Several degenerative diseases have been established to be associated with chronic exposure to ROS, which leads to increased production of free radicals and oxidative damage to mtDNA. Long-term exposure of human cells to ROS may initiate a vicious cycle to result in the decrease of the capacity of stress response, decrease in ATP synthesis, and further increase of ROS production of the cell. These will, in turn, elicit more serious consequences of oxidative damage and cell death in affected tissues when ROS reaches above a threshold. Experimental data from this and other laboratories have supported the contention that mutation and oxidative damage to mtDNA and mitochondrial respiratory function decline are important contributors to human aging and age-related progression of mitochondrial diseases. Further study on changes in the structure and function of mitochondria and mtDNA in cell response to oxidative stress is warranted to gain new insights into the molecular mechanisms of pathogenesis and age-accelerated progression of clinical symptoms in patients with mitochondrial diseases. The information thus obtained will be of great use for future development of antioxidant therapy and other regimens of treatment for a better management of these debilitating human diseases.

Acknowledgments

This work was supported jointly by a grant from the National Science Council (NSC92-2321-B-010-011-YC) and by an extramural grant NHRI-EX93-9120BN from the National Health Research Institutes, Taiwan.

References

1. Chance B, Sies H, Boveris A. Hydroperoxide metabolism in mammalian organs. *Physiol. Rev.* 59: 527–605 (1979).
2. Hockenbery DM, Oltvai ZN, Yin XM, Milliman C, Korsmeyer SJ. Bcl-2 functions in an antioxidant pathway to prevent apoptosis. *Cell* 75: 241–251 (1993).
3. Allen RG, Balin AK. Oxidative influence on development and differentiation: an overview of a free radical theory of development. *Free Radic. Biol. Med.* 6: 631–661 (1989).
4. Fraga CG, Shigenaga MK, Park JW, Degan P, Ames BN. Oxidative damage to DNA during aging: 8-hydroxy-2′-deoxyguanosine in rat organ DNA and urine. *Proc. Natl. Acad. Sci. USA* 87: 4533–4537 (1990).

5. Stadtman ER. Protein oxidation and aging. *Science* 257: 1220–1224 (1992).
6. Rikans LE, Hornbrook KR. Lipid peroxidation, antioxidant protection and aging. *Biochim. Biophys. Acta* 1362: 116–127 (1997).
7. Fridovich I. Superoxide anion radical ($O_2^{-\bullet}$), superoxide dismutases, and related matters. *J. Biol. Chem.* 272: 18515–18517 (1997).
8. Halliwell B. *Free Radicals in Biology and Medicine*, 3rd edn. Clarendon Press, Oxford, 1999.
9. Turrens JF. Superoxide production by the mitochondrial respiratory chain. *Biosci. Rep.* 17: 3–8 (1997).
10. Richter C, Gogvadze V, Laffranchi R, Schlapbach R, Schweizer M, Suter M, Walter P, Yaffee M. Oxidants in mitochondria: from physiology to diseases. *Biochim. Biophys. Acta* 1271: 67–74 (1995).
11. Lu CY, Wang EK, Lee HC, Tsay HJ, Wei YH, Increased expression of manganese-superoxide dismutase in fibroblasts of patients with CPEO syndrome. *Mol. Genet. Metab.* 80: 321–329 (2003).
12. Yen MY, Kao SH, Wang AG, Wei YH. Increased 8-hydroxy-2′-deoxyguanosine in leukocyte DNA in Leber's hereditary optic neuropathy. *Invest. Ophthalmol. Vis. Sci.* 45: 1688–1691 (2004).
13. Nohl H, Hegner D. Do mitochondria produce oxygen radicals *in vivo*? *Eur. J. Biochem.* 82: 563–567 (1978).
14. Yakes FM, van Houten B. Mitochondrial DNA damage is more extensive and persists longer than nuclear DNA damage in human cells following oxidative stress. *Proc. Natl. Acad. Sci. USA* 94: 514–519 (1997).
15. Wallace DC, Ye JH, Neckelmann SN, Singh G, Webster KA, Greenberg BD. Sequence analysis of cDNAs for the human and bovine ATP synthase beta subunit: mitochondrial DNA genes sustain seventeen times more mutations. *Curr. Genet.* 12: 81–90 (1987).
16. Wallace DC. Mitochondrial diseases in man and mouse. *Science* 283: 1482–1488 (1999).
17. Schon EA, Manfredi G. Neuronal degeneration and mitochondrial dysfunction. *J. Clin. Invest.* 111: 303–312 (2003).
18. Wei YH, Lee HC. Mitochondrial DNA mutations and oxidative stress in mitochondrial diseases. *Adv. Clin. Chem.* 37: 83–128 (2003).
19. Zeviani M, Spinazzola A. Mitochondrial disorders. *Curr. Neurol. Neurosci. Rep.* 3: 423–432 (2003).
20. Morgan-Hughes JA, Hanna MG. Mitochondrial encephalomyopathies: the enigma of genotype versus phenotype. *Biochim. Biophys. Acta* 1410: 125–145 (1999).

21. Melov S, Coskun P, Patel M, Tuinstra R, Cottrell B, Jun AS, Zastawny TH, Dizdaroglu M, Goodman SI, Huang TT, Miziorko H, Epstein CJ, Wallace DC. Mitochondrial disease in superoxide dismutase 2 mutant mice. *Proc. Natl. Acad. Sci. USA* 96: 846–851 (1999).
22. Pang CY, Lee HC, Wei YH. Enhanced oxidative damage in human cells harboring A3243G mutation of mitochondrial DNA: implication of oxidative stress in the pathogenesis of mitochondrial diabetes. *Diabetes Res. Clin. Pract.* 54 (Suppl 2): S45–S56 (2001).
23. Robinson BH. Human complex I deficiency: clinical spectrum and involvement of oxygen free radicals in the pathogenicity of the defect. *Biochim. Biophys. Acta* 1364: 271–286 (1998).
24. Luo X, Pitkanen S, Kassovska-Bratinova S, Robinson BH, Lehotay DC. Excessive formation of hydroxyl radicals and aldehydic lipid peroxidation products in cultured skin fibroblasts from patients with complex I deficiency. *J. Clin. Invest.* 99: 2877–2882 (1997).
25. Ihara Y, Hayabara T, Namba R, Nobukuni K, Mori A. Free radical, lipid peroxide and antioxidant in mitochondrial encephalomyopathy. *Rinsho Shinkeigaku* 34: 593–595 (1994).
26. Barrientos A, Moraes CT. Titrating the effects of mitochondrial complex I impairment in the cell physiology. *J. Biol. Chem.* 274: 16188–16197 (1999).
27. Piccolo G, Banfi P, Azan G, Rizzuto R, Bisson R, Sandona D, Bellomo G. Biological markers of oxidative stress in mitochondrial myopathies with progressive external ophthalmoplegia. *J. Neurol. Sci.* 105: 57–60 (1991).
28. Pitkänen S, Robinson BH. Mitochondrial complex I deficiency leads to increased production of superoxide radicals and induction of superoxide dismutase. *J. Clin. Invest.* 98: 345–351 (1996).
29. Ohkoshi N, Mizusawa H, Shiraiwa N, Shoji S, Harada K, Yoshizawa K. Superoxide dismutases of muscle in mitochondrial encephalomyopathies. *Muscle Nerve* 18: 1265–1271 (1995).
30. Brambilla L, Cairo G, Sestili P, O'Donnel V, Azzi A, Cantoni O. Mitochondrial respiratory chain deficiency leads to overexpression of antioxidant enzymes. *FEBS Lett.* 418: 247–250 (1997).
31. Rusanen H, Majamaa K, Hassinen IE. Increased activities of antioxidant enzymes and decreased ATP concentration in cultured myoblasts with the 3243A $\rightarrow$ G mutation in mitochondrial DNA. *Biochim. Biophys. Acta* 1500: 10–16 (2000).
32. Mitsui T, Kawai H, Nagasawa M, Kunishige M, Akaike M, Kimura Y, Saito S. Oxidative damage to skeletal muscle DNA from patients with mitochondrial encephalomyopathies. *J. Neurol. Sci.* 139: 111–116 (1996).

33. Filosto M, Tonin P, Vattemi G, Spagnolo M, Rizzuto N, Tomelleri G. Antioxidant agents have a different expression pattern in muscle fibers of patients with mitochondrial diseases. *Acta Neuropathol.* 103: 215–220 (2002).
34. Kunishige M, Mitsui T, Akaike M, Kawajiri M, Shono M, Kawai H, Matsumoto T. Overexpressions of myoglobin and antioxidant enzymes in ragged-red fibers of skeletal muscle from patients with mitochondrial encephalomyopathy. *Muscle Nerve* 28: 484–492 (2003).
35. Orr WC, Mockett RJ, Benes JJ, Sohal RS. Effects of overexpression of copper-zinc and manganese superoxide dismutases, catalase, and thioredoxin reductase genes on longevity in *Drosophila melanogaster*. *J. Biol. Chem.* 278: 26418–26422 (2003).
36. Chen Q, Ames BN. Senescence-like growth arrest induced by hydrogen peroxide in human diploid fibroblast F65 cells. *Proc. Natl. Acad. Sci. USA* 91: 4130–4134 (1994).
37. Amstad P, Moret R, Cerutti P. Glutathione peroxidase compensates for the hypersensitivity of Cu,Zn-superoxide dismutase overproducers to oxidant stress. *J. Biol. Chem.* 269: 1606–1609 (1994).
38. Ceballos I, Delabar JM, Nicole A, Lynch RE, Hallewell RA, Kamoun P, Sinet PM. Expression of transfected human Cu,Zn superoxide dismutase gene in mouse L cells and NS20Y neuroblastoma cells induces enhancement of glutathione peroxidase activity. *Biochim. Biophys. Acta* 949: 58–64 (1988).
39. de Haan JB, Cristiano F, Iannello R, Bladier C, Kelner MJ, Kola I. Elevation in the ratio of Cu/Zn-superoxide dismutase to glutathione peroxidase activity induces features of cellular senescence and this effect is mediated by hydrogen peroxide. *Hum. Mol. Genet.* 5: 283–292 (1996).
40. Li N, Oberley TD, Oberley LW, Zhong W. Inhibition of cell growth in NIH/3T3 fibroblasts by overexpression of manganese superoxide dismutase: mechanistic studies. *J. Cell. Physiol.* 175: 359–369 (1998).
41. Wenk J, Brenneisen P, Wlaschek M, Poswig A, Briviba K, Oberley TD, Scharffetter-Kochanek K. Stable overexpression of manganese superoxide dismutase in mitochondria identifies hydrogen peroxide as a major oxidant in the AP-1-mediated induction of matrix-degrading metalloprotease-1. *J. Biol. Chem.* 274: 25869–25876 (1999).
42. Li Y, *et al.* Dilated cardiomyopathy and neonatal lethality in mutant mice lacking manganese superoxide dismutase. *Nat. Genet.* 11: 376–381 (1995).
43. Williams MD, van Remmen H, Conrad CC, Huang TT, Epstein CJ, Richardson A. Increased oxidative damage is correlated to altered mitochondrial function in heterozygous manganese superoxide dismutase knockout mice. *J. Biol. Chem.* 273: 28510–28515 (1998).

44. Melov S, Schneider JA, Day BJ, Hinerfeld D, Coskun P, Mirra SS, Crapo JD, Wallace DC. A novel neurological phenotype in mice lacking mitochondrial manganese superoxide dismutase. *Nat. Genet.* 18: 159–163 (1998).
45. Ho Y-S, Magnetat J-L, Bronson RT, Cao J, Gargano M, Sugawara M, Funk CD. Mice deficient in cellular glutathione peroxidase develop normally and show no increased sensitivity to hyperoxia *J. Biol. Chem.* 272: 16644–16651 (1997).
46. Cheng WH, Ho YS, Ross DA, Valentine BA, Combs GF, Lei XG. Cellular glutathione peroxidase knockout mice express normal levels of selenium-dependent plasma and phospholipid hydroperoxide glutathione peroxidases in various tissues. *J. Nutr.* 127: 1445–1450 (1997).
47. de Haan JB, Bladier C, Griffiths P, Kelner M, O'Shea RD, Cheung NS, Bronson RT, Silvestro MJ, Wild S, Zheng SS, Beart PM, Hertzog PJ, Kola I. Mice with a homozygous null mutation for the most abundant glutathione peroxidase, Gpx1, show increased susceptibility to the oxidative stress-inducing agents paraquat and hydrogen peroxide. *J. Biol. Chem.* 273: 22528–22536 (1998).
48. de Haan JB, Bladier C, Lotfi-Miri M, Taylor J, Hutchinson P, Crack PJ, Hertzog P, Kola I. Fibroblasts derived from Gpx1 knockout mice display senescent-like features and are susceptible to H_2O_2-mediated cell death. *Free Radic. Biol. Med.* 36, 53–64 (2004).
49. Esposito LA, Melov S, Panov A, Cottrell BA, Wallace DC. Mitochondrial disease in mouse results in increased oxidative stress. *Proc. Natl. Acad. Sci. USA* 96: 4820–4825 (1999).
50. Brenneisen P, Briviba K, Wlaschek M, Wenk J, Scharffetter-Kochanek K. Hydrogen peroxide (H_2O_2) increases the steady-state mRNA levels of collagenase/MMP-1 in human dermal fibroblasts. *Free Radic. Biol. Med.* 22: 515–524 (1997).
51. Wallace DC. A mitochondrial paradigm of metabolic and degenerative diseases, aging, and cancer: a dawn for evolutionary medicine. *Ann. Rev. Genet.*, Epub ahead of print (2005).
52. Slupphaug G, Kavli B, Krokan HE. The interacting pathways for prevention and repair of oxidative DNA damage. *Mutat. Res.* 531: 231–251 (2003).
53. Grollman AP, Moriya M. Mutagenesis by 8-oxoguanine: an enemy within. *Trends Genet.* 9: 246–249 (1993).
54. Takao M, Aburatani H, Kobayashi K, Yasui A. Mitochondrial targeting of human DNA glycosylases for repair of oxidative DNA damage. *Nucleic Acids Res.* 26: 2917–2922.

55. Tomkinson AE, Bonk RT, Linn S. Mitochondrial endonuclease activities specific for apurinic/apyrimidinic sites in DNA from mouse cells. *J. Biol. Chem.* 263: 12532–12537 (1988).
56. Croteau DL, ap Rhys CM, Hudson EK, Dianov GL, Hansford RG, Bohr VA. An oxidative damage-specific endonuclease from rat liver mitochondria. *J. Biol. Chem.* 272: 27338–27344 (1997).
57. Souza-Pinto NC, Croteau DL, Hudson EK, Hansford RG, Bohr VA. Age-associated increase in 8-oxo-deoxyguanosine glycosylase/AP lyase activity in rat mitochondria. *Nucleic Acids Res.* 27: 1935–1942 (1999).
58. Kang D, Nishida J, Iyama A, Nakabeppu Y, Furuichi M, Fujiwara T, Sekiguchi M, Takeshige K. Intracellular localization of 8-oxo-dGTPase in human cells, with special reference to the role of the enzyme in mitochondria. *J. Biol. Chem.* 270: 14659–14665.
59. Tsutsui H, Ide T, Shiomi T, Kang D, Hayashidani S, Suematsu N, Wen J, Utsumi H, Hamasaki N, Takeshita A. 8-oxo-dGTPase, which prevents oxidative stress-induced DNA damage, increases in the mitochondria from failing hearts. *Circulation* 104: 2883–2885 (2001).
60. Aburatani H, Hippo Y, Ishida T, Takashima R, Matsuba C, Kodama T, Takao M, Yasui A, Yamamoto K, Asano M. Cloning and characterization of mammalian 8-hydroxyguanine-specific DNA glycosylase/apurinic, apyrimidinic lyase, a functional mutM homologue. *Cancer Res.* 57: 2151–2156 (1997).
61. Nishioka K, Ohtsubo T, Oda H, Fujiwara T, Kang D, Sugimachi K, Nakabeppu Y. Expression and differential intracellular localization of two major forms of human 8-oxoguanine DNA glycosylase encoded by alternatively spliced OGG1 mRNAs. *Mol. Biol. Cell* 10: 1637–1652 (1999).
62. Takao M, Zhang QM, Yonei S, Yasui A. Differential subcellular localization of human MutY homolog (hMYH) and the functional activity of adenine: 8-oxoguanine DNA glycosylase. *Nucleic Acids Res.* 27: 3638–3644 (1999).
63. Ohtsubo T, Nishioka K, Imaiso Y, Iwai S, Shimokawa H, Oda H, Fujiwara T, Nakabeppu Y. Identification of human MutY homolog (hMYH) as a repair enzyme for 2-hydroxyadenine in DNA and detection of multiple forms of hMYH located in nuclei and mitochondria. *Nucleic Acids Res.* 28: 1355–1364 (2000).
64. Thyagarajan B, Padua RA, Campbell C. Mammalian mitochondria possess homologous DNA recombination activity. *J. Biol. Chem.* 271: 27536–27543 (1996).
65. LeDoux SP, Wilson GL, Beecham EJ, Stevnsner T, Wassermann K, Bohr VA. Repair of mitochondrial DNA after various types of DNA damage in Chinese hamster ovary cells. *Carcinogenesis* 13: 1967–1973 (1992).

66. Clayton DA, Doda JN, Friedberg EC. The absence of a pyrimidine dimer repair mechanism in mammalian mitochondria. *Proc. Natl. Acad. Sci. USA* 71: 2777–2781 (1974).
67. Snyderwine EG, Bohr VA. Gene- and strand-specific damage and repair in Chinese hamster ovary cells treated with 4-nitroquinoline 1-oxide. *Cancer Res.* 52: 4183–4189 (1992).
68. Sancar A. DNA excision repair. *Annu. Rev. Biochem.* 65: 43–81 (1996).
69. Melov S, Doctrow SR, Schneider JA, Haberson J, Patel M, Coskun PE, Huffman K, Wallace DC, Malfroy B. Lifespan extension and rescue of spongiform encephalopathy in superoxide dismutase 2 nullizygous mice treated with superoxide dismutase-catalase mimetics. *J. Neurosci.* 21: 8348–8353 (2001).
70. Doctrow SR, Huffman K, Marcus CB, Musleh W, Bruce A, Baudry M, Malfroy B. Salen-manganese complexes: combined superoxide dismutase/catalase mimics with broad pharmacological efficacy. *Adv. Pharmacol.* 38: 247–269 (1997).
71. Jung C, Rong Y, Doctrow S, Baudry M, Malfroy B, Xu Z. Synthetic superoxide dismutase/catalase mimetics reduce oxidative stress and prolong survival in a mouse amyotrophic lateral sclerosis model. *Neurosci. Lett.* 304: 157–160 (2001).
72. Malfroy B, Doctrow SR, Orr PL, Tocco G, Fedoseyeva EV, Benichou G. Prevention and suppression of autoimmune encephalomyelitis by EUK-8, a synthetic catalytic scavenger of oxygen-reactive metabolites. *Cell Immunol.* 177: 62–68 (1997).
73. Melov S, Schneider JA, Day BJ, Hinerfeld Rong Y, Doctrow SR, Tocco G, Baudry M. EUK-134, a synthetic superoxide dismutase and catalase mimetic, prevents oxidative stress and attenuates kainate-induced neuropathology. *Proc. Natl. Acad. Sci. USA* 96: 9897–9902 (1999).
74. Ernster L, Dallner G. Biochemical, physiological and medical aspects of ubiquinone function. *Biochim. Biophys. Acta* 1271: 195–204 (1995).
75. Bresolin N, Bet L, Binda A. Clinical and biochemical correlations in mitochondrial myopathies treated with coenzyme Q_{10}. *Neurology* 38: 892–899 (1988).
76. Liou CW, Huang CC, Lin TK, Tsai JL, Wei YH. Correction of pancreatic β-cell dysfunction with coenzyme Q_{10} in a patient with mitochondrial encephalomyopathy, lactic acidosis and stroke-like episodes syndrome and diabetes mellitus. *Eur. Neurol.* 43: 54–55 (2000).
77. Mashima Y, Kigasawa K, Wakakura M, Oguchi Y. Do idebenone and vitamin therapy shorten the time to achieve visual recovery in Leber hereditary optic neuropathy? *J. Neuroophthalmol.* 20: 166–170 (2000).

78. Rötig A, de Lonlay P, Chretien D, Foury F, Koenig M, Sidi D, Munnich A, Rustin P. Frataxin expansion causes aconitase and mitochondrial iron–sulfur protein deficiency in Friedreich ataxia. *Nat. Genet.* 17: 215–217 (1997).
79. Huynen MA, Snel B, Bork P, Gibson TJ. The phylogenetic distribution of frataxin indicates a role in iron-sulfur cluster protein assembly. *Hum. Mol. Genet.* 10: 2463–2468 (2001).
80. Piemonte F, Pastore A, Tozzi G, Tagliacozzi D, Santorelli FM, Carrozzo R, Casali C, Damiano M, Federici G, Bertini E. Glutathione in blood of patients with Friedreich ataxia. *Eur. J. Clin. Invest.* 31: 1007–1011 (2001).
81. Schulz JB, Dehmer T, Schols L, Mende H, Hardt C, Vorgerd M, Burk K, Matson W, Dichgans J, Beal MF, Bogdanov MB. Oxidative stress in patients with Friedreich ataxia. *Neurology* 55: 1719–1721 (2000).
82. Rustin P, Rötig A, Munnich A, Sidi D. Heart hypertrophy and function are improved by idebenone in Friedreich's ataxia. *Free Radic. Res.* 36: 467–470 (2002).
83. Liu CY, Lee CF, Hong CH, Wei YH. Mitochondrial DNA mutation and depletion increase the susceptibility of human cells to apoptosis. *Ann. N.Y. Acad. Sci.* 1011: 133–145 (2004).

22 Oxidative Stress and Respiratory Disease

Rosario Maselli and Girolamo Pelaia

1. Introduction

The respiratory system is remarkably susceptible to oxidative stress because of its peculiar anatomical and functional properties, mainly related to the large area exposed to the external environment. Therefore, the cellular/tissue injury triggered by the oxidant burden generated by air pollutants in association with cigarette smoking plays a pivotal role in the pathogenesis of several lung disorders,[1,2] including chronic obstructive pulmonary disease (COPD), asthma, acute respiratory distress syndrome (ARDS), idiopathic pulmonary fibrosis (IPF), cystic fibrosis, and lung cancer.

In particular, inhaled oxidants such as ozone and nitrogen dioxide cause sequestration of inflammatory cells into the pulmonary microcirculation, thus leading to their accumulation within air spaces.[3] Cigarette smoke, which contains many oxidants and free radicals in both its gaseous and particulate phases, significantly contributes to recruit macrophages into the respiratory bronchioles, as well as to increase neutrophil numbers within lung microvessels.[4,5] Once recruited and activated, macrophages, neutrophils, and eosinophils produce and release reactive oxygen species (ROS) such as hydroxyl radicals ($OH^\bullet$) and superoxide anion ($O_2^{-\bullet}$), the latter being rapidly converted to hydrogen peroxide (H_2O_2) by superoxide dismutase (SOD). In neutrophils, the powerful oxidant hypoclorous acid (HOCL) is generated by myeloperoxidase from H_2O_2 in the presence of chloride ions. ROS are also released by airway epithelium, which may stimulate inflammatory cells directly, thereby contributing to propagation and amplification of lung oxidative stress.[6]

ROS are highly reactive and, therefore, oxidize the phospholipid content (lipid peroxidation) of cell membranes thus impairing their function. Moreover, ROS damage DNA and also severely alter protein structure by interacting with some amino acids (methionine, tyrosine, and cysteine). Airway epithelial cells, lung endothelial cells, and type II pneumocytes are particularly susceptible to oxidant injury. In the respiratory system, the cellular responses to oxidative damage operate within the pathological context of various lung diseases, many of which share the common feature represented by a significant imbalance between the harmful action of ROS and the protective effects of antioxidant defenses. With regard to the latter, a central role is played by the ubiquitous tripeptide glutathione (GSH), which provides an effective intra- and extracellular shield against oxidative stress, thereby protecting the membrane integrity of lung epithelial cells from free radical-mediated injury.[7] Furthermore, GSH is involved in modulation of the inflammatory and immune processes characterizing several respiratory disorders. In this regard, it is noteworthy that GSH levels are decreased in the epithelial lining fluid of patients with idiopathic pulmonary fibrosis, ARDS, and cystic fibrosis.[7] Therefore, a low pulmonary concentration of GSH can significantly contribute to the local oxidant/antioxidant imbalance, thus remarkably enhancing the noxious action of free radicals against the respiratory system.

The aim of this chapter is to outline the contribution of oxidative stress to the induction and progression of several relevant lung diseases.

2. Oxidative Stress and Asthma

Current evidence suggests that the chronic bronchial inflammation typical of asthma is also characterized by an increased oxidative stress in the airways.[8,9] Moreover, some epidemiological studies indicate that asthma may be associated with air pollution and a low dietary intake of antioxidants.[10,11] Indeed, higher levels of H_2O_2 are detectable in the exhaled breath of asthmatic patients with respect to control subjects,[12] especially after allergen exposure and during disease exacerbations. The latter are frequently associated with infections of airway epithelial cells by rhinoviruses, which are able to induce an intracellular generation of oxidants and the subsequent production of proinflammatory adhesion molecules and cytokines.[13] Several different cells involved in asthmatic inflammation, including eosinophils, neutrophils, monocytes/macrophages, and bronchial epithelial cells, are capable of producing and releasing high amounts of ROS. In particular, eosinophil peroxidase (EPO) and neutrophil myeloperoxidase (MPO) actively participate in ROS generation, and the concentrations of both EPO and MPO are remarkably increased in peripheral blood, induced sputum, and bronchoalveolar lavage fluid (BALF) of patients with stable asthma.[9] EPO-generated oxidants may interact with reactive nitrogen species (RNS) present into the bronchial lumen thus leading to protein nitration and enhanced nitrotyrosine expression,[14] detectable in airway inflammatory and structural cells.

ROS and RNS can evoke some peculiar features of asthma such as airway smooth muscle hyperresponsiveness to various contractile agonists, increased vascular permeability, and epithelial shedding. In asthmatic patients, there is a clear correlation between superoxide anion production from neutrophils and airway smooth muscle contraction induced by inhaled methacholine, as well as between oxidant generation by eosinophils and bronchial inflammatory responses to allergen challenge. Moreover, it has been demonstrated in animal models of allergic bronchial inflammation that a synthetic catalytic antioxidant, administered by intratracheal instillation, significantly attenuated antigen-induced airway eosinophilia.[15] With regard to oxidant-induced cytotoxicity, bronchial epithelial cells obtained from asthmatic patients were found to be more susceptible, with respect to normal subjects, to H_2O_2-induced apoptosis.[16] Furthermore, we have recently shown, in primary cultures of human bronchial epithelial cells, that H_2O_2 dramatically enhances cell death via phosphorylation of mitogen-activated protein kinases (MAPK).[17] Activation of these signal transducing enzymes is also responsible for airway epithelial cell death caused by peroxynitrite ($ONOO^-$),[18] a powerful oxidant agent that originates from the reaction of superoxide anion with nitric oxide (NO). In fact, MAPK mediate the cellular effects of oxidative stress and other biological stimuli (e.g., proinflammatory cytokines, growth factors), thereby significantly contributing to relevant aspects of asthma pathogenesis and evolution such

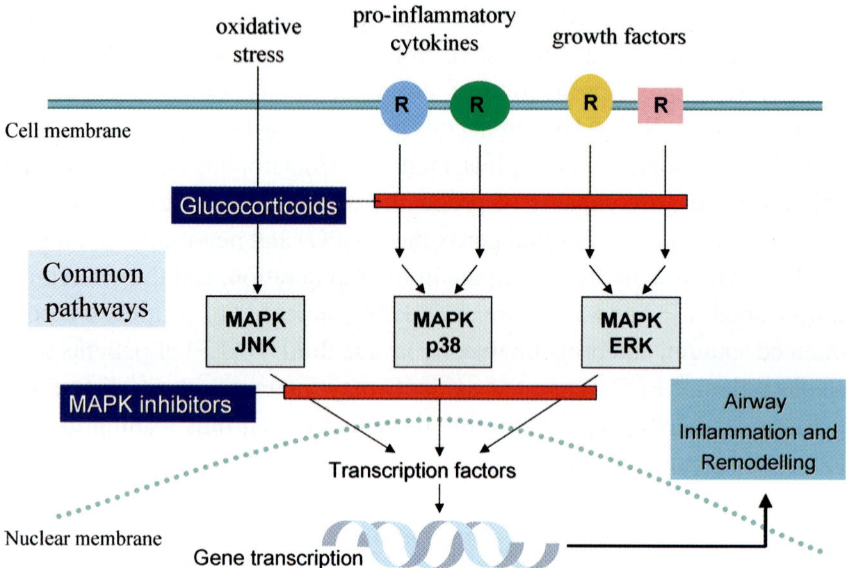

Fig. 1. Oxidative stress and activation of MAPK signaling pathways in the airways. MAPK activation, induced by either oxidative stress or cytokines/growth factors interacting with their receptors (R), as well as MAPK catalytic functions, may be inhibited by glucocorticoids and MAPK inhibitors, respectively, which can thus modulate airway inflammation and remodeling.

as airway inflammation and remodeling (Fig. 1). On the other hand, H_2O_2 can also trigger MAPK activation in pulmonary endothelial cells,[19] and this molecular mechanism could perhaps contribute to the angiogenic component of the bronchial remodeling occurring in asthma.

3. Oxidative Stress and COPD

Oxidative stress plays a key role in the development of the chronic, barely reversible airflow limitation that characterizes COPD. In fact, the major cause of COPD is cigarette smoking, which represents a rich source of oxidant agents. Furthermore, other factors involved in COPD pathogenesis and progression, such as air pollutants, occupational dusts, and respiratory infections, also have the ability to produce oxidative stress. Smokers and patients with COPD are subjected to a remarkable oxidant burden, as documented by the high concentrations of exhaled H_2O_2, which become even higher during disease exacerbations.[8] One of the most important sources of exhaled H_2O_2 is probably superoxide anion, produced in high quantities by alveolar macrophages from smokers. Increased levels of lipid peroxides, including 8-isoprostane and hydrocarbons such as ethane and pentane, are also detectable in the exhaled air condensate of patients with COPD.[20] Lipid peroxidation products positively correlate with airway obstruction, thus suggesting that oxidative stress is closely associated with the progressive decline in lung function occurring in COPD.[21] Moreover, oxidative inactivation of the antiproteinase α-1-antitrypsin favors the increase in elastase burden, which is responsible for the development of pulmonary emphysema.

Oxidants largely contribute to the inflammatory process underlying COPD by inducing the production of several mediators and cytokines such as tumor necrosis factor-α (TNF-α) and interleukin-8 (IL-8). In this regard, we have reported that H_2O_2 elicits a concentration-dependent increase in the amount of IL-8 released from bronchial epithelial cells, and this effect resulted to be at least in part mediated by MAPK activation.[17] Indeed, the IL-8 gene is regulated by the transcription factors nuclear factor-κB (NF-κB) and activator protein-1 (AP-1),[22] whose activation is controlled by MAPK.[23] With regard to MAPK-dependent, transcriptional regulation of IL-8 gene, a crucial role is played by the influences of oxidative stress on chromatin remodeling. In particular, it has been shown in pulmonary alveolar epithelial cells that H_2O_2 is able to stimulate the enzymatic activity of histone acetyl transferases (HATs).[24] As a consequence, the enhanced acetylation of the basic lysine residues of nucleosome core histones H3 and H4 neutralizes histone-positive charges, thus markedly reducing their electrostatic interactions with negatively charged DNA.[25] The subsequent DNA unwinding around nucleosomes facilitates NF-κB and AP-1 binding to their cognate promoter sites in target genes, which otherwise result to be hardly accessible because of the tight DNA supercoiling. MAPK exert a key function in mediating oxidant-induced histone acetylation, which is responsible for the increased expression of proinflammatory cytokines and chemokines. Indeed, oxidative stress-dependent activation of ERK and JNK MAPK has been found to be associated with an enhanced HAT activity of co-activator macromolecular complexes such as CBP/p300 and ATF-2.[26] Furthermore, p38 MAPK promotes the so-called H3 phosphoacetylation, consisting of the p38-catalyzed phosphorylation of a specific serine residue

(Ser10) of histone H3, which facilitates its interactions with HATs.[27] The subsequent acetylation of Lys14 located within the H3 amino-terminal tail results in a remarkable increase in gene transcription. In particular, H3 phosphoacetylation leads to an increased recruitment of NF-κB to its binding sites present in the IL-8 gene promoter.[27] H_2O_2 is also able to induce, in a time-dependent manner, the acetylation of histone H4 and the closely related synthesis of IL-8 by both bronchial and alveolar epithelial cells.[28,29] In other cell types such as alveolar macrophages, it has also been shown that H_2O_2 and cigarette smoke can stimulate IL-8 secretion by inhibiting the activity of histone deacetylase (HDAC) enzymes.[30] HDACs indeed repress gene transcription by deacetylating core histones, thus enhancing chromatin condensation and DNA supercoiling.[31] In particular, oxidative stress might impair HDAC activity by enhancing, in the presence of high NO levels, the production of peroxynitrite and the subsequent nitration of tyrosine residues on HDAC or associated proteins. This mechanism could also contribute to explain the low therapeutic efficacy, observed in COPD patients when compared to asthmatics, of inhaled glucocorticoids, whose anti-inflammatory actions are largely dependent on their ability to recruit and activate HDACs.[32]

Whatever are the molecular mechanisms implicated in the oxidant-induced synthesis of IL-8, whose levels are increased in the sputum obtained from COPD patients,[33] this chemokine exerts a powerful chemoattraction on neutrophils. The latter play a pivotal role, together with oxidant-activated alveolar macrophages, in the pathogenesis and progression of COPD, which is characterized by increased neutrophil amounts in both lung and peripheral blood. In fact, there is a relationship between circulating neutrophil numbers and airflow limitation, which is also correlated with the presence of neutrophils in the lungs.[21] Furthermore, ROS production from peripheral blood neutrophils is increased during exacerbations of COPD, and neutrophil myeloperoxidase expression is positively correlated with cigarette smoking.[8,34] On the other hand, the intratracheal administration of a catalytic antioxidant elicited, in rats exposed to tobacco smoke, a significant decrease in BAL neutrophils and macrophages, detected at 2 days and 8 weeks, respectively.[35]

4. Oxidative Stress and Interstitial Lung Diseases

Oxidative stress plays an important role in the pathophysiology of interstitial lung diseases such as idiopathic pulmonary fibrosis (IPF), which is characterized by a decreased antioxidant capacity in both BALF and plasma.[36] An imbalance between oxidants and antioxidants is also involved in the pathogenesis of sarcoidosis, whose more advanced stages are characterized by interstitial pulmonary fibrosis. Indeed, alveolar macrophages isolated from patients with either IPF or sarcoidosis generate high levels of superoxide anion.[37] These patients also exhibit enhanced BAL concentrations of oxidative stress biomarkers such as 8-isoprostane.[38] Moreover, in experimental animal models, a pre-treatment with antioxidant agents may be able to inhibit lung fibrosis induced by bleomycin administration.[39]

The increased oxidative burden associated with pulmonary fibrosis, arising from an excessive release of ROS from inflammatory cells such as macrophages and neutrophils, may significantly affect both proliferation and apoptosis of fibroblasts and alveolar epithelial cells, respectively.[40] In particular, the latter show an enhanced tendency to undergo cell death during the onset and development of IPF, a disease characterized by an increased fibroblast growth and extracellular matrix deposition. Indeed, proliferation of lung fibroblasts seems to be related to an oxidant/antioxidant imbalance, and very low intracellular levels of the antioxidant glutathione (GSH) are detectable in IPF.[40] In fact, GSH may contribute to suppress fibroblast proliferation, as well as to protect alveolar epithelial cells from oxidative injury.

Moreover, oxidative stress appears to be also capable of influencing the immune response, and via these interferences may be further implicated in the pathogenesis of interstitial lung diseases, most of which are immunologically mediated. In fact, oxidative stress may affect the functions of lymphocytes and dendritic cells by inducing the expression of costimulatory molecules, thus possibly leading to persistent antigen presentation and chronic tissue damage.[40] Both oxidants and antioxidants such as GSH are also involved in the regulation of T helper (Th) differentiation, thereby eventually contributing to the immune response underlying IPF, which seems to be linked to a Th2 phenotype.[41]

5. Oxidative Stress and ARDS

ARDS is a very severe respiratory disease, characterized by a diffuse alveolar damage affecting both pulmonary endothelial and epithelial cells, which represents the extreme end of a wide spectrum of lung injuries resulting in an extensive disruption of the blood–gas barrier. These pathological features originate from an acute inflammatory process, dominated by neutrophil infiltration, that leads to impaired gas exchange and severe hypoxemia, often refractory to oxygen therapy. ARDS patients are subjected to a remarkable oxidative burden, caused by several factors such as the respiratory burst of inflammatory cells, the high concentrations of inspired oxygen, and possibly the therapeutic use of inhaled NO.[42] Indeed, increased amounts of oxidatively modified proteins are detectable in BALF from subjects with ARDS, who also have high levels of lipid peroxidation products in both plasma and exhaled breath.[42,43] Moreover, an excess of H_2O_2 can be found in the exhaled breath condensate of such patients, who also exhibit elevated concentrations of ROS and RNS in lung lining fluid. These histotoxic agents are responsible for a serious damage of vascular endothelium and type I alveolar epithelial cells, thus leading to the development and progression of ARDS. On the other hand, although some antioxidants systems are upregulated in ARDS, the lung lining fluid from ARDS patients is characterized by low levels of GSH, which also appears to be predominantly in its oxidized state.[44,45] Furthermore, dietary antioxidants are depleted in these patients, thus implying that the antioxidant shield is largely overwhelmed by oxidative stress. All these findings have thereby prompted the experimental evaluation of the potentially therapeutic effects of several antioxidants. In this regard, it has been recently observed in animal models that vitamin E, a naturally occurring antioxidant, is able to exert a significant protection against lipopolysaccharide-induced acute lung injury.[46]

6. Oxidative Stress and Cystic Fibrosis

Cystic fibrosis (CF) is a genetic disorder characterized by a defective ion transport in exocrine cells of the lungs, pancreas, and sweat glands, which causes an excessive thickness of secretions. These alterations are responsible for pancreatic insufficiency and recurrent pulmonary infections, the latter leading to a chronic respiratory disease that is the most frequent cause of death for patients with CF. Oxidative stress is increased in CF,[47] as shown by high levels of plasma hydroperoxides and lipoperoxidation products. Indeed, elevated concentrations of isoprostanes, some of the most reliable biomarkers of oxidative stress, are detectable in patients with stable disease. Moreover, the occurrence of an enhanced oxidative damage to DNA is shown by the presence of increased urinary levels of 8-hydroxyguanosine.[48] CF patients are thus subjected to a high oxidant burden, mainly because of a massive ROS release from activated neutrophils which colonize the lungs as a result of recurrent respiratory infections.[49] These patients also exhibit decreased antioxidant defenses, probably due to malabsorption of vitamin E and β-carotene. Therefore, dietary supplementation with high doses of antioxidants, such as selenomethionine, β-carotene, and vitamins A, C, and E, may significantly improve pulmonary function.[50] These improvements appear to be correlated with the increased plasma concentrations of β-carotene and selenium, thus suggesting that a re-equilibrium in the oxidant/antioxidant balance may positively affect the clinical outcome of CF patients.

7. Oxidative Stress and Lung Cancer

Oxidative stress may be implicated in lung carcinogenesis via several mechanisms, mainly related to DNA damage and disruption of genomic integrity. Therefore, given the importance of this topic, the reader is referred to other two chapters of this book, entitled "Oxidative Damage to DNA and its Repair" (Chapter 7) and "Oxidative Stress and Multistage Carcinogenesis" (Chapter 9).

8. Conclusions

Oxidative stress significantly contributes to the pathophysiology of several different lung diseases. However, the specific molecular sensors of oxidative stress, as well as the precise cascade of biochemical events leading to oxidant-mediated pulmonary damage, are still not fully defined.

For all these reasons, a remarkable interest surrounds the experimental investigations aimed at further elucidating the cellular mechanisms underlying the effects of oxidative stress in the respiratory system. Such studies acquire a particular relevance also for their potential therapeutic impact, in that they may contribute to identify pharmacological targets suitable for the development of new antioxidant treatments. In this regard, MAP kinases play a key role as signal transduction pathways activated by oxidative stress, thus suggesting that their pharmacological modulation may represent a possible strategy for indirect antioxidant intervention (Fig. 1).

References

1. Barnes PJ. Reactive oxygen species and airway inflammation. *Free Radic. Biol. Med.* 9: 235–243 (1990).
2. Maselli R, Grembiale RD, Pelaia G, Cuda G. Oxidative stress and lung diseases. *Monaldi Arch. Chest Dis.* 57: 180–181 (2002).
3. Aris RM, Christian D, Hearne PQ, Kerr K, Finkbeiner WE, Balmes JR. Ozone-induced airway inflammation in human subjects as determined by airway lavage and biopsy. *Am. Rev. Respir. Dis.* 148: 1363–1372 (1993).
4. Pryor WA, Prier DG, Church DF. Electron-spin resonance study of mainstream and sidestream cigarette smoke: nature of the free radicals in gasphase smoke and in cigarette tar. *Environ. Health Perspect.* 47: 345–355 (1983).
5. MacNee W, Wiggs BB, Berzberg AS, Hogg JC. The effect of cigarette smoking on neutrophil kinetics in human lungs. *N. Engl. J. Med.* 321: 924–928 (1989).
6. Rochelle LG, Fischer BM, Adler KB. Concurrent production of reactive oxygen and nitrogen species by airway epithelial cells *in vitro*. *Free Radic. Biol. Med.* 24: 863–868 (1998).
7. Rahman I, MacNee W. Oxidative stress and regulation of glutathione in lung inflammation. *Eur. Respir. J.* 16: 534–554 (2000).
8. MacNee W. Oxidative stress and lung inflammation in airways diseases. *Eur. J. Pharm.* 429: 195–207 (2001).
9. Caramori G, Papi A. Oxidants and asthma. *Thorax* 59: 170–173 (2004).
10. Hatch GE. Asthma, inhaled oxidants, and dietary antioxidants. *Am. J. Clin. Nutr.* 61: 625S–630S (1995).
11. Sheppard L, Levy D, Norris G, Larson TV, Koenig JQ. Effects of ambient air pollution on non-elderly asthma hospital admission in Seattle, Washington, 1987–1994. *Epidemiology* 10: 23–30 (1999).

12. Emelyanov A, Fedoseev G, Abulimity A, Rudinski K, Fedulov A, Karabanov A, Barnes PJ. Elevated concentrations of exhaled hydrogen peroxide in asthmatic patients. *Chest* 120: 1136–1139 (2001).
13. Papi A, Papadopoulos NG, Stanciu LA, Bellettato CM, Pinamonti S, Degitz K, Holgate ST, Johnston SL. Reducing agents inhibit rhinovirus-induced up-regulation of the rhinovirus receptor intercellular adhesion molecule-1 (ICAM-1) in respiratory epithelial cells. *FASEB J.* 16: 1934–1936 (2002).
14. MacPherson JC, Comhair SA, Erzurum SC, Klein DF, Lipscomb MF, Kavuru MS, Samoszuk MK, Hazen SL. Eosinophils are a major source of nitric oxide-derived oxidants in severe asthma: characterization of pathways available to eosinophils for generating reactive nitrogen species. *J. Immunol.* 166: 5763–5772 (2001).
15. Chang L-Y, Crapo JD. Inhibition of airway inflammation and hyperreactivity by an antioxidant mimetic. *Free Radic. Biol. Med.* 33: 379–386 (2002).
16. Bucchieri F, Puddicombe SM, Lordan JL, Richter A, Buchanan D, Wilson SJ, Ward J, Zummo G, Howarth PH, Djukanovich R, Holgate ST, Davies DE. Asthmatic bronchial epithelium is more susceptible to oxidant-induced apoptosis. *Am. J. Respir. Cell Mol. Biol.* 27: 179–185 (2002).
17. Pelaia G, Cuda G, Vatrella A, Gallelli L, Fratto D, Gioffrè V, D'Agostino B, Caputi M, Maselli R, Rossi F, Costanzo FS, Marsico SA. Effects of hydrogen peroxide on MAPK activation, IL-8 production and cell viability in primary cultures of human bronchial epithelial cells. *J. Cell Biochem.* 93: 142–152 (2004).
18. Nabeyrat E, Jones GE, Fenwick PS, Barnes PJ, Donnelly LE. Mitogen-activated protein kinases mediate peroxynitrite-induced cell death in human bronchial epithelial cells. *Am. J. Physiol. Lung. Cell Mol. Physiol.* 284: L1112–1120 (2003).
19. Pelaia G, Cuda G, Vatrella A, Grembiale RD, De Sarro GB, Maselli R, Costanzo FS, Avvedimento VE, Rotiroti D, Marsico SA. Effects of glucocorticoids on activation of c-Jun N-terminal, extracellular signal-regulated, and p38 MAP kinases in human pulmonary endothelial cells. *Biochem. Pharmacol.* 62: 1719–1724 (2001).
20. Habib MP, Clements NC, Garewal HS. Cigarette smoking and ethane exhalation in humans. *Am. J. Respir. Crit. Care Med.* 151: 1368–1372 (1995).
21. Boots AW, Haenen GRMM, Bast A. Oxidant metabolism in chronic obstructive pulmonary disease. *Eur. Respir. J.* Suppl 46: 14s–27s (2003).
22. Hoffmann E, Dittrich-Breiholz O, Holtmann H, Kracht M. Multiple control of interleukin-8 gene expression. *J. Leukoc. Biol.* 72: 847–855 (2002).

23. Zhou L, Tan A, Iasvovskaia S, Li J, Lin A, Hershenson MB. Ras and mitogen-activated protein kinase kinase kinase-1 coregulate activator protein-1- and nuclear factor-mediated gene expression in airway epithelial cells. *Am. J. Respir. Cell Mol. Biol.* 28: 762–769 (2003).
24. Rahman I, Gilmour PS, Jimenez LA, MacNee W. Oxidative stress induces histone acetylation in alveolar epithelial cells (A549). *Am. J. Respir. Crit. Care Med.* 163: A61 (2001).
25. Cheung P, Allis CD, Sassone-Corsi P. Signaling to chromatin through histone modifications. *Cell* 103: 263–271 (2000).
26. Rahman I. Oxidative stress, transcription factors and chromatin remodelling in lung inflammation. *Biochem. Pharmacol.* 64: 935–942 (2002).
27. Saccani S, Pantano S, Natoli G. p38-marking of inflammatory genes for increased NF-κB recruitment. *Na. Immunol.* 3: 69–75 (2002).
28. Gilmour PS, Rahman I, Donaldson K, MacNee W. Histone acetylation regulates epithelial IL-8 release mediated by oxidative stress from environmental particles. *Am. J. Physiol. Lung Cell Mol. Physiol.* 284: L533–L540 (2003).
29. Tomita K, Barnes PJ, Adcock IM. The effect of oxidative stress on histone acetylation and IL-8 release. *Biochem. Biophys. Res. Commun.* 301: 572–577 (2003).
30. Ito K, Lim S, Caramori G, Chung KF, Barnes PJ, Adcock IM. Cigarette smoking reduces histone deacetylase 2 expression, and inhibits glucocorticoid actions in alveolar macrophages. *FASEB J.* 15: 1110–1112 (2001).
31. Ayer DE. Histone deacetylases: transcriptional repression with SINers and NuRDs. *Trends Cell Biol.* 9: 193–198 (1999).
32. Barnes PJ, Ito K, Adcock IM. Corticosteroid resistance in chronic obstructive pulmonary disease: inactivation of histone deacetylase. *Lancet* 363: 731–733 (2004).
33. Beeh KM, Kornmann O, Buhl R, Culpitt SV, Giembycz MA, Barnes PJ. Neutrophil chemotactic activity of sputum from patients with COPD: role of interleukin 8 and leukotriene B4. *Chest* 123: 1240–1247 (2003).
34. Aaron SD, Angel JB, Lunau M, Wright K, Fex C, Le Saux N, Dales RE. Granulocyte inflammatory markers and airway infection during acute exacerbation of chronic obstructive pulmonary disease. *Am. J. Respir. Crit. Care Med.* 163: 349–355 (2001).
35. Crapo JD. Oxidative stress as an initiator of cytokine release and cell damage. *Eur. Respir. J.* 22 (Suppl 44): 4s–6s (2003).
36. Rahman I, Skwarska E, Henry M, Davis M, O'Connor CM, Fitzgerald MX, Greening A, MacNee W. Systemic and pulmonary oxidative stress in idiopathic pulmonary fibrosis. *Free Radic. Biol. Med.* 27: 60–68 (1999).

37. Schaber T, Rau M, Stephan H, Lode H. Increased number of alveolar macrophages expressing surface molecules of the CD11/CD18 family in sarcoidosis and idiopathic pulmonary fibrosis is related to the production of superoxide anions by these cells. *Am. Rev. Respir. Dis.* 147: 1507–1513 (1993).
38. Montuschi P, Ciabattoni G, Paredi P, Pantelidis P, du Bois RM, Kharitonov SA, Barnes PJ. 8-Isoprostane as a biomarker of oxidative stress in interstitial lung diseases. *Am. J. Respir. Crit. Care Med.* 158: 1524–1527 (1998).
39. Oury TD, Thakker K, Menache M, Chang LY, Crapo JD, Day BJ. Attenuation of bleomycin-induced pulmonary fibrosis by a catalytic antioxidant metalloporphyrin. *Am. J. Respir. Cell Mol. Biol.* 25: 164–169 (2001).
40. Mastruzzo C, Crimi N, Vancheri C. Role of oxidative stress in pulmonary fibrosis. *Monaldi Arch. Chest Dis.* 57: 173–176 (2002).
41. Wallace WA, Ramage EA, Lamb D, Howie SE. A type 2 (Th2-like) pattern of immune response predominates in the pulmonary interstitium of patients with cryptogenic fibrosing alveolitis (CFA). *Clin. Exp. Immunol.* 101: 436–441 (1995).
42. Quinlan GJ, Upton RL. Oxidant/antioxidant balance in acute respiratory distress syndrome. *Eur. Respir. Mon.* 20: 33–46 (2002).
43. Chow C-W, Herrera Abreu MT, Suzuki T, Downey GP. Oxidative stress and acute lung injury. *Am. J. Respir. Cell Mol. Biol.* 29: 427–431 (2003).
44. Pacht ER, Timerman AP, Lykens MG, Merola AJ. Deficiency of alveolar fluid glutathione in patients with sepsis and the adult respiratory distress syndrome. *Chest* 100: 1397–1403 (1991).
45. Bunnell E, Pacht ER. Oxidized glutathione is increased in the alveolar fluid of patients with the adult respiratory distress syndrome. *Am. Rev. Respir. Dis.* 148: 1174–1178 (1993).
46. Rocksen D, Ekstrand-Hammarstrom B, Johansson L, Bucht A. Vitamin E reduces transendothelial lung injury in endotoxin-induced airway inflammation. *Am. J. Respir. Cell Mol. Biol.* 28: 199–207 (2003).
47. Brown RK, Kelly FJ. Evidence for increased oxidative damage in patients with cystic fibrosis. *Pediatr. Res.* 36: 487–493 (1994).
48. Brown RK, McBurney A, Lunec J, Kelly FJ. Oxidative damage to DNA in patients with cystic fibrosis. *Free Radic. Biol. Med.* 18: 801–806 (1995).
49. Sen CK. Oxygen toxicity and antioxidants: state of the art. *Indian J. Physiol. Pharmacol.* 39: 177–196 (1995).
50. Wood LG, Fitzgerald DA, Lee AK, Garg ML. Improved antioxidant and fatty acid status of patients with cystic fibrosis after antioxidant supplementation is linked to improved lung function. *Am. J. Clin. Nutr.* 77: 150–159 (2003).

23 Oxidative Stress and Human Reproduction

Ashok Agarwal and Shyam Allamaneni

1. Introduction

Human reproduction is a complex process involving interactions between many organs. Any disruption to this interactive system, whether in a man or woman, can result in an inability to have a biological child. Infertility can be defined as a lack of pregnancy after one year of regular unprotected intercourse. Approximately 15–20% of couples of reproductive age are infertile, which can be attributed equally to both male and female factors. In this chapter, we discuss how our understanding of oxidative stress as a cause of male infertility has evolved and provide information regarding its role in female infertility. Treatment strategies to counteract oxidative stress are also presented.

2. Oxidative Stress and Male Infertility

Defective sperm function is the most prevalent cause of male infertility and is difficult to treat. The etiology of sperm dysfunction is poorly understood despite an enormous amount of published research on the subject. It is of utmost importance to identify the factors/conditions that affect normal sperm function. Free radical-induced oxidative damage to spermatozoa is one such condition that has gained considerable attention for its role in inducing poor sperm function and infertility.

In men, free radicals support normal physiologic functioning of spermatozoa, but they can also lead to pathological conditions.[1–3] The presence of free radicals in the spermatozoa was reported by McLeod 50 years ago. Human spermatozoa rely on physiological levels of reactive oxygen species (ROS) for hyperactivation, capacitation, and acrosome reaction. Spermatozoa are vulnerable to perioxidative damage from high levels of oxygen free radicals because their plasma membrane contains polyunsaturated fatty acids; these acids help maintain membrane fluidity.[2] High levels of ROS can induce lipid peroxidation and damage sperm DNA, which in turn increases sperm membrane permeability, causes morphological abnormalities, and impairs fertility.[3,4]

3. ROS and Physiological Role

A minimal amount of ROS is needed during the fertilization process. *In vitro* experiments have shown that ROS plays a significant role in capacitation, hyperactivation, acrosome reaction, and oocyte fusion. It also acts as second messenger molecule and transmits signals by increasing the influx of calcium ions, which leads to increased production of ATP through a series of chain reactions.

Before sperm can undergo acrosome reaction and fuse with the oocyte, hyperactivation of the spermatozoa must occur via capacitation. According to *in vitro* experiments, adding minimal amounts of hydrogen peroxide to spermatozoa increases capacitation. On the other hand, antioxidant enzymes such as catalase and superoxide inhibit capacitation.[5] ROS may play a role in the acrosome reaction through its action on phospholipase A_2; it also helps in binding of spermatozoa to the zona pellucida by inhibiting tyrosine phosphatase activity and thus enhancing tyrosine phosphorylation.[6] Tyrosine phosphorylation is essential for interaction and binding between spermatozoal membrane molecules and ZP 3 proteins on the zona pellucida. Further research is needed to determine which radical is specifically involved in this process, what concentrations are needed, and the specific mechanisms that lead to the limited physiological production of ROS. Whether male infertility in some patients is result of the inability of spermatozoa to produce ROS radicals is one question that warrants investigation.

4. ROS and Pathological Mechanisms of Cell Injury

ROS affects most biomolecules including lipids, proteins, and nucleic acids. In some conditions, their action results in further production of free radicals. The extent of oxidative stress-induced damage depends on the amount, exposure duration, and type of ROS involved (e.g., hydrogen peroxide, superoxide ion, hydroxyl radical, etc.) as well as on factors in the surrounding environment such as temperature, oxygen tension, and the composition of seminal fluid including ions, proteins, and ROS scavengers.[7] Metal ions such as iron play an important catalytic role in the action of ROS. Spermatozoa are unable to repair the damage induced by excessive ROS because they lack the cytoplasmic enzyme systems that are required to accomplish this repair.

4.1. *Lipid peroxidation*

Polyunsaturated fatty acids are susceptible to attack by oxidants because of the presence of double bonds. The spermatozoa membrane contains large amounts of polyunsaturated fatty acids,[2] which maintain its fluidity. Peroxidation of these fatty acids leads to the loss of membrane fluidity and a reduction in the activity of membrane enzymes and ion channels. As a result, the normal cellular mechanisms that are required for fertilization are inhibited. It is possible to measure the extent of peroxidative damage by estimating the stable end-products of lipid peroxidation such as malondialdehyde.[8]

Lipid peroxidation in spermatozoa is a self-propagating reaction unless counteracted by seminal antioxidants. Once ROS acts on membrane lipids, alkyl and peroxyl lipd radicals are formed. These radicals, if not quenched by antioxidants, will act on other lipids in the membrane until all of them have undergone peroxidative damage.

4.2. *DNA damage*

DNA bases and phosphodiester backbones are other sites that are susceptible to peroxidative damage by ROS. High levels of ROS mediate the DNA fragmentation that is commonly observed in the spermatozoa of infertile men.[9,10] Normally, sperm DNA is protected from oxidative insult by its specific compact organization and by antioxidants in the seminal plasma. Spermatozoa are unique in that they cannot repair DNA and depend on the oocyte for repair after fertilization.[11] Various types of DNA abnormalities occur in sperm that have been exposed to ROS artificially. These abnormalities include base modification, production of base-free sites, deletions, frame shifts, DNA cross-links, and chromosomal rearrangements.[4,12] Patients with high levels of oxidative stress in their seminal fluid were found to have sperm with multiple single and double DNA strand breaks.[13] A biomarker for oxidative DNA damage, 8-hydroxy-2-deoxyguanosine, can be used to determine the extent of ROS-induced DNA damage.

4.3. *Apoptosis*

ROS may also initiate a chain of reactions that ultimately lead to apoptosis. Apoptosis is a natural process in which the body removes old and senescent cells; it is a process of programmed cell death. In human germ cells, apoptosis may help remove abnormal germ cells and prevent their overproduction. Multiple extrinsic and intrinsic cell factors control the process of apoptosis. In a study from our center, levels of ROS were positively associated with apoptosis in mature spermatozoa. Levels of caspases, which are proteases involved in apoptosis, correlated with levels of ROS. Our results also showed that apoptosis could be induced in cell cultures with H_2O_2, which further supports the theory that ROS is involved in apoptosis. The process of apoptosis may also be accelerated by ROS-induced DNA damage and ultimately may lead to a decline in sperm count.[14]

5. ROS and Body Defense Mechanisms

Because ROS have both physiological and pathological functions, the human body developed defense systems to maintain their levels within a certain range. Whenever ROS levels become pathologically elevated, antioxidants begin to work and help minimize the oxidative damage, repair it, or prevent it altogether. The male genital tract is rich in both enzymatic and non-enzymatic antioxidants. Catalase, superoxide dismutase, and glutathione peroxidase/reductase are enzymatic antioxidants that prevent ROS from acting on cellular molecules.[14]

Multiple non-enzymatic antioxidants forms are present in the semen such as vitamin C, vitamin E, urate, pyruvate, glutathione, taurine, and hypotaurine.[3] Vitamins C and E act as chain-breaking antioxidants and thus prevent the propagation of the peroxidative process. Because spermatozoa lack cytoplasmic enzymes, they often are unable to prevent oxidative damage. This is one of the features that make spermatozoa highly susceptible to peroxidative damage. Most cytoplasmic enzymes are extruded during the final stages of the sperm maturation process, which enables sperm to attain their characteristic morphology.[6] Nature compensated for this deficiency by providing an array of antioxidants in the seminal plasma.

6. Oxidative Stress Measurement

6.1. *Reactive oxygen species*

6.1.1. *Chemiluminescence assay*

The chemiluminescence assay is most commonly used method to measure ROS in semen.[15] Luminol (5-amino-2,3-dihydro-1,4-phthalazinedione) and lucigenin (bis-*N*-methylacridinium nitrate) are commonly used as probes. Luminol measures both intracellular and extracellular ROS including $O_2^{-\bullet}$, H_2O_2 and OH^-.[8] It provides an overall measurement of ROS in a given sample. On the other hand, lucigenin specifically measures only extracellular ROS particularly $O_2^{-\bullet}$ and OH^-.

The chemical reagents that are involved in the chemiluminescence assay are extremely light sensitive. Either photon counting or current counting luminometers are used to measure the luminescence. The results can be expressed as counted photon per minute (cpm), relative light units (RLU), and millivolts per second (mV/s).

6.1.2. *Flowcytometry*

Flow cytometry can also be used to measure ROS in spermatozoa.[16] An individual intracellular ROS radical can be identified separately using a low number of cells. 2′, 7′-dichlorofluorscein-diacetate and hydroethidine are used to detect H_2O_2 and $O_2^{-\bullet}$, respectively.

Other methods are available to directly measure ROS including the nitroblue tetrazolium technique, ferricytochrome C reduction method, and electron spin resonance method.[8]

6.1.3. *Indirect methods for ROS measurement*

Unlike the direct methods for measuring ROS, indirect methods measure the stable end-products of the peroxidative process. Malondialdehyde and other stable end-products of lipid peroxidation can be estimated with the thiobarbituric acid assay.[17] 8-Hydroxy-2-deoxyguanosine, an end-product of oxidative damage to DNA, is also used to determine the extent of peroxidative damage.[4]

6.2. *Antioxidants*

It is possible to measure levels of individual antioxidants and the total antioxidant status of the semen. The enhanced chemiluminescence assay and calorimetric assay are techniques that are commonly used to measure total antioxidant capacity (TAC). The results are expressed as molar trolox equivalents. Other methods can be used to measure TAC such as oxygen radical absorbance capacity, ferric reducing ability, and the phycoerythrin fluorescence-based assay.[18]

6.3. *ROS–TAC score*

To accommodate for the variations in both ROS and TAC values, a composite score has been developed using principal component analysis.[19] Fertile men tend to have high ROS–TAC scores whereas infertile men generally have significantly lower scores. ROS can also be directly measured in neat semen, thereby offering yet another measure of oxidative stress.

7. Sources of ROS

Human semen consists of mature and immature spermatozoa, round cells, leukocytes, epithelial cells, and seminal plasma. Morphologically abnormal

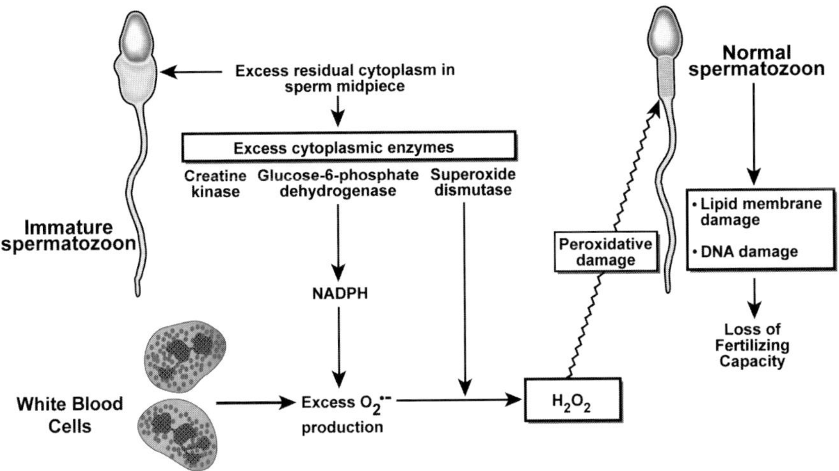

Fig. 1. Sources of reactive oxygen species in male reproductive tract and mechanisms of injury to mature spermatozoa.

spermatozoa and leukocytes are the major sources of ROS in the human reproductive tract (Fig. 1).

7.1. *Generation of ROS by spermatozoa*

Spermatozoal intracellular mechanisms may generate ROS at the level of plasma membrane (NADPH-oxidase system)[20] and mitochondria (NADPH-dependent oxido-reductase).[21] Human spermatozoa generate $O_2^{-\bullet}$,[17] which spontaneously or enzymatically dismutates to H_2O_2. In the presence of metal ions (iron) $O_2^{-\bullet}$, H_2O_2 produces OH^-. ROS production is elevated in patients who have a large percentage of spermatozoa with excess residual cytoplasm in the midpiece. The occurrence of spermatozoa with excess residual cytoplasm in the midpiece occurs because of defective spermatogenesis. The presence of cytoplasmic enzymes such as glucose-6-phosphate dehydrogenase and creatine phosphokinase is linked with defective sperm function. Oxidative damage can also affect morphologically normal mature spermatozoa — the damage may occur in the epididymis and seminiferous tubules where they are in close contact with the immature, ROS-producing spermatozoa.[22]

7.2. *Generation of ROS by leukocytes*

Extracellular ROS is produced by leukocytes in prostatic and seminal vesicle secretions.[23,24] During inflammation and infection, activated leukocytes can produce ROS in amounts 100-fold higher than non-activated leukocytes.[25] The importance of leukocyte contamination in producing ROS is well observed in Percoll-washed spermatozoa where a small number of leukocytes produce ROS. Increased levels of seminal leukocytes may also stimulate human spermatozoa to produce ROS. Such stimulation may be mediated via direct cell–cell contact or by soluble products released by leukocytes.[23]

8. Mechanisms of Male Fertility Potential Impairment

ROS impair the fertilizing potential of men by affecting various mechanisms that sperm use to fertilize ovum and contribute to embryo development.[26] ROS may affect the quality and number of spermatozoa reaching the ovum in the female reproductive tract by decreasing sperm motility and count. In addition, ROS impair the fertilization process by preventing the initiation of sperm–oocyte fusion events.[11] Finally, ROS can impair embryo development and affect the health of offspring by damaging sperm DNA.[4]

8.1. *Decreased motility*

For sperm to reach the ovum, adequate motility is essential. Spermatozoa have developed physiological mechanisms to achieve this purpose. Levels of ROS correlate inversely with motility.[27,28] Peroxidative damage to the sperm membrane can itself impair motility. But damage to axonemal proteins has also been shown to be a cause of impaired sperm motility. Excessive ROS causes ATP to deplete rapidly resulting in decreased phosphorylation of axonemal proteins.[29]

8.2. *Decreased sperm count*

ROS plays a part in the apoptosis of spermatozoa by activating caspases. Under normal conditions, abnormal sperm undergo apoptosis, which minimizes their proliferation. The severity of oligozoospermia has been correlated with excessive levels of ROS.[30] ROS may stimulate the process of apoptosis, resulting in the death of spermatozoa and decreased sperm count.[14] Patients with a low sperm count have a reduced chance of initiating a pregnancy.

8.3. *Decreased sperm–oocyte fusion*

The effect of ROS on sperm fertilizing capacity cannot be quantified by measuring routine semen parameters. It is possible that the levels of ROS needed to impair sperm–oocyte fusion events are lower than those required to affect sperm motility. Rather, the damage can be estimated by assessing sperm fusion capacity and measuring ROS levels *in vitro*. The inability of sperm to fuse with an oocyte appears to be due to the effects of ROS on the sperm membrane. The lipid peroxidation process results in a loss of membrane fluidity due to disorganization of membrane architecture. As a result, spermatozoa are unable to initiate the necessary biochemical reactions associated with acrosome reaction, zona pellucida binding, and oocyte penetration.[31,32]

8.4. *Sperm DNA damage*

Spermatozoal DNA is another important site of action by which ROS can affect the ability of a man to father a biological child. The percentage of sperm with DNA damage is negatively correlated with the fertilization rate.[10] The damaged DNA in spermatozoa may also affect embryo development.[33] Oocytes can repair DNA damage to some extent, but when the damage is severe, embryo death and abortions can occur. The effect of ROS on DNA integrity has become the focus of recent attention due to widespread use of assisted reproduction techniques (ART) such as intracytoplasmic injection (ICSI). In natural pregnancy, oxidative damage to the sperm membrane ensures that spermatozoa with damaged DNA lose their ability to fertilize an oocyte. With ICSI, sperm with DNA damage can potentially be injected into an oocyte.[1]

9. Clinical Diagnoses of Infertility and ROS

Irrespective of the clinical diagnosis, the presence of seminal OS in infertile men suggests that it plays a role in the pathophysiology of infertility via several mechanisms that act in synergism to impair sperm characteristics and functional capacity.[30] When an infertile man is diagnosed with certain specific pathologies such as male accessory gland infection, spinal cord injury, or varicocele — or when the patient has undergone vasectomy reversal — there is a good chance that oxidative stress is one of the causes of his infertility. Elevated levels of ROS and depressed levels of TAC are associated with varicocele.[34] These changes may be related to the functional sperm abnormalities and infertility that are commonly seen in these patients. A history of smoking is associated with high levels of oxidative stress.

10. Oxidative Stress and Female Infertility

Understanding the role of ROS in female infertility is still in the early stages. The presence of oxidative and antioxidant systems in various female reproductive tissues suggests that oxidative stress is a cause of infertility and certain reproductive diseases[35] such as endometriosis[36,37] and hydrosalpinx.[36] ROS and antioxidants have been detected in follicular fluid,[38–40] hydrosalpingeal fluid, tubal fluid, oocytes, and embryos.[41] Oxidative stress may also be involved in the etiology of defective embryo development.

10.1. *ROS and follicular fluid*

Graffian follicle contains the potential sources of ROS like large numbers of macrophages, neutrophils, and metabolically active granulosa cells. Although many studies have found ROS in follicular fluid,[38–40] levels are usually lower than those found in the serum.[39] Follicular fluid contains high levels of antioxidants, which protect oocytes from ROS-induced damage. ROS levels in follicular fluid may be used as markers for predicting the success of *in vitro* fertilization (IVF).

10.2. *ROS and endometriosis*

The molecular mechanisms involved in the implantation of endometrial cells on the peritoneum have long been a topic of research. Under normal conditions, ROS may facilitate cell implantation and development.[42] In peritoneal cavity, ROS may be produced by red blood cells, macrophages, endometrial cells and debris from menstrual reflux.

Studies of women with endometriosis have suggested that peritoneal macrophages are responsible for increased production of ROS or increased expression of xanthine oxidase in endometrial cells.[43,44] In addition, levels of oxidatively modified substances in peritoneal fluid and ectopic endometrial tissue tend to be high, which further supports the theory that ROS plays a role in endometriosis.[45] Furthermore, expressions of defensive antioxidant enzymes such as superoxide dismutase and glutathione peroxidase are altered in endometrial tissue in patients with endometriosis. Finally, such patients also have low levels of vitamin E in the peritoneal fluid.[36]

10.3. *ROS and idiopathic female infertility*

Elevated levels of ROS in peritoneal fluid may be the cause of infertility in some women who do not have any other obvious cause. Elevated levels can damage the ovum after its release from the ovary, the zygote/embryo, and most importantly, spermatozoa. As discussed previously, spermatozoa are very sensitive to oxidative stress. Studies have compared ROS levels in peritoneal fluid between women undergoing laparoscopy for infertility evaluation and fertile women undergoing tubal ligation. Levels of ROS in the peritoneal fluid were significantly higher in the patients with idiopathic infertility compared with the fertile women.[46]

10.4. *ROS and hydrosalpingeal fluid*

A study from our lab demonstrated the presence of ROS, antioxidants, and lipid peroxidation products in hydrosalpingeal fluid (HSF).[46] The mouse embryo blastocyst development rate is higher when they are incubated with HSF and low ROS levels than when incubated with HSF and very low ROS levels. Oxidative stress may be the mechanism of embryotoxicity in patients with hydrosalpinx.

11. Oxidative Stress and Embryo Development

The effect of oxidative stress on early embryonic development is another area of intense research. ROS may originate from embryo metabolism and from the surrounding environment.[47,48] ROS not only alters most types of cellular molecules but also induces early embryonic developmental block and retardation.[41] Multiple mechanisms of embryo protection against ROS exist.[49,50]

According to a study from our lab, ROS levels in day 1 culture media can help predict whether fertilization, embryo development, and pregnancy will be successful.[51] In our study, ROS levels in day 1 culture media correlated well with fertilization and embryo development in patients undergoing IVF and ICSI. They also related with pregnancy in ICSI but not in IVF.

12. Oxidative Stress and Assisted Reproduction

DNA damage induced by oxidative stress has important clinical implications in the context of assisted reproduction. Spermatozoa selected for ART most likely originate from an environment experiencing oxidative stress, and a large percentage of these sperm may have damaged DNA.[3] There is a strong possibility that spermatozoa with damaged DNA may be used during ART,[4] which can negatively affect the ART success rate and increase the risk of spontaneous abortion or offspring with genetic disorders. ROS levels in mature spermatozoa correlate significantly with the fertilizing potential of spermatozoa.[52,53] Estimating ROS levels may help predict the success rate of assisted reproduction procedures.

13. Treatment Strategies

Once seminal oxidative stress is diagnosed, treatment plans must focus on identifying and eliminating the source of ROS.[54] In most cases, oxidative stress appears to be due to increased generation of ROS rather than a depletion of antioxidants. Differentiating between a spermatozoal and leukocyte source of ROS can significantly affect therapeutic strategies. The underlying etiological factor for abnormal leukocyte infiltration (e.g., leukocytospermia, inflammation, infection, smoking) should be determined. When abnormal spermatozoa with excessive cytoplasm are detected, semen analysis should be performed after a full spermatogenic cycle. This will help distinguish between a temporary disturbance in spermatogenesis and a permanent defect in spermatogenesis.

When a specific cause is identified, medical and surgical management options should be considered to eliminate the source of ROS. Patients with male accessory gland infection should be treated with antibiotics. Anti-inflammatory agents may help patients with persistent leukocytospermia and elevated levels of cytokines. Varicocelectomy may remove an unknown stimulus of ROS generation. Antioxidant supplementation may or may not be effective depending on the pathology of the infertility. After treating the primary cause, patients should be advised to take antioxidant supplementation. Antioxidants should be started directly when a specific etiology cannot be identified (idiopathic infertility). Even though there is no definitive consensus on the use of antioxidants, many *in vitro* and *in vivo* studies have shown that they improve semen quality and fertility.[54]

In ART procedures, sperm preparation techniques separate mature spermatozoa and thus minimize the interaction between ROS producing cells in semen (e.g., leukocytes, immature abnormal spermatozoa) and normal spermatozoa. Density gradient separation and swim-up methods are commonly used sperm preparation methods. Adding antioxidants to the sperm preparation media and *in vitro* media may help prevent ROS-induced damage and preserves the quality of spermatozoa during ART procedures.

References

1. Aitken RJ. The Amoroso Lecture. the human spermatozoon — a cell in crisis? *J. Reprod. Fertil.* 115: 1–7 (1999).
2. Jones R, Mann T, Sherins R. Peroxidative breakdown of phospholipids in human spermatozoa, spermicidal properties of fatty acid peroxides, and protective action of seminal plasma. *Fertil. Steril.* 31: 531–537 (1979).

3. Saleh RA, Agarwal A. Oxidative stress and male infertility: from research bench to clinical practice. *J. Androl.* 23: 737–752 (2002).
4. Agarwal A, Said TM. Role of sperm chromatin abnormalities and DNA damage in male infertility. *Hum. Reprod. Update* 9: 331–345 (2003).
5. de Lamirande E, Gagnon C. Human sperm hyperactivation and capacitation as parts of an oxidative process. *Free Radic. Biol. Med.* 14: 157–166 (1993).
6. Aitken J, Fisher H. Reactive oxygen species generation and human spermatozoa: the balance of benefit and risk. *Bioessays* 16: 259–267 (1994).
7. Agarwal A, Saleh R. Role of oxidants in male infertility: rationale, significance, and treatment. *Urol. Clin. North Am.* 29: 817–827 (2002).
8. Sharma RK, Agarwal A. Role of reactive oxygen species in male infertility. *Urology* 48: 835–850 (1996).
9. Kodama H, Yamaguchi R, Fukuda J, Kasai H, Tanaka T. Increased oxidative deoxyribonucleic acid damage in the spermatozoa of infertile male patients. *Fertil. Steril.* 68: 519–524 (1997).
10. Sun JG, Jurisicova A, Casper RF. Detection of deoxyribonucleic acid fragmentation in human sperm: correlation with fertilization *in vitro*. *Biol. Reprod.* 56: 602–607 (1997).
11. Aitken RJ, Baker MA, Sawyer D. Oxidative stress in the male germ line and its role in the aetiology of male infertility and genetic disease. *Reprod. Biomed. Online* 7: 65–70 (2003).
12. Duru N, Morshedi M, Oehninger S. Effects of hydrogen peroxide on DNA and plasma membrane integrity of human spermatozoa. *Fertil. Steril.* 74: 1200–1207 (2000).
13. Twigg JP, Irvine DS, Aitken RJ. Oxidative damage to DNA in human spermatozoa does not preclude pronucleus formation at intracytoplasmic sperm injection. *Hum. Reprod.* 13: 1864–1871 (1998).
14. Sikka SC. Role of oxidative stress and antioxidants in andrology and assisted reproductive technology. *J. Androl.* 25: 5–18 (2004).
15. Kobayashi H *et al.* Quality control of reactive oxygen species measurement by luminol-dependent chemiluminescence assay. *J. Androl.* 22: 568–574 (2001).
16. Marchetti C, Obert G, Deffosez A, Formstecher P, Marchetti P. Study of mitochondrial membrane potential, reactive oxygen species, DNA fragmentation and cell viability by flow cytometry in human sperm. *Hum. Reprod.* 17: 1257–1265 (2002).
17. Alvarez JG, Touchstone JC, Blasco L, Storey BT. Spontaneous lipid peroxidation and production of hydrogen peroxide and superoxide in human

spermatozoa. Superoxide dismutase as major enzyme protectant against oxygen toxicity. *J. Androl.* 8: 338–348 (1987).
18. Said TM *et al.* Enhanced chemiluminescence assay versus colorimetric assay for measurement of the total antioxidant capacity of human seminal plasma. *J. Androl.* 24: 676–680 (2003).
19. Sharma RK, Pasqualotto FF, Nelson DR, Thomas AJ, Jr., Agarwal A. The reactive oxygen species-total antioxidant capacity score is a new measure of oxidative stress to predict male infertility. *Hum. Reprod.* 14: 2801–2807 (1999).
20. Aitken RJ, Buckingham D, West K, Wu FC, Zikopoulos K, Richardson DW. Differential contribution of leucocytes and spermatozoa to the generation of reactive oxygen species in the ejaculates of oligozoospermic patients and fertile donors. *J. Reprod. Fertil.* 94: 451–462 (1992).
21. Gavella M, Lipovac V. NADH-dependent oxidoreductase (diaphorase) activity and isozyme pattern of sperm in infertile men. *Arch. Androl.* 28: 135–141 (1992).
22. Gil-Guzman E *et al.* Differential production of reactive oxygen species by subsets of human spermatozoa at different stages of maturation. *Hum. Reprod.* 16: 1922–1930 (2001).
23. Ochsendorf FR. Infections in the male genital tract and reactive oxygen species. *Hum. Reprod. Update* 5: 399–420 (1999).
24. Shekarriz M, Sharma RK, Thomas AJ, Jr., Agarwal A. Positive myeloperoxidase staining (Endtz test) as an indicator of excessive reactive oxygen species formation in semen. *J. Assist. Reprod. Genet.* 12: 70–74 (1995).
25. Plante M, de Lamirande E, Gagnon C. Reactive oxygen species released by activated neutrophils, but not by deficient spermatozoa, are sufficient to affect normal sperm motility. *Fertil. Steril.* 62: 387–393 (1994).
26. Aitken RJ *et al.* Relative impact of oxidative stress on the functional competence and genomic integrity of human spermatozoa. *Biol. Reprod.* 59: 1037–1046 (1998).
27. Armstrong JS, Rajasekaran M, Chamulitrat W, Gatti P, Hellstrom WJ, Sikka SC. Characterization of reactive oxygen species induced effects on human spermatozoa movement and energy metabolism. *Free Radic. Biol. Med.* 26: 869–880 (1999).
28. Iwasaki A, Gagnon C. Formation of reactive oxygen species in spermatozoa of infertile patients. *Fertil. Steril.* 57: 409–416 (1992).
29. de Lamirande E, Gagnon C. Reactive oxygen species and human spermatozoa. II. Depletion of adenosine triphosphate plays an important role in the inhibition of sperm motility. *J. Androl.* 13: 379–386 (1992).

30. Pasqualotto FF, Sharma RK, Nelson DR, Thomas AJ, Agarwal A. Relationship between oxidative stress, semen characteristics, and clinical diagnosis in men undergoing infertility investigation. *Fertil. Steril.* 73: 459–464 (2000).
31. Aitken RJ, Irvine DS, Wu FC. Prospective analysis of sperm–oocyte fusion and reactive oxygen species generation as criteria for the diagnosis of infertility. *Am. J. Obstet. Gynecol.* 164: 542–551 (1991).
32. Griveau JF, Le Lannou D. Reactive oxygen species and human spermatozoa: physiology and pathology. *Int. J. Androl.* 20: 61–69 (1997).
33. Sakkas D, Mariethoz E, Manicardi G, Bizzaro D, Bianchi PG, Bianchi U. Origin of DNA damage in ejaculated human spermatozoa. *Rev. Reprod.* 4: 31–37 (1999).
34. Hendin BN, Kolettis PN, Sharma RK, Thomas AJ, Jr., Agarwal A. Varicocele is associated with elevated spermatozoal reactive oxygen species production and diminished seminal plasma antioxidant capacity. *J. Urol.* 161: 1831–1834 (1999).
35. Agarwal A, Saleh RA, Bedaiwy MA. Role of reactive oxygen species in the pathophysiology of human reproduction. *Fertil. Steril.* 79: 829–843 (2003).
36. Bedaiwy MA, Falcone T, Goldberg J, Attaran M, Nelson D, Agarwal A. Prediction of endometriosis with serum and peritoneal fluid markers: a prospective controlled trial. *Fertil. Steril.* 77(Suppl 1): S5 (2002).
37. Murphy AA, Santanam N, Parthasarathy S. Endometriosis: a disease of oxidative stress? *Semin. Reprod. Endocrinol.* 16: 263–273 (1998).
38. Attaran M *et al.* The effect of follicular fluid reactive oxygen species on the outcome of *in vitro* fertilization. *Int. J. Fertil. Womens Med.* 45: 314–320 (2000).
39. Jozwik M, Wolczynski S, Szamatowicz M. Oxidative stress markers in preovulatory follicular fluid in humans. *Mol. Hum. Reprod.* 5: 409–413 (1999).
40. Paszkowski T, Clarke RN, Hornstein MD. Smoking induces oxidative stress inside the Graafian follicle. *Hum. Reprod.* 17: 921–925 (2002).
41. Guerin P, El Mouatassim S, Menezo Y. Oxidative stress and protection against reactive oxygen species in the pre-implantation embryo and its surroundings. *Hum. Reprod. Update* 7: 175–189 (2001).
42. Bedaiwy MA, Falcone T. Peritoneal fluid environment in endometriosis. Clinicopathological implications. *Minerva Ginecol.* 55: 333–345 (2003).
43. Ota H, Igarashi S, Hatazawa J, Tanaka T. Endothelial nitric oxide synthase in the endometrium during the menstrual cycle in patients with endometriosis and adenomyosis. *Fertil. Steril.* 69: 303–308 (1998).
44. Zeller JM, Henig I, Radwanska E, Dmowski WP. Enhancement of human monocyte and peritoneal macrophage chemiluminescence activities in

women with endometriosis. *Am. J. Reprod. Immunol. Microbiol.* 13: 78–82 (1987).

45. Van Langendonckt A, Casanas-Roux F, Donnez J. Oxidative stress and peritoneal endometriosis. *Fertil. Steril.* 77: 861–870 (2002).
46. Bedaiwy MA *et al.* Relationship between oxidative stress and embryotoxicity of hydrosalpingeal fluid. *Hum. Reprod.* 17: 601–604 (2002).
47. Goto Y, Noda Y, Mori T, Nakano M. Increased generation of reactive oxygen species in embryos cultured *in vitro. Free Radic. Biol. Med.* 15: 69–75 (1993).
48. Nasr-Esfahani MH, Winston NJ, Johnson MH. Effects of glucose, glutamine, ethylenediaminetetraacetic acid and oxygen tension on the concentration of reactive oxygen species and on development of the mouse preimplantation embryo *in vitro. J. Reprod. Fertil.* 96: 219–231 (1992).
49. Guyader-Joly C, Guerin P, Renard JP, Guillaud J, Ponchon S, Menezo Y. Precursors of taurine in female genital tract: effects on developmental capacity of bovine embryo produced *in vitro. Amino Acids* 15: 27–42 (1998).
50. Paszkowski T, Clarke RN. The Graafian follicle is a site of L-ascorbate accumulation. *J. Assist. Reprod. Genet.* 16: 41–45 (1999).
51. Bedaiwy MA *et al.* Differential growth of human embryos *in vitro*: role of reactive oxygen species. *Fertil. Steril.* 82: 593–600 (2004).
52. Sukcharoen N, Keith J, Irvine DS, Aitken RJ. Predicting the fertilizing potential of human sperm suspensions *in vitro*: importance of sperm morphology and leukocyte contamination. *Fertil. Steril.* 63: 1293–1300 (1995).
53. Zorn B, Vidmar G, Meden-Vrtovec H. Seminal reactive oxygen species as predictors of fertilization, embryo quality and pregnancy rates after conventional *in vitro* fertilization and intracytoplasmic sperm injection. *Int. J. Androl.* 26: 279–285 (2003).
54. Agarwal A, Nallella KP, Allamaneni SSR, Said TM. Role of antioxidants in treatment of male infertility: an overview of the literature. *Reprod. Biomed. Online* 8: 616–627 (2004), www.rbmonline.com/Article/1284.

24 Oxidative Stress and Multistage Carcinogenesis

Prabhat C. Goswami and Keshav K. Singh

1. Introduction

Reactive oxygen species (ROS) are oxygen-containing molecules that have higher chemical reactivity than ground-state molecular oxygen. ROS including superoxide, hydrogen peroxide, hydroxyl radical, singlet molecular oxygen, and organic hydroperoxides are constantly generated intracellularly as by-products of aerobic metabolism and have traditionally been thought of as unwanted and toxic products of living in an aerobic environment.[1] Increased levels of ROS can cause oxidative stress, leading to damage to nucleic acid, proteins, and cell membranes and subsequently cell death. However, recent evidence suggests that the physiological levels of ROS production are tightly regulated and serve a signaling function.[2–5] Increasing evidence suggests that ROS may play a critical role in a wide number of human pathophysiological processes including cancer, autoimmune disorders, neuronal degeneration, atherosclerosis, fibrosis, wound healing, and aging. Cancer is a disease of uncontrolled proliferation of cells that express varying degrees of fidelity to their precursor cell of origin.[6] Both genotoxic (agents causing direct damage to DNA) and non-genotoxic, also known as epigenetic (non-DNA reactive agents, influencing cell proliferation, and cell death processes), agents are known to influence the carcinogenesis process.[7]

Carcinogenesis is a multistage process that has been experimentally classified into three main stages: initiation, promotion, and progression.

The initiation process involves mutations in cellular DNA that could result in activation of growth promoting genes (oncogenes) and/or inactivation of growth inhibitory genes (anti-oncogenes, also known as tumor suppressor genes). In addition to mutations, gene amplification and chromosomal translocations are two other well-known processes resulting in oncogene activation. Sequential genetic events during carcinogenesis of human colon cancer suggest multiple genetic alterations are associated with the development of cancer.[8] Promotion is a cellular selection and clonal expansion process, including mitogenesis of initiated cells.[9] While promotion occurs over long periods of time, it is also a reversible process. For example, the incidence of lung cancer in individuals who quit smoking is comparable to that of non-smokers.[10] Promotion could be caused by a variety of agents, including constituents of cigarette smoke, dietary fat, alcoholic beverages, dietary caloric intake, synthetic estrogens, and environmental carcinogens such as asbestos and halogenated hydrocarbons. The final stage, progression, is an irreversible process of additional genetic damage resulting in genetic instability, changes in nuclear ploidy, and disruption of chromosome integrity. These molecular events lead to transformation of a benign lesion into a malignant tumor, capable of invading adjacent tissues and metastasizing to distant sites.[6]

Increased DNA synthesis and cellular proliferation, as well as inhibition in cell death, are necessary for each stage of the carcinogenesis process. While inhibition in DNA synthesis is expected to inhibit proliferation, we and others have shown reversal of hydroxyurea and aphidicolin induced inhibition in DNA synthesis, in fact, accelerates cell proliferation in subsequent daughter generations.[11–13] Perturbations in cellular growth combined with accelerated proliferation could make daughter cells more susceptible to progressive accumulation of mutations. As such, continuous propagation of mutations in subsequent generations could result in an initiated preneoplastic cell that may clonally expand to a neoplasm.[14,15] Furthermore, non-genotoxic agents could also aid in selective clonal expansion of "spontaneously initiated cells."[16] These multistage processes suggest cancer is rarely caused by a single exposure to carcinogen acting on its own.[17] It is postulated that both endogenous and exogenous factors that influence damage to cellular macromolecules, cellular proliferation, and cellular death processes contribute to carcinogenesis.

2. Intracellular Reactive Oxygen Species, Antioxidants, and Carcinogenesis

ROS are generated in mitochondria as a by-product of normal respiration, and in other subcellular locations as a function of biochemical oxidation and reduction (redox) reactions. The superoxide anion ($O_2^{\bullet -}$) is the one electron reduction product of oxygen. This reaction is mediated enzymatically by NADPH and xanthine oxidases, and non-enzymatically by redox reactive compounds such as the semi-ubiquinone compound of the mitochondrial electron transport chain (Fig. 1). It is estimated that 4–5% of molecular oxygen is converted to ROS, primarily $O_2^{\bullet -}$, during mitochondrial oxidative metabolism. The superoxide anion is converted into hydrogen peroxide by superoxide dismutase antioxidant enzymes, and non-enzymatically to hydrogen peroxide and singlet oxygen.[18,19] In the presence of transition metals (e.g., ferrous or cuprous ions), hydrogen peroxide can undergo Fenton

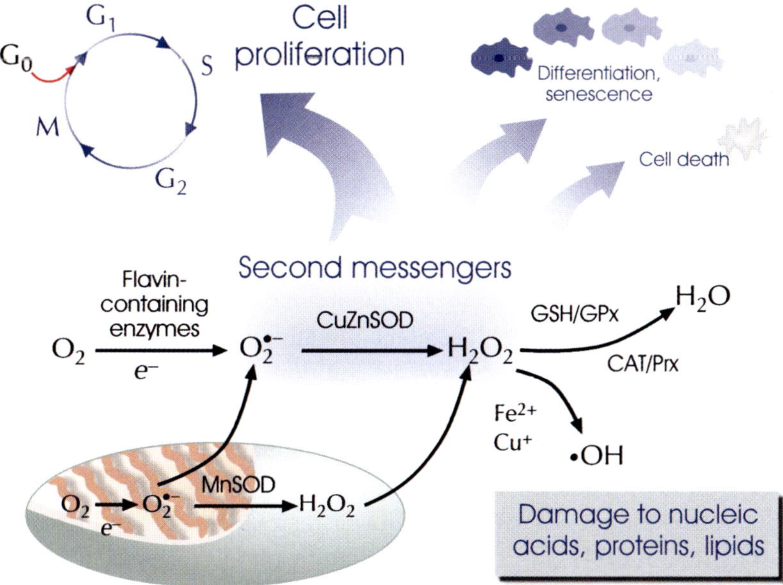

Fig. 1. A schematic diagram of intracellular ROS generation and their neutralization by antioxidant. ROS can serve as a second messenger regulating cell proliferation, differentiation, senescence, and cell death.

and Haber–Weiss reactions to form the highly reactive hydroxyl radical.[20] A hydroxyl radical can damage nucleic acids, lipids, and proteins, which could alter cellular functions and viability.

2.1. *Antioxidants*

In general, under normal physiological conditions cells have an adequate antioxidant defense system to neutralize ROS. Intracellular antioxidant defenses are primarily enzymatic and include superoxide dismutase (SOD), glutathione peroxidase (GPx), and catalase (CAT). SOD converts superoxide to hydrogen peroxide, and CAT and GPx convert hydrogen peroxide to water (Fig. 1). There are two intracellular forms of SOD, CuZnSOD (also known as SOD1) found in the cytoplasm and nucleus, and MnSOD (also known as SOD2) found in mitochondria.[21,22] A third form of SOD, extracellular SOD (EcSOD, also known as SOD3), is found in the plasma membrane.[23] Deletion mutation of the MnSOD gene in mice resulted in death within 5–21 days after birth, while deletions of CuZnSOD and EcSOD were non-lethal.[24–26] Different isozymes of GPx are found in most subcellular compartments, while CAT is found primarily in peroxisomes and cytoplasm.[27]

Intracellular non-enzymatic small molecular weight antioxidants include vitamins E, C, and A, β-carotene, cysteine, and glutathione among others.[28] Glutathione is the most abundant small molecular weight antioxidant inside the cell, present in both its reduced form (GSH) and oxidized form, glutathione disulfide (GSSG). Glutathione disulfide is reduced back to glutathione by NADPH-dependent glutathione reductase as well as thioredoxin/glutaredoxin pathways. In addition, glutathione has multiple functions including modulation of thiol-dependent cysteine containing enzymes, inhibition of membrane lipid peroxidation, and as a co-factor for glutathione peroxidase antioxidant enzyme.[29,30] Because intracellular GSSG concentration is significantly lower than GSH, a small increase in the oxidation of GSH could result in a significant increase in intracellular GSSG levels.[31] In general, under normal physiological conditions the concentrations of GSH and GSSG within the cell are tightly regulated. As such, fluctuations in the GSH/GSSG ratio are used as indicators of changes in intracellular reduction and oxidation (redox) reactions. The physiological concentrations of GSH and GSSG are maintained via alterations in GSH synthesis and/or elimination of GSSG from cells.[32] GSH synthesis is regulated by γ-glutamylcysteine synthase (γ-GCS) enzyme, which is activated following a decrease in GSH levels. Once the physiological concentration of GSH is re-established, γ-GCS enzyme is shut-off via a feedback mechanism.[33] Furthermore, cellular uptake of GSH is controlled by glutathione transferase (γ-GT), which produces hydrogen peroxide, which, in turn, is postulated to regulate GSH mediated inhibition of apoptosis and maintenance of tumor cell proliferation.[34,35]

Thus, each subcellular compartment in mammalian cells is protected by an array of antioxidants in order to maintain a balance between prooxidant production and antioxidant capacity. As such, oxidative stress occurs when the intracellular antioxidants (enzymatic and/or non-enzymatic) are unable to neutralize the prooxidants.

2.2. *ROS and carcinogenesis*

In recent years, increasing evidence suggests both oxygen- and organic-free radical intermediates could contribute to the multiple stages of carcinogenesis.[9,25,36,37] Such an influence could be mediated via genotoxic effects resulting in oxidative DNA adducts due to redox cycling processes, non-genotoxic effects such as changes in gene expression, or both. Frequently, cancer cells are found to be under oxidative stress and produce higher levels of ROS. The rate of hydrogen peroxide production in cancer cells was measured to be approximately 0.5 nmol/10^4 cells per hour.[38] Superoxide levels in blood samples of leukemia patients were higher compared to normal controls,[39] suggesting cancer cells are inherently under oxidative stress. However, the mechanisms responsible for increased ROS levels in cancer cells are not fully understood. Increased glycolytic activity (Warburg effect), defective mitochondrial electron transport chain (respiration injury), and aberrant proliferation are all postulated hypotheses for enhanced ROS levels in cancer cells contrasted to normal cells.[40]

Supporting the fact that cancer cells have higher ROS levels, numerous studies both *in vitro* and *in vivo* have shown altered antioxidant enzyme levels in cancer cells. MnSOD, the most widely studied antioxidant enzyme, has been found to be decreased in a number of primary tumors and tumor-derived cell lines.[41] Accordingly, ectopic expression of MnSOD in cancer cells has been shown to slow tumor cell growth *in vitro* and in nude mice.[42–48] Furthermore, overexpression of CuZnSOD has been shown to inhibit human glioma tumor cell growth.[49] While these reports clearly demonstrate reduced MnSOD expression in a number of human cancers, including glioma, oral squamous carcinoma, prostate carcinoma, and breast cancer, other reports in the literature show increased MnSOD expression in human cancers of gastric, central nervous system, lung, leukemia, mesothelioma, and squamous cell cancers of the larynx and oral cavity.[39,50–54] These differences could be due to differences in the assays used to measure antioxidant enzyme activities, as well as lack of comparisons with matched pair of normal cells. When assays were performed with matched control tissues, MnSOD expression was found to be increased in oral squamous cell carcinoma compared to normal human epithelium.[55] We have shown previously that overexpression of MnSOD is associated with mitochondrial dysfunction and increased resistance to apoptosis induced by a variety of oxidative agents. These results suggest that MnSOD overexpression provides cell survival advantages.[56] These observations clearly demonstrate MnSOD expression is altered in cancer contrasted to normal cells and support the hypothesis that alterations in MnSOD expression contribute to cancer cells increased ROS levels.

The mechanisms regulating abnormal MnSOD gene expression in cancer cells are not fully understood. Polymorphism at position 16 in the mitochondrial target sequence resulting in the replacement of an alanine with a valine is believed to alter the conformation of the leader sequence, thereby inhibiting the translocation of MnSOD to the mitochondria.[57] The alanine variant of MnSOD correlates with an increased risk for breast cancer.[58] Ho and Crapo reported amino acid substitution Ile58Thr in MnSOD.[59] The enzymatic activity of the Ile-58 form of MnSOD protein in transfected MCF7 human breast cancer cells was found to be threefold higher than the Thr variant.[60] Although additional intronic polymorphisms of MnSOD and mutations in the 5′-untranslated region have been identified,[61,62] it is not clear if these mutations affect MnSOD expression and/or protein function. Furthermore, because no mutations within the coding sequences for both MnSOD and CuZnSOD were found in colon and prostate cancer,[62,63] additional studies are necessary to investigate the mechanisms for mRNA regulation and translational/post-translational control of SOD enzyme activity. In fact, MnSOD in human pancreatic cancer is found to be tyrosine nitrated and this post-translational modification is associated with decreased MnSOD enzyme activity.[64–66] In support of this observation, we have found increased MnSOD enzyme activity in phosphatase treated protein extract isolated from NIH3T3 mouse fibroblasts cells (unpublished observation). These results strongly suggest post-translational modification of MnSOD protein could be a major regulatory pathway controlling MnSOD enzyme activity, which warrants elaborate additional studies.

Although polymorphic variants of other antioxidant enzymes have been found, only glutathione peroxidase 1 (GPx1) and glutathione transferases (GT) polymorphic variants are associated with cancer.[67] An amino acid change at position 197 (Pro–Leu) of GPx1 protein has been shown to be associated with human lung cancer.[68] GT-M1 null phenotype has been correlated to increased incidence of lung cancer in heavy smokers and for colorectal cancer.[69–71] Two single nucleotide substitutions (A–G and C–T) resulting in the amino acid changes I105V and A114V of GT-P were also found to be associated with overexpression of GT-P in a variety of human cancer.[72] GT-T1 null phenotype is associated with enhanced susceptibility to colon cancer and astrocytoma.[73,74] These observations suggest higher levels of cellular oxidants, if left unbalanced due to altered antioxidant enzyme gene expression and/or changes in other non-enzymatic reducing agents, could result in ROS induced damage to cellular macromolecules, which could then influence the initiation, promotion, and progression pathways of carcinogenesis.

3. ROS Dependent Damage to Cellular Macromolecules and Carcinogenesis

ROS can induce many forms of base damage in DNA, including base modification, loss of base (apurinic/apyrimidinic site), single- and double-strand breaks, DNA–protein cross-links, and deoxyribose oxidation. DNA damage can induce a number of biological responses, including changes in transcription, replication errors, activation of cell signaling pathways, aberrant cell proliferation, and genomic instability. While superoxide and hydrogen peroxide do not damage DNA directly, the hydroxyl radical causes a variety of lesions in all four bases of DNA.[75] For ROS-dependent modification of DNA, the hydroxyl radical must be generated in a proximal region of DNA. This is made possible by hydrogen peroxide, a readily diffusible ROS and precursor of hydroxyl radical formation. Although hydrogen peroxide itself does not attack DNA, its presence near DNA initiates Fenton chemistry such that the hydroxyl radical is now available in close proximity of DNA for damage to occur. Similar to hydrogen peroxide, peroxynitrite is a strong intracellular oxidant, formed from coupling of nitric oxide and superoxide, and is readily taken up by cells through active transport mechanisms.[76] The DNA damaging capability of peroxynitrite is believed to cause mutations associated with inflammation.[77] Another ROS, singlet oxygen, has been shown to selectively damage guanine.[78]

One of the most abundant and widely studied oxidative modification of DNA bases involves the C-8 hydroxylation of guanine, 8-oxo-7,8-dihydro-2′-deoxyguanosine (8-oxodG or 8-OHdG). This oxidative lesion in DNA produces site-specific G to T transversion and dose-dependent increase in cellular transformation.[79] Transversion of G to T is a common mutation found in many of the growth stimulatory (oncogenes) and inhibitory (tumor suppressor) genes.[80] ROS can also introduce 8-oxodG in dGTP of the cellular dNTP pool. During DNA replication the 8-oxodG is incorporated into DNA opposite to dC or dA on the template strand, which would result in A:T to C:G transversions.[81] In addition to 8-oxodG being a potent mutagen, this oxidative modification in DNA also interferes with binding of methylase and inhibits the methylation of adjacent cytosine.[82] Cytosine-hypomethylation is known to be associated with the development of cancer.[83] Additional ROS-dependent oxidative modification of DNA include thymine glycol, 8-oxo-adenine, 5-hydroxy-deoxycytidine, uracil analogs, and 8-nitroguanine among others.[81,84,85] Although 8-nitroguanine could induce G:C to T:A transversions, the possibility of this reaction *in vivo* is low because this lesion is unstable.

ROS-dependent DNA damage can occur both in the nucleus and mitochondria. In fact, it has been suggested that mitochondrial DNA (mtDNA) is more susceptible to ROS-dependent DNA damage because mtDNA is (a) in close proximity to the mitochondrial electron transport chain, (b) not protected by histones, and (c) less efficient in damage repair.[86] Considering tumor cells are more glycolytic than normal cells, mutations in mtDNA encoding for complexes I, III, IV, and V could affect the electron transport chain, resulting in increased ROS production and subsequently affecting tumor cells energy (ATP) production.[87] Mutations in mtDNA (complexes I, III, IV, and V) found in many human tumors support the hypothesis that ROS-dependent damage to mtDNA could cause cancer.[88–90] Furthermore, it has been suggested that the integration of fragments of mtDNA into nuclear DNA could result in oncogene activation.[91] In addition, ROS-dependent damage to nuclear encoded mtDNA could also affect mitochondrial biogenesis, which could subsequently result in increased leakage of ROS from the electron transport chain.

Although ROS-induced DNA damage is detrimental, cells have an adequate repair system to remove lesions from DNA. Nucleotide excision, base excision, homologous and non-homologous repairs are the four major DNA damage repair pathways in cells. Among these, base excision repair removes 8-oxodG[92] and is the only known major repair pathway in mitochondria.[93] Differential expression of mitochondrial and nuclear DNA glycosylase (OGG1), a repair enzyme that removes oxidized bases, with an organism's age further suggests DNA repair fidelity differs in mitochondria compared to nuclei.[94] Indeed, our study suggests that altered level of ROS leads to increased genomic instability in the nucleus.[95,96] Thus, defects in the DNA repair pathway could propagate DNA damage, in turn leading to genomic instability and development of neoplasia.

Furthermore, ROS-mediated damage to cellular membrane could lead to lipid peroxidation, which could result in reactive electrophiles such as epoxides and aldehydes.[97] Malondialdehyde (MDA), a by-product of lipid peroxidation, forms adducts with dG, dA, and dC.[98] MDA–DNA adducts appear to be mutagenic as they induce mutations and thyroid tumors in rat,[99] and alter cell proliferation within *in vitro* cell culture system.[100]

Besides damage to cellular macromolecules, ROS can interfere with cell-to-cell communication, also known as gap junction, pathways. Gap junctions are intercellular conduits made up of connexin hexamers, allowing passage of low molecular weight compounds of less than 1 kDa. Gap junctions maintain a steady level of low molecular weight growth regulatory compounds among cell populations. Disruption in cell-to-cell communication is postulated to be one of the primary steps during tumor promotion.[101] Tumor promoters (e.g., hydrogen peroxide, 12-*o*-tetradecanoylphorbol-13-acetate, paraquat, DDT, etc.) are known to inhibit cell-to-cell communication; using antioxidants to reverse this inhibition restores gap junction functions.[102–104] It has been postulated that blockage of cell-to-cell communication by ROS would be a selective advantage for preneoplastic cell's clonal expansion because the initiated cell will no longer be under the growth regulatory control of the surrounding network of normal cells.[101]

4. Oxidative Stress, Epigenetic Processes, and Carcinogenesis

Epigenetic processes such as DNA hypo- and hyper-methylation contribute to the development of neoplasia by altering gene expression.[105,106] Methylation at position 5 of cytosine is a natural event following DNA synthesis. While both strands of DNA are symmetrically methylated, initially the newly replicated strand is hemimethylated following replication. DNA methyl transferases transfer methyl groups from S-adenosylmethionine to cytosine residues of the newly replicated strand.[107] Therefore, a defect in DNA methyl transferase activity or S-adenosylmethionine cycle (perhaps due to changes in cysteine pool) could result in hypomethylated DNA, which, in turn, could enhance gene expression in subsequent daughter generations. Hypomethylation of c-myc, c-fos, and c-H-ras protooncogenes have been shown to be associated with hepato-carcinogenesis in rodents.[108,109] In contrast, hypermethylation of DNA would be expected to inhibit gene expression (gene silencing); such an inhibition for tumor suppressor genes would favor aberrant cell proliferation. Tumor suppressor genes such as retinoblastoma gene and cyclin dependent kinase inhibitors ($p14^{ARF}$ and $p16^{ink4a}$) are known to be hypermethylated in bladder and lung cancer.[110–113] A possible role of ROS signaling in hypermethylation of $p16^{ink4a}$ during nickel-induced carcinogenesis[114] suggests oxidative stress could influence epigenetic processes.

5. ROS Signaling and Cell Proliferation

The concept of an ROS-signaling pathway during cell division dates back to 1931 when Louis Rapkine first reported a periodic increase in "soluble"-SH groups during the sea urchin mitotic cycle.[115] Additional evidence for the "Rapkine cycle" was provided later by Kawamura and Dan in 1958,[116] demonstrating localized increase in protein-thiols staining during prophase and metaphase followed by a dramatic decrease in telophase of the sea urchin mitotic cycle. While these were significant observations, this field of research was essentially dormant until recently, when a number of studies reported the possible role of ROS signaling in many cellular pathways, including cell proliferation. Previous studies had shown treatment of cells with sublethal levels of oxidants stimulated cell division and the expression of growth related gene products.[2,117] ROS and hydrogen peroxide have been shown to operate as key signaling molecules in the cascades triggered by the platelet derived growth factor (PDGF), epidermal growth factor (EGF), cytokine and antigen receptors, and are required for proliferative responses to oncogenic Ras.[2,3,117,118] Superoxide generated from NADPH-dependent reduction of the herbicide paraquat showed a differential proliferation response in Syrian hamster embryo fibroblasts.[119] Lower levels of superoxide were growth stimulatory with increased thymidine incorporation while higher levels of superoxide were toxic to these fibroblasts. Low levels of superoxide (0.2–1.1 nmol/hour/4 $\times$ 10^4 cells) generated from the xanthine oxidase reactions in cultured fibroblasts isolated from the skin and palmer fascia of patients with Dupuytren's contracture also showed increased thymidine uptake and cell numbers.[4] In addition, decreased MnSOD protein levels during S-phase compared to G_0-phase in NIH 3T3 fibroblasts further supports the idea that intracellular redox state could regulate progression during the cell cycle.[120] It has been demonstrated that overexpression of PhGPx (GPx4) in human breast cancer cells (MCF7) inhibits proliferation primarily due to a delay in progression from G_1 to S.[121] This suggests lipid peroxidation modulated signaling pathways could also regulate proliferation. Since antioxidants antagonize these signaling cascades, these studies suggest that fluctuations in intracellular redox state caused by changes in ROS levels could regulate redox-sensitive biochemical processes within the cell.

In support of this idea, research has demonstrated that thiol antioxidants induce changes in the intracellular redox state to a more reducing environment, which then inhibits DNA synthesis and proliferation in both human and mouse fibroblasts.[122–125] Cells released from the thiol antioxidant induced growth delay showed a transient increase in prooxidant level prior to S-entry. The re-occurrence of this redox event in subsequent

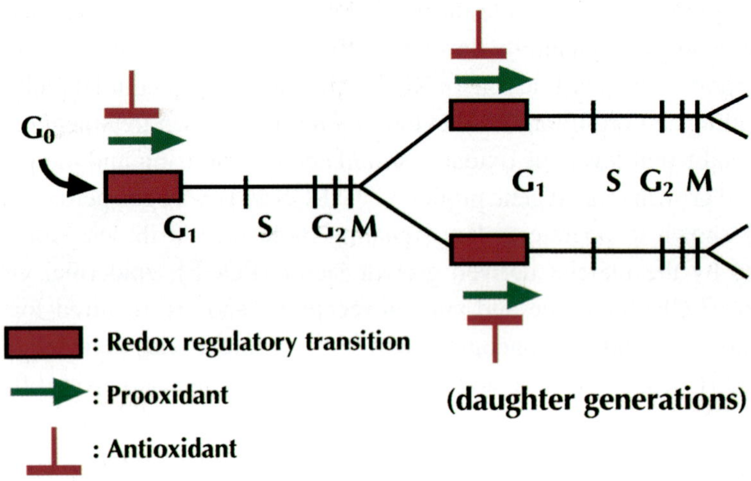

Fig. 2. A schematic illustration of a redox cycle within the mammalian cell cycle: prooxidants would initiate progression from G_1 to S while antioxidants would inhibit these processes. Once the redox event is initiated the cells would complete the present cell cycle and repeat the process in G_1 of the daughter generation.

daughter generations suggests a redox-sensitive checkpoint could regulate cell progression from G_0/G_1 to S in normal cells (Fig. 2).[122] In many ways such a redox-sensitive regulation in G_1 to S progression resembles the "Restriction Point."[126] Withdrawal of growth factors after the restriction point does not affect transit through the remainder of the cell cycle, while withdrawal of growth factors before the restriction point halts progression from G_0/G_1 to S. Similarly, manipulating the intracellular redox state toward a more reducing environment in cells in which the prooxidant event had already occurred would not be expected to affect cells' transit through the remainder of G_1, S, G_2, and M phases of the cell cycle. In contrast, such a manipulation prior to the prooxidant event would inhibit progression into S. It has been postulated that tumor cells' aberrant proliferation is associated with a loss in regulation of the restriction point. In support of this idea, we have previously reported that the thiol antioxidant-dependent redox sensitivity of progression from G_0/G_1 to S phase in human non-malignant breast epithelial cells is lost in breast cancer cells.[127] Thiol antioxidants are also known to induce apoptosis preferentially in cancer cells compared to non-transformed cells.[128,129] These results support the hypothesis that redox-sensitive signaling events may act as a mechanistic bridge to coordinate metabolic and gene expression pathways in preparation for cells entry into the S phase. Disruption of such a controlling mechanism during transformation could contribute toward the growth abnormalities seen in cancer progression. It would be of interest to determine whether the restriction point and redox-sensitive checkpoint map to the same or different region of the G_1 phase.

Progression from G_0/G_1 to S is largely regulated by the D-type cyclins (in particular cyclin D1) in association with the cyclin-dependent kinases (CDK) CDK4/6. This involves promoting the synthesis and stability of the cyclin subunit as well as decreasing the levels of cyclin-dependent kinase inhibitors (CKIs: p21, p27, p16). Cyclin/CDK kinase complex is activated upon removal of inhibitory serine and threonine phosphates from CDK by Cdc25 phosphatases. Active cyclin D1/CDK4,6 kinase complex partially phosphorylates the retinoblastoma (Rb) protein, which causes the release of the E2F family of proteins initiating transcription of E2F-mediated gene expression during G_1 to S transition.[130] Under non-stressed growth conditions, sequential biochemical events follow the checkpoint functions that monitor the efficacy of the preceding steps.[131] Manipulations of intracellular redox state with thiol-antioxidant are known to affect cyclin D1/CDK kinase,[122,123,132] Cdc25 phosphatase activities,[133,134] p21 and p27 expression,[122,127,135] and pRb phosphorylation.[122,136] Furthermore, recent work from Toren Finkel's laboratory has demonstrated the redox sensitivity of Cdc25 phosphatase activities and identified cysteine residues at amino acid positions 330 and 377 that are sensitive to changes in intracellular redox environment.[134] We have shown previously that irradiation, a classical generator of ROS, inhibits expression of the G_2-cell cycle checkpoint and DNA repair gene, topoisomerase IIα.[11,137] Irradiation-induced inhibition in topoisomerase IIα expression is primarily regulated by changes in its mRNA stability. Topoisomerase IIα mRNA stability was sensitive to redox-dependent interactions of RNA-binding proteins to its 3′-untranslated sequence region.[138,139] These results further support the hypothesis that intracellular redox state could influence cell cycle checkpoint gene expression via redox-sensitive interactions of proteins to nucleic acids.

Redox-dependent modifications of specific cysteine residues in transcription factors (AP1, NFκB, and p53) have been shown to affect their DNA binding activities.[140–142] AP-1 transcription factor consists of Jun (c-Jun, JunB, JunD), Fos (FosB, Fra-1, Fra-2), Maf, and ATF family of proteins, which can bind to both TPA and cAMP responsive elements in the promoter sequence of a number of proliferation associated genes.[143] Because cyclin D1 promoter sequence has AP1 binding sites, redox modulation of AP1 transcription factor DNA binding activity could alter cyclin D1 expression, which in turn would influence cell proliferation. JunB and c-Jun are also known to inhibit cyclin-dependent kinase inhibitors, $p21^{Waf1}$ and $p16^{INK4a}$,[144,145] and inhibition of $p21^{Waf1}$ and $p16^{INK4a}$ would be expected to stimulate proliferation. Redox-dependent activation of NFκB has been shown to be mediated via S-thiolation at cys62 of the p50 subunit.[141] Active NFκB complexes are dimers consisting of the Rel family proteins of p50 (NFκB1), p52 (NFκB2), c-Rel, v-Rel (p65), and RelB. NFκB is kept in the cytoplasm by binding to the inhibitory IκB protein and upon mitogenic stimuli IκB dissociates from NFκB, which facilitates NFκB's translocation to the nucleus.[146,147] Redox-dependent mixed disulfide formation of p53 with GSH inhibits p53 DNA binding activity.[142] Although many of the redox modifications in transcription factor DNA binding activities were observed *in vitro*, additional studies are necessary to verify the generality of this phenomenon *in vivo*. Activation of transcription factors is mediated via redox modulation of mitogen-activated protein (MAP) kinase signaling pathways.[148] MAP kinases are serine/threonine kinases that include p38 kinases, c-jun N-terminal kinases (JNK), and extracellular signal-regulated kinases (ERK). Exposure of cells to hydrogen peroxide has been shown to activate protein kinase C[149] and protein kinase B/Akt.[150] Hydrogen peroxide is also known to dissociate thioredoxin from MAP kinase (apoptosis signal regulating kinase, ASK1) and sensitizes cells to apoptosis.[151] It is, however, not clear how redox modulations of the same signaling pathways could lead to diverse biological endpoints, e.g., cell proliferation versus cell death.

In summary, while high levels of ROS are deleterious to cellular macromolecules, physiological levels of ROS generated from the mitochondrial electron transport chain and cellular biochemical redox reactions are essential regulating the various redox-sensitive signaling pathways controlling cell proliferation. A disruption in these ROS-mediating signaling pathways could contribute to aberrant proliferation, which is a hallmark of cancer cell growth. Indeed, intracellular redox-state-dependent alterations in protein's functions in many ways are analogous to phosphorylation/dephosphorylation events except that protein modification occurs on cysteines, arginine, histidine, methionine, and/or metal cofactors rather than on serine, threonine, or tyrosine residues. Although hypothetical at present, it is possible that both redox and phosphorylation/dephosphorylation modifications of proteins (a putative "redox/phos switch") could act in concert during activation (or inactivation) of key biological processes. Such a hypothetical binary switch concept, methyl/phos (acetyl/phos and ubiquitin/phos), has been proposed recently by Fischle *et al.*[152] for the original "histone code hypothesis." Experimental verifications of such an interesting hypothesis could have much broader implications in the near future for our understanding of various signaling cascades that act in concert in performing key biological regulatory processes. Furthermore, a better understanding of the relationship between oxidative stress and carcinogenesis could help in the development of antioxidant-based strategies for cancer prevention.

Acknowledgments

The authors would like to thank Dr Larry W Oberley for his valuable suggestions and continuous encouragement during writing of this review. We also thank Ms Kellie Bodeker for her valuable editorial assistance. For space limitations, we apologize to those authors whose research findings were not included in this review article. This work was supported by American Cancer Society grant IRG 77-004-25 to P.C.G.; NIH PPG CA66081 to L.W.O.; NIH RO1-097714 and Elsa Pardee Foundation to K.K.S.

References

1. Finkel T. Oxygen radicals and signaling. *Curr. Opin. Cell Biol.* 10: 248–253 (1998).
2. Sundaresan M, Yu ZX, Ferrans VJ, Irani K, Finkel T. Requirement for generation of H_2O_2 for platelet-derived growth factor signal transduction. *Science* 270: 296–299 (1995).

3. Bae YS, Kang SW, Seo MS, Baines IC, Tekle E, Chock PB, Rhee SG. Epidermal growth factor (EGF)-induced generation of hydrogen peroxide. Role in EGF receptor-mediated tyrosine phosphorylation. *J. Biol. Chem.* 272: 217–221 (1997).
4. Murrell GA, Francis MJ, Bromley L. Modulation of fibroblast proliferation by oxygen free radicals. *Biochem. J.* 265: 659–665 (1990).
5. Burdon RH, Rice-Evans C. Free radicals and the regulation of mammalian cell proliferation. *Free Radic. Res. Commun.* 6: 345–358 (1989).
6. Rubin E, Farber JL. Neoplasia. In: *Pathology*, 2nd edn. J.B. Lippincott, Philadelphia, 1994, pp. 143–198.
7. Williams GM, Weisburger JH. Carcinogen risk assessment. *Science* 221: 6 (1983).
8. Fearon ER, Vogelstein B. A genetic model for colorectal tumorigenesis. *Cell* 61: 759–767 (1990).
9. Guyton KZ, Kensler TW. Oxidative mechanisms in carcinogenesis. *Br. Med. Bull.* 49: 523–544 (1993).
10. Li F, Schneider JA, Kanton AF. Cancer epidemiology. In: Holland JF, Frei E, Bost RC Jr., Kufe DW, Morton DL, Weichselbaum RR. *Cancer Medicine*, 3rd edn. Lea & Febiger, Philadelphia, 1993, 322–329.
11. Goswami PC, Hill M, Higashikubo R, Wright WD, Roti Roti JL. The suppression of the synthesis of a nuclear protein in cells blocked in G2 phase: identification of NP-170 as topoisomerase II. *Radiat. Res.* 132: 162–167 (1992).
12. Goswami PC, He W, Higashikubo R, Roti Roti JL. Accelerated G1-transit following transient inhibition of DNA replication is dependent on two processes. *Exp. Cell Res.* 214: 198–208 (1994).
13. Tolmach LJ, Labanowska J. Kinetics of the development of accelerated cell-cycle transit resulting from inhibition of DNA replication in the previous cycle. *Cell Tissue Kinet.* 23: 125–135 (1990).
14. Pitot HC, Goldsworthy T, Moran S. The natural history of carcinogenesis: implications of experimental carcinogenesis in the genesis of human cancer. *J. Supramol. Struct. Cell Biochem.* 17: 133–146 (1981).
15. Butterworth BE. Consideration of both genotoxic and nongenotoxic mechanisms in predicting carcinogenic potential. *Mutat. Res.* 239: 117–132 (1990).
16. Ames BN, Gold LS. Too many rodent carcinogens: mitogenesis increases mutagenesis. *Science* 249: 970–971 (1990).
17. Doll R. Chronic and degenerative disease: major causes of morbidity and death. *Am. J. Clin. Nutr.* 62: 1301S–1305S (1995).

18. McCord JM. The evolution of free radicals and oxidative stress. *Am. J. Med.* 108: 652–659 (2000).
19. Droge W. Free radicals in the physiological control of cell function. *Physiol. Rev.* 82: 47–95 (2002).
20. Chance B, Sies H, Boveris A. Hydroperoxide metabolism in mammalian organs. *Physiol. Rev.* 59: 527–605 (1979).
21. McCord JM, Fridovich I. Superoxide dismutase. An enzymic function for erythrocuprein (hemocuprein). *J. Biol. Chem.* 244: 6049–6055 (1969).
22. Weisiger RA, Fridovich I. Mitochondrial superoxide simutase. Site of synthesis and intramitochondrial localization. *J. Biol. Chem.* 248: 4793–4796 (1973).
23. Oury TD, Ho YS, Piantadosi CA, Crapo JD. Extracellular superoxide dismutase, nitric oxide, and central nervous system O_2 toxicity. *Proc. Natl. Acad. Sci. USA* 89: 9715–9719 (1992).
24. Reaume AG, Elliott JL, Hoffman EK, Kowall NW, Ferrante RJ, Siwek DF, Wilcox HM, Flood DG, Beal MF, Brown RH Jr., Scott RW, Snider WD. Motor neurons in Cu/Zn superoxide dismutase-deficient mice develop normally but exhibit enhanced cell death after axonal injury. *Nat. Genet.* 13: 43–47 (1996).
25. Li Y, Trush MA. Oxidative stress and its relationship to carcinogen activation. In: Cutler R, Mori A, Packer L, Bertram J. *Oxidative Stress and Aging*, 1st edn. Birkhauser Verlag, Switzerland, 1995, p. 396.
26. Carlsson LM, Jonsson J, Edlund T, Marklund SL. Mice lacking extracellular superoxide dismutase are more sensitive to hyperoxia. *Proc. Natl. Acad. Sci. USA* 92: 6264–6268 (1995).
27. Peeters-Joris C, Vandevoorde AM, Baudhuin P. Subcellular localization of superoxide dismutase in rat liver. *Biochem. J.* 150: 31–39 (1975).
28. Clarkson PM, Thompson HS. Antioxidants: what role do they play in physical activity and health? *Am. J. Clin. Nutr.* 72: 637S–646S (2000).
29. Finkel T. Redox-dependent signal transduction, *FEBS Lett.* 476: 52–54 (2000).
30. Klatt P, Lamas S. Regulation of protein function by S-glutathiolation in response to oxidative and nitrosative stress. *Eur. J. Biochem.* 267: 4928–4944 (2000).
31. Meister A, Anderson ME. Glutathione. *Annu. Rev. Biochem.* 52: 711–760 (1983).
32. Schafer FQ, Buettner GR. Redox environment of the cell as viewed through the redox state of the glutathione disulfide/glutathione couple. *Free Radic. Biol. Med.* 30: 1191–1212 (2001).

33. Soltaninassab SR, Sekhar KR, Meredith MJ, Freeman ML. Multi-faceted regulation of gamma-glutamylcysteine synthetase. *J. Cell. Physiol.* 182: 163–170 (2000).
34. Perego P, Gatti L, Carenini N, Dal Bo L, Zunino F. Apoptosis induced by extracellular glutathione is mediated by H_2O_2 production and DNA damage. *Int. J. Cancer* 87: 343–348 (2000).
35. Perego P, Paolicchi A, Tongiani R, Pompella A, Tonarelli P, Carenini N, Romanelli S, Zunino F. The cell-specific anti-proliferative effect of reduced glutathione is mediated by gamma-glutamyl transpeptidase-dependent extracellular pro-oxidant reactions. *Int. J. Cancer* 71: 246–250 (1997).
36. Cerutti PA. Prooxidant states and tumor promotion. *Science* 227: 375–381 (1985).
37. Trush MA, Kensler TW. Role of free radicals in carcinogen activation. In: Sies H (ed.) *Oxidative Stress: Oxidant and Antioxidants*. Academic Press, London, 1991 pp. 277–318.
38. Szatrowski TP, Nathan CF. Production of large amounts of hydrogen peroxide by human tumor cells. *Cancer Res.* 51: 794–798 (1991).
39. Devi GS, Prasad MH, Saraswathi I, Raghu D, Rao DN, Reddy PP. Free radicals antioxidant enzymes and lipid peroxidation in different types of leukemias. *Clin. Chim. Acta* 293: 53–62 (2000).
40. Sun Y. Free radicals, antioxidant enzymes, and carcinogenesis. *Free Radic. Biol. Med.* 8: 583–599 (1990).
41. Oberley TD, Oberley LW. Antioxidant enzyme levels in cancer. *Histol. Histopathol.* 12: 525–535 (1997).
42. Church SL, Grant JW, Ridnour LA, Oberley LW, Swanson PE, Meltzer PS, Trent JM. Increased manganese superoxide dismutase expression suppresses the malignant phenotype of human melanoma cells. *Proc. Natl. Acad. Sci. USA* 90: 3113–3117 (1993).
43. Li Y, *et al.* Dilated cardiomyopathy and neonatal lethality in mutant mice lacking manganese superoxide dismutase. *Nat. Genet.* 11: 376–381 (1995).
44. Lam EW, Zwacka R, Engelhardt JF, Davidson BL, Domann FE Jr., Yan T, Oberley LW. Adenovirus-mediated manganese superoxide dismutase gene transfer to hamster cheek pouch carcinoma cells. *Cancer Res.* 57: 5550–5556 (1997).
45. Liu R, Oberley TD, Oberley LW. Transfection and expression of MnSOD cDNA decreases tumor malignancy of human oral squamous carcinoma SCC-25 cells. *Hum. Gene Ther.* 8: 585–595 (1997).

46. Zhong W, Oberley LW, Oberley TD, St Clair DK. Suppression of the malignant phenotype of human glioma cells by overexpression of manganese superoxide dismutase. *Oncogene* 14: 481–490 (1997).
47. Li N, Oberley TD, Oberley LW, Zhong W. Overexpression of manganese superoxide dismutase in DU145 human prostate carcinoma cells has multiple effects on cell phenotype. *Prostate* 35: 221–233 (1998).
48. Darby Weydert CJ, Smith BB, Xu L, Kregel KC, Ritchie JM, Davis CS, Oberley LW. Inhibition of oral cancer cell growth by adenovirus MnSOD plus BCNU treatment. *Free Radic. Biol. Med.* 34: 316–329 (2003).
49. Zhang Y, Zhao W, Zhang HJ, Domann FE, Oberley LW. Overexpression of copper zinc superoxide dismutase suppresses human glioma cell growth. *Cancer Res.* 62: 1205–1212 (2002).
50. Ho C-MJ, Zheng S, Comhair SA, Farver C, Erzurum SC. Differential expression of manganese superoxide dismutase and catalase in lung cancer. *Cancer Res.* 61: 8578–8585 (2001).
51. Cobbs CS, Levi DS, Aldape K, Israel MA. Manganese superoxide dismutase expression in human central nervous system tumors. *Cancer Res.* 56: 3192–3195 (1996).
52. Kahlos K, Anttila S, Asikainen T, Kinnula K, Raivio KO, Mattson K, Linnainmaa K, Kinnula VL. Manganese superoxide dismutase in healthy human pleural mesothelium and in malignant pleural mesothelioma. *Am. J. Respir. Cell Mol. Biol.* 18: 570–580 (1998).
53. Malafa M, Margenthaler J, Webb B, Neitzel L, Christophersen, M. MnSOD expression is increased in metastatic gastric cancer. *J. Surg. Res.* 88: 130–134 (2000).
54. Piyathilake CJ, Bell WC, Oelschlager DK, Heimburger DC, Grizzle WE. The pattern of expression of Mn and Cu-Zn superoxide dismutase varies among squamous cell cancers of the lung, larynx, and oral cavity. *Head Neck* 24: 859–867 (2002).
55. Yang J, Lam EW, Hammad HM, Oberley TD, Oberley LW. Antioxidant enzyme levels in oral squamous cell carcinoma and normal human oral epithelium. *J. Oral Pathol. Med.* 31: 71–77 (2002).
56. Park SY, Chang I, Kim JY, Kang SW, Park SH, Singh K, Lee MS. Resistance of mitochondrial DNA-depleted cells against cell death: role of mitochondrial superoxide dismutase. *J. Biol. Chem.* 279: 7512–7520 (2004).
57. Rosenblum JS, Gilula NB, Lerner RA. On signal sequence polymorphisms and diseases of distribution. *Proc. Natl. Acad. Sci. USA* 93: 4471–4473 (1996).

58. Ambrosone CB, Freudenheim JL, Thompson PA, Bowman E, Vena JE, Marshall JR, Graham S, Laughlin R, Nemoto T, Shields PG. Manganese superoxide dismutase (MnSOD) genetic polymorphisms, dietary antioxidants, and risk of breast cancer. *Cancer Res.* 59: 602–606 (1999).
59. Ho YS, Crapo JD. Isolation and characterization of complementary DNAs encoding human manganese-containing superoxide dismutase. *FEBS Lett.* 229: 256–260 (1988).
60. Zhang HJ, Yan T, Oberley TD, Oberley LW. Comparison of effects of two polymorphic variants of manganese superoxide dismutase on human breast MCF-7 cancer cell phenotype. *Cancer Res.* 59: 6276–6283 (1999).
61. Emahazion T, Jobs M, Howell WM, Siegfried M, Wyoni PI, Prince JA, Brookes AJ. Identification of 167 polymorphisms in 88 genes from candidate neurodegeneration pathways. *Gene* 238: 315–324 (1999).
62. Xu Y, Krishnan A, Wan XS, Majima H, Yeh CC, Ludewig G, Kasarskis EJ, St Clair DK. Mutations in the promoter reveal a cause for the reduced expression of the human manganese superoxide dismutase gene in cancer cells. *Oncogene* 18: 93–102 (1999).
63. Bostwick DG, Alexander EE, Singh R, Shan A, Qian J, Santella RM, Oberley LW, Yan T, Zhong W, Jiang X, Oberley TD. Antioxidant enzyme expression and reactive oxygen species damage in prostatic intraepithelial neoplasia and cancer. *Cancer* 89: 123–134 (2000).
64. Vickers SM, MacMillan-Crow LA, Green M, Ellis C, Thompson JA. Association of increased immunostaining for inducible nitric oxide synthase and nitrotyrosine with fibroblast growth factor transformation in pancreatic cancer. *Arch. Surg.* 134: 245–251 (1999).
65. MacMillan-Crow LA, Thompson JA. Immunoprecipitation of nitrotyrosine-containing proteins. *Methods Enzymol.* 301: 135–145 (1999).
66. Macmillan-Crow LA, Cruthirds DL. Invited review: manganese superoxide dismutase in disease. *Free Radic Res.* 34: 325–336 (2001).
67. Forsberg L, de Faire U, Morgenstern R. Oxidative stress, human genetic variation, and disease. *Arch. Biochem. Biophys.* 389: 84–93 (2001).
68. Ratnasinghe D, Tangrea JA, Andersen MR, Barrett MJ, Virtamo J, Taylor PR, Albanes D. Glutathione peroxidase codon 198 polymorphism variant increases lung cancer risk. *Cancer Res.* 60: 6381–6383 (2000).
69. Seidegard J, Pero RW, Markowitz MM, Roush G, Miller DG, Beattie EJ. Isoenzyme(s) of glutathione transferase (class Mu) as a marker for the susceptibility to lung cancer: a follow up study. *Carcinogenesis* 11: 33–36 (1990).
70. Seidegard J, Vorachek WR, Pero RW, Pearson WR. Hereditary differences in the expression of the human glutathione transferase active on trans-stilbene

oxide are due to a gene deletion. *Proc. Natl. Acad. Sci. USA* 85: 7293–7297 (1988).

71. Zhong S, Wyllie AH, Barnes D, Wolf CR, Spurr NK. Relationship between the GSTM1 genetic polymorphism and susceptibility to bladder, breast and colon cancer. *Carcinogenesis* 14: 1821–1824 (1993).
72. Hayes JD, Pulford DJ. The glutathione S-transferase supergene family: regulation of GST and the contribution of the isoenzymes to cancer chemoprotection and drug resistance. *Crit. Rev. Biochem. Mol. Biol.* 30: 445–600 (1995).
73. Chenevix-Trench G, Young J, Coggan M, Board P. Glutathione S-transferase M1 and T1 polymorphisms: susceptibility to colon cancer and age of onset. *Carcinogenesis* 16: 1655–1657 (1995).
74. Elexpuru-Camiruaga J, *et al.* Susceptibility to astrocytoma and meningioma: influence of allelism at glutathione S-transferase (GSTT1 and GSTM1) and cytochrome P-450 (CYP2D6) loci. *Cancer Res.* 55: 4237–4239 (1995).
75. Wiseman H, Halliwell B. Damage to DNA by reactive oxygen and nitrogen species: role in inflammatory disease and progression to cancer. *Biochem. J.* 313 (Pt 1): 17–29 (1996).
76. Radi R. Peroxynitrite reactions and diffusion in biology. *Chem. Res. Toxicol.* 11: 720–721 (1998).
77. Marnett LJ. Oxyradicals and DNA damage. *Carcinogenesis* 21: 361–370 (2000).
78. Devasagayam TP, Steenken S, Obendorf MS, Schulz WA, Sies H. Formation of 8-hydroxy(deoxy)guanosine and generation of strand breaks at guanine residues in DNA by singlet oxygen. *Biochemistry* 30: 6283–6289 (1991).
79. Zhang H, Xu Y, Kamendulis LM, Klaunig JE. Morphological transformation by 8-hydroxy-2′-deoxyguanosine in Syrian hamster embryo (SHE) cells. *Toxicol. Sci.* 56: 303–312 (2000).
80. Hussain SP, Harris CC. Molecular epidemiology of human cancer: contribution of mutation spectra studies of tumor suppressor genes. *Cancer Res.* 58: 4023–4037 (1998).
81. Wang D, Kreutzer DA, Essigmann JM. Mutagenicity and repair of oxidative DNA damage: insights from studies using defined lesions. *Mutat. Res.* 400: 99–115 (1998).
82. Weitzman SA, Turk PW, Milkowski DH, Kozlowski K. Free radical adducts induce alterations in DNA cytosine methylation. *Proc. Natl. Acad. Sci. USA* 91: 1261–1264 (1994).
83. Counts JL, Goodman JI. Hypomethylation of DNA: an epigenetic mechanism involved in tumor promotion. *Mol. Carcinog.* 11: 185–188 (1994).

84. Kreutzer DA, Essigmann JM. Oxidized, deaminated cytosines are a source of C $\rightarrow$ T transitions *in vivo*. *Proc. Natl. Acad. Sci. USA* 95: 3578–3582 (1998).
85. Loeb LA, Preston BD. Mutagenesis by apurinic/apyrimidinic sites. *Annu. Rev. Genet.* 20: 201–230 (1986).
86. Singh G, Sharkey SM, Moorehead R. Mitochondrial DNA damage by anti-cancer agents. *Pharmacol. Ther.* 54: 217–230 (1992).
87. Nakashima RA, Paggi MG, Pedersen PL. Contributions of glycolysis and oxidative phosphorylation to adenosine 5′-triphosphate production in AS-30D hepatoma cells. *Cancer Res.* 44: 5702–5706 (1984).
88. Schumacher HR, Szekely IE, Patel SB, Fisher DR. Mitochondria: a clue to oncogenesis? *Lancet* 2: 327 (1973).
89. Cavalli LR, Liang BC. Mutagenesis, tumorigenicity, and apoptosis: are the mitochondria involved? *Mutat. Res.* 398: 19–26 (1998).
90. Tamura G, Nishizuka S, Maesawa C, Suzuki Y, Iwaya T, Sakata, K, Endoh Y, Motoyama T. Mutations in mitochondrial control region DNA in gastric tumours of Japanese patients. *Eur. J. Cancer* 35: 316–319 (1999).
91. Shay JW, Werbin H. New evidence for the insertion of mitochondrial DNA into the human genome: significance for cancer and aging. *Mutat. Res.* 275: 227–235 (1992).
92. Fortini P, Parlanti E, Sidorkina OM, Laval J, Dogliotti E. The type of DNA glycosylase determines the base excision repair pathway in mammalian cells. *J. Biol. Chem.* 274: 15230–15236 (1999).
93. Dianov GL, Souza-Pinto N, Nyaga SG, Thybo T, Stevnsner T, Bohr VA. Base excision repair in nuclear and mitochondrial DNA. *Prog. Nucleic Acid Res. Mol. Biol.* 68: 285–297 (2001).
94. de Souza-Pinto NC, Hogue BA, Bohr VA. DNA repair and aging in mouse liver: 8-oxodG glycoxylase activity increase in mitochondrial but not in nuclear extracts. *Free Radic. Biol. Med.* 30: 916–923 (2001).
95. Rasmussen AK, Chatterjee A, Rasmussen LJ, Singh KK. Mitochondria-mediated nuclear mutator phenotype in *Saccharomyces cerevisiae*. *Nucleic Acids Res.* 31: 3909–3917 (2003).
96. Delsite RL, Rasmussen LJ, Rasmussen AK, Kalen A, Goswami PC, Singh KK. Mitochondrial impairment is accompanied by impaired oxidative DNA repair in the nucleus. *Mutagenesis* 18: 497–503 (2003).
97. Janero DR. Malondialdehyde and thiobarbituric acid-reactivity as diagnostic indices of lipid peroxidation and peroxidative tissue injury. *Free Radic. Biol. Med.* 9: 515–540 (1990).

98. Stone K, Ksebati MB, Marnett LJ. Investigation of the adducts formed by reaction of malondialdehyde with adenosine. *Chem. Res. Toxicol.* 3: 33–38 (1990).
99. *NTP Toxicology and Carcinogenesis Studies of Malonaldehyde, Sodium Salt (3-Hydroxy-2-propenal, Sodium Salt) (CAS No. 24382-04-5) in F344/N Rats and B6C3F1 Mice (Gavage Studies).* Environmental Health Information Service, November 1988.
100. Ji C, Rouzer CA, Marnett LJ, Pietenpol JA. Induction of cell cycle arrest by the endogenous product of lipid peroxidation, malondialdehyde. *Carcinogenesis* 19: 1275–1283 (1998).
101. Klaunig JE, Hartnett JA, Ruch RJ, Weghorst CM, Hampton JA, Schafer LD. Gap junctional intercellular communication in hepatic carcinogenesis. *Prog. Clin. Biol. Res.* 340D: 165–174 (1990).
102. Cerutti P, Ghosh R, Oya Y, Amstad P. The role of the cellular antioxidant defense in oxidant carcinogenesis. *Environ. Health Perspect.* 102 (Suppl 10) 123–129 (1994).
103. Upham BL, Kang KS, Cho HY, Trosko JE. Hydrogen peroxide inhibits gap junctional intercellular communication in glutathione sufficient but not glutathione deficient cells. *Carcinogenesis* 18: 37–42 (1997).
104. Ruch RJ, Klaunig JE. Antioxidant prevention of tumor promoter induced inhibition of mouse hepatocyte intercellular communication. *Cancer Lett.* 33: 137–150 (1986).
105. Counts JL, Goodman JI. Alterations in DNA methylation may play a variety of roles in carcinogenesis. *Cell* 83: 13–15 (1995).
106. Baylin SB. Tying it all together: epigenetics, genetics, cell cycle, and cancer. *Science* 277: 1948–1949 (1997).
107. Hergersberg M. Biological aspects of cytosine methylation in eukaryotic cells. *Experientia* 47: 1171–1185 (1991).
108. Wainfan E, Poirier LA. Methyl groups in carcinogenesis: effects on DNA methylation and gene expression. *Cancer Res.* 52: 2071s–2077s (1992).
109. Simile MM, Pascale R, De Miglio MR, Nufris A, Daino L, Seddaiu MA, Gaspa L, Feo F. Correlation between S-adenosyl-L-methionine content and production of c-myc, c-Ha-ras, and c-Ki-ras mRNA transcripts in the early stages of rat liver carcinogenesis. *Cancer Lett.* 79: 9–16 (1994).
110. Salem C, Liang G, Tsai YC, Coulter J, Knowles MA, Feng AC, Groshen S, Nichols PW, Jones PA. Progressive increases in *de novo* methylation of CpG islands in bladder cancer. *Cancer Res.* 60: 2473–2476 (2000).

111. Stirzaker C, Millar DS, Paul CL, Warnecke PM, Harrison J, Vincent PC, Frommer M, Clark SJ. Extensive DNA methylation spanning the Rb promoter in retinoblastoma tumors. *Cancer Res.* 57: 2229–2237 (1997).
112. Myohanen SK, Baylin SB, Herman JG. Hypermethylation can selectively silence individual p16ink4A alleles in neoplasia. *Cancer Res.* 58: 591–593 (1998).
113. Esteller M, Cordon-Cardo C, Corn PG, Meltzer SJ, Pohar KS, Watkins DN, Capella G, Peinado MA, Matias-Guiu X, Prat J, Baylin SB, Herman JG. p14ARF silencing by promoter hypermethylation mediates abnormal intracellular localization of MDM2. *Cancer Res.* 61: 2816–2821 (2001).
114. Govindarajan B, Klafter R, Miller MS, Mansur C, Mizesko M, Bai X, LaMontagne K Jr., Arbiser JL. Reactive oxygen-induced carcinogenesis causes hypermethylation of p16(Ink4a) and activation of MAP kinase. *Mol. Med.* 8: 1–8 (2002).
115. Rapkine L. Su les processus chimiques au cours de la division cellulaire. *Ann. Physio. Physiochem. Biol.* 7: 382–418 (1931).
116. Kawamura N, Dan K. A cytochemical study of the sulfhydryl groups of sea urchin eggs during the first cleavage. *J. Biophys. Biochem. Cytol.* 4: 615–619 (1958).
117. Irani K, Xia Y, Zweier JL, Sollott SJ, Der CJ, Fearon ER, Sundaresan M, Finkel T, Goldschmidt-Clermont PJ. Mitogenic signaling mediated by oxidants in Ras-transformed fibroblasts. *Science* 275: 1649–1652 (1997).
118. Lo YY, Cruz TF. Involvement of reactive oxygen species in cytokine and growth factor induction of c-fos expression in chondrocytes. *J. Biol. Chem.* 270: 11727–11730 (1995).
119. Nicotera TM, Privalle C, Wang TC, Oshimura M, Barrett JC. Differential proliferative responses of Syrian hamster embryo fibroblasts to paraquat-generated superoxide radicals depending on tumor suppressor gene function. *Cancer Res.* 54: 3884–3888 (1994).
120. Oberley TD, Schultz JL, Li N, Oberley LW. Antioxidant enzyme levels as a function of growth state in cell culture. *Free Radic. Biol. Med.* 19: 53–65 (1995).
121. Wang HP, Schafer FQ, Goswami PC, Oberley LW, Buettner GR. Phospholipid hydroperoxide glutathione peroxidase induces a delay in G1 of the cell cycle. *Free Radic Res.* 37: 621–630 (2003).
122. Menon SG, Sarsour EH, Spitz DR, Higashikubo R, Sturm M, Zhang H, Goswami PC. Redox regulation of the G1 to S phase transition in the mouse embryo fibroblast cell cycle. *Cancer Res.* 63: 2109–2117 (2003).

123. Sekharam M, Trotti A, Cunnick JM, Wu J. Suppression of fibroblast cell cycle progression in G1 phase by N-acetylcysteine. *Toxicol. Appl. Pharmacol.* 149: 210–216 (1998).
124. Kim KY, Rhim T, Choi I, Kim SS. N-acetylcysteine induces cell cycle arrest in hepatic stellate cells through its reducing activity. *J. Biol. Chem.* 276: 40591–40598 (2001).
125. Laragione T, Bonetto V, Casoni F, Massignan T, Bianchi G, Gianazza E, Ghezzi P. Redox regulation of surface protein thiols: identification of integrin alpha-4 as a molecular target by using redox proteomics. *Proc. Natl. Acad. Sci. USA* 100: 14737–14741 (2003).
126. Pardee AB. A restriction point for control of normal animal cell proliferation. *Proc. Natl. Acad. Sci. USA* 71: 1286–1290 (1974).
127. Menon SG, Coleman MC, Walsh SA, Spitz DR, Goswami PC. Redox regulation of the G1 to S transition in the mouse embryo fibroblast cell cycle. *Antioxid. Redox Signal.* 7: 711–718 (2005).
128. Havre PA, O'Reilly S, McCormick JJ, Brash DE. Transformed and tumor-derived human cells exhibit preferential sensitivity to the thiol antioxidants, N-acetyl cysteine and penicillamine. *Cancer Res.* 62: 1443–1449 (2002).
129. Hernandez-Saavedra D, McCord JM. Paradoxical effects of thiol reagents on Jurkat cells and a new thiol-sensitive mutant form of human mitochondrial superoxide dismutase. *Cancer Res.* 63: 159–163 (2003).
130. Nevins JR. E2F: a link between the Rb tumor suppressor protein and viral oncoproteins. *Science* 258: 424–429 (1992).
131. Hartwell LH, Weinert TA. Checkpoints: controls that ensure the order of cell cycle events. *Science* 246: 629–634 (1989).
132. Liu M, Wikonkal NM, Brash DE. Induction of cyclin-dependent kinase inhibitors and G(1) prolongation by the chemopreventive agent N-acetylcysteine. *Carcinogenesis* 20: 1869–1872 (1999).
133. Dunphy WG, Kumagai A. The cdc25 protein contains an intrinsic phosphatase activity. *Cell* 67: 189–196 (1991).
134. Savitsky PA, Finkel T. Redox regulation of Cdc25C. *J. Biol. Chem.* 277: 20535–20540 (2002).
135. Wang W, Furneaux H, Cheng H, Caldwell MC, Hutter D, Liu Y, Holbrook N, Gorospe M. HuR regulates p21 mRNA stabilization by UV light. *Mol. Cell. Biol.* 20: 760–769 (2000).
136. Yamauchi A, Bloom ET. Control of cell cycle progression in human natural killer cells through redox regulation of expression and phosphorylation of retinoblastoma gene product protein. *Blood* 89: 4092–4099 (1997).

137. Goswami PC, Roti Roti JL, Hunt CR. The cell cycle-coupled expression of topoisomerase IIalpha during S phase is regulated by mRNA stability and is disrupted by heat shock or ionizing radiation. *Mol. Cell. Biol.* 16: 1500–1508 (1996).
138. Goswami PC, Higashikubo R, Spitz DR. Redox control of cell cycle-coupled topoisomerase II alpha gene expression. *Methods Enzymol.* 353: 448–459 (2002).
139. Goswami PC, Sheren J, Albee LD, Parsian A, Sim JE, Ridnour LA, Higashikubo R, Gius D, Hunt CR, Spitz DR. Cell cycle-coupled variation in topoisomerase IIalpha mRNA is regulated by the 3′-untranslated region. Possible role of redox-sensitive protein binding in mRNA accumulation. *J. Biol. Chem.* 275: 38384–38392 (2000).
140. Abate C, Patel L, Rauscher FJ III, Curran T. Redox regulation of fos and jun DNA-binding activity *in vitro*. *Science* 249: 1157–1161 (1990).
141. Pineda-Molina E, Klatt P, Vazquez J, Marina A, Garcia de Lacoba M, Perez-Sala D, Lamas S. Glutathionylation of the p50 subunit of NF-kappaB: a mechanism for redox-induced inhibition of DNA binding. *Biochemistry* 40: 14134–14142 (2001).
142. Wu HH, Thomas JA, Momand J. p53 protein oxidation in cultured cells in response to pyrrolidine dithiocarbamate: a novel method for relating the amount of p53 oxidation *in vivo* to the regulation of p53-responsive genes. *Biochem. J.* 351: 87–93 (2000).
143. Chinenov Y, Kerppola TK. Close encounters of many kinds: Fos-Jun interactions that mediate transcription regulatory specificity. *Oncogene* 20: 2438–2452 (2001).
144. Passegue E, Wagner EF. JunB suppresses cell proliferation by transcriptional activation of p16(INK4a) expression. *EMBO J.* 19: 2969–2979 (2000).
145. Bakiri L, Lallemand D, Bossy-Wetzel E, Yaniv M. Cell cycle-dependent variations in c-Jun and JunB phosphorylation: a role in the control of cyclin D1 expression. *EMBO J.* 19: 2056–2068 (2000).
146. Pahl HL. Activators and target genes of Rel/NF-kappaB transcription factors. *Oncogene* 18: 6853–6866 (1999).
147. Baeuerle PA, Lenardo M, Pierce JW, Baltimore D. Phorbol-ester-induced activation of the NF-kappa B transcription factor involves dissociation of an apparently cytoplasmic NF-kappa B/inhibitor complex. *Cold Spring Harb. Symp. Quant. Biol.* 53 (Pt 2): 789–798 (1988).
148. Xia Z, Dickens M, Raingeaud J, Davis RJ, Greenberg ME. Opposing effects of ERK and JNK-p38 MAP kinases on apoptosis. *Science* 270: 1326–1331 (1995).

149. Gopalakrishna R, Anderson WB. Ca^{2+}- and phospholipid-independent activation of protein kinase C by selective oxidative modification of the regulatory domain. *Proc. Natl. Acad. Sci. USA* 86: 6758–6762 (1989).
150. Konishi H, Matsuzaki H, Tanaka M, Takemura Y, Kuroda S, Ono Y, Kikkawa U. Activation of protein kinase B (Akt/RAC-protein kinase) by cellular stress and its association with heat shock protein Hsp27. *FEBS Lett.* 410: 493–498 (1997).
151. Tobiume K, Matsuzawa A, Takahashi T, Nishitoh H, Morita K, Takeda K, Minowa O, Miyazono K, Noda T, Ichijo H. ASK1 is required for sustained activations of JNK/p38 MAP kinases and apoptosis. *EMBO Rep.* 2: 222–228 (2001).
152. Fischle W, Wang Y, Allis CD. Binary switches and modification cassettes in histone biology and beyond. *Nature* 425: 475–479 (2003).

149. [illegible] activation [illegible] selective [illegible] of the [illegible] pathway. Proc. Natl. Acad. Sci. USA [illegible]

150. [illegible]: Activation of [illegible] (ASK1) [illegible] and its association with [illegible] (1997).

151. Tobiume K, Matsuzawa A, Takahashi T, Nishitoh H, Morita K, Takeda K, Minowa O, Miyazono K, Noda T, Ichijo H: ASK1 is required for sustained activations of JNK/p38 MAP kinases and apoptosis. EMBO Rep 2: 222–228 (2001).

152. [illegible]: Binary switches and modification cascades in [illegible] (1995).

25 Oxidative Stress and Cancer Cachexia

Giovanni Mantovani and Clelia Madeddu

1. Oxidative Stress in Cancer: Causes and Pathophysiologic Mechanisms

Oxidation is the transfer of electrons from one atom to another and represents an essential part of aerobic life and normal metabolism, since oxygen is the ultimate electron acceptor in the electron flow system that produces energy in the form of ATP.[1] However, problems may arise when the electron flow becomes uncoupled (transfer of unpaired single electrons), generating free radicals: the oxygen-centered free radicals are known as reactive oxygen species (ROS). In addition to the ROS radicals, in living organisms, there are also other ROS non-radicals. It is accepted that ROS play different roles *in vivo*. Some are positive and are related to their involvement in energy production, phagocytosis, regulation of cell growth and intercellular signalling, and synthesis of biologically important compounds.[2] However, ROS may be very damaging, since they can attack lipids in cell membranes, proteins in tissues or enzymes, carbohydrates, and DNA to induce oxidations, which cause membrane damage, protein modification including enzymes, and DNA damage. This oxidative damage is considered to play a causative (pivotal) role in aging and several degenerative diseases, such as heart diseases, cataracts, cognitive dysfunction, and cancer.[3] Humans have evolved with antioxidant systems to protect against free radicals. These systems include some antioxidants produced in the body, namely endogenous, and others supplied from the diet, namely exogenous. Endogenous antioxidants include enzymatic defences, such as Se-glutathione peroxidase

(GPx), catalase, and superoxide dismutase, which metabolize superoxide, hydrogen peroxide, and lipid peroxides, hence preventing the formation of the toxic $OH^{\bullet}$, as well as non-enzymatic defences, such as glutathione, histidine-peptides, the iron-binding proteins transferrin and ferritin, lipoic acid, reduced CoQ_{10}, melatonin, urate, and plasma protein thiols, with the last two accounting for the major contribution to the radical-trapping capacity of plasma.

Several mechanisms may lead to oxidative stress (OS) in cancer patients. The first one is the altered energy metabolism which may account for symptoms such as anorexia/cachexia, nausea, and vomiting, which prevent a normal nutrition and thereby a normal supply of nutrients such as glucose, proteins, and vitamins, leading eventually to accumulation of free radicals, which are known as ROS, such as hydroxyl radicals, superoxide radicals, and others. The second mechanism is a non-specific chronic activation of the immune system with an excessive production of proinflammatory cytokines, which in turn may increase the ROS production.[4] Indeed, a chronic inflammatory condition associated with increased OS has been suggested as one of the triggering mechanisms behind the tumor-induced immune suppression.[5]

Cyclooxygenase-2 (COX-2) is an enzyme catalyzing the synthesis of prostaglandins (PGs) from arachidonic acid. Cells contain genes coding for two isoforms of COX (COX-1 and COX-2). COX-1 is expressed constitutively in most tissues and appears to be responsible for the production of PGs that mediate normal physiological functions, such as maintenance of the integrity of the gastric mucosa and regulation of renal blood flow. In contrast, COX-2 is undetectable in most normal tissues: it is induced by cytokines, growth factors, oncogenes, and tumor promoters, and it contributes to the synthesis of PGs in inflammed and neoplastic tissues.[6] It has been well demonstrated that dysregulation of COX-2 expression correlates with development of gastrointestinal cancers: several studies reported that COX-2 expression is increased in human colorectal adenocarcinomas such as has been detected in 80–90% of colorectal adenocarcinomas and in 40–50% of premalignant adenomas.[7] Several studies suggest that COX-2, by inducing the PGE2 synthesis, contributes to the development of certain types of tumors. PGs appear to be important in the pathogenesis of cancer because they affect mitogenesis, cell adhesion, immune surveillance, and apoptosis. Cancers such as cancer of the head and neck, breast, lung, and colon form more PGs than the normal tissues from which they arise.[8,9] Recently, several studies have reported that the chronic inflammation that occurs in patients with advanced cancer may be attributable to OS, which can adversely affect the immune functions. Indeed, free oxygen radicals produced by macrophages were able to inhibit non-specific and tumor-specific cytotoxicity and downregulate signal molecules.[10–12] Macrophage-derived nitric oxide reduces the phosphorylation and activation of JAK3/STAT5 signal transduction protein thus inhibiting the proliferative response of T cells to IL-2.[13] Therapeutic interventions aimed to protect the immune system in cancer patients from OS-induced cell damage may enhance their immune competence.

A third mechanism may be the result of the use of antineoplastic drugs: many of them, particularly alkylating agents and cisplatin, are able to produce an excess of ROS and therefore lead to OS.[14]

Moreover, OS reduces the rate of cell proliferation and when it occurs during chemotherapy, it may interfere with the cytotoxic effects of antineoplastic drugs, which depend on rapid cell cycle and proliferation of cancer cells.[15] Many anticancer drugs such as alkylating agents and especially platinum agents are highly reactive electrophilic compounds. Other anticancer drugs such as doxorubicin bind iron in the tissues and thus generate ROS and thereby may induce cardiotoxicity.[16] Several studies demonstrated that chemotherapy and radiation therapy are associated with increased formation of ROS and depletion of critical plasma and tissue antioxidants.[17] Cisplatin-combination chemotherapy induces a fall in the plasma total antioxidant status, which may reflect a failure of the physiological antioxidant defense mechanisms against oxidative damage induced by commonly used anticancer drugs. This probably results from a consumption of antioxidants caused by chemotherapy induced-oxidative stress as well as by the renal loss of water-soluble, small molecular weight antioxidants.[18]

Thus, the hypothesis may arise that the body redox systems, which include antioxidant enzymes and low molecular weight antioxidants, may be dysregulated in cancer patients and that this imbalance might enhance disease progression.

To counteract ROS and OS several approaches have been tried both in experimental systems and in humans. Among the most used antioxidant agents there are ALA, cysteine-containing compounds, amifostine, GSH, and vitamins. ALA is present in human cells in a bound lipoillysine form, in mitochondrial proteins that play a central role in oxidative metabolism: it has recently gained considerable attention as an antioxidant.[19] It has been reported to have beneficial effects in disorders associated with OS, inducing a substantial increase in cellular reduced glutathione and restoring severely glutathione deficient cells.[20] Within drug-related antioxidant pharmacology ALA is a model compound that enhances understanding of the mode of action of antioxidants in drug therapy.

Among the cysteine-containing compounds, the carboxycysteine-lysine salt appears to be one of the most interesting: the cysteine is a known precursor for glutathione synthesis that has been shown to act on redox balance and to be capable of significantly improving the antioxidant potential by elevating reduced glutathione levels.[21] Carboxycysteine-lysine salt protects alpha 1 antitripsin from inactivation by hypochlorous acid: in fact, having a chemical structure similar to methionine, it competes with the latter against the oxidative activity of ROS. The carboxycysteine-lysine salt is able to protect DNA from the ROS activity by concentrations of 2.5 mM.

Amifostine, an analog of cysteamine, is a phosphorilated aminothiol prodrug that is dephosphorilated at the tissue site by membrane-bound alkaline phosphatase to its active metabolite, the free thiol, WR-1065. WR-1065 is the form of the drug that is rapidly taken up into cells and it is the major cytoprotective metabolite. Oxidation of WR-1065 forms the symmetrical disulfide, WR-33278, which is structurally similar to the naturally occurring polyamine, spermine, and indeed it shares certain biochemical properties with the polyamines that may contribute to some of the pharmacologic and clinical properties associated with amifostine.

GSH is a key molecule in the redox body homeostasis. OS induces the transformation of GSH into GSSG by the action of GPx: GSSG may in turn be transformed into glutathione protein mixed disulfide or reduced back to GSH by glutathione reductase. During cancer growth, the glutathione redox status (GSH/GSSG) decreases in blood of tumor-bearing animals and humans, too. This effect is mainly due to an increase in GSSG levels. Two reasons may explain this increase: (1) the increase in peroxide production by the tumor that changes affecting the glutathione-related and the antioxidant enzyme activities, and can lead to GSH oxidation within the red blood cells, and (2) an increase of GSSG release from different tissues into the blood. The GSH/GSSG ratio in blood also decreases in patients bearing breast or colon cancers and this change associates with higher GSSG levels, especially in advanced stage of cancer progression.[22]

Antioxidant vitamins, which include vitamin A, vitamin C, and vitamin E, are hypothesized to decrease cancer risk and prevent tissue damage by trapping organic free radicals and/or deactivating reactive oxygen molecules.[23] Many studies have been carried out attempting at demonstrating a preventive role for vitamins as antioxidant agents against cancer and other diseases. The discrepancies between the results of these studies may be explained by the type of population studied (general or high-risk subjects), the different doses of supplementation (nutritional levels or higher), the number of antioxidant tested (one, two, or more), and the type of administration (alone or in balanced association). So, it appears that their preventive effect may be related to multiple nutrients consumed at nutritional doses and in combination, and optimal effect may be expected with a combination of nutrients at levels similar to those found in a healthy diet.[24]

Antioxidant vitamins, which include vitamin A, vitamin C, and vitamin E, are hypothesized to prevent cancer progression by trapping organic free radicals and/or deactivating reactive oxygen molecules.[23,25]

In three of our previous studies we demonstrated, in advanced-stage cancer patients, (1) the ability of antioxidant agents ALA and NAC to restore *in vitro* several important T cell functions,[26] (2) low levels of GPx activity,[27] and (3) the ability of different antioxidant agents, used alone or in combination, to reduce *in vivo* ROS levels and to increase the GPx activity.[28,29]

2. Cancer Cachexia

2.1. *Epidemiology and pathophysiology*

The anorexia/cachexia syndrome is one of the most common causes of death among patients with cancer.[30] The term "cachexia" derives from the Greek "kakòs," which means bad, and "hexis," meaning condition. The characteristic clinical picture of anorexia, tissue wasting, loss of body weight accompanied by a decrease in muscle mass and adipose tissue, and poor performance status that often precedes death has been named cancer-related anorexia/cachexia (CACS).[31–34] Unlike starvation, bodyweight loss in patients with cancer arises equally from loss of muscle and fat, characterized by increased catabolism of skeletal muscle and decreased protein synthesis.[35] Catabolic factors capable of direct breakdown of muscle and adipose tissue appear to be secreted by cachexia-inducing tumors and may play an active role in the process of tissue degeneration.[35] At the time of diagnosis, 80% of patients with upper gastrointestinal cancers and 60% of patients with lung cancer have already experienced substantial weight loss.[36] The prevalence of cachexia increases from 50% to more than 80% before death and in more than 20% of patients cachexia is the main cause of death.[36]

Since the 1980s, the earlier concepts explaining CACS have been replaced by a more complex insight which stresses the interaction between metabolically active molecules produced by the tumor itself and the host immune response.

2.2. *Metabolic abnormalities*

In addition to reduced food intake, important abnormalities in carbohydrate, protein, and lipid biochemistry and metabolism and changes in energy metabolism have been observed, which may account for CACS. The most important carbohydrate abnormalities are insulin resistance, increased glucose synthesis, gluconeogenesis, and Cori cycle activity, and decreased glucose tolerance and turnover. The main pathological changes of protein metabolism include increased protein turnover, muscle catabolism, and liver and tumour protein synthesis, while muscle protein synthesis is decreased. The main abnormalities found in lipid metabolism are enhanced lipid mobilisation, decreased lipogenesis, decreased lipoprotein lipase activity, elevated triglycerides, decreased high-density lipoproteins, increased venous glycerol, and decreased glycerol clearance from the plasma.[34,37,38]

2.3. *Proinflammatory cytokines*

CACS may result from circulating factors produced by the tumor, or by the host immune system in response to the tumor, such as cytokines released by lymphocytes and/or monocytes/macrophages. A number of proinflammatory cytokines, including interleukin (IL)-1, IL-6, tumor necrosis factor α (TNFα), interferon (IFN)α, and IFNγ, have been implicated in the pathogenesis of cachexia associated with human cancer. IL-1 and TNFα have been proposed as mediators of the host's response to inflammation.[39] Chronically elevated levels of these factors, either alone or in combination, are capable of reproducing the different features of CACS.[40–43] More direct evidence of a cytokine involvement in CACS is provided by the observations that cachexia in experimental animal models[44–46] can be relieved by the administration of specific cytokine antagonists. Additional factors and mechanisms thought to play a central role in CACS are the presence of a chronic systemic inflammatory state, circulating tumor-derived lipolytic and proteolytic factors, increased futile energy-consuming cycles, such as the Cori cycle, and a decreased food intake. In addition to chronic proinflammatory factors, circulating factors, such as lipid- and protein-mobilizing factors (LMFs and PMFs), may play a role in the development of CACS.

2.4. *Systemic inflammation*

There is evidence that a chronic, low-grade, tumor-induced activation of the host immune system, which shares numerous characteristics with the "acute-phase response" found after major traumatic events and septic shock, is involved in CACS. The acute-phase response is a systemic reaction to tissue injury, typically observed during inflammation, infection, or trauma, characterized by a series of hepatocyte-derived plasma proteins known as acute-phase reactants, including C-reactive protein, fibrinogen, complement factors B and C3, and by reduced synthesis of albumin and transferrin. An acute-phase response is observed in patients with cancer. In fact, the cytokines IL-1, IL-6, and TNFα are regarded as the major mediators of acute-phase protein induction in the liver.

2.5. *Decreased food intake*

Malnutrition may be considered one hallmark of cancer cachexia and is associated with anorexia, that is, loss of appetite and/or decreased food intake. Appetite is a complex function resulting from the contribution of peripheral and central nervous afferents in the ventral hypothalamus. Stimulation of the medial hypothalamic nucleus inhibits feeding, while stimulation of the lateral nucleus promotes food intake. Among peripheral afferents, oral stimulation by pleasant tastes elicits eating, whereas gastric distention inhibits it. There is evidence that proinflammatory cytokines such as IL-1, IL-6, and TNFα are involved in cancer-related anorexia and decreased food intake, but these cytokines do not seem to be the only mediators of CACS. Since multiple factors are involved in the control of food intake, it is possible that there are also many factors contributing to the tumor-associated anorexia. Indeed, anorexigenic compounds are either released by the tumor into the circulation or the tumor itself may induce metabolic changes resulting in the release of such substances by host tissues. Changes in tryptophan levels in patients with cancer result in increased brain serotonin synthesis and, thus, serotonergic activity, which leads to reduced food intake. Other factors could be involved in promoting the inhibitory afferents to the hypothalamus by stimulating serotonergic and catecolaminergic fibers, such as increased lactate and fatty acid blood levels, both of which are associated with tumor burden.

2.6. *Role of leptin and neuropeptides*

Proinflammatory cytokines, proposed as mediators of CACS, may have a central role in long-term inhibition of feeding by mimicking the hypothalamic effect of excessive negative feedback signaling from leptin. This could be via continuous stimulation of anorexigenic neuropeptides such as serotonin- and corticotropin-releasing factor, as well as by inhibition of the neuropeptide Y orexigenic network consisting of opioid peptides and galanin, and the recently identified melanin-concentrating hormone, orexin, and agouti-related peptide. An important role in stimulating feeding was demonstrated for ghrelin and the growth hormone secretagogue analogs[47] that have a mechanism of action opposite to that of leptin. Such abnormalities in the hypothalamic neuropeptide loop in tumor-bearing animals lead to the development of CACS.

3. Mechanisms Linking Oxidative Stress and Cachexia in Cancer

Regarding the mechanisms linking oxidative stress and cachexia in cancer, the following evidences should be taken into account:

1. In a murine model of muscle wasting and cachexia, TNFα has been shown to induce OS and nitric oxide synthase. Obviously, as previously reported, TNFα is one of the main cytokines involved in CACS. Moreover, TNFα-induced cachexia could be prevented with the antioxidants D-α tocopherol or the NOS inhibitor nitro-L-arginine.[48]
2. An enhanced protein degradation is seen in skeletal muscle of cachectic mice administered TNFα, which appears to be mediated by OS. There is some evidence that this may be a direct effect and is associated with an increase in total cellular ubiquitin-conjugated muscle proteins. Another cytokine, IL-6, may play a role in muscle wasting in certain animal tumors, possibly through both lysosomal (cathepsin) and non-lysosomal (proteasome) pathways.[49]
3. A high rate of glycolytic activity and lactate production is commonly seen in the skeletal muscle tissue in practically all catabolic conditions, including cancer,[50,51] burn injuries,[52] and sepsis.[53] Importantly, it was found even in well-nourished cancer patients, i.e., relatively early in the catabolic process.[54] Because the glycolytic metabolism is normally suppressed by ATP generated by the mitochondrial oxidative energy metabolism, the high glycolytic activity suggests that the capacity of the mitochondrial energy metabolism is too weak to meet the cellular demand for ATP. The mitochondrion is known to be exquisitely sensitive against reactive oxygen intermediates[55,56] but generates superoxide radicals and hydrogen peroxide, especially if its transmembrane potential (i.e., the energy state) is low.[57–59] This generates a potentially vicious circle unless contained by protective mechanisms. In addition, mitochondria were found to produce nitric oxide (NO),[60,61] which is also potentially damaging for mitochondria.[61–64] Therefore, it makes sense that mitochondria require normally adequate concentrations of antioxidants and radical scavengers, such as GSH.[65,66] Spermine is another

important scavenger of ROS[67] that was found to exert protective effects on mitochondria.[68–70] Among other claims, it was claimed that spermine strongly inhibits the induction of mitochondrial NO synthase.[71]

4. Some characteristic biochemical changes are typically found in all catabolic conditions tested thus far. These changes include, among others, a conspicuous increase in the plasma glutamate level,[72] which is similarly found in cancer patients,[33,73,74] HIV/SIV infection,[75,76] non-insulin-dependent diabetes mellitus,[77] amyotrophic lateral sclerosis,[78] and old age.[77] Even in healthy human subjects, episodes with elevated plasma glutamate levels were significantly correlated with a decrease in body cell mass.[79] Whether the increase in plasma glutamate is merely an epiphenomenon in the wasting process or directly involved in the pathogenetic mechanism remains to be determined. In addition, the elevated plasma glutamate levels have been shown to be associated with a decreased muscular uptake of glutamate and a corresponding decrease in i.m. glutamate and GSH levels.[72,77,80]
5. The biochemical changes seen in some murine tumor models (such as the transplantable fibrosarcoma MCA-105) also include the decrease in the plasma albumin level. This phenomenon is associated with practically all catabolic conditions and has been widely used as a quantitative measure of cachexia.[81,82] The decrease in albumin was found to be strongly correlated with a decrease in body cell mass and with the probability of survival. A recent study on cancer cachexia and senescence revealed a linkage between the decrease in plasma albumin and the increase in the plasma cystine/acid soluble thiol ratio, an indicator of the redox state.[83] Treatment of cancer patients with NAC caused not only a shift in the redox state to more reducing conditions but also a relative increase in plasma albumin and body cell mass.[83]
6. In the skeletal muscle of tumor bearing mice a significant impairment of mitochondrial respiratory chain activity (mito.RCA) is observed: a similar impairment of mitochondrial integrity was found in a TNFα-induced model of cachexia and a decreased mito.RCA may also explain the abnormally high glycolytic activity and muscular lactate production in catabolic conditions. An experimental study by Ushmorov *et al.*[84] on cachectic murine models showed that the decreased mito.RCA is attenuated by ornithine. The mechanism of this effect may be explained

tentatively by the fact that ROS compromise the mitochondrial integrity and function and that the ornithine derivative spermine exerts protective effects on mitochondria. It has also been reported that spermine is an effective inhibitor of the induction of NO synthase and that NO, in turn, is a strong inhibitor of mitochondrial functions. A role of NO in cachexia was suggested recently by studies on TNFα-induced murine model of cachexia. In this model, skeletal muscle wasting was prevented by treatment with antioxidants or with the NO synthase inhibitor nitro-L-arginine.

Our study[27] investigated the OS by assessing glutathione peroxidase (GPx) levels and superoxide dismutase and the serum levels of proinflammatory cytokines. We correlated them with the most important clinical indices of cancer patients such as stage of disease and ECOG PS with the aim of finding the prognostic role for disease outcome. We found that GPx was significantly lower in cancer patients than controls and the serum proinflammatory cytokines IL-6 and TNFα were significantly higher in cancer patients than controls. Moreover, GPx activity decreased significantly in stage IV/ECOG II-III, whilst a direct correlation between stage/ECOG PS and serum levels of IL-6 was observed. In conclusion, our study was the first that showed that antioxidant enzymes activity, which is considered a surrogate marker for the body oxidative stress, and proinflammatory cytokines, which are considered the most important surrogate marker for cancer cachexia, strictly correlated with the most important clinical parameters of cancer disease.

4. Treatment Approaches of CACS/OS in Cancer: An Innovative Approach Beyond Current Treatment

Cancer, mainly in its advanced stage, is characterized by complex biological and clinical symptoms that are critical for disease progression and therefore prognosis. Among these, a very important role is played by CACS and OS. In light of their role in the pathophysiology and the course of the neoplastic disease, an innovative approach, with an effective therapy able to counteract their onset and/or evolution, is critical in the aim of improving the prognosis of patients with cancer. The aim of our approach is to prevent and/or cure CACS/OS via administration of an integrated nutritional and pharmacological treatment. Prevention can take place only when biochemical and laboratory symptoms of CACS/OS are present in patients with advanced cancer, whereas the condition can be cured when the clinical symptoms are already present. Based upon several previously published studies and clinical experience,[4,85,86] an innovative approach has been developed. The integrated treatment consists of:

- A diet with high polyphenol content (400 mg) obtained by alimentary sources (onions, apples, oranges, red wine, green tea) or orally supplemented with tablets.
- Oral pharmaconutritional support enriched with N-3 PUFA (EPA 1.1 g, DHA 0.46 g, 310 kcal/can, 2 cans/day).
- Oral progestagen (medroxyprogesterone acetate 500 mg/day).
- Antioxidant treatment (alpha lipoic acid 300 mg/day orally, carbocysteine lysine salt 2.7 g/day orally, vitamin E 400 mg/day orally, vitamin A 30,000 IU/day orally, and vitamin C 500 mg/day orally).
- Selective COX-2 inhibitor (celecoxib 200 mg/day orally).
- With or without anti-TNFα monoclonal antibody (mAb).

The polyphenols, in particular quercetin, have been included for their high activity as antioxidants.[87] The oral dietary supplement has the objective to integrate the energetic/proteic intake with the supplementation of $n - 3$ PUFA, which is able to inhibit cytokine production (TNFα).

The treatment with medroxyprogesterone acetate has the objective to inhibit the cytokine production and to act positively on patients cenestesis: our previous experimental and clinical experience with MPA supports this choice.[86] The selected antioxidant treatment has been demonstrated to be effective in reducing blood levels of ROS and increasing blood levels of physiological antioxidant enzymes.[26–28] The COX-2 selective inhibitor Celecoxib has been chosen for its ability, demonstrated both in experimental and in clinical studies, to inhibit cancer-related inflammatory mediators (PGE2), angiogenesis, and therefore cancer progression. The anti-TNFα mAb is now under approval in the United States for the treatment of neoplastic cachexia: a multicenter randomized clinical trial is currently under way to test its effectiveness in cachectic pancreatic cancer patients. The first two agents of the integrated treatment (pharmaco-nutritional support containing PUFA and progestagen) have already been found effective when administered alone. The efficacy of the above cited antioxidant treatment has been already demonstrated in one of our recent studies.[28] Clinical data on the efficacy of selective COX-2 inhibitors in the treatment of CACS and OS have not yet been published.

A non-randomized phase II pilot study has been recently started in our institution with the aim to evaluate the effects of the above cited treatment on latent (preclinical) or early clinical phase of CACS/OS in advanced cancer patients. The study plans to include 40 patients (this number of patients is adequate according to the two-stage Simon design for phase II studies): the treatment duration is 16 weeks and the evaluation is completed in 24 weeks. Eligibility criteria: cancer patients with locoregionally advanced or metastatic disease (stage III–IV), with tumor of different sites, especially those inducing early CACS/OS (i.e., head and neck and gastrointestinal, mainly pancreatic, cancer). In this phase II pilot study there is not a control arm, but as a calibration arm we will consider a sample of 40 age/sex/clinical situation and biological parameters well matched patients who for mechanical obstruction or other clinically relevant causes cannot be submitted to planned treatment.

The endpoints of the phase II study are: efficacy and tolerability.

1. *Efficacy parameters*:
   - the correction of body composition, i.e., the increase of lean body mass (LBM);
   - the correction of weight loss;
   - the improvement of appetite;
   - the decrease of resting energy expenditure (kcal/day) calculated by indirect calorimetry;
   - the correction of the abnormal laboratory parameters of CACS/OS;
   - the improvement of quality of life (QL);
   - the improvement of performance status according to ECOG scale.
2. *Tolerability parameters*:
   - the absence of significant side effects and the compliance by patients.

If the phase II pilot study will be effective on the basis of the assessed parameters and well tolerated, namely without important side effects, an open phase III study will be carried out. Three different arms of treatment will be compared to no treatment (controls) in three groups of patients:

A. A first group of 80 patients in whom the clinical and/or laboratory symptoms of CACS are prevalent (patients with loss of body weight and/or pathological values of inflammatory cytokines and/or leptin) will be randomly assigned to receive either treatment A or no treatment. Treatment A will consist of diet with high polyphenols content + pharmaco-nutritional support containing $n - 3$ PUFA + synthetic progestagen + selective COX-2 inhibitor.
B. A second group 80 of patients in whom the clinical and/or laboratory symptoms of OS are prevalent (patients with pathological values of ROS and/or antioxidant enzymes) will be randomly assigned to receive either treatment B or no treatment. Treatment B will consist of diet with high polyphenols content + pharmaco-nutritional support containing $n - 3$ PUFA + antioxidant agents (for hospitalized patients the antioxidant treatment will be integrated with reduced glutathione i.v. + selective COX-2.
C. A third group of 80 patients in whom symptoms of both CACS and OS are present will be randomly assigned to receive either treatment C or no treatment. Treatment C will consist of treatments A + B.

Hypothesizing a mean difference before and after treatment (increase of LBM and QL, and decrease of cytokines) of 25% and a standard deviation between mean (m) and $2m$, considering an alpha type error 0.005 and a beta type error of 0.20, 80 patients will be enrolled for each arm.

4.1. *Preliminary results of the phase II study*

The rationale and the initial data for putting together such combination therapy is to enable a comprehensive evaluation of its effectiveness while in the subsequent phase III of the study we will select the single and/or the coupled agents which will demonstrate to be the most effective.

To date, 16 patients have been enrolled (eight head and neck, four breast, one ovarian, one lung, one stomach, and one pancreatic cancer; all stage IV). Patient characteristics have been reported in Table 1. Ten patients are presently evaluable, five are too early and one was withdrawn from the

Table 1. Patient characteristics.

		No.	%
Patients enrolled		16	
Male/female		9/7	
Age			
Mean ± SD:	57.9 ± 8.3		
Range:	44–76		
Weight			
Mean ± SD:	53.5 ± 13.6		
Range:	36–76		
BMI			
Mean ± SD:	21.2 ± 5.7		
Range:	14.4–31.6		
BMI <18.57		7	43.75
BMI 18.5–25		7	37.5
BMI 25–30		2	12.5
Tumor site			
Breast		4	25
Head and neck		8	50
Ovary		1	6.25
Lung		1	6.25
Stomach		1	6.25
Pancreas		1	6.25
Stage			
IV		16	100
ECOG PS			
0		1	6.25
1		5	31.25
2		9	56.25
3		1	6.25

study. Several nutritional (weight, LBM) and laboratory parameters (serum levels of TNFα, IL-6, leptin, and blood levels of ROS, GPx and SOD) have been evaluated after 1, 2, and 4 months of treatment. Four patients have been evaluated after 4 months of treatment, seven patients after 2 months, and ten patients after 1 month (Table 2). As for LBM a mean increase of

Table 2. Nutritional and laboratory parameters evaluated after 1, 2, and 4 months of treatment.

Parameters	Baseline	After 1 month, 10 patients	p Value	After 2 months, 7 patients	p Value	After 4 months, 4 patients	p Value
Weight (kg)	51.7 ± 13.2	52.6 ± 13.6	NS	56.8 ± 15.1	NS	59.8 ± 23.8	NS
Lean body mass (kg)	32.8 ± 12	35.0 ± 11.4	**0.05**	38.3 ± 10.5	**0.05**	36.6 ± 17.6	NS
ROS (FORT U)	481.8 ± 134.9	411.7 ± 60.2	NS	425.0 ± 21.6	NS	381.7 ± 98.3	NS
GPx (U/l)	8347.6 ± 4029.7	6587.3 ± 3159.5	NS	8623.7 ± 3272.1	NS	8897.0 ± 1162.6	NS
SOD (U/ml)	96.4 ± 74.7	76.3 ± 13.7	NS	94.7 ± 54.6	NS	99.7 ± 62.7	NS
IL-6 (pg/ml)	17.3 ± 7.4	19.9 ± 11.8	NS	11.4 ± 3.9	NS	7.3 ± 3.2	NS
TNFα (pg/ml)	59.4 ± 47.9	34.4 ± 17.3	**0.007**	23.1 ± 4.9	**0.002**	12.8 ± 7.3	NS
Leptin (ng/ml)	2.7 ± 2.7	3.4 ± 2.6	NS	25.7 ± 36.3	NS	32.2 ± 23.9	NS

Data are reported as mean ± standard deviation (SD). Significance was considered at 0.05 level ($p < 0.05$) as calculated with Student' t-test for paired data (post-treatment values versus baseline).

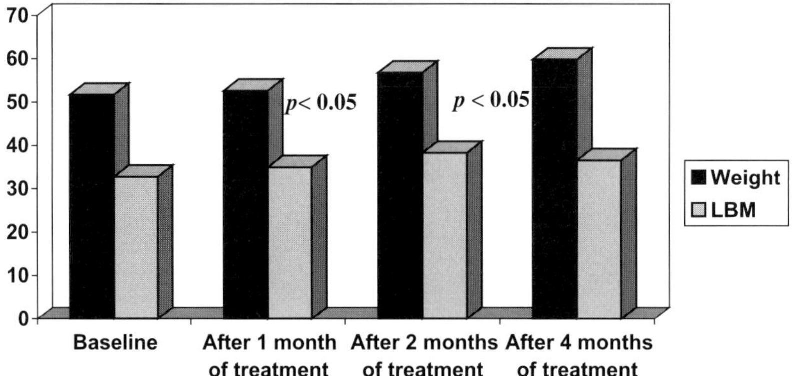

Fig. 1a. Weight and LBM after 1, 2, and 4 months of treatment. Data are reported as mean values. Significance was considered at 0.05 level ($p < 0.05$)* as calculated with Student's t-test for paired data (post-treatment values versus baseline).

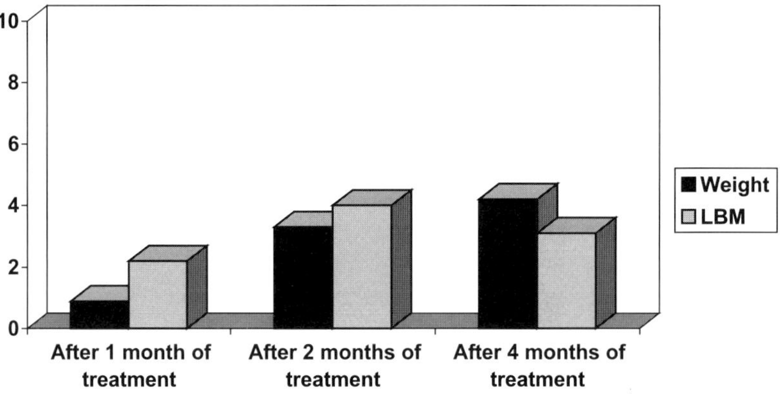

Fig. 1b. Weight and LBM change after 1, 2, and 4 months of treatment as compared to baseline (0).

2.2 kg (9.9%) after 1 month and 4.0 kg (19.5%) after 2 months ($p < 0.05$ versus baseline for both) have been registered (Figs. 1a and 1b). As for proinflammatory cytokines a mean decrease of TNFα has been registered (34.4 $\pm$ 17.3 pg/ml after 1 month and 35.5 $\pm$ 37.5 after 2 months of treatment: $p < 0.05$ versus baseline for both) (Fig. 2). As for QL, seven patients

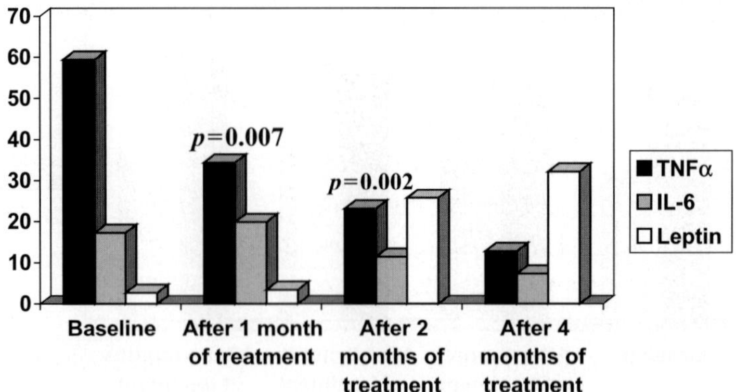

Fig. 2. Serum levels of TNFα (pg/ml), IL-6 (pg/ml), and leptin (ng/ml) after 1, 2, and 3 months of treatment. Data are reported as mean values. Significance was considered at 0.05 level ($p < 0.05$) as calculated with Student's t-test for paired data (post-treatment values versus baseline.)

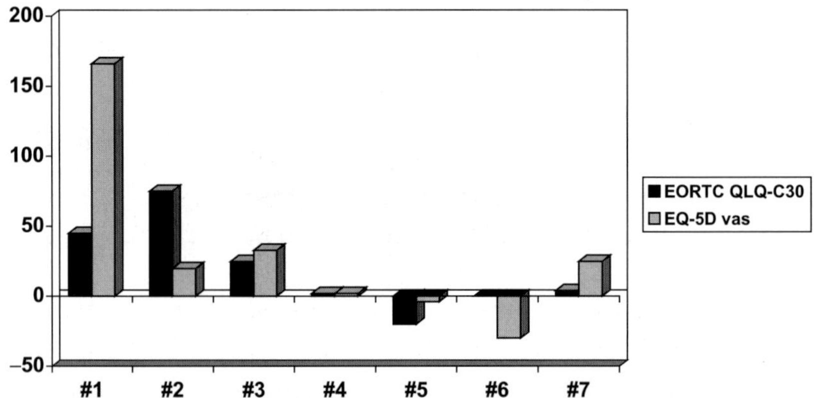

Fig. 3. QL by EORTC QTQ-C30 and EQ-5D vas in seven patients after 1 month of treatment. Bars represent the percent change of each patient score versus baseline (0). Increase, improvement of QL; decrease, worsening of QL.

have been assessed after 1 month of treatment: a mean improvement of 27% by EORTC QLQ-C30 and 13% by EQ-5Dvas have been registered. The analysis of QL of each patient by EORTC QLQ-C30 and EQ-5Dvas is reported in Fig. 3. The study is in progress until the accrual will be completed.

5. CACS/OS in Cancer: Where Will We Go From Here?

In recent years, we have come to a better understanding of cancer cachexia: it may be considered as a multifactorial complication of cancer resulting from a complex interaction of major central nervous system (CNS) and metabolic abnormalities attributable to a combination of tumor by-products and host cytokine release, co-morbidities, and psychological factors rather than a simple increase in energy consumption by the tumor and malnutrition on the part of the patient. Under normal circumstances, both humans and animals respond to malnutrition with a complex neuroendocrine mechanism that eventually leads to an increase in appetite, a relative sparing of lean body mass and consuming of fat stores, and an overall decrease in the normal resting energy expenditure.[88–92] Cachexia refers instead to a pathological state of malnutrition where appetite diminishes in conjunction with an increase in resting energy expenditure and a relative wasting of lean body mass. The resulting malnutrition and the loss of lean body mass worsens the quality of life and also affects recovery by decreasing tolerance to therapy and increasing complications. Therefore, it would be best to concentrate the efforts on early therapeutic intervention and consider the severity of clinical features as ranging from mild anorexia to severe cachexia. So far, attempts at drug therapy for cachexia with a variety of agents have had limited success. The most widely used agents, megestrol/medroxyprogesterone acetate, have been successful to a certain extent in reversing weight loss although this occurs as a result of an increase in the fat mass and water retention rather than the preservation of lean body mass. Megestrol/medroxyprogesterone acetate are generally recommended for long-term (longer than 2–3 months) use whereas glucocorticoids may be considered useful for a shorter period for appetite stimulation.[30,93] Glucorticoids have been shown to act rapidly on appetite, and they also show an improvement in fatigue and general sense of well-being. Furthermore, there also seems to be evidence for recommending anti-serotoninergic drugs, prokinetic agents, branched-chain aminoacids (BCAA), eicosopentaenoic acid (EPA), and thalidomide, which act on the feeding regulatory feedback to increase appetite, and inhibit tumor- and host-derived catabolic factors such as cytokines. Most of these second-line drugs have different sites and/or mechanisms of action. Therefore, these agents could be used to replace first-line drugs in case of failure depending on the cause of cachexia or the patient general conditions. Appetite stimulants could remove anorexia with mild side effects at doses that would be able to stabilize weight loss for a certain period of time.[30] A prokinetic agent should be used in case of early satiety or opioid-induced nausea. BCAA and EPA could be used for the nutritional support.[94] Most of the above suggested treatments have not received enough evaluation as yet to be recommended as any more than second-line treatments; nevertheless, they could be used not only on an individual basis but also in randomized controlled studies. Furthermore, several new promising drugs are soon to be tested in clinical trials:[95–102] they include melanocortin antagonists, growth hormone secretagogues (synthetic agonists of ghrelin, a newly identified orexigenic peptide), and cytokine antagonists or inhibitors. These agents could lead to the development of a combined drug therapy that may, at the same time, address the different aspects of cancer cachexia and target more specific pharmacological interventions, an approach that has been demonstrated to be highly effective in the management of other cancer-related symptoms such as chemotherapy-induced nausea and cancer pain.

The issues to be considered methodologically for this combined approach include the best way to assess the degree of CACS, the appropriate characterization by measuring all possible contributing factors (a CACS staging system), and the best ways to assess caloric intake, nutrition status, function, and well-being in these patients.

The above reported innovative treatment approach of CACS based on multiple components, each targeted at different factors involved, will be effective both in improving objective clinical symptoms such as lean body mass and subjective symptoms such as quality of life. It is to be taken into account that the treatment consists mainly of diet, relatively low-cost pharmaco-nutritional support and low-cost drugs; therefore, it may be considered as having a favourable cost–benefit profile while achieving an optimal patient compliance. As shown in previous studies, both physicians and patients look for more effective treatments for the most important clinical problems of CACS. Caregivers report that it is difficult to cope with patients who progressively lose weight and strength whilst persistently refusing adequate food intake. Selection criteria for cachexia need to be carefully defined and not just in terms of tumor type and extent, but also in terms of the mechanism inducing cachexia with the hope that the clearly defined patient subgroups will help to better identify those more likely to benefit from the available therapies. Cancer cachexia treatment should also address and focus on the symptomatic advantages in terms of quality of life rather than just on nutritional aspects, since the survival of these patients may be very short at this stage of disease. Effective and timely communication with patients and their relatives is a prerequisite for a comprehensive treatment approach. Ultimately, the main aim must be to eradicate the belief that cachexia is an unavoidable consequence of advanced cancer.

References

1. Davies KJ. Oxidative stress: the paradox of aerobic life. *Biochem. Soc. Symp.* 61: 1–31 (1993).
2. Halliwell B *et al.* Antioxidants and human disease: a general introduction. *Nutr. Rev.* 55: S44–S52 (1997).
3. Halliwell BE, Gutteridge JMC. Protection against oxidants in biological systems: the superoxide theory of oxygen toxicity. In: Halliwell B, Gutteridge JMC (eds.) *Free Radicals in Biology and Medicine.* Clarendon Press, Oxford, 1989, pp. 86–179.
4. Mantovani G *et al.* Cytokine activity in cancer-related anorexia/cachexia: role of megestrol acetate and medroxyprogesterone acetate. *Semin. Oncol.* 25: 45–52 (1998).
5. Malmberg KJ *et al.* A short-term dietary supplementation of high doses of vitamin E increases T helper 1 cytokine production in patients with advanced colorectal cancer. *Clin. Cancer Res.* 8: 1772–1778 (2002).
6. Herscman HR. Prostaglandin synthase 2. *Biochim. Biophys. Acta* 1299: 125–140 (1996).
7. Sano H *et al.* Expression of cyclooxygenase-1 and -2 in human colorectal cancer. *Cancer Res.* 55: 3785–3789 (1995).
8. Lupulescu A. Prostaglandins, their inhibitors and cancer. *Prostaglandins Leukot. Essent. Fatty Acids* 54: 83–94 (1996).
9. Bennett A *et al.* The production of prostanoids in human cancers, and their implications for tumor progression. *Prog. Lipid Res.* 25: 539–542 (1986).
10. Kono K *et al.* Hydrogen peroxide secreted by tumor-derived macrophages down-modulates signal-transducing ς molecules and inhibits tumor-specific T-cell and natural killer cell-mediated cytotoxicity. *Eur. J. Immunol.* 26: 1308–1313 (1996).

11. Aoe T *et al.* Activated macrophages induce structural abnormalities of the T cell receptor-CD3 complex. *J. Exp. Med.* 181: 1881–1886 (1995).
12. Otjuji M *et al.* Oxidative stress by tumor-derived macrophages suppresses the expression of CD3 ς chain of T-cell receptor complex and antigen-specific T-cell responses. *Proc. Natl. Acad. Sci. USA* 93: 13119–13124 (1996).
13. Bingisser RM *et al.* Macrophage-derived nitric oxide regulates T-cell activation via reversible disruption of the Jak3/STAT5 signaling pathway. *J. Immunol.* 160: 5729–5734 (1998).
14. Weijl NI *et al.* Free radicals and antioxidants in chemotherapy-induced toxicity. *Cancer Treat. Rev.* 23: 209–240 (1997).
15. Conklin KA. Dietary antioxidants during cancer chemotherapy: impact on chemotherapeutic effectiveness and development of side effects. *Nutr. Cancer* 37: 1–18 (2000).
16. Erhola M *et al.* Effects of anthracyclin-based chemotherapy on total plasma antioxidant capacity in small lung cancer patients. *Free Radic. Biol. Med.* 21: 383–390 (1996).
17. Sabitha KE, Shyamaladevi CS. Oxidant and antioxidant activity changes in patients with oral cancer and treated with chemotherapy. *Oral Oncol.* 35: 273–277 (1999).
18. Weijl NI *et al.* Cisplatin combination chemotherapy induces a fall in plasma antioxidants of cancer patients. *Ann. Oncol.* 9: 1331–1337 (1988).
19. Packer L, Witt EH, Tritschler HJ. Alpha-Lipoic acid as a biological antioxidant. *Free Radic. Biol. Med.* 19: 227–250 (1995).
20. Han D *et al.* Lipoic acid increases *de novo* synthesis of cellular glutathione by improving cysteine utilization. *BioFactors* 6: 321–338 (1997).
21. Beher J *et al.* Antioxidative and clinical effects of high-dose N-acetylcysteine in fibrosing alveolitis. Adjunctive therapy to maintenance immunosuppression. *Am. J. Respir. Crit. Care Med.* 156: 1897–1901 (1997).
22. Navarro J *et al.* Changes in glutathione status and the antioxidant system in blood and in cancer cells associate with tumor growth *in vivo*. *Free Radic. Biol. Med.* 26: 410–418 (1999).
23. McCall MR, Frei B. Can antioxidant vitamins materially reduce oxidative damage in humans? *Free Radic. Biol. Med.* 26: 1034–1053 (1999).
24. Hercberg S *et al.* The potential role of antioxidant vitamins in preventing cardiovascular diseases and cancers. *Nutrition* 14: 513–520 (1998).
25. Frei B, Stocker R, Ames BN. Antioxidant defenses and lipid peroxidation in human blood plasma. *Proc. Natl. Acad. Sci. USA* 85: 9748–9752 (1998).

26. Mantovani G *et al.* Restoration of functional defects in peripheral blood mononuclear cells isolated from cancer patients by thiol antioxidants alpha-lipoic acid and N-acetyl cysteine. *Int. J. Cancer* 86: 842–847 (2000).
27. Mantovani G *et al.* Quantitative evaluation of oxidative stress, chronic inflammatory indexes and leptin in cancer patients: correlation with stage and performance status. *Int. J. Cancer* 98: 84–91 (2002).
28. Mantovani G *et al.* The impact of different antioxidant agents alone or in combination on reactive oxygen species, antioxidant enzymes and cytokines in a series of advanced cancer patients at different sites: correlation with disease progression. *Free Radic. Res.* 37: 213–233 (2003).
29. Mantovani G *et al.* Reactive oxygen species, antioxidant mechanisms, and serum cytokine levels in cancer patients: impact of an antioxidant treatment. *J. Environ. Pathol. Toxicol. Oncol.* 22(1): 17–28 (2003).
30. Nelson KA. The cancer anorexia-cachexia syndrome. *Semin. Oncol.* 27: 64–68 (2000).
31. Heber D, Byerley LO, Chi J. Pathophysiology of malnutrition in the adult cancer patient. *Cancer* 58(8): 1867–1873 (1986).
32. Bruera E. Clinical management of anorexia and cachexia in patients with advanced cancer. *Oncology* 49(2): 35–42 (1992).
33. Brennan MR. Uncomplicated starvation versus cancer cachexia. *Cancer Res.* 37: 2359–2364 (1977).
34. Nelson K, Walsh D. Management of the anorexia/cachexia syndrome. *Cancer Bull.* 43: 403–406 (1991).
35. Tisdale MJ. Cancer cachexia: metabolic alterations and clinical manifestations. *Nutrition* 13(1): 1–7 (1997).
36. Bruera E. ABC of palliative care. Anorexia, cachexia and nutrition. *Br. Med. J.* 315(7117): 1219–1222 (1997).
37. Devereaux DF *et al.* Intolerance to administered lipids in tumor bearing animals. *Surgery* 100: 292–297 (1984).
38. Vlassara H *et al.* Reduced plasma lipoprotein lipase activity in patients with malignancy-associated weight loss. *Horm. Metab. Res.* 18(10): 698–703 (1986).
39. Moldawer LL *et al.* Circulating interleukin 1 and tumor necrosis factor during inflammation. *Am. J. Physiol.* 253(6): R922–R928 (1987).
40. Strassmann G *et al.* Evidence for the involvement of interleukin-6 in experimental cancer cachexia. *J. Clin. Invest.* 89(5): 1681–1684 (1992).
41. Busbridge J, Dascombe MJ, Hoopkins S. Acute central effects of interleukin-6 on body temperature, thermogenesis and food intake in the rat. *Proc. Nutr. Soc.* 38: 48A (1989).

42. Gelin J *et al.* Role of endogenous tumor necrosis factor alfa and interleukin 1 for experimental tumor growth and the development of cancer cachexia. *Cancer Res.* 51(1): 415–421 (1991).
43. McLaughlin CL *et al.* Food intake and body temperature responses of rat to recombinant interleukin 1 beta and a tripeptide interleukin 1 beta antagonist. *Physiol. Behav.* 52(6): 1155–1160 (1992).
44. Noguchi Y *et al.* Are cytokines possible mediators of cancer cachexia? *Surg. Today* 26(7): 467–475 (1996).
45. Sherry BA, Gelin J, Fong Y. Anticachectin/tumor necrosis factor alpha antibodies attenuate development of cancer cachexia. *Cancer Res.* 51: 415–421 (1991).
46. Matthys P, Billiau A. Cytokines and cachexia. *Nutrition* 13(9): 763–770 (1997).
47. Horvath TL *et al.* Minireview: ghrelin and the regulation of energy balance — a hypothalamic perspective. *Endocrinology* 142: 4163–4169 (2001).
48. Buck M, Chojkier M. Muscle wasting and dedifferentiation induced by oxidative stress in a murine model of cachexia is prevented by inhibitors of nitric oxide synthesis and antioxidants. *EMBO J.* 15: 1753–1765 (1996).
49. Tisdale MJ. Loss of skeletal muscle in cancer: biochemical mechanism. *Front. Biosci.* 6: D164–D174 (2001).
50. Shaw JHF, Wolfe RR. Glucose and urea kinetics in patients with early and advanced gastrointestinal cancer: the response to glucose infusion and TPN. *Surgery (St. Louis)* 101: 181–186 (1987).
51. Tayek JA. A review of cancer cachexia and abnormal glucose metabolism inhumans with cancer. *J. Am. Coll. Nutr.* 11: 445–456 (1992).
52. Wilmore DW, Aulick LH. Metabolic changes in burned patients. *Surg. Clin. North Am.* 58: 1173–1187 (1978).
53. Roth E *et al.* Metabolic disorders in severe abdominal sepsis: glutamine deficiency in skeletal muscle. *Clin. Nutr.* 1: 25–41 (1982).
54. Striebel J-P *et al.* Aminosa üreaufnahme und-abgabe kolorektaler Karzinome des Menschen. *Infusionstherapie* 13: 92–104 (1986).
55. Richter C, Kass GEN. Oxidative stress in mitochondria: its relationship to cellular Ca21 homeostasis, cell death, proliferation, and differentiation. *Chem. Biol. Interact.* 77: 1–23 (1991).
56. Viràg L, Salzman AL, Szabò C. Poly(ADP-Ribose) synthetase activation mediates mitochondrial injury during oxidant-induced cell death. *J. Immunol.* 161: 3753–3759 (1998).
57. Loschen G *et al.* Superoxide radicals as precursors of mitochondrial hydrogen peroxide. *FEBS Lett.* 42: 68–72 (1974).

58. Kroemer G *et al.* The biochemistry of programmed cell death. *FASEB J.* 9: 1277–1287 (1995).
59. Chandel NS *et al.* Mitochondrial reactive oxygen species trigger hypoxia-induced transcription. *Proc. Natl. Acad. Sci. USA* 95: 11715–11720 (1998).
60. Tatoyan A, Giulivi C. Purification and characterization of a nitric-oxide synthase from rat liver mitochondria. *J. Biol. Chem.* 273: 11044–11048 (1998).
61. Giulivi C. Functional implications of nitric oxide produced by mitochondria in mitochondrial metabolism. *Biochem. J.* 332: 673–679 (1998).
62. Schweizer M, Richter C. Nitric oxide potently and reversibly de-energizes mitochondria at low oxygen tension. *Biochem. Biophys. Res. Commun.* 204: 169–175 (1994).
63. Kurose I *et al.* Nitric oxide mediates Kupffer cell-induced reduction of mitochondrial energization in hepatoma cells. A comparison with oxidative burst. *Cancer Res.* 53: 2676–2682 (1993).
64. Buck M, Chojkier M. Muscle wasting and dedifferentiation induced by oxidative stress in a murine model of cachexia is prevented by inhibitors of nitric oxide synthesis and antioxidants. *EMBO J.* 15: 1753–1765 (1996).
65. Jain A *et al.* Glutathione deficiency leads to mitochondrial damage in brain. *Proc. Natl. Acad. Sci. USA* 88: 1913–1917 (1991).
66. Meister A. Mitochondrial changes associated with glutathione deficiency. *Biochim. Biophys. Acta* 1271: 35–42 (1995).
67. Ha HC *et al.* The natural polyamine spermine functions directly as a free radical scavenger. *Proc. Natl. Acad. Sci. USA* 95: 11140–11145 (1998).
68. Madsen KL *et al.* Role of ornithine decarboxylase in enterocyte mitochondrial function and integrity. *Am. J. Physiol.* 270: G789–G797 (1996).
69. Igarashi K *et al.* Inhibition of the growth of various human and mouse tumor cells by 1,15-bis(ethylamino)-4,8,12-triazapentadecane. *Cancer Res.* 55: 2615–2619 (1995).
70. Tassani V *et al.* Inhibition of mitochondrial permeability transition by polyamines and magnesium: importance of the number and distribution of electric charges. *Biochem. Biophys. Res. Commun.* 207: 661–667 (1995).
71. Szabò C *et al.* The mechanism of the inhibitory effect of polyamines on the induction of nitric oxide synthase: role of aldehyde metabolites. *Br. J. Pharmacol.* 113: 757–766 (1994).
72. Hack V *et al.* Abnormal glutathione and sulfate levels after interleukin 6 treatment and in tumor-induced cachexia. *FASEB J.* 10: 1219–1226 (1996).
73. Dröge W *et al.* Plasma glutamate concentration and lymphocyte activity. *J. Cancer Clin. Oncol.* 114: 124–128 (1988).

74. Eck H-P, Drings P, Dröge W. Plasma glutamate levels, lymphocyte reactivity and death rate in patients with bronchial carcinoma. *J. Cancer Clin. Oncol.* 115: 571–574 (1989).
75. Eck H-P *et al.* Metabolic disorder as an early consequence of simian immunodeficiency virus infection in rhesus macaques. *Lancet* 338: 346–347 (1991).
76. Dröge W *et al.* Abnormal amino acid concentrations in the blood of patients with acquired immune deficiency syndrome (AIDS) may contribute to the immunological defect. *Biol. Chem. Hoppe-Seyler* 369: 143–148 (1988).
77. Hack V *et al.* Elevated venous glutamate levels in (pre)catabolic conditions result at least partly from a decreased glutamate transport activity. *J. Mol. Med.* 74: 337–343 (1996).
78. Plaitakis A, Caroscio JT. Abnormal glutamate metabolism in amyotrophiclateral sclerosis. *Ann. Neurol.* 22: 575–579 (1987).
79. Kinscherf R *et al.* Low plasma glutamine in combination with high glutamate levels indicate risk for loss of body cell mass in healthy individuals: the effect of N-acetylcysteine. *J. Mol. Med.* 74: 393–400 (1996).
80. Gross A *et al.* Elevated hepatic g-glutamylcysteine synthetase activity and abnormal sulfate levels in liver and muscle tissue may explain abnormal cysteine and glutathione levels in SIV-infected rhesus macaques. *AIDS Res. Hum. Retroviruses* 12: 1639–1641 (1996).
81. Rothschild MA, Oratz M, Schreiber SS. *Serum albumin. Hepatology* 8: 385–401 (1988).
82. Tayek JA. Albumin synthesis and nutritional assessment. *Nutr. Clin. Pract.* 3: 219–221 (1988).
83. Hack V *et al.* The redox state as a correlate of senescence and wasting and as a target for therapeutic intervention. *Blood* 92: 59–67 (1998).
84. Ushmorov A *et al.* Differential reconstitution of mitochondrial respiratory chain activity and plasma redox state by cysteine and ornithine in a model of cancer cachexia. *Cancer Res.* 59(14): 3527–3534 (1999).
85. Mantovani G *et al.* Megestrol acetate in neoplastic anorexia/cachexia: clinical evaluation and comparison with cytokine levels in patients with head and neck carcinoma treated with neoadjuvant chemotherapy. *Int. J. Clin. Lab. Res.* 25(3): 135–141 (1995).
86. Mantovani G *et al.* Medroxyprogesterone acetate reduces the *in vitro* production of cytokines and serotonin involved in anorexia/cachexia and emesis by peripheral blood mononuclear cells of cancer patients. *Eur. J. Cancer* 33(4): 602–607 (1997).
87. Higdon JV, Frei B. Tea catechins and polyphenols: health effects, metabolism, and antioxidant functions. *Crit. Rev. Food Sci. Nutr.* 43(1): 89–143 (2003).

88. Schwartz MW *et al.* Hypothalamic response to starvation: implications for the study of wasting disorders. *Am. J. Physiol.* 269(5): 949–957 (1995).
89. Schwartz MW, Seeley RJ. Neuroendocrine responses to starvation and weight loss. *N. Engl. J. Med.* 336(25): 1802–1811 (1997).
90. Inui A. Feeding and body-weight regulation by hypothalamic neuropeptides — mediation of the actions of leptin. *Trends Neurosci.* 22(2): 62–67 (1999).
91. Marks DL, Ling N, Cone RD. Role of the central melanocortin system in cachexia. *Cancer Res.* 61(4): 1432–1438 (2001).
92. Ahima RS *et al.* Role of leptin in the neuroendocrine response to fasting. *Nature* 382(6588): 250–252 (1996).
93. Loprinzi CL *et al.* Randomized comparison of megestrol acetate versus dexamethasone versus fluoxymesterone for the treatment of cancer anorexia/cachexia. *J. Clin. Oncol.* 17(10): 3299–3306 (1999).
94. Nitenberg G, Raynard B. Nutritional support of the cancer patient: issues and dilemmas. *Crit. Rev. Oncol. Hematol.* 34(3): 137–168 (2000).
95. Mantovani G *et al.* Managing cancer-related anorexia/cachexia. *Drugs* 61(4): 499–514 (2001).
96. Inui A. Cancer anorexia-cachexia syndrome: are neuropeptides the key? *Cancer Res.* 59(18): 4493–4501 (1999).
97. Kotler DP. Cachexia. *Ann. Intern. Med.* 133(8): 622–634 (2000).
98. MacDonald N. Cachexia-anorexia workshop: introduction. *Nutrition* 16(10): 1007–1008 (2000).
99. Lechan RM, Tatro JB. Hypothalamic melanocortin signaling in cachexia. *Endocrinology* 142(8): 3288–3291 (2001).
100. Argiles JM *et al.* Cancer cachexia: a therapeutic approach. *Med. Res. Rev.* 21(1): 83–101 (2001).
101. Asakawa A *et al.* Ghrelin is an appetite-stimulatory signal from stomach with structural resemblance to motilin. *Gastroenterology* 120(2): 337–345 (2001).
102. Inui A. Ghrelin. An orexigenic and somatotrophic signal from the stomach. *Nat. Rev. Neurosci.* 2(8): 551–560 (2001).

26 Oxidative Stress in Cancer-Prone Diseases

Giovanni Pagano

1. Introduction

Several conditions of prooxidant states[a] have been reported in the recent decades for a wide range of genetic diseases,[1–18] providing a consistent basis for the interpretation of the phenotypes of several genetic diseases.[19,20]

A major focus in the studies of genetic diseases has assumed that gaining knowledge about the genotypic defects would shed light into diseases in the prospect of gene therapy. To date, a number of genes have been cloned, yet this prospect has remained elusive. On the other hand, studies of metabolic imbalances in several genetic disorders have been continued and, in some cases, have taken advantage from the studies of the functions of gene products, implying the role(s) of a prooxidant state in a given disease as, e.g., Fanconi anemia (FA)[7,8,21–27] (see below).

Some selected cancer-prone disorders will be considered, by focusing on the occurrence of prooxidant states in their phenotypes. These disorders include a set of chromosomal instability syndromes, aging-related disorders, and hereditary cancer syndromes.[6–10,14,15,20,28,29]

As there are well-established links of oxidative stress, cancer, and ageing,[3–6,28–32] the scenario is envisioned that prooxidant states may play analogous, though distinct roles in the pathogenesis of these diseases. Thus,

[a]Prooxidant states[1,2] may be defined as a number of cellular imbalances between reactive oxygen species (ROS) formation and a set of antioxidant systems. A prooxidant state commonly relates to a deficiency in coping with oxidative stress due to excess ROS formation and/or to lower-than-normal levels of antioxidant systems.

the examination of their phenotypic analogies may shed valuable insights into the pathogenesis of these diseases as well as of cancer and aging in general.

2. Chromosomal Instability Syndromes

Chromosomal instability syndromes are characterized by susceptibility to chromosomal breakages, increased frequency of breaks, and interchanges occurring either spontaneously or following exposure to various DNA-damaging agents.[6,29,33,34] They are inherited as autosomal recessive disorders, and show an increased tendency to develop malignancies. The diseases in this group have different genotypes and clinical manifestations, and include FA, ataxia telangiectasia (AT), Nijmegen breakage syndrome (NBS), Bloom syndrome (BS), and xeroderma pigmentosum (XP).[6,29,33–35] Two exceptions in this group of disorders are made by Cockayne syndrome and trichothiodystrophy that fail to show excess cancer risk.[17,36–38] The inability to repair a particular type of DNA damage has been associated to the phenotype of these disorders, also referred to as DNA repair disorders.[7,34,35,38,39] The abnormal sensitivity of these cells to oxidative stress may underly the definition and diagnosis of these diseases. For example, the exposures to bleomycin (in AT cells) and to mitomycin C (MMC) and other agents in FA cells have been associated to redox-dependent toxicity mechanisms.[20,21,40–44]

2.1. *Fanconi anemia*

This disorder is characterized by progressive bone marrow impairment, and by peculiar chromosomal rearrangements sensitive to some defined clastogens commonly referred to as "crosslinkers."[45–48] The major clinical features include myelopoietic failure, a high incidence of myelogenous leukemias and other malignancies,[46] and a set of clinical findings, such as recurring malformations (upper limbs, heart, digestive tract, and kidneys), insulin-resistant diabetes, other endocrinopathies, and abnormalities in skin pigmentation.[49,50] Mutations that lead to FA fall into 11 complementation groups.[47,51–53] Diagnosis is performed by excess FA cell sensitivity to either diepoxybutane (DEB) or mitomycin C (MMC), which induce high rates of chromosomal breaks and typical aberrations.[45] A set of studies has related FA phenotype to oxidative stress.[11,12,20,41,54–66] The available evidence for a prooxidant state in FA phenotype is summarized in Table 1. Initially confined to biochemical and cytogenetic investigations,[11,12,54–58] this evidence has been extended recently to the functions of the proteins encoded by some FA genes (FANCA, FANCC, FANCG),[22–27] with possible involvement of other FA gene products (reviewed in Refs. 67 and 68). The product of the FA gene C (FANCC) has been shown to associate with redox-related activities, namely NADPH cytochrome P450 reductase (RED)[22] and glutathione S-transferase (GSTP1).[23] The transcription pattern in *FANCC* defective versus corrected cells provided evidence for FANCC-associated regulation of proteins related to "inflammatory response," NFκB, cyclooxygenase-2, and HSP70, yet no involvement of transcripts related to DNA repair.[26] Concurrent results were obtained in another recent study that identified 69 proteins as direct interactors of FANCA, FANCC, or FANCG. These proteins were associated with transcription regulation, signaling, oxidative metabolism, and intracellular transport.[25]

A study of thc FANCG protein function provided evidence for interaction with a P450 protein, cytochrome P450 2E1 (CYP2E1), an activity also known to be involved in redox biotransformation of xenobiotics.[24] An early study reported on the abnormal regulation of xenobiotics biotransformation in FA cells showing excess sensitivity to cyclophosphamide[69] without S-9 metabolic activation, unlike non-FA cells,[70] suggesting a constitutive expression of Phase 1 activities for xenobiotics biotransformation.

A pioneering report by Nordenson[11] first suggested a relationship of the FA phenotype with a prooxidant state. Subsequent studies have provided a substantial body of evidence, as summarized in Table 1. FA cells are characterized by: (i) excess oxidative DNA damage (8-hydroxy-2′-deoxyguanosine, 8-OHdG) in H_2O_2-exposed FA cells;[54] (ii) increased sensitivity to oxygen and free iron;[12,62,64] (iii) correction of chromosomal abnormalities[11,61,63] and of apoptotic propension[68] by either antioxidant enzymes or by low molecular weight antioxidants; (iv) excess plasma levels of clastogenic factor and of tumor necrosis factor-α (TNF-α);[58,59,71] (v) involvement of redox-active cytokines, as TNF-α and interferon-γ (IFN-γ)[71,72] and of inducible nitric oxide synthase (iNOS);[73] and (vi) an

Table 1. Outline of the evidence for the involvement of oxidative stress in Fanconi anemia.

Endpoints	Materials	References
Antioxidants enzymes, hypoxia, and low molecular weight antioxidants as protection factors	Primary FA lymphocytes	11,12, 61–64
	fancc(−/−) bone marrow cells	68
↑ 8-OHdG	*fanca*(−/−) cell lines; leukocytes	54,55
↑ Leukocyte chemiluminescence	Leukocytes (FA patients and relatives)	56,57
↓ Catalase activity	FA fibroblast cell lines	54
↑ TNF-α and clastogenic factor		58,59
↓ Thioredoxin expression		60
Premature senescence by hypoxia-reoxygenation (through p53, and up-regulating p21)	*fancc*(−/−) mouse bone marrow cells	201
Functions of FA proteins in redox-related pathways		
FANCC	↓ NADPH Cyt P-450 reductase (RED)	22
	↑ Glutathione S-transferase (GSTP1)	23
FANCG	Cytochrome P450 2E1 (CYP2E1):	24
	↑ In *fancg(−/−)* cells; (↓) in corrected cells	
	↑ 8-OHdG in H_2O_2- or MMC-exposed *fancg(−/−)* cells	
FANCA, FANCC, and FANCG	Interactions with redox-related proteins	25–27

involvement of thioredoxin, which corrects MMC and DEB sensitivity in FA cells, and has lower-than-normal levels in FA fibroblasts.

An established line of evidence has related FA cell sensitivity to MMC, DEB, and other xenobiotics [cisplatin, 8-methoxypsoralen + UVA (PUVA), and hexavalent chromium], all characterized by redox-related toxicity mechanisms, including bioreductive biotransformation, redox coupling, glutathione metabolism, and induction of oxidative DNA damage.[42–44] This evidence arises from a number studies conducted on several organisms and cell systems, and stands against the opinion that MMC and other FA-related xenobiotics exert their toxicities as DNA "crosslinkers," which, in turn, are associated with the current opinion of FA as a DNA repair deficiency disorder.[26,45–48,52,53]

A series of studies utilizing an *ex vivo* approach to investigate the "fingerprints" of oxidative stress in white blood cells (WBC), plasma, and urine provided evidence that the abnormalities in redox pathways belong to FA's clinical phenotype and are not cell culture artifacts. Rumyantsev *et al.* first reported that freshly drawn WBC from FA patients produced excess ROS (detected by luminol-dependent chemiluminescence, LDCL).[56,57] This finding suggested the involvement of $HO^{\bullet}$ and $HO^{\bullet}$-like radicals in circulating WBC from FA patients. To a lesser extent, yet significantly above control values, WBC from FA heterozygotes (parents) also displayed excess ROS formation.[56,57]

These data have subsequently been confirmed and extended by Degan *et al.*, who provided evidence for a threefold association of ROS formation versus the accumulation of oxidative DNA damage (8-OHdG) in WBC, and versus spontaneous chromosomal instability.[55] A recent study has confirmed excess leukocyte levels of 8-OHdG, corresponding to excess 8-OHdG urinary levels.[74] This latter finding casts some doubts about the *in vivo* relevance of a deficiency in DNA repair, which would imply lower-than-normal excretion of damaged DNA bases.[74,75]

Clastogenic factor (*cf*) has also been detected in plasma from FA patients, siblings, and parents.[58] *Cf* is a product of plasma ultrafiltration, which increases the frequency of chromosomal breakages in cells from healthy donors.[9] The detection of *cf* in plasma from irradiated subjects, and from patients with other cancer-prone disorders, and the loss of clastogenic activity by SOD or low molecular weight free radical scavengers associates *cf* to a mixture of secondary radicals.[9,58]

Another indicator of ROS-related plasma component, TNF-α, has been found in FA patients in significantly increased levels versus control plasma.[59,71,72] Since TNF-α is a recognized effector of ROS release from phagocytes, its elevated levels can be associated with phagocyte activation.[31]

In a recent study a set of oxidative stress markers were evaluated in 56 FA patients and their parents.[74] Oxidative DNA damage (8-OHdG) in WBC and in urine was increased in FA patients, to a significantly higher extent in female than in male patients, and in patients aged $\leq$15 years, but not in patients aged 16 to 29 years. Female FA patients also displayed a highly significant excess in spontaneous chromosomal instability versus male patients. The same female:male ratio was detected both for 8-OHdG levels (WBC and urine) and for spontaneous chromosomal instability, thus suggesting that chromosomal breaks might be directly associated with oxidative DNA damage. Plasma levels of methylglyoxal, deriving from carbohydrate and amino acid oxidative degradation, were measured, showing a significant increase in untransplanted young FA patients ($\leq$15 years) and in parents, but neither in transplanted patients, nor in patients aged 16–29 years. A dramatic age-related difference was observed in glutathione, as young patients ($\leq$15 years) showed a significant increase in the GSSG:GSH ratio, unlike older patients, showing a decrease in the GSSG:GSH ratio versus controls of the respective age groups. No changes were observed in vitamin C, vitamin E, and uric acid plasma levels. The results suggested the occurrence of an *in vivo* prooxidant state in FA patients with gender and age distinctions, and with proficient excretion of oxidized DNA bases.[74]

Together, the available information points to the occurrence of a prooxidant state in FA. This body of evidence is compatible with the complex clinical phenotype of FA, including cancer proneness, bone marrow impairment, malformations, endocrinopathies, and abnormalities in skin pigmentation, as far as each of these clinical features may be caused by prooxidant states based on an extensive literature background.[4,19,20,28,30,76–85] Thus, it may be suggested that all these clinical endpoints may be ascribed, through different mechanisms, to a prooxidant state as a pervasive dysmetabolic condition, as depicted in Fig. 1.

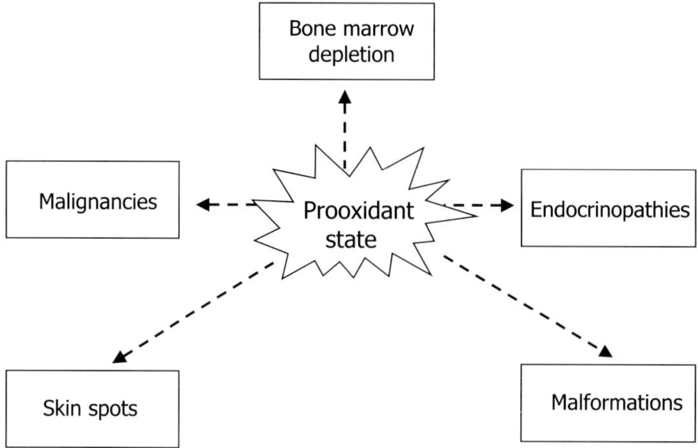

Fig. 1. Oxidative stress as a central event related to the occurrence of the clinical abnormalities observed in FA.

Further investigations on the role of oxidative stress in FA are warranted, as information obtained will be relevant not only to the pathogenesis of FA but also in a range of related disorders.

2.2. *Ataxia telangiectasia*

Ataxia telangiectasia (AT) is a rare autosomal recessive disorder characterized by cerebellar degeneration and neuromotor impairment, immunodeficiency, sterility, increased risk of cancer, and genomic instability.[86–91] No treatment exists and lifespan is about 20 years. Further clinical features are dilated blood vessels, growth retardation, and early aging.[92] Chromosomal instability is associated with a high sensitivity to ionizing radiation and radiomimetic chemicals.[89,90,93] The AT gene (ATM) is located to chromosome 11q22–23.[86,87] The ATM protein is a multifunctional protein kinase [phosphatidylinositol-3′ (PI-3) kinase], involved in the regulation of cellular responses to double-strand DNA breaks (DSB).[86,87] A set of evidence has demonstrated that ATM is involved also in other processes that maintain cellular homeostasis, with a direct involvement of oxidative stress in AT phenotype.[7,8,20,21,91,94–99]

A pioneering study by Shiloh *et al.*[90] reported an increased sensitivity of AT cells to DNA-damaging agents via free radical mechanisms. Some antioxidant enzymes, e.g., catalase,[94] were reported to display abnormal expression, and a defect in glutathione metabolism[95] was observed. An increased sensitivity of AT cells to TPA-activated neutrophils and to ROS generated by the xanthine/xanthine oxidase system was reported.[96]

Extensive studies of the ATM protein functions suggested abnormalities in redox pathways, as demonstrated by: (i) the hypersensitivity of AT cells to ROS inducers, (ii) premature cell aging, and (iii) degeneration of post-mitotic cells.[90,97–99] The agents causing AT cell hypersensitivity are ROS generators, including $O_2^{\bullet-}$, and H_2O_2. Moreover, a role for nitric oxide (NO) in the differential loss of Purkinje cells in AT has been suggested.[97]

A recent paper by Browne *et al.*[100] reported on the successful use in ATM-deficient mice of a synthetic catalytic antioxidant, the salen–manganese compound EUK-189, with both catalase and superoxide dismutase activities. EUK-189 is known to cross the blood–brain barrier and has been shown to be neuroprotective in animal models characterized by oxidative damage. Treatment with EUK-189 corrected the neurobehavioral deficit in ATM-deficient mice.[100]

Two recent studies conducted on cells from ATM-deficient mice showed that: (i) an antioxidant (isoindoline nitroxide) prevented Purkinje cell death in ATM-deficient mice and enhanced dendritogenesis to wild-type levels,[97] and (ii) desferrioxamine increases AT, but not normal cell resistance, to *t*-butyl hydroperoxide.[103] By analyzing the levels of some lipid peroxidation products and the oxidative DNA damage (8-OHdG) in plasma and WBC from patients with AT, Reichebach *et al.* reported a significant increase in oxidative damage to lipids and DNA.[101]

Together, the dataset obtained from studies of ATM functions, AT cells, ATM knock-out mice, and AT patients have provided evidence for a major role of a prooxidant state in AT, which is expected to contribute to the AT phenotype. Further clinical studies are warranted both in providing further information on the *in vivo* manifestations of oxidative stress and in prompting clinical studies aimed at mitigating the AT-associated oxidative stress and, possibly, disease progression.

2.3. *Xeroderma pigmentosum*

Xeroderma pigmentosum (XP) is an autosomal recessive disorder characterized by enhanced sensitivity to sunlight and very high incidence of skin tumors, and neurological symptoms.[103] XP is genetically heterogeneous and is classified into seven complementation groups (XPA–XPG) that correspond to genetic alterations in one of seven genes involved in defects in the nucleotide excision repair (NER) machinery.[104] Though the main deficiency in XP is recognized in repairing UV-induced DNA damage,[103,104] also abnormalities in redox pathways were reported to contribute to XP phenotype.[15,16,38,105–108]

A decreased catalase activity in fibroblasts XP patients was first reported by Vuillaume *et al.*,[15,16] who observed a number of defects in ROS-detoxifying activities. A catalase deficiency in XP was reported, since cell lines affected by a related disorder, tricothiodystrophy (TTD), have normal catalase activity,[38] suggesting that the difference in catalase expression between XP and TTD cells could be related to cancer proneness, which is exhibited by XP but not by TTD.[38] Oxidative damage was investigated in nuclear and mitochondrial DNA (mtDNA) in XP (group A) cells,[109] which display their defect in repairing oxidative lesions both in nuclear DNA and in mtDNA.[106,109]

Lachaise *et al.* reported on the relationship between catalase deficiency and the post-translational modification of transaldolase, which regulates NADPH levels and influences the catalase activity regulated in XP and SV40-transformed cells.[110] Transaldolase activity was found to be increased in XP and SV40-transformed fibroblasts, consistent with the lower-than-normal catalase expression.[110]

A study by Arbault *et al.* provided evidence for excess superoxide and hydrogen peroxide fibroblasts from XPA and XPD strains, whereas nitric oxide production was decreased XP cells versus normal fibroblasts.[109]

Some papers have reported on comparative data on the alterations of oxidative stress parameters in XP and other disorders (e.g., Cockayne syndrome), and showed minor, if any, oxidative stress-related changes in XP cells.[111,112] Unlike FA and AT, however, the information gathered so far on the involvement of oxidative stress in XP has been mostly investigated in fibroblast cultures, with the lack of data arising from *ex vivo* materials, e.g., freshly collected cells or biological fluids from XP patients. Unpublished data from a recent study (the EUROS Project, European Research on Oxidative Stress, #BMH4-CT98-3107) attempted to fill this gap, yet the limited number of recruited patients requires more extensive information on an *in vivo* increase in oxidative DNA damage and on other oxidative stress biomarkers.

It may be concluded that XP phenotype includes some features involved in a redox imbalance, firstly an abnormal catalase expression. However, further investigations are expected to clarify the *in vivo* relevance of a prooxidant state in the XP clinical phenotype.

2.4. *Bloom syndrome*

Bloom syndrome (BS) is a very rare autosomal recessive disorder, characterized by a sensitivity to sunlight with telangiectasia in face skin, severe growth retardation, immunodeficiency, and very high frequency of malignancies of several cell types and sites.[113] The cytogenetic analysis of BS cells shows excess breakages with quadriradials (from homologous chromosomes), and a marked increase in sister chromatid exchanges (SCE).[113] BS phenotype has been related to oxidative stress since the early report by Emerit and Cerutti,[5] who detected clastogenic activity in fibroblast cultures from BS patients; this activity could be removed by addition of SOD. Another major abnormality in ROS detoxification was observed in BS fibroblasts and lympholastoid cells, consisting of increased SOD and decreased catalase activities, which together result in excess H_2O_2 formation.[114] It is interesting to note that bromodeoxy-uridine, the reagent used to induce SCE, amplifies ROS-related DNA damage.[115]

The deficient gene in BS encodes the BLM protein, characterized as a gene product is a 3′–5′ DNA helicase, with a homology to the RecQ helicases.[116] Moreover, BLM protein possesses an ATPase activity that is strongly stimulated by either single- or double-stranded DNA. The role of BLM in DNA repair is a universally shared opinion, since its DNA helicase activity is assumed to play an exclusive role in maintaining DNA integrity.[120–123] Nevertheless, the concomitant ATPase activity of the BLM protein may also suggest its function in redox homeostasis, since a body of literature associates ATPase with oxidative stress.[119,120] A functional or physical interaction of BLM with the p53/p21 system was established in several studies.[121–123] In turn, p53 is related to the induction of redox-controlling genes, resulting in the production of ROS.[124–126] A recent paper reported on the p53-dependent upregulation of manganese superoxide dismutase (MnSOD) and glutathione peroxidase 1 (GPx).[126] An extensive analysis of altered mRNA profiles in human lung epithelial cells in response to hydrogen peroxide showed a pattern of transcriptional and/or post-transcriptional response to oxidative stress, which functionally related to activation of the p53/p21 pathway.[121] Another indirect link of BLM protein with a redox imbalance may be suggested by a recent report on the physical association of BLM with ATR [ataxia telangiectasia and rad3(+) related] protein since, in turn, ATR is activated by hyperoxia and relates to p53 induction.[127]

Lymphoblastoid cells from BS patients exhibited excess cytogenetic toxicity of redox-bioactivated quinones, MMC, and 4-nitroquinoline oxide (4NQO) in terms of micronuclei induction, thus suggesting an imbalance in redox-related detoxification pathways, in analogy with MMC sensitivity in FA cells.[115]

Together, the *in vitro* studies provide circumstantial evidence for a deficiency of redox pathways in BS cellular phenotype. However, the lack of information on the *in vivo* implications of any prooxidant state in BS requires *ad hoc* investigations aimed at evaluating any redox abnormalities in freshly drawn cells and biological fluids from suitable numbers of BS patients. Given the very low incidence of this disorder, these prospect studies appear a quite challenging task.

3. Progeroid Syndromes

Progeroid syndromes are a composite group of genetic diseases associated with early aging and, in several cases, with cancer proneness.[128] These have been classified into two categories: segmental progeroid syndromes, which involve multiple aspects of the senescent phenotype, and unimodal progeroid syndromes, in which predominantly one aspect of the phenotype is involved.[128] Two different examples of segmental progeroid syndromes will be discussed: the Werner syndrome (WS, an autosomal recessive disease) and the Down syndrome (trisomy 21).[129–132] Examples of unimodal progeroid syndromes included familial hypercholesterolemia (accelerated atherogenesis),[133] and XP (discussed in Sec. 2.3). To a different extent for each of these disorders, an involvement of a prooxidant state has been established or is, at least, strongly suggested by the available literature generally related to aging, cancer, and atherogenesis.[4,13,134,135]

3.1. *Down syndrome*

DS (trisomy 21) is by far the most frequent genetic disorder in humans, and is associated with a clinical phenotype including neurological and cognitive disturbances, immunodeficiency, early aging, and excess rate of malignancies (especially lymphocytic leukemia).[131,132] DS has long been investigated in respect of the phenotypic consequences of the triple gene dosages related to trisomy 21.[13,14,136–138] The presence of an extra copy of chromosome 21 involves a composite pattern of phenotypic abnormalities, related to the known DNA sequence of the genes residing in chromosome 21.[132,139,140]

The overexpression of Cu,ZnSOD (SOD1) in DS was first established in the 1970s[141] and has been subsequently investigated in a number of studies utilizing several approaches (*in vitro*, *ex vivo*, and animal models).[14,142–148] This literature has provided evidence for a major role of oxidative stress in DS clinical phenotype. Moreover, the over-expression of SOD1 [not of MnSOD (SOD2)][139] was reported to cause an increased ratio of SOD/(catalase + glutathione peroxidase),[149] although increased catalase and glutathione-related activities were reported in cells from DS patients.[13,136,141] Other studies reported under-expression of peroxiredoxin 2 in DS fetal brains.[140,146]

Direct evidence for increased oxidative stress in DS patients was provided by significant increases in oxidative DNA damage (urinary 8-OHdG) and in lipid peroxidation in DS patients.[147,150–154] Recent reports showed elevated levels of the isoprostane 8,12-iso-iPF2alpha-VI, a specific marker of lipid peroxidation in urine from subjects with DS compared with those of matched controls.[153] Excess plasma levels of uric acid and allantoin were reported in DS patients, accompanied by lower-than-normal levels of xanthine and hypoxanthine.[152,154]

A clinical study of dietary supplementation with alpha-lipoic acid and L-cysteine to DS patients showed a significant increase in thiol group levels and in total antioxidant status of serum versus basal values, while serum ROS levels were significantly decreased.[148]

Trisomy 16 in mice was established as an animal model for human trisomy 21, as the chromosome 16 in mice encodes SOD1, and the mice affected by trisomy 16 share many phenotypic resemblances with DS, with defects including abnormalities in cholinergic neurons, decreased cell proliferation in fetal brain, and T cell-dependent immunodeficiency.[141–143,145] Transgenic mice overexpressing human SOD1 undergo severe abnormalities in neuromuscular junctions as observed in aging mice and rats, and in DS patients.[14,145] Moreover, the SOD1 transgenic mice show altered macrophage functions,[155] and increased thymic and bone marrow apoptosis.[144]

Neuronal cells from human DS fetal brain undergo degeneration and apoptosis, unlike normal neurons which remain viable and proceed through differentiation.[137,156] The intracellular content of ROS in DS neurons is three- to fourfold elevated versus control cells, and lipid peroxidation is enhanced prior to apoptotic death. Neuronal degeneration can be prevented by treatment with catalase or low molecular weight scavengers.[137]

The information accumulated so far provides convincing evidence for the occurrence of a prooxidant state DS phenotype, unconfined to SOD1 overexpression. In summary, it can be inferred that enhanced $O_2^{\bullet -}$ dismutation leads to excess H_2O_2 levels and consequently to further radical reactions, e.g., including $HO^{\bullet}$ formation and lipid peroxidation. Further investigations are required to ascertain the composite dysmetabolic scenario associated with DS pathogenesis and to specific phenotypic features, as, e.g., leukemia and accelerated aging.

3.2. *Werner syndrome*

WS is a very rare autosomal recessive disorder, associated with premature aging with early symptoms in the second decade (adult progeria), propensity to increased cancer risk, high diabetes incidence, and a number of complications affecting various organs and systems (heart and vessels, eyes, and joints); it is characterized by genomic instability (translocation mosaicism and extensive deletions).[128,157–159] WS is caused by mutations in the WRN gene, encoding a 160 kDa protein (WRN), which has 3′–5′exonuclease, DNA helicase, and DNA-dependent ATPase activities.[158,159] The gene functionally interacts with a DNA polymerase, required for DNA replication and DNA repair, with the recognition that WS-associated genetic defect is related to the maintenance of DNA integrity.[160] The illness always presents a progressive, invalidating course, which cannot be prevented and is only relieved by palliative treatments.

A direct relationship of WRN with redox pathways may rely on its ATPase activity,[161,162] due to the extensive evidence associating ATPase with oxidative stress including, e.g., oxidative DNA damage, glutathione balance, and the induction of diabetes, a recognized oxidative stress-related condition.[76]

Some recent studies reported that WRN colocalizes with the ATR kinase after replication fork arrest, suggesting that WRN and ATR collaborate to prevent genome instability during the S phase.[163,164] In turn, the ATR-Chk1 pathway is activated by hyperoxia and phosphorylates p53, which relates to the induction of redox-controling genes resulting in the production of ROS,[127,165,166] thus suggesting multiple links of WRN functions with redox pathways.

Another line of evidence relates to the excess sensitivity of WS cells to a set of redox-active xenobiotics, including bleomycin, 4-nitroquinoline-*N*-oxide (4NQ), camptothecin (CPT), 8-methoxypsoralen (MOP), and mitomycin C (MMC).[167–171] Their toxicity mechanisms, though different, relate to oxidative stress,[42–44,172,173] providing hints for a deficiency in WS cells in coping with an endogenous prooxidant state in WS. An involvement of oxidative stress in WS cells was suggested by Kashino *et al.*,[18] who reported increased lifespan and a reduced rate of telomere shortening in WS cells exposed to ascorbic acid.

No studies were reported by evaluating the effects of an extensive set of low molecular weight antioxidants in WS cells, nor of antioxidant enzymes, with the exception of an early study by Nordenson.[174] Also, no published data are available evaluating any *in vivo* prooxidant state in body fluids or blood cells from WS patients. Recent data from the EUROS Project suggest the occurrence of an *in vivo* prooxidant state in three WS patients, to be verified on a more extensive number of patients.[175] The results showed exceedingly high levels of leukocyte 8-OHdG, GSSG: GSH ratio, and of plasma levels of glyoxal, methylglyoxal, uric acid and ascorbic acid.[175] Together, the analytical data from this study, and a review of the literature on WRN functions support the view that WS clinical phenotype should be compatible with an *in vivo* prooxidant state.[176]

4. Hereditary Cancer Syndromes

Hereditary cancer syndromes have been investigated in recent years by genetic analysis, and involve predisposition to tumors of the colon, breast, ovary, endometrium, thyroid, and other endocrine glands.[177] These hereditary cancer susceptibility syndromes include, among many others, hereditary non-polyposis colorectal cancer (HNPCC), familial adenomatous polyposis (FAP), hereditary breast and ovarian cancer (HBOC), and multiple endocrine neoplasia type 2 (MEN 2).[177–182]

Most of hereditary cancer syndromes have their origin in inherited mutations in tumor suppressor genes. Two specific tumor suppressor genes, *BRCA1* and *BRCA2*, have been associated to breast cancer and ovarian cancer, accounting for approximately 7–10% of cases, and to other malignanincies, e.g., pancreatic and prostatic cancer.[182–185]

Approximately 1–5% of colorectal cancer is attributable to mutations in five tumor suppressor genes (HNPCC and FAP). Mutations in the RET oncogene are involved in the MEN 2 hereditary cancer syndrome, and are responsible for approximately 20% of thyroid medullary carcinomas. The RET oncogene represents an exception as an oncogene, rather than a tumor suppressor gene, is involved in an autosomal dominant inherited cancer syndrome.[180]

The hereditary cancer syndromes are mostly related with susceptibility to multi-organ cancer, though usually limited to specific organs. For example, HNPCC is associated with excess risk of endometrial cancer, and stomach, biliary tract, urinary tract, and ovary cancers.[174,181] Mutations in *BRCA1* and *BRCA2*, also involved in FA, both increase the risk of breast and of ovarian cancer that are observed with excess prevalence in FA heterozygotes.[184,185] Wild-type BRCA1 and BRCA2 proteins can correct MMC hypersensitivity in FA cells;[48,186] in turn, this finding might suggest a possible involvement of BRCA2 in redox pathways due to the redox-related toxicity mechanisms of MMC. The monoubiquitination of FANCD2 occurs during the S phase of the cell cycle, and colocalization with BRCA1 and RAD51 in S-phase-specific nuclear foci occurs following exposure to MMC.[48,186] The FANCD2/BRCA1 and FANCD2/RAD51 complexes were suggested to participate in DNA repair by homologous recombination.[187] Not surprisingly, the interactions of BRCA2/FANCD1 with FANCG, and the direct involvement of FANCG in redox pathways are consistent with the finding that both BRCA1 and BRCA2 are also involved in the repair of oxidative DNA damage.[188] Thus, BRCA1 and BRCA2 may both be involved in DNA repair and in cell protection against oxidative damage.[67]

Implications of redox pathways in hereditary cancer syndromes have been reported for colon carcinogenesis, both involving HNPCC and FAP.[189–193] A series of studies by Bartsch and coworkers provided evidence for an association of colorectal cancer and FAP with oxidative stress endpoints including oxidative DNA damage and lipid peroxidation, measured by etheno (ε)–DNA adducts deriving from trans-4-hydroxy-2-nonenal, generated as the major aldehyde by lipid peroxidation (LPO) of omega-6 PUFAs.[191,192] A further aspect of the involvement of oxidative stress in colon carcinogenesis and in FAP was shown by Schmid *et al.* to be related to the role(s) of cyclooxygenases (COX).[191] Reactive intermediates formed during the arachidonic acid cascade, notably by COX-2, which is upregulated in polyps of FAP patients, may promote various stages from polyp toward adenoma and carcinoma sequence. Etheno–DNA adducts can be derived from reactive intermediates generated during arachidonic acid metabolism and lipid peroxidation.[191] Bras *et al.* reported on the occurrence of a prooxidant state in FAP patients, measured by excess levels of thiobarbituric acid reactive products and by lower-than-normal levels of ascorbic acid and tocopherol, suggesting an imbalance in the prooxidant/antioxidant status in FAP patients,[193] which may contribute toward innovative prevention and therapy in FAP patients.

5. Conclusions and Outlook in Future Research

The state-of-the-art supports the view that some selected cancer-prone genetic disorders and some cancer genetic diseases provide a mechanistic interplay between the molecular and clinical features relating these diseases, and specific imbalances in redox pathways. Far from being a matter of academic curiosity, the recognition that some diseases are associated with a cellular and/or organismal prooxidant state may imply both a theoretical reappraisal and practical consequences in the clinical management of a given disorder.

The major alternative interpretation for the phenotype of most of the diseases dicussed herein relies on deficiencies in the maintainance of DNA stability and/or in DNA repair pathways. The real *in vivo* relevance of DNA repair deficiency may be viewed as a controversial issue. In the case of FA, the sensitivity to "crosslinkers" of FA cells has been associated with the established view of a deficiency in DNA repair, yet this opinion both conceals the redox toxicity mechanisms of the FA-associated xenobiotics, and disregards the extensive body of evidence relating FA phenotype with oxidative stress. By leaving apart the subject of the respective contributions of the deficiencies in DNA repair and/or redox pathways in the disorders discussed here, it may be worth addressing future efforts in clinical research trying to compensate the prooxidant state observed in each of these disorders.

A major question should be addressed in the design of clinical trials based on the use of pharmaceutical and/or nutraceutical devices to compensate or mitigate the prooxidant state observed in a given disorder and, hence, the clinical phenotype and disease progression, i.e., whether, and to what extent, an adjustment of the biochemical imbalance seen in terms of a prooxidant state may be effective in counteracting, or delaying, the progression of clinical symptoms and the onset of life-threatening complications (e.g., malignancies). Some obliged steps toward the implementation of these clinical trials reside in adequate information on the *in vivo* manifestations of a prooxidant state for a given disorder. This should be achieved by means of a combined set of surrogate biomarkers of oxidative stress, encompassing several oxidative stress-related events [oxidative DNA damage, oxidative alterations of other molecules (carbohydrates, proteins, lipids), key antioxidant systems (low molecular weight, enzymes, glutathione, thioredoxin)]. This complex information is expected to arise from measurements of oxidative stress parameters in freshly drawn body fluids and blood cells, whereas only accessory information might be obtained from cultured cells, especially from immortalized cells that may provide misleading information versus the "real," *in vivo* biochemical asset. Due to the necessary complexity of the dataset to be obtained, and due to the logistic difficulties arising from patient recruitment (especially for rare and very rare diseases), one may foresee a quite long course before adequate information becomes available.

Another aspect to be highlighted in the prospect of conducting clinical trials based on the use of "antioxidants" in chemoprevention or therapy of oxidative stress-related disorders relies on monitoring any changes occurring in the redox endpoints that are targeted for being ameliorated. Thus, for any given disease to be investigated in these clinical studies, a selection of endpoints should be evaluated along with treatment, thus providing stepwise information on the benefits, if any, in terms of correcting the endpoint(s) to be evaluated. This strategy may be regarded as a potentially informative approach, compared to previous proposals of utilizing "antioxidants" based on their claimed safety, and expecting that the treatment would result in a detectable improvement of the patient's clinical conditions. On the other hand, a reliable evaluation of the clinical course requires suitably extensive recruitment groups, and long-term observation; hence, the only chance of providing predictive information relies on the interim observation of the compensation, if any, of the redox parameters to be monitored. Based on the experience achieved to date, apparently unrelated factors should be taken into account when designing studies and monitoring the analytical endpoints, i.e., dietary habits, and other factors involved in affecting the *in vivo* redox balance (e.g., sex hormone secretion).[194–197]

A last, yet most relevant aspect relates to the ethical issues involved in decision-making about the prerequisites for undertaking studies of the possible benefits of compensating a redox imbalance with the goal of ameliorating the clinical course of disease. Provided that either a medical or a rehabilition device is available, as in the cases of FA (hematopoietic stem cell transplantation) or DS (psychosocial management), more thorough caveats may be raised to start an experimental protocol, before an adequate dataset is available on the specific redox imbalances. In the opposite condition, patients affected by AT, BS, or WS are currently lacking any cure, and their prognosis is invariably fatal. Moreover, obtaining a suitable dataset from *ex vivo* materials from these patients may be faced with insurmountable obstacles, either due to the major anatomical location of redox imbalance (cerebellum in AT), or due to the extreme rarity of the disease (BS and WS). In such cases, bioethicists and decision makers might be encouraged to undertake clinical trials in human patients based on some recent animal studies carried out in ATM knockout mice by using different classes of antioxidant chemicals,[100,198,199] with promising results that might prove beneficial in AT patients.

In conclusion, an involvement of oxidative stress in several cancer-prone disorders has become well established in a consistent body of evidence encompassing *in vitro*, animal, and *in vivo* studies. Further information is required on the disease-specific prooxidant states occurring in patients' organisms, and this approach requires huge organizational efforts and suitable resources. Nevertheless, this approach may be regarded as a *sine qua non* for undertaking controlled clinical trials.

6. Note Added in Proof

Unlike the other FA complementation groups, associated with an autosomal inheritance, FA complementation group B was reported by Meetei *et al.* to display X-linked inheritance.[200] Zhang *et al.* have reported recently that bone marrow progenitor cells from *fancc*(−/−) mice show enhanced sensitivity to hypoxia-reoxygenation, a recognized source of oxidative stress, in terms of apoptotic response, thus providing evidence for a redox deficiency in an FA mouse model.[201]

References

1. Cerutti P. *Science* 227: 375–381 (1985).
2. Gille JJ, Wortelboer HM, Joenje H. *Hum. Genet.* 77: 28–31 (1987).
3. Fraga CG, Shigenaga MK, Park J-W, Degan P, Ames BN. *Proc. Natl. Acad. Sci. USA* 87: 4533–4537 (1990).
4. Floyd RA. *Carcinogenesis* 9: 1447–1450 (1990).
5. Emerit I. *Free Radic. Biol. Med.* 16: 99–109 (1994).
6. Duker NJ. *Am. J. Med. Genet.* 115: 125–129 (2002).
7. Barzilai A, Rotman G, Shiloh Y. *DNA Repair (Amst.)* 1: 3–25 (2002).
8. Barlow C, Dennery PA, Shigenaga MK, Smith MA, Morrow JD, Roberts LJ II, Wynshaw-Boris A, Levine RL. *Proc. Natl. Acad. Sci. USA* 96: 9915–9919 (1999).
9. Emerit I, Cerutti P. *Proc. Natl. Acad. Sci. USA* 78: 1868–1872 (1981).
10. Poot M, Hoehn H, Nicotera TM, Rüdiger HW. *Free Radic. Res. Commun.* 7: 179–187 (1989).
11. Nordenson I. *Hereditas* 86: 147–150 (1977).
12. Joenje H, Arwert F, Eriksson AW, de Koning H, Oostra AB. *Nature* 290: 142–143 (1981).

13. Kedziora J, Bartosz G. *Free Radic. Biol. Med.* 4: 317–330 (1988).
14. Groner Y, Elroy-Stein O, Avraham KB, Schickler M, Knobler H, Minc-Golombo D, Bar-Peled O, Yarom R, Rotshenker S. *Biomed. Pharmacother.* 48: 231–240 (1994).
15. Vuillaume M, Decroix Y, Calvayrac R, Vallot R, Best-Belpomme M. *C. R. Seances Acad. Sci. III* 296: 845–850 (1983).
16. Vuillaume M, Calvayrac R, Best-Belpomme M, Tarroux P, Hubert M, Decroix Y, Sarasin A. *Cancer Res.* 46: 538–544 (1986).
17. Tuo J, Jaruga P, Rodriguez H, Bohr VA, Dizdaroglu M. *FASEB J.* 17: 668–674 (2003).
18. Kashino G, Kodama S, Nakayama Y, Suzuki K, Fukase K, Goto M, Watanabe M. *Free Radic. Biol. Med.* 35: 438–443 (2003).
19. Frenkel K. *Environ. Health Perspect.* 81: 45–54 (1989).
20. Pagano G, Korkina LG, Brunk UT, Chessa L, Degan P, Del Principe D, Kelly FJ, Malorni W, Pallardó F, Pasquier F, Scovassi I, Zatterale IA, Franceschi C. *Med. Hypotheses* 51: 253–266 (1998).
21. Takao N, Li Y, Yamamoto K. *FEBS Lett.* 472: 133–136 (2000).
22. Kruyt FA, Hoshino T, Liu JM, Joseph P, Jaiswal AK, Youssoufian H. *Blood* 92: 3050–3056 (1998).
23. Cumming RC, Lightfoot J, Beard K, Youssoufian H, O'Brien PJ, Buchwald M. *Nat. Med.* 7: 814–820 (2001).
24. Futaki M, Igarashi T, Watanabe S, Kajigaya S, Tatsuguchi A, Wang J, Liu JM. *Carcinogenesis* 23: 67–72 (2002).
25. Reuter TY, Medhurst AL, Waisfisz Q, Zhi Y, Herterich S, Hoehn H, Gross HJ, Joenje H, Hoatlin ME, Mathew CG, Huber PA. *Exp. Cell Res.* 289: 211–221 (2003).
26. Zanier R, Briot D, Villard JA, Sarasin A, Rosselli F. *Oncogene* 23: 5004–5013 (2004).
27. Park SJ, Ciccone SL, Beck BD, Hwang B, Freie B, Clapp DW, Lee SH. *J. Biol. Chem.* 279: 30053–30059 (2004).
28. Ames BN. *Free Radic. Res. Commun.* 7: 121–128 (1989).
29. Heim S, Johansson B, Mertens F. *Mutat. Res.* 221: 39–51 (1989).
30. Vuillaume M. *Mutat. Res.* 186: 43–72 (1987).
31. Hebbel RP, Miller WJ. *Am. J. Hematol.* 29: 222–225 (1988).
32. Wiseman H, Halliwell B. *Biochem. J.* 313: 17–29 (1996).
33. Taylor AM. *Best Pract. Res. Clin. Haematol.* 14: 631–644 (2001).
34. Carney JP. *Curr. Opin. Immunol.* 11: 443–447 (1999).
35. Vessey JC, Norbury CJ, Hickson ID. *Prog. Nucleic Acid Res. Mol. Biol.* 63: 189–221 (1999).

36. Rapin I, Lindenbaum Y, Dickson DW, Kraemer KH, Robbins JH. *Neurology* 55: 1442–1449 (2000).
37. Itin HP, Sarasin A, Pittelkow MR. *J. Am. Acad. Dermatol.* 44: 891–920 (2001).
38. Vuillaume M, Daya-Grosjean L, Vicens P, Pennetier JL, Tarroux P, Baret A, Calvayrac R, Taieb A, Sarasin A. *Carcinogenesis* 13: 321–328 (1992).
39. Futaki M, Liu JM. *Trends Mol. Med.* 7: 560–565 (2001).
40. Cohen MM, Simpson SJ, Pazos L, *Cancer Res.* 41: 1817–1823 (1981).
41. Clarke AA, Philpott NJ, Gordon-Smith EC, Rutherford TR. *Br. J. Haematol.* 96: 240–247 (1997).
42. Dusre L, Rajagopalan S, Eliot HM, Covey JM, Sinha BK. *Cancer Res.* 50: 648–652 (1990).
43. Pritsos CA, Sartorelli AC. *Cancer Res.* 46: 3528–3532 (1986).
44. Pagano G, Manini P, Bagchi D. *Environ. Health Perspect.* 111: 1699–1703 (2003).
45. Auerbach AD, Buchwald M, Joenje H. In: Vogelstein B, Kinzier KW (eds.) *The Genetic Basis of Human Cancer*. McGraw-Hill, New York, 1998, pp. 317–322.
46. Alter BP. *Am. J. Hematol.* 53: 99–110 (1996).
47. Taniguchi T, D'Andrea AD. *Int. J. Hematol.* 75: 123–128 (2002).
48. Howlett NG, Taniguchi T, Olson S, Cox B, Waisfisz Q, De Die-Smulders C, Persky N, Grompe M, Joenje H, Pals G, Ikeda H, Fox EA, D'Andrea AD. *Science* 297: 606–609 (2002).
49. Wajnrajch MP, Gertner JM, Huma Z, Popovic J, Lin K, Verlander PC, Dev Batish S, Giampietro PF, Davis JG, New MI, Auerbach AD. *Pediatrics* 107: 744–754 (2001).
50. Morrell D, Chase CL, Kupper LL, Swift M. *Diabetes* 35: 143–147 (1986).
51. Ahmad SL, Hanaoka F, Kirk SH. *BioEssays* 24: 439–448 (2002).
52. Meetei AR, de Winter JP, Medhurst AL, Wallisch M, Waisfisz Q, van de Vrugt HJ, Oostra AB, Yan Z, Ling C, Bishop CE, Hoatlin ME, Joenje H, Wang W. *Nat. Genet.* 35: 165–170 (2003).
53. Levitus M, Rooimans MA, Steltenpool J, Cool NFC, Oostra AB, Mathew CG, Hoatlin ME, Waisfisz Q, Arwert F, De Winter JP, Joenje H. *Blood* 103: 2498–2503 (2004).
54. Takeuchi T, Morimoto K. *Carcinogenesis* 14: 1115–1120 (1993).
55. Degan P, Bonassi S, De Caterina M, Korkina LG, Pinto L, Scopacasa F, Zatterale A, Calzone R, Pagano G. *Carcinogenesis* 16: 735–742 (1995).

56. Rumyantsev AG, Samochatova EV, Afanas'ev IB, Korkina LG, Suslova TB, Cheremisina ZP, Maschan AA, Durnev AD, Lurye BL. *Ter. Arkh.* 61: 32–36 (1989).
57. Korkina LG, Samochatova EV, Maschan AA, Suslova TB, Cheremisina ZP, Afanas'ev IB. *J. Leukoc. Biol.* 52: 357–362 (1992).
58. Emerit L, Levy A, Pagano G, Pinto L, Calzone R, Zatterale A. *Hum. Genet.* 96: 14–20 (1995).
59. Schulz JC, Shahidi NT. *Am. J. Hematol.* 42: 196–201 (1993).
60. Kontou M, Adelfalk C, Ramirez MH, Ruppitsch W, Hirsch-Kauffmann M, Schweiger M. *Oncogene* 21: 2406–2412 (2002).
61. Nagasawa H, Little JB. *Carcinogenesis* 4: 795–798 (1983).
62. Hoehn H, Kubbies M, Poot M, Rabinovitch PS, In: Schroeder-Kurt TM, Auerbach AD, Obe G (eds.) *Fanconi Anemia: Clinical, Cytogenetic and Experimental Aspects.* Springer-Verlag, Berlin, 1989, pp. 161–173.
63. Dallapiccola B, Porfirio B, Mokini V, Alimena G, Isacchi G, Gandini E. *Hum. Genet.* 69: 62–65 (1985).
64. Poot M, Gross O, Epe B, Pflaum M, Hoehn H. *Exp. Cell Res.* 222: 262–268 (1996).
65. Ruppitsch W, Meisslitzer C, Hirsch-Kauffmann M, Schweiger M. *FEBS Lett.* 422: 99–102 (1998).
66. Pagano G, Youssoufian H. *BioEssays* 25: 589–595 (2003).
67. Pagano G, Degan P, d'Ischia M, Kelly FJ, Nobili B, Pallardó FV, Zatterale A. *Eur. J. Haematol.* 75: 93–100 (2005).
68. Saadatzadeh MR, Bijangi-Vishehsaraei K, Hong P, Bergmann H, Haneline LS. *J. Biol. Chem.* 279: 16805–16812 (2004).
69. Joenje H, Oostra AB. *Cancer Genet. Cytogenet.* 22: 339–345 (1986).
70. Madle S. *Mutat. Res.* 85: 347–356 (1981).
71. Dufour C, Corcione A, Svahn J, Haupt R, Poggi V, Nandor Bekassy A, Scime R, Pistorio A, Pistoia V. *Blood* 102: 2053–2059 (2003).
72. Pearl-Yafe M, Halperin D, Halevy A, Kalir H, Bielorai B, Fabian I. *Biochem. Pharmacol.* 65: 833–842 (2003).
73. Hadjur S, Jirik FR. *Blood* 101: 3877–3884 (2003).
74. Pagano G, Degan P, d'Ischia M, Kelly FJ, Pallardó FV, Zatterale A, Anak SS, Akişık EE, Beneduce G, Calzone R, De Nicola E, Dunster C, Lloret A, Manini P, Nobili B, Saviano A, Vuttariello E, Warnau M. *Carcinogenesis* 25: 1899–1909 (2004).
75. Loft S, Fischer-Nielsen S, Jeding IB, Vistisen K, Poulsen HE. *J. Toxicol. Environ. Health* 40: 391–404 (1993).
76. Vlassara H, Palace MR. *J. Intern. Med.* 251: 87–101 (2002).

77. Wells-Knecht KJ, Zyzak DV, Lichtfield JE, Thorpe SR, Baynes JW. *Biochemistry* 34: 3702–3709 (1995).
78. Smith MT. *Eur. J. Haematol. Suppl.* 60: 107–110 (1996).
79. Sheader EA, Benson RS, Best L. *Biochem. Pharmacol.* 61: 1381–1386 (2001).
80. Gredilla R, Barja G, Lopez-Torres M. *Free Radic. Res.* 35: 417–425 (2001).
81. Evans LM, Davies JS, Anderson RA, Ellis GR, Jackson SK, Lewis MJ, Frenneaux MP, Rees A, Scanlon MF. *Eur. J. Endocrinol.* 142: 254–262 (2000).
82. Prota G. *Melanins and Melanogenesis*. Academic Press, New York, 1992.
83. Memoli S, Napolitano A, d'Ischia M, Misuraca G, Palumbo A, Prota G. *Biochim. Biophys. Acta* 1346: 61–68 (1997).
84. Wells PG, Kim PM, Laposa RR, Nicol CJ, Parman T, Winn LM. *Mutat. Res.* 396: 65–78 (1997).
85. Hansen JM, Harris KK, Philbert MA, Harris C, *J. Pharmacol. Exp. Ther.* 300: 768–776 (2002).
86. Gatti RA, Berkel F, Boder E, Braedt G, Charmley P, Concannon P, Ersoy F, Fouroud T, Jaspers NGJ, Lange K, Lathrop GM, Leppert M, Nakamura Y, O'Connel P, Paterson M, Salser W, Sanal O, Silver J, Sparkes RS, Susi E, Weeks DE, Wei S, White R, Yoder F. *Nature* 336: 577–580 (1988).
87. Savitsky K, Bar-Shira A, Gilad S, Rotman G, Ziv Y, Vanagaite L, Tagle DA, Smith S, Uziel T, Sfez S, Ashkenazi M, Pecker I, Frydman M, Harnik R, Patanjali SR, Simmons A, Clines GA, Sartiel A, Gatti RA, Chessa L, Sanal O, Lavin MF, Jaspers NGJ, Taylor MR, Arlett CF, Miki T, Weissman SM, Lovett M, Collins FS, Shiloh YA. *Science* 268: 1749–1753 (1995).
88. Shackelford RE, Innes CL, Sieber SO, Heinloth AN, Leadon SA, Paules RS. *J. Biol. Chem.* 276: 21951–21959 (2001).
89. Shiloh Y, Parshad R, Frydman M, Sanford KK, Portnoi S, Ziv Y, Jones G. *Hum. Genet.* 84: 15–18 (1985).
90. Shiloh Y, Tabor E, Becker Y. *Carcinogenesis* 4: 1317–1322 (1983).
91. Watters DJ. *Redox Rep.* 8: 23–29 (2003).
92. Spacey SD, Gatti RA, Bebb G. *Can. J. Neurol. Sci.* 27: 184–191 (2000).
93. Bates PR, Lavin MF. *Mutat. Res.* 218: 165–170 (1989).
94. Sheridan RB III, Huang PC. *Mutat. Res.* 61: 381–386 (1979).
95. Meredith MJ, Dodson JL. *Cancer Res.* 47: 4576–4581 (1987).
96. Yi M, Rosin MP, Anderson CK. *Cancer Lett.* 54: 43–50 (1990).
97. Chen P, Peng C, Luff J, Spring K, Watters D, Bottle S, Furuya S, Lavin MF. *J. Neurosci.* 23: 11453–11460 (2003).
98. Kamsler A, Daily D, Hochman A, Stern N, Shiloh Y, Rotman G, Barzilai A. *Cancer Res.* 61: 1849–1854 (2001).

99. Ward AJ, Olive PL, Burr AH, Rosin MP. *Environ. Mol. Mutagen.* 24: 103–111 (1994).
100. Browne SE, Roberts LJ II, Dennery PA, Doctrow SR, Beal MF, Barlow C, Levine RL. *Free Radic. Biol. Med.* 36: 938–942 (2004).
101. Shackelford RE, Manuszak RP, Johnson CD, Hellrung DJ, Steele TA, Link CJ, Wang S. *DNA Repair* (*Amst.*) 2: 971–981 (2003).
102. Reichenbach J, Schubert R, Schindler D, Muller K, Bohles H, Zielen S. *Antioxid. Redox Signal.* 4: 465–469 (2002).
103. Nishigori C, Hattori Y, Toyokuni S. Role of reactive oxygen species in skin carcinogenesis. *Antioxid. Redox Signal* 6: 561–570 (2004).
104. Gratchev A, Strein P, Utikal J, Sergij G. *Exp. Dermatol.* 12: 529–536 (2003).
105. Crawford D, Zbinden I, Monet R, Cerutti P. *Cancer Res.* 48: 2132–2134 (1988).
106. Brooks PJ, Wise DS, Berry DA, Kosmoski JV, Smerdon MJ, Somers RL, Mackie H, Spoonde AY, Ackerman EJ, Coleman K, Tarone RE, Robbins JH. *J. Biol. Chem.* 275: 22355–22362 (2000).
107. Driggers WJ, Grishko VI, LeDoux SP, Wilson GL. *Cancer Res.* 56: 1262–1266 (1996).
108. Hoffschir F, Daya-Grosjean L, Petit PX, Nocentini S, Dutrillaux B, Sarasin A, Vuillaume M. *Free Radic. Biol. Med.* 24: 809–816 (1998).
109. Arbault S, Sojic N, Bruce D, Amatore C, Sarasin A, Vuillaume M. *Carcinogenesis* 25: 509–515 (2004).
110. Lachaise F, Martin G, Drougard C, Perl A, Vuillaume M, Wegnez M, Sarasin A, Daya-Grosjean L. *Free Radic. Biol. Med.* 30: 1365–1373 (2001).
111. Balajee AS, Dianova I, Bohr VA. *Nucleic Acids Res.* 27: 4476–4482 (1999).
112. Runger TM, Epe B, Moller K. *Rec. Res. Cancer Res.* 139: 31–42 (1995).
113. German J, Bloom D, Passarge E. *Clin. Genet.* 15: 361–367 (1979).
114. Nicotera TM, Notaro J, Notaro S, Schumer J, Sandberg AA. *Cancer Res.* 49: 5239–5243 (1989).
115. Poot M, Hoehn H, Nicotera TM, Rüdiger HW. *Free Radic. Res. Commun.* 7: 179–187 (1989).
116. Karow JK, Chakraverty RK, Hickson ID. *J. Biol. Chem.* 272: 30611 (1997).
117. Ababou M, Dutertre S, Lecluse Y, Onclercq R, Chatton B, Amor-Gueret M. *Oncogene* 19: 5955–5963 (2000).
118. van Brabant AJ, Stan R, Ellis NA. *Annu. Rev. Genomics Hum. Genet.* 1: 409–459 (2000).
119. Yang S, Zhu H, Li Y, Lin H, Gabrielson K, Trush MA, Diehl AM. *Arch. Biochem. Biophys.* 378: 259–268 (2000).
120. Duchen MR. *Cell Calcium* 28: 339–348 (2000).

121. Collister M, Lane DP, Kuehl BL. *Carcinogenesis* 19: 2115–2120 (1998).
122. Davalos AR, Campisi J. *J. Cell Biol.* 162: 1197–1209 (2003).
123. Garkavtsev IV, Kley N, Grigorian IA, Gudkov AV. *Oncogene* 20: 8276–8280 (2001).
124. Wang XW, Tseng A, Ellis NA, Spillare EA, Linke SP, Robles AI, Seker H, Yang Q, Hu P, Beresten S, Bemmels NA, Garfield S, Harris CC. *J. Biol. Chem.* 276: 32948–32955 (2001).
125. Liu G, Chen X. *Oncogene* 21: 7195–7204 (2002).
126. Hussain SP, Amstad P, He P, Robles A, Lupold S, Kaneko I, Ichimiya M, Sengupta S, Mechanic L, Okamura S, Hofseth LJ, Moake M, Nagashima M, Forrester KS, Harris CC. *Cancer Res.* 64: 2350–2356 (2004).
127. Das KC, Dashnamoorthy R. *Am. J. Physiol. Lung Cell Mol. Physiol.* 286: L87–97 (2004).
128. Martin GM. *Natl. Cancer Inst. Monogr.* 60: 241–247 (1982).
129. Oshima J. *Bioessays* 22: 894–901 (2000).
130. Shen JC, Loeb LA. *Trends Genet.* 16: 213–220 (2000).
131. Hayes A, Batshaw ML. *Pediatr. Clin. North Am.* 40: 523–535 (1993).
132. Capone GT. *J. Dev. Behav. Pediatr.* 22: 40–59 (2001).
133. Naoumova RP, Thompson GR, Soutar AK. *Curr. Opin. Lipidol.* 15: 413–422 (2004).
134. Nourooz-Zadeh J, Smith CC, Betteridge DJ. *Atherosclerosis* 156: 435–441 (2001).
135. de Nigris F, Lerman A, Ignarro LJ, Williams-Ignarro S, Sica V, Baker AH, Lerman LO, Geng YJ, Napoli C. *Trends Mol. Med.* 9: 351–359 (2003).
136. Brooksbank BW, Balasz R. *Exp. Brain Res.* 16: 37–44 (1984).
137. Busciglio J, Yankner BA. *Nature* 378: 776–779 (1995).
138. de Haan JB, Susil B, Pritchard M, Kola I. *J. Neural. Transm. Suppl.* 67: 67–83 (2003).
139. Gulesserian T, Seidl R, Hardmeier R, Cairns N, Lubec G. *J. Investig. Med.* 49: 41–46 (2001).
140. Sanchez-Font MF, Sebastia J, Sanfeliu C, Cristofol R, Marfany G, Gonzalez-Duarte R. *Cell Mol. Life Sci.* 60: 1513–1523 (2003).
141. Sinet PM, Allard D, Lejeune J, Jerome H. *C. R. Acad. Sci. D* 278: 3267–3270 (1974).
142. Epstein CJ, Cox DR, Epstein LB. *Ann. N.Y. Acad. Sci.* 450: 157–168 (1985).
143. Epstein CJ, Avraham KB, Lovett M, Smith S, Elroy-Stein O, Rotman G, Bry C, Groner Y. *Proc. Natl. Acad. Sci. USA* 84: 8044–8048 (1987).
144. Peled-Kamar M, Lotem J, Okon E, Sachs L, Groner Y. *EMBO J.* 14: 4985–4993 (1995).

145. Reaume AG, Elliott JL, Hoffman EK, Kowall NW, Ferrante RJ, Siwek DF, Wilcox HM, Flood DG, Beal MF, Brown RH Jr., Scott RW, Snider WD. *Nat. Genet.* 13: 43–47 (1996).
146. Kim SH, Fountoulakis M, Cairns N, Lubec G. *J. Neural. Transm. Suppl.* 61: 223–235 (2001).
147. Jovanovic SV, Clements D, MacLeod K. *Free Radic. Biol. Med.* 25: 1044–1048 (1998).
148. Gualandri W, Gualandri L, Demartini G, Esposti R, Marthyn P, Volonte S, Stangoni L, Borgonovo M, Fraschini F. *Int. J. Clin. Pharmacol. Res.* 23: 23–30 (2003).
149. Muchová J, Šustrová M, Garaiová I, Liptáková A, Blažiček P, Kvasnička P, Pueschel S, Duračková Z. *Free Radic. Biol. Med.* 31: 499–508 (2001).
150. Gulesserian T, Engidawork E, Fountoulakis M, Lubec G. *J. Neural. Transm. Suppl.* 61: 71–84 (2001).
151. Balcz B, Kirchner L, Cairns N, Fountoulakis M, Lubec G. *J. Neural Transm. Suppl.* 61: 193–201 (2001).
152. Nagyova A, Sustrova M, Raslova K. *Physiol. Res.* 49: 227–231 (2000).
153. Pratico D, Iuliano L, Amerio G, Tang LX, Rokach J, Sabatino G, Violi F. *Ann. Neurol.* 48: 795–798 (2000).
154. Žitňanová I, Korytar P, Aruoma OI, Sustrová M, Garaiová I, Muchová J, Kalnovičová T, Pueschel S, Ďuracková Z. *Clin. Chim. Acta* 341: 139–146 (2004).
155. Mirochnitchenko O, Inouye M. *J. Immunol.* 156: 1578–1586 (1996).
156. Ratan RR, Baraban JM. *Clin. Exp. Pharmacol. Physiol.* 22: 309–310 (1995).
157. Chen L, Oshima J. *J. Biomed. Biotechnol.* 2: 46–54 (2002).
158. Bohr VA, Cooper M, Orren D, Machwe A, Piotrowski J, Sommers J, Karmakar P, Brosh R. *Exp. Gerontol.* 35: 695–702 (2000).
159. von Kobbe C, Karmakar P, Dawut L, Opresko P, Zeng X, Brosh RM Jr., Hickson ID, Bohr VA, *J. Biol. Chem.* 277: 22035–22044 (2002).
160. Imamura O, Fujita K, Itoh C, Takeda S, Furuichi Y, Matsumoto T, Werner T. *Oncogene* 21: 954–963 (2002).
161. Salvemini D, Cuzzocrea S, *Curr. Opin. Investig. Drugs* 3: 886–895 (2002).
162. Geromel V, Kadhom N, Cebalos-Picot I, Ouari O, Polidori A, Munnich A, Rotig A, Rustin P. *Hum. Mol. Genet.* 10: 1221–1228 (2001).
163. Pichierri P, Rosselli F, Franchitto A. *Oncogene* 22: 1491–1500 (2003).
164. Pichierri P, Franchitto A. *Bioessays* 26: 306–313 (2004).
165. Davis T, Singhrao SK, Wyllie FS, Haughton MF, Smith PJ, Wiltshire M, Wynford-Thomas D, Jones CJ, Faragher RG, Kipling D. *J. Cell Sci.* 116: 1349–1357 (2003).

166. Hammond EM, Dorie MJ, Giaccia AJ. *J. Biol. Chem.* 278: 12207–12213 (2003).
167. Cheng WH, von Kobbe C, Opresko PL, Arthur LM, Komatsu K, Seidman MM, Carney JP, Bohr VA. *J. Biol. Chem.* 279: 21169–21176 (2004).
168. Poot M, Gollahon KA, Rabinovitch PS. *Hum. Genet.* 104: 10–14 (1999).
169. Poot M, Yom JS, Whang SH. *FASEB J.* 15: 1224–1226 (2001).
170. Poot M, Gollahon KA, Emond MJ, Silber JR, Rabinovitch PS. *FASEB J.* 17: 757–758 (2002).
171. Honma M, Tadokoro S, Sakamoto H, Tanabe H, Sugimoto M, Furuichi Y, Satoh T, Sofuni T, Goto M, Hayashi M. *Mutat. Res.* 520: 15–24 (2002).
172. Nunoshiba T, Demple B. *Cancer Res.* 53: 3250–3252 (1993).
173. Lauricella M, Calvaruso G, Carabillo M, D'Anneo A, Giuliano M, Emanuele S, Vento R, Tesoriere G. *FEBS Lett.* 499: 191–197 (2001).
174. Nordenson I. *Hereditas* 87: 151–154 (1977).
175. Pagano G, Zatterale A, Degan P, d'Ischia M, Kelly FJ, Pallardó FV, Calzone R, Dunster C, Giudice A, Lloret A, Manini P, Masella R, Vuttariello E, Kılınç Y, Warnau M. *Free Radic. Res.* 39: 529–533 (2005).
176. Pagano G, Zatterale A, Degan P, d'Ischia M, Kelly FJ, Pallardó FV, Kodama S. *Biogerontology* 6 (2005), in press.
177. Frank TS. *Arch. Pathol. Lab. Med.* 125: 85–90 (2001).
178. Offit K, Levran O, Mullaney B, Mah K, Nafa K, Batish SD, Diotti R, Schneider H, Deffenbaugh A, Scholl T, Proud VK, Robson M, Norton L, Ellis N, Hanenberg H, Auerbach AD. *J. Natl. Cancer Inst.* 95: 1548–1551 (2003).
179. Zawacki KL. *AACN Clin. Issues* 13: 523–539 (2002).
180. Bordi C. *Dig. Liver Dis.* 36 (Suppl 1): S31–34 (2004).
181. Fearnhead NS, Wilding JL, Bodmer WF. *Br. Med. Bull.* 64: 27–43 (2002).
182. Cowgill SM, Muscarella P. *Am. J. Surg.* 186: 279–286 (2003).
183. The Breast Cancer Linkage Consortium. *J. Natl. Cancer Inst.* 91: 1310–1316 (1999).
184. Malander S, Ridderheim M, Masback A, Loman N, Kristoffersson U, Olsson H, Nilbert M, Borg A. *Eur. J. Cancer* 40: 422–428 (2004).
185. Kirchhoff T, Kauff ND, Mitra N, Nafa K, Huang H, Palmer C, Gulati T, Wadsworth E, Donat S, Robson ME, Ellis NA, Offit K. *Clin. Cancer Res.* 10: 2918–2921 (2004).
186. Moynahan ME, Cui TY, Jasin M. *Cancer Res.* 61: 4842–4850 (2001).
187. Hussain S, Witt E, Huber PA, Medhurst AL, Ashworth A, Mathew CG. *Hum. Mol. Genet.* 12: 2503–2510 (2003).

188. Le Page F, Randrianarison V, Marot D, Cabannes J, Perricaudet M, Feunteun J, Sarasin A. *Cancer Res.* 60: 5548–5552 (2000).
189. Bartsch H, Nair J. *Cancer Detect. Prev.* 26: 308–312 (2002).
190. Bartsch H, Nair J, Owen RW. *Biol. Chem.* 383: 915–921 (2002).
191. Schmid K, Nair J, Winde G, Velic I, Bartsch H. *Int. J. Cancer* 87: 1–4 (2000).
192. Frank A, Seitz HK, Bartsch H, Frank N, Nair J. *Carcinogenesis* 25: 1027–1031 (2004).
193. Bras A, Sanches R, Cristovao L, Fidalgo P, Chagas C, Mexia J, Leitao N, Rueff J. *Eur. J. Cancer Prev.* 8: 305–310 (1999).
194. Schmidt AJ, Krieg JC, Vedder H. *J. Neurosci. Res.* 67: 544–550 (2002).
195. Aragno M, Parola S, Brignardello E, Mauro A, Tamagno E, Manti R, Danni O, Boccuzzi G. *Diabetes* 49: 1924–1931 (2000).
196. Ginsburg GS, O'Toole M, Rimm E, Douglas PS, Rifai N. *Clin. Chim. Acta* 305: 131–139 (2001).
197. Giannattasio A, Girotti M, Williams K, Hall L, Bellastella A. *J. Endocrinol. Invest.* 20: 439–444 (1997).
198. Gatei M, Shkedy D, Khanna KK, Uziel T, Shiloh Y, Pandita TK, Lavin MF, Rotman G. *Oncogene* 20: 289–294 (2001).
199. Schubert R, Erker L, Barlow C, Yakushiji H, Larson D, Russo A, Mitchell JB, Wynshaw-Boris A. *Hum. Mol. Genet.* 13: 1793–1802 (2004).
200. Meetei AR, Levitus M, Xue Y, Medhurst AL, Zwaan M, Ling C, Rooimans MA, Bier P, Hoatlin M, Pals G, de Winter JP, Wang W, Joenje H. *Nature Genet.* 36: 1219–1224 (2004).
201. Zhang X, Li J, Sejas DP, Pang Q. *Blood* 106: 75–85 (2005).

27 Iron-Induced Carcinogenesis

Shinya Toyokuni

1. Introduction

"Redox cycling" is a characteristic of transition metals such as iron and copper. Iron is an essential metal involved in oxygen transport mediated by hemoglobin in mammals and in the activity of various enzymes including catalase. Both deficiency and overload may cause such serious conditions in humans as microcytic anemia and hemochromatosis, respectively. Thus, iron metabolism is finely regulated. Recently, our understanding of iron metabolism has been enormously elaborated by several new findings such as the discovery of iron transporters, messenger RNA-based regulation of "iron metabolism-associated" genes, and the cloning of the hemochromatosis gene *HFE*. Furthermore, there is a growing body of evidence that suggests a role of iron in carcinogenesis. Our laboratory extensively investigated the carcinogenic processes in an animal model by the use of an iron chelate, ferric nitrilotriacetate, and the precise molecular mechanisms are now being elucidated. This chapter describes recent new findings associated with iron metabolism, and focuses on the mechanism of iron-induced carcinogenesis.

2. Fenton Chemistry and "Catalytic" Iron

Iron present in heme or iron–sulfur clusters or closely associated with proteins plays an important role in a variety of physiological cellular functions such as oxygen transport, energy metabolism, electron transport, and modulation of H_2O_2 levels. On the other hand, non-protein bound "free" or "catalytic" iron functions for damaging reactions.[1]

Iron is the most abundant transition metal in the human body (approximately 2–6 g).[2] Redox cycling of iron is closely associated with the production of reactive oxygen species (ROS). A British chemist, Fenton reported in as early as 1894 that ferrous sulfate and H_2O_2 cause the oxidation of tartaric acid, resulting in a beautiful violet color on the addition of caustic alkali.[3] This was the basis for the discovery of the Fenton reaction, which produces hydroxyl radicals (•OH), the most damaging chemical species in the biological system (Eq. (1)).

$$\mathrm{Fe(II)} + \mathrm{H_2O_2} \rightarrow \mathrm{Fe(III)} + \bullet\mathrm{OH} + \mathrm{OH^-} \qquad (1)$$

In order to understand the involvement of this chemical reaction in biological systems, the concept of "catalytic" or "free" iron proposed by Gutteridge[1] is vital. "Catalytic" iron has the following two characteristics: (1) redox activity and (2) diffusibility. In biological environments at neutral pH, the reduction potential of Fe(III) is +772 mV, close to that of the water/oxygen couple, which is +818 mV.[4] However, Fe(III) dissolves in water at a very low concentration (10^{-17} M) at neutral pH. Most Fe(III) precipitates as iron hydroxides at neutral pH.[5] On the other hand, iron chelated with citrate, ADP, ATP, or GTP can remain as "catalytic" iron at neutral pH.[6] In these iron chelates, at least one of the six ligands of iron is left free to produce catalytic activity.[7] It was suggested that the fewer the number of ligands involved in chelation, the higher the preservation of catalytic activity for ROS production.[8] This is further related to the redox potential of the iron chelate; in the redox potential between +460 mV and − 160 mV, the ferrous state gives a Fenton reaction, whereas the ferric state can be reduced by $O_2^{\cdot -}$.[9]

3. Catalytic Iron in the Biological Environment

Only a limited amount of data is currently available concerning the localization of "catalytic" iron in the cytoplasm or nuclei of cells due to a deficiency in appropriate technology. It has been believed that there exists a minute cellular "labile" pool of iron that is solubilized via chelation to low molecular weight biomolecules such as citrate and adenine nucleotides.[10,11] This pool of iron is considered to be at least partly responsible for the pathological generation of free radicals.

On the other hand, more data are available regarding extracellular "free" iron. The clinical significance of "non-transferrin plasma iron" ("catalytic" iron) has been previously discussed.[12] Plasma transferrin acts as a considerable reserve for coping with increasing amounts of incoming iron via iron transporters. However, in acute iron poisoning, "catalytic" iron concentrations ranging from 128 to over 800 μmol/l have been documented, exceeding by several times the total binding capacity of transferrin.[13] Similarly, in severe idiopathic hemochromatosis and Bantu siderosis, acute episodes of abdominal pain and shock have been observed in individuals with extremely high serum iron measurements exceeding 2000 μmol/l.[14]

Another important concept regarding iron-dependent oxidative damage is that of a "site-specific" mechanism. Fe(III) ions that are loosely bound to biological molecules such as DNA and proteins can undergo cyclic reduction and oxidation. This concept is different from that of "catalytic" iron in that the iron is not diffusible, and may explain the concentration of free radical damage to specific sites and possible "multi-hit" effects on the molecules at such sites.[15]

4. Iron Transporters

To consider the effect of iron status in the human body, how iron crosses the cellular membrane is a critical issue. There was until recently little molecular information available on the mechanisms of how metal ions are absorbed into circulation in mammals. In the presence of oxygen, Fe(III) is more stable than Fe(II). However, there are situations in which Fe(II) is required in organisms. The uptake and transport of iron under physiological conditions require specific mechanisms since Fe(III) has very low solubility at neutral pH, as described previously.[5] Therefore, the reduction of iron has been considered necessary for iron absorption. While the process of transferrin receptor-mediated endocytosis has been well established,[16–18] this was not the pathway by which iron in the diet is taken up into circulation from the outer environment, namely duodenum.

In 1997, mouse Nramp2 (natural resistance-associated macrophage protein 2)/DMT1 (divalent metal transporter 1; DCT1, divalent cation transporter 1) was identified as an iron transporter by studying *mk* mice, which show microcytic anemia, with a genetic approach. The anemia of *mk* mice was unresponsive to increased dietary iron, and iron injections did not reverse the anemia, suggesting a block of iron entry into red blood cell precursors as well.[19] It was of interest that Nramp2 is a homolog of Nramp1, which mediates the natural resistance to infection with intracellular parasites, affecting the capacity of macrophages to destroy ingested intracellular parasites early during infection.[20] Independently, this gene was identified with an expression cloning technique from a duodenal cDNA library prepared from rats with iron deficiency. This insightful approach was based on the idea that mRNA for iron transporter would be overexpressed in such a situation. These experiments further revealed that DMT1 transports not only Fe(II) but also Zn(II), Mn(II), Cu(II), Co(II), Cd(II), and Pb(II). Furthermore, this transporter was expressed in other organs such as kidney, liver, brain, heart, lung, and testis, although to a lesser extent (Fig. 1).[21]

Intestinal epithelial cells have two different iron transporters, one in the apical membrane and one in the basolateral membrane, as indicated by the findings that in *sla* mice normal uptake of iron into the villus cells is seen,

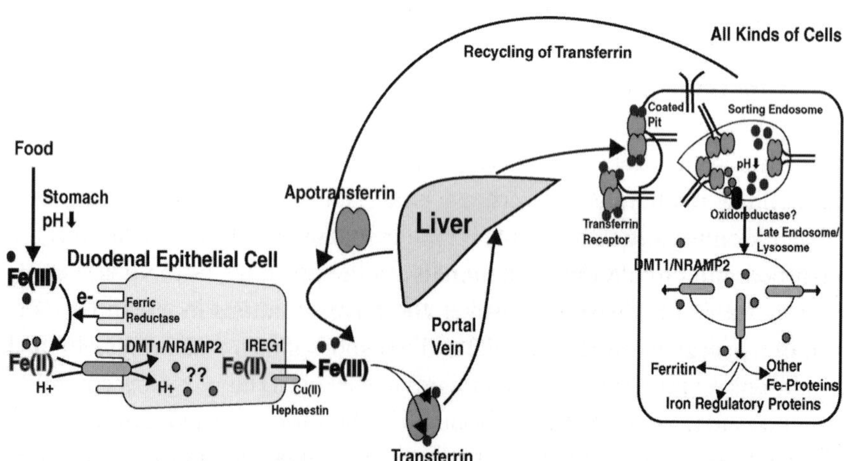

Fig. 1. Current understanding of iron absorption and transport in mammals. DMT1, divalent metal transporter 1; NRAMP2, natural resistance-associated macrophage protein 2; IREG1, iron-regulated transporter 1.[76]

via a process mediated by DMT1/Nramp2, but there is impaired release of iron into the bloodstream (Fig. 1). Recent attempts to clone the basolateral membrane transporter suggest that it consists of at least two subunits, one for Fe(II) transport and the other for oxidation of Fe(II) back to Fe(III).[22] Finally, in 2000, a novel duodenal iron-regulated transporter, Ireg1, implicated in the basolateral transfer of iron to the portal vein, was cloned.[23] This transporter was reported independently from two other laboratories as ferroportin 1 (FP1)[24] and metal transporter protein 1 (MTP1).[25] In contrast to Nramp2/DMT1, Ireg1 (FP1, MTP1) was expressed in the duodenum, reticuloendothelial system, pregnant uterus, and embryonic muscle and central nervous system cells.[25]

Thus, the author believes that, based on these major breakthroughs, a variety of novel findings can be expected regarding pathological conditions associated with iron metabolism during the next few years.

5. Post-transcriptional Regulation of Iron Metabolism

The expression of proteins that modulate the iron metabolism of mammalian cells is controlled by the intracellular levels of iron. This regulation is mediated mainly at a post-transcriptional level, namely by specific messenger RNA (mRNA)–protein interactions in the cytoplasm. Particular hairpin structures, called iron-responsive elements (IREs), in the respective mRNA are recognized by the transacting proteins, called iron-regulatory proteins (IRPs), that can control the efficiency of mRNA translation and stability. IREs are present not only in the 5′ untranslated region (UTR) of the ferritin heavy- and light-chains,[26,27] 5-aminolaevulinic acid synthase,[28–30] and mammalian mitochondrial aconitase,[30] but also in the 3′ UTR of transferrin receptor (TfR) mRNA[31] (Fig. 2). Recently, it was found that one of the two splice variants form of DMT1/Nramp2 contains 3′ UTR IREs with a higher affinity to IRP1.[32]

The predicted interaction of IRP-1 with the TfR IRE was convincingly demonstrated in cells treated with iron chelator to remove iron, and a clear correlation was shown between iron deprivation and the induction of TfR mRNA and protein.[33] It has now been established that IRP-1 plays a dual role as an IRE-binding form without a [4Fe–4S] cluster in iron deficiency,

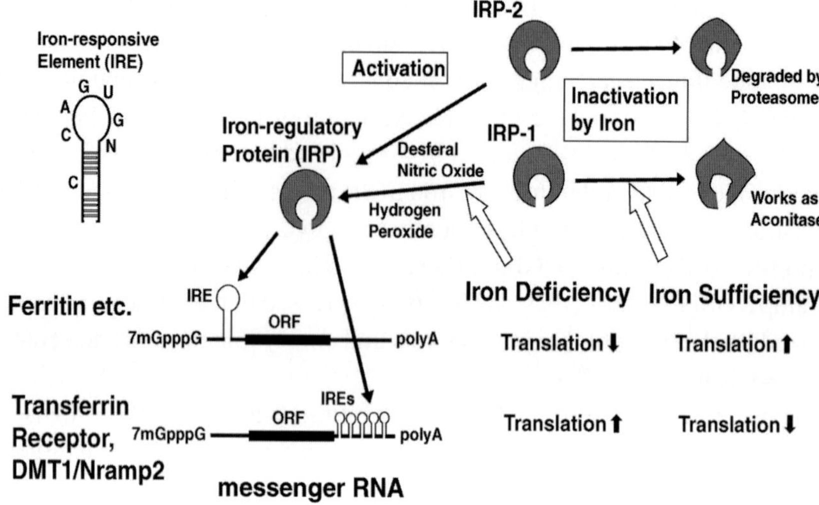

Fig. 2. Post-transcriptional regulation of iron metabolism by iron-regulatory proteins. Binding of iron-regulatory proteins to iron-responsive element in messenger RNA plays a key role in the post-trasncriptional regulation of iron-associated proteins. ORF, open reading frame. Desferal is an iron chelator that inactivates catalytic iron.[76]

and as a cytoplasmic aconitase with a [4Fe–4S] cluster in iron sufficiency. In iron deficiency, while translation of ferritin is blocked by the interaction of IRE and IRP-1 in the 5′ UTR region, the mRNA of TfR is stabilized by the same interaction in the 3′ UTR region. Furthermore, it was found that signals other than iron level can regulate IRP-1 and IRP-2 and modulate iron metabolism. Nitric oxide or oxidative stress transforms an inactive form of IRP-1 with a [4Fe–4S] cluster to an active form with a damaged [4Fe–4S] cluster, although the time required for the transformation is different ($\sim$15 vs. $<$1 h, respectively). The molecular mechanism of this activation has been studied in detail[34,35] (Fig. 2).

6. Hemochromatosis

Hereditary hemochromatosis is a genetic iron overload disorder that in the past could hardly be diagnosed until the progressive accumulation of iron, mainly in the form of ferritin and hemosiderin, caused solid organ injury, particularly to the liver, heart, and endocrine pancreas (especially insulin-secreting β-cells). The disease has been diagnosed on the basis of a classic triad: (1) a micronodular pigmented liver cirrhosis in all cases; (2) diabetes mellitus in about 75–80% of the cases; and (3) skin pigmentation in about 75–85% of the cases. However, the disease can now be discovered much earlier by biochemical analysis of blood before cirrhosis and other organ injuries have developed.[36]

Recently, *HFE*, the gene responsible for hereditary hemochromatosis, was identified by a positional cloning approach. HFE is related to major histocompatibility complex class I proteins, and is mutated in hereditary hemochromatosis.[37] Two point mutations, C282Y and H63D, have been linked to the majority of disease cases.[38] Hereditary hemochromatosis is usually inherited in an autosomal-recessive manner. Interestingly, it was reported that a mutation in the gene encoding ferroportin is associated with autosomal-dominant type of hemochromatosis.[39,40]

The structure of the protein was analyzed by X-ray crystallography,[41] and it was observed that HFE binds to the transferrin receptor (TfR), a receptor by which cells acquire iron-loaded transferrin, and that in cases of hemochromatosis this interaction is disrupted.[42] Intestinal crypt cells express HFE and TfR, whereas mature villus cells express Nramp2/DMT1, but not HFE. These results lead to a speculation that HFE and TfR together sense serum iron in crypt cells. It was proposed that HFE and TfR in crypt cells regulate the expression of the proteins involved in iron absorption in villus cells, including Nramp2/DMT1, via the IRE/IRP system.[43]

It is of note that one of the major causes of death today in hereditary hemochromatosis is either hepatic failure with cirrhosis or hepatocellular carcinoma.[44] Indeed, 219, 240, or 92.9 times greater risk was shown for primary hepatocellular carcinoma in hemochromatosis patients than in the age-matched control population in three independent studies.[45–47] In general, hepatocellular carcinoma is preceded by cirrhosis. A high incidence of cancers originating from other organs (esophageal cancer, skin melanoma, etc.) has also been reported.[47–50] Furthermore, cases of hepatocellular carcinoma have been reported in the absence of cirrhosis[51,52] and after reversal of cirrhosis with therapy.[53] These facts suggest that irreversible genetic alteration have occurred early in the course of the disease.

It has been suggested that consistent lipid peroxidation is one of the important factors for the etiology of the high incidence of hepatocarcinogenesis in hereditary hemochromatosis. The suggested mechanisms include increased lysosomal membrane fragility and peroxidative damage of organelles such as microsomes and mitochondria.[54] It was shown that the serum "catalytic" form of iron in advanced hemochromatosis patients exists largely as complexes with citrate.[55] We showed that ferric citrate efficiently induces oxidative single- and double-strand breaks in plasmid DNA *in vitro*.[56] Historical aspects of the association of iron with human and animal carcinogenesis have been reviewed previously.[57,58]

7. Target Genes in Fenton Reaction-Induced Carcinogenesis

After years of studies on the basis of carcinogenesis, it is well established that major alterations in cancer exist in the genome DNA. ROS may cause DNA damage, leading to an error of the genome information. This is defined as a mutation, a genetic change, and includes point mutations, deletions, and additions as well as chromosomal translocations. These events may cause activation of oncogenes (proliferation-associated genes), and inactivation of tumor suppressor genes, which are basically classified into two categories, caretakers (DNA repair genes) and gatekeepers (cell cycle inhibitors).[59] The caretakers usually take good care of our genome DNA and maintain its integrity. It is estimated that roughly 130,000 damage events may occur per day, per genome in the rat.[60] However, in the case of excessive oxidative stress such as in the situation of iron overload, accidents or mistakes might occur in the processes of repair or replication of DNA.

In contrast to the strictly selective antigen–antibody interactions, free radical reactions have been considered to reveal no such specificity, especially *in vitro*. For example, the second-order rate constant for the reaction of hydroxyl radical with a DNA base, guanine, is $1.0 \times 10^{10} M^{-1} s^{-1}$.[61] Thus, it may be hypothesized that the genome is randomly injured and that there is no specific target genes in Fenton reaction-induced cancer. We doubted this hypothesis, and used a genetic study to examine whether there is any target gene in ferric nitrilotriacetate (Fe-NTA)-induced renal cell carcinoma (Fig. 3). This model has been developed in our laboratory, and induces

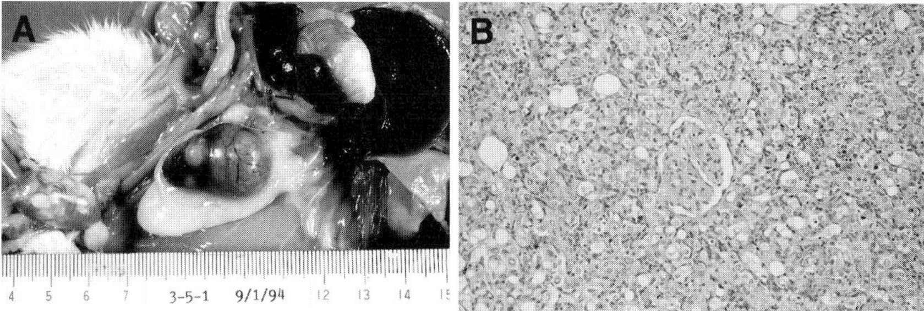

Fig. 3. Ferric nitrilotriacetate-induced renal cell carcinoma in rats. (A) Macroscopic view: renal cell carcinoma occupies half of the right kidney together with daughter nodules. (B) Histology of renal cell carcinoma: atypical cells forming glandular structure are invading the renal parenchyma, leaving one normal glomerulus in the center.

Fenton reaction specifically in the lumina of renal proximal tubules. After repeated intraperitoneal administration of Fe-NTA, renal cell carcinoma is observed in more than 90% of the treated rats. Detailed data on this model have been summarized elsewhere.[57,58,62]

We have used polymerase chain reaction (PCR) to scan the whole genome of Fe-NTA-induced renal cell carcinoma in F_1 hybrid rats in search of allelic losses with microsatellite polymorphic markers. A preliminary experiment revealed a significantly elevated frequency of allelic loss (>30%) on rat chromosomes 5 and 8. We then focused on chromosome 5. Microsatellite markers in the chromosomal areas around rat chromosome 5q32 showed allelic loss in more than 40% of the tumors.[63] Common allelic loss suggests the presence of a target tumor suppressor gene, according to Knudson's "two hit theory"[64] that both the alleles need to be mutated or methylated to inactivate the tumor suppressor gene. Thus, allelic loss is one of the rate-controlling steps in the process of this inactivation.

We searched for candidate genes from the map position. $p15^{INK4B}$ (*p15*) and $p16^{INK4A}$ (*p16*) tumor suppressor genes were the candidate genes at the map position indicated. We then evaluated whether these two genes are among the targets for carcinogenesis by Southern blot analysis, PCR/single-strand conformation polymorphism analysis, and Northern blot analysis, as well as methylation-specific PCR analysis.[65] We found that 44% of the renal cell carcinomas showed allelic loss of *p15* or *p16* (*p16* only, 38%); in 38% of the tumors *p15* or *p16* was inactivated; tumors with high-grade pathology had a high inactivation frequency. There were three patterns in the inactivation: homozygous deletion, point mutation with allelic loss, and methylation of the promoter region. This was the first report that showed the presence of any target gene in a Fenton reaction- or oxidative stress-induced cancer model.[66] The biological significance of these findings is immense, since *p16* is associated not only with the Retinoblastoma protein pathway as a cyclin-dependent kinase 4 and 6 inhibitor, but also with the *p53* pathway via *p19* ARF and MDM2.[66,67]

Therefore, allelic loss of *p16* appears a key event in our Fenton reaction-induced carcinogenesis model. The next question was when the allelic loss occurs during carcinogenesis. To answer this question, we studied the alteration of the number of alleles of *p16* in the renal proximal tubules. Fluorescent *in situ* hybridization experiments were performed at a single-cell resolution by the use of touch preparations of excised kidney. We clearly demonstrated that allelic loss of *p16* occurs quite early in carcinogenesis (1–3 weeks after the start of the experiment) and is gene-specific.[68] This fact is probably associated with which portion of the genome is susceptible to the attack of ROS and the start origin of DNA replication at the S-phase. These might differ depending on the kinds of cells and the conditions under which the cells are placed.

Our results may help explain the recent findings that homozygous deletion of *p16* but not methylation of the *p16* promoter is a genetic target in the pathogenesis of smoking-induced human lung cancer[69] and that a higher incidence of *p16* deletion is observed in cultured cells than in primary tumors.[70] In both of these conditions, cells have been exposed to high levels of ROS.

Two studies on cancers induced in hereditary haemochromatosis were performed quite recently. The mutation spectrum of the *p53* tumor suppressor gene was studied using tissues of hemochromatosis-associated hepatocellular carcinoma. In a British study, 60% A:T to G:C and 40% A:T to T:A mutations were observed[71] whereas 45% G:C to C:G, 33% A:T to C:G, 11% G:C to A:T at CpG, and 11% G:C to T:A mutations were observed in an American study.[72] These mutation spectra suggest that etheno-deoxyguanine or -deoxyadenine DNA adducts may be responsible for the DNA damage. These DNA modifications are produced by the reaction of DNA bases with lipid peroxidation products, and the increased formation of such modifications is observed in the livers of hereditary hemochromatosis patients.[73]

8. Non-Genetic Alterations in Iron-Induced Carcinogenesis

Can we explain all the mechanisms of iron-induced carcinogenesis with genetic alterations? Apparently, this is not true. Non-genetic changes are also important. We have performed differential display analysis between the control kidney and Fe-NTA-induced RCCs, and observed an elevated expression of annexin 2 (Anx2).[74] Messenger RNA and protein levels of Anx2 were increased time-dependently in the rat kidney after Fe-NTA administration as well as in LLC-PK1 cells after exposure to H_2O_2. The latter was inhibited by pretreatment with *N*-acetylcysteine, pyrrolidine dithiocarbamate, or catalase. Immunohistochemistry revealed negligible staining in the normal renal proximal tubules, but strong staining in regenerating proximal tubules, karyomegalic cells, and RCCs. Metastasizing RCCs showed higher Anx2 protein levels. Anx2 was phosphorylated at serine and tyrosinc rcsiducs in these cells and coimmunoprecipitated with phosphorylated actin. Overexpresison of Anx2 induced a higher cell proliferation rate in LLC-PK1 cells. In contrast, a decrease in proliferation leading to apoptosis was observed after Anx2 antisense treatment to cell lines established from Fe-NTA-induced RCCs. These results suggested that Anx2 is regulated by redox status, and that persistent operation of this adaptive mechanism plays a role in the proliferation and metastasis of oxidative stress-induced cancer (Fig. 4).[75] Anx2 is just an example, and many more genes are regulated by redox status. These non-genetic changes in concert with genetic changes appear to contribute toward selective proliferation of cells chronically exposed to iron.

9. Conclusions

Iron plays an important role in free radical-induced tissue damage and carcinogenesis. Clinical features of iron overload are seen in hemochromatosis. In the past few years, our understanding of iron metabolism, the

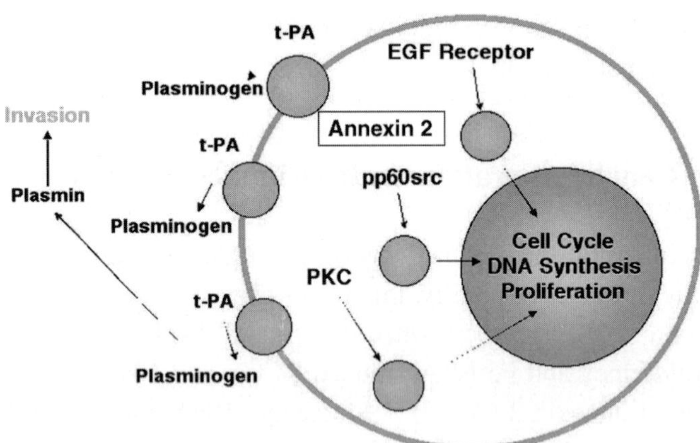

Fig. 4. Significance of annexin 2 in iron-induced carcinogenesis. EGF, epidermal growth factor; PKC, protein kinase C; t-PA, tissue plasminogen activator. Annexin 2 is a substrate for kinases and a receptor for tissue-type plasminogen activator and plasminogen, and is regulated by redox status. See text for details.

molecular mechanism of hemochromatosis, and iron-induced carcinogenesis has been enormously expanded. Especially, we have introduced a novel concept of "vulnerable sites in the genome by Fenton reaction." This concept may also be applied to protein modifications by aldehydes, another key reaction of Fenton reaction-associated covalent modification. If target genes or proteins are to be identified in each of Fenton reaction-associated diseases, these would greatly contribute to the prevention and therapy of the diseases.

Acknowledgments

This work was supported in part by a Grant-in-Aid from the Ministry of Education, Science, Sports and Culture of Japan, and a Grant-in-Aid for Cancer Research from the Ministry of Health, Labour and Welfare of Japan.

References

1. Gutteridge JMC *et al.* Superoxide-dependent formation of hydroxyl radicals and lipid peroxidation in the presence of iron salts: detection of "catalytic"

iron and anti-oxidant activity in extracellular fluids. *Biochem. J.* 206: 605–609 (1982).

2. Wriggleworth JM, Baum H. In: Jacobs A, Worwood M (eds.) *Iron in Biochemistry and Medicine, II*. Academic Press, London, 1980, pp. 29–86.
3. Fenton HJH. Oxidation of tartaric acid in presence of iron. *J. Chem. Soc.* 65: 899–910 (1984).
4. Thauer R *et al.* Energy conservation in chemotrophic anaerobic bacteria. *Bacteriol. Rev.* 41: 100–180 (1977).
5. Lippard SJ, Berg JM. *Principles of Bioorganic Chemistry*. University Science Books, Mill Valley, CA, 1994.
6. Gutteridge JMC. Superoxide-dependent formation of hydroxyl radicals from ferric-complexes and hydrogen peroxide: an evaluation of fourteen iron chelators. *Free Radic. Res. Commun.* 9: 119–125 (1990).
7. Graf E *et al.* Iron-catalyzed hydroxyl radical formation: stringent requirement for free iron coordination site. *J. Biol. Chem.* 259: 3620–3624 (1984).
8. Toyokuni S, Sagripanti JL. Iron-mediated DNA damage: sensitive detection of DNA strand breakage catalyzed by iron. *J. Inorg. Biochem.* 47: 241–248 (1992).
9. Geisser P. *Iron Therapy: With Special Emphasis on Oxidative Stress*. Georg Thieme Verlag, Stuttgart, 1996.
10. Mulligan M *et al.* Non-ferritin, non-heme iron pools in rat tissues. *Int. J. Biochem.* 18: 791–798 (1986).
11. Weaver J, Pollack S. Low-Mr iron isolated from guinea pig reticulocytes as AMP-Fe and ADP-Fe complexes. *Biochem. J.* 261: 787–792 (1989).
12. Hershko C, Peto TEA. Anotation: non-transferrin plasma iron. *Br. J. Haematol.* 66: 149–151 (1987).
13. Reynolds LG, Klein M. Iron-poisoning: a preventable hazard of childhood. *S. Afr. Med. J.* 67: 680–683 (1985).
14. Buchannan WM. Shock in Bantu siderosis. *Am. J. Clin. Pathol.* 55: 401–406 (1971).
15. Chevion M. A site-specific mechanism for free radical induced biological damage: the essential role of redox-active transtion metals. *Free Radic. Biol. Med.* 5: 27–37 (1988).
16. Dautry-Varsat A *et al.* pH and the recycling of transferrin during receptor-mediated endocytosis. *Proc. Natl. Acad. Sci. USA* 80: 2258–2262 (1983).
17. Harding C *et al.* Receptor-mediated endocytosis of transferrin and recycling of the transferrin receptor in rat reticulocytes. *J. Cell. Biol.* 97: 329–339 (1983).
18. Ponka P *et al.* Function and regulation of transferrin and ferritin. *Semin. Hematol.* 35: 35–54 (1998).

19. Fleming M *et al.* Microcytic anaemia mice have a mutation in Nramp2, a candidate iron transporter gene. *Nat. Genet.* 16: 383–386 (1997).
20. Vidal S *et al.* Natural resistance to infection with intracellular parasites: isolation of a candidate for Bcg. *Cell* 73: 469–485 (1993).
21. Gunshin H *et al.* Cloning and characterization of a mammalian proton-coupled metal-ion transporter. *Nature* 388: 482–488 (1997).
22. Vulpe C *et al.* Hephaestin, a ceruloplasmin homologue implicated in intestinal iron transport, is defective in the sla mouse. *Nat. Genet.* 21: 195–199 (1999).
23. McKie A *et al.* A novel duodenal iron-regulated transporter, IREG1, implicated in the basolateral transfer of iron to the circulation. *Mol. Cell.* 5: 299–309 (2000).
24. Donovan A *et al.* Positional cloning of zebrafish ferroportin1 identifies a conserved vertebrate iron exporter. *Nature* 403: 776–781 (2000).
25. Abboud S, Haile D. A novel mammalian iron-regulated protein involved in intracellular iron metabolism. *J. Biol. Chem.* 275: 19906–19912 (2000).
26. Hentze M *et al.* Identification of the iron-responsive element for the translational regulation of human ferritin mRNA. *Science* 238: 1570–1573 (1987).
27. Hentze M *et al.* A cis-acting element is necessary and sufficient for translational regulation of human ferritin expression in response to iron. *Proc. Natl. Acad. Sci. USA* 84: 6730–6734 (1987).
28. May B *et al.* Molecular regulation of 5-aminolevulinate synthase. Diseases related to heme biosynthesis. *Mol. Biol. Med.* 7: 405–421 (1990).
29. Cox T *et al.* Human erythroid 5-aminolevulinate synthase: promoter analysis and identification of an iron-responsive element in the mRNA. *EMBO J.* 10: 1891–1902 (1991).
30. Dandekar T *et al.* Identification of a novel iron-responsive element in murine and human erythroid delta-aminolevulinic acid synthase mRNA. *EMBO J.* 10: 1903–1909 (1991).
31. Casey J *et al.* Iron-responsive elements: regulatory RNA sequences that control mRNA levels and translation. *Science* 240: 924–928 (1988).
32. Gunshin H *et al.* Iron-dependent regulation of the divalent metal ion transporter. *FEBS Lett.* 509: 309–316 (2001).
33. Koeller D *et al.* A cytosolic protein binds to structural elements within the iron regulatory region of the transferrin receptor mRNA. *Proc. Natl. Acad. Sci. USA* 86: 3574–3578 (1989).
34. Hentze M, Kuhn L. Molecular control of vertebrate iron metabolism: mRNA-based regulatory circuits operated by iron, nitric oxide, and oxidative stress. *Proc. Natl. Acad. Sci. USA* 93: 8175–8182 (1996).

35. Wardrop S *et al.* Nitrogen monoxide activates iron regulatory protein 1 RNA-binding activity by two possible mechanisms: effect on the [4Fe–4S] cluster and iron mobilization from cells. *Biochemistry* 39: 2748–2758 (2000).
36. Cotran RS *et al. Robbins Pathologic Basis of Disease*, 6th edn. W.B. Saunders, Philadelphia, 1999.
37. Feder J *et al.* A novel MHC class I-like gene is mutated in patients with hereditary haemochromatosis [see comments]. *Nat. Genet.* 13: 399–408 (1996).
38. Lyon E, Frank E. Hereditary hemochromatosis since discovery of the HFE gene. *Clin. Chem.* 47: 1147–1156 (2001).
39. Njajou O *et al.* A mutation in SLC11A3 is associated with autosomal dominant hemochromatosis. *Nat. Genet.* 28: 213–214 (2001).
40. Montosi G *et al.* Autosomal-dominant hemochromatosis is associated with a mutation in the ferroportin (SLC11A3) gene. *J. Clin. Invest.* 108: 619–623 (2001).
41. Lebron J *et al.* Crystal structure of the hemochromatosis protein HFE and characterization of its interaction with transferrin receptor. *Cell* 93: 111–123 (1998).
42. Parkkila S *et al.* Association of the transferrin receptor in human placenta with HFE, the protein defective in hereditary hemochromatosis. *Proc. Natl. Acad. Sci. USA* 94: 13198–13202 (1997).
43. Waheed A *et al.* Association of HFE protein with transferrin receptor in crypt enterocytes of human duodenum. *Proc. Natl. Acad. Sci. USA* 96: 1579–1584 (1999).
44. Milman N *et al.* Clinically overt hereditary hemochromatosis in Denmark 1948–1985: epidemiology, factors of significance for long-term survival, and causes of death in 179 patients. *Ann. Hematol.* 80: 737–744 (2001).
45. Niederau C *et al.* Survival and causes of death in cirrhotic and in non-cirrhotic patients with primary hemochromatosis. *N. Engl. J. Med.* 313: 1256–1262 (1985).
46. Bradbear RA *et al.* Cohort study of internal malignancy in genetic hemochromatosis and other chronic non-alcoholic liver diseases. *J. Natl. Cancer Inst.* 75: 81–84 (1985).
47. Hsing AW *et al.* Cancer risk following primary hemochromatosis: a population-based cohort study in Denmark. *Int. J. Cancer* 60: 160–162 (1995).
48. Ammann RW *et al.* High incidence of extrahepatic carcinomas in idiopathic hemochromatosis. *Scand. J. Gasrtoenterol.* 15: 733–736 (1980).
49. Tiniakos G, Williams R. Cirrhotic process, liver cell carcinoma and extrahepatic malignant tumors in idiopathic hemochromatosis. *Appl. Pathol.* 6: 128–138 (1988).

50. Mallory M, Kowdley K. Hereditary hemochromatosis and cancer risk: more fuel to the fire? *Gastroenterology* 121: 1253–1254 (2001).
51. Fellows IW *et al.* Hepatocellular carcinoma in primary hemochromatosis in the absence of cirrhosis. *Gut* 29: 1603–1609 (1988).
52. Kew MD. Pathogenesis of hepatocellular carcinoma in hereditary hemochromatosis: occurrence in noncirrhotic patients. *Hepatology* 6: 1086–1087 (1990).
53. Blumberg RS *et al.* Primary hepatocellular carcinoma in idiopathic hemochromatosis after reversal of cirrhosis. *Gastroenterology* 95: 1399–1402 (1988).
54. Niemela O *et al.* Hepatic lipid peroxidation in hereditary hemochromatosis and alcoholic liver injury. *J. Lab. Clin. Med.* 133: 451–460 (1999).
55. Grootveld M *et al.* Non-transferrin-bound iron in plasma or serum from patients with idiopathic hemochromatosis: characterization by high performance liquid chromatography and nuclear magnetic resonance spectroscopy. *J. Biol. Chem.* 264: 4417–4422 (1989).
56. Toyokuni S, Sagripanti JL. Induction of oxidative single- and double-strand breaks in DNA by ferric citrate. *Free Radic. Biol. Med.* 15: 117–123 (1993).
57. Toyokuni S. Iron-induced carcinogenesis: the role of redox regulation. *Free Radic. Biol. Med.* 20: 553–566 (1996).
58. Okada S. Iron-induced tissue damage and cancer: the role of reactive oxygen free radicals. *Pathol. Int.* 46: 311–332 (1996).
59. Vogelstein B, Kinzler KW. *The Genetic Basis of Human Cancer*. McGraw-Hill, New York, 1998.
60. Bernstein C. In: Halliwell B, Aruoma OI (eds.) *DNA and Free Radicals*, 1st edn. Ellis Horwood, Chichester, UK, 1993, pp. 193–210.
61. Halliwell B, Gutteridge JMC. *Free Radicals in Biology and Medicine*, 3rd edn. Clarendon Press, Oxford, 1999.
62. Toyokuni S. Reactive oxygen species-induced molecular damage and its application in pathology. *Pathol. Int.* 49: 91–102 (1999).
63. Tanaka T *et al.* High incidence of allelic loss on chromosome 5 and inactivation of $p15^{INK4B}$ and $p16^{INK4A}$ tumor suppressor genes in oxystress-induced renal cell carcinoma of rats. *Oncogene* 18: 3793–3797 (1999).
64. Knudson AG Jr. *et al.* Mutation and childhood cancer: a probabilistic model for the incidence of retinoblastoma. *Proc. Natl. Acad. Sci. USA* 72: 5116–5120 (1975).
65. Herman JG *et al.* Methylation-specific PCR: a novel PCR assay for methylation status of CpG islands. *Proc. Natl. Acad. Sci. USA* 93: 9821–9826 (1996).
66. Kamijo T *et al.* Functional and physical interactions of the ARF tumor suppressor with p53 and Mdm2. *Proc. Natl. Acad. Sci. USA* 95: 8292–8297 (1998).

67. Tao W, Levine AJ. P19(ARF) stabilizes p53 by blocking nucleo-cytoplasmic shuttling of Mdm2. *Proc. Natl. Acad. Sci. USA* 96: 6937–6941 (1999).
68. Hiroyasu M *et al.* Specific allelic loss of p16INK4A tumor suppressor gene after weeks of iron-mediated oxidative damage during rat renal carcinogenesis. *Am. J. Pathol.* 160: 419–424 (2002).
69. Sanchez-Cespedes M *et al.* Increased loss of chromosome 9p21 but not p16 inactivation in primary non-small cell lung cancer from smokers. *Cancer Res.* 61: 2092–2096 (2001).
70. Zhang S *et al.* Higher frequency of alterations in the p16/CDKN2 gene in squamous cell carcinoma cell lines than in primary tumors of the head and neck. *Cancer Res.* 54: 5050–5053 (1994).
71. Vautier G *et al.* p53 mutations in british patients with hepatocellular carcinoma: clustering in genetic hemochromatosis. *Gastroenterology* 117: 154–160 (1999).
72. Marrogi A *et al.* Oxidative stress and p53 mutations in the carcinogenesis of iron overload-associated hepatocellular carcinoma [record supplied by publisher]. *J. Natl. Cancer. Inst.* 93: 1652–1655 (2001).
73. Nair J *et al.* Lipid peroxidation-induced etheno-DNA adducts in the liver of patients with the genetic metal storage disorders Wilson's disease and primary hemochromatosis. *Cancer Epidemiol. Biomarkers Prev.* 7: 435–440 (1998).
74. Tanaka T *et al.* Expression of stress-response and cell proliferation genes in renal cell carcinoma induced by oxidative stress. *Am. J. Pathol.* 156: 2149–2157 (2000).
75. Tanaka T *et al.* Redox regulation of annexin 2 and its implications for oxidative stess-induced renal carcinogenesis and metastasis. *Oncogene* 23: 3980–3989 (2004).
76. Toyokuni S. Iron and carcinogenesis: from Fenton reaction to target genes. *Redox Rep.* 7: 189–197 (2002).

28 Copper and Carcinogenesis

Theophile Theophanides and Jane Anastassopoulou

1. General Aspects

Copper metal has a $3d^{10}4s^1$ electronic configuration, where all 3d orbitals are filled and only a single electron occupies the 4s orbital. However, by loss of two electrons, one from the 3d orbital and one from the 4s orbital, Cu^{2+} becomes a d^9 system. Therefore, Cu^{2+} behaves as a transition element, since it has a partially filled d-shell with an unpaired electron, and thus paramagnetic, while Cu^+ is a d^{10} and diamagnetic.[1] These are interesting properties of copper in its reactions of oxidation–reduction and complex formation with ligands, such as proteins and enzymes. Copper and iron are the most likely transition elements of the periodic table, for biological cells to form hydroxyl free radicals (•OH) via the Fenton and Haber–Weiss reactions.[2–4] However, copper is scarcer than iron, which is the most abundant metal in earth's crust. Copper is present *in vivo* in low concentrations and binds to enzymes, in the tissues and body fluids in cells. It is located in proteins, ceruloplasmin, and albumin.[1] These transition metal ions are mobilized following myocardial ischemia and may play an essential role in redox-active catalytic reactions producing free oxygen radicals.[5] Free radicals are atoms or molecules and ions that contain one or more unpaired electrons.

The role of copper and oxygen in the evolution of life was to participate in the formation of amino acids, carbohydrates, purines, pyrimidines, nucleic acids, and fatty acids, as a catalyst in the reaction of ammonia, plus water and methane at the origin of life. In biological evolution copper coordination chemistry must have played an important role by solubilizing copper according to the following reactions:

$$H_2S + 2Cu^+ \rightarrow Cu_2S \text{ (insoluble)} + 2H^+ \quad (1)$$

$$Cu^+ \rightarrow Cu^{++} + e^- \text{(soluble)} \quad (2)$$

Biomineralization of copper by fungus called *Penicillium ochro-chloron* was found and published recently.[6] Copper was obtained as copper phosphate and oxalate salts within the matrix of small fugal mycelia beads.

Monovalent Cu^+ is a softer acid than Cu^{2+} and is complexed by sulfur aminoacids, preferentially. Copper participates in several catalytic biochemical reactions. Reactions that may be catalyzed by copper are extracellular oxidases, hormone synthases, synthesis of connective tissues, metabolism, oxygen transport, etc. Copper is present in biological systems as an active center in proteins or enzymes. In all these systems copper has been observed as Cu^{2+} or Cu^+. Cu^{3+} has also been proposed, but it is not very stable. It has been found only in small peptides.[1]

Copper bound to proteins can react with H_2O_2 to yield hydroxyl radicals (•OH), which oxidize the amino acid residue at the metal binding site. This is its role in oxidative stress leading to diseases. The mechanism of •OH production was proposed originally through the Haber–Weiss reaction[3,4]

$$O_2^{\bullet -} + H_2O_2 \rightarrow {}^{\bullet}OH + OH^- + O_2 \quad (3)$$

The one-electron reduction of molecular oxygen leads to the formation of superoxide anion radical ($O_2^{\bullet -}$) as follows:

$$O_2 + e^- \rightarrow O_2^{\bullet -} \quad (4)$$

Furthermore, the two- or four-electron reduction of molecular oxygen leads, in the presence of protons, to the formation of hydrogen peroxide and water,[7] i.e., the peroxide anion O_2^{2-} and oxide anion O^{2-}, respectively:

$$O_2 + 2e^- \xrightarrow{2H^+} H_2O_2 \quad (5)$$

$$H_2O_2 \xrightarrow{e^-} \bullet OH \xrightarrow{e^-} H_2O \quad (6)$$

The blue oxidases, the copper containing enzymes, catalyze the transfer of four electrons to form reducing substrates of O_2 with the formation of water.

It is known that the superoxide anion radical ($O_2^{\bullet -}$) is the major reactive oxygen species (ROS) generated in mitochondria, producing H_2O_2. Several biologically important molecules, such as glyceraldehydes, adrenalin, and noradrenalin are oxidized in the presence of molecular oxygen to produce superoxide anions.[8,9]

It was found that traces of soluble iron or copper could catalyze the transformation of $O_2^{\bullet -}$ produced in $O_2^{\bullet -}$-driven Fenton reactions:

$$O_2^{\bullet -} + Cu^{2+} \rightarrow Cu^{+} + O_2 \quad (7)$$

$$Cu^{+} + H_2O_2 \rightarrow Cu^{2+} + {}^{\bullet}OH + OH^{-} \quad (8)$$

Equations (7) and (8) take place during the metabolism of oxygen.[8,9] The above reactions could take place also with $Fe^{2+} \rightleftarrows Fe^{3+}$ in oxidation–reduction reactions of proteins.[10] The produced superoxide anion ($O_2^{\bullet -}$) is a free radical and reacts with Cu^{2+} compounds to form Cu^{+} compounds (Fig. 1).

The tetrahedral geometry stabilizes the Cu^{+} site relatively to Cu^{2+} and assists the electron transfer. The reduction of Cu^{2+} to Cu^{+} with reaction of the superoxide anion ($O_2^{\bullet -}$) takes place in all the systems of elimination of oxidative stress due to the presence of $O_2^{\bullet -}$. Protein oxidation induced by ROS implies the oxidation of certain amino acid residues of a protein. The involvement of a transition metal copper in the mechanism of protein oxidation could take place through the following steps:[11]

(i) Metal binds to protein

$$Cu^{2+} + \text{protein} \rightarrow Cu^{2+} \text{ (protein bound)} \quad (9)$$

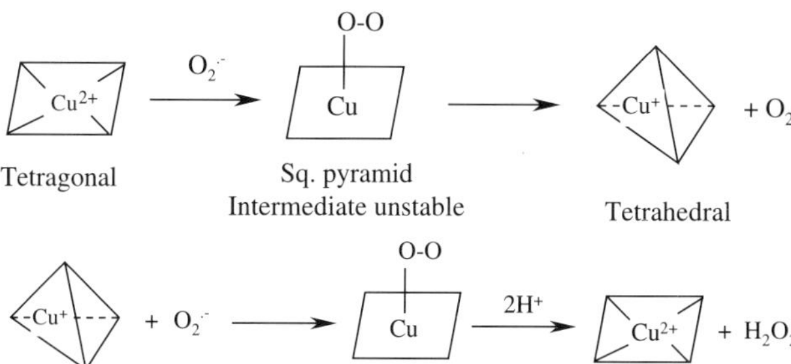

Fig. 1. The rearrangement of square geometry of Cu^{2+} into tetrahedral geometry of Cu^{+} and inversely. Cu–Zn–SOD is believed to react similarly, where copper is the active site.

(ii) The copper–protein complexes could react with the oxygen free radicals as follows:

$$Cu^{2+} \text{ (protein bound)} + O_2^{\bullet -} \rightarrow Cu^{+} \text{(protein bound)} + O_2 \quad (10)$$

The above reaction is a reduction of the coordinated copper(II) being reduced *in situ* by $O_2^{\bullet -}$ to a new complex with protein in which the most likely planar copper(II) is rearranged into tetrahedral copper(I) (see Fig. 1). This oxidation–reduction reaction takes place on the copper atom as active site. The transfer of an electron from superoxide anion to copper(II) cation is easier to take place when copper(II) is bound to protein, because the binding reduces the reduction potential of copper and allows the reaction to take place.

(iii) In acid media the inverse reaction is observed:

$$Cu^{+} \text{ (protein bound)} + O_2^{\bullet -} + 2H^{+} \rightarrow Cu^{2+} \text{(protein bound)} + H_2O_2 \quad (11)$$

(iv) Finally, hydroxyl radicals are produced:

$$Cu^{+} \text{(protein bound)} + H_2O_2 \rightarrow Cu^{2+} + {}^{\bullet}OH + OH^{-} + \text{protein} \quad (12)$$

The overall reaction leads to hydroxyl free radical production via a protein-bound copper(II). The transfer of an electron from superoxide anions to copper(II) and back to oxygen yields the reactive intermediate species, which is taking place with the aid of the protein. These ROS have both endogenous and exogenous origin and are used pathophysiologically and pharmacologically for the normal function or metabolism of most mammalian cells. ROS are also destructive unless tightly controlled by the cells' defenses to repair injuries caused by oxidative stress.[12] The control of ROS leads to a balance that is obtained through enzymes (SOD) and antioxidants, such as vitamins (A,C,E), thiols, etc.

The above reactions do take place when the cells or organs are exposed to high concentration of copper; however, *in vivo* it is not so certain if they take place and at what conditions. It was reported that *in vivo* accumulation of copper may act as a promoting factor for the development of liver cancer in LEC (Long–Evans Cinnamon) rats by creating a selective growth environment.[13,14] This would happen by increasing the content of copper via copper binding to proteins. Copper accumulation and changes in copper-related gene expression may contribute in liver hyperplasia.[15] Tumor suppression protein p53 mRNA and subcellular localization are altered by changes in cellular copper Hep G2 cells. It was confirmed that copper toxicity is correlated with apoptotic cell death. It is known that copper is highly toxic in excess and results in cellular damage.[16] A mechanism of copper incorporation into human ceruloplasmin has been proposed.[17] It was shown in the latter report that copper toxicity caused hepatic damage, which could lead to the development of hepatocarcinoma. Similarly, copper deficiency increased hepatotype tumorigenesis.[18]

2. Molecular Mechanisms of DNA Damage Induced by Organic Compounds in the Presence of Copper

A molecular mechanism of DNA damage induced by procarbazine in the presence of copper(II) has been published recently.[19] The presence of copper(II) is essential for the damage, since the presence of other metal ions, for example, iron(III), cobalt(II), nickel(II), manganese(II), and magnesium(II), did not cause DNA damage. It is suggested that a Cu^{+}-specific chelator is formed with procarbazine after reduction of Cu^{2+} to Cu^{+}. The lesions on DNA were found at the cytosine–guanine level interacting with the 5′-ACG-3′ sequence, complementary to codon 273 of the p53 suppressor gene. Double base lesions were also found at 5′-ACG-3′ and 5′-TG-3′ sequences. The conclusion was that oxidative DNA damage plays an important role in antitumor effects in mutagenesis, as well as in carcinogenesis induced by procarbazine and Cu^{2+}, since they increased significantly the formation of 8-oxo-7, 8-dihydro-2-deoxyguanosine. However, the Cu^{+}-specific intermediate does not have to be a chelating complex. The free radical mechanisms in cancer formation should occur through the role of oxidative DNA damage initiating carcinogenesis, because active oxygen species have been known to be mutagenic and thus could play a role in cancer formation. Point mutation due to oxidants at the G and C bases produces modifications of these bases, which would lead to activation of carcinogenesis.[20–27]

Copper(II) binds directly with a covalent bond to guanine and cytosine by blocking the sites N7(G) of DNA forming a more stable bond-DNA.[28]

Several studies involving interaction of copper metal ions with nucleic acids and components of nucleic acids showed the formation of very stable copper adducts of GMP, IMP, CMP interacting with Cu^{2+} either at the N7(G) and N3(C) sites or the phosphate anions.[29–39] It is well known that the G–C bases in both p53 and retinoblastoma tumor suppressor genes are targets of attacks for activating point mutations and oxidative DNA damage.[16] Both oncogenes and tumor suppression genes represent targets for mutation by oxidative exposure to oxidative stress.[16] It seems that copper(II) has a dual role in oxidative DNA damage: (1) it generates ROS by autoxidation of carcinogens with formation of Cu^+ intermediates and (2) It activates $H_2O_2$to form with organic radicals, such as quinone derivatives and reactive Cu^+ complexes (Fig. 2).

It seems that in the initial step Cu^{2+} can react with an electron giving Cu^+ and a second electron reacts with molecular oxygen producing $O_2^{\bullet -}$, which can dismutate yielding hydrogen peroxide [Eq. (5)] or quinone derivative and leading to DNA damage.

Benzene is a carcinogen in humans and exposure to benzene causes leukemia, lymphoma, and carcinomas of mammary gland and liver in humans and in animals.[40,41] It has been found that benzene metabolites are very toxic.[42,43] The presence of free Cu^{2+} is necessary in the reductive

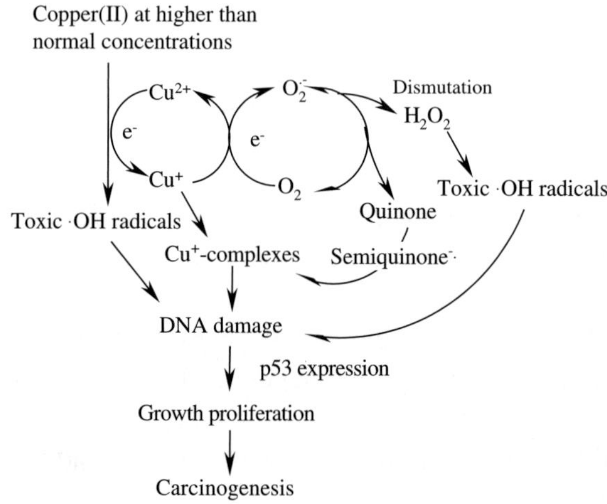

Fig. 2. Mechanism of DNA damage induced by high concentrations of copper leading to cancer.[1]

process Cu^{2+}–Cu^{+} in order to perform, for instance, the oxidation of benzene to *o*-*p*-benzoquinone.[44] The same has been observed in various phenolic derivatives, which also induced oxidative DNA damage similar to benzene metabolites[40–46] in the presence of Cu^{2+}. In addition, many aromatic nitro and amino compounds caused carcinogenesis through Cu^{2+}-mediated oxidative DNA damage induced by metabolites of binuclear and mononuclear aromatic amines. Benzoyl peroxide is widely used as an additive to initiate polymerization of monomers, as well as in acne treatment.[47] However, it has been reported that it acts as a tumor promoter and progressor.[48] Therefore, it does not act in polymerization as initiator, but most likely as a metabolite, which in the presence of Cu^{+} caused DNA damage specifically at 5′-G of GG sequences in double-stranded DNA. ESR spin trapping experiments[21,49] showed that the benzoyloxyl radical was formed through Cu^{2+}-mediated decomposition of benzoyl peroxide, which reduced DNA damage. Interested readers are directed to the references for more in-depth coverage of material available on this topic.

3. The Importance of Chemical Redox Potentials of Copper Complexes

It is known that many non-heme metalloproteins have long been found to participate in biological redox reactions. The interesting thing in these metalloproteins as compared to simple metal complexes is (1) their absorption and electron spin resonance spectra and (2) their abnormal redox potentials. The copper–protein complexes, such as ceruloplasmin and albumin, include in their active center a copper cation. The action of these proteins is lost when the copper cation is removed from the protein. Copper alternates in these proteins between Cu^{+} and Cu^{2+} as it functions. The redox potential of many of these proteins is in the range of +0.3 to +0.4 V, compared to −0.5 to +0.2 V for simple copper complexes. The oxidation–reduction chemical potentials of aquated copper are as follows:

$$Cu^{+}_{aq} + e^{-} \rightarrow Cu^{0}_{metal}, \qquad E^{0} = 0.52\,V \tag{13}$$

$$Cu^{2+}_{aq} + e^{-} \rightarrow Cu^{+}_{aq}, \qquad E^{0} = 0.15\,V \tag{14}$$

$$\text{Total}: \quad 2Cu^{+}_{aq} \leftrightarrow Cu^{0}_{metal} + Cu^{2+}_{aq}, \qquad E^{0} = 0.37\,V \tag{15}$$

aq = aquated with four water molecules. Cu^{+}_{aq} is tetrahedral and Cu^{2+}_{aq} is tetragonal.

It is shown that the redox potential for the aqueous Cu^{+}/Cu^{2+} pair is quite low (150 mV) compared to copper sites in proteins. It is believed that the tetrahedral coordination of copper(I) proteins is responsible for the higher redox potential.[50]

Unfortunately, most Cu^{2+}-complex redox chemical potentials for proteins are not known and their interpretation is not clear, because the detailed geometry of the copper coordination site is not known, and furthermore the abundance of hydrophobic residues closest to the copper site may cause changes in the redox potentials. The charge distribution in the environment of the redox centre may determine the redox potential.[50–53] The equilibrium constant of the redox reaction of transformation of hydrated Cu^{+} to hydrated Cu^{2+} is:

$$k = \frac{[Cu^{2+}]}{[Cu^{+}]} = 10^{6} \tag{16}$$

The equilibrium constant indicates that these redox reactions of copper(I) to copper(II) are very fast reactions. Therefore, the role of copper *in vivo* reactions is first to form complexes and then to give reactions allowed by oxidation–reduction chemical potentials involving the copper ion. This is how copper is transported into the tissues from square planar for copper(II) to tetrahedral for copper(I). The common coordination number of 6 with octahedral geometry is observed in all the simple complexes of copper(II). On the bases of the value of k and the dissociation constant k_a of the copper complex, copper could be eliminated by zinc, if in excess, from the human organs as in the therapy of Wilson's disease.[54]

The chemistry of copper dictates its biochemistry. It is known that unbound or free copper(II) is not very abundant in the human body. Almost all copper(II) cations in our body are bound by forming a complex either to transport proteins (ceraloplasmin, albumin) and storage proteins (in metallothioneins) or copper containing enzymes, such as the copper metalloenzymes.[55] Model copper metalenzymes could also mimic metalloenzymes and their enzymatic activity.[56–62] These model copper compounds may imitate the enzymatic activity of metalenzymes and their participation in the oxygen metabolism. Other transition metals, such as

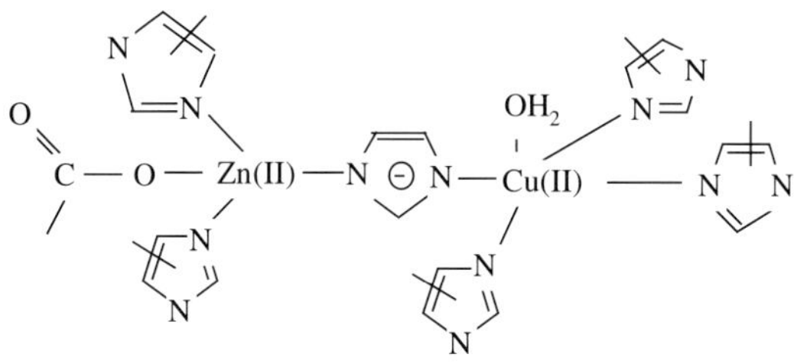

Fig. 3. The active site of Cu–Zn–SOD, X-ray structure.[64]

iron, zinc, and manganese are also involved in oxygen metabolism. In these model compounds copper is coordinated to nitrogen or sulfur and the copper atom is located at a specific environment in which the lipophilic part of the ligands could affect the bound copper.[54]

The copper coordination compounds could also mimic SOD-like products. SOD a metalloprotein containing copper(II) and Zinc(II) is a homodimeric enzyme located in eukaryotes (Fig. 3).[63]

The Cu^{2+} and Zn^{2+} cations bind to nitrogens of histidine rings and the imidazole bridge between Cu^{2+} and Zn^{2+}. Cu–Zn–SOD enzyme has a high molecular weight of the order of 30,000 Da, consisting of two units of about 15,000 Da each.

Cu–Zn–SOD catalyzes the dismutation reaction of superoxide to hydrogen peroxide and oxygen, and finally to water and thus it protects the cell from the side products of oxidation according to reaction (17):

$$2O_2^{\bullet-} \xrightarrow{2H^+} H_2O_2 + O_2 \rightarrow H_2O \tag{17}$$

Theoretical calculations showed that the catalytically active center of Cu–Zn–SOD is the copper(II) cation.[65] The importance of oxidants and cellular redox state on cell proliferation, apoptosis, and angiogenesis has been confirmed by numerous investigations.

4. The Role of Copper and Oxidative Stress in Diseases and Cancer

Copper imbalances in humans lead to diseases such as Wilson's disease,[54] Mankes syndrome,[66] and neurodegeneration.[67] Among the metals, transition metals and especially copper plays a crucial role in life, since as we mentioned earlier it participates in oxidation–reduction reactions that generate ROS (Eqs. (3) and (4)), which cause damage to lipids, proteins, and DNA.

On the other hand, transition metal ions are important for biological systems because they undergo single-electron redox exchanges. They may be "free" and "chelated," or "bound" in proteins. Chelators may be free molecular entities (metabolites, coenzymes) or prosthetic groups in heteroproteins (e.g., porphyrin in hemoproteins). They are able to combine and react with molecular oxygen (dioxygen) and/or oxygen-derived reactive species. This ability to combine with molecular oxygen (O_2), the hydroperoxyl anion (superoxide anion, $O_2^{\bullet -}$), the hydroperoxyl radical ($HO_2^{\bullet}$), or hydrogen peroxide (H_2O_2) in complex formation allows nature to control and handle oxygen chemistry in normal metabolic processes. Iron and copper are endogenous factors that contribute to oxidative stress that accompanies various pathological states. Copper(II) was shown to bind to DNA with higher affinity than any other divalent cation studied, which also explains why H_2O_2-dependent DNA oxidation has been reported to be 50 times faster than that of iron.[68]

The formation of coordination complexes with DNA may provide an advantageous active site for a reaction of a highly reactive oxygen species, such as the free hydroxyl radicals. The variation in the redox behavior of the transition metal ion by its coordination sphere, which can be octahedral, square planar, or tetrahedral, is considerable and accounts for the broad range of interactions with oxygen species that are observed in biological systems. If, for any reason, a complex between a copper metal ion and an oxygen species is destabilized, then ROS may be liberated and cause oxidative damage, which can affect all levels of biological organisation, thus leading to disease. The role of free radicals in tumor promotion through oxidative stress in the later stages of carcinogenesis has been shown.[69] Tumor promotion *in vivo* takes place through a series of complex molecular events leading to DNA damage.[19] It has been shown that differential oxidative stress induced by a skin tumor promoter, such as benzoyl peroxide, was inhibited by a biomimetic superoxide dismutase, copper(II) (3,5-diisopropyl salicylate)$_2$, whereas the corresponding zinc analog did not inhibit chemiluminescence as a noninvasive method of estimation of overall oxidative stress.[70] Endogenous copper compounds catalyzed ROS production from various organic carcinogens, resulting in oxidative DNA damage,[20] which means that copper-mediated oxidative DNA damage plays an important role in chemical carcinogenesis. Copper(II) is an essential cation for chromatin and is known to accumulate in heteromatic regions.[71] Copper(II) accumulates in the liver tissues of LEC rats and spontaneously develops hepatocellular carcinomas and hereditary hepatitis.[13]

It seems that there is a difference between free copper ions, most likely as aquated cations $[Cu(H_2O)_6]^{2+}$ and bound copper(II) cations forming complexes. Free aquated copper(II) cations are more reactive to participate in ROS generation under certain conditions, whereas bound copper cations, as in complexes with protein carriers and transporters, may be eliminated to minimize levels of free copper cations transformed in protein complexes. It has been shown that Cu^{2+} cations in the presence of H_2O_2 induced DNA damage at thymine and guanine bases by generation of ROS in phosphate buffer, whereas DNA damage was induced at polyguanines in bicarbonate buffer.[72] It has been reported that Cu^{2+} cations bind to nucleosomes with a binding constant of $4–5 \times 10^4\,M^{-1}$ [73] by forming very stable complexes. Moreover, it has been found that Cu^{2+} in the presence of H_2O_2 formed complexes with DNA fragments, which was enhanced by packing DNA as in nucleosome.[74]

The function of copper cations as an integral component of Cu–Zn superoxide dismutase is well established. SOD is indispensable to oxygen-metabolizing organisms and performs antioxidant functions in varied tissues and fluids. The vital role of copper in the biosynthesis of bone and connective tissues is established. Copper is linked in carcinogenesis, because it has been found that serum levels of copper are often elevated in animals and human cancer. Conversely, in many studies with varied types of tumours it has been demonstrated that with remission usually comes a decrease in serum copper levels to normal.[75–79] Extensive DNA damage in the presence of Cu^{2+} has been demonstrated in the case of *N*-acetylcysteine, which has induced damage to DNA by cleaving DNA, which was enhanced by piperidine treatment.[80]

Deoxyribose phosphate breakage and base modifications were observed (Figs. 4 and 5), indicating the participation of Cu^+ and H_2O_2 in DNA damage. The role of transition metals in oxidative DNA damage is to generate

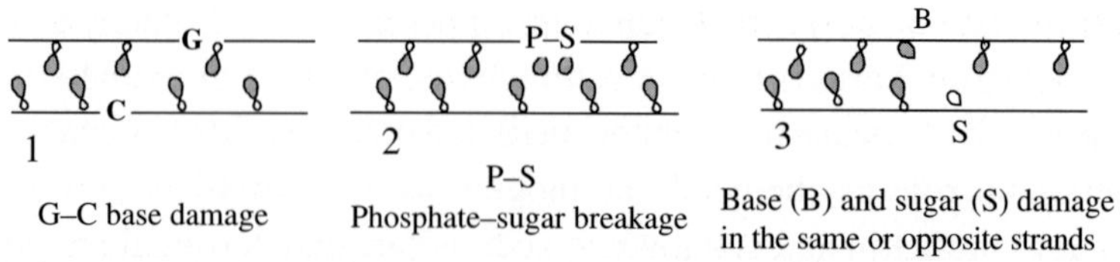

Fig. 4. Patterns of DNA damage from free radical attack: (1) base damage (G–C) leading to mutations, (2) phosphate–sugar damage leading to single-strand break (ssb) or double-strand breaks (dsb), and (3) base and sugar damage.

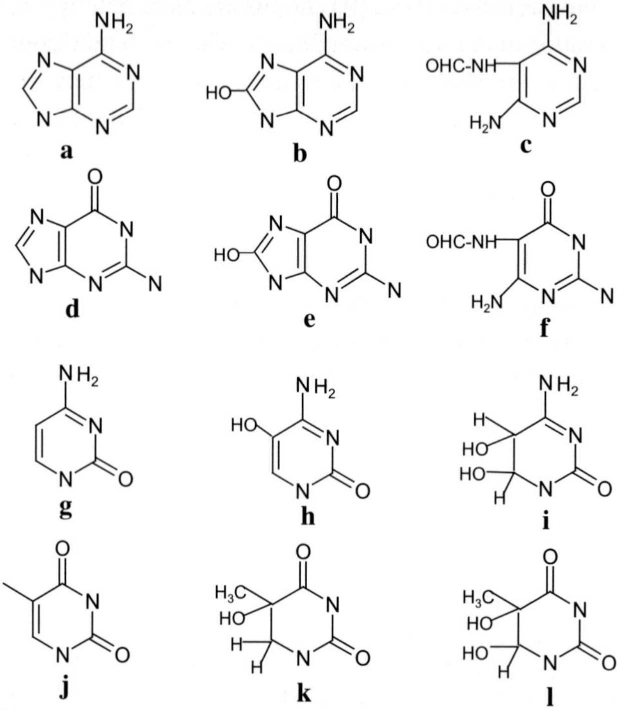

Fig. 5. DNA bases and some of the products resulting from free radical attack on DNA: (a) adenine, (b) 8-hydroxyadenine, (c) 4,6-diamino-5-formamidopyrimidine, (d) guanine, (e) 8-hydroxyguanine, (f) 2,6-diamino-4hydroxy-5-formamidopyrimi-dine, (g) cytosine, (h) 5-hydroxycytosine, (i) cytosine glycol, (j) thymine, (k) 5-hydroxy-6-hydrothymine, and (l) thymine glycol (*cis* and *trans*).

ROS (Eqs. (3) and (4)), which can damage bases in DNA, and in particular the most reactive bases in G-C levels of DNA. DNA damage includes breaks (single-strand break, ssb, or double-strand breaks, dsb) (Fig. 4), depurination, and depyrimidation and chemical modification of bases or sugars. The damage results from the addition of hydroxyl radicals to double bonds C4=C5 and C8=N7 of purines and C5=C6 of pyrimidines and abstractions of hydrogen atoms from base–sugar moiety or sugar-phosphate group.[81–84]

Epidemiological studies on the biochemistry of copper suggest that the copper metal as well as others may play an important role in carcinogenesis.[79] In a number of studies investigating the relation of this metal with cancer risk in humans was found to be significant. However, the relation is not conclusive evidence. The study on serum iron, copper, and zinc concentrations and risk of cancer mortality in US adults indicated an inverse association of cancer mortality with serum iron transferin serum and serum copper. In fact, people with the highest level of serum iron transferin serum or serum copper had a high risk of dying. A case–cohort epidemiological study showed that there is a U-shaped relationship between plasma copper levels and risk of breast cancer.[84] The pathological conditions that may have a free radical component are the hypo-, hyper-oxygenations and reperfusion after ischemia, immune reactions, radiation injuries, atherosclerosis, chemical carcinogenesis, cancer, diabetes, parkinsonism, smoking air pollution, and drug-induced reactions.

5. Conclusions

Depending on concentration there is evidence that exposure to excess copper can damage cells and organs. The effect of excess copper on cells leads to acute damage to the cell membrane and leakage of internal enzymes, which initiates and promotes cell death. The removal of copper(II) from ceruloplasmin and serum albumin, the proteins which complex with copper(II) *in vivo* by biological antioxidants is the defense mechanism used to prevent high concentrations of copper in the body and maintain a physiological balance. However, under pathological conditions the physiological balance is lost. If a large amount of toxic organic substances is present, such as benzene and quinones, excess of superoxide is produced, which in the presence of copper leads to a redox cycle and thus increasing the hydroxyl radical production causing DNA or protein damage.

References

1. Theophanides T, Anastassopoulou J. *Crit. Rev. Oncol. Hematol.* 42: 57–64 (2002).
2. Fenton HJH, Jackson H. *J. Chem. Soc. Trans. (Lond.)* 75: 1–11 (1899).
3. Haber F, Weiss J. *Naturwissenschaften* 20: 948–950 (1932).
4. Haber F, Weiss J. *Proc. R. Soc. (London) A* 147: 332–352 (1934).
5. Chevrion M *et al. Proc. Natl. Acad. Sci. USA* 90: 1102–1106 (1993).
6. Crusberg TC. *Microsc. Anal.* 18: 11–13 (2004).
7. Czapski G, Ilan YA. *Photochem. Photobiol.* 28: 651–653 (1978).
8. Halliwell B, Gutteridge JMC. *Free Radicals in Biology and Medicine*, 3rd edn. Oxford University Press, London, 1999, p. 28.
9. Davis MD *et al. Eur. J. Biochem.* 173: 345–347 (1988).
10. Stadtman ER. *Free Radic. Biol. Med.* 9: 315–325 (1990).
11. Bonomo RP *et al.* In: Russo N, Salahub R, Witko M (eds.) *Metal–Ligand Interactions*. Kluwer Academic Publishers, The Netherlands, 2004, pp. 21–40.
12. Manzl C *et al. Toxicology* 196: 57–64 (2004).
13. Suzuki K *et al. Carcinogenesis* 14: 1881–1884 (1993).
14. Sawaki M *et al. Carcinogenesis* 15: 1833–1837 (1994).
15. Eagon PK *et al. Carcinogenesis* 20: 1091–1096 (1999).
16. Narayanan VS, Fitch CA, Levenson CW. *J. Nutr.* 131: 1427–1432 (2001).
17. Hellman NE *et al. J. Biol. Chem.* 277: 46632–46638 (2002).
18. Davis CD, Newman S. *Cancer Lett.* 159: 57–62 (2000).
19. Ogawa K *et al. Mutat. Res.* 539: 145–155 (2003).
20. Kawanishi S, Hiraku Y, Murata M, Oikawa S. *Free Radic. Biol. Med.* 32: 822–832 (2002).
21. Kawanishi S, Hiraku Y, Oikawa S. *Mutat. Res.* 488: 65–76 (2001).
22. Slaga TJ, Klein-Szanto AJ, Triplett LL, Yotti LP, Trosko KE. *Science* 213: 1023–1025 (1981).
23. Hiraku Y, Yamashaki M, Kawanishi S. *FEBS Lett.* 432: 13–16 (1998).
24. Hazlewood C, Davies MJ. *Arch. Biochem. Biophys.* 2: 79–91 (1996).
25. Ahmad A, Asad SF, Sing S, Hadi SM. *Cancer Lett.* 154: 29–37 (2000).
26. Johnson MA, Fischer JG, Kays SE. *Crit. Rev. Food Sci. Nutr.* 32: 1–31 (1992).
27. Iwamoto *et al. Arch. Biochem. Biophys.* 416: 155–163 (2003).

28. Eichhorn GI. *Inorganic Chemistry*. Elsevier, Amsterdam, 1975, pp. 1191–1243.
29. Pouskouleli G, Kourounakis P, Theophanides T. *Inorg. Chim. Acta* 18: 5–8 (1976).
30. Theophanides T. In: Theophanides T (ed.) *Infrared and Raman Spectroscopy of Biological Molecules*. D. Reidel Publishing Co, Dordrecht, 1979, pp. 185–204.
31. Makrigiannis G, Papagiannakopoulos P, Theophanides T. *Inorg. Chim. Acta*. 46: 263–269 (1980).
32. Tajmir-Riahi HA, Theophanides T. *Inorg. Chim. Acta*. 80: 223–230 (1983).
33. Theophanides T. *Int. J. Quantum Chem*. l. XXVI: 933–941 (1984).
34. Scherer E, Tajmir-Riahi HA, Theophanides T. *Inorg. Chim. Acta*. 92: 285–292 (1984).
35. Theophanides T, Tajmir-Riahi HA. In: Rentzepis PM, Capellos C (eds.) *Chemical Reaction Dynamics*. Mathematical and Physical Sciences 184, D. Ridel, Dordrecht, 1986, pp. 551–563.
36. Theophanides T, Anastassopoulou J. In: Schmid ED *et al.* (eds.) *Spectroscopy of Biological Molecules — New Advances*. John Willey & Sons Ltd, Chichester, 1988, pp. 433–438.
37. Theophanides T, Anastassopoulou J. In: La Mesa C *et al.* (eds.) *Equilibria in Soluzione, Aspetti Teorici, Sperimentali ed Applicitivi*. Mara Editore, Italy, 1988, pp. 122–140.
38. Theophanides T. In: Escribano R. (ed.) *Curso de Espectroscopia Infrarroja por Transformada de Fourier*. Escuela de Verano Universidad de Zaragoza, Jasa Huesca, 1989, pp. 257–270.
39. Theophanides T. In: Theophanides T (ed.) *Spectroscopy of Inorganic Bioactivators*, Vol. 280. Kluwer Academic Publishers, Dordrecht, 1989, pp. 265–272.
40. Yardley-Jones A, Anderson D, Parke DV. *Br. J. Ind. Med.* 48: 437–444 (1991).
41. Sørensen M, Skov H, Autrup H, Hertel O, Soft S. *Sci. Total Environ.* 309: 69–80 (2003).
42. Souĉek P, Filipcova P, Gut I. *Biochem. Pharmacol.* 27: 2333–2292 (1994).
43. Kowalówka-Zawieja J, Zielńska-Psuja B, Plewka A. *Toxicology* 188: 161–170 (2003).
44. Gabriel J *et al. Appl. Catal. B Environ.* 51: 157–162 (2004).
45. Vestergaard S, Loft S, Møller P. *Free Radic. Biol. Med.* 32: 481–484 (2002).
46. IARC Working Group. *Benzene in IARC Monographs on the Evaluation of Carcinogenic Risk of Chemicals and its Metabolism of Chemicals to Humans*, Suppl. 7. IARC, Lyon, 1987, pp. 120–122.
47. Kraus AL *et al. Regul. Toxicol. Pharmacol.* 21: 87–107 (1995).

48. Slaga TJ *et al. Science* 213: 1023–1024 (1988).
49. Hazlewood C, Davies MJ. *Arch. Biochem. Biophys.* 32: 79–91 (1996).
50. Messerschmidt A. *Struct. Bonding* 90: 37–68 (1998).
51. Sykes AG. *Adv. Inorg. Chem.* 36: 377–380 (1985).
52. Canters GW, Gilardi G. *FEBS Lett.* 325: 39 (1993).
53. Sykes AG. *Struct. Bonding* 75: 175–224 (1990).
54. Brewer GJ. *Expert Opin. Pharmacother.* 2: 1473–1477 (2001).
55. Cherian MG *et al. Toxicol. Appl. Pharmacol.* 126: 1–5 (1994).
56. Anastassopoulou J, Theophanides T, Paleos CM. In: Bertoluzza A *et al.* (eds.) *Spectroscopy of Biological Molecules — State of the Art.* Societa Editrice ESCULAPIO, Bologna, Italy, 1989, pp. 247–248.
57. Anastassopoulou J, Paleos CM, Theophanides T, Behnam V, Bertrand M. In: Bal W, Jezierski A (eds.) *Proceedings in II Symposium on Inorganic Biochemistry and Molecular Biophysics.* Wroclaw, 1989, pp. 13–18.
58. Anastassopoulou J, Alix A, Marx J, Paleos CM, Theophanides T. In: Anastassopoulou J *et al.* (eds.) *Metal Ions in Biology and Medicine*, Vol. 2 Libbey Eurotext, Paris, 1992, pp. 94–95.
59. Paleos CM, Tsiourvas D, Malliaris A, Anastassopoulou J, Theophanides T, In: Salahub D, Russo N (eds.) *Metal-Ligand Interactions: From Atoms, to Clusters, to Surfaces.* Kluwer Academic Publishers, Dordrecht, 1992, p. 397.
60. Anastassopoulou J *et al. J. Mol. Struct.* 415: 225–232 (1997).
61. Peppas E, Anastassopoulou J, Theophanides T. *J. Mol. Struct.* 559: 219 (2000).
62. Ragazos J, Anastassopoulou J, Theophanides T. In: Merlin JC, Turrell S, Huvenne JP (eds.) *Spectroscopy of Biological Molecules.* Kluwer Academic Publishers, 1995, pp. 153–154.
63. Roberfroid M, Calderon PB. *Free Radicals and Oxidation Phenomena in Biological Systems.* M. Dekker, Inc., New York, 1994, Chap. 5, pp. 193–236.
64. Solomon EI, Penfield KW, Wilcox DE. *Struct. Bonding* 53: 1–57 (1983).
65. Szilágyi I, Nagy G, Hernadi K, Ladádi I, Pálinkó I. *J. Mol. Struct. (Theochem).* 666–667; 451–445 (2003).
66. Harrison MD, Damerson CT. *J. Biochem. Mol. Toxicol.* 7: 64–69 (2001).
67. Waggoner DJ, Barthnika TB, Gitlin JD. *Neurobiol. Dis.* 6: 221–230 (1999).
68. Burkitt MJ. *Meth. Enzymol.* 234: 66–80 (1994).
69. Cerutti PAA. *Lancet* 344: 862–866 (1994).
70. Duran HA, de Rey BM. *Carcinogenesis* 12: 2047–2052 (1991).
71. Saucier MA, Wang X, Re RN, Brown J, Bryan SE. *J. Inorg. Chem.* 41: 117–124 (1991).
72. Midorikawa K, Kawanishi S. *FEBS Lett.* 495: 187–190 (2001).
73. Gelatashvili ES, Sigua KI, Sapojnikova NA. *Biochemistry* 70: 207–210 (1998).

74. Liang Q, Dedon PC. *Chem. Res. Toxicol.* 14: 416–422 (2001).
75. Liender MC. *Mutat. Res.* 475: 141–152 (2001).
76. de Hartog GJM, Haenen GRMM, Vegt E, van der Vijgh WJF, Bast A. *Chem. Biol. Interact.* 145: 33–39 (2003).
77. Strausak D, Mercer JF, Dieter HH, Stremmel W, Multhaup G. *Brain Res. Bull.* 55: 175–185 (2001).
78. Kinnula VL, Crapo JD. *Free Radic. Biol. Med.* 36: 718–744 (2004).
79. Wu T, Sempos C, Freudenheim JL, Muti P, Smit E. *Ann. Epidemiol.* 14: 195–201 (2004).
80. Oikawa S, Yamada K, Yamashita N, Tada-Oikawa S, Kawanishi S. *Carcinogenesis* 20: 1485–1490 (1999).
81. Anastassopoulou J. In: Theophanides T (ed.) *Spectroscopy of Inorganic Bioactivators*. D. Reidel Publishing Co, Dordrecht, 1989, pp. 273–276.
82. Anastassopoulou J, *Magnes. Res.* 5: 101–105 (1992).
83. Anastassopoulou J, In: Russo N, Anastassopoulou J, Barone M (eds.) *Topics in Molecular Organization and Engineering-Properties and Chemistry of Biomolecular Systems*. Kluwer Academic Publishers, Dordrecht, 1994, pp. 23–28.
84. Overvad K *et al. Am. J. Epidemiol.* 137: 409–414 (1993).

29 Arsenic, Oxidative Stress, and Carcinogenesis

Michael F. Hughes and Kirk T. Kitchin

1. Background

The metalloid arsenic is a natural contaminant of air, water, soil, and food. Arsenic is also used in many commercial, industrial, and medicinal products. For example, arsenic is used in semiconductors, as a pesticide, and as a chemotherapeutic agent. Thus, the sources of exposure to arsenic are both natural and anthropogenic. Concern over exposure to arsenic has increased, because of its pervasiveness in the environment and its human carcinogenicity. A major public health problem is the contamination by inorganic arsenic (iAs) of groundwater that is the primary source of drinking water for many populations worldwide including Bangladesh, India, and Mexico.[1,2] The mechanism of action of arsenic-induced carcinogenicity is, however, not known. A definitive understanding of this mechanism will reduce the uncertainty in the risk assessment for this metalloid and aid in setting cost-effective exposure limits.

Although arsenic exposure causes cancer in humans, it is used to treat certain forms of cancer. Arsenic trioxide has been recently used to treat human acute promyelocytic leukemia with great success.[3] Arsenic can induce many biological effects, among them apoptosis in some situations, and this may be the mechanism of its anti-leukemic effect.

Arsenic and its role in environmental and human health has recently been reviewed by the International Agency for Research on Cancer (IARC),[4] World Health Organization,[5] and the National Research Council of the

United States of America.[6,7] Shorter reviews on various aspects of arsenic include those on exposures of arsenic throughout the world,[1] arsenicals in the environment,[8] metabolism of arsenic,[9–12] toxicity, genotoxicity, and carcinogenicity of arsenic,[1,13–15] the effect of arsenic on molecular mechanism such as signal transduction pathways[16–19] and heat shock response,[20] and human risks.[21]

1.1. *Chemistry and structure*

More than 200 arsenic compounds have been identified in the environment and many of these are bound to sulfur and iron in soil. Arsenic exists in inorganic and organic forms and in different oxidation states. The oxidation states of arsenic are −III, 0, III, and V. In the case of arsenic in drinking water, the arsenicals of interest include arsenate (iAs^V, $As^V(O)O_3^{3-}$) and arsenite (iAs^{III}, $As^{III}O_3^{3-}$). These arsenicals are metabolized to monomethylarsonic acid ($MMAs^V$, $CH_3As^V(O)(OH)_2$), monomethylarsonous acid ($MMAs^{III}$, $CH_3As^{III}(OH)_2$), dimethylarsinic acid ($DMAs^V$, $(CH_3)_2As^V(O)OH$)), dimethylarsinous acid ($DMAs^{III}$, $(CH_3)_2As^{III}OH$)), and trimethylarsine oxide ($TMAs^VO$, $(CH_3)_3As^V(O)$)). Arsenate is an oxyanion and is chemically similar to phosphate. At physiological pH, the pentavalent arsenicals are ionized, whereas the trivalent arsenicals are essentially unionized. The difference between the ionization potential of the pentavalent and trivalent arsenicals impacts their cellular uptake and perhaps their toxic effects.

1.2. *Metabolism of arsenic*

The mammalian metabolism of iAs has an important role in its eventual disposition and potential toxicological effects.[9–12] Arsenic is metabolized by a sequential two-electron reduction of pentavalent arsenic and the oxidative methylation of trivalent arsenic. The metabolism of iAs^V and iAs^{III} follows the basic scheme shown below:

$$iAs^V + 2e^- \rightarrow iAs^{III} + CH_3^+ \rightarrow MMAs^V + 2e^- \rightarrow MMAs^{III} + CH_3^+ \rightarrow DMAs^V + 2e^- \rightarrow DMAs^{III} + CH_3^+ \rightarrow TMAs^VO$$

The reduction of pentavalent arsenic can occur non-enzymatically with thiols such as glutathione.[22,23] Recently, it has been reported[24,25] that purine nucleotide phosphorylase catalyzes the *in vitro* reduction of iAs^{V}. This enzyme, however, does not appear to have a significant role in iAs^{V} reduction *in vivo*.[26] An $MMAs^{V}$ reductase has been partially purified from human liver and is from the omega class of glutathione *S*-transferase.[27] A methyltransferase catalyzes the oxidative methylation of trivalent arsenic to pentavalent methylated arsenic. The enzyme requires as cofactors a thiol and *S*-adenosylmethionine. Arsenic methyltransferases have been partially purified from rabbit, hamster, and rhesus monkey liver.[28–31] From rat liver, Lin *et al.*[32] isolated an As^{III} methyltransferase that catalyzes the methylation of iAs^{III} to $DMAs^{V}$. This enzyme also methylates $MMAs^{III}$. The cDNA sequence analysis of this enzyme shows it has a high degree of homology with the human arsenic (+3 oxidation state) methyltransferase.

Once iAs is absorbed *in vivo*, it is rapidly methylated and excreted in the urine by most mammalian species. $DMAs^{V}$ is the primary metabolite of iAs excreted, but the other trivalent and pentavalent inorganic and organic arsenicals are also eliminated but in smaller amounts. Differences in the disposition of iAs exist between and within mammalian species.[9,12] For example, guinea pigs and the marmoset and rhesus monkeys do not methylate iAs.[9] The rat is unique in that it rapidly methylates iAs, but retains arsenic longer than other species. Rat erythrocytes have a greater uptake and accumulation of $DMAs^{III}$ than the erythrocytes of other species.[33] Humans tend to excrete more MMAs (both III and V) and less DMAs than other species. This has fostered the interpretation that MMAs accounts for the increased human sensitivity toward the toxic effects of arsenic. There also appears to be a variation in methylation of iAs among several human populations.[9,12]

1.3. *Toxicity of arsenic*

The oxidation state of arsenic is the most important determinant of its toxic effect. The trivalent forms of arsenic are more potent than the pentavalent forms. For example, the acute toxicity of iAs^{III} in the mouse is more than twofold greater than iAs^{V} (8 versus 22 mg As/kg).[34] Humans appear to be more sensitive to the acute toxicity of iAs. The LD_{50} of iAs in humans is 1–3 mg As/kg.[35]

The mechanism of the toxic effect of iAs^{III} has been thought to involve its binding to critical thiol groups in proteins and altering their function. Trivalent arsenicals react directly with thiol groups.[22,23] But there may be a role for oxidative stress in arsenic-induced toxicity. Human fibroblasts are more sensitive to the toxicity of iAs^{III} *in vitro* than Chinese hamster ovary cells.[36,37] The hamster cells have higher levels of glutathione peroxidase and catalase than the fibroblasts, suggesting a role for reactive oxygen species (ROS) in arsenic-induced toxicity.[37]

A recent paper by Samikkannu *et al.*[38] lends further support for a role of oxidative stress in arsenic toxicity. The activity of pyruvate dehydrogenase (PDH), which contains a critical vicinal dithiol, was inhibited by iAs^{III} to a greater extent in HL60 cells than purified PDH. Phenylarsine oxide, a trivalent organic arsenical, showed higher reactivity with vicinal dithiols within the cells than iAs^{III}. Hydrogen peroxide was produced in the cells by iAs^{III}, but not by phenylarsine oxide. Exogenously added antioxidants, but not dithiols, reduced the PDH inhibitory effect of iAs^{III} in the cells. In contrast, the inhibitory effect of PDH by phenylarsine oxide was reduced by dithiols, but not antioxidants. Samikkannu *et al.*[38] suggested that iAs^{III} generates ROS, which inhibit PDH and potentially other important proteins. PDH inhibition occurs at levels of arsenic much lower than required if the mechanism was by direct binding of arsenic to critical thiol groups.

Phosphate may be replaced by iAs^{V} in *in vitro* biochemical reactions.[15] Arsenolysis, the uncoupling of ATP formation by iAs^{V}, may occur at the substrate level during glycolysis, and at the mitochondrial level during oxidative phosphorylation. Whether this occurs *in vivo* is not known. However, in rabbit and human erythrocytes, iAs^{V} but not iAs^{III} reduces cellular ATP levels.[39,40] The inability of cells to generate ATP because of arsenolysis would lead to a toxic event.

The methylation of arsenic has generally been regarded a detoxication reaction. This premise was based on the evidence that the primary metabolites of iAs, pentavalent methylated arsenicals, are not retained in tissues, are rapidly excreted (by most species), and have lower acute toxicity than iAs. However, the view that the methylation of arsenic is solely a detoxication reaction has changed. Trivalent methylated arsenicals, once thought at best to be fleeting intermediates of arsenic metabolism, have been detected in urine of individuals exposed to iAs.[41,42] $MMAs^{III}$ and $DMAs^{III}$ are potent toxicants *in vitro* and *in vivo*. $MMAs^{III}$ was more cytotoxic than iAs^{III} to rat and human cells, while $DMAs^{III}$ was as potent as iAs^{III}.[43] $MMAs^{III}$ has a lower ip LD_{50} than iAs^{III} in the hamster.[44] Thus, the methylation of arsenic may be a double-edge sword, in that oxidative methylation of trivalent arsenic decreases its toxicity and facilitates its excretion, but the reduction of methylated pentavalent arsenic enhances its toxic effect.

1.4. *Carcinogenicity of arsenic*

1.4.1. *Human*

Inorganic arsenic is classified by the IARC and the US Environmental Protection Agency (US EPA) as a human carcinogen. This classification is primarily based on the results of epidemiology studies of populations exposed to iAs via inhalation or ingestion of drinking water contaminated with iAs. There is an association between occupational inhalation exposure of iAs to copper smelter workers[45] and arsenic pesticide manufacturers and lung cancer mortality.[46,47] Chronic exposure to iAs in drinking water can result in the development of cancer.[4–7] Studies from Taiwan[48,49] showed there was a high prevalence of skin cancer in a population that ingested iAs-contaminated drinking water from artesian wells. Additional studies of the Taiwanese and other populations have reported that internal cancer (bladder, lung, kidney) can develop after chronic ingestion of iAs-contaminated drinking water.[50,51] The US EPA recently lowered the arsenic drinking water standard in the United States from 50 to 10 μg/l after a re-evaluation[6,7] of the Taiwanese epidemiological and other data.

1.4.2. *Animal*

Many of the initial studies that investigated the carcinogenicity of iAs in animal models gave negative or equivocal results. These studies entailed long-term exposure to iAs either in the drinking water or diet of rodents and dogs, or continuous oral administration to primates.[15] In the 1980s, several studies reported the development of lung tumors in rats after intratracheal administration of iAs.[15] But the high mortality and the method of administration of arsenic in these studies have raised questions on the relevancy of these results.

More recent studies have examined the carcinogenicity of $DMAs^{V}$ in drinking water[52,53] and $MMAs^{V}$ in the diet[54] or drinking water[55] in rodents. Only $DMAs^{V}$ in the ppm dose range was carcinogenic, with development of bladder tumors in rats.

Other investigators have used genetically modified animals to study arsenic-induced carcinogenicity. K6/ODC transgenic mice, which overexpress ornithine decarboxylase in the skin, develop skin tumors after drinking water exposure to iAs^{III}, $DMAs^{V}$[56] or $MMAs^{III}$ (Chen *et al.*, unpublished). TG.AC mice, which have a mutated v-Ha-*ras* oncogene and are a model for genetically initiated skin, develop skin tumors after exposure to iAs^{III} in drinking water followed by a period of dermal application of 12-*O*-tetradecanoylphorbol-13-acetate (TPA).[57] No evidence of organ-specific tumors in p53 heterozygous (+/−) knockout or wild-type C57BL/6J mice was observed after long-term exposure to $DMAs^{V}$ in drinking water.[58] However, in both strains of $DMAs^{V}$-exposed mice, nonorgan-specific tumors (primarily malignant lymphomas) appeared earlier than in non-treated mice of both strains. There was also a significant increase in the tumor multiplicity in the high dose group of the knockout mice and a significant increase in the incidence and multiplicity of tumors in the $DMAs^{V}$-exposed wild-type mice.

Arsenic is a transplacental carcinogen in mice. Pregnant C3H mice were exposed to iAs^{III} in drinking water from gestation days 8 to 18.[59] After birth, the offspring received no additional treatment. Liver and adrenal tumors developed in male offspring in a dose-related manner, while similar results were observed in the ovaries and lungs of female offspring. Other offspring of iAs^{III}-exposed mice were topically treated with TPA.[60] Tumors were promoted in the liver of male offspring and lungs in the offspring of both sexes.

Arsenic is a cocarcinogen for mouse skin.[61] Mice exposed to iAs^{III} in drinking water (10 ppm) for 26 weeks and ultraviolet (UV) radiation had a greater than twofold increase in the number of tumors compared to mice exposed to UV radiation alone. The tumors that developed were primarily squamous cell carcinomas and in the co-exposed group the tumors appeared earlier and were more invasive than the tumors of mice exposed only to UV radiation. Mice exposed only to iAs^{III} did not develop tumors.

$DMAs^V$ is a multi-organ tumor promoter in rodents.[14,15,62] In rats, tumors in bladder, kidney, liver, and thyroid gland are promoted by $DMAs^V$ administered in drinking water in initiation-promotion assays. In mice, tumors in lung and skin are promoted by $DMAs^V$. Rat hepatic preneoplastic positive foci (glutathione *S*-transferase placental form) are induced by $MMAs^V$, $DMAs^V$, and $TMAs^VO$.[63] In K6/ODC transgenic mice, $DMAs^V$ promotes skin tumor development after initiation of the skin with a topical application of 7,12-dimethylbenz[*a*]anthracene.[64]

1.4.3. *Mechanism of arsenic-induced carcinogenicity*

Despite a large body of peer-reviewed literature on the subject, the mechanism of arsenic-induced carcinogenicity is not known.[4–7,14,15] Several theories have been proposed, because of the reactive arsenic species that are formed *in vivo* and the number of organs and biochemical systems affected by arsenic. More than one mechanism may operate and some of these mechanisms may work together. The proposed mechanisms of arsenic-induced carcinogenicity include genotoxicity, inhibition of DNA repair, altered DNA methylation, cell proliferation (altered growth signals), and oxidative stress. The remainder of this chapter will focus on the evidence that supports the role of oxidative stress in arsenic-induced carcinogenicity.

2. Oxidative Stress Induced by Arsenic

2.1. *Detection of radicals — in vitro*

Some of the most convincing evidence that arsenic is an oxidative stressor is the detection of radical species by electron spin resonance (ESR) spectroscopy *in vitro* and *in vivo* in the presence of arsenic. Oxygenated radicals adducted to the spin trap 5-5-dimethyl-1-pyrroline-*N*-oxide (DMPO) have been detected *in vitro* with $DMAs^V$ and $DMAs^{III}$[65,66] and in human–hamster hybrid cells[67] and porcine endothelial cells[68] exposed to iAs^{III}. Pretreatment of the cells with superoxide dismutase (SOD) inhibited arsenic-induced formation of the radical adduct, suggesting that superoxide anion is formed and then is converted to the hydroxyl radical.

Fluorescent probes such as 2′,7′-dichlorofluoroscein diacetate are used to assess the formation of oxidants. The probes can pass through cell membranes and are oxidized by ROS to a fluorescent form that can be detected and quantified. Human,[69] human–hamster hybrid,[67] and Chinese hamster ovary cells[70] incubated with iAs^{III} and fluorescent probes show an increased intensity of fluorescence with increased dose of arsenic. These radicals are detected within 5 minutes of treatment with arsenic, showing the rapidity of the formation of the ROS within the cells. The fluorescence was inhibited by the antioxidant butylated hydroxytoluene and the free radical scavenger dimethyl sulfoxide that were added along with arsenic. Gurr *et al.*[70] reported that nitric oxide synthase inhibitors decreased the intracellular level of iAs^{III}-induced oxidants. This suggests that reactive nitrogen species are also formed in the presence of arsenic.

2.2. *Detection of radicals — in vivo*

The formation of the hydroxy radical, detected via formation of the 2,3-hydroxybenzoic acid adduct from sodium salicylate, was observed in the striatum of female and male rats exposed to iAs^{III}.[71] This was accomplished by inserting a microdialysis probe into awake and freely moving rats, and then infusing iAs^{III} (100 μM) into the brain. Microdialysis samples were collected and analyzed by liquid chromatography and electrochemical detection. A significant increase in the concentration of 2,3-dihydroxybenzoic acid was observed in both female (by 112%) and male (by 49%) rats infused with iAs^{III}. Interestingly, female rats had a higher basal level of 2,3-dihydroxybenzoic acid formation than did male rats (92 versus 59 pmol/ml). The noted increase in 2,3-dihydroxybenzoic acid varied considerably among animals in a particular treatment group as well as between treatment groups. The formation of the adduct was not attributed to any cell type within the brain. There was also no dose–response relationship, as all doses of administered iAs^{III} gave the same response (approximately 100% of control levels). This unique study provides direct evidence that iAs^{III} exposure increased the formation of hydroxy radical *in vivo*.

2.3. *Oxidative DNA damage*

The lesions 8-oxo-2′-deoxyguanosine (8-oxodG)[72] and 8-hydroxy-2′-deoxyguanosine (8-OHdG),[73] biomarkers for oxidative stress, are observed in DNA isolated from cells *in vitro*, rodents and humans exposed to arsenic. Arsenic-exposed rodents excrete these oxidative lesions in urine. The presence of these lesions may lead to base-pair substitutions (G to T and A to C)[74] during DNA synthesis. These lesions may arise from arsenic which generates ROS that damage DNA. Alternatively, arsenic may interfere with the systems that protect against the oxidative lesions forming or their repair. The oxidative DNA lesions may also form by a photooxidation process that does not involve ROS.[75]

2.3.1. *In vitro*

In human–hamster hybrid cells incubated with iAs^{III}, there is a dose-dependent formation of 8-OHdG, indicating oxidative DNA damage was being induced.[76] The induction of 8-OHdG by iAs^{III} in these cells is reduced during the concurrent exposure to catalase or SOD, suggesting the involvement of H_2O_2 or superoxide anion.

2.3.2. *In vivo — animal*

Mice (ddY male) administered an equimolar acute oral dose of $DMAs^V$ or iAs^{III} show an increase in urinary 8-oxodG levels.[77] The levels increased significantly with administered dose of $DMAs^V$. The levels observed with iAs^{III} were slightly elevated over control, but were not significantly different. In this same study, $DMAs^V$ was given to mice at a dose of 400 ppm in their drinking water for 4 weeks. This dose promotes tumors in mouse lung. A significant increase in 8-oxodG levels was observed in the lungs and liver of the male mice and skin of female hairless mice.

$DMAs^V$ administered orally to rats over 4 weeks induced 8-OHdG formation in kidney, but the increase was not dose-dependent.[78] Maximum induction was observed at 10 mg/kg, but decreased at the higher concentration of 20 mg/kg.

2.3.3. *In vivo — human*

Samples of skin neoplasm and keratosis from individuals exposed to iAs and individuals not exposed to iAs but afflicted with Bowen's disease (a form of intraepidermal carcinoma) were examined by immunohistochemistry for oxidative DNA damage.[79] In skin samples of individuals exposed to iAs, 22 out of the 28 (78%) were 8-OHdG positive. Only one out of 11 Bowen's disease samples (9%) from the individuals not exposed to iAs gave a positive reaction with the 8-OHdG antibody. In addition, in the iAs-exposed group, four out of five deparaffined skin tumor samples tested showed detectable levels of arsenic by neutron activation analysis.

In another study,[80] 28 out of 28 skin tumors from individuals exposed to iAs stained positively with a 8-oxodG monoclonal antibody. The skin tumors were collected from an area of China that has a long history of non-ferrous metal production and arsenic exposures were from air, soil, drinking water, and mining activities. The tumor types included 17 squamous cell carcinomas and 11 basal cell epitheliomas. In arsenic-unrelated skin tumor samples, the positive staining rate was three out of 20 samples. Interestingly, in all arsenic exposed subjects every keratosis and normal skin sample stained positively for 8-oxodG.

2.4. *Signal transduction and gene expression*

Arsenic activates several signal transduction pathways that regulate gene expression.[16–19,81] In these multi-component pathways, such as the phosphorylation cascade involving mitogen-activated protein kinases, extracellular signals are transmitted into the cell that responds in some manner. In the nucleus, the response may be the binding of a regulatory protein, called a transcription factor, to a specific DNA site. The DNA sequence regulated by the transcription factor is then transcribed. This process is called transcriptional activation. Transcription factors that are activated by arsenic include activator protein-1 (AP-1), nuclear factor kappa B (NF-κB), and NF-E2-related factor-2 (Nrf2).[82–87] AP-1 and NF-κB have roles in cell proliferation, differentiation, and transformation, events that encompass carcinogenesis. Antioxidant responses of the cell are influenced by Nrf2.

Transcriptional activation of genes is a tightly controlled process and is influenced by the oxidation state of the cell.[88] Polyphenols found in tea, which are antioxidants, inhibit iAs^{III}-induced AP-1 transcriptional activity and AP-1 DNA binding activity.[89] The expression of Nrf2, which regulates genes that respond to oxidative stress, is enhanced by arsenic with the involvement of H_2O_2.[90]

2.5. *Stress proteins*

A number of proteins, termed stress proteins, are induced by arsenic. These proteins include metallothionein, ubiquitin, heme oxygenase, and heat shock proteins (from 27 to 110 kDa).[20] Many of these proteins are constitutively expressed at low levels to maintain cellular homeostasis and the protein induction is an adaptive response to a stressor. The induced stress proteins protect and repair susceptible protein targets and assist in DNA repair.

Heme oxygenase, which exists in three forms, is an inducible stress proteins. *In vitro* studies with human skin fibroblasts showed that heme oxygenase is induced by iAs^{III}, UVa radiation, and H_2O_2.[91] In addition, the induction of this protein by iAs^{III} in these cells is inhibited by the oxygen radical scavengers sodium azide and dimethyl sulfoxide.[69] Heme oxygenase-1 (HO-1), the major isoform of the enzyme that breaks down heme into biliverdin, carbon monoxide, and Fe, is induced more effectively by iAs^{III} than iAs^{V}, and not at all by $MMAs^{V}$ or $DMAs^{V}$.[92] Rodents administered iAs^{III} that had the highest levels of hepatic iAs also had the greatest induction of hepatic HO-1.[93,94] The induction occurs within 2 h after exposure to iAs^{III}. HO-1 tissue levels fall as the tissue levels of iAs also decline.

2.6. *Apoptosis*

Arsenic can induce apoptosis, programmed cell death, in many cell types.[81] Arsenite induces apoptosis in Chinese hamster ovary cells by a mechanism that appears to involve the generation of H_2O_2.[95] In NIH3T3 cells, iAs^{III}, but not iAs^{V}, increased intracellular peroxide levels.[96] Only iAs^{III} was able to induce apoptosis in these cells. Antioxidants such as *N*-acetylcysteine and polyphenols found in tea, catalase, and the spin trap DMPO can prevent iAs^{III}-induced apoptosis *in vitro*.[95–99] In mouse epidermal JB6 cells, the induction of apoptosis may involve activation of AP-1 transcription and DNA binding activity.[97] Selective inhibitors of this signal transduction pathway inhibited iAs^{III}-induced apoptosis in these cells. The dose of arsenic is critical in initiating apoptosis. At low submicromolar doses of arsenic, telomerase activity, which maintains chromosomal telomere length and thereby preserves chromosomal stability, is increased.[99] Thus, cell proliferation may occur. At mid-micromolar doses of arsenic, telomerase activity is decreased, leading to chromosomal instability and apoptosis is induced.[98,99]

2.7. *Biochemical indicators of oxidative stress*

2.7.1. *In vitro*

In human fibroblasts, iAs^{III} modulates cellular antioxidant defense mechanisms.[69] The levels of glutathione, measured 24 h after exposure of iAs^{III} (5 μM) to the cells, was significantly increased. The increased glutathione may be a mechanism of cellular protection. The activities of superoxide dismutase and catalase were significantly increased and decreased, respectively. Glutathione peroxidase activity was significantly decreased at the highest dose (10 μM).

2.7.2. *In vivo — animal*

Animals administered arsenic in their drinking water for extended periods show biochemical signs of oxidative stress. Male Wistar rats exposed to iAs^{III} (100 ppm) (1–4 months) have elevated levels of lipid peroxide, decreased levels of non-enzymatic antioxidants (e.g., reduced glutathione), and decreased activity of antioxidant enzymes (e.g., SOD) compared to control rats.[100,101] These biochemical indicators of oxidative stress were observed in blood, brain, kidney, and liver of iAs^{III}-exposed rats. The oxidative stress can be lessened, but not completely, by treating the animals with antioxidants (ascorbic acid, α-tocopherol) or chemical antagonists (*N*-acetylcysteine, meso-2,3-dimercaptosuccinic acid) that bind arsenic. However, treatment with antioxidants, antagonists, or their combination, will further improve the oxidative stress in the tissue.

There is a clear temporal pattern of increasing oxidative stress in mice exposed to arsenic. Male mice were administered water from a well in India that contained 3.2 ppm arsenic.[102,103] Several members of a family that had ingested this water exhibited clinical features of arsenic toxicity. After 2 months of arsenic exposure, there was a pattern of compensatory response in the mice to the initial oxidative stress (increased hepatic glutathione, glucose-6-phosphate dehydrogenase, glutathione reductase, and glutathione peroxidase). However, by 4–6 months of arsenic exposure, only glutathione reductase activity was elevated, while the hepatic glutathione concentration and activities of glutathione peroxidase and glucose-6-phosphate dehydrogenase were significantly decreased. By 9 months of arsenic exposure, increased thiobarbituric acid reactive substances (TBARS) and decreased catalase activity became evident. By 12 months of arsenic exposure, hepatic toxicity became evident. Of the 16 study parameters, only one (total serum protein) remained unchanged throughout the full time course of the arsenic exposure.

2.7.3. *In vivo — human*

Humans exposed to elevated levels of arsenic in drinking water (>400 ppb) show signs of oxidative stress in blood cells.[87,104] Some of the individuals exposed to high levels of arsenic in these studies displayed signs of arsenic toxicity, including skin and vascular disorders. Human serum TBARS was positively correlated with total serum arsenic and inversely correlated with whole blood non-protein sulfhydryl.[87] Whole blood showed a positive correlation with reactive oxidants in plasma and an inverse relationship with the level of plasma antioxidant capacity.[104] There was no significant association between levels of plasma reactive oxidants and antioxidant capacity.

3. Arsenic-Induced Oxidative Stress and Cancer

Cancer is a multi-event process that can take many years to develop. To better understand this process, the pathogenesis of cancer has been classified into three stages, initiation, promotion, and progression.[105] Initiation is the process whereby DNA in a somatic cell is irreversibly mutated. During promotion, there is clonal expansion of the initiated cell. Progression refers to the malignant conversion of the clonally expanded cells into higher states of malignancy and is characterized by karyotypic instability. Oxidative stress may have a role in each of these three stages in the development of cancer.[106–108] Because arsenic is carcinogenic, and there is evidence that it is an oxidative stressor, one of the proposed mechanisms of arsenic-induced carcinogenicity is oxidative stress.[109]

3.1. *Initiation*

Arsenic is not a point mutagen as are many of the classical carcinogens such as the nitrosamines and polycyclic aromatic hydrocarbons. In most standard mutagenicity assays that test for point mutations, the results with arsenic are negative.[13] However, arsenic induces DNA damage such as strand breaks and DNA–protein crosslinks *in vitro* and *in vivo*.[13] Large deletion mutations are observed in human–hamster hybrid cells incubated with iAs^{III}.[67,76,110] Arsenic induces chromosomal aberrations, sister chromatid exchanges (SCE), and formation of micronuclei. In addition, arsenic is a co-mutagen, enhancing the effect of several known mutagens including methyl methanesulfonate[111] and UV radiation.[112] The lack of a point mutagenic effect of arsenic has raised questions whether or not arsenic is an initiator. However, it is clear that arsenic is genotoxic,[13] which may lead to an initiating event. In addition, $DMAs^{V}$ is a complete carcinogen in rat bladder,[52,53] which suggests that this arsenical has initiating activity.

3.1.1. *In vitro genotoxicity and oxidative stress*

A role for ROS in arsenic-mediated genotoxicty was suggested by Nordenson and Beckman,[109] who observed that superoxide dismutase decreased the number of SCE in cultured human lymphocytes induced by iAs^{III}. Catalase also decreased the number of sister chromatid exchanges in one of two experiments.

Trivalent methylated arsenicals damage DNA with the involvement of ROS. In the phage X174 DNA nicking assay, it appears that ROS are the intermediates in the DNA nicking ability of $MMAs^{III}$ and $DMAs^{III}$.[66] The pentavalent arsenicals iAs^{V}, $MMAs^{V}$, and $DMAs^{V}$ did not nick DNA.[110,111]

$DMAs^{III}$ damages DNA *in vitro* by a proposed dimethylated arsenic peroxide intermediate, forming *cis*-thymine glycol.[112] From experiments with $^{18}O_2$, it was proposed that $DMAs^{III}$ reacts with molecular oxygen to form a dimethylated arsenic peroxide. One oxygen of the peroxide reacts with thymine to form thymine 5,6-epoxide while the other stays with $DMAs^{III}$ to form $DMAs^{V}$. The thymine epoxide is then hydrolyzed to *cis*-thymine glycol.

Induction of micronuclei by iAs^{III} was greater in a Chinese hamster ovary (CHO) cell line (XRS-5) that had five- to sixfold lower levels of catalase and glutathine peroxidase than parental CHO cells.[95,113] The addition of catalase and glutathione peroxidase to the XRS-5 cells in the presence of iAs^{III} decreased the formation of micronuclei in these cells. This implicates H_2O_2 in having a role in the induction of micronuclei in these iAs^{III}-treated cells.

While not a point mutagen, iAs^{III} is a gene and chromosomal mutagen in human-hybrid cells.[67,114] Intragenic and multi-locus mutations, primarily large multi-locus deletions, occur in the hybrid cells treated with iAs^{III}. The effect is dose-dependent and is reduced when the cells are concurrently treated with the radical scavenger dimethyl sulfoxide. The genotoxic effect is increased when the cells are pretreated with buthionine *S–R* sulfoximine, which depletes non-protein sulfhydryls, primarily GSH, within the cells.

3.1.2. *In vivo genotoxicity and oxidative stress*

DNA single-strand breaks are detected in the lung of mice administered $DMAs^{V}$.[115] These breaks are not found in other tissues of mice and occur approximately 12 h after the administration of $DMAs^{V}$. Based on results from *in vitro* experiments in this same study, the authors suggested that $DMAs^{V}$ was metabolized to dimethylarsine, which further reacted with molecular oxygen to form a dimethylarsenic peroxyl radical. This peroxyl radical then interacted with the DNA to induce the single strand breaks.

Garlic and mustard oil have been reported to have biological effects including antioxidant properties. Therefore, these two agents were examined as possible antagonists to arsenic-induced micronuclei in mouse bone marrow. Antagonism of arsenic-induced micronuclei was demonstrated for both garlic[116] and mustard oil.[117] This experimental result of antagonism could have occurred via either chelation of trivalent arsenicals or by inhibition of arsenic-induced oxidative stress.

3.2. *Promotion*

Of the three classifications of the pathogenesis of cancer, most of the current evidence supports arsenic as a promoter, with the involvement of oxidative stress. Prooxidant states within cells are induced by tumor promoters,[105] and there is ample evidence that arsenic is an oxidative stressor. Tumor promoters modulate the antioxidant systems of cells,[105] and this occurs with arsenic as observed in rodents and humans in its modulation of antioxidants such as glutathione and antioxidant enzymes such as SOD. Ornithine decarboxylase, the rate-limiting enzyme in polyamine biosynthesis and a marker for promotion, is induced by iAs^{III} and $DMAs^{V}$ in rat liver.[118,119] There is a strong correlation between the inherent capacity of tumor-promoting compounds to induce ODC and their tumor-promoting ability.[105] While there is minimal evidence that iAs^{III} is a promoter, there is an extensive amount of evidence that its primary metabolite, $DMAs^{V}$, is a multi-organ tumor promoter.

Promotion involves the expansion or proliferation of initiated cells. Arsenic induces cellular proliferation, and this may occur by mitogenesis or cellular toxicity followed by regeneration. Cohen and colleagues[120–122] propose that the hyperplasia induced in rat urinary bladder by dietary $DMAs^{V}$ is a non-DNA reactive event and is due to cellular toxicity followed by regeneration. It is not known what causes the cellular toxicity, but it may be due to arsenic-induced oxidative stress.

In rats exposed to $DMAs^{V}$ in their drinking water, there is a significant increase in the 2-bromo-2′-deoxyuridine labeling index, a measure of cellular proliferation, in morphologically normal bladder epithelium.[53] Cyclooxygenase-2 and 8-OHdG, markers of oxidative stress, were significantly increased in the bladder of the treated rats. Rats administered $TMAs^{V}O$ in their drinking water have a higher incidence of hepatic adenomas than control rats.[122] The development of these tumors was associated with a significantly higher level of 8-OHdG and proliferating cell nuclear antigen (PCNA) in liver of treated (200 ppm) than control animals. Increased PCNA is indicative of cellular proliferation. Thus, in rats exposed to arsenic, there are results associating tumor development with oxidative stress and cellular proliferation.

3.3. *Progression*

Progression is the least understood of the three classifications, particularly with arsenic-induced carcinogenesis. Tumor initiators have a role in the malignant conversion of tumors[124] and arsenic may have initiating activity. $DMAs^{V}$ is a complete carcinogen in rat urinary bladder.[52,53] This conversion may occur by a clastogenic effect, in the chromosomal region of a tumor suppressor gene or a protooncogene. The tumor suppressor gene $p27^{kip1}$ is downregulated in papillomas and transitional cell carcinomas of urinary bladder of rats exposed to $DMAs^{V}$ in their drinking water.[53] Arsenic is a clastogen, and the most potent forms for this effect *in vitro* appear to be $MMAs^{III}$ and $DMAs^{III}$.[125] As described previously, ROS may have a role in this genotoxic event, and the chromosomal damage may lead to the progression of the initiated cell in the body to a cancerous state.

4. Potential Mechanism of Arsenic-Induced Oxidative Stress

Just as the mechanism of arsenic-induced carcinogenicity is not known, the same dilemma exists for the mechanism of arsenic-induced oxidative stress. As with the carcinogenicity of arsenic, there are several potential mechanisms for ROS formation by arsenic and more than one mechanism may be effective.

4.1. *Redox cycling*

Unlike forms of iron and copper that undergo redox cycling, the pentavalent and trivalent forms of arsenic differ by two electrons. If arsenic undergoes redox cycling, the mechanism of transfer of electrons to oxygen is probably different from what occurs with iron and copper. In the review by Del Razo *et al.*,[20] it was proposed that the spontaneous oxidation of iAs^{III} to iAs^{V} is an exergonic reaction and that under physiological conditions H_2O_2 is formed. However, this may be a futile cycle, because the H_2O_2 formed in the reaction would oxidize iAs^{III} to iAs^{V}. Alternatively, molecular oxygen (about 0.25 mM *in vivo*) drives trivalent arsenicals to pentavalency;

glutathione (about 2 mM in many organs) and similar reducing agents drive pentavalent arsenicals to trivalency.

4.2. *Formation of arsine*

Yamanaka and Okada[131] proposed that dimethylarsine is formed in mice administered $DMAs^V$. The expired air of mice administered $DMAs^V$ (1.5 gm/kg) was passed through a solution of 5% H_2O_2, which would oxidize expired arsines. Analysis of this solution showed the presence of a small amount of $DMAs^V$, indicating that the mice expired dimethylarsine. These investigators propose that the DNA strand breaking ability of $DMAs^V$, which occurs *in vitro* and *in vivo*, begins with the reduction of $DMAs^V$ to dimethylarsine. An electron is transferred from dimethylarsine to molecular oxygen, forming a dimethylarsenic radical, superoxide anion, and a positive hydrogen ion. The dimethylarsenic radical then reacts with molecular oxygen to form a peroxyl radical. A dimethyl arsenic peroxyl radical, adducted to the spin trap DMPO, was detected by ESR in an incubation of dimethylarsine with molecular oxygen.[119] This peroxyl radical may have toxicological activity, because exogenously added SOD and catalase did not completely diminish the dimethylarsine-induced DNA strand breaks.

4.3. *Release of iron from ferritin*

In vitro studies[132,133] have shown that iron from horse spleen and human liver ferritin is released by all tested arsenicals, but most strongly by $DMAs^{III}$. The released iron can generate activated oxygen by the Haber–Weiss reaction and damage DNA. A strong synergistic interaction of released iron resulted from joint exposure to $DMAs^{III}$ and ascorbic acid; the latter a well-known endogenous releaser of ferritin iron. Experiments performed under anaerobic conditions showed that $DMAs^{III}$ released iron without requiring molecular oxygen.

4.4. *Stimulation of NAD(P)H oxidase*

NAD(P)H oxidase is a multi-component enzyme found in phagocytes and vascular endothelial cells.[134] In activated phagocytes, the cytosolic components of this enzyme translocate to the plasma membrane and associate with membrane-bound components. This complex generates superoxide anion to assist in microbial killing. Vascular endothelial cells have a low-activity NADPH oxidase, and the superoxide anion produced is a source of second messengers. Recent studies have shown that low levels of iAs^{III} ($<5\,\mu M$) stimulate NADPH oxidase in vascular endothelial cells producing superoxide anion[135,136] and elicit DNA strand breaks.[135] NADPH oxidase inhibitors decrease the iAs^{III}-dependent stimulation of this enzyme. SOD and catalase decrease the DNA damaging effect from the stimulation of NADPH oxidase by iAs^{III}. Arsenic is a well-known atherogen in humans and its stimulation of NADPH oxidase, by increasing superoxide anion levels, may be the mechanism for this vascular effect. Whether this has an effect on the carcinogenicity of arsenic is not known.

4.5. *Inhibition of redox enzymes*

Glutathione reductase and thioredoxin reductase are both flavoproteins of the nucleotide-disulfide oxidoreductase family. Both of these enzymes have redox-active dithiol groups at the catalytic site and can channel electrons from NADPH to proteins and other molecules for ensuing reductions. These enzymes partially maintain the redox status of the cell. Inhibition of these enzymes may result in a state of oxidative stress within the organism.

4.5.1. *In vitro inhibition of redox enzymes*

Trivalent arsenicals and arsinothiols (trivalent As bound to a thiol such as glutathione) are effective inhibitors of purified yeast glutathione reductase.[10] Some trivalent methylated arsenicals and arsinothiols are more potent inhibitors than iAs^{III}. These same arsenicals are also potent inhibitors of purified mouse liver thioredoxin reductase and its activity in primary cultured rat hepatocytes.[10] In hepatocytes treated with $MMAs^{III}$, the peak cellular concentration of MMAs occurred at the time of peak inhibition of cellular thioredoxin activity.

4.5.2. *In vivo inhibition of redox enzymes*

Male New Zealand rabbits were exposed to 5 mg/l iAs^{V} in their drinking water for 18 weeks.[137] Overall, the arsenic exposed animals consumed

182 mg of iAs^V per animal and achieved elevations of 1, 29, and 39 times higher concentrations of total arsenic in their blood, urine, and hair, respectively, than did control animals. No overt signs of toxicity were observed in the arsenic treated animals. The concentration of hepatic glutathione was not affected by iAs^V treatment to the rabbits. However, the hepatic thioredoxin reductase and glutathione reductase activities were decreased by 30 and 20%, respectively, in the iAs^V-exposed animals.

Arsenic inhibits enzymes that are important in maintaining the redox status of cells. Additional studies are required to determine if inhibition of these enzymes has a role in arsenic-induced carcinogenesis.

5. Summary

At this point in time, there is substantial evidence for oxidative stress being a major contributor to arsenic carcinogenesis. The type of supportive data that is presently available includes (1) decreases in cellular antioxidants, (2) increases in concentration of free radical species, and (3) oxidative DNA lesions such as 8-HOdG.

Antioxidant defenses are diminished after cellular systems, rodents and humans are exposed to arsenicals. These include decreased glutathione,[102,103,138] decreased total serum antioxidants, and decreased activities of SOD,[100,101] glutathione peroxidase,[102,103] and glutathione and thioredoxin reductases.[10]

Oxidative stressors are increased after cells, rodents, and humans are exposed to arsenicals. These ROS and free radicals include superoxide radical, hydroxy radical, hydrogen peroxide, nitric oxide, and the two free radicals containing arsenic (dimethylarsenic radical and dimethylarsenic peroxyl radical).[66–71,119]

So far, the biological effects of diminished antioxidants and increased free radicals and ROS have mostly been observed in 8-OHdG and 8-oxodG. Arsenic exposures have been linked to increased 8-OHdG and 8-oxodG in many cases.[53,63,73,76–80,128] Formation of *cis*-thymine glycol has also been observed after exposure to arsenic.[116]

Other biological effects of arsenic leading to neoplasia that could be due to oxidative stress are changes in signal transduction pathways,[16–19] which may lead to cell proliferation, induction of heme oxygenase,[93] and other stress proteins[20] and genotoxicity (clastogenicity, micronuclei).[13] So far, little experimental or epidemiological evidence links arsenic exposure to specific gene mutations and final tumor endpoints.

Through oxidative DNA damage and eventual base changes, the carcinogenesis process may start through mutations in oncogene and tumor suppressor genes. This is a mechanism in which arsenic can be an initiator of carcinogenesis. Oxidative stress-induced clastogenesis is a second way arsenic could cause cancer.

Arsenicals, particularly $DMAs^V$, have been shown to promote carcinogenesis in experimental two-step initiation–promotion protocols in rat urinary bladder,[139] liver,[124] kidney,[140] and thyroid.[140] Promotion of carcinogenesis by $DMAs^V$ has also been demonstrated in mouse lung[141] and skin.[142] Thus, using the endpoint of tumors in experimental animals, promotion of carcinogenesis by $DMAs^V$ is now well established as a possible mechanism of arsenic carcinogenesis.

From about 1990 onward, the oxidative stress theory of arsenic carcinogenesis has gathered much positive, supporting data. It is now a robust theory with more detail available to support the possible genetic and cellular progressions from a normal state to neoplasia. However, other viable theories of arsenic carcinogenesis have also gathered additional support during this time interval. Some of the stronger alternative theories of arsenic carcinogenesis include chromosomal abnormalities, altered growth factors, enhanced cell proliferation and promotion of carcinogenesis. The latter three can temporally and causally be connected as in growth factors → cell proliferation → promotion → cancer. Another appealing mechanistic combination is oxidative stress → clastogenesis → cancer.

A more holistic view would be that the many different arsenicals, particularly the trivalent species that are presently known to be formed *in vivo* at concentrations near the micromolar range act via several various mechanisms during the development of neoplasia.

Acknowledgments

This article has been reviewed in accordance with the policy of the National Health and Environmental Effects Research Laboratory, US Environmental

Protection Agency, and approved for publication. Approval does not signify that the contents necessarily reflect the views and policies of the Agency, nor does mention of trade names or commercial products constitute endorsement or recommendation for use.

References

1. Mandal BK, Suzuki KT. *Talanta* 58: 201–235 (2002).
2. Nordstrom DK. *Science* 296: 2144–2146 (2002).
3. Bachleitner-Hofmann T, Kees M, Gisslinger H. *Leuk. Lymphoma* 43: 1535–1540 (2002).
4. *IARC Monographs on the Evaluation of Carcinogenic Risks to Humans: Some Drinking-Water Disinfectants and Contaminants, Including Arsenic*, Vol. 84. International Agency for Research on Cancer, Lyon, France, 2004.
5. *Arsenic and Arsenic Compounds*, 2nd edn. Environmental Health Criteria Document 224, International Programme in Chemical Safety, World Health Organization, 2001.
6. National Research Council, *Arsenic in Drinking Water.* National Academy Press, Washington, DC, 1999.
7. National Research Council, *Arsenic in Drinking Water: 2001 Update*. National Academy Press, Washington, DC, 2001.
8. Cullen WR, Reimer J. *Chem. Rev.* 89: 713–764 (1989).
9. Vahter M. *Toxicol. Lett.* 112–113: 209–217 (2000).
10. Thomas DJ, Styblo M, Lin S. *Toxicol. Appl. Pharmacol.* 176: 127–144 (2001).
11. Styblo M *et al. Environ. Health Perspect.* 110(Suppl. 5): 767–771 (2002).
12. Vahter M. *Toxicology* 181–182: 211–217 (2002).
13. Basu A, Mahata J, Gupta S, Giri AK. *Mutat. Res.* 488: 171–194 (2001).
14. Kitchin KT. *Toxicol. Appl. Pharmacol.* 172: 249–261 (2001).
15. Hughes MF. *Toxicol. Lett.* 133: 1–16 (2002).
16. Yang C, Frenkel K. *J. Environ. Pathol. Toxicol. Oncol.* 21: 331–342 (2002).
17. Bernstam L, Nriagu J. *J. Toxicol. Environ. Health Part B* 3: 293–322 (2000).
18. Simeonova PP, Luster MI. *J. Environ. Pathol. Toxicol. Oncol.* 19: 281–286 (2000).
19. Haung C, Ke Q, Costa M, Shi X. *Mol. Cell. Biochem.* 255: 57–66 (2004).
20. Del Razo LM. *et al. Toxicol. Appl. Pharmacol.* 177: 132–147 (2001).
21. Byrd DM *et al. Int. Arch. Occup. Health* 68: 484–494 (1996).

22. Scott N, Hatelid KM, MacKenzie NE, Carter DE. *Chem. Res. Toxicol.* 6: 102–106 (1993).
23. Delnomdedieu M, Basti MM, Otvos JD, Thomas DJ. *Chem.–Biol. Interact.* 90: 139–155 (1994).
24. Radabaugh TR, Sampayo-Reyes A, Zakharyan RA, Aposhian HV. *Chem. Res. Toxicol.* 15: 692–698 (2002).
25. Gregus Z, Nemeti B. *Toxicol. Sci.* 70: 13–19 (2002).
26. Nemeti B, Csanaky I, Gregus Z. *Toxicol. Sci.* 74: 22–31 (2003).
27. Zakharyan R *et al. Chem. Res. Toxicol.* 14: 1051–1057 (2001).
28. Zakharyan R, Wu Y, Bogdan GM, Aposhian HV. *Chem. Res. Toxicol.* 8: 1029–1038 (1995).
29. Zakharyan R *et al. Toxicol. Appl. Pharmacol.* 158: 9–15 (1999).
30. Wildfang E, Zakharyan RA, Aposhian HV. *Toxicol. Appl. Pharmacol.* 152: 366–375 (1998).
31. Wildfang E, Radabaugh TR, Aposhian HV. *Toxicology* 168: 213–222 (2001).
32. Lin S *et al. J. Biol. Chem.* 277: 10795–10803 (2002).
33. Shiobara Y, Ogra Y, Suzuki KT. *Chem. Res. Toxicol.* 14: 1446–1452 (2001).
34. Bencko V *et al.* In: Fouts JR, Gut I (eds.) *Industrial and Environmental Xenobiotics: In Vitro Versus In Vivo Biotransformation and Toxicity*. Excerpta Medica, Oxford, 1978, pp. 312–316.
35. Ellenhorn MJ. *Ellenhorn's Medical Toxicology: Diagnosis and Treatment of Human Poisoning*. Williams & Wilkins, Baltimore, 1997, p. 1540.
36. Lee TL, Ko JL, Jan KY. *Toxicology* 56: 289–299 (1989).
37. Lee TC, Ho IC. *Environ. Health Perspect.* 102(Suppl. 3): 101–105 (1994).
38. Samikkannu T *et al. Chem. Res. Toxicol.* 16: 409–414 (2003).
39. Delnomdedieu M, Styblo M, Thomas DJ. *Chem.–Biol. Interact.* 98: 69–83 (1995).
40. Winski SL, Carter DE. *J. Toxicol. Environ. Health A* 53: 345–355 (1998).
41. Aposhian HV *et al. Chem. Res. Toxicol.* 13: 693–697 (2000).
42. Mandal BK, Ogra Y, Suzuki KT. *Chem. Res. Toxicol.* 14: 371–378 (2001).
43. Styblo M *et al. Arch. Toxicol.* 74: (2000) 289–299.
44. Petrick JS, Jagadish B, Mash EA, Aposhian HV. *Chem. Res. Toxicol.* 14: 651–656 (2001).
45. Lee-Feldstein A. *J. Occup. Med.* 28: 296–302 (1986).
46. Mabuchi K, Lilienfeld A, Snell L. *Arch. Environ. Health* 34: 312–319 (1979).
47. Ott MG, Holder BB, Gordon HL. *Arch. Environ. Health* 29: 250–255 (1974).
48. Tseng WP *et al. J. Natl. Cancer Inst.* 40: 453–463 (1968).
49. Tseng WP *et al. Environ. Health Perspect.* 19: 109–119 (1977).
50. Smith AH *et al. Environ. Health Prespect.* 97: 259–267 (1992).

51. Bates MN, Smith AH, Cantor KP. *Am. J. Epidemiol.* 141: 523–530 (1995).
52. Wei M, Wanibuchi H, Yamamoto S, Li W, Fukushima S. *Carcinogenesis* 20: 1873–1876 (1999).
53. Wei M *et al. Carcinogenesis* 23: 1387–1397 (2002).
54. Arnold LL *et al. Toxicology* 190: 197–219 (2003).
55. Shen J *et al. Toxicol. Appl. Pharmacol.* 193: 335–345 (2003).
56. Chen Y *et al. Toxicol. Lett.* 116: 27–35 (2000).
57. Germolec DR *et al. Mutat. Res.* 386: 209–218 (1997).
58. Salim EI *et al. Carcinogenesis* 24: 335–342 (2003).
59. Waalkes MP, Ward JM, Liu J, Diwan BA. *Toxicol. Appl. Pharmacol.* 186: 7–17 (2003).
60. Waalkes MP, Ward JM, Diwan BA. *Carcinogenesis* 25: 133–141 (2004).
61. Rossman TG, Uddin AM, Burns FJ, Bosland MC. *Toxicol. Appl. Pharmacol.* 176: 64–71 (2001).
62. Kenyon EM, Hughes MF. *Toxicology* 160: 227–236 (2001).
63. Nishikawa T *et al. Int. J. Cancer* 100: 136–139 (2002).
64. Morikawa T *et al. Jpn. J. Cancer Res.* 91: 579–581 (2000).
65. Yamanaka K *et al. Biochem. Biophys. Res. Commun.* 168: 58–64 (1990).
66. Nesnow S *et al. Chem. Res. Toxicol.* 15: 1627–1634 (2002).
67. Liu SX *et al. Proc. Natl. Acad. Sci. USA* 98: 1643–1648 (2001).
68. Barchowsky A *et al. Free Radic. Biol. Med.* 27: 1405–1412 (1999).
69. Lee TC, Ho IC. *Arch. Toxicol.* 69: 498–504 (1995).
70. Gurr JR, Liu F, Lynn S, Jun KY. *Mutat. Res.* 416: 137–148 (1998).
71. Garcia-Chavez E *et al. Brain Res.* 976: 82–89 (2003).
72. Cooke MS, Evans MD, Herbert KE and Lunec J. *Free Radic. Res.* 32: 281–397 (2000).
73. Kasai H. *Mutat. Res.* 387: 147–163 (1997).
74. Cheng KC *et al. J. Biol. Chem.* 267: 166–172 (1992).
75. Kasai H, Yamaizumi Z, Berger M, Cadet J. *J. Am. Chem. Soc.* 114: 9692–9654 (1992).
76. Kessel M *et al. Mol. Cell. Biochem.* 235/235: 301–308 (2002).
77. Yamanaka K *et al. Biochem. Biophys. Res. Commun.* 287: 66–70 (2001).
78. Vijayaraghavan M *et al. Cancer Lett.* 165: 11–17 (2001).
79. Matsui M *et al. J. Invest. Dermatol.* 113: 26–31 (1999).
80. An Y *et al. Cancer Lett.* 214: 11–18 (2004).
81. Bode AM, Dong Z. *Crit. Rev. Oncol. Hematol.* 42: 5–24 (2002).
82. Cavigelli M *et al. EMBO J.* 15: 6269–6279 (1996).
83. Parrish AR *et al. Toxicol. Sci.* 50: 98–105 (1999).
84. Haung C *et al. Mol. Cell. Biochem.* 222: 29–34 (2001).

85. Liu J *et al. Toxicol. Sci.* 61: 314–320 (2001).
86. Li M, Cai JF, Chiu JF. *J. Cell. Biochem.* 87: 29–38 (2002).
87. Pi J *et al. Environ. Health Perspect.* 110: 331–336 (2002).
88. Arrigo A-P. *Free Radic. Biol. Med.* 27: 936–944 (1999).
89. Chen NY, Ma WY, Yang CS, Dong Z. *J. Environ. Pathol. Toxicol. Oncol.* 19: 287–295 (2000).
90. Pi J *et al. Exp. Cell Res.* 290: 234–245 (2003).
91. Keyse SM, Tyrell RM. *Proc. Natl. Acad. Sci. USA* 86: 99–103 (1989).
92. Brown JL, Kitchin KT, George M. *Teratog. Carcinog. Mutagen.* 17: 71–84 (1997).
93. Kitchin KT *et al. Teratog. Carcinog. Mutagen.* 19: 385–402 (1999).
94. Kenyon EM, Del Razo LM, Hughes MF, Kitchin KT. *Toxicology* 206: 389–401 (2005).
95. Wang TS, Kou CF, Jan KY, Huang H. *J. Cell. Physiol.* 169: 256–268 (1996).
96. Chen YC, Lin-Shian SY, Lin JK. *J. Cell. Physiol.* 177: 324–333 (1998).
97. Chen NY, Ma WY, Yang CS, Dong Z. *J. Environ. Pathol. Toxicol. Oncol.* 19: 287–295 (2000).
98. Liu L *et al. J. Biol. Chem.* 278: 31998–32004 (2003).
99. Zhang TC, Schmitt MT, Mumford JL. *Carcinogenesis* 24: 1811–1817 (2003).
100. Flora SJ. *Clin. Exp. Pharmacol. Physiol.* 26: 865–869 (1999).
101. Ramanathan K, Balakumar BS, Panneerselvam C. *Hum. Exp. Toxicol.* 21: 675–680 (2002).
102. Santra A, Chowdhury A, Mazumder DN. *Indian J. Gastroenterol.* 19: 112–115 (2000).
103. Santra A *et al. J. Toxicol. Clin. Toxicol.* 38: 395–405 (2000).
104. Wu MM *et al. Environ. Health Perspect.* 109: 1011–1017 (2001).
105. Pitot HC, Dragan YP. In: Klaassen CD (ed.) *Casarett & Doull's Toxicology: The Basic Science of Poisons*. McGraw Hill, New York, 1996, pp. 201–267.
106. Klaunig JE *et al. Environ. Health Perspect.* 106(Suppl. 1): 289–295 (1998).
107. Athar M. *Indian J. Exp. Biol.* 40: 656–667 (2002).
108. Klaunig JE, Kamendulis LM. *Annu. Rev. Pharmacol. Toxicol.* 44: 239–267 (2004).
109. Kitchin KT, Ahmad S. *Toxicol. Lett.* 137: 3–13 (2003).
110. Hei TK, Liu SX, Waldren C. *Proc. Natl. Acad. Sci. USA* 95: 8103–8107 (1998).
111. Lee TC, Wang-Wuu S, Huang RY, Lee KCC, Jan KY. *Cancer Res.* 46: 1854–1857 (1986).
112. Rossman TG. *Mutat. Res.* 91: 207–211 (1981).
113. Nordenson I, Beckman L. *Hum. Hered.* 41: 71–73 (1991).

114. Mass MJ *et al. Chem. Res. Toxicol.* 14: 355–361 (2001).
115. Andrewes P, Kitchin KT, Wallace K. *Chem. Res. Toxicol.* 16: 994–1003 (2003).
116. Yamanaka K *et al. Toxicol. Lett.* 143: 145–153 (2003).
117. Wang TS, Huang H. *Mutagenesis* 9: 253–257 (1994).
118. Wang TS *et al. Toxicology* 121: 229–237 (1997).
119. Yamanaka K, Hasegawa A, Sawamura R, Okada S. *Biochem. Biophys. Res. Commun.* 165: 43–50 (1989).
120. Das T, Roychoudhury A, Sharma A, Talukder G. *Environ. Mol. Mutagen.* 21: 383–338 (1993).
121. Choudhury AR, Das T, Sharma A. *Cancer Lett.* 121: 45–52 (1997).
122. Cerutti PA. *Science* 227: 375–381 (1985).
123. Brown JL, Kitchin KT. *Cancer Lett.* 98: 227–231 (1996).
124. Wanibuchi H *et al. Jpn. J. Cancer Res.* 88: 1149–1154 (1997).
125. Arnold LL *et al. Carcinogenesis* 20: 2171–2179 (1999).
126. Cohen SM, Yamamoto S, Cano M, Arnold LL. *Toxicol. Sci.* 59: 68–74 (2001).
127. Cohen SM *et al. Chem. Res. Toxicol.* 15: 1150–1157 (2002).
128. Shen J *et al. Carcinogenesis* 24: 1827–1835 (2003).
129. Hennings H *et al. Nature* 304: 67–69 (1983).
130. Kligerman AD *et al. Environ. Mol. Mutagen.* 42: 192–205 (2003).
131. Yamanaka K, Okada S. *Environ. Health Perspect.* 102(Suppl. 3): 37–40 (1994).
132. Ahmad S, Kitchin KT, Cullen WR. *Arch. Biochem. Biophys.* 382: 195–202 (2000).
133. Ahmad S, Kitchin KT, Cullen WR. *Toxicol. Lett.* 133: 47–57 (2002).
134. Babior BM. *Blood* 5: 1464–1476 (1999).
135. Lynn S, Gurr JR, Lai HT, Jan KY. *Circ. Res.* 86: 514–519 (2000).
136. Smith KR, Klei LR, Barchowsky A. *Am J. Physiol Lung Cell. Mol. Physiol.* 280: L442–L449 (2001).
137. Nikaido M *et al. Environ. Toxicol.* 18: 306–311 (2003).
138. Ahmad S, Anderson WL, Kitchin KT. *Cancer Lett.* 139: 129–135 (1999).
139. Wanibuchi H *et al. Carcinogenesis* 17: 2435–2439 (1996).
140. Yamamoto S *et al. Cancer Res.* 55: 1271–1276 (1995).
141. Yamanaka K *et al. Carcinogenesis* 17: 767–770 (1996).
142. Yamanaka K *et al. Cancer Lett.* 152: 79–85 (2000).

30 Estrogen-Induced Carcinogenesis: Importance of Oxidative Stress

Hari K. Bhat

1. Introduction

Studies *in vitro*, in experimental animals, and in women provide compelling evidence that estrogens contribute to the development of breast cancer.[1–17] The federal government has added steroidal estrogens to the list of known human carcinogens.[18] The clinical trials of estrogen plus progestin treatment therapy have been terminated due to an increased breast cancer risk and a lack of overall benefit to patients.[19] Epidemiological studies strongly suggest that sex hormones are involved in the development of a variety of human cancers.[1–12] There is increasing evidence of elevated breast cancer risk with increases in total lifetime exposure of women to estrogens.[1,5,9,11,12] Although early cohort studies failed to identify an association between serum estrogen levels and breast cancer risk (probably due to lack of proper detection methods),[20,21] more recent epidemiological results reveal strong associations between breast cancer risk and plasma or urinary estrogen levels.[22,23] This finding is consistent with increased risk associated with hormone replacement studies seen in most large studies and in meta analysis.[5,11,24–26] This concept of tumor induction by estrogens is supported by breast cancer risk factors such as early menarche, late menopause, obesity, and high mean values of serum estrogen.[8,9] Risk of breast cancer is significantly increased among women who are currently using estrogen alone or in combination with progestin as compared with postmenopausal women who have never used hormones.[5,11,12] Estrogen medications, e.g. oral contraceptives, have been estimated to increase breast cancer risk by approximately 3% per year of intake.[27] Also, late menarche, early menopause, and pregnancy at a young age, in theory, decrease the risk of breast cancer by reducing the lifetime exposure to estrogens.[28] Similarly, ovariectomy before 35 years of age also reduces breast cancer risk.[29]

The above-mentioned studies suggest a link between estrogens and cancer. The carcinogenic activity of estrogenic compounds has now been recognized by the International Agency for Research on Cancer, which has classified estrogens as human carcinogens.[30,31] The mechanism(s) whereby estrogens cause cancer has not been conclusively established and certain aspects remain controversial. This mechanism is currently being investigated in rodent models of hormonal carcinogenesis. Natural female sex hormone βE2 and synthetic estrogen DES induce tumors in rats, mice, and hamsters.[13–17] It must be noted that *not* all estrogens are tumorigenic in animal models.[32–34] Carcinogenic and noncarcinogenic estrogens, however, differ in their metabolic activation profiles.[33–35] Therefore, it is predicted that estrogen metabolism may play a key role in the development of hormonal carcinogenesis.

2. Animal Models of Estrogen-Induced Carcinogenesis

The estrogen-induced hamster renal tumor model is one of the well-established and useful models of hormonal carcinogenesis. In this animal model, estrogen alone is sufficient for the induction and promotion of tumors (Fig. 1). Subcutaneous implantation of βE2 for about 6 months induces target-organ-specific kidney tumors with ~80–100% tumor incidence.[13,14,32] The shared characteristics between human breast and uterine cancers, and the estrogen-induced hamster kidney tumors point to a common mechanistic origin. These include: (1) direct covalent binding of estrogen quinone metabolites to DNA, (2) enhancement of endogenous DNA adducts by chronic estrogen exposure, and (3) chromosomal damage/aberration induced by estrogens or by reactive estrogen quinone metabolites.[33,36–53] A specific estradiol-4-hydroxylase activity has been identified in organs that are prone to estrogen-induced hyperplasia or cancer. These include rat pituitary, mouse uterus, and

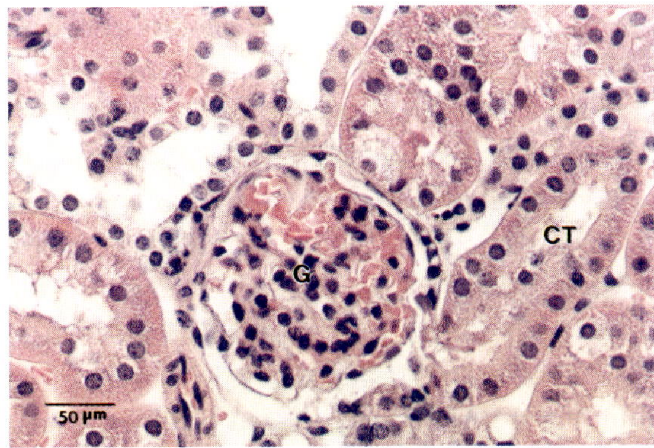

Fig. 1a. Paraffin section of an untreated male Syrian hamster kidney stained with hematoxylin and eosin. Normal kidney architecture with normal convoluted tubules (CT) and glomerulus (G) is observed. Magnification = 40×. (*Courtesy*: Bhat *et al.*, *Proc. Natl. Acad. Sci. USA*, 100, 3913–3918, 2003.)

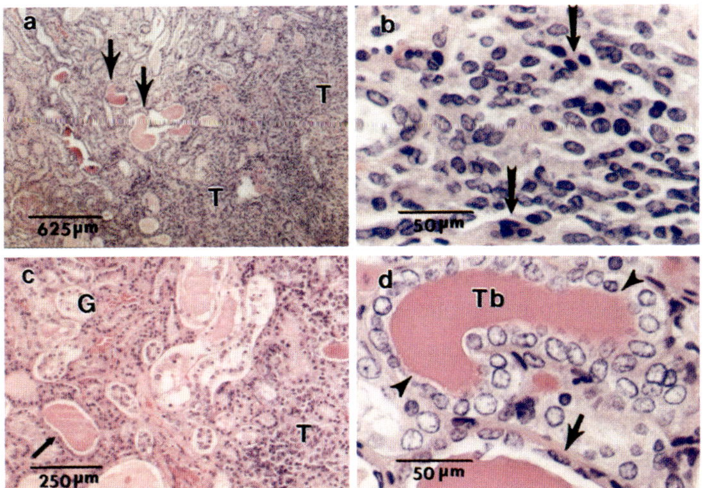

Fig. 1b. Paraffin section of a tumor-bearing kidney stained with hematoxylin and eosin. The tumors were induced by treatment of male Syrian hamsters with βE2 for 7 months. (a) An abnormal kidney architecture with tumor nodules (T) and congestion of scattered convoluted tubules (arrow) within the tumor nodules can be observed. (b and c) The tumor nodules are composed of a combination of round to spindled hyperchromatic cells (b, arrows), and in some of the tumor nodules (T), entrapped and atrophic glomeruli (G) are present (c). Many of the congested tubules (Tb) are filled with pink eosinophilic deposits (arrow in c, arrow head in d) and are lined by somewhat flattened epithelial cells (d, arrow). Magnification: a = 4×; b = 40×; c = 10×; d = 40×. (*Courtesy*: Bhat *et al.*, *Proc. Natl. Acad. Sci. USA*, 100, 3913–3918, 2003.)

hamster kidney.[54–56] However, the enzyme activity could not be detected in livers of these species.[54–56] Elevated estradiol-4-hydroxylase activity has been identified in human myometrium[39] as well as in MCF-7 breast cancer cells.[57] Increased 4-hydroxyestradiol (4-OHE2) formation in myometrial precursor cells is postulated to mediate benign tumor growth and blastocyst implantation, based upon physiological studies in the mouse uterus.[58] Predominant 4-hydroxylation of βE2 by microsomes of neoplastic human breast tissue, as compared with non-neoplastic breast tissue, has also been demonstrated.[40] Several studies have indicated that 4-hydroxylation of βE2 plays an important role in estrogen-induced carcinogenesis.[33,34,39,40] Furthermore, 4-OHE2 is as carcinogenic as the parent βE2 in the hamster kidney tumor model.[33,34,59] Genomic instability, induced in a variety of species (hamster, mouse, rat) at different tissue sites, using either synthetic or natural steroid hormones for tumor formation,[43,60] closely resembles genomic instability found in hormone-related/associated human cancers.[60] It is important to note that in post-menopausal women, mesenchymal cells of the breast are the major source of estrogen, either as such or after the conversion of androgens to estrogens by aromatase.[61] It is equally important to note that in the hamster tumor model, mesenchymal cells play an important role in the origin of the estrogen-induced and estrogen-dependent renal neoplasm.[13,62,63] Thus, it is evident that there exists a strong similarity between the hamster tumor model of hormonal carcinogenesis and hormone-associated human cancers, which points to a common mechanistic origin.

Although the estrogen-induced hamster renal tumor model supports the role of estrogens in carcinogenesis, it is sometimes criticized as not being a good model system because estrogen use is not associated with renal tumors in humans. In recent years, the mechanism of estrogen-induced carcinogenesis has been studied using a rodent model that is relevant to human breast cancers: the female ACI rat model of breast cancer. A βE2-induced ACI rat model of breast cancer developed by Shull *et al.* in 1997 is now being used as a representative system to study the mechanism of estrogen-induced breast carcinogenesis.[16,17] The propensity of the ACI rats to develop mammary carcinomas has been recognized for a long time,[64,65] but Shull showed in 1997 that mammary carcinomas can be induced in female ACI rats with βE2.[16] Continuous treatment with βE2 of female ACI rats results in 100% mammary tumor incidence within 197 days (Fig. 2).[16,66] The first palpable

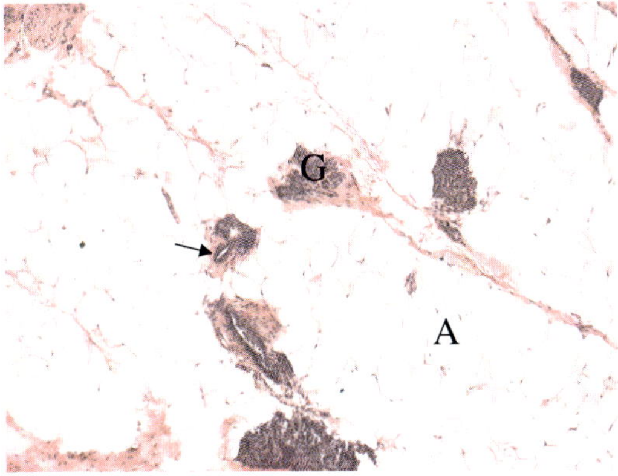

Fig. 2a. Paraffin section of a normal mammary gland tissue and surrounding fat from a control female ACI rat stained with hematoxylin and eosin. Female ACI rats were implanted with 20 mg pellet of cholesterol and euthanized after 46 weeks of treatment. Please note the normal adipose cells (A), glands (G), and ducts (arrow) of the mammary tissue. Magnification 10×. (*Courtesy*: Valerie Turan and Kenneth Reuhl, Rutgers University, New Jersey, USA.)

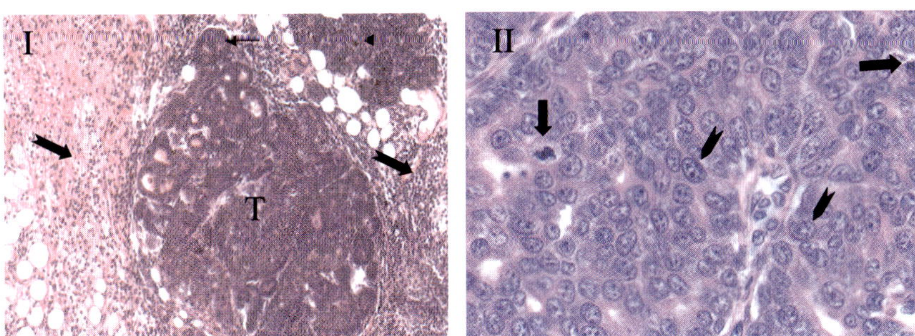

Fig. 2b. Paraffin section of a multifocal mammary adenocarcinoma from a female ACI rat stained with hematoxylin and eosin. Female ACI rats were implanted with a 20 mg pellet containing cholesterol and 2 mg βE2 and euthanized after 46 weeks of treatment. Please note a large focus of mammary adenocarcinoma (T), invasive tumor areas (thin arrows), and marked secondary inflammation (notched arrows) (2b-I). Numerous mitotic figures (arrows) and large nuclei with decreased amount of cytoplasm and prominent nucleoli (notched arrow heads) can be observed (2b-II). Magnification: a $= 5\times, b = 20\times$. (*Courtesy*: Valerie Turan and Kenneth Reuhl, Rutgers University, New Jersey, USA.)

tumors are observed between 143 and 145 days. All mammary tumors have been classified as carcinomas, and invasive features have been observed. Mammary tumors have not been observed in ovary-intact female ACI rats that were not treated with βE2. The majority of tumors show features of intraductal carcinoma of the comedo type. The disadvantage of the ACI rat model is that pituitary tumors have also been observed in 100% of βE2 treated rats (in contrast with the hamster model, where βE2 causes only target organ-specific kidney tumors). In spite of this drawback, it is probably more useful and more relevant to characterize the mechanism of hormone-induced carcinogenesis in the rat model as the target tumor organ is the breast.

3. Mechanisms of Estrogen-Induced Carcinogenesis

3.1. *Estrogen metabolism and resultant oxidative stress as the proposed mechanism of estrogen-induced cancer*

Several studies of estrogen-induced carcinogenesis indicate that tumor induction is dependent on the generation of βE2 metabolites.[51–58,67–71] Since hormones like βE2 are essential in estrogen-induced and estrogen-dependent tumors, it is postulated that hormonal activity of estrogens is necessary but not sufficient to induce tumors. Since these tumors are estrogen-induced and estrogen-dependent (if estrogen is withdrawn, tumors will regress), estrogens and their metabolic products are considered to be important for tumor development. βE2 is mainly metabolized to 2- and 4-OHE2 (generally known as catechol estrogens) in target organs of estrogen-induced cancer.[51,54–56] Elevated estradiol-4-hydroxylase activity has been shown in organs prone to estradiol-induced hyperplasia or cancer in rodents, humans, and human breast cancer cell lines.[39,40,54–58]

Several lines of evidence support the role of oxidative stress in tumor formation.[33,34,72–75] Treatment of Syrian hamster embryo cells with DES in the presence of an exogenous metabolic activation system enhances the frequency of morphological transformation of cells; furthermore, this treatment elicits unscheduled DNA synthesis and mutations.[41] Exposure of Syrian hamster embryo cells to catechol estrogens not only induces a higher frequency of morphological transformation than βE2, but it also causes chromosome aberrations.[41–44] Different types of oxidative stress-mediated changes have been reported in the target organs of hamsters and rats *in vivo* after treatment with DES or with βE2 and its carcinogenic metabolite 4-OHE2. These include: (1) 8-hydroxylation of guanine residues[36,46]; (2) single-strand breaks[47]; (3) increases in levels of lipid hydroperoxides and lipid hydroperoxide-induced DNA adducts[48–50]; and (4) damage to mitochondrial DNA.[53] These data are consistent with previous reports of free radical-mediated genotoxicity, manifested as single strand breaks of DNA induced by estrone-3,4-quinone in MCF-7 cells.[76] Support for the role of oxidative stress in tumor formation is also provided by increases in tumor incidence and in the number of tumor nodules in hamsters treated with a combination of iron-enriched diet and βE2 (iron participates in the generation of hydroxy radicals).[77] Metabolic activation of estrogens to reactive intermediates is postulated to be required for the carcinogenic process, analogous to the metabolic activation of hydrocarbons and other non-steroidal estrogen carcinogens.[33–35,46–50,74–79] Catechol estrogens are orthohydroquinones, that are capable of undergoing metabolic redox cycling.[67–72] Metabolic redox cycling between catechol estrogens and their corresponding quinones generates oxidative stress and potentially harmful free radicals (Fig. 3). Catechol quinone DNA adducts of 4-OHE2 have been shown to be formed in the female ACI rat mammary gland after injection of 4-OHE2 into the rat mammary gland and excision of the mammary gland 1 h post-treatment.[80] βE2 is a good catechol progenitor and has strong estrogenic potential; its use results in ~80–100% tumor incidence in the hamster kidney and rat breast.[13,14,16,17] 17α-Ethinylestradiol (αEE) is a strong estrogen but a very weak catechol progenitor and this results in only a 10% tumor incidence in the hamster model after 9 months of continuous exposure.[32–34,81,82] Liehr *et al.* using a V-79 cell carcinogenicity assay, found that low doses of βE2 (in the 10^{-10} and 10^{-12} molar ranges) cause a 3.8–4.2-fold increase in rate of genetic mutations.[83] In other experiments, Russo *et al.* administered βE2 to MCF-10F benign breast cells *in vitro* in doses ranging from 0.007 nM to 1 μM and found that even very low βE2 concentrations induce loss of heterozygosity (LOH) at chromosomal sites at which human breast cancers commonly exhibit LOH.[84,85] They also demonstrated neoplastic

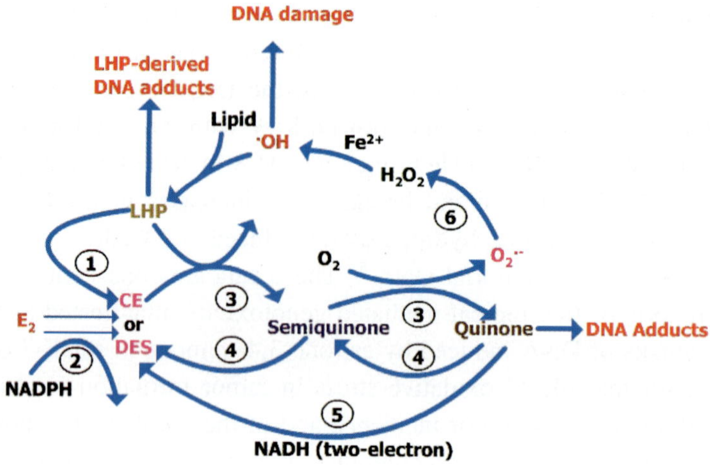

Fig. 3. Proposed mechanism of the formation of reactive oxygen species by steroid estrogens. Steroid estrogens (E2) are converted to catechol estrogens (CE) by hydroperoxide or NADPH-dependent cytochrome P450-mediated oxidation (1, 2). CEs and DES are oxidized by organic hydroperoxide-dependent microsomal enzymes to semiquinones and quinones (3). Quinone metabolites may be reduced by NADPH or NADH-dependent cytochrome P450 reductase (4, 5). This metabolic redox cycling may generate superoxide radicals. Hydrogen peroxide, formed from superoxide by superoxide dismutase (6), may be reduced by Fe^{2+} to hydroxyl radicals. Thus potentially harmful reactive oxygen species may be generated that may result in different types of DNA, protein or lipid damage.

transformation in these cells by demonstrating anchorage-independent colony formation and loss of duct differentiation. Damage to mtDNA has been demonstrated in βE2-induced hamster renal tumors.[53] Estrogen-mediated oxidative DNA damage in mammary gland epithelia included the induction of 8-hydroxydeoxyguanine (8-OHdG), both *in vitro* and *in vivo*, thereby suggesting a role of oxidative stress in the initiation and/or progression of breast neoplasia.[36,72,86–92] The induction of kidney tumors in Syrian hamsters has been shown to be decreased by using inhibitors of estrogen metabolism or free radical scavengers,[93,94] indicating the role of oxidative stress mediated by estrogen metabolism in estrogen-induced carcinogenesis. Taken together, these data support the concept that, in addition to hormonal stimulus, oxidative stress that is present due to metabolic activation and free radical generation of carcinogenic estrogens plays a critical role in tumor development.

3.2. *Estrogen metabolism/oxidative stress and human breast cancers*

Cancer may develop only in those estrogen-sensitive organs that synthesize hydroxy metabolites of estrogen at the target site of carcinogenesis. These hydroxylated estrogens may elicit biological activities distinct from βE2, most notably an oxidant stress response induced by free radicals generated by metabolic redox cycling reactions. It has recently been shown that hydroxylated and O-methylated estrogens account for nearly 95% of the total estrogen content in normal human breast and in human breast tumor tissue, with no difference in O-methylated estrogen levels between the tumor and control groups.[95] Levels of 4-OHE2, a carcinogenic metabolite of βE2 in animal models, have been shown to be increased ~20-fold in breast tumor tissue compared with normal or non-tumorigenic breast tissue.[95] Rogan *et al.* have recently reported similar findings.[96] 4-OHE2 may undergo metabolic redox cycling between its catechol and quinone metabolites and generate potentially harmful free radicals and oxidative stress[33–35,39,40,73,74] that can cause cellular DNA damage, induce cell proliferation, and initiate tumorigenesis.[72,74] Cytochrome P4501B1 (Cyp1B1) mRNA levels have been found to be highest in the human breast tissue among all the Cyps analyzed.[97] This is consistent with the fact that Cyp1B1 is primarily an extrahepatic enzyme and is the main enzyme responsible for the conversion of βE2 into 4-OHE2, a catechol metabolite of βE2.[98–100] The presence of Cyp1B1 in the breast tissue will result in the formation of 4-OHE2 from βE2. Although not confirmed to be carcinogenic in the human breast, 4-OHE2 has been observed to have a strong carcinogenic activity in a Syrian hamster kidney tumor model and induces uterine tumors in mice.[15,59] Local activation of estrogen to potentially reactive metabolites in the breast tissue may play a role in initiating and promoting the carcinogenic process. Redox cycling between quinone and unstable semiquinone causes hydroxyl radical formation, the most potent reactive oxygen species that when formed at the target site can lead to hydroxylated nucleotide bases, e.g. 8-OHdG formation and permanent mutations if not repaired. It is possible that the reactive oxygen metabolites produced in the liver and other organs, and transported via the blood could be responsible for damage in the breast. This is unlikely, though, because concentration of unconjugated catechol estrogens is very low in systemic circulation.[101,102] Therefore it is unlikely that these 2- and 4-hydroxy estrogen metabolites will have any significant interaction with ERs or DNA in tissues distant from where they are produced. Rather, their effects are likely to be exerted in the tissue in which they are synthesized.

3.3. *Receptor-mediated hormonal effects of estrogens and estrogen-induced proliferation*

The epigenetic mechanism of carcinogenesis through hormone receptor-mediated events has been accepted for a long time. The most commonly held hypothesis is that estrogens bind to ERα (or ERβ) and stimulate the transcription of genes involved in cell proliferation.[103,104] Estrogens primarily elicit their responses by binding to their cognate receptors and then through the interaction of the receptor-ligand complex with the estrogen response elements (EREs) on estrogen-responsive genes.[105–108] With each cycle of new DNA synthesis during mitosis, there is a chance of an error in DNA replication. If not repaired, these errors in replication result in point mutations. As the process continues, several mutations accumulate.[33,71] When these mutations involve critical regions of genes needed for cellular proliferation, DNA repair, apoptosis, and neoplastic transformation results.[109] This mechanistic construct would explain why anti-estrogens reduce the risk of development of breast cancer.

Some studies have also proposed that the induction of breast cancer is caused by a covalent bond formation of 16α-hydroxyestrone, a metabolite of estrone with ER.[51,52] This receptor modification would result in a permanent uncontrolled stimulation of cell proliferation by receptor-mediated processes.[51,52,110] This hypothesis implies a correlation of high levels of 16α-hydroxyestrone with the induction of breast cancer. Over the years, however, this hypothesis has not been substantiated.

However, during the last decade experimental evidence has accumulated which suggests that the estrogen-dependent tumor growth via ERs as the *sole* contribution of estrogens in tumor development is unlikely. One of the confounding observations is that in mammary glands either normal[111–116] or malignant[117] cells that express proliferation markers do not express ERα.[111,112,117] Because more than 90% of the ERβ-bearing mammary cells do not proliferate, and because 55–70% of the dividing cells have neither ERα nor ERβ, it is clear that the presence of these receptors in epithelial cells is not a prerequisite for estrogen-mediated proliferation.[112] Furthermore, the Syrian hamster embryo cells used for mechanistic studies of hormonal carcinogenesis do not express measurable levels of ERs.[118–120] Therefore, the induction of aneuploidy and cell transformation by estrogens in these cells may not solely depend on hormone receptors. In the untreated male hamster kidney, only a limited number of cells express ERα.[13,121] ERα in this tissue is upregulated after sub-chronic exposure to βE2.[13,121] In the crossbred ER knockout/Wnt-1 expressing mice, the onset of mammary cancer was delayed but not eliminated suggesting that Wnt-1 proto-oncogene expression in these animals induces mammary cancer regardless of ER status.[122] It is suggested that the direct mitogenic effect of estrogens on mammary epithelial cells may be acquired during breast cancer development.[123]

Alternatively, oxidative stress may modify the ability of ERα to bind to EREs and thereby modify subsequent gene expression. It has been shown that in one-third of human breast cancer patients, ERα is unable to bind to its cognate ERE.[124,125] This can be partially rectified by treatment with a thiol reducing agent, suggesting that ER DNA interaction is sub ject to redox modulation.[124] This has also been reported to be the case for other zinc-finger-type proteins and transcriptional activators.[126] Treatment of recombinant ERα DNA-binding domain or ERα-enriched extracts from CHO and MCF-7 cells with oxidative stress-inducing chemicals such as H_2O_2 and menadione produces a dose-dependent loss of ER–DNA-binding capacity.[124] These results suggest that DNA binding and transactivation are highly sensitive intracellular ERα functions that are impaired by oxidative stress in some ERα-positive human breast tumors and suggest that oxidative stress can modify estrogen-dependent gene expression. It has recently been shown that 4-hydroxyequilenin, a major metabolite of equine estrogens present in estrogen replacement formulations, induces 8-OHdG formation in ERα-containing cell lines.[127] This damage is increased by agents that catalyze redox cycling or deplete glutathione, and decreased by an ERα antagonist tamoxifen, suggesting that the mechanism of DNA damage induced by equine catechol estrogens could involve oxidative stress and ERs may play a role in this process.[127] Free radical formation in human breast cancer cell line MCF-7 has been shown after the addition of estrone 3,4-quinone, the *o*-quinone form of 3,4-catechol estrogen.[128] Patel and Bhat have shown that physiological levels of βE2 can increase 8-iso prostaglandin $F_{2\alpha}$ ($PGF_{2\alpha}$) (a known marker of oxidative stress) levels in MCF-7 cells.[129] It has also been demonstrated that co-treatment of tumor cells with βE2 and α-naphthoflavone (an inhibitor of metabolic activation of βE2) results in the inhibition of βE2-induced increase in $PGF_{2\alpha}$ levels, which suggests that oxidative stress is created as a result of metabolic activation of estrogens.[129] Additionally, Mobley and Brueggemier have recently shown in human breast cancer cell lines that βE2 is capable of inducing an increase in sensitivity to oxidative DNA damage through an ER-mediated mechanism.[130] It appears therefore that oxidative stress may be produced in an ER-dependent or independent manner. Oxidative stress may alter expression of genes and cause loss of normal cellular control. Reactive oxygen species and metabolic activation have been known to modulate gene expression.[131–135]

In an attempt to show that both oxidative stress and receptor-mediated effects are required in estrogen-induced carcinogenesis, Bhat *et al.* used an estrogen-induced hamster renal tumor model, a well-established animal model of hormonal carcinogenesis that shares many biochemical and molecular characteristics with human breast and uterine cancers.[136,137] Hamsters were implanted with 25-mg pellets of βE2, 17α-estradiol (αE2), αEE, menadione, a combination of αE2 and αEE, or a combination of αEE and menadione for 7 months. Different estrogens used in this study differed in their carcinogenic, metabolic activation and hormonal potential.[32,54,138,139] Menadione was used as a test chemical to produce oxidative stress which has been shown to induce oxidative stress both *in vitro* as well as *in vivo*.[140–142] As expected, the group treated with βE2 developed target organ-specific kidney tumors (Fig. 1b). The kidneys of hamsters treated with αE2, αEE, or menadione alone did not show any gross evidence of tumors. Kidneys of hamsters treated with a combination of αE2 and αEE showed vascular congestion of glomeruli, foci with abnormal tubules, and first signs of proliferation in the interstitial cells (Fig. 4). Kidneys of hamsters treated with a combination of menadione and αEE showed foci of tumors with congested tubules and atrophic glomeruli (Fig. 5). Chronic treatment of hamsters with a combination of a chemical known to produce oxidative stress and a poorly carcinogenic estrogen that

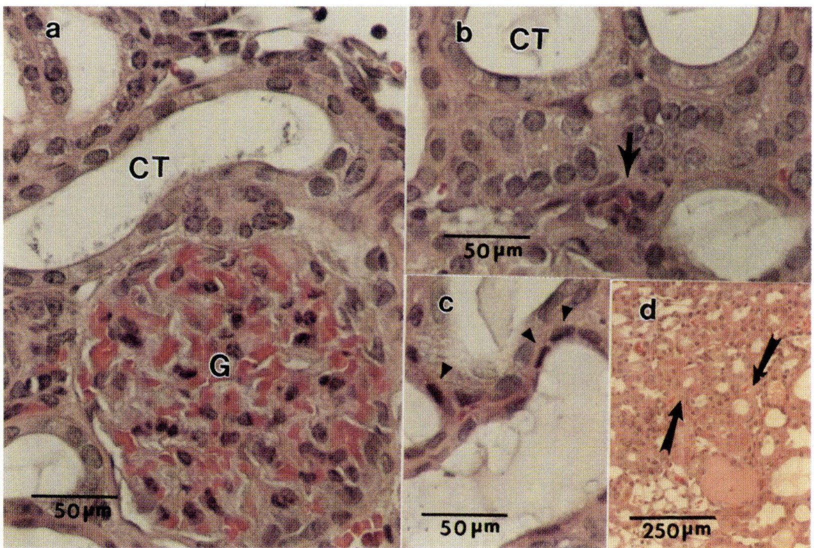

Fig. 4. Paraffin section of a male hamster kidney stained with hematoxylin and eosin. Male Syrian hamsters were treated with a combination of αEE and αE2 for 7 months. (a) Vascular congestion of glomeruli (G) and convoluted tubules (CT) is observed. (b) Kidneys contain foci where there are atypical collections of both interstitial cells (arrow) and convoluted tubules (CT). (c) Some of the tubules contain cuboidal cells that have scant cytoplasm and irregular, slightly pleomorphic hyperchromatic nuclei (arrowheads). (d) Some slightly crowded renal collecting tubules (arrows) are also observed in kidneys of hamsters treated with a combination of αEE and αE2 for 7 months. Magnification: a–c = 40×; d = 10×. (*Courtesy*: Bhat *et al.*, *Proc. Natl. Acad. Sci. USA*, 100, 3913–3918, 2003.)

is metabolized to catechol estrogens to a lesser extent than βE2 resulted in tumor formation. Thus, these data provide evidence that oxidant stress plays a crucial role in estrogen-induced carcinogenesis. No evidence of hemosiderin was observed in kidney sections of hamsters treated with menadione or menadione plus αEE, suggesting that the histopathological effects of menadione are not through its effects on iron homeostasis.[136,143] Tumors were not detected in the groups treated with αE2, αEE, or menadione alone. These chemicals either lack or have weak estrogenic potential or are poor catechol progenitors.[138,139] It appears that both estrogenic potential and oxidative stress caused by metabolic redox cycling of estrogen metabolites are essential for estrogen-induced carcinogenesis, since,

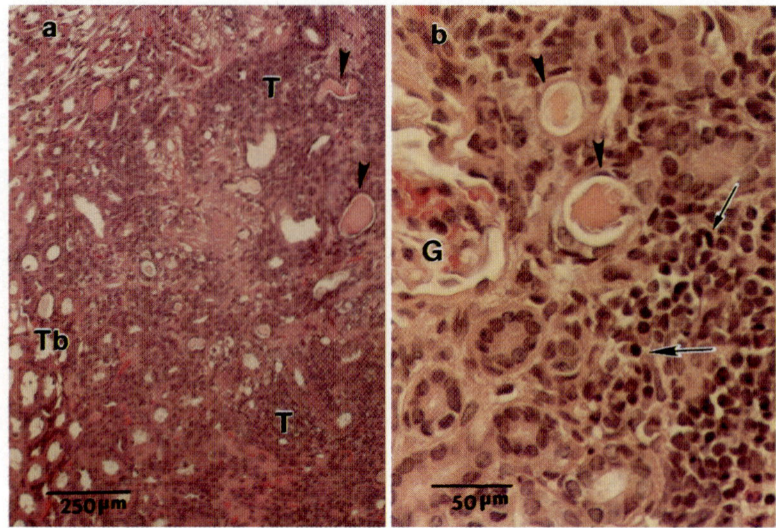

Fig. 5. Paraffin section of a tumor-bearing kidney stained with hematoxylin and eosin. The tumors were induced by treatment of male Syrian hamsters with a combination of αEE and menadione for 7 months. (a) Sections of the kidney demonstrate foci of tumor (T) with congested renal tubules (Tb and arrowheads). (b) The tumor is comprised of hyperchromatic cells with nuclear crowding (arrows). Congested renal tubules (arrow heads) and atrophied glomeruli (G) are also seen entrapped within the tumor nodule. Magnification a $= 10\times$; b $= 40\times$. (*Courtesy*: Bhat *et al.*, *Proc. Natl. Acad. Sci. USA*, 100, 3913–3918, 2003.)

if estrogen is withdrawn, tumors regress.[14] The hormonal effects of estrogens may promote the development of tumors. In the hamster renal tumor model, chronic treatment with αEE results in poor tumor incidence (about 10%) after a prolonged treatment of 9–10 months, compared with βE2, which takes only about 6 months to induce tumors with incidence rates near 100%. αEE has about 30% of the potential to form catechol estrogens compared to βE2.[139] This means that αEE still has some, albeit low, potential to produce oxidative stress. Thus, αEE is a poor carcinogen in the hamster model.

A more than twofold increase in $PGF_{2\alpha}$, an established marker of oxidative stress *in vitro* and *in vivo*[144,145] has been detected in tumor-bearing kidney homogenates of hamsters treated with βE2 for 7 months compared with untreated controls (Fig. 6).[136] Kidney homogenates of hamsters treated with αEE for 7 months did not show any increase in $PGF_{2\alpha}$ levels compared

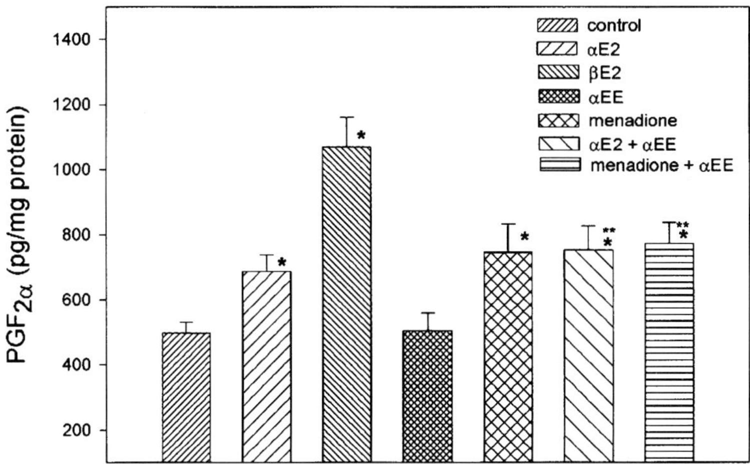

Fig. 6. 8-iso-Prostaglandin $F_{2\alpha}$ ($PGF_{2\alpha}$) levels in kidney homogenates of hamsters treated with αE2, βE2, αEE, menadione, αE2 + αEE, or menadione + αEE for 7 months. A >two-fold increase in $PGF_{2\alpha}$ is detected in βE2-treated tumor-bearing kidneys of hamsters. The fold increases in $PGF_{2\alpha}$ are 1.38, 1.50, 1.52, and 1.55, respectively, for kidneys of hamsters treated with αE2, menadione, αE2 + αEE, and menadione + αEE compared with untreated controls. $PGF_{2\alpha}$ and protein were analyzed from 10 kidney homogenates from each group, and data are expressed as mean $PGF_{2\alpha}$ pg/mg protein ± SEM. $^{*}p < 0.05$ compared with untreated controls by an unpaired t-test, $^{**}p < 0.05$ compared to αEE treated group by an unpaired t-test. (*Courtesy*: Bhat *et al.*, *Proc. Natl. Acad. Sci. USA*, 100, 3913–3918, 2003.)

with untreated controls (Fig. 6). As expected, menadione treatment resulted in an increase in kidney levels of $PGF_{2\alpha}$ compared with untreated controls. There were no significant differences in $PGF_{2\alpha}$ levels among αE2-, menadione-, and menadione + αEE-treated groups.

Tumors were clearly seen in kidneys of hamsters treated with a combination of αEE and menadione. This treatment group also showed a significant increase in $PGF_{2\alpha}$ levels compared with the αEE-treated group and compared with untreated controls. αE2 treatment leads to $PGF_{2\alpha}$ formation at reduced levels compared with βE2. This may indicate that αE2 catechols may be methylated faster than βE2 catechols, thus making them available at reduced levels for catechol quinone redox cycling. Treatment of hamsters with αEE did not result in increased $PGF_{2\alpha}$ formation. αEE is known to inhibit cytochrome P450 activity and, therefore, catechol estrogen formation.[146,147] The reduced ability of αEE to form catechol estrogens has been suggested to be responsible for the poor carcinogenic potential of αEE.[139]

In summary, the contributing role of steroid hormones in promoting the growth of certain malignancies, most notably breast and endometrial carcinomas, has been recognized for years. However, the mechanism of tumorigenic transformation is not yet fully understood. This complex process may combine endocrine aspects, such as receptor-mediated cell proliferation, with oxidative stress-mediated events (Fig. 7).

4. Conclusions

Long-term exposure to estradiol increases the risk of breast cancer in a variety of animal species, as well as in women.[1–17] Epidemiological studies suggest a strong correlation between estrogen use and incidence of breast cancer.[1–12] The mechanisms responsible for this effect have not been firmly established. Available data suggest that the mechanism of tumor formation by estrogens is more complex than previously considered. Oxidative stress is created as a result of the metabolic activation of carcinogenic estrogens to catechol estrogens and redox cycling between catechol estrogens and their corresponding quinones (Fig. 3). Some of the recent studies provide strong evidence that oxidative stress plays a critical role in estrogen-induced tumorigenesis, and that the oxidant potential of different estrogens is associated with their potential to form catechol estrogens.

17β-Estradiol is converted into 2-OHE2 and 4-OHE2 by P450 mediated processes.[57,98–100] However, 2-OHE2 and 4-OHE2 differ in their carcinogenic potential. Catechol quinone DNA adducts of 4-OHE2 have been shown to be formed in the female ACI rat mammary gland.[148] Although not proven to be carcinogenic in human breast cancers, 4-OHE2 levels have been shown to be significantly increased in human breast cancers compared to non-tumor tissue.[39,95,96] It has also been reported that 4-OHE2 level is elevated in human endometrial and breast cancers in comparison to normal tissue.[39] It is toxicologically active and appears to play a role in tumorigenesis, because it generates free radicals from reductive–oxidative cycling with the corresponding semiquinone and quinone forms, which can cause cellular damage.[47,149] Picomole amounts of 4-OHE2 have been obtained

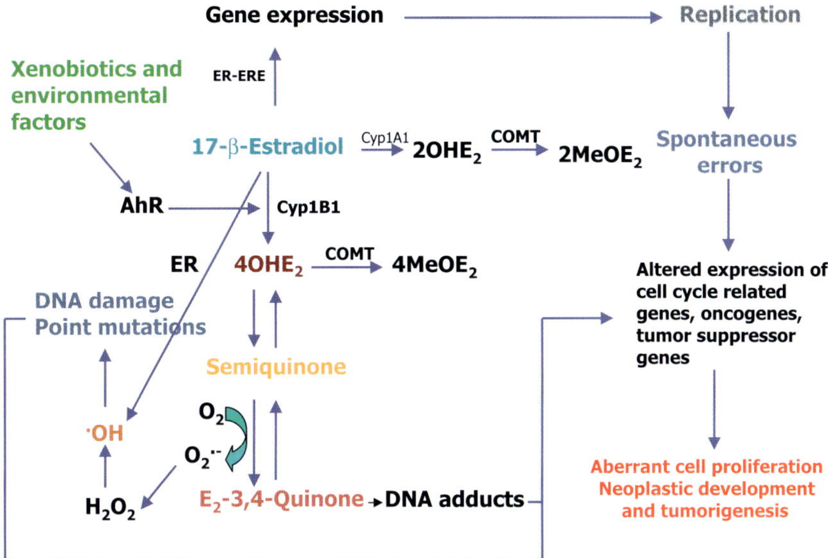

Fig. 7. Proposed mechanism of estrogen-induced carcinogenesis. The mechanism of estrogen-induced carcinogenesis seems to be complex. 17β-Estradiol can be metabolically activated to 2-OHE2 and 4-OHE2 by Cyp1A1 and Cyp1B1, respectively. 4-OHE2 (and 2-OHE2) can be converted into their respective quinones via semiquinone intermediates. This redox cycling can lead to the formation of superoxide radical. 2-OHE2 and 4-OHE2 can be methylated by catechol-*O*-methyltransferase (COMT) and thus not available for redox cycling. H_2O_2 formed from superoxide radical by superoxide dismutase can be further converted into hydroxyl radical by an iron-catalyzed Fenton reaction. The hydroxyl radical can also be produced by an ER-dependent pathway. The hydroxyl radical produced can damage DNA and cause point mutations. E2-quinones can also lead to DNA adduct formation. DNA damage as a result of adduct formation, point mutations, etc., is suggested to lead to altered expression of cell cycle-related genes, oncogenes, and tumor suppressor genes. 17β-Estradiol can induce gene expression via ER-ERE-dependent mechanisms. Spontaneous errors during replication can result in altered expression of genes. Xenobiotics and other environmental factors can also alter estrogen metabolizing enzyme Cyp1B1 via aryl hydrocarbon (AhR) receptor-mediated processes. Thus, oxidative stress created as a result of the metabolic activation of estrogens to catechol estrogens and subsequent redox cycling of catechol estrogens to quinone metabolites generates reactive oxygen species and free radicals, which act in concert with receptor-mediated processes to produce altered expression of genes critical in the cellular control of proliferation, and finally results in aberrant cell proliferation, neoplastic development and tumorigenesis.

from breast tumor samples in ERKO/Wnt-1 mice but not their methoxy conjugates nor the 2-OHE2 or their methoxy conjugates.[150] These results are consistent with the hypothesis that mammary tumor development is primarily initiated by metabolism of estrogens to 4-OHE2, and then, to catechol estrogen-3,4-quinones, which can redox cycle to produce ROS and may react with DNA to induce oncogenic mutations.[150]

On the contrary, evidence for the role of 2-OHE2 in breast carcinogenesis is lacking and may even support a protective role for this metabolite in breast cancer risk.[74] Some studies suggest that treatment of rodents with certain inducers of estradiol 2-hydroxylation may decrease spontaneous tumorigenesis in estrogen-sensitive tissues.[151] It is also important to note that 2-OHE2 has antiproliferative and anticarcinogenic effects.[152–154] *In vitro*, 2-OHE2 exhibits a growth inhibitory effect on MCF-7 breast cancer cells.[155] In addition, 2-OHE2 has little tumorigenic activity in the Syrian hamster tumor model.[59] 4-OHE2 and 2-OHE2 have been shown to affect gene regulation differently.[156] In two ovarian cancer cell lines OVCAR-3 and A2780-CP70, 4-OHE2 has been shown to induce hypoxia-inducible factor 1α (HIF-1α) and vascular endothelial growth factor A (VEGF-A) expression but not by 2-OHE2.[156] Overexpression of HIF-1α occurs in most human cancers.[157] The expression and activity of HIF-1α are correlated with tumorigenicity and angiogenesis in nude mice.[158] In addition, certain estrogen-induced tumors have also been associated with an increase in the expression of VEGF-A and its receptors.[159] It has also been shown that only 4-OHE2 and not 2-OHE2 metabolite is capable of inducing 8-OHdG in MCF-7 cells.[160] It must be noted however that 2-OHE2 has been shown to induce uterine tumors in mice although only 12% compared to 66% with 4-OHE2 treatment.[149] This differential mechanism of 4-OHE2 vs. 2-OHE2-induced carcinogenesis needs to be explored.

4-Hydroxyestradiol may also affect tumorigenesis via ER-mediated processes. 4-OHE2 does bind ERα, but has a lower affinity for ERα than βE2.[161] It is also possible that 4-OHE2 has its own receptor different from βE2 as has been suggested recently.[162] Furthermore, it is known that 2-OHE2 is methylated faster than 4-OHE2[139,163] and thus removed out of circulation before it has chance to produce reactive oxygen species. It is also known that 2-OHE2 inhibits the methylation of 4-OHE2,[164] thus making it available for a longer time. It is important to point out that estrogenic effects, most likely through receptor-mediated events, cannot be discounted in estrogen-mediated carcinogenesis.

Additionally, it is possible that oxidative stress may modify the ability of ERα to bind to its ERE usually located within the promoter region of estrogen-responsive target genes and thereby modify subsequent gene expression.[105–108] Endogenous cleavage of 67 kD ER and formation of an $\sim$50 kD nuclear receptor product has been suggested to be associated with the progression to hormonally-independent breast tumors in some murine models.[165] It has been suggested that truncated DNA binding ER may compete for available target gene EREs, interfering with normal receptor regulated gene transcription. It has been shown that in one-third of human breast cancer patients, ERα is unable to bind to its cognate ERE.[124,125] Oxidant (H_2O_2, menadione) exposure to cultured CHO or MCF-7 cells impairs the ability of endogenous ER to bind DNA and transactivate an ER-responsive reporter gene, demonstrating that extracellular redox stress can modulate intracellular ER function.[124] Treatment of MCF-7 cells with physiological levels of βE2 has been shown to increase the sensitivity to DNA damage as measured by 8-OHdG formation.[130] A two- to fourfold increase in PGF2α levels has been shown in cancer cell lines following treatment with 10 nM βE2.[129] Decrease in oxidative stress may also be reflected by an increase in antioxidant defense enzymes and/or catechol methyltransferase, the enzyme responsible for methylation of catechol estrogens and thus for the removal of catechol estrogens from redox cycling. Decrease in antioxidant defense enzymes has been shown *in vitro* and *in vivo* following βE2 treatment.[137,166] Thus, it is concluded that oxidative stress generated as a result of metabolic redox cycling of carcinogenic estrogens between their catechol estrogen and quinone metabolites plays an important role in estrogen-induced carcinogenesis.

References

1. Henderson BE, Ross RK, Pike MC. Hormonal chemoprevention of cancer in women. *Science* 259: 633–638 (1993).
2. IARC Monographs on the Evaluation of the Carcinogenic Risk of Chemicals to Humans. *Sex Hormones* (II), Vol. 21, pp. 139–362 (1979). International Agency for Research on Cancer, IARC, Lyon.

3. Henderson BE, Feigelson HS. Hormonal carcinogenesis. *Carcinogenesis* 21: 427–433 (2000).
4. Ross RK, Paganini-Hill A, Wan PC, Pike MC. Effect of hormone replacement therapy on breast cancer risk: estrogen versus estrogen plus progestin. *J. Natl. Cancer Inst.* 92: 328–332 (2000).
5. Schairer C, Lubin J, Troisi R, Sturgeon S, Brinton L, Hoover R. Menopausal estrogen and estrogen-progestin replacement therapy and breast cancer risk. *JAMA* 283: 485–491 (2000).
6. Verloop J, Rookus MA, Van Leeuwen FE. Prevalence of gynecologic cancer in women exposed to diethylstilbestrol *in utero*. *New Engl. J. Med.* 342: 1838–1839 (2000).
7. Lipman ME. Endocrine responsive cancers. In: Williams RH (ed.) *Textbook of Endocrinology*. WB Saunders & Co, Philadelphia, 1985, pp. 1309-1326.
8. Marshall E. Epidemiology: search for a killer. Focus shifts from fat to hormones. *Science* 259: 618–621 (1993).
9. Key TJ. Serum oestradiol and breast cancer risk. *Endocr. Relat. Cancer* 6: 175–180 (1999).
10. Service RF. New role of estrogen in cancer. *Science* 279: 1631–1633 (1998).
11. Steinberg KK, Smith SJ, Thacker SB, Stroup DF. Breast cancer risk and duration of estrogen use — the role of study design in meta-analysis. *Epidemiology* 5: 415–421 (1994).
12. Colditz GA, Hankinson SE, Hunter DJ, Willett WC, Manson JE, Stampfer MJ, Hennekens C, Rosner B, Speizer FE. The use of estrogens and progestins and the risk of breast cancer in post-menopausal women. *New Engl. J. Med.* 332: 1589–1593 (1995).
13. Bhat HK, Hacker HJ, Bannasch P, Thompson EA, Liehr JG. Localization of estrogen-receptors in interstitial cells of hamster kidney and in estradiol-induced renal tumors as evidence of the mesenchymal origin of this neoplasm. *Cancer Res.* 53: 5447–5451 (1993).
14. Kirkman H. Estrogen induced tumors of the kidney in the Syrian hamster. Growth characteristics in the Syrian hamsters. *Natl. Cancer Inst. Monogr.* 1: 1–57 (1959).
15. Newbold PR, Bullock BC, McLachlan JA. Uterine adenocarcinoma in mice following developmental treatment with estrogens: a model for hormonal carcinogenesis. *Cancer Res.* 50: 7677–7681 (1990).
16. Shull JD, Spady TJ, Snyder MC, Johansson SL, Pennington KL. Ovary-intact, but not ovariectomized female ACI rats treated with 17β-estradiol rapidly develop mammary carcinoma. *Carcinogenesis* 18: 1595–1601 (1997).

17. Harvell DM, Strecker TE, Tochacek XB, Pennington KL, McComb RD, Roy SK, Shull JD. Rat strain-specific actions of 17β-estradiol in the mammary gland: correlation between estrogen-induced lobuloalveolar hyperplasia and susceptibility to estrogen-induced mammary cancers. *Proc. Natl. Acad. Sci. USA* 97: 2779–2784 (2000).
18. NIEHS Press Release. New federal report on carcinogens lists estrogen therapy, ultraviolet, wood dust, NIEHS PR # 02-11, December 11, 2002.
19. Writing Group for the Women's Health Initiative Investigators. Risks and benefits of estrogen plus progestin in healthy post-menopausal women: principal results from the women's health initiative randomized controlled trial. *JAMA* 288: 321–333 (2002).
20. Wysowski DK, Comstock GW, Helsing KJ, Lau HL. Sex hormone levels in serum in relation to the development of breast cancer. *Am. J. Epidemiol.* 125: 791–799 (1987).
21. Garland CF, Friedlander NJ, Barrett-Connor E, Khaw KT. Sex hormones and post-menopausal breast cancer: a prospective study in an adult community. *Am. J. Epidemiol.* 135: 1220–1230 (1992).
22. Adlecreutz H, Gorbach SL, Goldin BR, Woods MN, Dwyer JT, Hamalainen E. Estrogen metabolism and excretion in Oriental and Caucasian women. *J. Natl. Cancer Inst.* 86: 1076–1082 (1994).
23. Toniolo PG, Levitz M, Zeleniuch-Jacquotte A, Banerjee Sigma, Koenig KL, Shore RE, Strax P, Pasternack BS. A prospective study of endogenous estrogens and breast cancer in post-menopausal women. *J. Natl. Cancer Inst.* 87: 190–197 (1995).
24. Collaborative Group on Hormonal Factors in Breast Cancer. Breast cancer and hormone replacement therapy: collaborative re-analysis of data from 51 epidemiological studies of 52,705 women with breast cancer and 108,411 women without breast cancer. *Lancet* 350: 1047–1059 (1997).
25. Magnusson C, Baron JA, Correia N, Bergstrom R, Adami HO, Persson I. Breast cancer risk following long-term oestrogen-progestin-replacement therapy. *Int. J. Cancer* 81: 339–344 (1999).
26. Sillero-Arenas M, Delgado-Rodriguez M, Rodrigues-Canteras R, Bueno-Cavanillas A, Galvez-Vargas R. Menopausal hormone replacement therapy and breast cancer: a meta-analysis. *Obstet. Gynecol.* 79: 286–294 (1992).
27. Pike M, Bernstein L, Spencer D. Exogenous hormones and breast cancer risk. In: Neiderhuber J (ed.) *Current Therapy in Oncology*. B.C. Decker, St. Louis, 1993, pp. 292–302.
28. Holzman D. Elusive estrogens may hold key to some cancer risk. *J. Natl. Cancer Inst.* 87: 1207–1209 (1995).

29. Clarke R. Introduction and overview: sex steroids in the mammary gland. *J. Mammary Gland Biol. Neoplasia* 5: 245–250 (2000).
30. Nelson R. Steroidal oestrogens added to a list of known human carcinogens. *Lancet* 360: 2053 (2002).
31. IARC Monographs on the Evaluation of Carcinogenic Risks to Humans. *Hormonal Contraception and Post-menopausal Hormone Therapy*, Vol. 72, pp. 474–530 (1992).
32. Li JJ, Li SA, Oberly TD, Parson JA. Carcinogenic activities of various steroidal and non-steroidal estrogens in hamster kidney: relation to hormonal activity and cell proliferation. *Cancer Res.* 55: 4347–4351 (1995).
33. Liehr JG. Is estradiol a genotoxic mutagenic carcinogen? *Endocr. Rev.* 21: 40–54 (2000).
34. Liehr JG. Genotoxicity of steroidal oestrogens oestrone and oestradiol: possible mechanism of uterine and mammary cancer development. *Hum. Reprod. Update* 7: 273–281 (2001).
35. Liehr JG, Roy D. Free radical generation of redox cycling by estrogens. *Free Radic. Biol. Med.* 8: 415–423 (1990).
36. Han X, Liehr JG. 8-Hydroxylation of guanine bases in kidney and liver DNA of hamsters treated with estradiol. Role of free radicals in estrogen-induced carcinogenesis. *Cancer Res.* 54: 5515–5517 (1994).
37. Han X, Liehr JG. Microsome-mediated 8-hydroxylation of guanine bases of DNA by steroid estrogens: correlation of DNA damage by free radicals with metabolic activation of quinones. *Carcinogenesis* 16: 2571–2574 (1995).
38. Wang MY, Liehr JG. Identification of fatty acid hydroperoxide cofactors in the cytochrome P450-mediated oxidation of estrogens to quinone metabolites. Role and balance of lipid peroxides during estrogen-induced carcinogenesis. *J. Biol. Chem.* 269: 284–291 (1994).
39. Liehr JG, Ricci MJ, Jefcoate CR, Hannigan EV, Hokanson JA, Zhu BT. 4-Hydroxylation of estradiol by human uterine myometrium and myoma microsomes: implications for mechanism of uterine tumorigenesis. *Proc. Natl. Acad. Sci. USA* 92: 9220–9224 (1995).
40. Liehr JG, Ricci MJ. 4-Hydroxylation of estrogens as marker of human mammary tumors. *Proc. Natl. Acad. Sci. USA* 93: 3294–3296 (1996).
41. Tsutsui T, Suzuki N, Maizumi H, McLachlan JA, Barrett JC. Alteration in diethylstilbestrol-induced mutagenicity and cell transformation by exogenous metabolic activation. *Carcinogenesis* 7: 1415–1418 (1986).
42. Tsutsui T, Tamura Y, Hagiwara M, Miyachi T, Hikiba H, Kubo C, Barett JC. Induction of mammalian cell transformation and genotoxicity by

2-methoxyestradiol, an endogenous metabolite of estrogens. *Carcinogenesis* 21: 735–740 (2000).

43. Banerjee SK, Banerjee S, Li SA, Li JJ. Induction of chromosome aberrations in Syrian hamster renal cortical cells by various estrogens. *Mutant Res.* 311: 191–197 (1994).
44. Tsutsui T, Tamura Y, Yagi E, Barrett JC. Involvement of genotoxic effects in the initiation of estrogen-induced cellular transformation: studies using Syrian hamster embryo cells treated with 17β-estradiol and eight of its metabolites. *Int. J. Cancer* 86: 8–14 (2000).
45. Yan ZJ, Roy D. Mutations in DNA polymerase mRNA of stilbene estrogen-induced kidney tumors in Syrian hamsters. *Biochem. Mol. Biol. Int.* 37: 175–183 (1995).
46. Roy D, Floyd RA, Liehr JG. Elevated 8-hydroxydeoxyguanosine levels in DNA of diethylstilbestrol-treated Syrian hamsters: covalent DNA damage by free radicals generated by redox cycling of diethylstilbestrol. *Cancer Res.* 51: 3882–3885 (1991).
47. Han X, Liehr JG. DNA single strand breaks in kidneys of Syrian hamsters treated with steroid estrogens. Hormone-induced free radical damage preceding renal malignancy. *Carcinogenesis* 15: 997–1000 (1994).
48. Wang MY, Liehr JG. Induction by estrogens of lipid peroxidation and lipid peroxide derived malonaldehyde DNA adducts in male Syrian hamsters: role of lipid peroxidation in estrogen-induced kidney carcinogenesis. *Carcinogenesis* 16: 1941–1945 (1995).
49. Ho SM, Roy D. Sex hormone-induced nuclear DNA damage and lipid peroxidation in the dorsolateral prostates of Noble rats. *Cancer Lett.* 84: 155–162 (1994).
50. Wang M, Dhingra K, Hittelman WN, Liehr JG, de Andrade M, Li D. Lipid peroxidation-induced putative malondialdehyde-DNA adducts in human breast tissues. *Cancer Epidemiol. Biomarkers Prev.* 5: 705–710 (1996).
51. Schineider J, Kinne D, Fracchia A, Pierce V, Anderson KE, Bradlov HL, Fishman J. Abnormal oxidative metabolism of estradiol in women with breast cancer. *Proc. Natl. Acad. Sci. USA* 79: 3047–3051 (1982).
52. Bradlov HL, Hershcopf RJ, Martucci CP, Fishman J. Estradiol 16β-hydroxylation in the mouse correlates with mammary tumor incidence and presence of murine mammary tumor virus: a possible model for the hormonal etiology of breast cancer in humans. *Proc. Natl. Acad. Sci. USA* 82: 6295–6299 (1985).

53. Bhat HK. Depletion of mitochondrial DNA and enzyme in estrogen-induced hamster kidney tumors: a rodent model of hormonal carcinogenesis. *J. Biochem. Mol. Toxicol.* 16: 1–9 (2002).
54. Weisz J, Bui QD, Roy D, Liehr JG. Elevated 4-hydroxylation of estradiol by hamster kidney microsomes: a potential pathway of metabolic activation of estrogens. *Endocrinology* 131: 655–661 (1992).
55. Bunyagidj C, McLachlan JA. Catechol estrogen formation in mouse uterus. *J. Steroid Biochem.* 31: 795–801 (1988).
56. Bui QD, Weisz J. Identification of microsomal, organic hydroperoxide-dependent catechol estrogen formation: comparison with NADPH-dependent mechanism. *Pharmacology* 36: 356–364 (1988).
57. Spink DC, Hayes CL, Young NR, Christou M, Sutter TR, Jefcote CR, Gierthy JF. The effects of 2,3,7,8-tetrachlorodibenzo-p-dioxin on estrogen metabolism in MCF-7 breast cancer cells: evidence for induction of novel 17β-estradiol-4-hydroxylase. *J. Steroid Biochem. Mol. Biol.* 51: 251–258 (1994).
58. Paria BC, Chakraborty C, Dey SK. Catechol estrogen formation in the mouse uterus and its role in implantation. *Mol. Cell. Endocrinol.* 69: 25–32 (1990).
59. Liehr JG, Fang WF, Sirbasku DA, Ari-Ulubelen A. Carcinogenicity of catechol estrogens in Syrian hamsters. *J. Steroid Biochem.* 24: 353–356 (1986).
60. Li JJ, Li SA, Davis MF, Tawfik O, Tekmal RR, Coe J. Genomic instability: an early common characteristic of solely hormone-induced carcinogenesis in different experimental models. *Proc. Amr. Assoc. Cancer Res.* 42: 880 (2001), Abstract # 4723.
61. Jones M. Local estrogen biosynthesis in males and females. *Endocr. Relat. Cancer* 6: 131–137 (1999).
62. Hacker HJ, Bannasch P, Liehr JG. Histochemical analysis of the development of estradiol-induced kidney tumors in male Syrian hamsters. *Cancer Res.* 48: 971–976 (1988).
63. Gonzales A, Oberly TD, Li JJ. Morphological and immunohistochemical studies of the estrogen-induced Syrian hamster renal tumor: probable cell of origin. *Cancer Res.* 49: 1020–1028 (1989).
64. Dunning WF, Curtis MR, Segaloff A. Strain differences in response to diethylstilbestrol and the induction of mammary gland and bladder cancer in the rat. *Cancer Res.* 7: 511–521 (1947).
65. Rothschild TC, Boylan ES, Calhoon RE, Vonderhaar BK. Transplacental effects of diethylstilbestrol on mammary development and tumorigenesis in female ACI rats. *Cancer Res.* 47: 4508–4516 (1987).

66. Li SA, Weroha SJ, Tawfik O, Li JJ. Prevention of solely estrogen-induced mammary tumors in female ACI rats by tamoxifen: evidence for estrogen receptor mediation. *J. Endocrinol.* 175: 297–305 (2002).
67. Liehr JG, Ulubelen AA, Strobel HW. Cytochrome P450-mediated redox cycling of estrogens. *J. Biol. Chem.* 261: 16865–16870 (1986).
68. Roy D, Liehr JG. Temporary decrease in renal quinone reductase activity by chronic administration of estradiol to male Syrian hamsters. Increased superoxide formation by redox cycling of estrogen. *J. Biol. Chem.* 263: 3646–3654 (1988).
69. MacLusky NJ, Barena ER, Clark CR, Naftolin I. In: Merriam GM, Lipset MP (eds.) *Catechol Estrogens*. Raven, New York, 1983, pp. 151–165.
70. Li SA, Klicka JK, Li JJ. Estrogen 2- and 4-hydroxylase activity, catechol estrogen formation, and implications for estrogen carcinogenesis in the hamster kidney. *Cancer Res.* 45: 181–185 (1985).
71. Liehr JG. Dual role of oestrogens as hormones and procarcinogens: tumour initiation by metabolic activation of oestrogens. *Eur. J. Cancer Prev.* 6: 3–10 (1997).
72. Yager JD, Liehr JG. Molecular mechanisms of estrogen carcinogenesis. *Ann. Rev. Pharmacol. Toxicol.* 36: 203–232 (1996).
73. Cavalieri EL, Rogan EG, Chakravarti D. Initiation of cancer and other diseases by catechol orto-quinones: a unifying mechanism. *Cell. Mol. Life Sci.* 59: 665–681 (2002).
74. Cavalieri EL, Stack DE, Devaneson PD, Todorovic R, Dwivedy I, Higginbotham S, Johansson SL, Patil KD, Gross ML, Gooden JK, Ramanathan R, Cerny RL, Rogan EG. Molecular origin of cancer: catechol estrogen 3,4-quinones as endogenous tumor initiators. *Proc. Natl. Acad. Sci. USA* 94: 10937–10942 (1997).
75. Stack DE, Cavalieri EL, Rogan EG. Catecholestrogens as procarcinogens: depurinating adducts and tumor initiation. *Adv. Pharmacol.* 42: 833–836 (1998).
76. Nutter LM, Ngo EO, Abul-Hajj YJ. Characterization of DNA damage induced by 3,4-estrone-o-quinone in human cells. *J. Biol. Chem.* 266: 16380–16386 (1991).
77. Wyllie S, Leihr JG. Enhancement of estrogen-induced renal tumorigenesis in hamsters by dietary iron. *Carcinogenesis* 19: 1285–1290 (1998).
78. Jan ST, Devanesan PD, Stack DE, Ramanathan R, Byun J, Gross ML, Rogan EG, Cavalieri EL. Metabolic activation and formation of DNA adducts of hexestrol, a synthetic nonsteroidal carcinogenic estrogen. *Chem. Res. Toxicol.* 11: 412–419 (1998).

79. Chakravati D, Pelling JC, Cavalieri EL, Rogan EG. Relating aromatic hydrocarbon-induced DNA adducts and c-H-ras mutations in mouse skin papillomas: the role of apurinic sites. *Proc. Natl. Acad. Sci. USA* 92: 10422–10426 (1995).
80. Li KM, Todorovic R, Devanesan P, Higginbotham S, Kofeler H, Ramanathan R, Gross ML, Rogan EG, Cavalieri EL. Metabolism and DNA binding studies of 4-hydroxyestradiol and estradiol-3,4-quinone *in vitro* and in female ACI rat mammary gland *in vivo*. *Carcinogenesis* 25: 289–297 (2004).
81. Li JJ, Gonzalez A, Banerjee S, Banerjee SK, Li SA. Estrogen carcinogenesis in the hamster kidney: role of cytotoxicity and cell proliferation. *Environ. Health Perspect.* 101(Suppl. 5): 259–264 (1993).
82. Li JJ, Li SA. Estrogen carcinogenesis in the hamster kidney: a hormone-driven multistep process. *Prog. Clin. Biol. Res.* 394: 255–267 (1996).
83. Kong LY, Szaniszlo P, Albrecht T, Liehr JG. Frequency and molecular analysis of hprt mutations induced by estradiol in Chinese hamster V79 Cells. *Int. J. Oncol.* 17: 1141–1149 (2000).
84. Lareef MH, Russo IH, Sheriff RS, Tahin Q, Russo J. Estrogen-receptor independent induction of loss of heterozygosity in human breast epithelial cells by estrogen and metabolites. *Breast Cancer Res. Treat.* 76(Suppl. 1): S102 (2002), Abstract # 383.
85. Russo J, Hu YF, Tahin Q, Mihaila D, Slater C, Lareef MH, Russo IH. Carcinogenicity of estrogens in human breast epithelial cells. *APMIS* 109: 39–52 (2001).
86. Cavalieri E, Frenkel K, Liehr JG, Rogan E, Roy D. Estrogens as endogenous genotoxic agents — DNA adducts and mutations. *J. Natl. Cancer Inst. Monogr.* 27: 75–93 (2000).
87. Yager JD. Endogenous estrogens as carcinogens through metabolic activation. *J. Natl. Cancer Inst. Monogr.* 27: 67–73 (2000).
88. Chen Y, Liu X, Pisha E, Constantinou AI, Hua Y, Shen L, van Breemen RB, Elguindi EC, Blond SY, Zhang F, Bolton JL. A metabolite of equine estrogens, 4-hydroxyequilenin, induces DNA damage and apoptosis in breast cancer cell lines. *Chem. Res. Toxicol.* 13: 342–350 (2000).
89. Jefcoate CR, Liehr JG, Santen RJ, Sutter TR, Yager JD, Yue W, Santner SJ, Tekmal R, Demers L, Pauley R, Naftolin F, Mor G, Berstein L. Tissue-specific synthesis and oxidative metabolism of estrogens. *J. Natl. Cancer Inst. Monogr.* 27: 95–112 (2000).
90. Liehr JG. 4-Hydroxylation of oestrogens as a marker for mammary tumours. *Biochem. Soc. Trans.* 27: 318–323 (1999).

91. Musarrat J, Arezina-Wilson J, Wani AA. Prognostic and aetiological relevance of 8-hydroxyguanosine in human breast carcinogenesis. *Eur. J. Cancer* 32A: 1209–1214 (1996).
92. Wani G, Milo GE, D'Ambrosio SM. Enhanced expression of the 8-oxo-7,8-dihydrodeoxyguanosine triphosphatase gene in human breast tumor cells. *Cancer Lett.* 125: 123–130 (1998).
93. Liehr JG. Vitamin C reduces the incidence and severity of renal tumors by estradiol and diethylstilbestrol. *Am. J. Clin. Nutr.* 54: 1256S–1260S (1991).
94. Liehr JG, Wheeler WJ. Inhibition of estrogen-induced renal carcinoma in Syrian hamsters by vitamin C. *Cancer Res.* 43: 4638–4642 (1983).
95. Castagnetta LAM, Granata OM, Traina A, Ravazzolo B, Amoroso M, Miele M, Bellavia V, Agostara B, Carruba G. Tissue content of hydroxyestrogens in relation to survival of breast cancer patients. *Clin. Cancer Res.* 8: 3146–3155 (2002).
96. Rogan EG, Badawi AF, Devanesan PD, Meza JL, Edney JA, West WW, Higginbotham SM, Cavalieri EL. Relative imbalances in estrogen metabolism and conjugation in breast tissue of women with carcinoma: potential biomarkers of susceptibility to cancer. *Carcinogenesis* 24: 697–702 (2003).
97. Modugno F, Knoll C, Kanbour-Shakir A, Romkes M. A potential role for the estrogen-metabolizing cytochrome P450 enzymes in human breast carcinogenesis. *Breast Cancer Res. Treat.* 82: 191–197 (2003).
98. Hayes CL, Spink DC, Spink BC, Cao JQ, Walker NJ, Sutter TR. 17 Beta-estradiol hydroxylation catalyzed by human cytochrome P450 1B1. *Proc. Natl. Acad. Sci. USA* 93: 9776–9781 (1996).
99. Spink DC, Spink BC, Cao JQ, Gierthy JF, Hayes CL, Li Y, Sutter TR. Induction of cytochrome P450 1B1 and catechol estrogen metabolism in ACHN human renal adenocarcinoma cells. *J. Steroid Biochem. Mol. Biol.* 62: 223–232 (1997).
100. Lee AJ, Cai MX, Thomas PE, Conney AH, Zhu BT. Characterization of the oxidative metabolites of 17beta-estradiol and estrone formed by 15 selectively expressed human cytochrome p450 isoforms. *Endocrinology* 144: 3382–3398 (2003).
101. Lipsett MB, Merriam GR, Kono S, Brandon DD, Pfeiffer DG, Merriam GR. Metabolic clearance of catechol estrogens. In: Merriam GR, Lipsett MB (eds.) *Catechol Estrogens*. Raven Press, New York, 1983, pp. 105–114.
102. Emons G, Merriam GR, Pfeiffer D, Loriaux DL, Ball P, Knuppen R. Metabolism of exogenous 4- and 2-hydroxyestradiol in the human male. *J. Steroid Biochem.* 28: 499–504 (1987).

103. Santen RJ. To block estrogen's synthesis or action: that is the question. *Clin. Endocrinol. Metab.* 87: 3007–3012 (2002).
104. Preston-Martin S, Pike MC, Ross RK, Jones PA, Henderson BE. Increased cell division as a cause of human cancer. *Cancer Res.* 50: 7415–7421 (1990).
105. Evans R. The steroid and thyroid hormone superfamily. *Science* 240: 889–895 (1988).
106. Yamamoto KR. Steroid receptor regulated transcription of specific genes and gene networks. *Ann. Rev. Genet.* 19: 209–252 (1985).
107. Green S, Chambon P. Nuclear receptors enhance our understanding of transcription regulation. *Trends Genet.* 4: 309–314 (1988).
108. Beato M. Gene regulation by steroid hormones. *Cell* 56: 335–344 (1989).
109. Hahn WC, Weinberg RA. Rules for making human tumor cells. *New Engl. J. Med.* 347: 1593–1603 (2002).
110. Swaneck GE, Fishman J. Covalent binding of the endogenous estrogen 16 alpha-hydroxyestrone to estradiol receptor in human breast cancer cells: characterization and intranuclear localization. *Proc. Natl. Acad. Sci. USA* 85: 7831–7835 (1988).
111. Russo J, Ao X, Grill C, Russo IH. Pattern of distribution of cells positive for estrogen receptor α and progesterone receptor in relation to proliferating cells in the mammary gland. *Breast Cancer Res. Treat.* 53: 217–227 (1999).
112. Saji S, Jensen EV, Nilsson S, Rylander T, Warner M, Gustafsson JA. Estrogen receptors alpha and beta in the rodent mammary gland. *Proc. Natl. Acad. Sci. USA* 97: 337–342 (2000).
113. Zeps N, Bentel JM, Papadimitriou JM, Dawkins HJ. Murine progesterone receptor expression in proliferating mammary epithelial cells during normal pubertal development and adult estrous cycle. Association with ER alpha and ER beta status. *J. Histochem. Cytochem.* 47: 1323–1330 (1999).
114. Soderquist G. Effects of sex steroids on proliferation in normal mammary tissue. *Ann. Med.* 30: 511–524 (1998).
115. Shoker BS, Jarvis C, Clarke RB, Anderson E, Hewlett J, Davies MP, Sibson DR, Sloane JP. Estrogen receptor-positive proliferating cells in the normal and precancerous breast. *Am. J. Pathol.* 155: 1811–1815 (1999).
116. Shoker BS, Jarvis C, Sibson DR, Walker C, Sloane JP. Oestrogen receptor expression in the normal and pre-cancerous breast. *J. Pathol.* 188: 237–244 (1999).
117. Clarke RB, Howell A, Potten CS, Anderson E. Dissociation between steroid receptor expression and cell proliferation in human breast. *Cancer Res.* 57: 4987–4991 (1997).

118. Barrett JC, Wong A, McLachlan JA. Diethylstilbestrol induces neoplastic transformation without measurable gene mutation at two loci. *Science* 212: 1402–1404 (1981).
119. Barrett JC, Tsutsui T. Mechanism of estrogen-associated carcinogenesis. In: Huff J, Boyd J, Barrett JC (eds.) *Cellular and Molecular Mechanisms of Hormonal Carcinogenesis: Environmental Influences.* Wiley-Liss, New York, 1996, pp. 105–112.
120. Korach KS, McLachlan JA. The role of the estrogen receptor in diethylstilbestrol toxicity. *Arch. Toxicol.* 58(Suppl. 8): 33–42 (1985).
121. Li JJ, Weroha SJ, Davis MF, Tawafik O, Hou X, Li SA. ER and PR in renomedullary interstitial cells during syrian hamster estrogen-induced tumorigenesis: evidence for receptor-mediated oncogenesis. *Endocrinology* 142: 4006–4014 (2001).
122. Bocchinfuso WP, Hively WP, Couse JF, Varmus HE, Korach KS. A mouse mammary tumor virus-Wnt-1 transgene induces mammary gland hyperplasia and tumorigenesis in mice lacking estrogen receptor-α. *Cancer Res.* 59: 1869–1876 (1999).
123. Planas-Silva MD, Donaher JL, Weinberg RA. Functional activity of ectopically expressed estrogen receptor is not sufficient for estrogen-mediated cyclin D1 expression. *Cancer Res.* 59: 4788–4792 (1999).
124. Liang X, Lu B, Scott GK, Chang C-H, Baldwin MA, Benz CC. Oxidant stress impaired DNA binding of estrogen receptor from human breast cancer. *Mol. Cell. Endocrinol.* 146: 151–161 (1998).
125. Scott GK, Kushner P, Vigne JL, Benz CC. Truncated forms of DNA-binding estrogen receptors in human breast cancer. *J. Clin. Invest.* 88: 700–706 (1991).
126. Sun Y, Oberley LW. Redox regulation of transcriptional activators. *Free Radic. Biol. Med.* 21: 335–348 (1996).
127. Liu X, Yao J, Pisha E, Yang Y, Hua Y, Van Breemen RB, Bolton JL. Oxidative DNA damage induced by equine estrogen metabolites: role of estrogen receptor α. *Chem. Res. Toxicol.* 15: 512–519 (2002).
128. Nutter LM, Wu YY, Ngo EO, Sierra EE, Guiterrez PL, Abul-Hajj YJ. An o-quinone form of estrogen produces free radicals in human breast cancer cells: correlation with DNA damage. *Chem. Res. Toxicol.* 7: 23–28 (1994).
129. Patel MM, Bhat HK. Differential oxidant potential of carcinogenic and weakly carcinogenic estrogens: involvement of metabolic activation and cytochrome P450. *J. Biochem. Mol. Toxicol.* 18: 37–42 (2004).

130. Mobley JA, Brueggemeier RW. Estrogen receptor-mediated regulation of oxidative stress and DNA damage in breast cancer. *Carcinogenesis* 25: 3–9 (2004).
131. Amstad PA, Krupitza G, Cerutti PA. Mechanism of c-fos induction by active oxygen. *Cancer Res.* 52: 3952–3960 (1992).
132. Maki A, Berezesky IK, Fargnoli J, Holbrook NJ, Trump BF. Role of (Ca2+)i in induction of c-fos, c-jun, and c-myc mRNA in rat PTE after oxidative stress. *FASEB J.* 6: 919–924 (1992).
133. Ding M, Li JJ, Leonard SS, Ye JP, Shi X, Colburn NH, Castranova V, Vallyanathan V. Vanadate-induced activation of activator protein-1: role of reactive oxygen species. *Carcinogenesis* 20: 663–668 (1999).
134. Vincent F, Corral M, Defer N, Adolphe M. Effects of oxygen free radical on articular chondrocyte in culture: c-myc and c-Ha-ras messenger RNAs and proliferation kinetics. *Exp. Cell Res.* 192: 333–339 (1991).
135. Bhat HK, Hacker HJ, Thompson EB, Liehr JG. Differential regulation by estrogen of c-fos in hamster kidney and estrogen-induced kidney tumor cells: receptor mediation versus metabolic activation. *Int. J. Oncol.* 7: 527–534 (1995).
136. Bhat HK, Calaf G, Hei TK, Loya T, Vadgama JV. Critical role of oxidative stress in estrogen-induced carcinogenesis. *Proc. Natl. Acad. Sci. USA* 100: 3913–3918 (2003).
137. Liehr JG. Hormone-associated cancer: mechanistic similarities between human breast cancer and estrogen-induced kidney carcinogenesis in hamsters. *Environ. Health Perspect.* 105: 565–569 (1997).
138. Korenmann SG. Comparative binding activity of estrogens and its relation to estrogen potency. *Steroids* 13: 163–177 (1969).
139. Zhu BT, Roy D, Liehr JG. The carcinogenic activity of ethinyl estrogens is determined by both their hormonal characteristics and by their conversion to catechol metabolites. *Endocrinology* 132: 577–583 (1993).
140. Thor H, Smith MT, Hartzell P, Bellomo G, Jewell SA, Orrenius S. The metabolism of menadione(2-methyl-1,4-napthoquinone) by isolated hepatocytes. A study of the implications of oxidative stress in intact cells. *J. Biol. Chem.* 257: 12419–12425 (1982).
141. Ngo EO, Sun TP, Chang JY, Wang CC, Chi KH, Cheng AL, Nutter LM. Menadione-induced DNA damage in a human tumor cell line. *Biochem. Pharmacol.* 42: 1961–1968 (1991).
142. Chang M, Shi M, Forman J. Exogenous glutathione protects endothelial cells from menadione toxicity. *Am. J. Physiol.* 262: L637–L643 (1992).

143. Calderaro M, Martins EA, Menehgini R. Oxidative stress by menadione affects cellular copper and iron homeostasis. *Mol. Cell. Biochem.* 126: 17–23 (1993).
144. Pratico D, Lawson JA, FitzGerald GA. Cyclooxygenase-dependent formation of the isoprostane, 8-epi-prostaglandin $F_{2\alpha}$. *Biol. Chem.* 270: 9800–9808 (1995).
145. Morrow JD, Hill KE, Burk RF, Nammour TM, Badr KF, Robberts LJ II. A series of prostaglandin F2-like compounds are produced *in vivo* in humans by a non-cyclooxygenase, free radical-catalyzed mechanism. *Proc. Natl. Acad. Sci. USA* 87: 9383–9387 (1980).
146. White INH, Muller-Eberhard U. Decreased liver cytochrome P450 in rats caused by norethindrone or ethinylestradiol. *Biochem. J.* 166: 57–64 (1977).
147. Oritz de Montellano PR, Kunze KL. Self-catalyzed inactivation of hepatic cytochrome P-450 by ethinylestradiol. *J. Biol. Chem.* 255: 5578–5585 (1980).
148. Li KM, Todorovic R, Devanson P, Higgginbotham S, Kofeler H, Ramanathan R, Gross ML, Rogan EG, Cavalieri EL. Metabolism and DNA binding studies of 4-hydroxyestradiol and estradiol-3,4-quinone *in vitro* and in female ACI rat mammary gland *in vivo*. *Carcinogenesis* 25: 289–297 (2004).
149. Newbold RR, Liehr JG. Induction of uterine adenocarcinoma in CD-1 mice by catechol estrogens. *Cancer Res.* 60: 235–237 (2000).
150. Yue W, Santen RJ, Wang J.-P, Li Y, Verderame MF, Bocchinfuso WP, Korach KS, Devanson P, Todorovic R, Rogan EG, Cavalieri EL. Genotoxic metabolites of estradiol in breast: potential mechanism of estradiol induced carcinogenesis. *J. Steroid Biochem. Mol. Biol.* 86: 477–486 (2003).
151. Hiraku Y, Yamashita N, Nishiguchi M, Kawanishi S. Catechol estrogens induce oxidative DNA damage and estradiol enhances cell proliferation. *Int. J. Cancer* 92: 333–337 (2001).
152. Fotsis T, Zhang Y, Pepper MS, Adlercreutz H, Montesano R, Nawroth PP, Schweigerer L. The endogenous oestrogen metabolite 2-methoxyoestradiol inhibits angiogenesis and suppresses tumor growth. *Nature* 368: 237–239 (1994).
153. Hughes RA, Harris T, Altmann E, McAllister D, Vlahos R, Robertson A, Cushman M, Wang Z, Stewart AG. 2-Methoxyestradiol and analogs as novel antiproliferative agents: analysis of three-dimensional quantitative structure–activity relationships for DNA synthesis inhibition and estrogen receptor binding. *Mol. Pharmacol.* 61: 1053–1069 (2002).

154. Seegers JC, Aveling ML, Van Aswegen CH, Cross M, Koch F, Joubert WS. The cytotoxic effects of estradiol-17 beta, catecholestradiols and methoxyestradiols on dividing MCF-7 and HeLa cells. *J. Steroid Biochem.* 32: 797–809 (1989).
155. Vandewalle B, Lefebvre J. Opposite effects of estrogen and catecholestrogen on hormone-sensitive breast cancer cell growth and differentiation. *Mol. Cell. Endocrinol.* 61: 239–246 (1989).
156. Gao N, Nester RA, Sarkar MA. 4-Hydroxy estradiol but not 2-hydroxyestradiol induces expression of hypoxia-inducible factor 1α and vascular endothelial growth factor A through phosphatidylinositol 3-kinase/Akt/FRAP pathway in OVCAR-3 and A2780-CP70 human ovarian carcinoma cells. *Toxicol. Appl. Pharmacol.* 196: 124–135 (2004).
157. Zhong H, Chiles K, Feldser D, Laughner E, Hanrahan C, Georgescu MM, Simons JW, Semenza GL. Modulation of hypoxia-inducible factor 1 alpha expression by the epidermal growth factor/phosphatidylinositol 3-kinase/PTEN/AKT/FRAP pathway in human prostate cancer cells: implications for tumor angiogenesis and therapeutics. *Cancer Res.* 60: 1541–1545 (2000).
158. Maxwell PH, Dachs GU, Gleadle JM, Nicholls LG, Harris AL, Stratford IJ, Hankinson O, Pugh CW, Ratcliffe PJ. Hypoxia-inducible factor-1 modulates gene expression in solid tumors and influences both angiogenesis and tumor growth. *Proc. Natl. Acad. Sci. USA* 94: 8104–8109 (1997).
159. Banerjee SK, Sarkar DK, Weston AP, De A, Campbell DR. Over expression of vascular endothelial growth factor and its receptor during the development of estrogen-induced rat pituitary tumors may mediate estrogen-initiated tumor angiogenesis. *Carcinogenesis* 18: 1155–1161 (1997).
160. Bianco NR, Perry G, Smith MA, Templeton DJ, Montano MM. Functional implications of antiestrogen induction of quinone reductase: inhibition of estrogen-induced deoxyribonucleic acid damage. *Mol. Endocrinol.* 17: 1344–1355 (2003).
161. Lottering ML, Haag M, Seegers JC. Effects of 17 beta-estradiol metabolites on cell cycle events in MCF-7 cells. *Cancer Res.* 52: 5926–5932 (1992).
162. Philips BJ, Ansell PJ, Newton LG, Harada N, Honda S-I, Ganjam VK, Rottinghaus GE, Welshons WV, Lubahn DB. Estrogen receptor-independent catechol estrogen binding activity: protein binding studies in wild-type, estrogen receptor-α KO, and aromatase KO mice tissues. *Biochemistry* 43: 6698–6708 (2004).

163. Zhu BT, Liehr JG. Inhibition of catechol O-methyltransferase-catalyzed O-methylation of 2- and 4-hydroxyestradiol by catecholamines. *Arch. Biochem. Biophys.* 304: 248–256 (1993).
164. Roy D, Weisz J, Liehr JG. 2-Hydroxyestradiol mediated inhibition of catechol O-methyl transferase catalyzed methylation of 4-hydroxyestradiol. *Carcinogenesis* 11: 459–462 (1990).
165. Sluyser M. Steroid/thyroid receptor-like proteins with oncogenic potential: a review. *Cancer Res.* 50: 451–458 (1990).
166. Liehr JG, Roy D, Gladek A. Mechanism of inhibition of estrogen-induced renal carcinogenesis in male Syrian hamsters by vitamin C. *Carcinogenesis* 10: 1983–1988 (1989).

31 Oxidative Stress in HIV Infection

Wulf Dröge

1. Introduction

Oxygen radicals (superoxide) and superoxide-derived "reactive oxygen species" (ROS) are constantly generated in almost all living tissues and play a role in various important physiological signaling processes.[1,2] However, ROS are chemically highly reactive molecules that can potentially damage vital tissue constitutents, such as DNA, proteins, and lipids.[3] "Oxidative stress" occurs if ROS rcach abnormally high concentrations. The pathology of oxidative stress may involve both oxidative tissue damage and the dysregulation of physiological signals. Superoxide can be formed from molecular oxygen by certain highly regulated enzymes such as NAD(P)H oxidases, or non-enzymatically by semi-ubiquinone in the mitochondrial respiratory chain and by a few other mechanisms.[2] Superoxide, in turn, is enzymatically converted into hydrogen peroxide by superoxide dismutases (SODs). Superoxide and hydrogen peroxide can give rise to additional types of ROS, some of which are chemically more aggressive than superoxide and hydrogen peroxide.

To ensure their function as signaling molecules, ROS are rapidly scavenged by various types of antioxidants such as glutathione, vitamin C, and vitamin E. Abnormally high concentrations of ROS (i.e., oxidative stress) may therefore result either from an increased production of ROS or by a decrease in cellular antioxidant concentrations.

In view of the difficulty to demonstrate and quantitate ROS directly in biological tissues, the evidence for oxidative stress is mostly indirect. It typically relies on the demonstration of products of lipid peroxidation and the decrease in the concentrations of antioxidants such as glutathione and antioxidative vitamins.

2. Evidence for Oxidative Stress in HIV Infection

That HIV infection may lead to oxidative stress was first suggested by the finding that intracellular glutathione, plasma cystine, and cysteine concentrations of HIV-infected patients are abnormally low.[4–6] The abnormal cysteine status and the decrease in intracellular glutathione levels of peripheral blood mononuclear cells from HIV-infected patients have been confirmed in numerous studies.[7–15] In addition, HIV-infected individuals were found to have abnormally low glutathione levels in the blood plasma and alveolar lining fluid[16] and significantly decreased plasma albumin levels.[17,18] Albumin is the quantitatively most important thiol-containing redox buffer of the plasma. As these changes were demonstrable not only in symptomatic but also in clinically asymptomatic HIV^+ subjects, they did not appear to result from the metabolic dysregulation that is typically seen in advanced disease. A decrease in cystine and glutathione was also demonstrated in simian immunodeficiency virus (SIV)-infected rhesus macaques.[19]

As glutathione is the quantitatively most important ROS scavenger, it was not surprising to see that the decrease in glutathione, cysteine, and albumin concentrations in HIV-infected subjects was associated with an increase in lipid peroxidation as conlcuded from increased concentrations of plasma malondealdehyde, plasma lipid peroxides, and breath pentane.[20–27] In addition, antioxidative vitamin levels, such as plasma concentrations of vitamin C and the β-carotene/vitamin A levels, were shown to be significantly decreased.[28–31] Decreased levels of α-tocopherol/vitamin E were found by some authors[32] but not by others.[30] One group found increased levels of oxidatively modified DNA bases, such as 8-hydroxyguanine, in HIV-infected subjects.[25]

3. Evidence for the Contribution of Oxidative Stress to the Pathogenesis of HIV Infection

The notion that oxidative stress may contribute to the pathogenesis of HIV infection was suggested by several reports showing (i) that ROS and/or

GSH depletion stimulate the signaling cascade that triggers virus replication, (ii) that GSH depletion inhibits certain lymphocyte functions in cell cultures, (iii) that cysteine supplementation was found to enhance immunological functions and to ameliorate disease progression in clincal trials, and (iv) that cysteine plays a role in the regulation of hepatic urea production, i.e., a major determinant of nitrogen balance.

3.1. *Enhancement of nuclear factor-κB (NF-κB) activity and virus replication*

A role of ROS in the regulation of gene expression was originally suggested by the finding that superoxide or low micromolar concentrations of hydrogen peroxide increase the production of the lymphokine interleukin-2 in activated T cells.[33] In line with this finding it was subsequently shown that antioxidant thiols inhibit the activation of the transcription factor NF-κB and the NF-κB-dependent expression of genes under the control of the HIV-LTR promoter in lymphoid cell cultures.[34–36] Thiol-containing antioxidants were found to inhibit HIV-1 replication both in acutely infected and latently infected cultured T cell lines and in a pro-monocytic cell line,[35–37] and a phosphodiester compound of vitamin E and vitamin C was found to inhibit the NF-κB-dependent transcription of genes under control of the HIV-1 promoter.[38] In line with these reports it was found that NF-κB activation and HIV-LTR activity are regulated by intracellular glutathione levels,[39,40] and that the activation of the transcription factor NF-κB is enhanced in certain T cell lines by hydrogen peroxide[41] or by a moderate pro-oxidative shift in the glutathione redox status.[42,43] The redox-responsive signaling cascades involved in lymphocyte activation have been analyzed in considerable detail.[2]

3.2. *Impairment of lymphocyte functions by glutathione depletion*

Whereas certain signaling cascades are enhanced or even induced by oxidative conditions, other lymphocyte functions such as lymphocyte proliferation are exquisitely sensitive to ROS and favored by relatively high levels of glutathione.[2] Studies of lymphocyte functions in cell cultures have been greatly facilitated by the empirical finding that lymphocyte cultures are strongly enhanced by thiol compounds.[43,45] Since 1970, immunologists have routinely been adding 2-mercaptoethanol to the cell culture medium when studying immunological responses of murine lymphocytes.[46] 2-Mercaptoethanol was later shown to enhance the cysteine supply to the lympoid cells and to increase thereby the intracellular glutathione concentration.[45] Even a moderate depletion of the intracellular glutathione pool by treatment with buthionine sulfoximine, a specific inhibitor of glutathione biosynthesis, causes a strong decrease in a variety of lymphocyte functions.[47] From these seemingly conflicting requirements for lymphocyte activation and proliferation, it is obvious that the immune system needs a delicately balanced intermediate level of glutathione. A study of 85 untreated healthy human subjects indicated that healthy subjects happen to have, on the average, optimal intracellular glutathione levels.[48] Individuals with glutathione levels near the median level of 25 nmol/mg protein were found to have, on the average, a significantly higher number of $CD4^+$ T cells than individuals with either lower or higher glutathione levels. This exquisite sensitivity of the lymphocyte population against changes in intracellular glutathione levels strongly suggests that the conspicuous glutathione depletion in HIV-infected individuals may play a causative role in the development of the immunological deficiency and disease progression.

3.3. *Clinical effects of cysteine supplementation*

The causative role of the conspicuous glutathione and cysteine depletion in the development of immunological dysfunctions in HIV infection has also been suggested by a series of clinical intervention studies. The free amino acid L-cysteine is relatively unstable and therefore not suited for clinical therapy. Cystine, i.e., the oxidized form, is poorly soluble in water and not readily taken up by the intestine. Most studies were therefore performed with the *N*-acetylated form of L-cysteine, which is relatively resistant to oxidation. It is a well-established drug in some Western countries for the treatment of chronic bronchitis and paracetamol intoxication.[49] In view of the existing pharmacological and toxicological data and its apparent safety in clinical medicine, *N*-acetyl-cysteine (NAC) has also been proposed for the treatment of HIV infection.[6,50] Results from several clinical studies of NAC by different laboratories revealed positive effects on several disease parameters. The therapeutic effect of NAC on immunological functions has been demonstrated in two randomized placebo-controlled studies in two groups of asymptomatic HIV-infected patients with or without anti-retroviral therapy, respectively.[17] In both studies, NAC treatment was found to cause amongst other positive effects the almost complete restoration of natural killer (NK) cell activity and a significant increase in the antigen-specific response to the recall-antigen tetanus toxoid (TET).[17] These findings were particularly satisfying as the restoration of immune functions is a widely accepted aim in the therapy of HIV infection. In line with this conclusion, NAC-treated HIV patients also showed a significantly improved two-year survival rate in an open label study.[14] A placebo-controlled trial with 3.2–8.0 g NAC per day for 8 weeks showed that whole blood glutathione levels were significantly increased.[14,51] Relatively low doses of NAC were also found to moderately decrease the plasma concentrations of TNF-α and to moderately slow the decrease in CD4 T cell counts.[9,52] Relatively small doses of NAC (600 mg per day) in combination with sodium selenite were studied in a randomized placebo-controlled trial by Look and colleagues[53] and were found to mediate a small but significant increase in the $CD4^+/CD8^+$ cell ratio together with a decrease in the absolute $CD8^+/CD38^+$ cell count after 6 and 12 weeks of treatment. An increase in absolute $CD4^+$ T cell numbers was also achieved in a randomized double-blind trial on the effects of a micronutrient mixture, including N-acetylcysteine, acetyl-L-carnitine, and α-lipoic acid, twice daily for 12 weeks.[54] Intravenous administration of NAC (3.0 g) for 15 days, in contrast, was found to be associated with a decrease in plasma p24 antigen without a substantial change in $CD4^+$ T cell numbers.[55] A relatively brief clinical study by Walker *et al.*[56] finally confirmed the safety of NAC for HIV^+ patients but failed to show significant therapeutic effects on viral load. Olivier[57] reported an increased tendency of lymphocytes from HIV-infected patients to undergo apoptosis and reported that NAC treatment ameliorated this process. This study, unfortunately, was not performed in a randomized double-blind fashion.

3.4. *Evidence for a role of cysteine in hepatic urea production and in the development of cachexia*

The loss of skeletal muscle tissue (cachexia) is another major clinical problem in HIV infection in addition to immunodeficiency. There are two lines of evidence that the hepatic availability of cysteine through its catabolism into sulfate and protons controls the hepatic urea production, i.e., a determining factor in the maintenance of nitrogen balance.[10,58–60] Studies of SIV-infected rhesus macaques and of mice with a transplanted fibrosarcoma showed consistently that the increase in muscular sulfate and the decrease in muscular glutathione levels were associated with a decrease in hepatic sulfate and a corresponding increase hepatic urea concentration.[58,59] Cysteine supplementation to the tumor-bearing mice yielded an increase in hepatic sulfate concentration and a corresponding decrease in hepatic urea levels.[10] As the urea cycle activity plays a decisive role in the breakdown of amino acids and the control of nitrogen balance, these results strongly suggest that a decrease in cysteine availability may contribute to the negative nitrogen balance that is commonly seen in all catabolic processes.

4. Loss of Cysteine as the Major Cause of Glutathione Depletion

The increase in lipid peroxidation and the decrease in antioxidant defenses as examplified by the decrease in glutathione and vitamin C levels is widely believed to result from an increased rate of ROS production. An increased rate of superoxide production might be explained by the dysregulation of cytokine levels and its effect on NADPH oxidase activation. Relatively large amounts of superoxide are typically produced by activated macrophages and neutrophils in inflamed tissues or by the xanthine oxidase reaction after ischemia and reperfusion.[2] However, there is no direct evidence for an increased rate of ROS production in HIV infection by any mechanism. Instead, there are several lines of evidence indicating that the massive decrease in plasma cysteine and intracellular glutathione concentrations of HIV-infected individuals is simply the consequence of excessive cysteine catabolism.[61] As the catabolism of cysteine yields sulfate (i.e., the salt of sulfuric acid), the net loss of cysteine can be easily demonstrated by the sulfate content of the urine.[61] It has also been shown that the peripheral tissues of the lower extremities of HIV-infected patients (i.e., mainly the skeletal muscle tissues) release substantial amounts of sulfate into the blood, indicating that the skeletal muscle tissue is the major site of elevated cysteine catabolism.[61] From the arterial venous differences of the plasma amino acid and sulfate concentrations of HIV^+ patients and healthy control subjects, it was estimated that the skeletal muscle tissue of a patient with a body weight of 70 kg produces, on the average, an *excessive* amount of sulfate equivalent to a daily catabolism of more than 5 g cysteine per day.[61] These findings were in line with studies on SIV-infected macaques, showing that the intracellular sulfate level in the skeletal muscle tissue was significantly increased and intracellular glutathione levels accordingly decreased.[59] The normal urinary daily sulfate excretion of healthy subjects was found to have a relatively small variability with a mean value of 1.88 ± 0.13 g corresponding to approximately 2.7 g cysteine per day.[61,62] The urinary sulfate excretion of clinically asymptomatic HIV^+ individuals without any anti-retroviral therapy, in contrast, showed a strong inter- and intra-individual variability and was, on the average, 4.8 g per day. An only slightly lower value was found for patients who had been treated with highly active anti-retroviral therapy (HAART). These data indicate that even asymptomatic HIV-infected subjects release, on the average, an *excess* of about 3 g sulfate per day corresponding to a *net* loss of approximately 4 g cysteine per day. It would be difficult for these patients to compensate this *excessive* loss of cysteine by an increased consumption of ordinary dietary proteins. In several earlier studies on protein-deficient diets in experimental animals the sulfur-containing amino acid cysteine and its precursor methionine were identified as the most limiting amino acids.[63–67] Taken together, these facts strongly suggested that the virus-induced cysteine deficiency may be a key factor in the pathogenesis of HIV disease and one of the causative factors leading to disease progression.

Importantly, the urinary sulfate excretion by early asymptomatic HIV-infected individuals was elevated more strongly than the excretion of urea, indicating that the excessive cysteine catabolism was associated with a net loss of glutathione, i.e., a substance with a relatively high sulfur/nitrogen ratio.[61] As the protein and glutathione content of the healthy human subject is relatively stable over time, the sulfur/nitrogen ratio in the urine of healthy subjects is obviously determined by the average sulfur/nitrogen ratio of the dietary proteins.

5. Concluding Remarks

Several lines of evidence support the conclusion that oxidative stress does occur in HIV infection and that it plays a role in the regulation of virus replication, in the development of immunodeficiency, and in disease progession. As there is no evidence for an increased rate of ROS production, it is reasonable to assume that increased concentrations of ROS may result mainly from the decrease in the concentrations of key antioxidants. Because glutathione is the quantitatively most important antioxidant and ROS scavenger, there is a strong possibility that the depletion of the glutathione pool alone may account for the increase in oxidative stress and the decreased concentrations of antioxidative vitamins as schematically illustrated in Fig. 1. The depletion of the glutathione pool appears to result from a decreased availability of the glutathione precursor cysteine as a consequence of an abnormal rate of intramuscular cysteine catabolism. This implies that the oxidative stress in HIV infection may be secondary to a dysregulation of biochemical processes related to cysteine catabolism. There is suggestive evidence that the decreased availability of cysteine may also enhance the hepatic urea production and may thus indirectly account for the development of a negative nitrogen balance, i.e., a key factor in AIDS-related cachexia. The cause and the mechanism of this abnormal cysteine catabolism are not known and clearly deserve more detailed investigations. In the absence of detailed information about these mechanisms, cysteine supplementation appears to be the method of choice to ameriorate the oxidative stress. Positive results have already been obtained in several clinical trials on the cysteine derivative *N*-acetylcysteine.

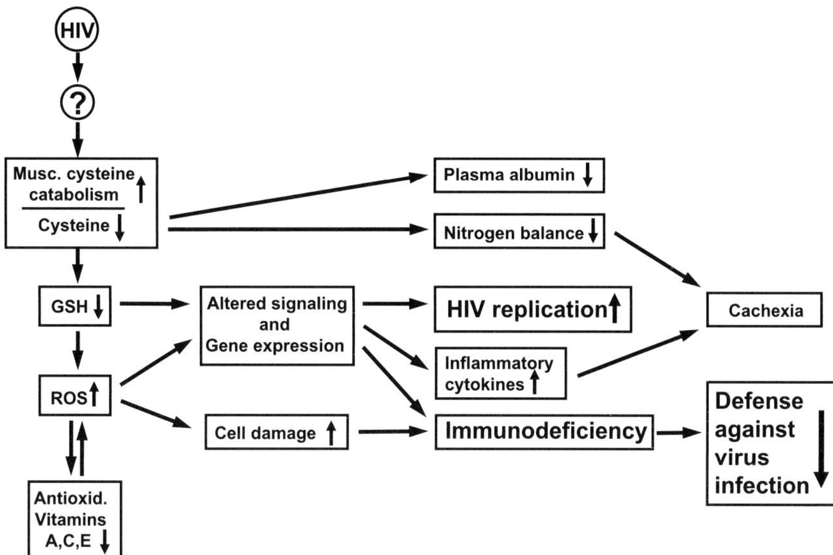

Fig. 1. Oxidative stress in HIV infection — Hypothetical scheme. A large body of evidence indicates that an abnormal increase in ROS concentrations (oxidative stress) plays a role in the regulation of virus replication, in the development of immunodeficiency, and in disease progression. It is reasonable to assume that the increased concentrations of ROS may result mainly from the decrease in the concentrations of the key antioxidant glutathione. The depletion of the glutathione pool is believed to account for the increase in ROS concentrations and indirectly for the decrease in the concentrations of antioxidative vitamins. The glutathione deficiency appears to result from a decreased availability of the glutathione precursor cysteine through an abnormal rate of intramuscular cysteine catabolism. Evidence from experimental animal studies suggest that a decreased availability of cysteine may also enhance the hepatic urea production and may thus indirectly account for the development of a negative nitrogen balance which is a key factor in AIDS-related cachexia. How HIV infection leads to the abnormal increase in cysteine catabolism is not known. This point deserves more detailed investigations.

References

1. Beckman KB, Ames BN. *Physiol. Rev.* 78: 547–581 (1998).
2. Dröge W. *Physiol. Rev.* 82: 47–95 (2002).
3. Harman D. *Proc. Natl. Acad. Sci. USA* 78: 7124–7128 (1981).

4. Dröge W *et al.* *Biol. Chem. Hoppe-Seyler* 369: 143–148 (1988).
5. Eck H-P *et al.* *Biol. Chem. Hoppe-Seyler* 370: 101–108 (1989).
6. Dröge W, Eck H-P, Mihm S. *Immunol. Today* 13: 211–214 (1992).
7. Staal FJ *et al.* *Lancet* 339: 909–912 (1992).
8. Hortin GL, Landt M, Powderly WG. *Clin. Chem.* 40: 785–789 (1994).
9. Åkerlund B *et al.* *Eur. J. Clin. Pharmacol.* 50: 457–461 (1996).
10. Hack V *et al.* *FASEB J.* 11: 84–92 (1997).
11. Walmsley SL *et al.* *AIDS* 11: 1689–1697 (1997).
12. Roederer M *et al.* *Int. Immunol.* 3: 933–937 (1991).
13. De Quay B, Malinverni R, Lauterburg BH. *AIDS* 6: 815–819 (1992).
14. Herzenberg LA *et al.* *Proc. Natl. Acad. Sci. USA* 94: 1967–1972 (1997).
15. Jahoor F *et al.* *Am. J. Physiol.* 276: E205–E211 (1999).
16. Pacht ER *et al.* *Chest* 112: 785–788 (1997).
17. Breitkreutz R *et al.* *J. Mol. Med.* 78: 55–62 (2000).
18. Madebo T, Lindtjørn B, Aukrust P, Berge RK. *Am. J. Clin. Nutr.* 78: 117–122 (2003).
19. Eck H-P, Stahl-Hennig C, Hunsmann G, Dröge W. *Lancet* 338: 346–347 (1991).
20. Sonnerborg A, Carlin G, Åkerlund B, Jarstrand C. *Scand. J. Infect. Dis.* 20: 287–290 (1988).
21. Halliwell B, Cross CE. *Arch. Intern. Med.* 151: 29–31 (1991).
22. Revillard JP, Vincent CMA. *J. Acquir. Immune Defic. Syndr.* 5: 637–638 (1992).
23. Favier A *et al.* *Chem–Biol. Interact.* 91: 165–180 (1994).
24. Malvy DJM *et al.* *Clin. Chim. Acta* 224: 89–94 (1994).
25. Jaruga P *et al.* *Free Radic. Biol. Med.* 32: 414–420 (2002).
26. Allard JP *et al.* *Am. J. Clin. Nutr.* 67: 143–147 (1998).
27. Aghdassi E, Allard JP. *Free Rad. Biol. Med.* 28: 880–886 (2000).
28. Bogden JD *et al.* *Ann. NY Acad. Sci.* 587: 189–195 (1990).
29. Lacey CJ *et al.* *Int. J. STD AIDS* 7: 485–489 (1996).
30. Treitinger A *et al.* *Eur. J. Clin. Invest.* 30: 454–459 (2000).
31. Simba RD, Graham NMH, Caiaffa WT. *Arch. Intern. Med.* 153: 2149–2154 (1993).
32. Javier JJ, Fodyce-Baum MK, Beach RS, *FASEB Proc.* 4: A940 (1990).
33. Roth S, Dröge W. *Cell. Immunol.* 108: 417–424 (1987).
34. Roederer M *et al.* *AIDS Res. Hum. Retroviruses* 7: 563–567 (1991).
35. Mihm S *et al.* *AIDS* 5: 497–503 (1991).
36. Raju P, Herzenberg LA, Herzenberg LA, Roederer M. *AIDS Res. Hum. Retroviruses* 10: 961–967 (1994).

37. Roederer M *et al. Proc. Natl. Acad. Sci. USA* 87: 4884–4888 (1990).
38. Hirano F *et al. Immunopharmacology* 39: 31–38 (1998).
39. Montano MA *et al. Proc. Natl. Acad. Sci. USA* 93: 12376–12381 (1996).
40. Staal FJ *et al. AIDS Res. Hum. Retroviruses* 9: 299–306 (1993).
41. Schreck R, Baeuerle PA. *Trends Cell. Biol.* 1: 39–42 (1991).
42. Galter D, Mihm S, Dröge W. *Eur. J. Biochem.* 221: 639–648 (1994).
43. Hehner SP *et al. J. Immunol.* 165: 4319–4328 (2000).
44. Meister A, Anderson ME. *Ann. Rev. Biochem.* 52: 711–760 (1983).
45. Ishii T, Sugita Y, Bannai S, *J. Cell. Physiol.* 133: 330–336 (1987).
46. Fanger MW, Hart DA, Wells JV, Nisonoff A. *J. Immunol.* 105: 1043–1045 (1970).
47. Dröge W *et al. FASEB J.* 8: 1131–1138 (1994).
48. Kinscherf R *et al. FASEB J.* 8: 448–451 (1994).
49. Cotgreave IA. *Adv. Pharmacol.* 38: 205–227 (1997).
50. Dröge W. In: *Project News*, No. 2. AIDS-Zentrum des Bundesgesundheitsamtes, Berlin, Germany, 1989, p. 4.
51. De Rosa SC *et al. Eur. Clin. Invest.* 30: 915–929 (2000).
52. Jarstrand C, Åkerlund B. *Chem–Biol. Interact.* 91: 141–146 (1994).
53. Look MP *et al. Eur. J. Clin. Invest.* 28: 389–397 (1998).
54. Kaiser J *et al. 11th Conference on Retroviruses and Opportunistic Infections*, 8–11 February 2004, San Francisco, Abstract No. 494.
55. Clotet B *et al. Int Conference on AIDS*, Vol. 8, B89 (1992), Abstract No. PoB 3013.
56. Walker RE *et al. Int. Conference on AIDS* (1992), Abstract No. MoB 0022.
57. Olivier R. *Meth. Enzymol.* 251: 270–278 (1995).
58. Hack V *et al. FASEB J.* 10: 1219–1226 (1996).
59. Gross A, Hack V, Stahl-Hennig C, Dröge W. *AIDS Res. Hum. Retroviruses* 12: 1639–1641 (1996).
60. Dröge W, Holm E. *FASEB J.* 11: 1077–1089 (1997).
61. Breitkreutz R *et al. AIDS Res. Hum. Retroviruses* 16: 203–209 (2000).
62. Dröge W, Breitkreutz R. *Proc. Nutr. Soc.* 59: 595–600 (2000).
63. Allison JB, Anderson JA, Seeley RD. *J. Nutr.* 33: 361–370 (1947).
64. Lubaszewska S, Pastuszewska B, Kielanowski J. *Z. Tierphysiol. Tierernahr. Futtermittelkd.* 31: 120–128 (1973).
65. Yoshida A, Moritoki K. *Nutr. Rep. Int.* 9: 159–168 (1974).
66. Okumura J, Muramatsu T. *Japan Poult. Sci.* 15: 69–73 (1978).
67. Webel DM, Baker DH. *Nutr. Res.* 19: 569–577 (1999).

32 Oxidative Stress and Breast Cancer

Jiyoung Ahn and Christine B. Ambrosone

1. Overview

1.1. *Breast cancer epidemiology*

Breast cancer is the most frequently diagnosed non-skin malignancy in women in the United States, with 213,910 cases expected in 2004,[1] and its incidence is gradually increasing. A woman who lives to be 90 years old has a 1 in 8 risk of being diagnosed with breast cancer in the United States.[2] Despite focused efforts over the last few decades to further understand the causes of breast cancer, little new information has been gained regarding its etiology. Risk factors that are "known" explain only approximately 40% of the variability in incidence.[3] The rest of the remaining risk for breast cancer remains a speculative or unknown realm. Estrogen exposure (e.g., early age at menarche, no or few children, late first full-term pregnancy, and hormone replacement therapy), family history of breast cancer, alcohol consumption, and physical activity have been considered as important risk factors, while data on other risk factors are inconsistent, including the potential effects of diet, smoking, and environmental factors on breast cancer risk.[4]

1.2. *Oxidative stress in breast cancer risk*

There is increasing evidence indicating that oxidative stress is involved in the pathogenesis of breast cancer. Exposures from endogenous and exogenous oxidant sources constantly produce reactive oxygen species (ROS) including superoxide radicals, hydrogen peroxide, and hydroxyl radicals *in vivo*. These ROS cause oxidative damage to biomolecules (e.g., DNA, protein, and lipids), and can cause genetic alterations, a process held in check only by the existence of multiple antioxidant systems that alter the balance between prooxidant cellular activity and antioxidant defenses. Sies defined oxidative stress as "a disturbance in the prooxidant–antioxidant balance in favor of the former,"[5] and the imbalance toward ROS may be related to carcinogenesis, either directly by damaging DNA or indirectly by causing abnormal signaling and cell cycle control. DNA double-strand breaks are probably the most dangerous of the many types of DNA damage that can be induced by direct ionization of DNA or indirectly via the generation of free radicals. In addition to DNA damage, ROS, particularly those generated by cancer therapy, induce mitochondrial changes and apoptosis,[6,7] whereby the mitochondrial membrane becomes permeable and the signaling cascade is triggered.[8,9]

Variability in exposure to factors that could impact levels of ROS, through endogenous processes or exogenous routes, will ultimately determine levels of oxidative stress in the breast, and many breast cancer risk factors can be linked through an oxidative stress mechanism, as described below. The role of oxidative stress in carcinogenesis has been widely demonstrated in *in vitro* studies and small human studies in relation to breast cancer risk,[10–12] and recent molecular epidemiologic studies of genetics and diet, hormonal factors, and environmental exposures also support a role for oxidative stress in DNA damage and subsequent breast carcinogenesis.

1.3. *Oxidative stress in cancer therapy*

In addition to the role of oxidative stress in cancer etiology, it is also likely to play an important role in outcomes after cancer therapy, not limited to breast cancer. Ionizing radiation and chemotherapeutic agents, including cyclophosphamide (CP) and anthracyclines, are often the most effective tools in breast cancer treatment. Experimental and clinical studies have shown that both radiation therapy and CP exert their cytotoxic effects to cancer cells primarily through increased formation of ROS.[13–15] The produced ROS can damage cells, proteins, and DNA or interact with other cellular molecules, producing secondary oxidation products, reactive molecules that contribute to cytotoxicity of cancer cells through the same mechanisms described above.

It is widely held that many chemotherapeutic agents and radiation therapy induce mitochondrial changes and apoptosis through mechanisms associated with ROS production.[6,7] As reviewed by Mignotte,[7] it has been well documented that oxidative stress provokes cell death as a result of massive cellular damage associated with lipid peroxidation and alterations of proteins and nucleic acids. Apoptosis occurs when, through a pathway of signaling, the mitochondrial membrane becomes permeable.[8,9] Mitochondria are the main site for ROS generation and are thought to be a major intracellular target for oxidative damage.[16] Anticancer agents can cause mitochondrial permeabilization through enhanced generation of ROS, and once the mitochondrial membrane barrier function is lost, a number of other factors contribute to cell death. While ROS, among other factors, induce or facilitate mitochondrial permeabilization, glutathione and antioxidant enzymes such as MnSOD, CAT, and GPX1 inhibit it.[8] In fact, experimental results indicate that MnSOD prevents the disruption of mitochondrial membrane potential.[17] Recently, it was shown that inhibition of SOD caused accumulation of superoxide radicals, leading to free-radical-mediated damage to mitochondrial membranes and apoptosis of cancer cells.[18] In a commentary on the study of MnSOD and apoptosis of cancer cells, Kastan and Cleveland[19] suggested that a promising way of treating some cancers could be by increasing levels of ROS and inhibition of SOD.

The majority of ROS-created lesions are rapidly repaired; however, unrepaired breaks may generate chromosomal aberrations and subsequent cancer cell death or may trigger intracellular apoptotic pathways.[20] Although greater protection of DNA and the mitochondria from ROS can prevent normal and tumor cell damage, it may weaken the effects of therapy upon the tumor and may reduce the likelihood of toxic skin reactions, therefore it may have poor prognostic result after breast cancer therapy. Furthermore, enhanced DNA repair capabilities will also prevent cell damage and death. Thus, interindividual variability resulting from polymorphisms in genes that protect cells from ROS and those that repair treatment-induced DNA damage will determine, to some degree, the efficacy of cancer treatment and the likelihood of severe treatment-related toxicity, as discussed below.

2. Biomarkers of Oxidative Stress

Numerous approaches have been used to evaluate levels of markers of oxidative stress in relation to breast cancer risk. Direct measurement of ROS is almost impossible due to the relatively short-term presence of the reactive intermediates;[21] thus, measurement of oxidative damage is a more common way to monitor oxidative stress. DNA adducts and 8-hydroxy-2-deoxyguanosine (8-OH-dG), resulting from direct DNA damage, and malondialdehyde (MDA) metabolites and adducts, caused by lipid peroxidation, are biomarkers commonly used in studies of breast cancer. Many studies have found that measures of oxidative stress, represented by these and other biomarkers, are consistently higher in tissue and body fluids from women with breast cancer compared with controls, although studies to date remain small.[22,23] Although it is quite clear that dietary change can alter the levels of some of the biomarkers, it is not clear whether they reflect processes in the initiation of a breast cancer or whether they are products of cancer.[24]

2.1. *DNA adducts*

The interaction of ROS with DNA generates bulky DNA adducts, and the measurement of these adducts is an indicator of oxidative stress. Since lipophilic aromatic compounds such as polycyclic aromatic hydrocarbons (PAHs) can be stored in the fatty tissues of the breast[25] and human mammary epithelial cells have a high capacity of metabolizing these compounds into DNA-binding species, DNA adducts could be useful biomarkers in the breast. As reviewed by Li D *et al.*, samples from breast cancer patients contained significantly higher levels of aromatic DNA adducts than did samples obtained from controls.[26] For example, a bulky benzo[*a*]pyrene (BP)-like adduct was detected in about 40% of the cancer patients, but in none of the controls.[26] Wang *et al.* evaluated MDA–DNA adducts, induced by an end product of lipid peroxidation, in normal breast tissue from breast cancer patients and that of healthy controls, and found that breast tissues from cancer patients exhibited significantly higher levels of the MDA–DNA adducts than those found in non-cancer controls.[27] The level of these adducts correlated with the presence of the BP-like adducts. These results indicate that DNA adducts resulting from oxidative stress can accumulate in human breast tissues and appear to be higher in women with breast cancer, perhaps due to greater exposures to sources of ROS, or to decreased detoxification and/or repair.

2.2. *8-Hydroxy-2-deoxyguanosine8-OH-dG*

The biomarker 8-hydroxy-2-deoxyguanosine (8-oxo-dG), a measure of oxidative damage to DNA, has been shown to be a valid indicator of oxidative stress.[28] The measurement of 8-oxo-dG from either human lymphocytes, breast tissue samples, or urine samples by either high-performance liquid chromatography (HPLC) or immunohistochemical assays have been developed successfully in human studies to reveal biologically significant differences between groups of individuals.[29] Oxidative DNA damage has been reported to be higher in tissue from women with breast cancer as compared with controls.[30] In addition, a significantly higher level of nuclear staining for 8-OH-dG was observed in samples adjacent to breast tumors compared to levels in tissues from women without breast cancer.[31] To date, most studies have been conducted in the context of case–control studies, and considering the long induction period of cancer, there is justifiable interest in determining whether biomarkers of DNA damage may be predictive of cancer risk. Furthermore, whether elevated levels of 8-oxo-dG is a result of increased oxidative stress or a failure of DNA repair is yet to be determined.[32]

2.3. *Autoantibodies to oxidized DNA*

The measurement of serum antibodies (Abs) that recognize 5-hydroxymethyl-2′deoxyuridine (HMdU), which is a product of thymine nucleotide oxidation, is also used as a biomarker of oxidative stress. ROS modification of DNA alters its immunogenicity leading to the generation of antibodies to ROS-DNA.[33] HMdU is measured in a simple enzyme-linked immunosorbent assay. Women healthy at blood donation but who were diagnosed 0.5–6 years later with breast or colorectal cancer exhibited significantly increased anti-HMdU Abs over the age-matched controls ($P < 0.001$).[34] Additional studies have shown that anti-HMdU Abs can be reduced by high levels of α-tocopherol,[35] and higher levels are associated with alcohol consumption, smoking, and GSTM1 null genotype.[36] Interestingly, Mooney and colleagues found that levels were higher among women than men, controlling for other factors known to be associated with ROS levels, suggesting that estrogens could impact oxidative stress levels and thus, HMdU Abs.[37]

2.4. *F2-isoprostanes*

The interaction of ROS with lipids results in lipid peroxidation, and the measurement of lipid peroxidation is considered a valid and sensitive indicator of oxidative stress.[38] The F2-isoprostanes are a unique series of prostaglandin-like compounds, formed *in vivo* when free radicals catalyze peroxidation of arachidonic acid, independent of the cyclooxygenase enzymes.[39] The measurement of F2-isoprostanes as an indicator of oxidative stress has been fairly well validated, and this biological marker is currently considered most appropriate for epidemiologic purposes, measuring total body oxidative stress.[40] Although it has been demonstrated that antioxidant supplementation decreases F2-isoprostane levels in smokers,[41,42] few studies have used F2-isoprostanes in the context of breast cancer risk. Djuric's group have analyzed F2-isoprostanes in human urine and plasma, and in breast nipple aspirate fluids,[43] finding that levels were higher in specimens from women with breast cancer, compared to those in normal controls.

2.5. *TBARS and aldehyde*

The TBARS assay is a simple spectrophotometric assay that measures a chromogen that is produced by the heating reaction of thiomarbituric acid (TBA) with malondialdehyde.[40] However, since this method does not measure free forms of MDA, but only forms generated by decomposition of peroxides during the heating process with acid, other compounds (sugars, amino acids, bilirubin) may react in this process.[40] Thus, generating artifact as well as lack of specificity is often a problem, and this biomarker tends to overestimate in the biological sample.[40] Using TBARS, there was one small study finding higher levels of TBARS in cancer tissue than adjacent normal tissues in breast cancer patients,[44] and another that noted TBARS levels to be lower in breast tissue from women with breast cancer compared to those with benign breast disease.[45]

Aldehyde is another stable end point of lipid peroxidation due to oxidative stress. 4-HNE (hydroxynonenal), propanol, and 4-hydroxyhexenal are often measured directly, using GC/MS or HPLC in tissue and urine samples. However, this biomarker is influenced by various conditions due to peroxide breakdown, such as the existence of transition metal.[40] To our knowledge, there have been no studies of these markers in relation to breast cancer.

3. Exogenous Factors Related to Oxidative Stress and Risk Factors of Breast Cancer

3.1. *Family history of breast cancer*

Perhaps the most consistent risk factor for breast cancer is diagnosis of the disease in a first degree relative. A family history of breast cancer may or may not imply genetic susceptibility, it may also be due to shared environments or lifestyle habits, or other less penetrant, more prevalent inherited factors. Among women with a family history of breast cancer, a proportion of them carry mutant alleles in *BRCA1* or *BRCA2*, which confer a high lifetime risk of breast cancer. The prevalence of deleterious *BRCA1* mutations is estimated to be 1/800 in the general population, but the two genes are believed to be responsible for most truly hereditary breast cancers.

Several mutations, such as 185delAG and 5382insC for *BRCA1* and 617delT for *BRCA2*, have been observed to occur, especially with higher frequency among Ashkenazi Jewish population.[46] Since these proteins are required for maintenance of chromosomal stability in mammalian cell and function in the biological response in DNA damage, mutations of these proteins are highly related to elevated risk of breast cancer.[47] BRCA1 is required for the transcription-coupled repair of oxidative damage.[48] Thus, poor repair due to mutations in *BRCA1*, combined with normal or higher levels of oxidative stress, could link these inherited mutations to breast cancer risk. This mutation is present in families with hereditary breast cancer, especially early onset of breast cancer, i.e., before the age of 35.[49]

3.2. *Reproductive and hormonal factors*

Estrogens have a role in the development and growth of breast cancer.[50] Estrogen promotes cell proliferative effects directly or indirectly, by production of growth factors or induction of enzymes or proteins involved in DNA synthesis.[51] Furthermore, the alkylation of cellular molecules and the generation of active free radicals that can damage DNA have both been implicated in the potential genotoxicity of estrogen and some of its metabolites, such as the catechol estrogens.[52] These semiquinone radicals have been shown to damage protein,[53] and to induce kidney tumors[54] in hamsters treated with estradiol. Evidence that these effects are through an oxidative stress mechanism comes from the observation that when hamsters were treated with estradiol, products of lipid peroxidation more than doubled in the kidney, and increases were noted in glutathione and glutathione peroxidase in the target tissue.[55] Thus, cumulative exposure of breast tissue to estrogen, as in early menarche, late menopause, and hormone replacement therapy, impact breast cancer risk through an oxidative stress mechanism.[56]

Mobley *et al.*[57] showed that treatment of calf thymus DNA with hydroxy estradiol resulted in damage (8-oxo-2′-deoxyguanosine), and that the presence of endogenous antioxidants such as glutathione, SOD, and catalase dramatically reduced the amount of DNA damage induced by the catechol estrogens. The authors note that extremely high levels of catechol estrogens were needed for observed DNA damage. However, Yoshie and Ohshima[58] found that DNA strand breakage occurred when plasmid DNA was incubated with both a catechol estrogen and a nitric oxide-releasing compound, both of which are formed in the human breast. Therefore, lower amounts of catechol estrogens used by Mobley would likely result in DNA damage in the presence of a nitric oxide-releasing compound. Estrogens have also been shown to have antioxidant capabilities.[59] The net effect (pro-oxidant or antioxidant) may be dependent upon levels of catechol estrogens, determined, in part, by catechol *O*-methyl transferase (COMT), or other enzymatic activities.

3.3. *Fruits and vegetables*

Increasing evidence indicates that breast cancer may be partly caused by oxidative damage coupled with a failure of antioxidants to protect breast tissue.[60] Fruits and vegetables are rich sources of a number of nutrients, including antioxidant vitamins such as carotenoids, the tocopherols, vitamin C, and flavonoids, and the inverse relationships with consumption of fruits and vegetables could be tied in through their antioxidant properties. Antioxidants have been proposed as providing an alternative substrate for oxidation, and thus they may be important in preventing the onset and/or the progression of breast cancer. However, a pooled analysis from eight cohort studies suggested only a weak or null association between fruit and vegetable intake and breast cancer.[61] Analysis of data from the Long Island Breast Cancer Study Project (LIBCSP), a large study with more than 2000 participants, showed that higher fruit and vegetable consumption was associated with decreased breast cancer risk among postmenopausal women (OR for the highest quintile compared with the lowest (95% CI) = 0.72 (0.53 to 0.99)), with weaker associations among premenopausal women.[62] Inconsistencies in study findings may be due to heterogeneity in study populations, and the putative protective effects of dietary antioxidants may only be noted among women with specific genetic profiles in genes that protect from oxidative stress. Thus, variability in genes that generate or protect from oxidative stress could modify associations between dietary antioxidants and breast cancer risk.

4. Genetic Polymorphisms of Enzymes Related to Oxidative Stress

In addition to exogenous sources of exposure factors that could increase or decrease oxidative load, ROS are endogenously generated by numerous enzymes (e.g., myeloperoxidase, nitric oxide synthase) or regulatory processes such as those stimulated by tumor necrosis factor and nuclear factor kappa-beta. On the other hand, endogenous defenses against ROS include glutathione peroxidases, catalase, and superoxide dismutases, which form the first line of defense against superoxide and hydrogen peroxide. UDP-glucuronsyltransferases (UGTs) and glutathione *S*-transferases

(GSTs) are phase II enzymes that also participate in detoxification of ROS, as a second defense line for oxidative stress. Many of these enzymes are polymorphic, and breast cancer risk related to oxidative stress could be impacted by this inter-individual variability.

4.1. *Gene polymorphisms that generate ROS*

4.1.1. *Myeloperoxidase*

Myeloperoxidase (MPO) is thought to function as an anti-microbial agent by catalyzing a reaction between hydrogen peroxide, produced by NADPH oxides, and chloride to generate hypochlorous acid (HOCl), a toxic oxidizing agent. HOCl further reacts with other biological molecules to generate secondary radicals, including highly reactive hydroxyl ions.[63] The enzyme is present in neutrophils, which invade inflamed tissues, including the breast, to combat infection and, presumably, to protect breast milk during lactation.[64] In addition to its presence in human breast milk, detection with immunohistochemistry has demonstrated the presence of MPO in breast tissue from women with cancer,[65] and *MPO* gene co-amplification has been observed with c-erB-2 in human breast carcinomas.[66]

A frequently occurring polymorphism in Caucasians in the promoter region of the *MPO* gene is a –463 G→A substitution, which is located in the consensus binding site of the SP1 transcription factor in the 5′ upstream region of the gene.[67] The *MPO G* wild-type allele confers higher transcriptional activation than the −463 A variant *in vitro*,[68] and the former has been associated with increased MPO mRNA and protein levels in myeloid leukemia cells.[69] In the Caucasian population, 8% were homozygous for the A alleles and 31% were heterozygous.[70] To date, five of nine control studies have found significantly reduced lung cancer risk associated with the A alleles, comparing with having the common type G allele. MPO may be particularly important in relation to breast cancer, as suggested by associations between MPO activity and estrogen levels. Lacrimal fluid peroxide activity is positively correlated with 17-beta estradiol plasma levels,[71] and intracellular MPO activity in neutrophills was higher in premenopausal women than postmenopausal women.[72] Circulating variations in MPO are dependent on estradiol levels during the menstrual cycle,[73] and hormone replacement therapy restores MPO release from neutrophils in menopausal women.[72] In addition, *MPO* genotype related to several diseases has been shown to be gender dependent, indicating that the gender difference in risk may be related to the possible effects of sex hormones on *MPO* gene expression. For example, GG genotype is a male risk factor in lung cancer, while it is a female risk factor in Alzheimer's disease and multiple sclerosis.[69,74] Furthermore, an *in vitro* study suggested that the A allele creates a putative estrogen receptor binding site.[75] Because of the presence of MPO in the breast and breast tumor tissues, its association with hormone levels and its ability to generate ROS, the polymorphism may be important in the oxidative stress pathway in human breast cancer. In the Long Island Breast Cancer Project, having at least one variant A allele was associated with an overall 17% reduction in breast cancer risk. Furthermore, when consumption of fruits and vegetables and specific dietary antioxidants were dichotomized at the median, inverse associations with either GA or AA genotypes were most pronounced among premenopausal women who consumed higher amounts of total fruits and vegetables (OR for AA genotype: 0.43, CI: 0.18–1.00).[76] Studies of *MPO* in relation to breast cancer survival have also shown that women with the variant (low activity) A allele had poorer survival than women with G, high activity alleles, indicating that greater generation of ROS may be associated with better tumor cell kill and better survival.[77]

4.1.2. *Tumor necrosis factor*

Tumor Necrosis Factor (TNF-α) is a cytokine acting in a paracrine or autocrine fashion on a wide variety of target cells. TNF-α triggers receptor-mediated processes yielding ROS and causing oxidative stress in mitochondria.[78] TNF-α was initially discovered through its antitumor activity; however, its overexpression has been implicated in mitogenic actions and supports the stimulation of the cancer cell proliferation process,[79] as well as the cancer cell survival pathway, supposedly via anti-apoptotic proteins. Furthermore, Chovolou *et al.*[80] demonstrated *in vitro* that overexpression of TNF-α decreases sensitivity to TNF-α induced apoptosis and downregulates MnSOD, indicating that a pro-oxidant signal linked to the downregulation of antioxidant defense may be associated with resistance to apoptosis induced by TNF-α. A study noted that higher levels of TNF-α

could result in more ROS in the mitochondria, causing oxidative stress and resultant DNA damage; conversely, low levels could be protective. In addition, the activities of the aromatase, estradiol 17β-hydroxysteroid dehydrogenase and estrogen sulfatase are all increased by IL-6 and TNF-α, indicating TNF-α is also involved the regulation of the enzyme, which further increase estrogen synthesis in breast tissue, and could relate to the risk of breast cancer.[81]

A −308 G→A polymorphism has been reported in the 5′ upstream region of the gene that directly affects the regulation of TNF-α, with the variant allele associated with higher constitutive inducible levels of TNF-α.[82] In a study of the *TNF-α* gene polymorphism in relation to both lymphoma and breast cancer in a Tunisian population,[83] Chouchane found that heterozygosity of the variant allele significantly increased cancer risk. The −308 G→A substitution was also associated with increased risk of prostate cancer,[84] oral cancer,[85] and uterine endometrial cancer.[86] On the other hand, one study evaluated associations between the *TNF-α*−308 polymorphism and breast cancer outcome, with null results.[87] However, the sample size of the study did not have enough power to detect statistically significant associations, and they did not adjust for any possible confounding factors.

4.1.3. *Nuclear factor kappa-beta*

Nuclear factor kappa-beta (NF-κB) is transcription factor responsible for modulating the expression of many genes involved in cell proliferation, differentiation, apoptosis, and metastasis.[88] NF-κB is a hetreodimeric complex of Rel family proteins which is physically confined to the cytoplasm of normal cells through its interaction with inhibitor of KappaB (Iκb) proteins.[89] It is activated upon stimulation of cells with a variety of signals, including oxidative stress. Constitutive activation of NF-κB is observed in a number of cancers, including breast cancer.[90] However, this NF-κB activation mechanism remains largely unknown.

Brantley *et al.* demonstrated that NF-κB positively regulates mammary epithelial proliferation, branching, and functions in maintenance of normal epithelial architecture during early post-natal development in the mouse model, indicating NF-κB may have an important role in the breast.[91] By sequencing the entire gene, several SNPs were identified, including 1837 T→C, 1867 GG/G, and 2584 G→T polymorphisms.[92] However, one small study showed no significant association between one of the variants and breast cancer risk.[93]

4.1.4. *Nitric oxide synthase*

Nitric oxide, an ROS, is generated by a family of nitric oxide synthase (NOS). Three isozymes of NOS have been found: endothelial (eNOS), neuronal (nNOS), and inducible form (iNOS).[94] nNOS is constitutively expressed; however, the inducible iNOS, found in epithelia and macrophage, is regulated by cytokines. Though both iNOS and eNOS are expressed at high levels in normal mammary epithelium, the expression of eNOS is downregulated and iNOS is absent in the breast carcinoma MCF-7 cell line.[95,96] Constitutively produced NO is an important mediator of numerous physiologic functions, including vasodilatation, smooth muscle relaxation, inhibition of platelet aggregation, and regulation of neurotransmission. However, the role of these enzymes and their product NO in the normal breast development and breast cancer is not clearly understood. Although there are no studies, to date, evaluating *NOS* polymorphisms in relation to breast cancer risk, associations have been evaluated in relation to risk of other cancers. A study in Korea found the distribution of *ecNOS* genotypes to vary between lung cancer cases and controls,[97] and a study of prostate cancer found that the glu→asp 298 polymorphism of *ecNOS* in intron 4 was associated with a threefold increase in risk.[98]

4.2. *Genetic polymorphisms that neutralize to ROS*

Catalase (CAT), glutathione peroxidases (GPX), and superoxide dismutase (SOD) are major enzymes that neutralize ROS, working together. SOD catalyzes the dismutation of two superoxide radicals ($O_2^{\bullet -}$), producing hydrogen peroxide (H_2O_2) and oxygen, and CAT and GPX1 remove the toxic H_2O_2 by converting them into water.

4.2.1. *Catalase*

Catalase is a heme enzyme that has a predominant role in controlling H_2O_2 concentrations in human cells, by converting H_2O_2 into H_2O and O_2.

Catalase induction was elicited by H_2O_2 in hamster tracheal epithelial cells[99] and human retinal pigment epithelial cells,[100] indicating a key role for catalase in antioxidant defense. It was also found to be inducible in both primary rat hepatocytes and rat hepatoma cell lines.[101] Acatalasemic mice that have blood and tissue levels of catalase that are approximately one-tenth that of normal mice and females are susceptible to spontaneous mammary carcinoma.[102] Because a preventive effect of vitamin E on human breast cancer is controversial, Ishii and colleagues used the acatalasemic mouse to test whether carcinogenesis could be prevented by vitamin E. In this study, acatalasemic mice developed mammary tumors after nine months of vitamin E deprivation, and 14 months after supplementation. Normal mice did not develop mammary tumors, regardless of diet. These data indicate that there could be important implications for the study of variability in CAT in relation to antioxidants and human breast cancer risk.

A common polymorphism has been identified in the promoter region of the *CAT* gene, a −262 C→T substitution on the 5′ region of the human *CAT* gene from the transcription start site.[103,104] The variant alters gene expression when incorporated upstream in a Luciferase reporter construct and transiently transfected in HepG2 (human liver) cells and K562 (human blood cells). Different patterns have also been detected on gel shift analysis.[103] This variability in CAT activity is thought to play a role in host response to oxidative stress and, indeed, variant *CAT* alleles appeared to be associated with increased risk of hypertension[104] and vitiligo,[105] both conditions being related to oxidative stress. Thus, the polymorphism in this gene could have important implications for breast cancer etiology. In the Long Island Breast Cancer Project, having CC genotype was associated with an overall 17% reduction in breast cancer risk. Furthermore, when consumption of fruits and vegetables and specific dietary antioxidants were dichotomized at the median, inverse associations with CC genotypes were most pronounced among women who consumed higher amounts of fruits (OR: 0.71, CI: 0.54–0.92).[106]

4.2.2. *Glutathione peroxidases*

Glutathione peroxidases are a family of enzymes that catalyze the reduction of H_2O_2 and organic hydroperoxides to water and alcohol, respectively. This enzyme is ubiquitously expressed in humans, being particularly abundant in erythrocytes, kidney, and liver.[107] Selenium-dependent glutathione peroxidase (GPX1) is present in the cytosol and in the mitochondria.[108] Knockout mice studies have shown that GPX1 is of critical importance in protection against oxidative stress generated by H_2O_2.[109] GPX1 is transcriptionally upregulated as an adaptive response to oxidative stress, and has been reported to inhibit breast cancer cell activities.[110]

An in-frame variable polyalanine (GCG) repeat polymorphism has been described, and the six alanine (ALA6) repeat allele also has a nucleotide substitution associated with C→T substitution. The ALA6 polymorphism was also found to be associated with increased risk of prostate cancer (OR: 1.67, 95% CI: 0.97–2.87).[111] Measurement of 8-hydroxydeoxyguanosine (8OHdG), a marker of oxidative damage in DNA from normal lung tissue, revealed a trend of less 8OHdG associated with one or two copies of the six alanine repeat (ALA6) allele,[112] indicating that the variant may protect DNA from ROS damage. The 197 C→T variant, another polymorphism in *GPX1*, recently has been found. An *in vitro* study showed that the GPX1 T allele was less responsive to the stimulation of GPX1 enzyme activity during selenium supplementation than the C allele,[113] indicating the risk associated with C→T *GPX1* polymorphism may differ to the response to the oxidative stress. In addition, T allele was associated with a greater than twofold increase in lung cancer risk in a prospective cohort study of lung cancer.[114] On case–control study, consisting of 101 stroke patients, and 214 control patients, in the Finnish/Swedish population showed no significant association of GPX1 activity with risk of stroke.

4.2.3. *Manganese superoxide dismutase*

Superoxide dismutases (SOD)s comprise a family of metalloenzymes that catalyze the conversion of two superoxide radicals ($O_2^{\bullet -}$) into hydrogen peroxide (H_2O_2) and oxygen. There are three known isoforms of SOD: MnSOD, CuZnSOD, and ECSOD. MnSOD differs from two other isoforms in that it exists in mitochondria and it forms a homotetramer instead of homodimer.[115] Though MnSOD is synthesized in the cytosol, it is post-transcriptionally modified for transport into the mitochondrion.[116] Since mitochondria consume over 90% of a cell's oxygen, MnSOD, existing in mitochondrion, is considered important in the oxidative stress defense.[115] MnSOD is induced with free radical challenge[101] and cigarette smoke.[117]

A T→C polymorphism of *MnSOD* in the mitochondrial targeting sequence results in a change of amino acids, thought to alter the secondary structure of the protein.[116] Rosenblum[118] suggests that the alteration might affect the cellular distribution of the enzyme and mitochondrial transport of MnSOD into the mitochondrion, where it would be biologically available. They further suggest that inefficient targeting of MnSOD could leave mitochondria without their full defense against superoxide radicals, which could lead to protein oxidation, as well as mitochondrial DNA mutations. Ambrosone *et al.* found that women who were homozygous for the variant allele had a fourfold increase in breast cancer risk in comparison to those with who were homozygous or heterozygous for the common allele (OR: 4.3, 95% CI: 1.7–10.8), particularly for premenopausal women.[119] Furthermore, risk was most pronounced among women below the median intake of fruits and vegetables, and of dietary ascorbic acid and α-tocopherol, with little increased risk for those with diets rich in these foods. In agreement with this, two other studies performed by Mitrunen and Egan provided support for these results, though odds ratio were not statistically significant and the effect size was smaller.[120,121] 8-OHdG, markers of oxidative damage, have also been shown to be higher among those with the *MnSOD* polymorphism.[122] In relation to prostate cancer, the Finish ATBC Study showed that men homozygous for the Ala allele had a 70% increase in risk over men homozygous for the Val allele (OR: 1.72, 95% CI: 0.96–3.08).[123] In the Physicians Health Study with 569 cases and 755 controls, investigators found that there was a significant interaction between prostate cancer risk, the MnSOD Ala allele, and low baseline plasma antioxidant levels, with those with AA genotypes and low antioxidants at almost a fourfold increased risk of prostate cancer,[124] similar to Ambrosone's results for breast cancer.

Since MnSOD works in conjunction with two other antioxidant enzymes, myeloperoxidase, catalase and glutathione peroxidase (i.e., these enzymes remove or generate the toxic hydrogen peroxide produced by the SODs), the interaction among these enzymes will help to fully understand the role of MnSOD in breast cancer prevention.

4.2.4. *Extracellular superoxide dismutase*

Extracellular SOD (EC-SOD) is the principle enzymatic scavenger of superoxide in the extracellular space, mostly found in plasma, lymph, and synovial fluid as well as tissues.[107] It is a tetramic glycoprotein, containing one Cu^{2+} and Zn^{2+}, per subunit, and the amino acid compositions are quite different from MnSOD and CuZnSOD.[125] EC-SOD, unlike Mn-SOD and CuZn-SOD, has heparin-binding capacity, and thus EC-SOD binds on the surface of endothelial cells through the heparin sulfate proteoglycan and eliminates the oxygen radicals from the NADP-dependent oxidative system of neutrophils.[126]

Molecular genetic studies have shown that a single base substitution causing substitution of glycine for arginine-213 in the heparin-binding domain of this enzyme causes extremely high plasma levels of EC-SOD.[127] This mutation is located in the region associated with the heparin affinity of the enzyme. The authors speculated that the amino acid substitution may result in a decrease of heparin affinity which favors the presence of EC-SOD in the serum. In a study of 242 healthy volunteers in Australia,[128] serum EC-SOD levels were found to be distributed in two discrete groups of low level (29.9–152.1 g/l) and high level (940.2–1798 g/l). All individuals within the high level group (3.3%) carried the R213G mutation, whereas none of the low-level EC-SOD volunteers did. Similar distribution of phenotype was observed in a large cohort ($n = 4925$) in Sweden,[127] where 4% had eightfold higher plasma levels of EC-SOD. All but one of the individuals in this group carried the R213G polymorphism. It is likely that those with high EC-SOD were homozygous for the variant allele. This genetic polymorphism has not been evaluated in relation to breast cancer risk.

4.2.5. *NAD(P)H: quinone oxidoreductase-1 (NQO1)*

NQO1 is a cystolic flavoenzyme that catalyzes two-electron reduction of various substrates, such as quinines, quinone-imines, nitro and azo compounds, utilizing NADPH as a cofactor. NQO1 can generate antioxidant forms of both vitamin E and ubiquinone after free radical attack. In fact, synthetic antioxidants and extracts of cruciferous vegetables, including broccoli, have been found to be potent inducers of NQO1.[129] NQO1 serves as an activating enzyme of some antitumor quinones, by two-electron reduction.[129] The capability to protect cells from oxidative challenge and the ability to reduce quinones via a two-electron mechanism, which precludes generation of reactive oxygen radicals, imply that NQO1 may play a significant role in the reduction of ROS, and NQO1 may play a role as a chemoprotective enzyme. NQO1 is a flavoprotein that functions as a homodimer, having each catalytic site per monomer. NQO1 is a highly inducible protein and the 5′ region contains an AP2, ARE, or EpRE (electrophile responsive element) and an XRE (xenobiotic responsive element). NQO1 is expressed in human epithelial and endothelial tissues and at high levels throughout many human solid tumors.

Traver *et al.* characterized a polymorphism in *NQO1*, a C-to-T substitution at position 609 of *NQO1* gene, which codes for a proline-to-serine change at residue 187.[130,131] In cells with a T/T genotype, NQO1 activity was not detected, and lack of activity corresponded to a lack of NQO1 protein,[132,133] due to the rapid degradation of the mutant form of NQO1 enzyme.[134] Moran *et al.* have shown that exposure to benzene metabolites does not induce NQO1 in individuals of the T/T genotype as it does in persons with the C/C genotype, and induces NQO1 to an intermediate degree in persons with the T/C genotype.[135] Therefore, the *NQO1* polymorphism has direct functional implications for the enzyme, with genotype a reliable indicator for enzyme activity. Although *NQO1* is a very logical candidate gene for examination of its relationship with breast cancer considering estrogen metabolism and oxidative stress linked to breast cancer etiology described above, few epidemiologic studies has evaluated the role of *NQO1* polymorphisms in breast cancer risk. Hamajima found that the TT genotype of *NQO1* C609T was associated with increased risk of lung cancer, but not with breast cancer.[136] Although *NQO1* has not been well examined in relation to breast cancer, a recent report found that the *NQO1* polymorphism might influence the development of different histologic types of breast cancer.[137]

4.2.6. *Glutathione S-transferases*

Glutathione *S*-transferases (GSTs) are a family of phase II enzymes that are involved in the detoxification of carcinogen metabolites and reactive oxidative products.[138] Thus, they are the second line of defense after SOD, CAT, and GPX. The GSTs comprise five classes, alpha, mu, pi, theta, and zeta, of which at least three are represented in both normal and breast tumor tissue.[139] Of these classes, the alpha class appears to possess the greatest peroxidase activity but enzymes of this class are expressed at low levels in both normal and breast tumor tissues.

The polymorphism of *GSTA1*, *GSTMI*, *GSTT1*, and *GSTP1* genes have been studied with risk of cancer. Glutathione *S*-transferase α is a primary hepatic GST, and *GSTA1*B* allele, which consists of several linked SNPs in the proximal region of the *GSTA1* gene, is associated with reduced expression levels of GSTA1 enzyme, compared to the common *GSTA1*A* allele. Although *GSTA1* has not been evaluated in relation to risk of breast cancer, there was significantly reduced hazard of death after breast cancer treatment for women with *GSTA1*B/*B* genotypes (hazard ratio (HR) = 0.3, 95% CI = 0.1–0.8).[140]

A substantial proportion of Caucasians have a homozygous deletion of the *GSTM1* and *GSTT1* genes, which results in lack of enzyme activity, with the *GSTM1* null polymorphism present in approximately 50% of the population.[141] As reviewed by Rebbeck,[142] studies have shown that individuals who possess the homozygous null allele are at increased risk of lung and bladder cancer, both of which are associated with exposure to chemical carcinogens. However, studies of possible associations between *GSTM1* and breast cancer risk have yielded inconsistent results.[143–146] While the western New York study and another study performed in Australia did not show an association between *GSTM1* and breast cancer,[147,148] Helzlsouer noted a more than twofold increased risk with the null allele of these genes.[144] Zheng *et al.* have also confirmed an association *GSTM1* and *GSTP1* null genotype with about 60% increased risk of breast cancer, respectively.[149]

For GSTP1 gene, two variant alleles, *GSTP1*B* and *GSTP1*C*, have been detected in comparison with the wild type allele *GSTP1*A*. These variant alleles have a point mutation at nucleotide 313, resulting in *isoleucine* → valine amino acid substitution. Since this site is located in close proximity to the hydrophobic binding site for electrophilic substitutes, the valine variant allele has been demonstrated to show an altered specific activity and affinity for electrophilic substrates.[150] In agreement with this, one study in Iceland showed weak associations between *GSTP1* polymorphisms and breast cancer risk.[151] Sweeney *et al.* demonstrated that women with the low-activity valine/valine genotype had better survival, compared with isoleucine/isoleucine after treatment for breast cancer (HR = 0.3, 95% CI = 0.1–1.0).[152]

4.3. *Oxidative stress through hormone metabolism*

The secondary metabolism of 17β-estradiol involves O-methylation by catechol-O-methyltransferase, conjugation to glucuronides and sulfates, and clearance of reactive semiquinones and quinones, reported to involve catechol oxidation coupled to glutathione conjugation.[153] Genetic polymorphisms in enzymes that may affect ultimate levels of ROS generated by the metabolism of steroid hormones that may impact breast cancer risk include catechol-O-methyltransferase and glucuronosyltransferases.

4.3.1. *Catechol-O-methyl transferase*

Catechol-O-methyl transferase (COMT) is an phase II enzyme that conjugates and inactivates the catechol estrogens, by transferring a methyl group from the methyl donor SAM to one hydroxyl moiety of the catechol ring of a substrate.[154,155] Because of the potential for the catechol estrogens, particularly the 4-hydroxy catechol, to bind to DNA and result in DNA damage,[156,157] and to undergo redox cycling to damaging quinones and semiquinones, the possible role of variable activity in the enzyme in relation to breast cancer risk is considered important.

An valine → methionine amino acid substitution at position 158/108 has been linked to decreased methylation activity of COMT,[158,159] with the trimodal distribution of COMT enzyme activity in the human population associated with high ($COMT^{Val/Val}$), intermediate ($COMT^{Val/Met}$), and low COMT ($COMT^{Met/Met}$) activities. Thus, it has been suggested that carrying this low activity, $COMT^{Met/Met}$ variant may be associated with increased risk for breast cancer. However, the epidemiological evidence have given discrepant results. Thompson and Ambrosone found that *COMT* Met allele was associated with increased risk in premenopausal women, with decreased risk among post-menopausal women.[160] A study in Taiwan showed increased risk of breast cancer particular in post-menopausal group and furthermore that combined "high-risk" genotypes for *COMT*, *CYP17*, and *CYP1A1* inferred the greatest risk of all.[161] A study in Korea showed increased risk of breast risk with low activity genotypes in both pre- and post-menopausal women.[162] In contrast to these studies, others have shown null or inverse associations between low-activity genotypes and breast cancer risk.[163–168]

4.3.2. *UDP-glucuronsyltransferases*

UDP-glucuronsyltransferases (UGTs) are also phase II enzymes, which catalyze the addition of the glycols group from a nucleotide sugar to small hydrophobic molecules, making them more easily excreted.[169] The UGTs are involved not only in the metabolism of many drugs and xenobiotics, but also are important in the biotransformation of important endogenous substrates, including estradiol.[170]

Three human liver UGTs (UGT2B7, 1A1, 1A3) have been shown to catalyze the glucuronidation of catechol estrogens and lead to their enhanced elimination.[171] UGT2B7 was shown to react with higher efficiency toward 4-hydroxyestrogenic catechols, whereas UGT1A1 showed higher activities toward 2-hydroxyestrogens.[171] Both of these enzymes are polymorphic. There are variable numbers of TA repeats in the promoter TATA box of *UGT1A1*, and they are inversely related to levels of gene expression.[172] Guillemette *et al.* demonstrated an association with breast cancer among African Americans. They showed that *UDP1A1* genotype of seven or eight repeats in the A(TA)nTAA motif in the TATA box versus that of 5/5, 5/6, and 6/6 was 80% increase of the risk (OR 1.8 CI = 1.0–3.1), and they further found the association was stronger for ER-breast cancer.[173] However, a subsequent study done by same group did not support a strong association with *UGT1A1* genotype and breast cancer in a Caucasian population.[174] On the contrary, Grant *et al.* have suggested that polymorphism of *UGT1A1* may function as a determinant of oxidative stress level, since *UGT1A1* has major role in determining circulating bilirubin, a known antioxidant. Thus, this polymorphism may be associated with risk of breast cancer through oxidative DNA damage.[175]

5. Summary

There is accumulating evidence that oxidative stress may contribute to breast cancer etiology, and that a number of breast cancer risk factors could be exerting their effects through generation of ROS, or by preventing oxidative damage. In the few studies that have examined gene–diet interactions, it is most encouraging to note that consumption of fruits and vegetables modified the effects of polymorphisms in genes related to production of or protection from ROS. Continued research in the potential mechanisms of oxidative stress in breast cancer etiology may further elucidate causal pathways, and also demonstrate the public health importance of dietary factors. Furthermore, investigation into the role of endogenous and exogenous oxidants and antioxidants in relation to breast cancer therapy may have clinical relevance for reduction of treatment-related toxicities and promotion of survival of breast cancer patients.

References

1. American Cancer Society. *Cancer Statistics*, 2004.
2. Feuer EJ, Wun LM, Boring CC, Flanders WD, Timmel MJ, Tong T. The lifetime risk of developing breast cancer. *J. Natl. Cancer Inst.* 85(11): 892–897 (1993).
3. Madigan MP, Ziegler RG, Benichou J, Byrne C, Hoover RN. Proportion of breast cancer cases in the United States explained by well-established risk factors. *J. Natl. Cancer Inst.* 87(22): 1681–1685 (1995).
4. Kelsey JL, Bernstein L. Epidemiology and prevention of breast cancer. *Annu. Rev. Public Health* 17: 47–67 (1996).
5. Sies H. *Oxidative Stress. Introductory Remarks* Academic Press, London, 1985, pp. 1–8.
6. Mancini M, Sedghinasab M, Knowlton K, Tam A, Hockenbery D, Anderson BO. Flow cytometric measurement of mitochondrial mass and function: a novel method for assessing chemoresistance. *Ann. Surg. Oncol.* 5(3): 287–295 (1998).
7. Mignotte B, Vayssiere JL. Mitochondria and apoptosis. *Eur. J. Biochem.* 252(1): 1–15 (1998).
8. Costantini P, Jacotot E, Decaudin D, Kroemer G. Mitochondrion as a novel target of anticancer chemotherapy. *J. Natl. Cancer Inst.* 92(13): 1042–1053 (2000).
9. Kroemer G, Petit P, Zamzami N, Vayssiere JL, Mignotte B. The biochemistry of programmed cell death. *FASEB J.* 9(13): 1277–1287 (1995).
10. Burrows CJ, Muller JG. Oxidative nucleobase modifications leading to strand scission. *Chem. Rev.* 98(3): 1109–1152 (1998).
11. Feig DI, Reid TM, Loeb LA. Reactive oxygen species in tumorigenesis. *Cancer Res.* 54(7 Suppl.): 1890s–1894s (1994).
12. Guyton KZ, Kensler TW. Oxidative mechanisms in carcinogenesis. *Br. Med. Bull.* 49(3): 523–544 (1993).

13. Sun J, Chen Y, Li M, Ge Z. Role of antioxidant enzymes on ionizing radiation resistance. *Free Radic. Biol. Med.* 24(4): 586–593 (1998).
14. Kim K, Smith PK. Childhood stress, behavioural symptoms and mother–daughter pubertal development. *J. Adolesc.* 21(3): 231–240 (1998).
15. Kong Q, Lillehei KO. Antioxidant inhibitors for cancer therapy. *Med. Hypotheses* 51(5): 405–409 (1998).
16. Richter C, Park JW, Ames BN. Normal oxidative damage to mitochondrial and nuclear DNA is extensive. *Proc. Natl. Acad. Sci. USA* 85(17): 6465–6467 (1988).
17. Mantymaa P *et al.* Induction of mitochondrial manganese superoxide dismutase confers resistance to apoptosis in acute myeloblastic leukaemia cells exposed to etoposide. *Br. J. Haematol.* 108(3): 574–581 (2000).
18. Huang P, Feng L, Oldham EA, Keating MJ, Plunkett W. Superoxide dismutase as a target for the selective killing of cancer cells. *Nature* 407(6802): 390–395 (2000).
19. Cleveland JL, Kastan MB. Cancer. A radical approach to treatment. *Nature* 407(6802): 309–311 (2000).
20. Ross GM. Induction of cell death by radiotherapy. *Endocr. Relat. Cancer* 6(1): 41–44 (1999).
21. Abuja PM, Albertini R. Methods for monitoring oxidative stress, lipid peroxidation and oxidation resistance of lipoproteins. *Clin. Chim. Acta.* 306(1–2): 1–17 (2001).
22. Musarrat J, Arezina-Wilson J, Wani AA. Prognostic and aetiological relevance of 8-hydroxyguanosine in human breast carcinogenesis. *Eur. J. Cancer* 32A(7): 1209–1214 (1996).
23. Djuric Z *et al.* Levels of 5-hydroxymethyl-2′-deoxyuridine in DNA from blood as a marker of breast cancer. *Cancer* 77(4): 691–696 (1996).
24. Institute of Medicine. *Dietary Reference Intakes for Vitamin C, Vitamin E, Selenium, and Carotenoids*. National Academy of Sciences, 2000.
25. Obana H, Hori S, Kashimoto T, Kunita N. Polycyclic aromatic hydrocarbons in human fat and liver. *Bull. Environ. Contam. Toxicol.* 27(1): 23–27 (1981).
26. Li D, Zhang W, Sahin AA, Hittelman WN. DNA adducts in normal tissue adjacent to breast cancer: a review. *Cancer Detect. Prev.* 23(6): 454–462 (1999).
27. Wang M, Dhingra K, Hittelman WN, Liehr JG, de Andrade M, Li D. Lipid peroxidation-induced putative malondialdehyde–DNA adducts in human breast tissues. *Cancer Epidemiol. Biomarkers Prev.* 5(9): 705–710 (1996).

28. Halliwell B. Why and how should we measure oxidative DNA damage in nutritional studies? How far have we come? *Am. J. Clin. Nutr.* 72(5): 1082–1087 (2000).
29. Gedik CM, Boyle SP, Wood SG, Vaughan NJ, Collins AR. Oxidative stress in humans: validation of biomarkers of DNA damage. *Carcinogenesis* 23(9): 1441–1446 (2002).
30. Li D *et al.* Oxidative DNA damage and 8-hydroxy-2-deoxyguanosine DNA glycosylase/apurinic lyase in human breast cancer. *Mol. Carcinog.* 31(4): 214–223 (2001).
31. Rozalski R, Gackowski D, Roszkowski K, Foksinski M, Olinski R. The level of 8-hydroxyguanine, a possible repair product of oxidative DNA damage, is higher in urine of cancer patients than in control subjects. *Cancer Epidemiol. Biomarkers Prev.* 11(10 Pt 1): 1072–1075 (2002).
32. Halliwell B. Effect of diet on cancer development: is oxidative DNA damage a biomarker? *Free Radic. Biol. Med.* 32(10): 968–974 (2002).
33. Ashok BT, Ali R. Binding of human anti-DNA autoantibodies to reactive oxygen species modified-DNA and probing oxidative DNA damage in cancer using monoclonal antibody. *Int. J. Cancer* 78(4): 404–409 (1998).
34. Frenkel K *et al.* Serum autoantibodies recognizing 5-hydroxymethyl-2′-deoxyuridine, an oxidized DNA base, as biomarkers of cancer risk in women. *Cancer Epidemiol. Biomarkers Prev.* 7(1): 49–57 (1998).
35. Hu JJ *et al.* Alpha-tocopherol dietary supplement decreases titers of antibody against 5-hydroxymethyl-2′-deoxyuridine (HMdU). *Cancer Epidemiol. Biomarkers Prev.* 8(8): 693–698 (1999).
36. Wallstrom P *et al.* Antibodies against 5-hydroxymethyl-2′-deoxyuridine are associated with lifestyle factors and GSTM1 genotype: a report from the Malmo Diet and Cancer cohort. *Cancer Epidemiol. Biomarkers Prev.* 12(5): 444–451 (2003).
37. Mooney LA *et al.* Gender differences in autoantibodies to oxidative DNA base damage in cigarette smokers. *Cancer Epidemiol. Biomarkers Prev.* 10(6): 641–648 (2001).
38. Meagher EA, FitzGerald GA. Indices of lipid peroxidation in vivo: strengths and limitations. *Free Radic. Biol. Med.* 28(12): 1745–1750 (2000).
39. Kelly FJ. Urinary F2-isoprostane metabolite analysis: a step closer to obtaining a reliable measure of oxidative stress? *Clin. Exp. Allergy* 31(3): 355–356 (2001).
40. Halliwell B. Lipid peroxidation, antioxidants and cardiovascular disease: how should we move forward? *Cardiovasc. Res.* 47(3): 410–418 (2000).

41. Dietrich M *et al.* Vitamin C supplementation decreases oxidative stress biomarker f2-isoprostanes in plasma of nonsmokers exposed to environmental tobacco smoke. *Nutr. Cancer* 45(2): 176–184 (2003).
42. Dietrich M *et al.* Antioxidant supplementation decreases lipid peroxidation biomarker F(2)-isoprostanes in plasma of smokers. *Cancer Epidemiol. Biomarkers Prev.* 11(1): 7–13 (2002).
43. Chen G, Djuric Z. Detection of 2,6-cyclolycopene-1,5-diol in breast nipple aspirate fluids and plasma: a potential marker of oxidative stress. *Cancer Epidemiol. Biomarkers Prev.* 11(12): 1592–1596 (2002).
44. Kumaraguruparan R, Subapriya R, Viswanathan P, Nagini S. Tissue lipid peroxidation and antioxidant status in patients with adenocarcinoma of the breast. *Clin. Chim. Acta* 325(1–2): 165–170 (2002).
45. Seven A *et al.* Breast cancer and benign breast disease patients evaluated in relation to oxidative stress. *Cancer Biochem. Biophys.* 16(4): 333–345 (1998).
46. Heisey RE, Carroll JC, Warner E, McCready DR, Goel V. Hereditary breast cancer. Identifying and managing BRCA1 and BRCA2 carriers. *Can. Fam. Physician* 45: 114–124 (1999).
47. Venkitaraman AR. A growing network of cancer-susceptibility genes. *N. Engl. J. Med.* 348(19): 1917–1919 (2003).
48. Gowen LC, Avrutskaya AV, Latour AM, Koller BH, Leadon SA. BRCA1 required for transcription-coupled repair of oxidative DNA damage. *Science* 281(5379): 1009–1012 (1998).
49. Carter RF. BRCA1, BRCA2 and breast cancer: a concise clinical review. *Clin. Invest. Med.* 24(3): 147–157 (2001).
50. Lupulescu A. Estrogen use and cancer incidence: a review. *Cancer Invest.* 13(3): 287–295 (1995).
51. Clemons M, Goss P. Estrogen and the risk of breast cancer. *N. Engl. J. Med.* 344(4): 276–285 (2001).
52. Nandi S, Guzman RC, Yang J. Hormones and mammary carcinogenesis in mice, rats, and humans: a unifying hypothesis. *Proc. Natl. Acad. Sci. USA* 92(9): 3650–3657 (1995).
53. Winter RB. Adolescent idiopathic scoliosis. *N. Engl. J. Med.* 314(21): 1379–1380 (1986).
54. Kirkman H, Robbins M. Estrogen-induced tumors of the kidney. V. Histology and histogenesis in the Syrian hamster. *Natl. Cancer Inst. Monogr.* 1: 93–139 (1959).

55. Roy D, Liehr JG. Changes in activities of free radical detoxifying enzymes in kidneys of male Syrian hamsters treated with estradiol. *Cancer Res.* 49(6): 1475–1480 (1989).
56. Hulka BS, Moorman PG. Breast cancer: hormones and other risk factors. *Maturitas* 38(1): 103–113 (2001).
57. Mobley JA, Bhat AS, Brueggemeier RW. Measurement of oxidative DNA damage by catechol estrogens and analogues in vitro. *Chem. Res. Toxicol.* 12(3): 270–277 (1999).
58. Yoshie Y, Ohshima H. Synergistic induction of DNA strand breakage by catechol-estrogen and nitric oxide: implications for hormonal carcinogenesis. *Free Radic. Biol. Med.* 24(2): 341–348 (1998).
59. Subbiah MT, Kessel B, Agrawal M, Rajan R, Abplanalp W, Rymaszewski Z. Antioxidant potential of specific estrogens on lipid peroxidation. *J. Clin. Endocrinol. Metab.* 77(4): 1095–1097 (1993).
60. Ambrosone CB. Oxidants and antioxidants in breast cancer. *Antioxid. Redox Signal.* 2(4): 903–917 (2000).
61. Smith-Warner SA *et al.* Intake of fruits and vegetables and risk of breast cancer: a pooled analysis of cohort studies. *J. Am. Med. Assoc.* 285(6): 769–776 (2001).
62. Gaudet MM, Britton JA, Kabat GC, Steck-Scott S, Eng SM, Teitelbaum SL, Terry MB, Neugut AI, Gammon MD. Fruits, vegetables, and micronutrients in relation to breast cancer modified by menopause and hormone receptor status. *Cancer Epidemiol. Biomarkers Prev.* 13(9): 1485–1494 (2004).
63. Klebanoff SJ. Oxygen metabolism and the toxic properties of phagocytes. *Ann. Intern. Med.* 93(3): 480–489 (1980).
64. Josephy PD. The role of peroxidase-catalyzed activation of aromatic amines in breast cancer. *Mutagenesis* 11(1): 3–7 (1996).
65. Samoszuk MK, Nguyen V, Gluzman I, Pham JH. Occult deposition of eosinophil peroxidase in a subset of human breast carcinomas. *Am. J. Pathol.* 148(3): 701–706 (1996).
66. Coene ED *et al.* Amplification units and translocation at chromosome 17q and c-erbB-2 overexpression in the pathogenesis of breast cancer. *Virchows Arch.* 430(5): 365–372 (1997).
67. Austin GE *et al.* Sequence comparison of putative regulatory DNA of the 5′ flanking region of the myeloperoxidase gene in normal and leukemic bone marrow cells. *Leukemia* 7(9): 1445–1450 (1993).
68. Piedrafita FJ, Molander RB, Vansant G, Orlova EA, Pfahl M, Reynolds WF. An Alu element in the myeloperoxidase promoter contains a composite

SP1-thyroid hormone–retinoic acid response element. *J. Biol. Chem.* 271(24): 14412–14420 (1996).

69. Reynolds WF, Chang E, Douer D, Ball ED, Kanda V. An allelic association implicates myeloperoxidase in the etiology of acute promyelocytic leukemia. *Blood* 90(7): 2730–2737 (1997).
70. London SJ, Lehman TA, Taylor JA. Myeloperoxidase genetic polymorphism and lung cancer risk. *Cancer Res.* 57(22): 5001–5003 (1997).
71. Liberati V, de Feo G, Madia F, Marcozzi G. Effect of oral contraceptives on lacrimal fluid peroxidase activity in women. *Ophthalmic. Res.* 34(4): 251–253 (2002).
72. Bekesi G *et al.* Induced myeloperoxidase activity and related superoxide inhibition during hormone replacement therapy. *BJOG* 108(5): 474–481 (2001).
73. Marcozzi FG, Madia F, Del Bianco G, Mattei E, de Feo G. Lacrimal fluid peroxidase activity during the menstrual cycle. *Curr. Eye Res.* 20(3): 178–182 (2000).
74. Nagra RM *et al.* Immunohistochemical and genetic evidence of myeloperoxidase involvement in multiple sclerosis. *J. Neuroimmunol.* 78(1–2): 97–107 (1997).
75. Reynolds WF *et al.* MPO and APOEepsilon4 polymorphisms interact to increase risk for AD in Finnish males. Neurology 55(9): 1284–1290 (2000).
76. Ahn J, Gammon MD, Santella, R. M., Gaudet MM, Britton JA, Teitelbaum SL, Terry MB, Neugut AI, Ambrosone, CB. Myeloperoxidase (MPO) genotype, fruit and vegetable consumption, and breast cancer risk. *Cancer Res.* 64(20): 7634–7639 (2004).
77. Ambrosone CB, Ahn J, Furberg H, Sweeney C, Trovato A. Polymorphisms in genes related to oxidative stress (MnSOD, MPO, CAT) and survival after treatment for breast cancer. *Cancer Res.* 65(3): 1105–1111 (2005).
78. Palladino MA, Jr *et al.* Characterization of the antitumor activities of human tumor necrosis factor-alpha and the comparison with other cytokines: induction of tumor-specific immunity. *J. Immunol.* 138(11): 4023–4032 (1987).
79. Shea-Eaton WK, Lee PP, Ip MM. Regulation of milk protein gene expression in normal mammary epithelial cells by tumor necrosis factor. *Endocrinology* 142(6): 2558–2568 (2001).
80. Chovolou Y, Watjen W, Kampkotter A, Kahl R. Resistance to tumor necrosis factor-alpha (TNF-alpha)-induced apoptosis in rat hepatoma cells expressing TNF-alpha is linked to low antioxidant enzyme expression. *J. Biol. Chem.* 278(32): 29626–29632 (2003).

81. Purohit A, Newman SP, Reed MJ. The role of cytokines in regulating estrogen synthesis: implications for the etiology of breast cancer. *Breast Cancer Res.* 4(2): 65–69 (2002).
82. Wilson AG, Symons JA, McDowell TL, McDevitt HO, Duff GW. Effects of a polymorphism in the human tumor necrosis factor alpha promoter on transcriptional activation. *Proc. Natl. Acad. Sci. USA* 94(7): 3195–3199 (1997).
83. Chouchane L, Ahmed SB, Baccouche S, Remadi S. Polymorphism in the tumor necrosis factor-alpha promotor region and in the heat shock protein 70 genes associated with malignant tumors. *Cancer* 80(8): 1489–1496 (1997).
84. Oh BR *et al.* Frequent genotype changes at -308, and 488 regions of the tumor necrosis factor-alpha (TNF-alpha) gene in patients with prostate cancer. *J. Urol.* 163(5): 1584–1587 (2000).
85. Chiu CJ *et al.* Association between genetic polymorphism of tumor necrosis factor-alpha and risk of oral submucous fibrosis, a pre-cancerous condition of oral cancer. *J. Dent. Res.* 80(12): 2055–2059 (2001).
86. Sasaki M *et al.* Frequent genotype changes at -308 of the human tumor necrosis factor-alpha promoter region in human uterine endometrial cancer. *Oncol. Rep.* 7(2): 369–373 (2000).
87. Park KS, Mok JW, Ko HE, Tokunaga K, Lee MH. Polymorphisms of tumour necrosis factors A and B in breast cancer. *Eur. J. Immunogenet.* 29(1): 7–10 (2002).
88. Rayet B, Gelinas C. Aberrant rel/nfkb genes and activity in human cancer. *Oncogene* 18(49): 6938–6947 (1999).
89. Ghosh S, May MJ, Kopp EB. NF-kappa B and Rel proteins: evolutionarily conserved mediators of immune responses. *Annu. Rev. Immunol.* 16: 225–260 (1998).
90. Nakshatri H, Bhat-Nakshatri P, Martin DA, Goulet RJ, Jr., Sledge GW, Jr. Constitutive activation of NF-kappaB during progression of breast cancer to hormone-independent growth. *Mol. Cell. Biol.* 17(7): 3629–3639 (1997).
91. Brantley DM *et al.* Nuclear factor-kappaB (NF-kappaB) regulates proliferation and branching in mouse mammary epithelium. *Mol. Biol. Cell.* 12(5): 1445–1455 (2001).
92. Shinohara Y *et al.* Novel single nucleotide polymorphisms of the human nuclear factor kappa-B 2 gene identified by sequencing the entire gene. *J. Hum. Genet.* 46(1): 50–51 (2001).
93. Curran JE, Weinstein SR, Griffiths LR. Polymorphic variants of NFKB1 and its inhibitory protein NFKBIA, and their involvement in sporadic breast cancer. *Cancer Lett.* 188(1–2): 103–107 (2002).

94. Khalkhali-Ellis Z, Hendrix MJ. Nitric oxide regulation of maspin expression in normal mammary epithelial and breast cancer cells. *Am. J. Pathol.* 162(5): 1411–1417 (2003).
95. Martin JH, Alalami O, van den Berg HW. Reduced expression of endothelial and inducible nitric oxide synthase in a human breast cancer cell line which has acquired estrogen independence. *Cancer Lett.* 144(1): 65–74 (1999).
96. Zeillinger R *et al.* Simultaneous expression of nitric oxide synthase and estrogen receptor in human breast cancer cell lines. *Breast Cancer Res. Treat.* 40(2): 205–207 (1996).
97. Cheon KT, Choi KH, Lee HB, Park SK, Rhee YK, Lee YC. Gene polymorphisms of endothelial nitric oxide synthase and angiotensin-converting enzyme in patients with lung cancer. *Lung* 178(6): 351–360 (2000).
98. Medeiros R *et al.* Endothelial nitric oxide synthase gene polymorphisms and genetic susceptibility to prostate cancer. *Eur. J. Cancer Prev.* 11(4): 343–350 (2002).
99. Shull S *et al.* Differential regulation of antioxidant enzymes in response to oxidants. *J. Biol. Chem.* 266(36): 24398–24403 (1991).
100. Tate DJ, Jr., Miceli MV, Newsome DA. Phagocytosis and H2O2 induce catalase and metallothionein gene expression in human retinal pigment epithelial cells. *Invest. Ophthalmol. Vis. Sci.* 36(7): 1271–1279 (1995).
101. Rohrdanz E, Kahl R. Alterations of antioxidant enzyme expression in response to hydrogen peroxide. *Free Radic. Biol. Med.* 24(1): 27–38 (1998).
102. Ishii K, Zhen LX, Wang DH, Funamori Y, Ogawa K, Taketa K. Prevention of mammary tumorigenesis in acatalasemic mice by vitamin E supplementation. *Jpn. J. Cancer Res.* 87(7): 680–684 (1996).
103. Forsberg L, Lyrenas L, de Faire U, Morgenstern R. A common functional C–T substitution polymorphism in the promoter region of the human catalase gene influences transcription factor binding, reporter gene transcription and is correlated to blood catalase levels. *Free Radic. Biol. Med.* 30(5): 500–505 (2001).
104. Goulas A *et al.* An association study of a functional catalase gene polymorphism, −262 C→T, and patients with Alzheimer's disease. *Neurosci. Lett.* 330(2): 210–213 (2002).
105. Casp CB, She JX, McCormack WT. Genetic association of the catalase gene (CAT) with vitiligo susceptibility. *Pigment. Cell. Res.* 15(1): 62–66 (2002).
106. Ahn J *et al.* Associations between breast cancer risk and the endogenous antioxidant catalase (CAT), fruit and vegetable consumption, and supplement use. *Am. J. Epidemiol.* 2005 (in press).

107. Forsberg L, de Faire U, Morgenstern R. Oxidative stress, human genetic variation, and disease. *Arch. Biochem. Biophys.* 389(1): 84–93 (2001).
108. Ursini F, Maiorino M, Gregolin C. Phospholipid hydroperoxide glutathione peroxidase. *Int. J. Tissue React.* 8(2): 99–103 (1986).
109. de Haan JB *et al.* Mice with a homozygous null mutation for the most abundant glutathione peroxidase, Gpx1, show increased susceptibility to the oxidative stress-inducing agents paraquat and hydrogen peroxide. *J. Biol. Chem.* 273(35): 22528–22536 (1998).
110. Gouaze V *et al.* Glutathione peroxidase-1 protects from CD95-induced apoptosis. *J. Biol. Chem.* 277(45): 42867–42874 (2002).
111. Kote-Jarai Z *et al.* Association between the GCG polymorphism of the selenium dependent GPX1 gene and the risk of young onset prostate cancer. *Prostate Cancer Prostatic. Dis.* 5(3): 189–192 (2002).
112. Hardie LJ *et al.* The effect of hOGG1 and glutathione peroxidase I genotypes and 3p chromosomal loss on 8-hydroxydeoxyguanosine levels in lung cancer. *Carcinogenesis* 21(2): 167–172 (2000).
113. Hu YJ, Diamond AM. Role of glutathione peroxidase 1 in breast cancer: loss of heterozygosity and allelic differences in the response to selenium. *Cancer Res.* 63(12): 3347–3351 (2003).
114. Ratnasinghe D *et al.* Glutathione peroxidase codon 198 polymorphism variant increases lung cancer risk. *Cancer Res.* 60(22): 6381–6383 (2000).
115. Borgstahl GE *et al.* Human mitochondrial manganese superoxide dismutase polymorphic variant Ile58Thr reduces activity by destabilizing the tetrameric interface. *Biochemistry* 35(14): 4287–4297 (1996).
116. Shimoda–Matsubayashi S, Matsumine H, Kobayashi T, Nakagawa-Hattori Y, Shimizu Y, Mizuno Y. Structural dimorphism in the mitochondrial targeting sequence in the human manganese superoxide dismutase gene. A predictive evidence for conformational change to influence mitochondrial transport and a study of allelic association in Parkinson's disease. *Biochem. Biophys. Res. Commun.* 226(2): 561–565 (1996).
117. Gilks CB, Price K, Wright JL, Churg A. Antioxidant gene expression in rat lung after exposure to cigarette smoke. *Am. J. Pathol.* 152(1): 269–278 (1998).
118. Rosenblum JS, Gilula NB, Lerner RA. On signal sequence polymorphisms and diseases of distribution. *Proc. Natl. Acad. Sci. USA* 93(9): 4471–4473 (1996).
119. Ambrosone CB *et al.* Manganese superoxide dismutase (MnSOD) genetic polymorphisms, dietary antioxidants, and risk of breast cancer. *Cancer Res.* 59(3): 602–606 (1999).

120. Mitrunen K *et al.* Association between manganese superoxide dismutase (MnSOD) gene polymorphism and breast cancer risk. *Carcinogenesis* 22(5): 827–829 (2001).
121. Egan KM, Thompson PA, Titus-Ernstoff L, Moore JH, Ambrosone CB. MnSOD polymorphism and breast cancer in a population-based case–control study. *Cancer Lett.* 199(1): 27–33 (2003).
122. Hong YC, Lee KH, Yi CH, Ha EH, Christiani DC. Genetic susceptibility of term pregnant women to oxidative damage. *Toxicol Lett.* 129(3): 255–262 (2002).
123. Woodson K *et al.* Manganese superoxide dismutase (MnSOD) polymorphism, alpha-tocopherol supplementation and prostate cancer risk in the alpha-tocopherol, beta-carotene cancer prevention study (Finland). *Cancer Causes Control* 14(6): 513–518 (2003).
124. Li H, Kantoff PW, Giovannucci E, Leitzmann MF, Gaziano M, Stampfer MJ. Manganese superoxide dismutase (MnSOD) polymorhism, prediagnostic plasma antioxidants and prostate cancer risk. *Cancer Res.* 65(6): 2498–2504 (2005).
125. Mitrunen K, Hirvonen A. Molecular epidemiology of sporadic breast cancer. The role of polymorphic genes involved in oestrogen biosynthesis and metabolism. *Mutat. Res.* 544(1): 9–41 (2003).
126. Fattman CL, Schaefer LM, Oury TD. Extracellular superoxide dismutase in biology and medicine. *Free Radic. Biol. Med.* 35(3): 236–256 (2003).
127. Marklund SL, Nilsson P, Israelsson K, Schampi I, Peltonen M, Asplund K. Two variants of extracellular-superoxide dismutase: relationship to cardiovascular risk factors in an unselected middle-aged population. *J. Intern. Med.* 242(1): 5–14 (1997).
128. Adachi T, Yamazaki N, Tasaki H, Toyokawa T, Yamashita K, Hirano K. Changes in the heparin affinity of extracellular-superoxide dismutase in patients with coronary artery atherosclerosis. *Biol. Pharm. Bull.* 21(10): 1090–1093 (1998).
129. Benson AM, Hunkeler MJ, Talalay P. Increase of NAD(P)H:quinone reductase by dietary antioxidants: possible role in protection against carcinogenesis and toxicity. *Proc. Natl. Acad. Sci. USA* 77(9): 5216–5220 (1980).
130. Traver RD *et al.* NAD(P)H:quinone oxidoreductase gene expression in human colon carcinoma cells: characterization of a mutation which modulates DT-diaphorase activity and mitomycin sensitivity. *Cancer Res.* 52(4): 797–802 (1992).
131. Traver RD *et al.* Characterization of a polymorphism in NAD(P)H: quinone oxidoreductase (DT-diaphorase). *Br. J. Cancer* 75(1): 69–75 (1997).

132. Siegel D, McGuinness SM, Winski SL, Ross D. Genotype–phenotype relationships in studies of a polymorphism in NAD(P)H:quinone oxidoreductase 1. *Pharmacogenetics* 9(1): 113–121 (1999).
133. Misra V, Grondin A, Klamut HJ, Rauth AM. Assessment of the relationship between genotypic status of a DT-diaphorase point mutation and enzymatic activity. *Br. J. Cancer* 83(8): 998–1002 (2000).
134. Siegel D, Anwar A, Winski SL, Kepa JK, Zolman KL, Ross D. Rapid polyubiquitination and proteasomal degradation of a mutant form of NAD(P)H:quinone oxidoreductase 1. *Mol. Pharmacol.* 59(2): 263–268 (2001).
135. Moran JL, Siegel D, Ross D. A potential mechanism underlying the increased susceptibility of individuals with a polymorphism in NAD(P)H:quinone oxidoreductase 1 (NQO1) to benzene toxicity. *Proc. Natl. Acad. Sci. USA* 96(14): 8150–8155 (1999).
136. Hamajima N *et al.* NAD(P)H: quinone oxidoreductase 1 (NQO1) C609T polymorphism and the risk of eight cancers for Japanese. *Int. J. Clin. Oncol.* 7(2): 103–108 (2002).
137. Siegelmann-Danieli N, Buetow KH. Significance of genetic variation at the glutathione S-transferase M1 and NAD(P)H:quinone oxidoreductase 1 detoxification genes in breast cancer development. *Oncology* 62(1): 39–45 (2002).
138. Mannervik B *et al.* Nomenclature for human glutathione transferases. *Biochem. J.* 282(Pt. 1): 305–306 (1992).
139. Forrester LM *et al.* Expression of glutathione S-transferases and cytochrome P450 in normal and tumor breast tissue. *Carcinogenesis* 11(12): 2163–2170 (1990).
140. Sweeney C *et al.* Association between a glutathione S-transferase A1 promoter polymorphism and survival after breast cancer treatment. *Int. J. Cancer* 103(6): 810–814 (2003).
141. Brockmoller J, Gross D, Kerb R, Drakoulis N, Roots I. Correlation between transstilbene oxide-glutathione conjugation activity and the deletion mutation in the glutathione *S*-transferase class mu gene detected by polymerase chain reaction. *Biochem. Pharmacol.* 43(3): 647–650 (1992).
142. Rebbeck TR. Molecular epidemiology of the human glutathione S-transferase genotypes GSTM1 and GSTT1 in cancer susceptibility. *Cancer Epidemiol. Biomarkers Prev.* 6(9): 733–743 (1997).
143. Bailey LR, Roodi N, Verrier CS, Yee CJ, Dupont WD, Parl FF. Breast cancer and CYPIA1, GSTM1, and GSTT1 polymorphisms: evidence of a lack of association in Caucasians and African Americans. *Cancer Res.* 58(1): 65–70 (1998).

144. Helzlsouer KJ *et al.* Association between glutathione S-transferase M1, P1, and T1 genetic polymorphisms and development of breast cancer. *J. Natl. Cancer Inst.* 90(7): 512–518 (1998).
145. Kelsey KT *et al.* Glutathione S-transferase class mu deletion polymorphism and breast cancer: results from prevalent versus incident cases. *Cancer Epidemiol. Biomarkers Prev.* 6(7): 511–515 (1997).
146. Zhong S, Wyllie AH, Barnes D, Wolf CR, Spurr NK. Relationship between the GSTM1 genetic polymorphism and susceptibility to bladder, breast and colon cancer. *Carcinogenesis* 14(9): 1821–1824 (1993).
147. Ambrosone CB *et al.* Cytochrome P4501A1 and glutathione S-transferase (M1) genetic polymorphisms and postmenopausal breast cancer risk. *Cancer Res.* 55(16): 3483–3485 (1995).
148. Ambrosone CB, Coles BF, Freudenheim JL, Shields PG. Glutathione-S-transferase (GSTM1) genetic polymorphisms do not affect human breast cancer risk, regardless of dietary antioxidants. *J. Nutr.* 129(2S Suppl.): 565S–568S (1999).
149. Zheng W, Wen WQ, Gustafson DR, Gross M, Cerhan JR, Folsom AR. GSTM1 and GSTT1 polymorphisms and postmenopausal breast cancer risk. *Breast Cancer Res. Treat.* 74(1): 9–16 (2002).
150. Zimniak P *et al.* Naturally occurring human glutathione S-transferase GSTP1-1 isoforms with isoleucine and valine in position 104 differ in enzymic properties. *Eur. J. Biochem.* 224(3): 893–899 (1994).
151. Gudmundsdottir K, Tryggvadottir L, Eyfjord JE. GSTM1, GSTT1, and GSTP1 genotypes in relation to breast cancer risk and frequency of mutations in the p53 gene. *Cancer Epidemiol. Biomarkers Prev.* 10(11): 1169–1173 (2001).
152. Sweeney C *et al.* Association between survival after treatment for breast cancer and glutathione S-transferase P1 Ile105Val polymorphism. *Cancer Res.* 60(20): 5621–5624 (2000).
153. Zhu BT, Conney AH. Is 2-methoxyestradiol an endogenous estrogen metabolite that inhibits mammary carcinogenesis? *Cancer Res.* 58(11): 2269–2277 (1998).
154. Axelrod J, Tomchick R. Enzymatic *O*-methylation of epinephrine and other catechols. *J. Biol. Chem.* 233(3): 702–705 (1958).
155. Guldberg HC, Marsden CA. Catechol-*O*-methyl transferase: pharmacological aspects and physiological role. *Pharmacol. Rev.* 27(2): 135–206 (1975).
156. Cavalieri EL *et al.* Molecular origin of cancer: catechol estrogen-3,4-quinones as endogenous tumor initiators. *Proc. Natl. Acad. Sci. USA* 94(20): 10937–10942 (1997).

157. Liehr JG. Hormone-associated cancer: mechanistic similarities between human breast cancer and estrogen-induced kidney carcinogenesis in hamsters. *Environ. Health Perspect.* 105(Suppl 3): 565–569 (1997).
158. Lachman HM, Papolos DF, Saito T, Yu YM, Szumlanski CL, Weinshilboum RM. Human catechol-*O*-methyltransferase pharmacogenetics: description of a functional polymorphism and its potential application to neuropsychiatric disorders. *Pharmacogenetics* 6(3): 243–250 (1996).
159. Dawling S, Roodi N, Mernaugh RL, Wang X, Parl FF. Catechol-*O*-methyltransferase (COMT)-mediated metabolism of catechol estrogens: comparison of wild-type and variant COMT isoforms. *Cancer Res.* 61(18): 6716–6722 (2001).
160. Thompson PA *et al.* Genetic polymorphisms in catechol-*O*-methyltransferase, menopausal status, and breast cancer risk. *Cancer Res.* 58(10): 2107–2110 (1998).
161. Huang CS, Chern HD, Chang KJ, Cheng CW, Hsu SM, Shen CY. Breast cancer risk associated with genotype polymorphism of the estrogen-metabolizing genes CYP17, CYP1A1, and COMT: a multigenic study on cancer susceptibility. *Cancer Res.* 59(19): 4870–4875 (1999).
162. Yim DS *et al.* Relationship between the Val158Met polymorphism of catechol-*O*-methyl transferase and breast cancer. *Pharmacogenetics* 11(4): 279–286 (2001).
163. Lavigne JA *et al.* An association between the allele coding for a low activity variant of catechol-*O*-methyltransferase and the risk for breast cancer. *Cancer Res.* 57(24): 5493–5497 (1997).
164. Millikan RC *et al.* Catechol-*O*-methyltransferase and breast cancer risk. *Carcinogenesis* 19(11):1943–1947 (1998).
165. Hamajima N *et al.* Limited association between a catechol-*O*-methyltransferase (COMT) polymorphism and breast cancer risk in Japan. *Int. J. Clin. Oncol.* 6(1): 13–18 (2001).
166. Bergman-Jungestrom M, Wingren S. Catechol-*O*-methyltransferase (COMT) gene polymorphism and breast cancer risk in young women. *Br. J. Cancer* 85(6): 859–862 (2001).
167. Mitrunen K *et al.* Polymorphic catechol-*O*-methyltransferase gene and breast cancer risk. *Cancer Epidemiol. Biomarkers Prev.* 10(6): 635–640 (2001).
168. Goodman JE *et al.* COMT genotype, micronutrients in the folate metabolic pathway and breast cancer risk. *Carcinogenesis* 22(10): 1661–1665 (2001).
169. Tukey RH, Strassburg CP. Human UDP-glucuronosyltransferases: metabolism, expression, and disease. *Annu. Rev. Pharmacol. Toxicol.* 40: 581–616 (2000).

170. de Wildt SN, Kearns GL, Leeder JS, van den Anker JN. Glucuronidation in humans. Pharmacogenetic and developmental aspects. *Clin. Pharmacokinet.* 36(6): 439–452 (1999).
171. Cheng Z, Radominska-Pandya A, Tephly TR. Cloning and expression of human UDP-glucuronosyltransferase (UGT) 1A8. *Arch. Biochem. Biophys.* 356(2): 301–305 (1998).
172. Hall D, Ybazeta G, Destro-Bisol G, Petzl-Erler ML, Di Rienzo A. Variability at the uridine diphosphate glucuronosyltransferase 1A1 promoter in human populations and primates. *Pharmacogenetics* 9(5): 591–599 (1999).
173. Guillemette C, Millikan RC, Newman B, Housman DE. Genetic polymorphisms in uridine diphospho-glucuronosyltransferase 1A1 and association with breast cancer among African Americans. *Cancer Res.* 60(4): 950–956 (2000).
174. Guillemette C *et al.* Association of genetic polymorphisms in UGT1A1 with breast cancer and plasma hormone levels. *Cancer Epidemiol. Biomarkers Prev.* 10(6): 711–714 (2001).
175. Grant DJ, Bell DA. Bilirubin UDP-glucuronosyltransferase 1A1 gene polymorphisms: susceptibility to oxidative damage and cancer? *Mol. Carcinog.* 29(4): 198–204 (2000).

33 Oxidative Stress and Photocarcinogenesis: Strategies for Prevention

Santosh K. Katiyar

1. Introduction

Oxidative processes and generation of reactive oxygen species (ROS) have been implicated in many disease processes, including cancer. The increased generation and decreased degradation of ROS may lead to oxidative stress and free radical-mediated injury in various tissues. The most reactive oxygen and radical species are the most damaging, the least likely to accumulate or move to other parts of the tissues, and difficult to detect. Although many free radical-mediated processes occur normally in biological systems, excessive or prolonged free radical challenges may result in the chronic or acute molecular, cellular, and tissue damage associated with aging and a wide variety of diseases including cancer in different organ systems. The relationship between oxidative stress and the neoplastic process is well defined and understood.[1–6] The skin, which is easily exposed to experimental and environmental agents containing or producing free radicals, is a useful model to study the role of ROS in skin diseases, including cancer, aging, and inflammatory diseases. Human skin is constantly exposed to a large number of physical and chemical environmental agents. Some of these agents produce adverse biological effects commonly through the generation of ROS in the skin. The major environmental and physical agent to which skin is constantly exposed is solar ultraviolet (UV) radiation. Exposure of the mammalian skin to UV plays a causal and decisive role in acute and chronic skin damage which results in the development of melanoma, non-melanoma skin cancers (NMSC), photoaging, and other inflammatory diseases of the skin. Sunburn, pigmentation, hyperplasia, immune suppression, and vitamin D synthesis represent acute responses of the skin to solar UV radiation, whereas photoaging and NMSC or photocarcinogenesis represent chronic damage. Since the role of oxidative stress in various diseases of the body and their possible preventive strategies is difficult to discuss and summarize at one place, this chapter focuses on the role of solar UV radiation induced oxidative stress and oxidative stress-mediated development of NMSC. We will also discuss the appropriate or affordable strategies which can minimize the effects of solar UV radiation. The author's research laboratory mainly focuses on the chemopreventive effect of dietary botanical supplements on UV-induced oxidative stress, and oxidative stress-mediated adverse biological effects, such as photocarcinogenesis, and these findings will be discussed in detail.

2. Solar UV Radiation and the Skin

Although many environmental and genetic factors contribute to the development of skin diseases, the most important and hazardous is chronic exposure to solar UV light. The UV radiation present in sunlight is mainly divided into three regions, short-wave UVC (200–290 nm), mid-range UVB (290–320 nm), and long-wave UVA (320–400 nm). The UVC spectrum is a potent mutagen and can induce immune suppression however it is absorbed by the stratospheric ozone layer, so its role in human pathogenesis is minimal. Reduction in stratospheric ozone layer allows an increase of UVB radiation to reach the Earth's surface.[7] The UV exposure to skin is responsible for the inflammatory responses, development of oxidative stress, and immunotoxicity in the open skin areas of the body. UVB is also mutagenic, and extensive epidemiological evidence has indicated that UVB spectrum is responsible for the induction of melanoma and NMSC.[8] Moreover, UVB radiations of the solar spectrum are responsible for sunburn, oxidative stress, and immune suppression. UVA, the major component of the UV portion of the solar spectrum, does cause premature aging of the skin, induce oxidative stress, and can suppress some immunological functions.[9,10]

Skin is much more than a passive physical barrier between the external environment and internal tissues. Therefore, skin is a first defense barrier organ of the body from external environmental pollutants, including environmental chemicals and solar UV radiation. Thus the major role of the skin is to provide a protective covering at this crucial interface between inside and outside. Morphologically, skin is a composite of a variety of cell types and organellar bodies, each of which has a particular function. The major function of the skin is protective, to protect the organism from the external environment. Achieving this goal has resulted in the evolution of a complex structure involving several different layers, each with particular properties. The major layers include the epidermis, the dermis, and the hypodermis (Fig. 1). The epidermis is a stratifying layer of epithelial cells that overlies the connective tissue layer, the dermis. The dermis is divided into papillary dermis and reticular dermis. The epidermis and dermis are supported by an internal layer of adipose tissue, called hypodermis. Skin cancer is mainly associated with the epidermal layer and its cell type. The major cell type of the epidermis is the keratinocytes. It comprises >90% of the cells of the epidermal layer. In laboratory animals like mouse, it is about two to three cell layers thick (Fig. 1, panels C and D), but in case of human skin, the epidermis is quite thick and comprises of about 8–15 cell layers

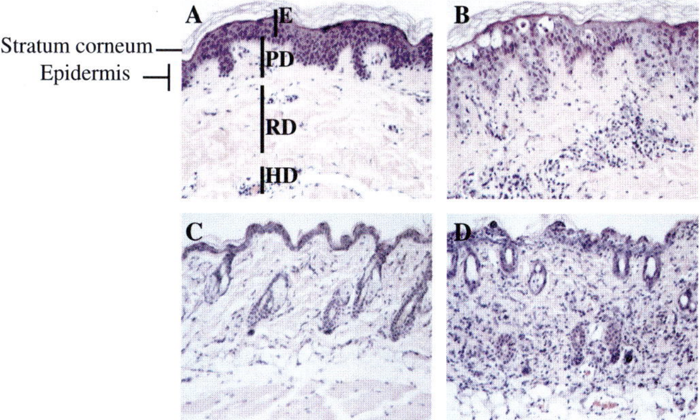

Fig. 1. Structure of the skin: human (panels A and B) and mouse (panels C and D). Panels A and C show the morphology of the normal skin. Panels B (human) and D (mouse) show the morphological changes in the skin 48 h after UV irradiation. Panels B and D also show the infiltration of leukocytes after UV irradiation compared with the non-UVB-irradiated skin (panels A and C). The human epidermis is thicker than that of mouse. E = epidermis, PD = papillary dermis, RD = reticular dermis, HD = hypodermis.

(Fig. 1, panels A and B). Thus human skin is comparatively more protective than mouse skin against environmental factors, including the effect of UV radiation. It is well documented that solar UV exposure to mammalian skin induces a number of pathologic conditions, such as sunburn cell formation, hyperplastic response, oxidative stress, and DNA damage which contribute to the development of skin diseases, for example, skin cancers.[10,11]

3. UV Radiation and Oxidative Stress

By definition, ROS are any species that are more reactive than ground-state molecular oxygen (O_2). Any atoms or molecules containing one or more unpaired electrons are chemically defined as free radicals.[12] Some of the ROS have an odd number of electrons and thus qualify as free radicals, such as superoxide anions, hydroxyl, hydroperoxyl, and peroxyl. The other ROS that contain an even number of electrons are not free radicals, but can form free radical species or can be produced by reactions involving free radicals, such as hydrogen peroxide (H_2O_2), and hypohalous acids (hypochlorous, hypobromous, and hypothiocyanous acids). Most of the oxygen in the body is used in cellular metabolism. Through a series of one-electron subtractions, molecular oxygen is, in sequence, changed to superoxide anion, hydrogen peroxide, hydroxyl radical, and finally to water. Most reactions occur in the mitochondria and are related to energy production. Cellular enzymes and controlled metabolic processes ordinarily keep oxidative damage to cells at a minimum. In times of increased oxidative stress, however, including high metabolic demands and outside stimulus such as solar UV light, smoking, and pollution-protective controls may not be adequate and oxidative damage may occur. The maximum damage occurs from free radicals, and occurs where they are created. Other reactive molecules, such as singlet oxygen and hydrogen peroxide, are not free radicals but are capable of initiating oxidative reactions and generating free-radical species. Most ROS, including free radicals, are potent oxidizing agents. Short-lived free radicals are especially reactive. Oxidative stress may develop when the balance between the rates of ROS generation and dissipation is so disrupted that excessive levels of free radicals may overwhelm the capacity of the natural antioxidant defense system and injure cells. Exposure of the skin to UV radiation results in generation of reactive oxygen species, such as singlet oxygen, peroxy radicals, superoxide anion, and hydroxyl radicals that damage cellular DNA and non-DNA cellular targets like proteins and lipids.[13–16] UV-induced ROS results in oxidative stress when their formation exceeds the antioxidant defense ability of the target cell. The induction of oxidative stress and imbalance of antioxidant defense system have been associated with the onset of several diseases including rheumatoid arthritis, inflammation, photoaging, immunotoxicity, and skin cancer. Thus, UV radiation is a critical major environmental oxidizing agent and hazardous to the human biological system.

UV exposure of the skin induces mainly the formation of H_2O_2, hydroxyl radicals, nitric oxide, and lipid peroxides. Formation of H_2O_2, lipid peroxides, hydroxyl radicals, and nitric oxide may create a state of oxidative stress in the skin which may act as a tumor initiator[10,17] and tumor promoter[10,18] by damaging macromolecules such as DNA, proteins, and lipids. Iwai *et al.*[19] suggested that UV-induced immune suppression might be mediated, at least in part, through ROS. To confirm their observations, they found that application of glutathione as an antioxidant to the skin during irradiation significantly reversed UV-induced immunosuppression. UV-induced immune suppression is considered as a risk factor for skin cancer development.[20,21]

4. Mechanism of UV-Induced Oxidative Stress: Double Hit Model of Keratinocytic Injury

Oxidative products produced by the inflammatory leukocytes have been proposed as the mediating agent(s) between inflammation and the development of tumor at the inflammatory site. We have observed that a single UV exposure (90 or 180 mJ/cm^2) to mouse skin induces infiltration of leukocytes. The peak time of infiltration ranges between 24 and 72 h post UV irradiation.[6] These infiltrating leukocytes were found to be the major source of H_2O_2 and nitric oxide production, and expression of inducible nitric oxide synthase.[6] As detailed in the schematic diagram of the skin (Fig. 2), UV irradiation to the skin induces inflammatory responses, chemotactic factors, and ROS (oxidative stress) within minutes. This is the first hit of keratinocytes by ROS generated after UV exposure. UV-induced chemotactic factors induce infiltration of leukocytes, mainly activated macrophages and neutrophils (CD11b+ cells) into the skin.[6,22] CD11b+ cells are the

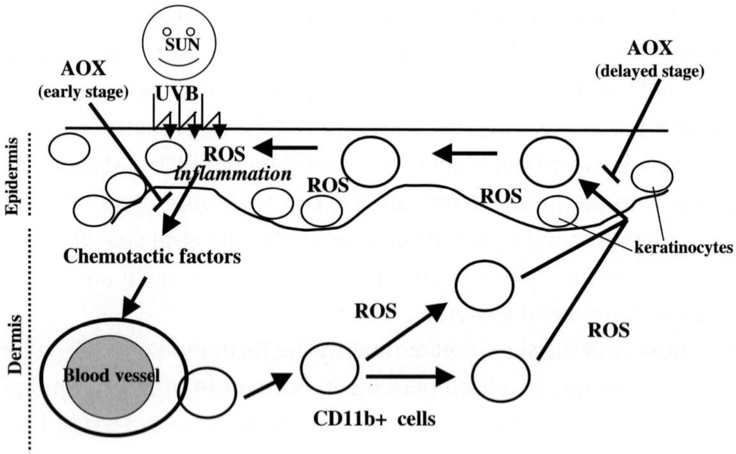

Fig. 2. The schematic diagram depicts the mechanism of UV-induced generation of oxidative stress in the skin. UV exposure induces inflammatory responses, chemotactic factors, and reactive oxygen species (ROS) at an early stages or time points. Inflammatory responses and chemotactic factors stimulate the infiltration of leukocytes in UV-irradiated skin. Infiltrating leukocytes, particularly activated macrophages and neutrophils (CD11b+ cells), are the major source of ROS at delayed stages or time points. Treatment of skin with antioxidant, topical or dietary supplement, may prevent UV-induced ROS generation at early stage, and also at delayed stage by inhibiting the infiltration of CD11b+ cells. Inhibition of UV-induced oxidative stress by antioxidant (AOX) could be an effective strategy to prevent the risk of photocarcinogenesis.

major source of oxidative stress,[23] and further enhance the oxidative stress potential at the UV-irradiated skin site which is injurious to the epidermal keratinocytes, and this constitutes injury to the epidermal keratinocytes second time after a single UV exposure. NMSC [squamous cell carcinoma (SCC) and basal cell carcinoma (BCC)] originates from epidermal layer, therefore is very important site for ROS attack. The use of antioxidant may reduce the oxidative stress at the early stage and, at delayed stage by inhibiting the infiltration of inflammatory leukocytes.

5. UV Induces Depletion of Cutaneous Antioxidant Defense

The skin possesses a wide range of interlinked antioxidant defense mechanisms to protect itself from UV-induced photooxidative damage; however, the capacity of these defensive systems is not unlimited, and it can be overwhelmed by excessive exposure to UV radiation.[24] Cellular integrity is maintained by antioxidant enzymes, including catalase, glutathione peroxidase, and glutathione reductase, which collectively neutralize hydrogen peroxide and lipid hydroperoxides, as shown in Fig. 3. In addition, superoxide dismutase dismutates superoxides (Fig. 3). The extracellular space in the skin is protected from superoxide anion by extracellular superoxide dismutase. Non-enzymic antioxidants such as glutathione and ascorbic acid in the aqueous phase and vitamin E and ubiquinol-10 in the lipid phase, particularly in membranes, neutralize the oxidant molecules. We and others have shown that antioxidant enzymes have been decreased after acute high dose of UV exposure and chronic exposure of the skin to UV radiation.[22,25–29] It has been shown that antioxidants, especially dietary antioxidants, can prevent the adverse effects of UV radiation on the antioxidant defense system and may protect against photocarcinogenesis, at least in animal models.[22,27] There are evidences that acute high dose of UV radiation or chronic exposure of skin to UV radiation induces depletion of antioxidant enzymes, and thus contributes towards the increase in the level of oxidative stress.[22,27]

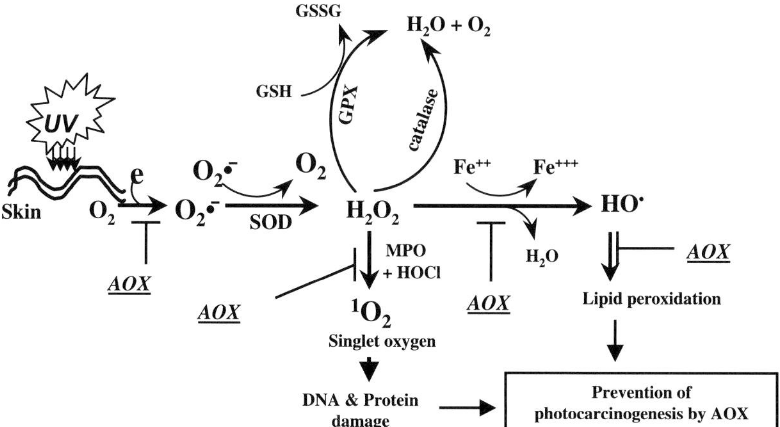

Fig. 3. The schematic diagram depicts the antioxidant defense system in the skin. Interaction of UV photons with the target cells in the skin induces the generation of ROS. Active target sites of antioxidant (AOX) are shown by blocking heads. These target sites may be involved in the reduction of UV-induced ROS generation in the skin by antioxidant treatment. Reduction of oxidative stress would contribute to protection against photocarcinogenesis.

Endogenous antioxidant glutathione appears to play a major role in the protection of cells against oxidative damage.[30] It is indicated by the fact that after depletion of human skin cells of glutathione, they become extremely sensitive to both UVB and UVA radiations.[31,32]

6. UV Induces DNA Damage

DNA may absorb UVB (290–320 nm), and directly induces changes between adjacent pyrimidine bases on one strand of DNA. Cyclobutane pyrimidine dimers, particularly thymine dimers or less commonly 6–4 photoproducts may be generated which are considered as an essential step in UV carcinogenesis.[11] The DNA strand breakage, thymine glycols, and 8-hydroxyguanine are all forms of oxidative DNA damage. Strand breakage of DNA is induced by both UVB and to a greater extent by UVA radiation[33] but is unlikely to be a premutagenic lesion. 8-hydroxyguanine, which is a premutagenic DNA lesion, has been observed after UVB radiation,[15,34] but the UV doses are so high that it is unlikely to be relevant. On the other hand, UVA radiation does induce 8-hydroxyguanine damage at biologically relevant UV doses. A close association exists between high oxidative stress, formation of 8-hydroxyguanine in DNA, and carcinogenesis.[15] The formation of lesions in DNA leads to: (i) loss of tumor suppressor gene function, (ii) amplification of cellular oncogenes, (iii) modulation of membrane-related growth signal pathways, and (iv) modulation in immune status. Evidence implicating DNA as the target for most of the effects of UV such as lethality, mutation, and malignant transformation.[36,37] The strategies, which can prevent UV-induced DNA damage, would result in the prevention of non-melanoma skin cancer.

7. UV Radiation and Skin Cancer

Following are the major factors which contribute to skin cancer incidence:

1. Genetic alterations, e.g., mutations like addition, deletion, and substitution, etc. in genome.
2. Environmental factors, e.g., UV radiation, pollutants like polycyclic aromatic hydrocarbons or toxic chemicals.

3. Dietary constituents, e.g., diet containing toxic ingredients, charcoal roasted meat, etc.

7.1. *Epidemiology of UV carcinogenesis*

Although several environmental, genetic, and dietary factors contribute to the development of skin cancers, the most important is the chronic exposure to solar UV radiation. Chronic exposure to solar UV radiation is responsible for approximately 1.3 million new cases of NMSC (SCC and BCC) each year in the United States.[38–42] These numbers are probably underestimates, because many skin cancers are treated or removed in clinics without being reported to cancer registries, and thus has a tremendous impact on public health and healthcare expenditures. NMSC is by far the most common type of malignancy, thus making UV light the most prevalent environmental carcinogen known.[38–40] The incidence of skin cancer is continuing to increase at an alarming rate, and this increase is expected to continue as the population ages, changing life style, and larger amounts of UV radiation reaching the surface of the Earth because of depletion of the ozone layer.[38–42] Epidemiologic data link melanoma to intense sunlight exposure in childhood, and provides support for a role of UVA spectrum (320–400 nm).[43] Outdoors laborers, such as fishermen and gardeners, were found to be prone to skin cancer, particularly on the sun-exposed areas of the body. Approximately 80% of NMSC occur on chronically sun-exposed areas of the body, such as the face, neck, and the dorsal surface of the arms. The incidence of these cancers in Caucasians has been seen to be higher in populations living closer to the equator. According to the American Cancer Society, one in five Americans will develop skin cancer in their life time.[41]

7.2. *Characteristics of UV radiation*

Skin cancers occur more frequently than all other cancers combined.[41] Whereas UVB (290–320 nm) is believed to interact directly with DNA to initiate signature mutations of basal and squamous cell carcinomas, UVA wavelengths (320–400 nm) are believed to interact indirectly, including the production of free radicals.[44,45] Free radicals indirectly damage DNA and cause protein damage, which contribute to other skin disorders like premature aging or photoaging of the skin. Also, UVB is important for tumor initiation, and UVA predominantly causes tumor promotion.[47] In contrast to UVB, UVA irradiation constitutes a severe oxidative stress.[47–50] At levels found in sunlight, UVA, in contrast to UVB, may be more than 10 times more effective at causing lipid peroxidation.[51] UVA is more cytotoxic than UVB.[46] In addition, UVA can inhibit DNA repair.[52] UV radiation can induce the expression of matrix metalloproteinase synthesis[53,54] that can augment the biologic aggressiveness of skin cancer. Sunlight contains about 20 times as much UVA as UVB. Whereas UVB is almost entirely (99%) absorbed in the epidermis, UVA is capable of reaching dermal layers,[55,56] and even affecting circulating blood cells.[57] Therefore, UVA is able to have a greater effect on the underlying cutaneous vasculature and supporting tissues than UVB. Window glass blocks most UVB irradiation but does not block UVA irradiation. This creates more problems for those who spend long hours in cars.[58] Without protection, their skin may be particularly susceptible to oxidative stress. Indeed, pilots who fly transcontinental routes at high altitudes without protection have an increased susceptibility to melanoma and NMSC.[59,60]

7.3. *Strategies to prevent UV-induced skin cancer or photocarcinogenesis*

Among Caucasian populations, tanned skin has become an important social signal of health and prosperity. The popularity of holidays in the sun, of outdoor activities, body-shaping, and the use of sun-beds for cosmetic purposes lead to an increased exposure to UV radiation. These social practices are fatal for human health. Thus the need to study cellular and molecular effects that UV radiation, especially UVB radiation, exerts on human skin has become more and more important. As mentioned, the populations in the northern hemisphere are increasingly being exposed to natural and artificial sources of UV radiation and therefore, there is an urgent need to develop new and effective photoprotective strategies which can protect skin from detrimental effects of UV radiation, including but not limited to UV-induced oxidative stress-mediated skin diseases such as melanoma and NMSC. Although there are many ways by which the adverse effects of overexposure to UV radiation can be minimized, a much more effective method of handling this problem is through preventive measures. Strategies to protect the skin from adverse UV effects can be separated into two categories: (i) endogenous sun protection, and (ii) exogenous sun protection. Endogenous sun protection includes thickening of the epidermis following UVB radiation, pigmentation, cellular scavenger systems, and DNA repair. Exogenous sun protection is the domain of sunscreens and the use of topical application of chemopreventive agents. Public healthcare practitioners recommend a variety of photoprotective measures or strategies, such as wearing protective clothing, reducing sun exposure particularly during peak hours of UV intensity from (10:00 AM to 4:00 PM), and using topical sunscreens. Additionally, the use of dietary botanicals is receiving considerable interest in the protection of skin from the adverse biological effects of solar UV radiation. The use of dietary supplements and antioxidants, such as green tea polyphenols, grape seed proanthocyanidins, and vitamins C and E are also supposed to be efficient in reduction of UV-induced effects on human health.

7.4. *Prevention of photocarcinogenesis by sunscreens: adequate or inadequate?*

Sunscreens are widely advocated as a means of reducing skin cancer risk. To protect the skin against harmful effects of solar UV radiation, sunscreens are commonly employed. Topical application of the sunscreens with the capacity to block the penetration of UV radiation, particularly UVB, is considered a major strategy for protection of the skin against UV-induced effects. It is considered that sunscreens have the ability to act as chemical and physical barriers that absorb, scatter, or reflect the damaging UVB radiation that impinges on the skin. Generally, the effectiveness of a sunscreen is expressed as the sun protection factor (SPF). SPF is traditionally assessed by its ability to inhibit the development of erythema 24 h after exposure of the skin to UV light. Topical sunscreens capable of preventing erythema have been assumed to protect against UV-induced carcinogenesis as well. However, the correlation between inflammation and tumorigenesis is not completely established. With our present understanding of the immunological and molecular events leading to skin cancer, the measurement of inhibition of UV-induced erythema might be insufficient as an indicator of protection from UV-induced carcinogenesis. The ability of a sunscreen to protect against erythema, the so-called SPF, although well characterized may not be an adequate measure of a sunscreen's ability to protect against other biological endpoints, particularly immune suppression.[61] There is considerable evidence regarding sunscreen protection against UV-induced sunburn,[62,63] immune suppression,[64–66] actinic keratosis,[67,68] and DNA damage,[69,70] but despite these published reports, the effectiveness of sunscreens in preventing or reducing skin cancer remains a controversial area. An SPF that measures protection against erythema or even edema has not been adequately correlated with sunscreen activity against many other biologic reactions induced by UV radiation. It has been suggested that to evaluate sunscreen efficacy it is important to use a panel of assays including immune protection factor (IPF), mutation protection factor (MPF), and protection against photocarcinogenesis.

The use of sunscreen is largely based on extrapolation from animal studies, as it is difficult to evaluate long-term protection in humans. Sunscreens reduce the erythematogenous capacity of UVB radiation through absorption or through reflexion of UV radiation. Although a tendency of using sunscreens with high SPF can be observed during the last two decades, sunscreens do not provide complete protection. Most of the sunscreen that is available in the United States at this time provides less protection against UVA, which is a major UV spectrum in sunlight for generating ROS, than UVB. Most importantly, sunscreens failed to be effective once damage to the skin or the cells have been induced following UVB exposure. Limited data indicate that sunscreens can inhibit actinic keratoses that are regarded as precursors of SCC.[67,71] A study conducted in Australia has shown that daily use of a SPF 16 sunscreen, over a period of 4.5 years, reduced the total number of SCC by 40% but not the number of people with the tumor. No protective effect was seen for basal cell carcinoma.[72] Some studies even show that sunscreen use is associated with an increased risk of melanoma.[73] Haywood *et al.* showed that sunscreens inadequately protect against UV-induced free radicals in skin, which are implicated in skin aging and melanoma.[74] Moreover, it is difficult to find an effective sunscreen that can provide full spectral protection against UV light (UVA+UVB). In addition, sunscreen ingredients may become free radicals themselves when activated by UV irradiation,[75] and sunscreen chemicals may be absorbed into the skin[76] to potentially cause harm. Despite the extensive use of sunscreens during the last two decades, the incidence of skin cancers is still increasing, and the role of sunscreens in protection against skin cancers is controversial. Sunscreen use has been shown to decrease the formation of actinic keratoses, which are linked to SCC.[67] Animal models have shown that sunscreens reduce the incidence of basal and squamous cell tumors,[17,77] which are UVB related; however, there have been several studies to suggest that sunscreen use is associated with increased risk of melanoma.[78,79] This may reflect inadequate sunscreen application;[80,81] lack of durability of the application; the lack of, or inadequacy of, UVA filters in sunscreen preparations combined with prolonged sunbathing;[78] the photo-instability of sunscreen filters that results in reduced protection; or the production of reactive free radicals or mutagens within the cream.[82–84] A link between sunscreen use and melanoma, however, is still debated[85] and unclear.[86] Therefore for these reasons, in addition to the use of sunscreens, the use of antioxidants, particularly dietary ingredients/supplements which have antioxidant properties, such as green tea polyphenols (GTP) and grape seed proanthocyanidins (GSP), may prove highly beneficial for the reduction of solar UV radiation induced oxidative stress, and oxidative stress mediated skin diseases, including NMSC.

7.5. *Chemoprevention of photocarcinogenesis by dietary antioxidants: an affordable strategy*

Chemoprevention refers to the use of agents to inhibit, reverse, or retard tumorigenesis following various mechanistic pathways. Numerous phytochemicals derived from edible plants have been reported to interfere with a specific stage of the carcinogenic process. Many population-based studies have highlighted the ability of macronutrients and micronutrients in vegetables, fruits, and beverages to reduce the risk of cancer, which is primarily associated with the development of oxidative stress especially in case of NMSC. As we have discussed that UV radiation-induced oxidative stress is involved in several skin diseases, particularly NMSC, the use of dietary antioxidants may have a better strategy to neutralize the effect of ROS or oxidative stress. In this reference, several laboratories have been involved in extensive experimental studies on *in vitro* and *in vivo* animal and human system to demonstrate the beneficial effects of dietary antioxidants, such as green tea polyphenols (GTP), grape seed proanthocyanidins (GSP), and resveratrol from grape skin, etc. against the inhibition of oxidative stress and other biomarkers of photocarcinogenesis. These effects are being discussed here with particular reference to GTP and GSP in detail as to demonstrate that how dietary antioxidants or dietary supplements can be useful for the prevention of melanoma and NMSC, which is a major health-related problem among Caucasians.

8. Dietary Antioxidants and Skin

The use of dietary supplements having antioxidant properties is receiving considerable interest to protect skin from adverse biological effects caused by the generation of ROS after the overexposure of UV light. These botanical supplements or dietary antioxidants hold promise for use as a complementary and alternative medicine. This interest has received attention particularly from researchers, pharmaceutical industries, and consumers. In this regard, the botanicals possessing antioxidant properties along with the anti-inflammatory and immunomodulatory effects are the most studied group of compounds. Extensive laboratory studies have been demonstrated the efficacy of naturally occurring botanicals in animal models related with protection against inflammation, oxidative stress and cancer. These botanicals or antioxidants are vitamin E,[87] GTP,[5,6] garlic,[88] ginger,[89] silymarin,[90,91] vitamin C,[87] all-*trans* retinoic acid,[92] and GSP,[93] etc.

Since oxidants play an important role in many skin disorders including the initiation, promotion, and progression stages of multistage skin carcinogenesis, the antioxidants can be targeted for intervention at these stages of multistage skin carcinogenesis or other skin disorders which are developed through the oxidative stress like aging of the skin.[5,10,94] Studies have shown that dietary and/or environmental mutagens and carcinogens, including solar UV light to which humans are constantly exposed, exert their adverse biological effects, at least in part, via the generation of ROS. The generation of ROS plays a major role in the induction of cancer, specifically, at the promotion stage of carcinogenesis.[94–98] Dietary intake of naturally occurring antioxidants, therefore, has been suggested as an important strategy against the toxic effects of mutagenic and carcinogenic agents.[95–98] We and others have demonstrated the chemoprotective effects of GTP and GSP against chemical tumor promotion as well as UV light-induced skin tumor promotion in animal models.[5,94,98–102] Therefore, we will specifically highlight the chemopreventive strategies by using dietary antioxidants, such as GTP and GSP.

8.1. *Green tea and its polyphenolic constituents*

Because of its characteristic aroma, flavor, and health benefits, tea, next to water, is the most popular beverage consumed worldwide. Tea is manufactured from the leaf and bud of the plant *Camellia sinensis* and is commercially available mainly in three forms: green tea, black tea, and oolong tea.[5,98–100,103] Of the total tea production, about 78% is consumed as black tea mainly in the Western countries and some Asian countries, while about 20% is consumed as green tea mainly in Asian countries, including Japan, China, Korea, and some parts of India. Approximately 2% is manufactured in the form of oolong tea, which is particularly produced and consumed in southeastern China.[5,99,103] The term "green tea" refers to the product manufactured from the fresh tea leaves by steaming and drying at elevated temperatures with care to avoid oxidation and polymerization of the epicatechin components present in green tea leaves.[103] Since most of the skin cancer chemopreventive studies on *in vivo* and *in vitro* models have been carried out with green tea, this chapter will highlight the investigations and beneficial effects of green tea against UV-induced oxidative stress, and oxidative stress-mediated skin cancer as a novel chemopreventive strategy.

The active constituents responsible for photoprotective efficacy in green tea are called epicatechins or epicatechin derivatives. These epicatechins are also commonly called as "polyphenols" and are easily soluble in water and organic solvents like acetone, ethanol, etc. The major epicatechins found in green tea are, (−)-epicatechin, (−)-epicatechin-3-gallate, (−)-epigallocatechin, and (−)-epigallocatechin-3-gallate (EGCG). There chemical structures are shown in Fig. 4. During processing of tea, these epicatechins get polymerized and form more complex polymerized molecules called theaflavins and thearubigins. This commercial production of tea is called as black tea, which is mainly used in Western countries

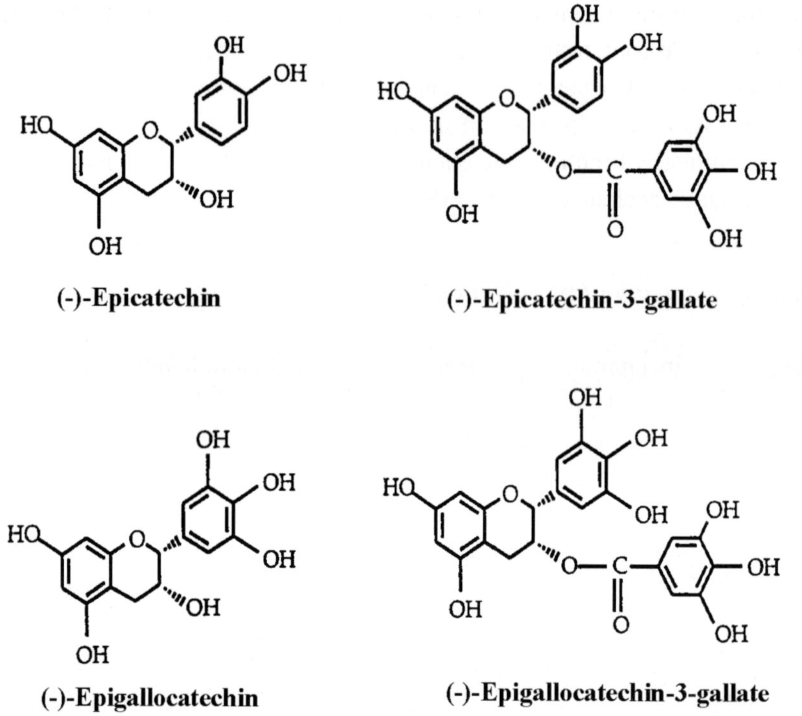

(-)-Epicatechin

(-)-Epicatechin-3-gallate

(-)-Epigallocatechin

(-)-Epigallocatechin-3-gallate

Fig. 4. Chemical structures of major epicatechin derivatives or polyphenolic constituents present in green tea. These epicatechins are also found in grape seeds as monomeric flavanols. When these monomers polymerize, they form dimers, trimers, tetramers, and oligomers, and are known as proanthocyanidins.

including United States. Experimental studies indicate that polyphenolic constituents or epicatechin derivatives from green tea are antioxidative and anti-inflammatory in nature, and have been shown to possess anti-carcinogenic effects in various *in vitro* and *in vivo* model systems.[98–103] These photoprotective effects are summarized below.

8.2. *Prevention of photocarcinogenesis or NMSC by green tea*

NMSC, including BCC and SCC, represent the most common malignant neoplasms in humans.[40–42] Various animal models have been employed to examine the anti-carcinogenic effects of green tea. It has been found that oral feeding of GTP in drinking water to laboratory animals resulted in significant protection against skin tumorigenesis when determined in terms of tumor incidence, tumor multiplicity, and tumor size per treatment group compared to that of non-GTP treated animals.[5,98–102] The water extract of green tea as a sole source of drinking water to mice afforded protection against UVB radiation-induced tumor initiation and tumor promotion stages,[104,105] and also induced partial regression of already established skin papillomas in female CD-1 mice.[106] Topical application of EGCG, a major constituent of GTP, inhibited photocarcinogenesis in BALB/cAnNHsd mice with no visible toxicity.[107] Mittal *et al.*[108] developed a cream-based formulation in hydrophilic ointment for the topical application of GTP. Topical application of GTP or EGCG in the term of hydrophilic cream or ointment to SKH-1 hairless mouse skin significantly inhibited UVB-induced tumorigenesis. The chemopreventive effect of this ointment-based treatment was found to be much superior than that of other vehicles used for GTP or EGCG application.[108] These results indicated that the use of EGCG or GTP with hydrophilic ointment might increase the concentration inside the cellular layers of the skin and/or absorption capacity of tea constituents. In addition to increased chemopreventive effect against photocarcinogenesis in these experiments, the treatment of EGCG also increased the latency period of tumor appearance by 8 weeks during the whole photocarcinogenesis protocol. The mechanism of photoprotective effects related with the antioxidant effect of GTP are summarized below.

8.3. *Prevention of UV-induced oxidative stress*

As we have discussed in this chapter, wavelengths in the UVB region of the solar spectrum (290–320 nm) are absorbed by the skin, producing erythema, burns, oxidative stress, and eventually may lead to skin cancer development.[109,110] UVA can penetrate much deeper in the dermis. Though, the skin possesses an elaborate antioxidant defense system to deal with UV-induced oxidative stress, excessive and chronic exposure to UV can overwhelm the cutaneous antioxidant capacity, leading to oxidative damage which may result in skin cancer induction. Reflecting the antioxidant potential of green tea, the addition of epicatechin derivatives (polyphenols from green tea) to mouse epidermal microsomes resulted in decreased photo-enhanced lipid peroxidation.[111] We showed that topical application of

EGCG or GTP before UV exposure to mouse and human skin significantly reduces UVB-induced nitric oxide and hydrogen peroxide production, and also leukocyte infiltration.[6,112,113] The infiltrating leukocytes are the major source of nitric oxide and hydrogen peroxide production which contribute to oxidative stress. EGCG has been shown to block UVB-induced leukocyte infiltration in mouse as well as in human skin, and thus may able to inhibit UVB-induced production of ROS.[6,113–115] Although ROS help the host to destroy invading microorganisms,[116] excessive and uncontrolled production can also damage host tissues and predispose it to various disease states.[116,117] Thus, the topical application of EGCG may prove an alternate strategy to ameliorate the harmful effects caused by UV exposure through decreased ROS production. EGCG application to mouse skin before UV exposure resulted in a decrease in the number of hydrogen peroxide producing and inducible nitric oxide synthase expressing cells, and reduction in the production of hydrogen peroxide and nitric oxide both in the epidermis and the dermis of UV-irradiated sites.[6] Similar observations were also found in Caucasian skin where EGCG was topically applied before UVB ($4 \times$ minimal erythema dose) exposure.[115] Additionally, treatment with EGCG was also found to inhibit UV-induced epidermal lipid peroxidation, and protect antioxidant enzymes in human skin.[115] Inhibition of UV-induced lipid peroxidation in human skin by EGCG is a characteristic feature that may prevent human skin from solar UV light-induced basal cell and squamous cell carcinogenesis. Based on the evidences of photoprotective effects of GTP/EGCG in animal and human systems, it appears that GTP or EGCG induces protective effects by acting at different active sites of ROS generating cascade, as shown in Fig. 3. Kim *et al.*[118] observed that EGCG application on guinea pigs skin inhibits UVB-induced lipid peroxidation and erythema response. These experimental observations suggest that green tea may have the potential to reduce the risk of UV-induced oxidative stress-mediated skin diseases in humans.

In continuation of our studies to determine the antioxidant potential of EGCG, we conducted *in vitro* experiments using normal human epidermal keratinocytes to determine the effects of EGCG against UVB-induced oxidative stress-mediated cell signaling events, which play a critical role in tumor promotion stage of carcinogenesis. In this study, application of

EGCG to normal human epidermal keratinocytes was found to inhibit UVB-induced intracellular production of hydrogen peroxide concomitant with the inhibition of UVB-induced oxidative stress-mediated phosphorylation of epidermal growth factor receptor and mitogen-activated protein kinase signaling pathways.[119] These observations indicate that EGCG could play an important role in the attenuation of oxidative stress-mediated cellular signaling responses, which are essentially involved in various skin disorders in humans. Very recently, we developed a cream-based formulation of EGCG and GTP for human use.[108] Topical application of EGCG and GTP in this formulation resulted in significantly high protection against UVB-induced depletion of glutathione peroxidase, catalase, and the level of endogenous glutathione content. Photoprotective effect on these antioxidant defense enzymes was also found when GTP was given in drinking water (0.2%, w/v) to mice.[27] These photoprotective effects were observed when mice were exposed to multiple exposures of UVB for 2 months.

Oxidation of some amino acids residues of proteins such as lysine, arginine, and proline leads to the formation of carbonyl derivatives that affects the nature and function of proteins.[120] Presence of carbonyl groups in proteins has become a widely accepted measure of oxidative damage of proteins under conditions of oxidative stress. Multiple exposure of UVB to the skin resulted in several fold increase in the level of protein carbonyls in comparison to non-UV exposed skin.[27] Topical application of EGCG and GTP significantly inhibited single or multiple UVB irradiation-induced protein oxidation in mice.[27] Vayalil *et al.*[121] observed that administration of GTP in drinking water resulted in reduction of protein oxidation at the UV-irradiated skin site. Treatment of HS68 human fibroblasts in culture system with GTP also prevented UV-induced oxidation of proteins, and thus supported the *in vivo* animal observations. The inhibition of UVB-induced protein oxidation by GTP would result in reduction of the photooxidative damage to the skin, and therefore would help to reduce the risk of skin cancer.

8.4. *Prevention of DNA photodamage*

Several studies have documented that UV irradiation to skin results in instantaneous cyclobutane pyrimidine dimers (CPDs) formation in DNA of target cells.[11] Most of the UV-induced CPD were found in the epidermis but a significant number of CPD were also observed in the dermis.[11] The presence of CPD in the dermis indicates the penetrating depth of UV light inside the skin. It has been found that UV exposure at less than one minimal erythema dose is sufficient to damage DNA in the human skin.[11] The topical application of GTP before UV exposure to human skin resulted in a dose-dependent inhibition of CPD formation.[122] Interestingly, treatment with GTP also resulted in the inhibition of UV-induced erythema. Observations also indicated that with the increase in exposure of UV dose, both erythema and CPD formation in the skin were increased. These observations reveal a direct relationship between CPD formation and erythema development. Because CPDs are instantaneously formed when DNA molecules absorb photons, and erythema develops in later stages, it seems that UV-induced CPDs mediate erythema development. Pharmacokinetic studies reveal that UV-induced DNA damage in human skin declines after 3–4 days of UV exposure. This may occur because cells with damaged DNA undergo apoptosis or the damaged DNA has been repaired. Histological observations of CPD staining indicate that topical treatment of GTP to human skin resulted in reduction of DNA damage following UV exposure in comparison to non-GTP treated skin sites.[122] Wei *et al.*[123] has shown that an aqueous extract of green tea scavenges H_2O_2 and inhibits UV-induced oxidative DNA damage in *in vitro* system. Zhao *et al.*[124] demonstrated that application of green tea extract to Epiderm, a reconstituted human skin equivalent, also inhibited psoralen-UVA- 8-methoxypsoralen–DNA adducts formation.[124] Treatment of skin with 5% green tea extract significantly inhibited DNA damage induced by a solar simulator when assessed by a ^{32}P-postlabeling technique.[125] These observations demonstrated the potential of green tea in the prevention of DNA damage.

9. Grape Seed Proanthocyanidins

Grape seeds are by-products of grapes (*Vitis vinifera*) formed during the industrial production of grape juice and wine. They are a potent source of proanthocyanidins which are mainly composed of dimers, trimers and oligomers of monomeric catechins,[126,127] as described below.

9.1. *Active constituents of GSP*

GSP is a complex mixture of monomers of epicatechins and the polymeric forms of epicatechins. Chemical composition of GSP constitutes approximately 89% proanthocyanidins and 6.6% monomeric flavanols. These monomeric flavanols are epicatechins, similar to those found in green tea, as shown in Fig. 4. Proanthocyanidins are formed when epicatechins are polymerized. Chemical analysis of GSP indicated that it contains dimers (6.6%), trimers (5.0%), tetramers (2.9%), and oligomers (74.8%). Monomeric flavanols are: (+)-catechin (2.5%), (−)-epicatechin (2.2%), (−)-epigallocatechin (1.4%), and (−)-epigallocatechin-3-gallate (0.5%).[93] GSP is stable at room temperature, and can be stored for more than a year at 4°C.

9.2. *Prevention of photocarcinogenesis by GSP*

The chemopreventive effect of dietary feeding of GSP has been evaluated by using photocarcinogenesis protocol in SKH-1 hairless mice.[97] Dietary feeding of GSP (0.2 and 0.5%, w/w) with control diet during photocarcinogenesis protocol resulted in a dose-dependent reduction in photocarcinogenesis when expressed in terms of percent of mice with tumors and tumor multiplicity compared with that of non-GSP-fed control animals. Feeding of GSP at the dose of 0.2 and 0.5% resulted in 20 and 35% inhibition of tumor incidence (% of mice with tumors), respectively, at the termination of the experiment at 24 weeks as compared to non-GSP fed animals. Non-GSP fed animals achieved 100% tumor incidence at 16th week of tumor promotion while GSP fed animals could not achieve 100% tumor incidence up to the end of 24th week. Further, feeding of GSP increased the latency period of tumors appearance.[97] Dietary feeding of 0.2 and 0.5% GSP in control diet to mice significantly inhibited tumor multiplicity by 46 and 65%, respectively, as compared to non-GSP fed animals, and also inhibited tumor size when expressed in terms of total tumor volume per group (66–78%) or tumor volume per tumor bearing mouse by 57–66%.

9.3. *Prevention of malignant conversion by GSP*

The photoprotective efficacy of GSP was also tested to determine whether dietary feeding of GSP prevents spontaneous malignant conversion of papillomas into carcinomas. Histological examinations indicated that 70% mice developed carcinoma in non-GSP-fed control mice compared to only 25% in GSP-fed group of mice. Thus, 45% prevention in terms of carcinoma incidence was observed by dietary feeding of GSP. When data were analyzed in terms of carcinoma multiplicity, it was found that GSP treatment resulted in prevention of UVB-induced transformation of benign papillomas to carcinomas by 61%. Further, GSP inhibited the growing size of carcinoma and also inhibited total carcinoma volume/group and average carcinoma volume/carcinoma by 75 and 36%, respectively, compared to non-GSP-fed group of mice.[93] These experimental observations support the efficacy of GSP as a chemopreventive agent, and a safe strategy to prevent oxidative stress-mediated skin cancer among high-risk human population.

9.4. *Prevention of UV-induced oxidative damage by GSP*

Since UV-induced oxidative stress is involved in the induction of melanoma and NMSC, it was determined whether dietary feeding of GSP prevents UV-induced oxidative damage in the skin. Lipid peroxidation plays an important role in oxidative stress-mediated diseases. It was observed that feeding of GSP to animals resulted in 66 and 57% reduction in UVB-induced epidermal lipid peroxidation when measured, respectively, at 24 and 48 h after UVB irradiation. Since lipid peroxidation is one of the hallmarks of oxidative damage, the antioxidant potential of GSP was further determined. Treatment with GSP (5–80 μg/ml) *in vitro* to epidermal microsomes resulted in inhibition (41–77%) of Fe^{3+}-induced lipid peroxidation in a dose-dependent manner. Further, antioxidant potential of GSP was compared with other known antioxidants, and it was found that treatment with equal doses (10 μg/ml) of EGCG, ascorbic acid (vitamin C), silymarin, BHT, vitamin E, and GSP to epidermal microsomes *in vitro* resulted in inhibition of Fe^{3+}-induced lipid peroxidation by 44, 58, 44, 67, 44, and 59%, respectively.[97] The data obtained from these experiments suggested that prevention of photocarcinogenesis in mice by GSP treatment could be associated with the prevention of UV-induced oxidative damage to lipids.

Acknowledgments

I thank my former and current colleagues and postdoctoral fellows for their outstanding contributions. The work in the author's laboratory was supported by funds from the National Institutes of Health (CA94593, CA89738, CA105368, ES11421), Cancer Research and Prevention Foundation, and funds from the Veterans Administration.

References

1. Pryor WA. The involvement of free radicals in chemical carcinogenesis. In: Cerutti PA, Nygaard OF, Simic MG (eds.) *Anticarcinogenesis and Radiation Protection.* Plenum Press, New York, 1987, p. 1.
2. Perchellet JP, Perchellet EM. Phorbol ester tumor promoters and multistage skin carcinogenesis. *ISI Atlas Sci. Pharmacol.* 2: 325 (1988).
3. Sun Y. Free radicals, antioxidant enzymes, and carcinogenesis. *Free Radic. Biol. Med.* 8: 583 (1990).
4. Tyrell RM. Ultraviolet radiation and free radical damage to skin. *Biochem. Soc. Symp.* 61: 47–53 (1995).
5. Katiyar SK, Elmets CA. Green tea polyphenolic antioxidants and skin photoprotection. *Int. J. Oncol.* 18: 1307–1313 (2001).
6. Katiyar SK, Mukhtar H. Green tea polyphenol (−)-epigallocatechin-3-gallate treatment to mouse skin prevents UVB-induced infiltration of leukocytes, depletion of antigen presenting cells and oxidative stress. *J. Leukoc. Biol.* 69: 719–726 (2001).
7. Van der Leun JC. Human health. In: Van der Leun JC, Tevini M (eds.) *United Nations Environmental Program Report on the Environmental Effects of Ozone Depletion.* EPA, Washington, DC, 1989.
8. Urbach F. Evidence of epidemiology of UV-induced carcinogenesis in man. *Natl. Cancer Inst. Monogr.* 50: 5–10 (1978).
9. Ullrich SE. Potential for immunotoxicity due to environmental exposure to ultraviolet radiation. *Hum. Exp. Toxicol.* 14: 89–91 (1995).
10. Mukhtar H, Elmets CA. Photocarcinogenesis: mechanisms, models and human health implications. *Photochem. Photobiol.* 63: 355–447 (1996).

11. Katiyar SK, Matsui MS, Mukhtar H. Kinetics of UV light-induced cyclobutane pyrimidine dimers in human skin *in vivo*: an immunohistochemical analysis of both epidermis and dermis. *Photochem. Photobiol.* 72: 788–793 (2000).
12. Moslen MT, Smith CV. *Free Radical Mechanisms of Tissue Injury*. CRC Press, Boca Raton, FL, 1992.
13. Cadet J, Berger M, Decarroz C, Wagner JR, Van Liet JE, Ginot YM, Vigny P. Photosensitized reactions of nucleic acids. *Biochimie* 68: 813–834 (1986).
14. Peak MJ, Ito A, Foote CS, Peak JG. Photosensitized inactivation of DNA by monochromatic 334-nm radiation in the presence of 2-thiouracil: genetic activity and backbone breaks. *Photochem. Photobiol.* 47: 809–813 (1988).
15. Beehler BC, Przybyszewski J, Box HB, Kulesz-Martin MF. Formation of 8-hydroxydeoxyguanosine within DNA of mouse keratinocytes exposed in culture to UVB and H_2O_2. *Carcinogenesis* 13: 2003–2007 (1992).
16. Berton TR, Mitchell DL, Fischer SM, Locniskar MF. Epidermal proliferation but not the quantity of DNA photodamage is corrected with UV-induced mouse skin carcinogenesis. *J. Invest. Dermatol.* 109: 340–347 (1997).
17. Kligman LH, Akin FJ, Kligman AM. Sunscreens prevent ultraviolet photocarcinogenesis. *J. Am. Acad. Dermatol.* 3: 30–35 (1980).
18. Katiyar SK, Korman NJ, Mukhtar H, Agarwal R. Protective effects of silymarin against photocarcinogenesis in a mouse skin model. *J. Natl. Cancer Inst.* 89: 556–566 (1997).
19. Iwai I, Hatao M, Naganuma M, Kumano Y, Ichihashi M. UVA-induced immune suppression through an oxidative pathway. *J. Invest. Dermatol.* 112: 19–24 (1999).
20. Yoshikawa T, Rae V, Bruins-Slot W, vand-den-Berg JW, Taylor JR, Streilein JW. Susceptibility to effects of UVB radiation on induction of contact hypersensitivity as a risk factor for skin cancer in humans. *J. Invest. Dermatol.* 95: 530–536 (1990).
21. Donawho CK, Muller HK, Bucana CD, Kripke ML. Enhanced growth of murine melanoma in ultraviolet-irradiated skin is associated with local inhibition of immune effector mechanisms. *J. Immunol.* 157: 781–786 (1996).
22. Katiyar SK, Afaq F, Perez A, Mukhtar H. Green tea polyphenol (−)-epigallocatechin-3-gallate treatment of human skin inhibits ultraviolet radiation-induced oxidative stress. *Carcinogenesis* 22: 287–294 (2001).
23. Mittal A, Elmets CA, Katiyar SK. CD11b+ cells are the major source of oxidative stress in UV radiation-irradiated skin: Possible role in photoaging and photocarcinogenesis. *Photochem. Photobiol.* 77: 259–264 (2003).

24. Berg RJW, de Gruijl FR, van der Leun JC. Interaction between ultraviolet A and ultraviolet B radiations in skin cancer induction in hairless mice. *Cancer Res.* 53: 4212–4217 (1993).
25. Fuchs J, Huflejt ME, Rothfuss LM, Wilson DS, Carcamo G, Packer L. Impairment of enzymic and non-enzymic antioxidants in skin by UVB radiation. *J. Invest. Dermatol.* 93: 769–773 (1989).
26. Shindo Y, Witt E, Han D, Packer L. Dose–response effects of acute ultraviolet irradiation on antioxidants and molecular markers of oxidation in murine epidermis. *J. Invest. Dermatol.* 104: 470–475 (1994).
27. Vayalil PK, Elmets CA, Katiyar SK. Treatment of green tea polyphenols in hydrophilic cream prevents UVB-induced oxidation of lipids and proteins, depletion of antioxidant enzymes and phosphorylation of MAPK proteins in SKH-1 hairless mouse skin. *Carcinogenesis* 24: 927–936 (2003).
28. Fuchs J, Huflejt ME, Rothfuss LM, Wilson DS, Carcamo G. Acute effects of near ultraviolet and visible light on the cutaneous antioxidant defense system. *Photochem. Photobiol.* 50: 739–744 (1989).
29. Steenvoorden DP, van Henegouwen GM. The use of endogenous antioxidants to improve photoprotection. *J. Photochem. Photobiol. B* 41: 1–10 (1997).
30. Meister A, Andersen ME. Glutathione. *Annu. Rev. Biochem.* 52: 711–760 (1983).
31. Tyrrell RM, Pidoux M. Endogenous glutathione protects human skin fibroblasts against the cytotoxic action of UVB, UVA and near-visible radiations. *Photochem. Photobiol.* 44: 561–564 (1986).
32. Tyrrell RM, Pidoux M. Correlation between endogenous glutathione content and sensitivity of cultured human skin cells to radiation at defined wavelengths in the solar UV range. *Photochem. Photobiol.* 47: 405–412 (1988).
33. Tyrrell RM. Damage and repair from non-ionizing radiations. In: Hurst A, Nasim A (eds.) *Repairable Lesions in Microorganisms*. Academic Press, London, 1984, pp. 85–124.
34. Maccubbin AE, Przybysweski J, Evans MS, Budzinski EE, Patrzyc HB, Kulesz-Martin M, Box HC. DNA damage in UVB-irradiated keratinocytes. *Carcinogenesis* 16: 1659–1660 (1995).
35. Floyd RA. The role of 8-hydroxyguanine in carcinogenesis. *Carcinogenesis* 11: 1447–1450 (1990).
36. Ananthaswamy HN, Pierceall WE. Molecular mechanism of ultraviolet radiation carcinogenesis. *Photochem. Photobiol.* 52: 1119–1136 (1990).
37. Elmets CA. Cutaneous photocarcinogenesis. In: Mukhtar H (ed.) *Pharmacology of the Skin*. CRC Press, Boca Raton, FL, 1992, p. 389.

38. Miller DL, Weinstock MA. Nonmelanoma skin cancer in the United States: incidence. *J. Am. Acad. Dermatol.* 30: 774–778 (1994).
39. Urbach F. Incidences of nonmelanoma skin cancer. *Dermatol. Clin.* 9: 751–755 (1991).
40. Johnson TM, Dolan OM, Hamilton TA, Lu MC, Swanson NA, Lowe L. Clinical and histologic trends of melanoma. *J. Am. Acad. Dermatol.* 38: 681–686 (1998).
41. *Cancer Facts and Figures 2001*. Publication No. 5008.01. American Cancer Society, Atlanta, GA, 2001.
42. O'Shaughnessy JA, Kelloff GJ, Gordon GB, Dannenberg AJ, Hong WK, Fabian CJ, Sigman CC, Bertagnolli MM, Stratton SP, Lam S, Nelson WG, Meyskens FL, Alberts DS, Follen M, Rustgi AK, Papadimitrakopoulou V, Scardino PT, Gazdar AF, Wattenberg LW, Sporn MB, Sakr WA, Lippman SM, Von Hoff DD. Treatment and prevention of intraepithelial neoplasia: an important target for accelerated new agent development. Recommendations of the American Association for Cancer Research task force on the treatment and prevention of intraepithelial neoplasia. *Clin. Cancer Res.* 8: 314–346 (2002).
43. Moan J, Dahlback A, Setlow RB. Epidemiologic support for an hypothesis for melanoma induction indicating a role for UVA radiation. *Photochem. Photobiol.* 70: 243–247 (1999).
44. Packer L. *Ultraviolet radiation (UVA, UVB) and skin antioxidants*. In: Rice-Evans CA, Burdon RH (eds.) *Free Radical Damage and Its Control*. Elsevier Science, Amsterdam, 1994.
45. Scharfettfer-Kochanek K, Wlaschek M, Brenneisen P, Schauen M, Blaudschun R, Wenk J. UV-induced reactive oxygen species in photocarcinogenesis and photoaging. *Biol. Chem.* 378: 1247–1257 (1997).
46. de Gruijl FR. Photocarcinogenesis: UVA versus UVB. *Methods Enzymol.* 319: 359–366 (2000).
47. Danpure HJ, Tyrrell RM. Oxygen-dependence of near UV (365 nm) lethality and the interaction of near UV and X-rays in two mammalian cell lines. *Photochem. Photobiol.* 23: 171–177 (1976).
48. Tyrrell RM. UVA (320–380 nm) radiation as an oxidative stress. In: Sies H (ed.) *Oxidative Stress, Oxidants and Antioxidants*. Academic Press, London, 1991, pp. 57–83.
49. Tyrell RM. Oxidant, antioxidant status and photocarcinogenesis: the role of gene activation. *Photochem. Photobiol.* 63: 380–386 (1996).

50. Gaboriau F, Demoulins-Giacco N, Tirache I, Morliere P. Involvement of singlet oxygen in ultraviolet A-induced lipid peroxidation in cultured human skin fibroblasts. *Arch. Dermatol. Res.* 287: 338–340 (1995).
51. Morliere P, Moysan A, Tirache I. Action spectrum for UV-induced lipid peroxidation in cultured human skin fibroblasts. *Free Radic. Biol. Med.* 19: 365–371 (1995).
52. Parsons PG, Hayward IP. Inhibition of DNA repair synthesis by sunlight. *Photochem. Photobiol.* 42: 287–293 (1985).
53. Scharffetter-Kochanek K, Wlaschek M, Briviba K, Sies H. Singlet oxygen induces collagenase expression in human skin fibroblasts. *FEBS Lett.* 331: 304–306 (1993).
54. Fisher GJ, Choi HC, Bata-Csorgo Z, Shao Y, Datta S, Wang ZQ, Kang S, Voorhees JJ. Ultraviolet irradiation increases matrix metalloproteinase-8 protein in human skin *in vivo*. *J. Invest. Dermatol.* 117: 219–226 (2001).
55. Gilchrest BA, Soter NA, Hawk JL, Barr RM, Black AK, Hensby CN, Mallet AL, Greaves MW, Parrish JA. Histologic changes associated with ultraviolet A-induced erythema in normal human skin. *J. Am. Acad. Dermatol.* 9: 213–219 (1983).
56. Parrish JA. Responses of skin to visible and ultraviolet radiation. In: Goldsmith LA (ed.) *Biochemistry and Physiology of the Skin*. Oxford University Press, New York, 1983, pp. 713–733.
57. Moller P, Wallin H, Holst E, Knudsen LE. Sunlight-induced DNA damage in human mononuclear cells. *FASEB J.* 16: 45–53 (2002).
58. Singer RS, Hamilton TA, Voorhees JJ. Griffiths CEM. Association of asymmetrical facial photodamage with automobile driving. *Arch. Dermatol.* 130: 121–123 (1994).
59. Rafnsson V, Hrafnkelsson J, Tulinius H. Incidence of cancer among commercial airline pilots. *Occup. Environ. Med.* 57: 175–179 (2000).
60. Hammar NL. Cancer incidence in airline and military pilots in Sweden 1961–1996. *Aviat. Space Environ. Med.* 73: 2–7 (2002).
61. Ullrich SE, Kim TH, Ananthaswamy HN, Kripke ML. Sunscreen effects on UV-induced immune suppression. *J. Invest. Dermatol. Symp. Proc.* 4: 65–69 (1999).
62. Meyers DP, Scott IR, Lowe NJ. Exposure to low levels of ultraviolet light B or ultraviolet light A induces cutaneous photodamage in human skin. In: Lowe NJ, Shaath NA, Pathak MA (eds.) *Sunscreens: Development, Evaluation, and Regulatory Aspects*. Marcel-Dekker, New York, 1997, pp. 101–115.

63. Kaidbey K, Gange RW. Comparison of methods for assessing photoprotection against ultraviolet A *in vivo*. *J. Am. Acad. Dermatol.* 16: 346–353 (1987).
64. Bestak R, Barnetson RS, Nearn MR, Halliday GM. Sunscreen protection of contact hypersensitivity responses from chronic solar-simulated ultraviolet irradiation correlates with the absorption spectrum of the sunscreen. *J. Invest. Dermatol.* 105: 345–351 (1995).
65. Damian DL, Halliday GM, Barnetson RS. Broad-spectrum sunscreens provide greater protection against ultraviolet radiation-induced suppression of contact hypersensitivity to a recall antigen in humans. *J. Invest. Dermatol.* 109: 146–151 (1997).
66. Roberts LK, Beasley DG. Commercial sunscreen lotions prevent ultraviolet-radiation-induced immune suppression of contact hypersensitivity. *J. Invest. Dermatol.* 105: 339–344 (1995).
67. Naylor MF, Boyd A, Smith DW, Cameron GS, Hubbard D, Neldner KH. High sun protection factor sunscreens in the suppression of actinic neoplasia. *Arch. Dermatol.* 131: 170–175 (1995).
68. Thompson SC, Jolley D, Marks R. Reduction of solar keratoses by regular sunscreen use. *N. Engl. J. Med.* 329: 1147–1151 (1993).
69. Freeman SE, Ley RD, Ley KD. Sunscreen protection against UV-induced pyrimidine dimers in DNA of human skin *in situ*. *Photodermatology* 5: 243–247 (1988).
70. van Praag MC, Roza L, Boom BW, Out-Luijting C, Henegouwen JB, Vermeer BJ, Mommaas AM. Determination of the photoprotective efficacy of a topical sunscreen against UVB-induced DNA damage in human epidermis. *J. Photochem. Photobiol. B.* 19: 129–134 (1993).
71. Thompson SC, Jolley D, Marks R. Reduction of solar keratoses by regular sunscreen use. *N. Engl. J. Med.* 329: 1147–1151 (1993).
72. Green A *et al.* Daily sunscreen application and betacarotene supplementation in prevention of basal cell and squamous cell carcinomas of the skin: a randomized controlled trial. *Lancet* 354: 723–729 (1999).
73. Weinstock MA. Do sunscreens increase or decrease melanoma risk: an epidemiologic evaluation? *J. Invest. Dermatol. Symp. Proc.* 4: 97–100 (1999).
74. Haywood R, Wardman P, Sanders R, Linge C. Sunscreens inadequately protect against ultraviolet A-induced free radicals in skin: implications for skin aging and melanoma? *J. Invest. Dermatol.* 121: 862–868 (2003).
75. Xu CX, Green A, Parisi A, Parsons PG. Photosensitization of the sunscreen octyl p-dimethylaminobenzoate by UVA in human melanocytes but not in keratinocytes. *Photochem. Photobiol.* 73: 600–604 (2001).

76. Cross SE, Jiang RY, Benson HAE, Roberts MS. Can increasing the viscosity of formulations be used to reduce the human skin penetration of the sunscreen oxybenzone? *J. Invest. Dermatol.* 117: 147–150 (2001).
77. Forbes PD, Davies RE, Sambuco CP, Urbach F. Inhibition of ultraviolet radiation-induced skin tumors in hairless mice by topical application of the sunscreen 2-ethyl hexyl-p-methoxycinnamate. *J. Toxicol. Cutaneous Ocul. Toxicol.* 8: 209–226 (1989).
78. Autier P *et al.* Melanoma and the use of sunscreens: an EORTC case–control study in Germany, Belgium and France. *Int. J. Cancer* 61: 749–755 (1995).
79. Azizi E, Iscovich J, Pavlotsky F, Shafir R, Luria I, Federenko L, Fuchs Z, Milman V, Gur E, Farbstein H, Tal O. Use of sunscreen is linked with elevated naevi counts in Israeli school children and adolescents. *Melanoma Res.* 10: 491–498 (2000).
80. Stokes R, Diffey B. How well are sunscreen users protected? *Photodermatol. Photoimmunol. Photomed.* 13: 186–188 (1997).
81. Wulf HC, Stender IM, Lock-Anderson J. Sunscreens used at the beach do not protect against erythema: a new definition of SPF is proposed. *Photodermatol. Photoimmunol. Photomed.* 13: 129–132 (1997).
82. Flindt-Hansen H, Nielsen CJ, Thune P. Measurements of the photodegradation of PABA and some PABA derivatives. *Photodermatol.* 5: 257–261 (1988).
83. Gasparro FP. The molecular basis of UV-induced mutagenicity of sunscreens. *FEBS Lett.* 336: 184–185 (1993).
84. Dunford R, Salinaro A, Cai L, Serpone N, Horikoshi S, Hidaka H, Knowland J. Chemical oxidation and DNA damage catalysed by inorganic sunscreen ingredients. *FEBS Lett.* 418: 87–90 (1997).
85. Rigel DS. The effect of sunscreen on melanoma risk. *Dermatol. Clin.* 20: 601–606 (2002).
86. Bigby M. The sunscreen and melanoma controversy. *Arch. Dermatol.* 135: 1526–1527 (1999).
87. Keller KL, Fenske NA. Uses of vitamins A, C, and E and related compounds in dermatology: a review. *J. Am. Acad. Dermatol.* 39: 611–625 (1998).
88. Reeve VE, Bosnic M, Rozinova E, Boehm-Wilcox C. A garlic extract protects from ultraviolet B (280–320 nm) radiation-induced suppression of contact hypersensitivity. *Photochem. Photobiol.* 58: 813–817 (1993).
89. Katiyar SK, Agarwal R, Mukhtar H. Inhibition of tumor promotion in SENCAR mouse skin by ethanol extract of *Zingiber officinale* rhizome. *Cancer Res.* 56: 1023–1030 (1996).

90. Katiyar SK, Korman NJ, Mukhtar H, Agarwal R. Protective effects of Silymarin against photocarcinogenesis in a mouse skin model. *J. Natl. Cancer Inst.* 89: 556–566 (1997).
91. Katiyar SK. Treatment of silymarin, a plant flavonoid, prevents ultraviolet light-induced immune suppression and oxidative stress in mouse skin. *Int. J. Oncol.* 21: 1213–1222 (2002).
92. Wang Z, Boudjelal M, Kang S, Voorhees JJ, Fisher GJ. Ultraviolet irradiation of human skin causes functional vitamin A deficiency, preventable by all-*trans* retinoic acid pre-treatment. *Nat. Med.* 5: 418–422 (1999).
93. Mittal A, Elmets CA, Katiyar SK. Dietary feeding of proanthocyanidins from grape seeds prevents photocarcinogenesis in SKH-1 hairless mice: relationship to decreased fat and lipid peroxidation. *Carcinogenesis* 24: 1379–1388 (2003).
94. Hursting SD, Slaga TJ, Fischer SM, DiGiovanni J, Phang JM. Mechanism-based cancer prevention approaches: targets, examples, and the use of transgenic mice. *J. Natl. Cancer Inst.* 91: 215–225 (1999).
95. Wattenberg LW. Inhibition of carcinogenesis by naturally occurring and synthetic compounds. In: Uroda Y, Shankel DM, Waters MD (eds.) *Antimutagenesis and Anticarcinogenesis, Mechanisms II*. Plenum, New York, 1990, pp. 155–166.
96. Ames BN. Dietary carcinogens and anticarcinogens. *Science* 221: 1256–1264 (1983).
97. Block G. Micronutrients and cancer: time for action? *J. Natl. Cancer Inst.* 85: 846–848 (1993).
98. Katiyar SK, Mukhtar H. Tea antioxidants in cancer chemoprevention. *J. Cell. Biochem. Suppl.* 27: 59–67 (1997).
99. Katiyar SK, Mukhtar H. Tea consumption and cancer. *World Rev. Nutr. Diet.* 79: 154–184 (1996).
100. Katiyar SK, Ahmad N, Mukhtar H. Green tea and skin. *Arch. Dermatol.* 136: 989–994 (2000).
101. Yang CS, Landau JM, Huang MT, Newmark HL. Inhibition of carcinogenesis by dietary polyphenolic compounds. *Annu. Rev. Nutr.* 21: 381–406 (2001).
102. Yang CS, Maliakal P, Meng X. Inhibition of carcinogenesis by tea. *Annu. Rev. Pharmacol. Toxicol.* 42: 25–54 (2002).
103. Hara Y. (ed.) *Green Tea, Health Benefits and Applications*. Marcel Dekker, New York, 2001.
104. Wang ZY, Huang MT, Ferraro T, Wong CQ, Lou YR, Iatropoulos M, Yang CS, Conney AH. Inhibitory effect of green tea in the drinking water on

tumorigenesis by ultraviolet light and 12-O-tetradecanoylphorbol-13-acetate in the skin of SKH-1 mice. *Cancer Res.* 52: 1162–1170 (1992).

105. Wang ZY, Agarwal R, Bickers DR, Mukhtar H. Protection against ultraviolet B radiation-induced photocarcinogenesis in hairless mice by green tea polyphenols. *Carcinogenesis* 12: 1527–1530 (1991).
106. Wang ZY, Huang MT, Ho CT, Chang R, Ma W, Ferraro T, Reuhl KR, Yang CS, Conney AH. Inhibitory effect of green tea on the growth of established skin papillomas in mice. *Cancer Res.* 52: 6657–6665 (1992).
107. Gensler HL, Timmermann BN, Valcic S, Wachter GA, Dorr R, Dvorakova K, Alberts DS. Prevention of photocarcinogenesis by topical administration of pure epigallocatechin gallate isolated from green tea. *Nutr. Cancer* 26: 325–335 (1996).
108. Mittal A, Piyathilake C, Hara Y, Katiyar SK. Exceptionally high protection of photocarcinogenesis by topical application of (−)-epigallocatechin-3-gallate in hydrophilic cream in SKH-1 hairless mouse model: relationship to inhibition of UVB-induced global DNA hypomethylation. *Neoplasia* 5: 555–565 (2003).
109. Kligman LH, Kligman AM. The nature of photoaging: its prevention and repair. *Photodermatology* 3: 215–227 (1986).
110. Parrish JA, Jaenicke KF, Anderson RR. Erythema and melanogenesis action spectra of normal human skin. *Photochem. Photobiol.* 36: 187–191 (1982).
111. Katiyar SK, Agarwal R, Mukhtar H. Inhibition of spontaneous and photo-enhanced lipid peroxidation in mouse epidermal microsomes by epicatechin derivatives from green tea. *Cancer Lett.* 79: 61–66 (1994).
112. Elmets CA, Singh D, Tubesing K, Matsui M, Katiyar SK, Mukhtar H. Cutaneous photoprotection from ultraviolet injury by green tea polyphenols. *J. Am. Acad. Dermatol.* 44: 425–432 (2001).
113. Katiyar SK, Matsui MS, Elmets CA, Mukhtar H. Polyphenolic antioxidant (−)-epigallocatechin-3-gallate from green tea reduces UVB-induced inflammatory responses and infiltration of leukocytes in human skin. *Photochem. Photobiol.* 69: 148–153 (1999).
114. Katiyar SK, Challa A, McCormick TS, Cooper KD, Mukhtar H. Protection of UVB-induced immunosuppression in mice by the green tea polyphenol (−)-epigallocatechin-3-gallate may be associated with alterations in IL-10 and IL-12 production. *Carcinogenesis* 20: 2117–2124 (1999).
115. Katiyar SK, Afaq F, Perez A, Mukhtar H. Green tea polyphenol (−)-epigallocatechin-3-gallate treatment to human skin inhibits ultraviolet radiation-induced oxidative stress. *Carcinogenesis* 22: 287–294 (2001).

116. Klebanoff SJ. Phagocytic cells: products of oxygen metabolism. In: Gallin JI, Goldstein IM, Goldstein S, Snyderman R (eds.) *Inflammation: Basic Principles and Clinical Correlates*. Raven Press, New York, 1988, pp. 391–444.
117. Halliwell B, Gutteridge JMC, Cross CE. Free radicals, antioxidants, and human disease: where are we now? *J. Lab. Clin. Med.* 119: 598–620 (1992).
118. Kim J, Hwang J-S, Cho Y-K, Han Y, Jeon Y-J, Yang K-H. Protective effects of (−)-epigallocatechin-3-gallate on UVA- and UVB-induced skin damage. *Skin Pharmacol. Appl. Skin Physiol.* 14: 11–19 (2001).
119. Katiyar SK, Afaq F, Azizuddin K, Mukhtar H. Inhibition of UVB-induced oxidative stress-mediated phosphorylation of mitogen-activated protein kinase signaling pathways in cultured human epidermal keratinocytes by green tea polyphenol (−)-epigallocatechin-3-gallate. *Toxicol. Appl. Pharmacol.* 176: 110–117 (2001).
120. Stadtman ER, Levine RL. Protein oxidation. *Ann. N. Y. Acad. Sci.* 899: 191–208 (2000).
121. Vayalil PK, Mittal A, Hara Y, Elmets CA, Katiyar SK. Green tea polyphenols prevent ultraviolet light-induced oxidative damage and matrix metalloproteinases expression in mouse skin. *J. Invest. Dermatol.* 122: 1480–1487 (2004).
122. Katiyar SK, Perez A, Mukhtar H. Green tea polyphenol treatment to human skin prevents formation of ultraviolet light B-induced pyrimidine dimers in DNA. *Clin. Cancer Res.* 6: 3864–3869 (2000).
123. Wei H, Ca Q, Rahn R, Zhang X, Wang Y, Lebwohl M. DNA structural integrity and base composition affect ultraviolet light-induced oxidative DNA damage. *Biochemistry* 37: 6485–6490 (1998).
124. Zhao JF, Zhang YJ, Jin XH, Athar M, Santella RM, Bickers DR, Wang ZY. Green tea protects against psoralen plus ultraviolet A-induced photochemical damage to skin. *J. Invest. Dermatol.* 113: 1070–1075 (1999).
125. Chatterjee ML, Agarwal R, Mukhtar H. Ultraviolet B radiation-induced DNA lesions in mouse epidermis: an assessment using a novel ^{32}P-postlabelling technique. *Biochem. Biophys. Res. Commun.* 229: 590–595 (1996).
126. Silva RC, Rigaud J, Cheynier V, Chemina A. Procyanidin dimers and trimers from grape seeds. *Phytochemistry* 30: 1259–1264 (1991).
127. Prieur C, Rigaud J, Cheynier V, Moutounet M. Oligomeric and polymeric procyanidins from grape seeds. *Phytochemistry* 36: 781–789 (1994).

34 Oxidative Stress and Coenzyme Q_{10} Therapy

Franklin L. Rosenfeldt, Silvana Marasco, Jee-Yoong Leong, and Salvatore Pepe

1. Introduction

Oxidative stress is being recognized increasingly as a major component of the pathophysiology of many diseases, especially those of the cardiovascular and nervous systems. Coenzyme Q_{10} (CoQ_{10}) is a lipid-soluble antioxidant and an integral component of the mitochondrial respiratory chain for oxidative energy production. CoQ_{10} is also known as ubiquinone because of its widespread occurrence (as CoQ_{10} or homolog) in all animals, plants, and most aerobic microorganisms. CoQ_{10} occurs in two forms: an oxidized form, ubiquinone, and a reduced form, ubiquinol. Ubiquinol is a potent antioxidant. Being lipid soluble, CoQ_{10} readily crosses cell membranes to enter cells. It is found in high concentrations in mitochondria, the main site of oxygen free radical production. It is highly effective as a cellular antioxidant. Tissue deficiencies of CoQ_{10} occur in aging and in diseases such as heart failure. In this chapter, we review the biochemistry of CoQ_{10} and its therapeutic action in a wide variety of states of oxidative stress.

2. Biochemistry of Coenzyme Q_{10}

CoQ_{10} comprises an aromatic carbon benzoquinone ring and an isoprene side chain (Fig. 1).

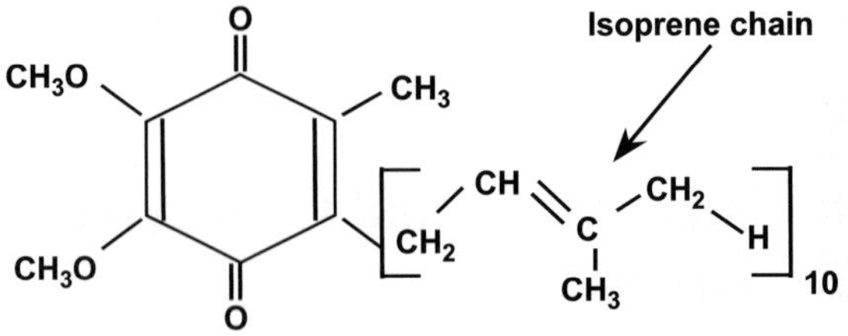

Fig. 1. Structure of coenzyme Q_{10} (ubiquinone).

In humans, there are 10 farsenyl units in the side chain, hence the name Q_{10}. In rats and fish, the side chain contains nine units and in microorganisms, six to nine units. CoQ_{10} levels vary in the body, with the highest levels occurring in organs with the highest metabolic rates such as the heart (Fig. 2).[1] Tissue CoQ_{10} levels diminish with advancing age.[2]

CoQ_{10} has a wide variety of functions (Table 1). CoQ_{10} is abundant particularly in the inner mitochondrial membrane where it is an essential redox component in coupling NADH-dehydrogenase (Complex 1) to cytochrome *bc1* or succinate dehydrogenase (Complex 2) to cytochrome *bc1* (Complex 3, ubiquinone cytochrome *c* oxidoreductase) by transferring free electrons.[3] Thus, CoQ_{10} facilitates a proton-motive Q cycle within the mitochondrial membrane, where CoQ_{10} is found as a semiquinone in addition to a fully reduced (ubiquinol, $CoQ_{10}H_2$) or oxidized (ubiquinone, CoQ_{10}) form. The production of a trans-membrane proton gradient across the inner mitochondrial membrane drives the reduction of oxygen to water at cytochrome *c* oxidase (Complex 4) and ultimately drives ATP synthase (Complex 5) to form ATP.

Improved preservation of mitochondrial ATP-generating capacity after ischemia and reperfusion has been reported for rabbit hearts pretreated with CoQ_{10}. These results corresponded to the improved post-ischemic preservation of myocardial contractile function and reduced creatine phosphokinase release in CoQ_{10} pretreated hearts.[5] Hano *et al.*[6] showed that CoQ_{10} pretreatment improved post-ischemic recovery of high-energy phosphates and contractile function in isolated rat hearts, while preventing calcium overload and preserving diastolic dysfunction. A more recent study, also using an isolated rat heart model, demonstrated that CoQ_{10} pretreatment improved

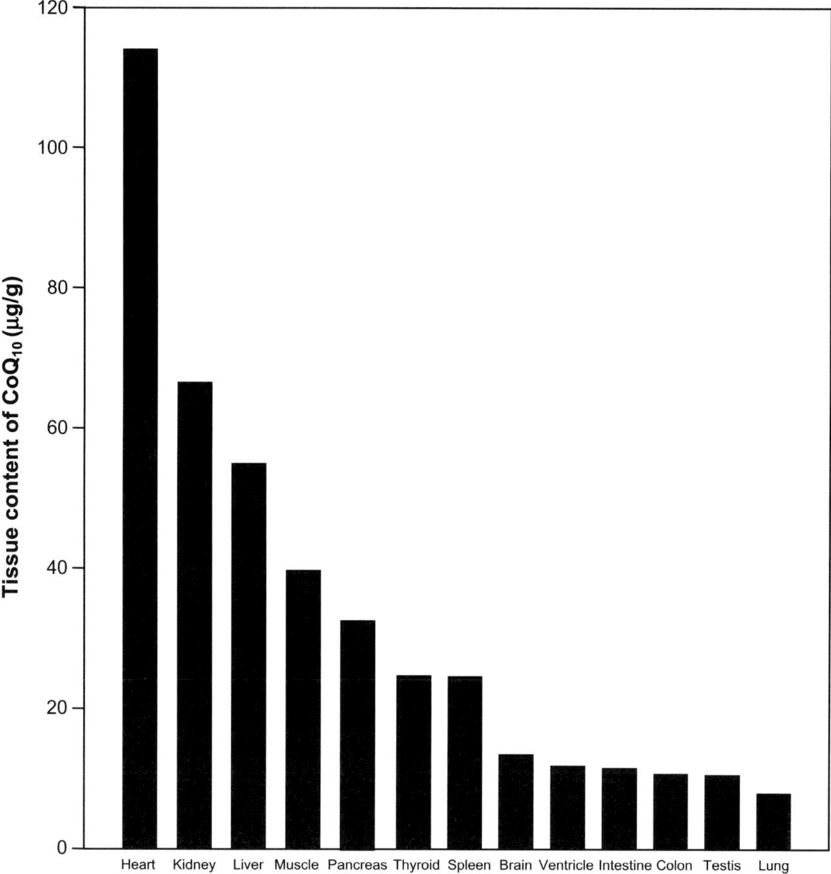

Fig. 2. Human organ tissue content of coenzyme Q_{10}.[1]

Table 1. Functions of coenzyme Q_{10}.[4]

Participation as electron carrier in the mitochondrial respiratory chain
Participation in extra-mitochondrial electron transport
Endogenously synthesized, lipid-soluble antioxidant
Regulation of mitochondrial permeability transition pore
Required for activation of mitochondrial uncoupling proteins
Regulation of the physiochemical properties of membranes
Modulation of the amount of β_2-integrins on the surface of blood monocytes
Improvement of endothelial dysfunction

diastolic function during reperfusion, maintained higher ATP levels, preserved coronary vasodilatation by sodium nitroprusside, and increased coronary flow.[7] Thus, CoQ_{10} is crucial for preservation of oxidative phosphorylation during conditions of metabolic stress.

CoQ_{10} also specifically binds to a site in the inner mitochondrial membrane that inhibits the mitochondrial permeability transition pore (MPTP).[8–10] The MPTP is a large conductance channel, which when opened can trigger collapse of mitochondrial proton-motive force and membrane potential leading to the disruption of ionic homeostasis and oxidative phosphorylation in cell death signaling pathways, particularly after ischemia and reperfusion.[11] CoQ_{10} protects creatine kinase and other key proteins from oxidative inactivation during reperfusion, a function crucial in preserving energy metabolism and cardiac performance.[12–16]

CoQ_{10} is carried mainly by lipoproteins in the circulation, predominantly in its reduced form, ubiquinol. Ubiquinol acts as an antioxidant in plasma lipoproteins, lowering the oxidation rate of dietary fatty acids transported in the lipoproteins.[17,18] Ubiquinol is oxidized to ubiquinone during its antioxidative action. Ubiquinone itself does not have any antioxidant activity. It is the reduced form, ubiquinol, which is responsible for the antioxidant properties of CoQ_{10}.[19,20]

CoQ_{10} has an important role in preventing the initiation and/or propagation of lipid peroxidation in plasma lipoproteins and membrane proteins. Ferrara *et al.*[21] demonstrated that chronic treatment with CoQ_{10} in rats protected against cardiac injury due to oxidative stress created by H_2O_2 in the heart. CoQ_{10} can inhibit lipid peroxidation in mitochondria,[22] protein oxidation,[23] and DNA oxidation.[24] After its antioxidative action, ubiquinone can be recycled to the antioxidant, active, reduced ubiquinol form via the mitochondrial Q cycle. CoQ_{10} importantly is also responsible for transforming vitamin E radicals to regenerate the reduced (active) α-tocopherol form of vitamin E.[25]

CoQ_{10} also plays a crucial role in extra-mitochondrial electron transfer such as that required to regulate NADH oxidoreductase activity in the plasma membrane,[26,27] and also has potential redox activity in both Golgi apparatus and lysosomes.[28]

3. Metabolism

CoQ_{10} incorporated into cellular membranes arises either from *de novo* synthesis or from dietary intake.

3.1. *Synthesis*

CoQ_{10} shares with cholesterol and dolichol a common metabolic pathway called the mevalonate pathway. The CoQ_{10} molecule comes from two sources (Fig. 3). The benzoquinone ring is derived from phenylalanine or tyrosine. This ring is also common to vitamin K. The 10-carbon,

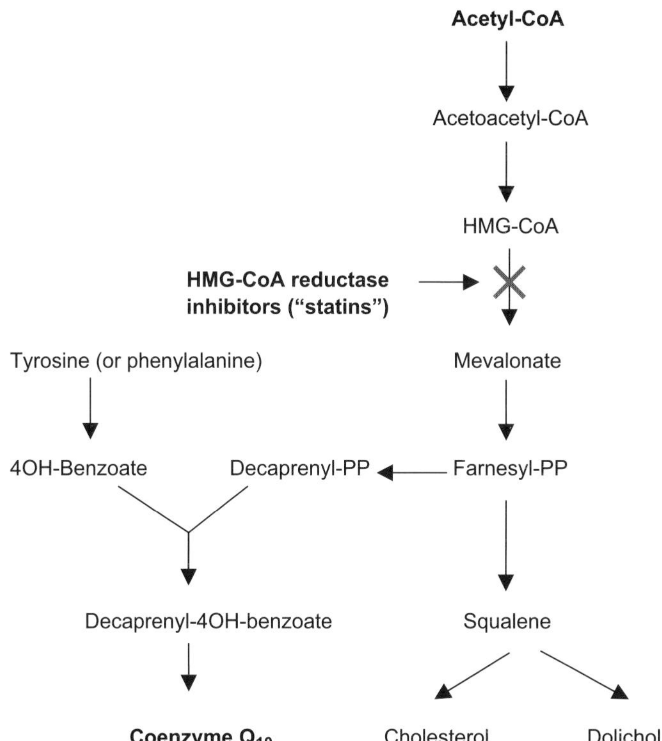

Fig. 3. Coenzyme Q_{10} synthesis pathway.

isoprenoid side chain is derived from acetyl CoA. The second step in the mevalonate pathway requires the enzyme 3-hydroxy-3-methylglutaryl coenzyme A reductase (HMG-CoA reductase). The commonly used cholesterol lowering drugs, the statins, inhibit HMG-CoA reductase. Thus, the statins not only reduce the synthesis of cholesterol but also of CoQ_{10} and dolichol.

Recently, it has been reported that three important genes are crucial to synthesis of CoQ_{10}. The CoQ_3 gene permits production of enzymes that catalyze two O-methylations whereas the CoQ_7 gene is crucial for processes leading to hydroxylation of the benzoquinone ring.[29,30] The CoQ_2 gene encodes for *p*-hydroxybenzoate:polyprenyl transferase, an enzyme that catalyzes the prenylation of *p*-hydroxybenzoate with an all-*trans* polyprenyl group thus forming the polyisoprenoid side chain.[31,32] Although the full molecular nature and sites responsible for *de novo* synthesis of CoQ_{10} are yet to be fully delineated there is evidence that CoQ_{10} is synthesized in the endoplasmic reticulum and Golgi system.[2]

3.2. *Dietary intake and distribution*

CoQ_{10} is poorly absorbed from food in the gut: only 10% of CoQ_{10} contained in a meal is absorbed.[33] Bioavailability from a standard oral dose is low, being only 2–4%,[34] however, it is improved when CoQ_{10} is in an oily suspension.[35] Water soluble gel formulations have been developed for improved CoQ_{10} absorption.[36,37]

Oral supplementation of CoQ_{10} leads to an elevation of plasma levels, with peak plasma CoQ_{10} levels occurring between 5 and 10 h after ingestion.[18] CoQ_{10} is absorbed slowly from the gastrointestinal tract, probably due to its high molecular weight and low water solubility. Following absorption from the gastrointestinal tract, CoQ_{10} is taken up by chylomicrons and transported to the liver for packaging into very low density lipoproteins (VLDL). From there it is transported to various tissues according to their requirement. Orally administered CoQ_{10} appears to have a low clearance rate from the plasma, and therefore has a relatively long plasma half-life of 34 ± 5 h, with excretion predominantly through the biliary tract. Approximately 90% of the steady-state serum concentration can be achieved after 4 days of dosing.

Analysis of the distribution of CoQ_{10} in the circulation shows that about 60% of CoQ_{10} is transported by LDL and less than 30% by HDL.[17] However, in the absence of significant exogenous supply of CoQ_{10}, individual tissues must rely on their own production as endogenously produced CoQ_{10} is not transported within the body or redistributed to any great degree. Although CoQ_{10} is present in a normal diet, with meat and poultry being the richest sources, endogenous production appears to be the main source in humans.[38] Whether it is in the diet or pharmaceutical supplementation, it is the oxidized form of CoQ_{10} that is ingested and absorbed. The CoQ_{10} is then reduced in the circulation, most likely in the red blood cells.[39] Thus, most CoQ_{10} in the blood is present as the reduced form ubiquinol, consistent with its activity as an antioxidant in the circulation.

In humans, the fate of exogenously administered CoQ_{10} once it reaches the circulation has not been completely elucidated. Work in rat hearts has shown that exogenously administered labelled CoQ_{10} is incorporated into subcellular organelles, especially in the inner membranes and matrix of mitochondria, within 72 h of administration.[40] It has also been demonstrated that incubation of beef heart submitochondrial particles in a CoQ_{10} solution leads to incorporation of CoQ_{10} in their membranes.[41] The same authors found that kinetic saturation with CoQ_{10} could not be achieved because of the intrinsic insolubility of the molecule, thus concluding that the upper limit of electron transfer from NADH is a function of CoQ_{10} solubility in the membrane phospholipids.

Our own investigations into the use of CoQ_{10} in cardiac surgery patients receiving oral CoQ_{10} (300 mg/day) demonstrated a fourfold increase in serum concentration, a 2.5-fold increase in concentration in atrial myocardium, and a 2.4-fold increase in concentration in atrial mitochondria in patients receiving oral CoQ_{10} (300 mg/day).[42]

4. Cardiovascular Disease, Oxidative Stress, and Therapy

Oxidative stress has been implicated in the pathogenesis of a wide variety of cardiovascular diseases including heart failure and atherosclerosis. This has led to the development of treatments for these diseases using antioxidants.

4.1. *Heart failure*

From the early 1990s, experimental and clinical evidence has been accumulating of the role of oxidative stress in the pathogenesis of heart failure. Increased myocardial levels of oxidative stress markers have been demonstrated in animal models of heart failure produced by coronary ligation,[43] pressure overload,[44] and rapid cardiac pacing.[45] Reactive oxygen species (ROS) are key pathophysiological mediators in myocardial remodeling in heart failure.[46] In clinical heart failure, there is also evidence of increased levels of oxidative stress markers such as malondialdehyde in serum,[47] and isoprostanes in urine.[48] Furthermore, the levels of these markers correlate with the severity of heart failure.

Studies in animals have shown the beneficial effect of antioxidant therapy for heart failure. Vitamin E in guinea pigs with pressure overload can prevent the transition from compensated hypertrophy to heart failure.[49] Similarly, probucol, a lipid-lowering agent with antioxidant actions, can protect against heart failure induced by adriamycin[50] and diabetes.[51] See Kukin and Fuster[52] for a detailed review.

There are multiple molecular, cellular, and neurohumorol mechanisms that contribute to the syndrome of heart failure and it is likely that oxidative stress is involved in some or all of these processes. There is no doubt that antioxidant therapy can attenuate oxidative stress. However, many of the early clinical trials of antioxidant therapy for heart failure were negative. This may be explained by ineffective agents being given in the wrong doses.[53] However, the results of using more potent antioxidants such as CoQ_{10} that have other beneficial actions have been more encouraging. CoQ_{10} treatment for heart failure has been claimed to ameliorate symptoms, improve quality of life, and reduce rates of hospitalization. However, most trials have been open label and in some, only 50% of patients took angiotensin converting enzyme (ACE) inhibitors that are now standard therapy for heart failure.

4.1.1. *Australian pilot study of coenzyme Q_{10} in heart failure*

We performed a randomized, double-blind placebo-controlled pilot trial of CoQ_{10} therapy in patients with class II and class III systolic heart failure.[54] This trial was designed in the pre-beta blocker era of heart failure therapy.

The aim of the trial was to determine the effect of CoQ_{10} in patients with heart failure due to ischemic or dilated cardiomyopathy who were on maximal non-beta blocker therapy. The inclusion criteria were New York Heart Association (NYHA) functional class II or III heart failure with an ejection fraction less than 40% and were receiving maximal therapy including ACE inhibitors. Patients were randomized double blind to 150 mg daily of oral CoQ_{10} or placebo for 3 months. Thirty-five patients completed the trial. There was a threefold increase in plasma CoQ_{10} levels in the treated group (0.7 ± 0.4 to $2.1 \pm 0.3\,\mu$g/ml) but no change in the placebo group. There were no differences in demographics or medications between groups. After 3 months of therapy, the NYHA class in the CoQ_{10} group ($n = 17$) showed a significant improvement of 0.5 class compared with placebo ($n = 18$) ($p = 0.01$) (Table 2).

The Specific Activities Scale (SAS) also showed a significant ($p = 0.004$) improvement in the CoQ_{10} group, but no change in the placebo group. The 6-min walk test distance showed a significant ($p = 0.047$) increase in the CoQ_{10} group with no change in the placebo group (between-group difference $p = 0.024$). For the Naughton Exercise Test, the difference in increase in exercise time approached significance in favor of the CoQ_{10} group ($p = 0.056$). There was a correlation between increase in exercise time and increase in serum CoQ_{10} level ($r^2 = 0.15$, $p = 0.024$). This study showed several benefits of CoQ_{10}, but due to small sample size, it was not powered to detect many important endpoints.

4.1.2. *Meta-analysis of randomized trials of coenzyme Q_{10} in heart failure*

A meta-analysis showing a beneficial effect of CoQ_{10} in heart failure was published in 1997.[55] To assess the effect of CoQ_{10} in heart failure in the current era, we conducted a meta-analysis of randomized trials of CoQ_{10} in heart failure published up to 2003.[56] Only prospective, randomized, double-blinded and placebo-controlled trials were included in this analysis. The analysis methodology used was fixed effects modeling. This technique combines results of trials weighted according to the sample size in each trial. The Review Manager ("Revman" version 4.04) and Metaview (version 4.0) software packages from the Cochrane collaboration were used for the statistical analyses. Nine trials were identified by Medline search

Table 2. Outcome variables in two treatment groups at baseline and after 3 months of therapy. The two far right columns show the statistical significance of the difference in response between the two groups over 3 months.

	Baseline			Three-month value				Difference between CoQ_{10} change and placebo change	
	Placebo	CoQ_{10}		Placebo		CoQ_{10}			
	($n = 18$)	($n = 17$)	p Value	($n = 18$)	p Value vs baseline	($n = 17$)	p Value vs baseline	Absolute difference	p Value
NYHA	2.7 ± 0.2	2.9 ± 0.06	0.91	2.7 ± 0.17	0.67	2.4 ± 0.12	0.001	−0.5	0.01
Canadian SAS	2.6 ± 0.1	2.7 ± 0.14	0.47	2.4 ± 0.2	0.38	2.3 ± 0.14	0.004	−0.2	0.29
Naughton Exercise time (sec)	533 ± 59	504 ± 53	0.89	500 ± 61	0.22	557 ± 50	0.14	+103.8	0.56
6 min walk distance (m)	345 ± 33	351 ± 25	0.72	328 ± 31	0.63	372 ± 23	0.046	+37.7	0.29
Fractional Shortening (FS%)	14 ± 1.1	15 ± 0.9	0.42	14 ± 1.1	0.38	17 ± 1.5	0.35	0.001	0.90
Serum CoQ_{10} level (μg/ml)	0.7 ± 0.05	0.7 ± 0.03	0.67	0.67 ± 0.07	0.34	2.13 ± 0.29	0.0001	+1.5	0.0001
Serum Creatinine mmol/L	0.1 ± 0.01	0.1 ± 0.01	0.21	0.14 ± 0.001	0.49	0.11 ± 0.01	0.85	−0.01	0.48

NYHA, New York Heart Association functional class; SAS, Specific Activities Scale.

Table 3. Summary of nine trials of CoQ_{10} in heart failure.

Reference	No. of subjects	Study design	CoQ_{10} daily dose and duration	Outcomes weighted mean difference
Hofman-Bang[57]	69	Crossover	100 mg for 3 months	EF rest: +14% EF exercise: −4.3% Max. exercise capacity: +6%* Life quality: +6%* Mortality: 0.74 (odds ratio)
Keogh[54]	35	Parallel	150 mg for 3 months	NYHA class: −13%* Exercise duration: +18% Mortality: 0
Khatta[58]	46	Parallel	200 mg for 6 months	EF rest: 0 Exercise duration: 0
Langsjoen[59]	19	Crossover	100 mg for 12 weeks	EF rest: +19%**
Morisco[60]	563	Parallel	2 mg/kg for 12 months	Mortality: 0.75 (odds ratio)
Permanetter[61]	25	Crossover	100 mg for 4 months	EF rest: +14% EF exercise: +6.2% Max. exercise capacity: +3% NHYA class: −6%
Munkholm[62]	22	Parallel	200 mg for 12 weeks	EF rest: −9%
Poggesi[63]	18	Crossover	100 mg for 2 months	EF rest: +14%**
Watson[64]	27	Crossover	100 mg for 12 weeks	EF rest: 0 Mortality: 0.14 (odds ratio)

$^{*}p < 0.05$, $^{**}p < 0.001$.

and were included in the meta-analysis. Parameters measured are listed in Table 3.

The only three parameters with adequate numbers of subjects for meaningful analysis were CoQ_{10} levels (five trials), ejection fraction at rest (seven trials), and mortality (five trials). Other parameters were measured in only two trials each. For CoQ_{10} levels (279 patients) the weighted mean difference was 1.4 μg/ml, representing an increase of 161%. For ejection fraction at rest (384 patients), the weighted mean difference showed a trend in favor of CoQ_{10}, of 1.9% (95% confidence limits −0.13 to 3.9%) (Fig. 4).

Several of the individual trials showed positive outcomes for some parameters such as symptom class and exercise capacity. It is clear overall that there were insufficient numbers of patients in the trials for meaningful results. We carried out sample size calculations to determine the number of patients necessary in a trial to detect significant differences in various parameters. We calculated that for a parallel (two group) study of ejection fraction at rest, to detect a 2% increase in ejection fraction with a power of 0.8 and an alpha of 0.05, 394 patients per group would be required, and to detect a 5% increase in ejection fraction 64 patients per group would be required. For mortality the current meta-analysis showed a slight reduction from 6.4 to 5.0% (1.4% absolute risk reduction) with an odds ratio of 0.76. We calculated that to detect a 2% reduction in mortality 2100 patients per group would be required.

We conclude that for ejection fraction measurements all trials to date (except Hofman-Bang *et al.*[57]) had insufficient subjects to detect a clinically meaningful difference of 5%. The meta-analysis showed a trend toward an improvement in ejection fraction. Furthermore, trials to detect a mortality difference would need to be prohibitively large, requiring 2000 or more patients per group. For the future, a reasonable expectation would be to conduct a multinational prospective, randomized trial containing 300–400 patients per group to make a more definitive conclusion as to the effects of CoQ_{10} on cardiac function and symptoms in cardiac failure. Such a trial, the "Q-symbio" trial is currently in progress.[65]

In light of the encouraging findings of the Australian trial, of the meta-analysis reported here, and of a previous meta-analysis,[55] it is not unreasonable to recommend to patients with symptomatic heart failure despite conventional therapy or those who are experiencing side effects of conventional therapy, to take 150–300 mg of CoQ_{10} daily.

4.1.3. *Statins cause CoQ_{10} deficiency*

The 3-hydroxy-3-methylglutaryl coenzyme A (HMG CoA) reductase inhibitors or "statins" are at present one of the most widely prescribed drugs in the Western world. These drugs lower cholesterol by inhibiting

Comparison: Co-enzymeQ$_{10}$ versus placebo for the treatment of heart failure
Outcome: Ejection fraction (rest) %

Study	Exp *n*	Exp. means (sd)	Cntr *n*	Cntr means (sd)	WMD (95% fixed)	Weight (%)	WMD (95% CL)
Hofman Bang	69	24.00 (12.00)	69	23.00 (12.00)		24.7	1.00 [−3.00,5.00]
Khatta	23	30.00 (9.40)	23	30.00 (8.90)		14.1	0.00 [−5.30,5.30]
Langsjoen	19	58.80 (12.60)	19	49.30 (14.60)		5.3	9.50 [0.83,18.17]
Munkholm	11	32.00 (11.00)	11	35.00 (8.00)		6.1	−3.00 [−11.04,5.03]
Permanetter	25	39.23 (13.08)	25	34.38(12.00)		8.2	4.85 [−2.12,11.81]
Pogessi	18	50.30 (6.40)	18	46.60 (5.90)		24.5	3.70 [−0.32,7.72]
Watson	27	31.00 (9.00)	27	31.00 (9.00)		17.2	0.00 [−4.80,4.80]
Total (95% CI)	192		192			100.0	1.86 [−0.13,3.85]

Chi-square 7.13 (df=6) Z=1.84

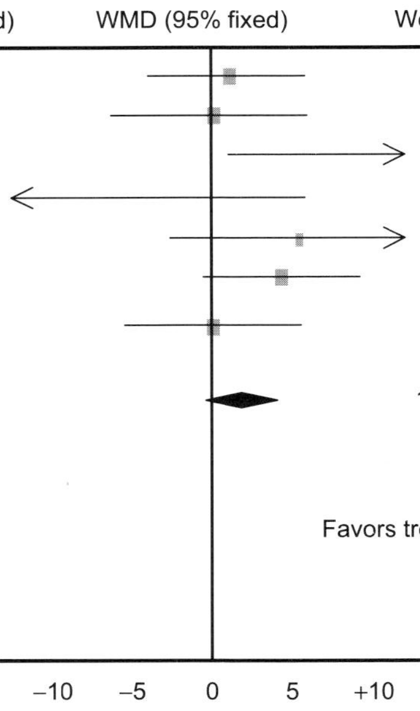

Favors control — Favors treatment

−10 −5 0 5 +10

Fig. 4. Effect of CoQ_{10} on ejection fraction at rest: weighted mean difference.

Table 4. Summary of results from nine studies of CoQ_{10} in heart failure.

Parameter	No. of studies	No. of patients	Weighted mean difference (95% CI)*	Change (%)
Serum CoQ_{10}	5	139	1.4 (1.3 to 1.5)	+161%
EF rest	7	384	1.9 (−0.13 to 3.9)	+5%
EF exercise	2	188	−0.5 (−3.9 to 2.9)	−5%
Maximum exercise capacity	2	198	14.2 (−3.9 to 12.4)	+5%
NYHA class	2	85	−0.09 (−0.037 to 0.18)	−5%
Mortality	5	836	0.76 (0.43 to 1.37) (odds ratio)	−5%
Exercise duration	2	81	1.0 (−0.54 to 2.54)	+5%

*None were statistically significant.

the enzyme HMG CoA reductase, a key enzyme in the synthetic pathway for cholesterol and also for CoQ_{10} (Fig. 3). From 1990 to 2003, 15 studies in humans have been published evaluating the effects of statins on CoQ_{10} metabolism.[66] Nine of these were randomized controlled trials, and eight of these nine demonstrated significant depletion of CoQ_{10} due to statin therapy. Of particular interest is a study by De Pinieux *et al.*[67] showing raised lactate to pyruvate ratios in statin-treated patients, indicating mitochondrial dysfunction, most likely induced by CoQ_{10}depletion. A study by Miyake *et al.*[68] of 97 noninsulin dependent diabetics treated with simvastatin showed a decrease in serum CoQ_{10} levels. Supplementation with CoQ_{10} caused a decrease in cardiothoracic ratios suggesting that statin-induced CoQ_{10} depletion had caused a depression in cardiac function, reversible by CoQ_{10} supplementation.

In summary, statins, especially the lipid-soluble types such as simvastatin, deplete body CoQ_{10} levels. This depletion may be particularly important in the elderly where CoQ_{10} levels are generally low. Adverse effects of statin-induced CoQ_{10} have been observed at a mitochondrial level and a clinical level and these effects can be corrected by concurrent administration of CoQ_{10}.

4.2. *Hypertension*

CoQ_{10} has been shown in laboratory and clinical studies to have an hypotensive effect. This finding encouraged researchers to conduct randomized

Table 5. Four positive placebo-controlled studies of coenzyme Q_{10} in hypertension.

Reference	No. of subjects	Daily dose (mg)	Duration (weeks)	Baseline BP (mmHg)	BP decrease systolic/diastolic (mmHg)
Yamagami[73]	20	100	12	167/97	19/16
Singh[74]	59	120	8	167/106	15/9
Burke[75]	83	120	12	165/81	18/2
Hodgson[76]	74	200	12	–	6/3

clinical trials of CoQ_{10} in hypertension. We have identified eight such studies in the literature, four of which were placebo controlled (Table 5) and four were not.[69–72] The four studies with placebo controls included between 20 and 83 patients. Subjects were treated for between 8 and 12 weeks with 100–200 mg CoQ_{10} per day. Significant decreases of 6–19 mmHg in systolic and 2–16 mmHg in diastolic blood pressure were seen. The four studies without placebo controls simply compared the blood pressure before and after treatment. Decreases in blood pressure ranged from 12 to 21 mmHg systolic, and pressure from 9 to 15 mmHg diastolic. Altogether in the eight studies the mean decrease in systolic blood pressure was 16 mmHg and diastolic blood pressure 10 mmHg.

One likely mechanism of action of CoQ_{10} in lowering blood pressure is the preservation of nitric oxide within the endothelium. ROS such as superoxide generated in the vasculature can reduce the available concentration of nitric oxide. Superoxide combines with nitric oxide to produce peroxynitrite. CoQ_{10} can scavenge ROS thus protecting nitric oxide from attack by ROS with a consequent presentation of nitric oxide-induced vasodilation. Thus, CoQ_{10} works by a different mechanism to other antihypertensive agents. Being devoid of significant side effects, CoQ_{10} may have a useful clinical role as an adjunct or alternative to conventional agents such as diuretics and ACE inhibitors in the treatment of hypertension. In support of this, in one study 50% of subjects treated with CoQ_{10} were able to cease at least one of their other hypertensive medications.[72] In conclusion, more large-scale prospective randomized clinical studies of CoQ_{10} in hypertension are indicated.

4.3. *Ischemic heart disease*

Because of the beneficial effect of CoQ_{10} on the efficiency of mitochondrial energy production,[42] it might be expected that CoQ_{10} would be effective in treating ischemic heart disease. Confirming this are two double blind placebo-controlled crossover trials of CoQ_{10} in patients with ischemic heart disease showing benefit in terms of a reduction in angina, improved exercise tolerance, and a reduction in ischemic changes on ECG.[77,78]

4.4. *Cardiac surgery*

From 1982 to 2004, at least eight controlled trials of CoQ_{10} in cardiac surgery have been published.[13,15,16,42,79–82] All but one of these have shown a beneficial effect of some kind. The one negative trial[15] used oral CoQ_{10} for just 12 h before surgery, which would have been an inadequate dosing duration to increase tissue levels. A prospective randomized placebo-controlled trial from our unit of 300 mg per day of oral CoQ_{10} for 2 weeks preoperatively in 121 coronary bypass or valve replacement procedures showed increased mitochondrial CoQ_{10} content, increased efficiency of mitochondrial energy production, and improved function in myocardial strips.[42]

5. Neurological Disease

5.1. *Parkinson's disease*

Parkinson's disease is a degenerative neurological disorder characterized by resting tremor, slowness of movement, and muscular rigidity. The main pathological feature is loss of dopaminergic neurons in the substantia nigra and the presence of hyaline material (Lewy bodies) in neurons in the substantia nigra and extranigral regions of the brain. In Parkinson's disease patients there is a selective decrease in Complex I activity in the mitochondrial electron transport chain in both the substantia nigra and platelets. CoQ_{10} content is reduced in both the serum and mitochondria isolated from platelets in patients with Parkinson's disease.[83] Furthermore, treatment of these patients with CoQ_{10} slows the progressive deterioration of function.[84]

5.2. *Friedreich's ataxia*

Friedreich's ataxia (FRDA) is an autosomal recessive degenerative disease (1 in 30,000 live births) characterized by progressive limb and gait ataxia, loss of deep tendon reflexes, loss of the sense of position and vibration in the lower limbs, dysarthria, and hypertrophic cardiomyopathy. The clinical features usually present in adolescence and are progressive. The pathological changes include loss of large sensory neurons in the dorsal root ganglia and degeneration of the dorsal columns of the spinal cord.

The genetic abnormality has been mapped to chromosome 9q13, which encodes the protein frataxin. The genetic abnormality accounting for 98% of cases is the expansion of a GAA triplet repeat in intron 1 of the FRDA gene. This results in decreased frataxin mRNA levels, which leads to lower levels of frataxin protein detected in skeletal muscle, cerebellum, and cerebral cortex in these patients.

The exact function of frataxin in humans is still unknown although evidence from yeast and mice indicate it has a key role in mitochondrial iron homeostasis. Endomyocardial biopsies in FRDA patients show deficient activity of the iron–sulfur (Fe–S) cluster containing proteins, namely complexes I, II, and III of the mitochondrial respiratory chain. It appears that mitochondrial iron accumulation in FRDA is a consequence of deregulation of a mitochondrial iron import system triggered by the decreased amount of frataxin, normally acting as a regulator of the mitochondrial iron homeostasis. Studies of skeletal muscle from these patients have demonstrated a profound deficit of mitochondrial ATP production. Current evidence suggests that this frataxin deficiency results in impaired mitochondrial respiratory chain function due to the mechanisms outlined above. In addition, increased oxidative damage is seen in these patients and is likely to be a secondary consequence of impaired respiratory chain function and increased free radical generation.

CoQ_{10} therapy in conjunction with vitamin E has been assessed in a small study of FRDA patients showing significant improvements in heart and skeletal muscle energetics after 6 months of therapy.[85] Idibenone, a short-chain analog of CoQ_{10}, is a potent free radical scavenger that crosses the blood–brain barrier, and has been recommended in the treatment of FRDA. However, a 1-year study of idibenone in 29 Friedreich ataxia patients showed a reduction in left ventricular hypertrophy but no improvement in neurological condition.[86]

5.3. *Huntington's disease*

Huntington's disease (HD) is an autosomal dominant movement disorder becoming clinically apparent between 20 and 50 years of age. The patients develop chorea, namely jerky hyperkinetic movements affecting all parts of the body. Pathologically there is atrophy of the caudate nucleus and putamen. The disease gene has been mapped to chromosome 4p. Studies in both rats and primates have replicated the pathological and clinical features of Huntington's disease by the administration of the toxin, 3-nitropropionic acid. The resulting striatal lesions are accompanied by focal increases in lactate confined to the basal ganglia and are attenuated by antioxidants. The development of transgenic mouse models has allowed further study in this area. Ferrante *et al.*[87] showed that administration of CoQ_{10} significantly delays the onset of motor deficits, cerebral atrophy, and neuronal inclusions. This work led on to a clinical trial of CoQ_{10} in 360 HD patients over a 30-month period. CoQ_{10} slowed progression on the total functional capacity scale by approximately 14% over the 30 months. There were also some benefits in neuropsychological tests examined as secondary endpoints. However, due to the insufficient sample size, none of these effects reached statistical significance.[88]

6. Oxidative Stress and CoQ_{10} Therapy in Physical Exercise

Vigorous physical exercise generates oxidative stress, especially in untrained individuals.[89] Physical training increases antioxidant reserve and this reduces the oxidative stress response to exercise, consequently antioxidant therapy has been recommended to enhance athletic performance.[90] CoQ_{10} has been used to reduce oxidative stress in exercise and improve physical performance. We identified 11 studies in which CoQ_{10} was tested for an effect on exercise capacity; six were positive and five showed no effect. Of the six positive trials (Table 6), four were in trained sports persons, athletes, cyclists, and skiers,[91–94] and two involved untrained

Table 6. Coenzyme Q_{10} in exercise — Studies showing a positive effect.

Reference	Subjects	No. enrolled	Oxygen consumption	Exercise capacity
Wyss[95]	Untrained	18	+7%*	+33%*
Zeppili[96]	Trained and untrained	19	+11%**	+10%**
Amadio[91]	Athletes	10	+18%**	—
Fiorella[92]	Athletes	22	—	+13%*
Bonetti[93]	Cyclists	28	0	+5%*
Ylikoski[94]	Skiers	18	+3%*	+5%**

$^{*}p < 0.05$; $^{**}p < 0.01$.

individuals.[95,96] Subjects ($n = 18$–28 per study) were given CoQ_{10}, 90–100 mg per day for 4–8 weeks. Benefits were observed in terms of improved maximum oxygen consumption, averaging 8% (range 3–18%) and improved exercise capacity, averaging 13% (range 5–33%). Five other trials failed to show any statistically significant benefit of CoQ_{10}.[97–101] Four of these were in trained sports persons and one in untrained individuals, and included 10–19 subjects with a duration of treatment of 4–8 weeks. Dosage and duration of therapy were similar in the two groups of studies.

In conclusion, it appears that a modest improvement in exercise capacity may be observed with CoQ_{10} supplementation but this is not a consistent finding. Inconsistencies in trial results may be due to small numbers of subjects enrolled and to differences in experimental design. In view of the indication of benefit in some studies, larger randomized trials in this area are indicated.

7. Summary and Conclusions

1. There is robust and increasing evidence that oxidative stress is an important contributor to the pathophysiology of cardiovascular diseases including heart failure, hypertension, and ischemic heart disease. The same is true of major neurological diseases such as Parkinson's disease, Friedrich's ataxia, and Huntington's disease.
2. Despite conclusive data of the efficacy of CoQ_{10} therapy in animal models of many human diseases, the results of prospective randomized

clinical trials while being encouraging have not been uniformly convincing.
3. Further research is indicated on the role of CoQ_{10} and other antioxidants in the treatment of the major cardiovascular and neurological diseases.
4. Oxidative stress is increased in physical exercise, especially in untrained individuals. CoQ_{10} can reduce exercise-induced oxidative stress and may improve physical performance.

8. Future Implications

Because of the encouraging evidence of the efficacy of CoQ_{10} in cardiovascular and neurological disease, both from clinical trials and from our own clinical experience over the last five years, we believe that this is a fruitful field for research and therapy. CoQ_{10} is a compound with both antioxidant and energy promoting actions at a cellular and mitochondrial level. Alpha-lipoic acid is another such compound. There is increasing laboratory[102] and clinical evidence[103] of the therapeutic efficacy of alpha-lipoic acid in oxidant-related diseases. In nature, antioxidants usually function as networks, each agent being regenerated by other members of the network.[104] We believe that therapy with groups of antioxidants is both logical and efficacious. We have completed a pilot trial of CoQ_{10} combined with alpha-lipoic acid, magnesium orotate, and omega-3 fatty acids in patients undergoing cardiac surgery.[105] The results were sufficiently encouraging to warrant the conduct of a prospective, randomized clinical trial of the same agents with the addition of selenium in cardiac surgery and neurosurgery patients. Also in progress is a multinational prospective randomized clinical trial of CoQ_{10} in advanced cardiac failure, the Q-symbio trial.[65] This trial is adequately powered to finally prove or disprove the clinical efficacy of CoQ_{10} in heart failure. The next few years should see major advances in our knowledge of the effect of CoQ_{10} and other antioxidants in the treatment of diseases where oxidative stress is a major factor.

References

1. Aberg F, Appelkvist EL, Dallner G, Ernster L. Distribution and redox state of ubiquinones in rat and human tissues. *Arch. Biochem. Biophys.* 295: 230–234 (1992).

2. Kalen A, Appelkvist EL, Dallner G. Age-related changes in the lipid compositions of rat and human tissues. *Lipids* 24: 579–584 (1989).
3. Mitchell P. Protonmotive redox mechanism of the cytochrome b-c1 complex in the respiratory chain: protonmotive ubiquinone cycle. *FEBS Lett.* 56: 1–6 (1975).
4. Ebadi M. Actions and functions of mitochondria and their ubiquinone (coenzyme Q_{10}). In: Ebadi M, Marwah J, Chopra R (eds.) *Mitochondrial Ubiquinone (Coenzyme Q_{10})*. Prominent Press, Scottsdale, AZ, 2001, pp. 1–111.
5. Nayler WG. The use of coenzyme Q_{10} to protect ischaemic heart muscle. In: Yamamura Y, Folkers K, Ito Y (eds.) *Biomedical and Clinical Aspects of Coenzyme Q*. Elsevier/North-Holland Biomedical Press, Amsterdam, 1980, pp. 409–424.
6. Hano O, Thompson-Gorman SL, Zweier JL, Lakatta EG. Coenzyme Q_{10} enhances cardiac functional and metabolic recovery and reduces Ca^{2+} overload during post-ischemic reperfusion. *Am. J. Physiol.* 266: H2174–H2181 (1994).
7. Whitman GJ, Niibori K, Yokoyama H, Crestanello JA, Lingle DM, Momeni R. The mechanisms of coenzyme Q_{10} as therapy for myocardial ischemia reperfusion injury. *Mol. Aspects Med.* 18(Suppl): S195–S203 (1997).
8. Fontaine E, Ichas F, Bernardi P. A ubiquinone-binding site regulates the mitochondrial permeability transition pore. *J. Biol. Chem.* 273: 25734–25740 (1998).
9. Walter L, Nogueira V, Leverve X, Heitz MP, Bernardi P, Fontaine E. Three classes of ubiquinone analogs regulate the mitochondrial permeability transition pore through a common site. *J. Biol. Chem.* 275: 29521–29527 (2000).
10. Papucci L, Schiavone N, Witort E *et al.* Coenzyme Q_{10} prevents apoptosis by inhibiting mitochondrial depolarization independently of its free radical scavenging property. *J. Biol. Chem.* 278: 28220–28228 (2003).
11. Di Lisa F, Canton M, Menabo R, Dodoni G, Bernardi P. Mitochondria and reperfusion injury. The role of permeability transition. *Basic Res. Cardiol.* 98: 235–241 (2003).
12. Crestanello JA, Kamelgard J, Lingle DM, Mortensen SA, Rhode M, Whitman GJ. Elucidation of a tripartite mechanism underlying the improvement in cardiac tolerance to ischemia by coenzyme Q_{10} pretreatment. *J. Thorac. Cardiovasc. Surg.* 111: 443–450 (1996).
13. Chello M, Mastroroberto P *et al.* Protection by coenzyme Q_{10} from myocardial reperfusion injury during coronary artery bypass grafting. *Ann. Thorac. Surg.* 58: 1427–1432 (1994).

14. Chen FU, Lin YT, Wu SC. Effectiveness of coenzyme Q_{10} on myocardial preservation during hypothermic cardioplegic arrest. *J. Thorac. Cardiovasc. Surg.* 107: 242–247 (1994).
15. Taggart DP, Jenkins M *et al.* Effects of short-term supplementation with coenzyme Q_{10} on myocardial protection during cardiac operations. *Ann. Thorac. Surg.* 61: 829–833 (1996).
16. Zhou M, Zhi Q, Yu D, Han J. Effects of coenzyme Q_{10} on myocardial protection during cardiac valve replacement and scavenging free radical activity *in vitro*. *J. Cardiovasc. Surg.* 40: 355–361 (1999).
17. Alleva R, Tomasetti M, Battino M, Curatola G, Littarru GP, Folkers K. The roles of coenzyme Q and vitamin E on the peroxidation of human low density lipoprotein subfractions. *Proc. Natl. Acad. Sci. USA* 92: 9388–9391 (1995).
18. Tomono Y, Hasegawa J, Seki T, Motegi K, Morishita N. Pharmacokinetic study of deuterium-labelled coenzyme Q_{10} in humans. *Int. J. Pharmacol. Ther. Toxicol.* 24: 536–541 (1986).
19. Frei B, Kim MC, Ames BN. Ubiquinol-10 is an effective lipid-soluble antioxidant at physiological concentrations. *Proc. Natl. Acad. Sci. USA* 87: 4879–4883 (1990).
20. Stocker R, Bowry VW, Frei B. Ubiquinol-10 protects human low density lipoprotein more efficiently against lipid peroxidation than does alpha-tocopherol. *Proc. Natl. Acad. Sci. USA* 88: 1646–1650 (1991).
21. Ferrara N, Abete P, Ambrosio G *et al.* Protective role of chronic ubiquinone administration on acute cardiac oxidative stress. *J. Pharmacol. Exp. Ther.* 274: 858–865 (1995).
22. Glinn MA, Lee CP, Ernster L. Pro- and anti-oxidant activities of the mitochondrial respiratory chain: factors influencing NAD(P)H-induced lipid peroxidation. *Biochem. Biophys. Acta* 1318: 246–254 (1997).
23. Ernst A, Stolzing A, Sandig G, Grune T. Antioxidants effectively prevent oxidation-induced protein damage in OLN 93 cells. *Arch. Biochem. Biophys.* 421: 54–60 (2004).
24. Tomasetti M, Littarru GP, Stocker R, Alleva R. Coenzyme Q_{10} enrichment decreases oxidative DNA damage in human lymphocytes. *Free Radic. Biol. Med.* 27: 1027–1032 (1999).
25. Constantinescu A, Maguire JJ, Packer L. Interactions between ubiquinones and vitamins in membranes and cells. *Mol. Aspects Med.* 15(Suppl): S57–S65 (1994).
26. Lawen A, Martinius RD, McMullen G *et al.* The universality of bioenergetic disease: the role of mitochondrial mutation and the putative inter-relationship

between mitochondria and plasma membrane NADH oxidoreductase. *Mol. Aspects Med.* 15: S13–S27 (1994).

27. Villalba JM, Navarro F, Gomez-Diaz C, Arroyo A, Bello RI, Navas P. Role of cytochrome b5 reductase on the antioxidant function of coenzyme Q in the plasma membrane. *Mol. Aspects Med.* 18(Suppl): S7–S13 (1997).
28. Crane FL, Sun IL, Barr R, Morrš DJ. Coenzyme Q in Golgi apparatus membrane redox activity and proton uptake. In: Folkers K, Yamamura Y (eds.) *Biomedical and Clinical Aspects of Coenzyme Q*. Elsevier, Amsterdam, 1984: pp. 77–86.
29. Vajo Z, King LM, Jonassen T, Wilkin DJ, Ho N, Munnich A, Clarke CA. Conservation of the *Caenorhabditis elegans* timing gene clk-1 from yeast to human: a gene required for ubiquinone biosynthesis with potential implications for aging. *Mamm. Genome* 10: 1000–1004 (1999).
30. Jonassen T, Clarke CF. Isolation and functional expression of human CoQ_3, a gene encoding a methyltransferase required for ubiquinone biosynthesis. *J. Biol. Chem.* 275: 12381–12387 (2000).
31. Ashby MN, Kutsunai SY, Ackerman S, Tzagoloff A, Edwards PA. CoQ_2 is a candidate for the structural gene encoding para-hydroxybenzoate: polyprenyltransferase. *J. Biol. Chem.* 267: 4128–4136 (1992).
32. Forsgren M, Attersand A, Lake S, Grunler J, Swiezewska E, Dallner G, Climent I. Isolation and functional expression of human CoQ_2, a gene encoding a polyprenyl transferase involved in the synthesis of CoQ. *Biochem. J.* 382: 519–526 (2004).
33. Weber C, Bysted A, Holmer G. Intestinal absorption of coenzyme Q_{10} in a meal or as capsules to healthy subjects. *Nutr. Res.* 17: 941–945 (1997).
34. Zhang Y, Aberg F, Appelkvist G, Dallner G, Ernster L. Uptake of dietary coenzyme Q supplement is limited in rats. *J. Nutr.* 125: 446–453 (1995).
35. Bhagavan HN, Chopra RK, Sinatra ST. Absorption and bioavailability of coenzyme Q_{10}. In: Ebadi M, Marwah J, Chopra R (eds.) *Mitochondrial Ubiquinone (Coenzyme Q_{10})*. Prominent Press, Scottsdale, AZ, 2001, pp. 143–149.
36. Chopra RK, Goldman R, Bhagavan HN. Relative bioavailability of coenzyme Q_{10} formulations. *J. Am. Pharm. Assoc.* 38: 262 (1998).
37. Chopra RK, Goldman R, Sinatra ST, Bhagavan HN. Relative bioavailability of coenzyme Q_{10} formulations in human subjects. *Int. J. Vitam. Nutr. Res.* 68: 109–113 (1998).
38. Weber C, Sejersgard Jakobsen T, Mortensen SA, Paulsen G, Holmer G. Antioxidative effect of dietary coenzyme Q_{10} in human blood plasma. *Int. J. Vit. Nutr. Res.* 64: 311–315 (1994).

39. Stocker R, Suarna C. Extracellular reduction of ubiquinone-1 and -10 by human Hep G2 and blood cells. *Biochem. Biophys. Acta* 88: 1646–1650 (1993).
40. Nakamura T, Sanma H, Himeno M, Kato K. Transfer of exogenous coenzyme Q_{10} to the inner membrane of heart mitochondria in rats. In: Yamamura Y, Folkers K, Ito Y (eds.) *Biochemical and Clinical Aspects of Coenzyme Q*. Elsevier/North-Holland Biochemical Press, Amsterdam, 1980, pp. 3–13.
41. Lenaz G, Fato R, Castelluccio C *et al.* An updating of the biochemical function of coenzyme Q in mitochondria. *Mol. Aspects Med.* 15(Suppl): S29–S36 (1994).
42. Rosenfeldt F, Marasco S, Lyon W *et al.* Coenzyme Q_{10} therapy before cardiac surgery improves mitochondrial function and *in vitro* contractility of myocardial tissue. *J. Thorac. Cardiovasc. Surg.* 129: 25–32 (2005).
43. Hill MF, Singal PK. Antioxidant and oxidative stress changes during heart failure subsequent to myocardial infarction in rats. *Am. J. Pathol.* 148: 291–300 (1996).
44. Dhalla AK, Singal PK. Antioxidant changes in hypertrophied and failing guinea pig hearts. *Am. J. Physiol.* 266: H1280–H1285 (1994).
45. Ide T, Tsutsui H, Kinugawa S *et al.* Direct evidence for increased hydroxyl radicals originating from superoxide in the failing myocardium. *Circ. Res.* 86: 152–157 (2000).
46. Singal PK, Dhalla AK, Hill M *et al.* Endogenous antioxidant changes in the myocardium in response to acute and chronic stress conditions. *Mol. Cell. Biochem.* 129: 179–186 (1993).
47. Belch JJ, Bridges AB, Scott N *et al.* Oxygen free radicals and congestive heart failure. *Br. Heart J.* 65: 245–248 (1991).
48. Cracowski JL, Tremel F, Marpeau C *et al.* Increased formation of F(2)-isoprostanes in patients with severe heart failure. *Heart* 84: 439–440 (2000).
49. Dhalla AK, Hill MF, Singal PK. Role of oxidative stress in transition of hypertrophy to heart failure. *J. Am. Coll. Cardiol.* 28: 506–514 (1996).
50. Singal PK, Siveski-Iliskovic N, Hill M *et al.* Combination therapy with probucol prevents Adriamycin-induced cardiomyopathy. *J. Mol. Cell. Cardiol.* 27: 1055–1063 (1995).
51. Kaul N, Siveski-Iliskovic N, Thomas TP *et al.* Probucol improves antioxidant activity and modulates development of diabetic cardiomyopathy. *Nutrition* 11: 551–554 (1995).
52. Kukin ML, Fuster V (eds.) *Oxidative Stress and Cardiac Failure*. Futura Publishing Company, Armonk, NY, 2003.

53. Cohn JN. Foreword. In: Kukin ML, Fuster V (eds.) *Oxidative Stress and Cardiac Failure*. Futura Publishing Company, Armonk, NY, 2003, pp. vii–viii.
54. Keogh A, Fenton S, Leslie C *et al.* Randomised double-blind, placebo-controlled trial of coenzyme Q_{10} therapy in class II and III systolic heart failure. *Heart Lung Circ. J.* 12: 135–141 (2003).
55. Soja A, Mortensen S. Treatment of congestive heart failure with coenzyme Q_{10} illuminated by meta-analysis of clinical trials. *Mol. Aspects Med.* 18(Suppl): S159–S168 (1997).
56. Rosenfeldt F, Hilton D, Pepe S, Krum H. Systematic review of effect of coenzyme Q_{10} in physical exercise, hypertension and heart failure. *Biofactors* 18: 91–100 (2003).
57. Hofman-Bang C, Rehnqvist N, Swedberg K, Wiklund I, Astrom H. Coenzyme Q_{10} as an adjunctive in the treatment of chronic congestive heart failure. The Q_{10} Study Group. *J. Card. Fail.* 1: 101–107 (1995).
58. Khatta M, Alexander BS, Krichten CM *et al.* The effect of coenzyme Q_{10} in patients with congestive heart failure. *Ann. Int. Med.* 132: 636–640 (2000).
59. Langsjoen PH, Vadhanavikit S, Folkers K. Response of patients in classes III and IV of cardiomyopathy to therapy in a blind and crossover trial with coenzyme Q_{10}. *Proc. Natl. Acad. Sci. USA* 82: 4240–4244 (1985).
60. Morisco C, Trimarco B, Condorelli M. Effect of coenzyme Q10 therapy in patients with congestive heart failure: a long-term multicenter randomized study. *Clin. Invest.* 71(Suppl): S134–S136 (1993).
61. Permanetter B, Rossy W, Klein G, Weingartner F, Seidl KF, Blomer H. Ubiquinone (coenzyme Q_{10}) in the long-term treatment of idiopathic dilated cardiomyopathy. *Eur. Heart J.* 13: 1528–1533 (1992).
62. Munkholm H, Hansen HH, Rasmussen K. Coenzyme Q_{10} treatment in serious heart failure. *Biofactors* 9: 285–289 (1999).
63. Poggesi L, Galanti G, Comeglio M, Toncelli L, Vinci M. Effect of coenzyme Q_{10} on left ventricular function in patients with dilative cardiomyopathy. *Curr. Ther. Res.* 49: 878–886 (1991).
64. Watson PS, Scalia GM, Galbraith A, Burstow DJ, Bett N, Aroney CN. Lack of effect of coenzyme Q_{10} on left ventricular function in patients with congestive heart failure. *J. Am. Coll. Cardiol.* 33: 1549–1552 (1999).
65. Mortensen SA. Overview of coenzyme Q_{10} as adjunctive therapy in chronic heart failure. Rationale, design and end-points of "Q-symbio" — A multinational trial. *Biofactors* 18: 79–89 (2003).

66. Langsjoen PH, Langsjoen AM. The clinical use of HMG CoA-reductase inhibitors and the associated depletion of coenzyme Q_{10}. A review of animal and human publications. *Biofactors* 18: 101–111 (2003).
67. De Pinieux G, Chariot P, Ammi-Said M *et al.* Lipid-lowering drugs and mitochondrial function: effects of HMG-CoA reductase inhibitors on serum ubiquinone and blood lactate/pyruvate ratio. *Br. J. Clin. Pharmacol.* 42: 333–337 (1996).
68. Miyake Y, Shouzu A, Nishikawa M *et al.* Effect of treatment with 3-hydroxy-3-methylglutaryl coenzyme A reductase inhibitors on serum coenzyme Q_{10} in diabetic patients. *Arzneimittelforschung* 49: 324–329 (1999).
69. Folkers K, Drzewoski J, Richardson PC, Ellis J, Shizukuishi S, Baker L. Bioenergetics in clinical medicine. XVI: reduction of hypertension in patients by therapy with coenzyme Q_{10}. *Res. Commun. Chem. Pathol. Pharmacol.* 31: 129–139 (1981).
70. Digiesi V, Cantini F, Bisi G, Guarino GC, Oradei A, Littarru GP. Mechanism of action of coenzyme Q_{10} in essential hypertension. *Curr. Ther. Res.* 5: 668–672 (1992).
71. Digiesi V, Cantini F, Oradei A *et al.* Coenzyme Q_{10} in essential hypertension. *Mol. Aspects Med.* 15(Suppl): S257–S263 (1994).
72. Langsjoen P, Willis R, Folkers K. Treatment of essential hypertension with coenzyme Q_{10}. *Mol. Aspects Med.* 15(Suppl): S265–S272 (1994).
73. Yamagami T, Shibata N, Folkers K. Bioenergetics in clinical medicine: studies on coenzyme Q_{10} and essential hypertension. *Res. Commun. Chem. Pathol. Pharmacol.* 11: 273–287 (1975).
74. Singh RB, Niaz MA, Rastogi SS, Shukla PK, Thakur AS. Effect of hyrdosoluble coenzyme Q_{10} on blood pressures and insulin resistance in hypertensive patients with coronary artery disease. *J. Hum. Hypertens.* 13: 203–208 (1999).
75. Burke BE, Neuenschwander R, Olson RD. Randomised double-blind, placebo-controlled trial of coenzyme Q_{10} in isolated systolic hypertension. *South. Med. J.* 94: 1112–1117 (2001).
76. Hodgson JM, Watts GF, Playford DA, Burke V, Croft KD. Coenzyme Q_{10} improves blood pressure and glycaemic control: a controlled trial in subjects with type 2 diabetes. *Eur. J. Clin. Nutr.* 56: 1137–1142 (2002).
77. Kamikawa T, Kobayashi A, Yamashita T *et al.* Effects of CoQ_{10} on exercise tolerance in chronic stable angina pectoris. *Am. J. Cardiol.* 56: 247 (1985).
78. Schardt F, Welzel D, Schiess W, Toda K. Effect of CoQ_{10} on ischemia-induced ST-segment depression: a double-blind, placebo controlled,

crossover study. In: Folkers K, Yamamura Y (eds.) *Biochemical and Clinical Aspects of CoQ_{10}*. Elsevier, Amsterdam, 1985, pp. 385–394.

79. Tanaka J, Tominaga R *et al.* Coenzyme Q_{10}: the prophylactic effect on low cardiac output following cardiac valve replacement. *Ann. Thorac. Surg.* 33: 145–151 (1982).
80. Shiguma S, Ohmori H, Kimura H *et al.* The protective effect of coenzyme Q_{10} on myocardial metabolism and hemodynamics in open heart surgery (in Japanese). *Kyobu Geka* 36: 268–271 (1983).
81. Sunamori M, Tanaka H, Maruyama T *et al.* Clinical experience of coenzyme Q_{10} to enhance intraoperative myocardial protection in coronary artery revascularization. *Cardiovasc. Drug. Ther.* 5: S297–S300 (1991).
82. Judy WV, Stogsdill WW *et al.* Myocardial preservation by therapy with coenzyme Q_{10} during heart surgery. *Clin. Invest.* 71: S155–S161 (1993).
83. Shults CW, Haas RH, Passov D, Beal MF. Coenzyme Q_{10} levels correlate with the activities of complexes I and II/III in mitochondria from Parkinsonian and non-Parkinsonian subjects. *Ann. Neurol.* 42: 261–264 (1997).
84. Shults CW, Oakes D, Kieburtz K *et al.* Effect of coenzyme Q_{10} in early Parkinson disease: evidence of slowing of the functional decline. *Arch. Neurol.* 59: 1541–1550 (2002).
85. Cooper JM, Schapira AHV. Friedreich's ataxia: disease mechanisms, antioxidant and coenzyme Q_{10} therapy. *Biofactors* 18: 163–171 (2003).
86. Mariotti C, Solari A, Torta D, Marano L, Fiorentini C, Di Donato S. Idebenone treatment in Friedreich patients: one-year long randomized placebo-controlled trial. *Neurology* 60: 1676–1679 (2003).
87. Ferrante RJ, Andreassen OA, Dedeoglu A *et al.* Therapeutic effects of coenzyme Q_{10} and remacemide in transgenic mouse models of Huntington's disease. *J. Neurosci.* 22: 1592–1599 (2002).
88. The Huntington Study Group. A randomized, placebo-controlled trial of coenzyme Q_{10} and remacemide in Huntington's disease. *Neurology* 57: 375–376 (2001).
89. Sjodin B, Hellsten Y, Apple FS. Biochemical mechanism for oxygen free radical formation during exercise. *Sports Med.* 10: 236–254 (1990).
90. Dekkers JC, van Doornen LJP, Kemper HCG. The role of antioxidant vitamins and enzymes in the prevention of exercise-induced muscle damage. *Sports Med.* 21: 213–238 (1996).
91. Amadio E, Palermo R, Peloni G, Littarru G. Effect of CoQ_{10} administration on VO_2max and diastolic function in athletes. In: Folkers K, Littarru GP, Yamagami T, (eds.) *Biochemical and Clinical Aspects of Coenzyme Q_{10}*. Elsevier, Amsterdam, 1991, pp. 525–533.

92. Fiorella PL, Bargossi AM, Grossi G *et al.* Metabolic effects of coenzyme Q_{10} treatment in high level athletes. In: Folkers K, Littarru GP, Yamagami T (eds.) *Biochemical and Clinical Aspects of Coenzyme Q_{10}*. Elsevier, Amsterdam, 1991, pp. 513–520.
93. Bonetti A, Solito F, Carmosino G, Bargossi AM, Fiorella PL. Effect of ubidecarenone oral treatment on aerobic power in middle-aged trained subjects. *J. Sports Med. Phys. Fitness* 40: 51–57 (2000).
94. Ylikoski T, Piirainen J, Hanninen O, Penttinen J. The effect of coenzyme Q_{10} on the exercise performance of cross-country skiers. *Mol. Aspects Med.* 18(Suppl): S283–S290 (1997).
95. Wyss V, Lubich T, Ganzit GP *et al.* Remarks on prolonged ubiquinone administration in physical exercise. In: Lenaz G, Bernabei O, Rabbi A, Battino M (eds.) *Highlights in Ubiquinone Research.* Taylor & Francis, London, pp. 303–308 (1990).
96. Zeppilli P, Merlino B, De Luca A *et al.* Influence of coenzyme Q_{10} on physical work capacity in athletes, sedentary people and patients with mitochondrial disease. In: Folkers K, Littarru GP, Yamagami T (eds.) *Biochemical and Clinical Aspects of Coenzyme Q_{10}*. Elsevier, Amsterdam, 1991.
97. Braun B, Clarkson PM, Freedson PS, Kohl RL. Effects of coenzyme Q_{10} supplementation on exercise performance, VO_2max, and lipid peroxidation in trained cyclists. *Int. J. Sport Nut.* 1: 353–365 (1991).
98. Porter DA, Costill DL, Zachwieja JJ *et al.* The effect of oral coenzyme Q_{10} on the exercise tolerance of middle-aged, untrained men. *Int. J. Sports Med.* 16: 421–427 (1995).
99. Weston B, Zhou S, Weatherby RP, Robson SJ. Does exogenous coenzyme Q_{10} affect aerobic capacity in endurance athletes? *Int. J. Sport. Nutr.* 7: 197–206 (1997).
100. Snider IP, Bazzarre TL, Murdoch SD, Goldfarb A. Effects of coenzyme athletic performance system as an ergogenic aid on endurance performance to exhaustion. *Int. J. Sport Nutr.* 2: 272–286 (1992).
101. Laakosenen R, Fogelholm M, Himberg JJ, Laakso J, Salorinne Y. Ubiquinone supplementation and exercise capacity in trained young and older men. *Eur. J. Appl. Physiol.* 72: 95–100 (1995).
102. Hagen TM, Ingersoll RT, Lykkesfeldt J *et al.* (R)-alpha-lipoic acid-supplemented old rats have improved mitochondrial function, decreased oxidative damage, and increased metabolic rate. *FASEB J.* 13: 411–418 (1999).
103. Ziegler D, Nowak H, Kempler P, Vargha P, Low PA. Treatment of symptomatic diabetic polyneuropathy with the antioxidant alpha-lipoic acid: a meta-analysis. *Diabet. Med.* 21: 114–121 (2004).

104. Cadenas E, Packer L. Antioxidants in health and disease. In: Packer L, Fuchs J (eds.) *Handbook of Antioxidants*, Vol. 3. Marcel Dekker, New York, 1996.
105. Hadj A, Esmore DS, Rowland MA, Lewin J, Rosenfeldt FL. Preoperative preparation for cardiac surgery utilising a combination of metabolic, physical and mental therapy. *Heart Lung Circ. J.* (2005), submitted.

35 Plant-Derived Antioxidants

Fazlul H. Sarkar and Yiwei Li

1. Introduction

As humans live in an aerobic environment, their exposure to reactive oxygen species (ROS) is continuous and unavoidable. The biological systems in the human body interact with the external environment to maintain an internal environment that favors survival, growth, differentiation, and reproduction. Although a number of defense systems have evolved to combat the accumulation of ROS, these defense systems are not always adequate to counteract the production of ROS, resulting in a state of oxidative stress.[1] It is important to note that oxidative stress has been linked to aging and a variety of chronic diseases such as atherosclerosis, neurodegenerative diseases, diabetes, pulmonary fibrosis, arthritis.[2,3] More importantly, oxidative stress could be carcinogenic because ROS can cause severe DNA damage, which plays an important role in carcinogenesis.[2,4] Once DNA damage occurs, DNA repair is a critical process in order to prevent mutagenesis. However, under oxidative stress, the repair of DNA damage can be inhibited by several redox-dependent metals, resulting in carcinogenesis.[4] Moreover, the activation of nuclear factor-kappa B (NF-κB) by ROS under oxidative stress has been known as a key event in carcinogenesis.[4] Therefore, antioxidants are important in combating cancers and some chronic diseases, which have been tightly linked with oxidative stress.

In nature, to resist oxygenic threat, antioxidants have evolved in parallel with our oxygenic atmosphere. Plants employ antioxidants to defend their structures against ROS produced during photosynthesis.[5] Plants, therefore, produce various antioxidant components, which could be beneficial for human health. A variety of plant-derived components have been found to reduce oxidative stress via the antioxidant mechanism. Among them, isoflavones, curcumin, epigallocatechin-3-gallate, indole-3-carbinol (I3C), resveratrol, lycopene, vitamin E, and vitamin C have shown more promising effects on the reduction of oxidative stress.[6–12] Most of them have been found to inhibit NF-κB activation stimulated by ROS.[13–20] Moreover, these antioxidants have shown their inhibitory effects on atherosclerosis, neurodegeneration, oncogenesis, cancer growth, and metastasis,[21–24] suggesting that they could be used as chemopreventive and/or chemotherapeutic agents for some chronic diseases and cancers.

2. Oxidative Stress and NF-κB Activation in Chronic Diseases and Cancers

It has been well known that NF-κB activation stimulated by ROS is a very important event in the development of some chronic diseases and cancers,[25,26] which are linked with oxidative stress. Under the situation of oxidative stress, ROS induces DNA damage and alters cell signal transduction pathways including the NF-κB pathway.[27] The direct addition of H_2O_2 to culture medium activates NF-κB in many types of cell lines.[28] In addition, it has been found that ROS in cells is increased in response to the agents that also activate NF-κB.[28,29] These findings suggest that oxidative stress activates NF-κB activity in cells.

NF-κB plays important roles in the physiological processes as well as in the defensive response to injury, infection, and other stress conditions.[30] The NF-κB family is composed of several proteins: RelA (p65), RelB, c-Rel, NF-κB1 (p50), and NF-κB2 (p52), each of which may form homo- or heterodimers.[31,32] In human cells without specific extracellular signal, NF-κB is sequestered in the cytoplasm through tight association with its inhibitors: IκB, which acts as NF-κB inhibitor, and p100 proteins, which serve as both inhibitors and precursors of NF-κB DNA-binding subunits.[31,33] NF-κB can be activated by many types of stimuli including tumor necrosis factor-α (TNF-α), ultraviolet radiation, H_2O_2, free radicals, etc. The activation of NF-κB occurs through phosphorylation of IκB by

IKKβ and/or phosphorylation of p100 by IKKα, leading to degradation of IκB and/or the processing of p100 into a small form (p52). This process allows two forms of activated NF-κB (p50–p65 and p52–RelB) to become free, translocate into nucleus, bind to NF-κB-specific DNA-binding sites, and regulate downstream gene transcription.[33,34]

In this way, NF-κB controls the expression of many genes that are involved in cellular physiological processes including stress response, inflammation, differentiation, cell growth, apoptosis, etc.[35–37] The disorder of these physiological processes has been demonstrated to be linked with the occurrence of some chronic diseases and cancers. It has been reported that overexpression of NF-κB protects cells from apoptosis and favors cell survival, while inhibition or absence of NF-κB induces apoptosis.[38] An *in vivo* study showed that mice lacking NF-κB p65 died embryonically from extensive apoptosis in the liver, suggesting the anti-apoptotic role of NF-κB.[39] The deregulated cell proliferation or inability of cells to undergo apoptotic cell death results in the development of cancers. NF-κB also promotes the expression of genes related to inflammation and degeneration, resulting in chronic inflammatory and degenerative diseases.[25,40,41] Therefore, the deregulated NF-κB under oxidative stress has been described as a major cause in cancers and some of the chronic diseases.[26,40]

3. NF-κB as a Preventive or Therapeutic Target in Inflammatory Diseases and Cancers

Inhibition of NF-κB activation stimulated by ROS is now widely recognized as a valid strategy to combat inflammatory disease.[25,42] However, it has become obvious that inhibition of NF-κB activity is not only desirable for the treatment of inflammation but also in cancer therapy.[43,44] Examination of the inflammatory microenvironment in neoplastic tissues has supported the hypothesis that inflammation is a cofactor in oncogenesis for a variety of cancers. Many anti-inflammation drugs and antioxidants inhibit NF-κB activity and induce apoptosis; therefore, they may also be desirable in the treatment of cancers.

Experimental studies have shown the cellular growth and anti-apoptotic activity of NF-κB in malignant cells.[45,46] It has been reported that NF-κB is constitutively activated in Hodgkin's tumor cells, whereas inhibition of NF-κB blocks the cell growth.[46] It has been demonstrated that NF-κB regulates growth and survival of multiple myeloma and that NF-κB is a novel therapeutic target in multiple myeloma.[47] Our data also showed that plant-derived antioxidant compounds including genistein, I3C, and 3,3′-diindolylmethane (DIM) inhibited the activity of NF-κB and the growth of cancer cells, and induced apoptosis in cancer cells,[13,17,48] suggesting that NF-κB is a target for cancer prevention and/or treatment.

Now it has become more obvious that inhibition of NF-κB activity is desirable in the prevention and treatment of cancers and inflammations. Thus, plant-derived antioxidants with NF-κB inactivation activity may serve as agents against cancers and some chronic diseases.

4. Plant-Derived Antioxidants Inhibiting Oxidative Stress and NF-κB Activation

4.1. *Isoflavones*

Isoflavones are a subclass of the more ubiquitous flavonoids and are much more narrowly distributed in soybeans. Genistein, daidzein, and glycitein are three main isoflavones found in soybeans. Genistein and daidzein have been found in relatively high concentration in soybeans and most soy-protein products, while much lower amounts of glycitein are present in soybeans. Experimental studies have revealed that isoflavones, particularly genistein, exert antioxidant effects on human cells. It has been reported that genistein protects cells against ROS by scavenging free radicals and reducing the expression of stress-response-related genes.[6,49] Isoflavones also stimulate antioxidant protein gene expression in Caco-2 cells.[50] Sierens *et al.*[51] have found that isoflavone supplementation reduces hydrogen peroxide-induced DNA damage in sperm, suggesting the antioxidant effects of isoflavone. In addition, it has been found that isoflavones and synthetic isoflavone derivatives suppress lipid peroxidation of human high-density lipoproteins, decrease oxidized low-density lipoproteins, and reduced atherosclerotic plaque thickness, suggesting their preventive and therapeutic effects on cardiovascular diseases.[52,53] Kawakami *et al.*[54] have also reported that soy isoflavones may reduce the risk of some cardiovascular diseases through their radical scavenging function and hypocholesterolemic action. Moreover, it has been demonstrated that genistein inhibits tumor promoter 12-*O*-tetradecanoylphorbol-13-acetate induced hydrogen peroxide production in human polymorphonuclear leukocytes and HL-60 cells, suggesting the inhibitory effect of genistein on carcinogenesis through antioxidant mechanism.[55]

4.1.1. *Inhibition of oxidative stress and NF-κB activation in vitro by soy isoflavone genistein*

Our laboratory has investigated whether genistein treatment could modulate NF-κB DNA binding activity in PC3 and LNCaP prostate cancer cells by electrophoresis mobility shift assay (EMSA). We found that 50 μM genistein treatment for 24–72 h significantly inhibited NF-κB DNA-binding activity in both cell lines.[13] We further investigated whether genistein could block NF-κB induction by oxidative stress inducers, H_2O_2 and TNF-α,[13] both of which have been previously shown to induce NF-κB DNA-binding activity. After treatment with H_2O_2 or TNF-α, we observed an increase in NF-κB DNA-binding activity in prostate cancer cell lines, as expected. However, when the cells were pre-treated with genistein for 24 h prior to stimulation with the inducing agent, genistein abrogated the induction of NF-κB DNA-binding activity elicited by either H_2O_2 or TNF-α. Western blot analysis of nuclear extracts showed similar results.[13] These results demonstrated that genistein not only reduced NF-κB DNA-binding activity in non-stimulated conditions, but inhibited NF-κB activation in cells under oxidative stress condition.

Other investigators also demonstrated similar effect of genistein on NF-κB in different types of cells. Baxa and Yoshimura[54] showed that genistein reduced NF-κB in T lymphoma cells via a caspase-mediated cleavage of IκBα. Tabary *et al.*[57] also found that genistein inhibited constitutive and inducible NF-κB activation and decreased interleukin-8 production in human cystic fibrosis bronchial gland cells. Our *in vitro* data along with results from other investigators suggested that genistein functions as an antioxidant, which could be a potent agent for the inhibition of oxidative stress and the prevention and/or treatment of cancers.

4.1.2. *Inhibition of oxidative stress and NF-κB activation in vivo by soy isoflavones*

Since our *in vitro* results showed inactivation of NF-κB by genistein treatment, we further investigated the effect of isoflavone supplementation on NF-κB activation *in vivo* in human volunteers.[14] The lymphocytes from healthy male subjects were harvested from peripheral blood and cultured for 24 h in the absence and presence of genistein. EMSA revealed that genistein treatment inhibited basal levels of NF-κB DNA-binding activity by 56% and abrogated TNF-α-induced NF-κB activity by 50%.[14] Furthermore, when human volunteers received 50 mg of soy isoflavone supplements (Novasoy™) twice daily for three weeks, TNF-α failed to activate NF-κB activity in lymphocytes harvested from these volunteers, while lymphocytes from these volunteers collected prior to soy isoflavone intervention showed activation of NF-κB DNA-binding activity upon TNF-α treatment *in vitro*.[14]

We further measured the levels of oxidative DNA damage in the blood of the six subjects before and after supplementation with Novasoy™. DNA was isolated from lymphocyte nuclei from the six subjects and analyzed for levels of 5-OHmdU, a modified DNA base that represents the endogenous status of cellular oxidative stress. We found that the mean value of 5-OHmdU was significantly decreased after three weeks of soy supplementation.[14] These results have demonstrated that isoflavone supplementation is very effective in reducing the level of 5-OhmdU, decreasing oxidative damage, and inhibition of NF-κB activation in humans *in vivo*, providing strong evidence that soy isoflavone functions as an antioxidant and that these effects of isoflavone may be responsible for its chemopreventive activity.

4.1.3. *The effects of soy isoflavone genistein on cancer cells*

The effects of isoflavone genistein on cancer cells have been widely studied in various cancer cells. The results from our laboratory and other investigators have revealed that genistein inhibits the growth of various cancer cells including leukemia, lymphoma, neuroblastoma, breast, prostate, lung, gastric, head, and neck cancer cells.[13,58–65] We and other investigators have also found that genistein induces apoptosis with modulation of expression of genes related to apoptotic processes.[49,61,63–65] Genistein has been shown to regulate the molecules in cell signaling pathways including Akt, NF-κB, MAPK, p53, AR, and ER pathways.[48,62] By microarray and reverse transcriptase-polymerase chain reaction analysis, we have also found that genistein regulates the expression of genes that are critically involved in the control of cell growth, cell cycle, apoptosis, cell signaling transduction, angiogenesis, tumor cell invasion, and metastasis,[66,67] suggesting its pleiotropic effects on cancer cells. These effects make isoflavone a promising agent against oxidative stress, some chronic diseases, and cancers.

4.2. *Indole-3-carbinol and 3,3′-diindolylmethane*

I3C is produced from naturally occurring glucosinolates contained in a wide variety of plants including members of the family Cruciferae, and particularly members of the genus *Brassica*. I3C is biologically active and it is easily converted *in vivo* to its dimeric product DIM. Under the acidic conditions of the stomach, I3C undergoes extensive and rapid self-condensation reactions to form several derivatives.[68] DIM is the major derivative and condensation product of I3C and it is also biologically active. The formation of DIM from I3C has been believed to be a likely prerequisite for I3C-induced anti-carcinogenesis. I3C and DIM have been shown to reduce oxidative stress and stimulate antioxidant response element-driven gene expression as antioxidants.[69,70] Furthermore, we and other investigators have found that I3C and DIM inhibit oncogenesis and cancer cell growth, and induce apoptosis in various cancer cells,[9,17,71–73] suggesting that I3C and DIM may serve as potent agents for prevention and/or treatment of cancers.

We have also investigated whether I3C treatment could inhibit NF-κB DNA-binding activity in prostate and breast cancer cells by EMSA.[17,73] Cancer cells were treated with 60 or 100 μmol/l I3C for 48 h or with 20 μg/l TNF-α for 10 min. Nuclear proteins were harvested from samples, incubated in DNA-binding buffer with ^{32}P labeled NF-κB consensus oligonucleotide, and subjected to 8% non-denatured polyacrymide gel. After drying the gel, autoradiography of the gel showed that TNF-α treatment stimulated NF-κB activation as expected; however, I3C significantly inhibited NF-κB DNA-binding activity in prostate and breast cancer cells, corresponding with the inhibition of cell proliferation and the induction of apoptosis by I3C in prostate and breast cancer cells.[17,73] These results suggest that inhibition of NF-κB activity by I3C may reduce the oxidative stress induced by ROS or TNF-α.

4.3. *Curcumin*

Curcumin is a compound from *Curcuma longa* (tumeric). *C. longa* is a plant widely cultivated in tropical regions of Asia and Central America. Turmeric extract from the rhizomes, commonly called curcuminoids, is mainly composed of curcumin. Curcumin has recently received considerable attention due to its pronounced anti-inflammatory, anti-oxidative, immunomodulating, anti-atherogenic, and anti-carcinogenic activities.[7,74–76]

Curcumin is a potent scavenger of oxygen free radicals such as hydroxyl radical and nitrogen dioxide radical.[77] It has been reported that curcumin inhibits lipid peroxidation in rat brain, liver, and lens, suggesting its antioxidant properties.[78–80] Chuang *et al.*[81] have shown that curcumin inhibits diethylnitrosamine-induced liver inflammation and activation of NF-κB in rats. Curcumin can also protect against inflammation-related changes. Administration of curcumin decreases the level of the prostanoids in alcohol toxicity model, suggesting its protective effects against inflammation.[82] It has been reported that curcumin inhibited IKK, suppressed both constitutive and inducible NF-κB activation, and potentiated TNF-induced apoptosis.[83] Curcumin also showed strong antioxidant and anticancer properties through regulating the expression of genes that require the activation of activator protein 1 and NF-κB.[84] It has been known that curcumin inhibits the growth of cancer cells, induces apoptosis, reduces cell survival signal protein Akt, and regulates the expression of genes related to anti-invasion.[15,85–87] In addition, NF-κB has been implicated in the development of drug resistance in cancer cells. Curcumin has been found to significantly inhibit chemotherapeutic agent doxorubicin-induced NF-κB activation,[88] suggesting its effect on reducing drug resistance and sensitizing cancer cell to chemotherapeutic agents.

4.4. *Epigallocatechin-3-gallate*

Consumption of green tea has been associated with human health including the prevention of cancer and heart disease. Green tea and its constituents have been studied both *in vitro* and *in vivo*. Green tea contains several catechins including epicatechin, epigallocatechin, epicatechin-3-gallate, and epigallocatechin-3-gallate (EGCG). However, EGCG has been believed to be the most potent for inhibition of oncogenesis and reduction of oxidative stress among these catechins.[24,89]

EGCG has been shown to have strong antioxidant activity. It has been reported that EGCG treatment resulted in a significant dose- and time-dependent inhibition of activation and translocation of NF-κB to the nucleus by suppressing the degradation of IκBα in the cytoplasm.[90,91] EGCG has also been shown to inhibit activation of IKK and phosphorylation of IκBα, corresponding with the inhibition of activation of NF-κB.[92,93] There are growing evidences showing that EGCG inhibits the proliferation of various cancer cells and induces apoptotic processes in cancer cells,[24,89] suggesting its inhibitory effects on cancers. It has been found that EGCG had a concurrent effect on two important transcription factors, such as p53 (stabilization of p53) and NF-κB (negative regulation of NF-κB activity), and also caused a change in the ratio of Bax/Bcl-2 in a manner that favors apoptosis.[94] Moreover, EGCG has been found to reduce the levels of matrix metalloproteinases, suppress angiogenesis, and inhibit invasion and metastasis.[95,96] In addition, EGCG also prevents oxidative modification of low density lipoproteins in human and the development of atherosclerosis in apoprotein E-deficient mice,[97,98] suggesting that EGCG may reduce the risk of cardiovascular diseases.

4.5. *Resveratrol*

Resveratrol (3,5,4′-trihydroxystilbene) is a phytoalexin present in a wide variety of plant species including grapes, mulberries, and peanuts. Relatively high quantities of resveratrol are found in grapes. The concentration of resveratrol in red wine and grape juice is in the range of 0.05–10 mg/l, depending on grape cultivar, geographical origin, and process methodology.[10] Resveratrol has been shown to have beneficial effects on the reduction of oxidative stress and the prevention of heart diseases, degenerative diseases, and cancers.[10,99,100]

Resveratrol has been reported to modulate lipoprotein metabolism and to inhibit platelet aggregation and coagulation,[101] suggesting its preventive effects on cardiovascular diseases. It has been found that resveratrol reduces DNA damage and formation of A2E-epoxidation, which is implicated in the degenerative disease.[102] Moderate wine consumption has been associated with decreased odds of developing age-related degenerations.[103] Experimental studies have shown that resveratrol inhibits the growth of various cancer cells and induces apoptotic cell death.[104–107] The induction of apoptosis by resveratrol has been believed to be mediated through p53-depenedent, Fas, MAPK, or ceramide signaling pathway.[104–107] Resveratrol also shows their inhibitory effects on the activity of NF-κB,[18] suggesting its role as antioxidant contributing to cancer prevention and/or treatment.

4.6. *Lycopene*

Tomatoes are rich in lycopene, which is the pigment principally responsible for the deep-red color of tomato and its products. Tomato products including ketchup, tomato juice, and pizza sauce are the richest sources of lycopene in the US diet. The consumption of tomatoes and tomato products containing lycopene have been shown to be associated with decreased risk of chronic diseases such as cardiovascular diseases and cancers.[11]

Lycopene is a potent antioxidant. It has been found that lycopene, as a biologically occurring carotenoid, exhibits high physical quenching rate constant with singlet oxygen, suggesting its high activity as antioxidant.[108] Sesso *et al.*[109] have found that higher plasma lycopene concentrations are associated with a lower risk of cardiovascular diseases in women. The prevention of lipid peroxidation by lycopene may be one of the reasons that lycopene reduces the risk of atherosclerosis and cardiovascular diseases.[110] In addition to the effect on cardiovascular disease, lycopene also shows beneficial effects on cancer prevention and treatment. Giovannucci *et al.*[111] have reported that frequent consumption of tomato products is associated with a lower risk of prostate cancer. The inverse associations between plasma lycopene and prostate cancer have also been reported.[112] Experimental studies also show that lycopene inhibits cell growth in breast, prostate, and endometrial cancer cells with regulation of cell cycle-related genes.[113,114] Clinical trial have revealed that lycopene supplements reduce tumor size and PSA level in localized prostate cancers,[115] suggesting its promising effects on prostate cancer treatment.

4.7. *Vitamins and others*

Vitamin E (α-tocopherol) is a lipid-soluble antioxidant distributed in green leaf vegetables, nuts, seeds, sunflower, and plant oils. Plant oils are the main dietary source of vitamin E. Vitamin E exerts potent antioxidant effect. It has been reported that vitamin E inhibits NF-κB activation and NF-κB-dependent transcription, and induces differentiation through reduction of NF-κB,[19,116,117] suggesting that vitamin E may exert its antioxidant effect through modulation of NF-κB. Vitamin E supplement has been associated with decreased risk of degenerative disease and cardiovascular disease.[118,119] Vitamin E also shows its inhibitory effects on carcinogenesis.[120] Vitamin E and its deriver have been known to inhibit cancer cell growth via modulating cell cycle regulatory and apoptotic machineries,[121,122] suggesting their inhibitory effects on cancers.

Vitamin C is a water-soluble antioxidant. The sources of vitamin C are fruits and vegetables, particularly orange, strawberry, citrus, kiwi, Brussels sprouts, and cauliflower.[5] It has been reported that vitamin C inhibits NF-κB activation by the inhibition of IκBα phosphorylation or the activation of p38 mitogen-activated protein kinase.[20,123]

In addition to vitamin E and C, vitamin A, ginseng, ubiquinone, ginkgo, and docosahexaenoic acid have also been known as antioxidants.[22] They may have some beneficial effects on human health, particularly in chronic diseases including cancers.

5. Conclusions

Oxidative stress has been linked to aging, some chronic diseases, and carcinogenesis. NF-κB plays important roles in oxidative stress and carcinogenesis. Therefore, targeting NF-κB may be a novel and important preventive or therapeutic strategy against some chronic diseases and cancers. The plant-derived components (isoflavones, curcumin, EGCG, I3C, resveratrol, lycopene, vitamin E, vitamin C, etc.) have been found to reduce oxidative stress and inhibit NF-κB activation. They may have inhibitory effects on atherosclerosis, neurodegeneration, oncogenesis, cancer cell growth, and progression. These effects make them strong candidates as chemopreventive or therapeutic agents against cardiovascular diseases, degenerative diseases, and cancers.

Acknowledgments

Our work cited in this chapter was partly funded by grants from the National Cancer Institute, NIH (5R01CA083695 and 5R01CA101870, and 1R01CA108535) awarded to F.H.S. and also partly supported by a grant from the Department of Defense (DOD Prostate Cancer Research Program DAMD17-03-1-0042 awarded to F.H.S.).

References

1. Finkel T, Holbrook NJ. *Nature* 408: 239–247 (2000).
2. Davies KJ. *Biochem. Soc. Symp.* 61: 1–31 (1995).
3. Beal MF. *Free Radic. Biol. Med.* 32: 797–803 (2002).
4. Galaris D. Evangelou A. *Crit. Rev. Oncol. Hematol.* 42: 93–103 (2002).
5. Benzie IF. *Comp. Biochem. Physiol. A* 136: 113–126 (2003).
6. Ruiz-Larrea MB, Mohan AR, Paganga G, Miller NJ, Bolwell GP, Rice-Evans CA. *Free Radic. Res.* 26: 63–70 (1997).
7. Miquel J, Bernd A, Sempere JM, Diaz-Alperi J, Ramirez A. *Arch. Gerontol. Geriatr.* 34: 37–46 (2002).
8. Rietveld A, Wiseman S. *J. Nutr.* 133: 3285S–3292S (2003).
9. Chung FL, Morse MA, Eklind KI, Xu Y. *Ann. N.Y. Acad. Sci.* 686: 186–201 (1993).
10. Fremont L. *Life Sci.* 66: 663–673 (2000).
11. Heber D, Lu QY. *Exp. Biol. Med. (Maywood)* 227: 920–923 (2002).
12. Urso ML, Clarkson PM. *Toxicology* 189: 41–54 (2003).
13. Davis JN, Kucuk O, Sarkar FH. *Nutr. Cancer* 35: 167–174 (1999).
14. Davis JN, Kucuk O, Djuric Z, Sarkar FH. *Free Radic. Biol. Med.* 30: 1293–1302 (2001).
15. Aggarwal BB, Kumar A, Bharti AC. *Anticancer Res.* 23: 363–398 (2003).

16. Gupta S, Hastak K, Afaq F, Ahmad N, Mukhtar H. *Oncogene* 23: 2507–2522 (2004).
17. Chinni SR, Li Y, Upadhyay S, Koppolu PK, Sarkar FH. *Oncogene* 20: 2927–2936 (2001).
18. Estrov Z, Shishodia S, Faderl S, Harris D, Van Q, Kantarjian HM, Talpaz M, Aggarwal BB. *Blood* 102: 987–995 (2003).
19. Calfee-Mason KG, Spear BT, Glauert HP. *J. Nutr.* 132: 3178–3185 (2002).
20. Carcamo JM, Pedraza A, Borquez-Ojeda O, Golde DW. *Biochemistry* 41: 12995–13002 (2002).
21. Vinson JA, Teufel K, Wu N. *J. Agric. Food. Chem.* 52: 3661–3665 (2004).
22. Grundman M, Grundman M, Delaney P. *Proc. Nutr. Soc.* 61: 191–202 (2002).
23. Fleischauer AT, Simonsen N, Arab L. *Nutr. Cancer* 46: 15–22 (2003).
24. Lambert JD, Yang CS. *J. Nutr.* 133: 3262S–3267S (2003).
25. Makarov SS. *Mol. Med. Today* 6: 441–448 (2000).
26. Karin M, Cao Y, Greten FR, Li ZW. *Nat. Rev. Cancer* 2: 301–310 (2002).
27. Owuor ED, Kong AN. *Biochem. Pharmacol.* 64: 765–770 (2002).
28. Dudek EJ, Shang F, Taylor A. *Free Radic. Biol. Med.* 31: 651–658 (2001).
29. Toledano MB, Leonard WJ. *Proc. Natl. Acad. Sci. USA* 88: 4328–4332 (1991).
30. Lenardo MJ, Baltimore D. *Cell* 58: 227–229 (1989).
31. Ghosh G, van Duyne G, Ghosh S, Sigler PB. *Nature* 373: 303–310 (1995).
32. Muller CW, Rey FA, Harrison SC. *Nat. Struct. Biol.* 3: 224–227 (1996).
33. Israel A. *Nature* 423: 596–597 (2003).
34. Chen ZJ, Parent L, Maniatis T. *Cell* 84: 853–862 (1996).
35. Karin M, Delhase M. *Semin. Immunol.* 12: 85–98 (2000).
36. Chen F, Castranova V, Shi X. *Am. J. Pathol.* 159: 387–397 (2001).
37. Barkett M, Gilmore TD. *Oncogene* 18: 6910–6924 (1999).
38. Beg AA, Baltimore D. *Science* 274: 782–784 (1996).
39. Beg AA, Sha WC, Bronson RT, Ghosh S, Baltimore D. *Nature* 376: 167–170 (1995).
40. Nichols TC, Fischer TH, Deliargyris EN, Baldwin AS Jr. *Ann. Periodontol.* 6: 20–29 (2001).
41. Mattson MP, Camandola S. *J. Clin. Invest.* 107: 247–254 (2001).
42. Yamamoto Y, Gaynor RB. *J. Clin. Invest.* 107: 135–142 (2001).
43. Bharti AC, Aggarwal BB. *Biochem. Pharmacol.* 64: 883–888 (2002).
44. Orlowski RZ, Baldwin AS. *Trends Mol. Med.* 8: 385–389 (2002).
45. Aggarwal BB. *Biochem. Pharmacol.* 60: 1033–1039 (2000).
46. Bargou RC, Emmerich F, Krappmann D, Bommert K, Mapara MY, Arnold W, Royer HD, Grinstein E, Greiner A, Scheidereit C, Dorken B. *J. Clin. Invest.* 100: 2961–2969 (1997).

47. Hideshima T, Chauhan D, Richardson P, Mitsiades C, Mitsiades N, Hayashi T, Munshi N, Dang L, Castro A, Palombella V, Adams J, Anderson KC. *J. Biol. Chem.* 277: 16639–16647 (2002).
48. Li Y, Sarkar FH. *Clin. Cancer Res.* 8: 2369–2377 (2002).
49. Zhou Y, Lee AS. *J. Natl. Cancer Inst.* 90: 381–388 (1998).
50. Kameoka S, Leavitt P, Chang C, Kuo SM. *Cancer Lett.* 146: 161–167 (1999).
51. Sierens J, Hartley JA, Campbell MJ, Leathem AJ, Woodside JV. *Teratog. Carcinog. Mutagen.* 22: 227–234 (2002).
52. Ferretti G, Bacchetti T, Menanno F, Curatola G. *Atherosclerosis* 172: 55–61 (2004).
53. Jiang F, Jones GT, Husband AJ, Dusting GJ. *J. Vasc. Res.* 40: 276–284 (2003).
54. Kawakami Y, Tsurugasaki W, Yoshida Y, Igarashi Y, Nakamura S, Osada K. *J. Agric. Food Chem.* 52: 1764–1768 (2004).
55. Wei H, Wei L, Frenkel K, Bowen R, Barnes S. *Nutr. Cancer* 20: 1–12 (1993).
56. Baxa DM, Yoshimura FK. *Biochem. Pharmacol.* 66: 1009–1018 (2003).
57. Tabary O, Escotte S, Couetil JP, Hubert D, Dusser D, Puchelle E, Jacquot J. *Am. J. Pathol.* 155: 473–481 (1999).
58. Constantinou A, Kiguchi K, Huberman E. *Cancer Res.* 50: 2618–2624 (1990).
59. Buckley AR, Buckley DJ, Gout PW, Liang H, Rao YP, Blake MJ. *Mol. Cell Endocrinol.* 98: 17–25 (1993).
60. Zhou HB, Chen JJ, Wang WX, Cai JT, Du Q. *World J. Gastroenterol.* 10: 1822–1825 (2004).
61. Alhasan SA, Pietrasczkiwicz H, Alonso MD, Ensley J, Sarkar FH. *Nutr. Cancer* 34: 12–19 (1999).
62. Gong L, Li Y, Nedeljkovic-Kurepa A, Sarkar FH. *Oncogene* 22: 4702–4709 (2003).
63. Li Y, Bhuiyan M, Sarkar FH. *Int. J. Oncol.* 15: 525–533 (1999).
64. Li Y, Upadhyay S, Bhuiyan M, Sarkar FH. *Oncogene* 18: 3166–3172 (1999).
65. Lian F, Bhuiyan M, Li YW, Wall N, Kraut M, Sarkar FH. *Nutr. Cancer* 31: 184–191 (1998).
66. Li Y, Sarkar FH. *J. Nutr.* 132: 3623–3631 (2002).
67. Li Y, Sarkar FH. *Cancer Lett.* 186: 157–164 (2002).
68. Verhoeven DT, Verhagen H, Goldbohm RA, van den Brandt PA, van Poppel G. *Chem. Biol. Interact.* 103: 79–129 (1997).
69. Nho CW, Jeffery E. *Toxicol. Appl. Pharmacol.* 198: 40–48 (2004).
70. Benabadji SH, Wen R, Zheng JB, Dong XC, Yuan SG. *Acta Pharmacol. Sin.* 25: 666–671 (2004).
71. Sarkar FH, Rahman KM, Li Y. *J. Nutr.* 133: 2434S–2439S (2003).

72. Firestone GL, Bjeldanes LF. *J. Nutr.* 133: 2448S–2455S (2003).
73. Rahman KW, Li Y, Sarkar FH. *Nutr. Cancer* 48: 84–94 (2004).
74. Banerjee M, Tripathi LM, Srivastava VM, Puri A, Shukla R. *Immunopharmacol. Immunotoxicol.* 25: 213–224 (2003).
75. Ramirez-Tortosa MC, Mesa MD, Aguilera MC, Quiles JL, Baro L, Ramirez-Tortosa CL, Martinez-Victoria E, Gil A. *Atherosclerosis* 147: 371–378 (1999).
76. Rao CV, Rivenson A, Simi B, Reddy BS. *Cancer Res.* 55: 259–266 (1995).
77. Tonnesen HH, Greenhill JV. *Int. J. Pharm.* 87: 79–87 (1992).
78. Reddy AC, Lokesh BR. *Toxicology* 107: 39–45 (1996).
79. Awasthi S, Srivatava SK, Piper JT, Singhal SS, Chaubey M, Awasthi YC. *Am. J. Clin. Nutr.* 64: 761–766 (1996).
80. Shukla PK, Khanna VK, Khan MY, Srimal RC. *Hum. Exp. Toxicol.* 22: 653–658 (2003).
81. Chuang SE, Cheng AL, Lin JK, Kuo ML. *Food Chem. Toxicol.* 38: 991–995 (2000).
82. Jayadeep VR, Arun OS, Sudhakaran PR, Menon VP. *J. Nutr. Biochem.* 11: 509–514 (2000).
83. Bharti AC, Donato N, Singh S, Aggarwal BB. *Blood* 101: 1053–1062 (2003).
84. Duvoix A, Morceau F, Delhalle S, Schmitz M, Schnekenburger M, Galteau MM, Dicato M, Diederich M. *Biochem. Pharmacol.* 66: 1475–1483 (2003).
85. Radhakrishna PG, Srivastava AS, Hassanein TI, Chauhan DP, Carrier E. *Cancer Lett.* 208: 163–170 (2004).
86. Chen HW, Yu SL, Chen JJ, Li HN, Lin YC, Yao PL, Chou HY, Chien CT, Chen WJ, Lee YT, Yang PC. *Mol. Pharmacol.* 65: 99–110 (2004).
87. Chaudhary LR, Hruska KA. *J. Cell Biochem.* 89: 1–5 (2003).
88. Chuang SE, Yeh PY, Lu YS, Lai GM, Liao CM, Gao M, Cheng AL. *Biochem. Pharmacol.* 63: 1709–1716 (2002).
89. Mukhtar H, Ahmad N. *Toxicol. Sci.* 52: 111–117 (1999).
90. Afaq F, Adhami VM, Ahmad N, Mukhtar H. *Oncogene* 22: 1035–1044 (2003).
91. Ahmad N, Gupta S, Mukhtar H. *Arch. Biochem. Biophys.* 376: 338–346 (2000).
92. Chen PC, Wheeler DS, Malhotra V, Odoms K, Denenberg AG, Wong HR. *Inflammation* 26: 233–241 (2002).
93. Yang F, Oz HS, Barve S, de Villiers WJ, McClain CJ, Varilek GW. *Mol. Pharmacol.* 60: 528–533 (2001).

94. Hastak K, Gupta S, Ahmad N, Agarwal MK, Agarwal ML, Mukhtar H. *Oncogene* 22: 4851–4859 (2003).
95. Kim HS, Kim MH, Jeong M, Hwang YS, Lim SH, Shin BA, Ahn BW, Jung YD. *Anticancer Res.* 24: 747–753 (2004).
96. Jung YD, Ellis LM. *Int. J. Exp. Pathol.* 82: 309–316 (2001).
97. Miura Y, Chiba T, Tomita I, Koizumi H, Miura S, Umegaki K, Hara Y, Ikeda M, Tomita T. *J. Nutr.* 131: 27–32 (2001).
98. Miura Y, Chiba T, Miura S, Tomita I, Umegaki K, Ikeda M, Tomita T. *J. Nutr. Biochem.* 11: 216–222 (2000).
99. Dong Z. *Mutat. Res.* 523–524: 145–150 (2003).
100. Ignatowicz E, Baer-Dubowska W. *Pol. J. Pharmacol.* 53: 557–569 (2001).
101. Olas B, Wachowicz B, Saluk-Juszczak J, Zielinski T. *Thromb. Res.* 107: 141–145 (2002).
102. Sparrow JR, Vollmer-Snarr HR, Zhou J, Jang YP, Jockusch S, Itagaki Y, Nakanishi K. *J. Biol. Chem.* 278: 18207–18213 (2003).
103. Obisesan TO, Hirsch R, Kosoko O, Carlson L, Parrott M. *J. Am. Geriatr. Soc.* 46: 1–7 (1998).
104. Laux MT, Aregullin M, Berry JP, Flanders JA, Rodriguez E. *J. Altern. Complement. Med.* 10: 235–239 (2004).
105. Scarlatti F, Sala G, Somenzi G, Signorelli P, Sacchi N, Ghidoni R. *FASEB J.* 17: 2339–2341 (2003).
106. Delmas D, Rebe C, Lacour S, Filomenko R, Athias A, Gambert P, Cherkaoui-Malki M, Jannin B, Dubrez-Daloz L, Latruffe N, Solary E. *J. Biol. Chem.* 278: 41482–41490 (2003).
107. Shih A, Davis FB, Lin HY, Davis PJ. *J. Clin. Endocrinol. Metab.* 87: 1223–1232 (2002).
108. Di Mascio P, Kaiser S, Sies H. *Arch. Biochem. Biophys.* 274: 532–538 (1989).
109. Sesso HD, Buring JE, Norkus EP, Gaziano JM. *Am. J. Clin. Nutr.* 79: 47–53 (2004).
110. Visioli F, Riso P, Grande S, Galli C, Porrini M. *Eur. J. Nutr.* 42: 201–206 (2003).
111. Giovannucci E, Rimm EB, Liu Y, Stampfer MJ, Willett WC. *J. Natl. Cancer Inst.* 94: 391–398 (2002).
112. Lu QY, Hung JC, Heber D, Go VL, Reuter VE, Cordon-Cardo C, Scher HI, Marshall JR, Zhang ZF. *Cancer Epidemiol. Biomarkers Prev.* 10: 749–756 (2001).
113. Nahum A, Hirsch K, Danilenko M, Watts CK, Prall OW, Levy J, Sharoni Y. *Oncogene* 20: 3428–3436 (2001).
114. Kim L, Rao AV, Rao LG. *J. Med. Food* 5: 181–187 (2002).

115. Kucuk O, Sarkar FH, Djuric Z, Sakr W, Pollak MN, Khachik F, Banerjee M, Bertram JS, Wood DP Jr. *Exp. Biol. Med. (Maywood)* 227: 881–885 (2002).
116. Hirano F, Tanaka H, Miura T, Hirano Y, Okamoto K, Makino Y, Makino I. *Immunopharmacology* 39: 31–38 (1998).
117. Sokoloski JA, Hodnick WF, Mayne ST, Cinquina C, Kim CS, Sartorelli AC. *Leukemia* 11: 1546–1553 (1997).
118. Dutta A, Dutta SK. *J. Am. Coll. Nutr.* 22: 258–268 (2003).
119. Fariss MW, Zhang JG. *Toxicology* 189: 129–146 (2003).
120. Omer B, Akkose A, Kolanci C, Oner P, Ozden I, Tuzlali S. *J. Natl. Cancer Inst.* 89: 972–973 (1997).
121. Ni J, Chen M, Zhang Y, Li R, Huang J, Yeh S. *Biochem. Biophys. Res. Commun.* 300: 357–363 (2003).
122. Gunawardena K, Murray DK, Meikle AW. *Prostate* 44: 287–295 (2000).
123. Bowie AG, O'Neill LA. *J. Immunol.* 165: 7180–7188 (2000).

36 Oxidative Stress and Cancer Therapy

Kevin Pong

1. Free Radical Scavengers

Quercetin (QC, Fig. 1) is a naturally occurring plant flavonoid that has been evaluated in a number of disease models, including cancer, atherosclerosis, and prostatitis. In preclinical studies, QC significantly enhanced the growth inhibitory activity of cytarabine in leukemia cells. The combination of QC and cytarabine also provided a synergistic effect on colony formation of acute lymphoid leukemia and acute myeloid leukemia cells.[1] QC has also been shown to inhibit growth in the MCF-7 breast cancer and U937 monoblastoid cells,[2,3] and induce late G1 phase arrest in human ovarian carcinoma cells,[4] Although the mechanism of action is unclear, it has been suggested that its activity is mediated by binding to type II estrogen binding sites.

In a phase I trial, QC was administered by intravenous (IV) infusion to 51 patients with cancer. Nine of the patients displayed inhibition of lymphocyte tyrosine kinase phosphorylation 1 h after administration. One patient with end-stage metastatic ovarian cancer had a reduction in serum CA 125 from 295 to 55 units/ml following two courses of 420 mg QC. Another patient with metastatic hepatocellular carcinoma had a sustained decrease in serum α-fetoprotein following treatment with 60 mg QC.[5]

QC 12 (Fig. 1), a water-soluble prodrug of quercetin, was developed by ML Laboratories, in an attempt to overcome the adverse events produced by dimethylsulfoxide, the solvent used for the dissolution of quercetin. When QC 12 was given orally to six cancer patients, no plasma quercetin could

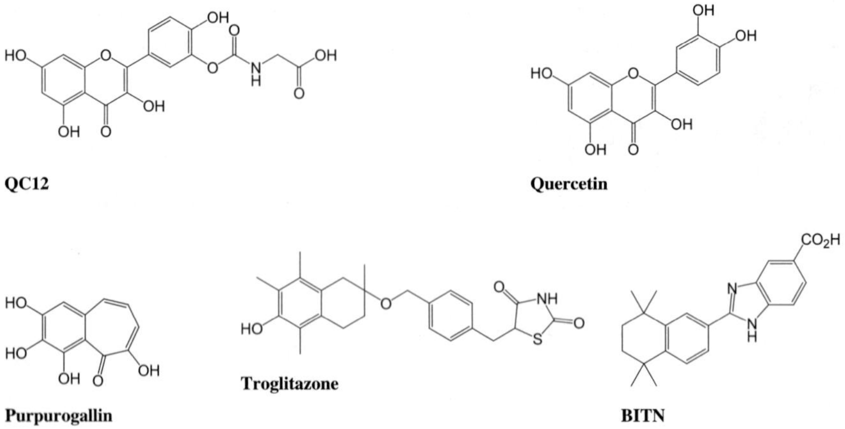

Fig. 1. Structures of free radical scavengers.

be detected, whereas detectable levels of quercetin were present in plasma following IV administration.[6] To date, there has been no development of QC 12 reported.

Troglitazone (TRO, Fig. 1) is a peroxisome proliferator-activated receptor-gamma agonist. In preclinical studies, TRO showed antiproliferative activity in cultured PC-3 prostate cancer cells. Treatment of PC-3 tumors in mice with TRO significantly inhibited proliferation. In addition, TRO induced necrosis in cultured human prostate cancers cells, which was not observed in normal prostate cells.[7] Although a phase II study in 41 men with advanced prostate cancer was conducted with TRO,[8] clinical development of this drug was later discontinued in the United States.

Purpurogallin (PPG, Fig. 1) is a natural product with antioxidant properties. Preclinical studies at the University of Toronto showed that PPG was able to inhibit DNA synthesis and oxidative stress in murine fibrosarcoma L-939 and human U-87 MG glioblastoma cells.[9] Although the preclinical data suggested a potential utility for PPG as an anticancer agent, no recent clinical development has been reported for this indication.

Benzimidazole tetranaphthalene (BITN, Fig. 1) is a retinoid compound that was synthesized by scientists at Ankara University, Turkey. BITN was found to be a more potent inhibitor of ethoxyresorufin O-deethylase

(EROD) and pentoxyresorufin O-depentylase (PROD) than retinoic acid (RA) and buthylated hydroxytoluen (BHT). Since EROD and PROD transform polycyclic hydrocarbons and aromatic amines to carcinogenic agents, BITN appears to be a more potent anticancer agent than RA and BHT.[10] Although the preclinical data suggested a potential utility for BITN as an anticancer agent, no recent clinical development has been reported for this indication.

2. Lipid Peroxidation Inhibitors

U-74500A (Fig. 2), developed at Pharmacia (now Pfizer), belongs to a series of 21 aminosteroids known as lazaroids. This class of compounds has been shown to inhibit the formation of free radicals and reverse oxidative damage and lipid peroxidation. Kim *et al.*[11] reported that U-74500A, in a dose-dependent manner, inhibited proliferation of human breast cancer cells. Although U-74500A also inhibited proliferation of mouse lymphocytes, its potency was significantly reduced, suggesting that human breast cancer cells are more sensitive to lazaroids than mouse lymphocytes. Similarly, human glioma cells exposed to U-74500A for 72 h showed marked reduction in proliferation. This reduction was enhanced with the co-administration of cisplatin.[12] Furthermore, these compounds were shown to be efficacious in models of neurodegenerative disorders,[13,14] myocardial infarction,[15] and organ transplantation.[16,17]

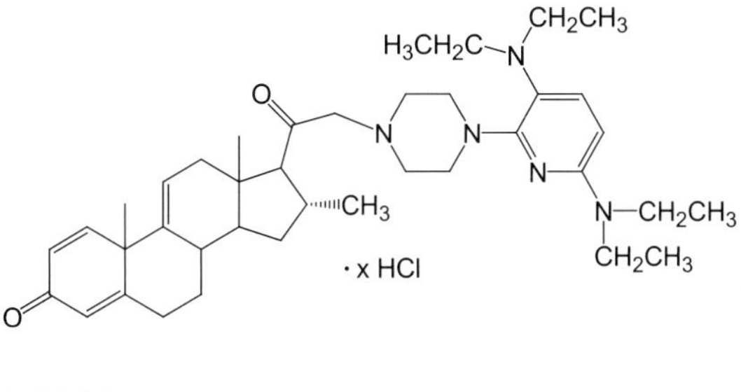

H_3CH_2C—N—CH_2CH_3

CH_3 · x HCl

N—CH_2CH_3 / CH_2CH_3

OH

O

U-74500A 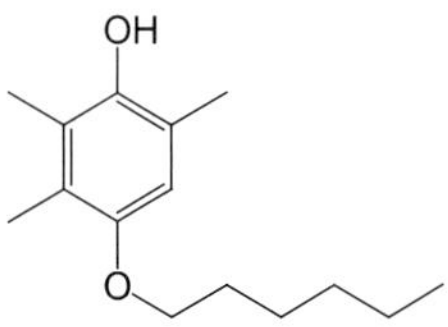 **HX 1171**

Fig. 2. Structures of lipid peroxidation inhibitors.

Although the preclinical data suggested a potential utility for U-74500A as an antiglioma agent, no recent clinical development has been reported for this indication.

HX 1171 (HTHQ, Fig. 2), developed by Nippon Hypox, is the most potent lipid peroxidation inhibitor from a series of hydroquinone monoalkyl ethers.[18] HTHQ was found to be a potent inhibitor of Glu-P-1 induced mutagenesis and hepatocarcinogenesis,[19,20] PhIP-induced mammary carcinogenesis in female rats,[21] DMBA-induced rat mammary tumor development,[22] PhIP-induced colon carcinogenesis,[23] and aminopyrine- and sodium nitrite-induced multi-organ carcinogenesis in rats.[24] Preclinical studies of HTHQ for cancer were discontinued for unspecified reasons.

3. SOD Mimetics

Endogenous free radical scavengers, such as the enzyme superoxide dismutase (SOD), catalytically destroy oxidants. Preclinical studies investigating the therapeutic utility of superoxide dismutase (SOD) in culture and animal disease models have yielded promising results.[25] A number of studies have investigated the clinical efficacy of SOD; however, the instability of the natural form of the enzyme, the immune response produced by the body, and the degradation of SOD enzymes by endogenous enzymes have limited the success and enthusiasm of developing a SOD therapeutic protein.[26] Because of these limitations, SOD mimetics have been developed as therapeutic agents, in this case, for cancer.

M 40403 (Fig. 3) is being developed by MetaPhore Pharmaceuticals as a candidate compound for oncology. M 40403 is a small molecule mimetic of SOD that removes free radicals at a greatly enhanced rate. Unlike naturally occurring SOD enzymes, the metal-based mimetic, in this case manganese, has a low molecular weight, is more stable, has a longer half-life, and does not induce an immune response.

Interleukin-2 (IL-2) is used to treat metastatic renal cell carcinoma and malignant melanoma. However, IL-2 induces hypotension, thereby limiting its dose. M 40403 has been shown to act synergistically with IL-2. More specifically, M 40403 reduced IL-2-induced hypotension, allowing the dose of IL-2 to be increased. Furthermore, subcutaneous implants of renal carcinoma in mice were also inhibited by the IL-2 and M 40403

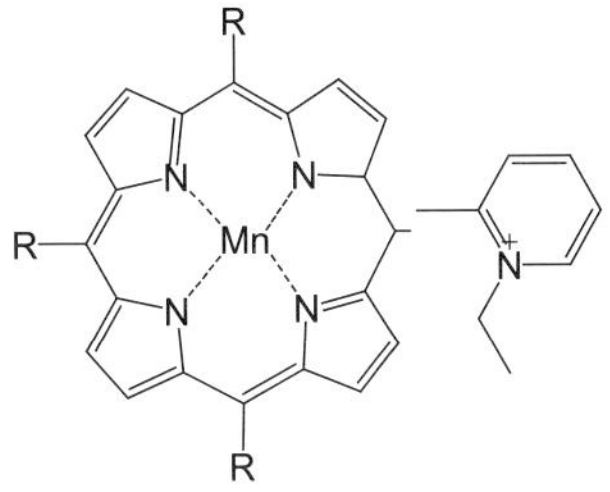

AEOL 10113 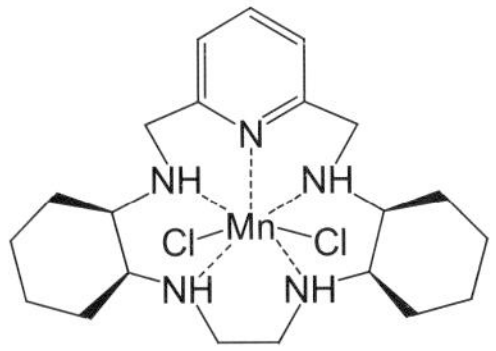 **M-40403**

Fig. 3. Structures of SOD mimetics.

combination therapy.[27] M 40403 has also been shown to be efficacious in models of arthritis,[28] ischemic injury,[29–31] and inflammatory pain.[32]

MetaPhore Pharmaceuticals has completed a phase I trial of IV administration of M 40403 in healthy human volunteers. There were no dose-limiting adverse events reported. A phase II trial of M 40403 in combination with IL-2 in patients with advanced skin cancer and end-stage kidney cancer is intended. This combination therapy may be an exciting and novel approach in treating cancer.[33]

AEOL 10113 (Fig. 3) is being developed by Incara Pharmaceuticals as an anticancer agent. In a mouse tumor model, treatment with AEOL 10113 reduced HIF-1 activation in tumors following radiation therapy (RT), preventing angiogenesis and delaying tumor growth (www.incara.com). In addition, AEOL 10113 has been shown to protect lung tissue from radiation-induced injury; RT is a key therapeutic approach in the treatment of thoracic tumors.[34] A phase I trial for cancer is planned for Q1 2005; however, Incara Pharmaceuticals is actively looking for a licensing partner for this indication.

4. Conclusions

Utility of broad-spectrum free radical scavengers and lipid peroxidation inhibitors have yielded mixed and disappointing results, in part, due to lack of robust efficacy or intolerable toxicity and adverse events (Table 1). However, small molecule SOD mimetics, like MetaPhore Pharmaceuticals' M 40403 and Incara Pharmaceuticals' AEOL 10113 appear to be well tolerated and are at least as potent as native enzyme, without the stability

Table 1. A partial list of antioxidant compounds, at various stages of development, for the treatment of cancer.

Company	Drug	Mechanism of action	Indication	Highest development status
Sankyo	Troglitazone	Free radical scavenger	Prostate cancer	Discontinued clinical
University of Birmingham (UK)	Quercetin	Free radical scavenger	Cancer	Phase I
Metaphore Pharmaceuticals	M-40403	SOD mimetic	Cancer	Phase I
Nippon Hypox	HX 1171	Lipid peroxidation inhibitor	Cancer	Discontinued preclinical
University of Toronto	Purpurogallin	Free radical scavenger	Cancer	Discontinued preclinical
Pharmacia (now Pfizer)	U74500A	Lipid peroxidation inhibitor	Glioma	Preclinical
ML Laboratories (UK)	QC 12	Free radical scavenger	Cancer	Preclinical
Ankara University (Turkey)	BITN	Free radical scavenger	Cancer	Preclinical
Aeolus Pharmaceuticals	AEOL-10113	SOD mimetic	Cancer	Preclinical

and size liabilities. In terms of their anticancer properties, M 40403 and AEOL 10113 are acting via different mechanisms of action, i.e., inhibition of IL-2-induced hypotension and antiangiogenesis properties. Structure–activity relationship studies may lead to the development of a SOD mimetic that possess both activities, thereby increasing its utility and potency in treating cancer. Taken together, SOD mimetics hold great promise in their potential utility as anticancer agents.

References

1. Teofili L, Pierelli L, Iovino MS, Leone G, Scambia G, De Vincenzo R, Benedetti-Panici P, Menichella G, Macri E, Piantelli M. The combination

of quercetin and cytosine arabinoside synergistically inhibits leukemic cell growth. *Leuk. Res.* 16: 497–503 (1992).
2. Scambia G, Ranelletti FO, Panici PB, De Vincenzo R, Bonanno G, Ferrandina G, Piantelli M, Bussa S, Rumi C, Cianfriglia M. Quercetin potentiates the effect of adriamycin in a multidrug-resistant MCF-7 human breast-cancer cell line: P-glycoprotein as a possible target. *Cancer Chemother. Pharmacol.* 34: 459–464 (1994).
3. Rong Y, Yang EB, Zhang K, Mack P. Quercetin-induced apoptosis in the monoblastoid cell line U937 *in vitro* and the regulation of heat shock proteins expression. *Anticancer Res.* 20: 4339–4345 (2000).
4. Shen F, Weber G. Synergistic action of quercetin and genistein in human ovarian carcinoma cells. *Oncol. Res.* 9: 597–602 (1997).
5. Ferry DR, Smith A, Malkhandi J, Fyfe DW, deTakats PG, Anderson D, Baker J, Kerr DJ. Phase I clinical trial of the flavonoid quercetin: pharmacokinetics and evidence for *in vivo* tyrosine kinase inhibition. *Clin. Cancer Res.* 2: 659–668 (1996).
6. Mulholland PJ, Ferry DR, Anderson D, Hussain SA, Young AM, Cook JE, Hodgkin E, Seymour LW, Kerr DJ. Pre-clinical and clinical study of QC12, a water-soluble, pro-drug of quercetin. *Ann. Oncol.* 12: 245–248 (2001).
7. Kubota T, Koshizuka K, Williamson EA, Asou H, Said JW, Holden S, Miyoshi I, Koeffler HP. Ligand for peroxisome proliferator-activated receptor gamma (troglitazone) has potent antitumor effect against human prostate cancer both *in vitro* and *in vivo. Cancer Res.* 58: 3344–3352 (1998).
8. Mueller E, Smith M, Sarraf P, Kroll T, Aiyer A, Kaufman DS, Oh W, Demetri G, Figg WD, Zhou XP, Eng C, Spegelman BM, Kantoff PW. Effects of ligand activation of peroxisome proliferators-activated receptor gamma in human prostate cancer. *Proc. Natl. Acad. Sci. USA* 97: 10990–10995 (2000).
9. Fung KP, Wu TW, Lui CP. Purpurogallin inhibits DNA synthesis of murine fibrosarcoma L-929 and human U-87 MG glioblastoma cells *in vitro. Chemotherapy* 42: 199–205 (1996).
10. Ates Z, Suzen S, Buyukbingol E, Can-Eke B, Iscan M. Effects of a benzimidazole compound on monooxygenase activities. *Farmaco* 52: 703–706 (1997).
11. Kim RS, Zaborniak CL, Begleiter A, LaBella FS. Antiproliferative properties of aminosteroid antioxidants on cultured cancer cells. *Cancer Lett.* 64: 61–66 (1992).
12. Savaraj N, Xu R. Cytotoxic effect of novel 21-amino steroid U-74500A alone and in combination with cisplatin in human glioma cells. *Proc. Am. Soc. Clin. Oncol.* 13: 179 (1994).

13. Hall ED. Novel inhibitors of iron-dependent lipid peroxidation for neurodegenerative disorders. *Ann. Neurol.* 32 (Suppl.): S137–S142 (1992).
14. Hall ED, McCall JM, Means ED. Therapeutic potential of the lazaroids (21-aminosteroids) in acute central nervous system trauma, ischemia, and subarachnoid hemorrhage. *Adv. Pharmacol.* 28: 221–268 (1994).
15. Levitt MA, Sievers RE, Wolfe CL. Reduction of infarct size during myocardial ischemia and reperfusion by lazaroid U-74500A, a nonglucocorticoid 21-aminosteroid. *J. Cardiovasc. Pharmacol.* 23: 136–140 (1994).
16. Du Z, Hicks M, Winlaw D, Macdonald P, Spratt P. Lazaroid U74500A enhances donor lung preservation in the rat transplant model. *Transplant. Proc.* 27: 3574–3577 (1995).
17. Nishida T, Morita S, Miyamoto K, Masuda M, Tominaga R, Kawachi Y, Yasui H. The effect of lazaroid (U74500A), a novel inhibitor of lipid peroxidation, on 24-our heart preservation. A study based on a working model using cross-circulated blood-perfused rabbit hearts. *Transplantation* 61: 194–199 (1996).
18. Hirose M, Satoh T. HTHQ. *Drug News Perspect.* 7: 167–170 (1994).
19. Hirose M, Iwata S, Ito E, Nihro Y, Takahashi S, Mizoguchi Y, Miki T, Satoh T, Ito N, Shirai T. Strong anti-mutagenic activity of the novel lipophilic antioxidant 1-O-hexyl-2,3,5-trimethylhydroquinone against heterocyclic amine-induced mutagenesis in the Ames assay and its effect on metabolic activation on 2-amino-6-methyldipyrido[1,2-a:3′,2′-d] imidazole (Glu-P-1). *Carcinogenesis* 16: 2227–2232 (1995).
20. Hirose M, Hasegawa R, Kimura J, Akagi K, Yoshida Y, Tanaka H, Miki T, Satoh T, Wakabayashi K, Ito N. Inhibitory effects of 1-O-hexyl-2,3,5-trimethylhydroquinone (HTHQ), green tea catechins and other antioxidants on 2-amino-6-methyldipyrido[1,2-a:3′,2′-d] imidazole (Glu-P-1)-induced rat hepatocarcinogenesis and dose-dependent inhibition by HTHQ of lesion induction by Glu-P-1 or 2-amino-3,8-dimethylimidazo[4,5-f] quinoxaline (MeIQx). *Carcinogenesis* 16: 3049–3055 (1995).
21. Hirose M, Akagi K, Hasegawa R, Yaono M, Satoh T, Hara Y, Wakabayashi K, Ito N. Chemoprevention of 2-amino-1-methyl-6-phenylimidazo [4,5-b]-pyridine (PhIP)-induced mammary gland carcinogenesis by antioxidants in F344 female rats. *Carcinogenesis* 16: 217–221 (1995).
22. Futakuchi M, Hirose M, Miki T, Tanaka H, Ozake M, Shirai T. Inhibition of DMBA-initiated rat mammary tumor development by 1-O-hexyl-2,3,5-trimethylhydroquinone, phenylethyl isothiocyanate, and novel synthetic ascorib acid derivatives. *Eur. J. Cancer Prev.* 7: 153–159 (1998).

23. Futakuchi M, Hirose M, Imaida K, Takahashi S, Ogawa K, Asamoto M, Miki T, Shirai T. Chemoprevention of 2-amino-1-methyl-6-phenylimidazo-[4,5-b] pyridine-induced colon carcinogenesis by 1-O-hexyl-2,3,5-trimethylhydroquinone after initiation with 1,2-dimethylhydrazine in F344 rats. *Carcinogenesis* 23: 283–287 (2002).
24. Yada H, Hirose M, Tamano S, Kawabe M, Sano M, Takahashi S, Futakuchi M, Miki T, Shirai T. Effects of antioxidant 1-O-hexyl-2,3,5-trimethylhydroquinone or ascorbic acid on caracinogenesis induced by administration of aminopyrine and sodium nitrite in a rat multi-organ carcinogenesis model. *Jpn. J. Cancer Res.* 93: 1299–1307 (2002).
25. Doctrow SR, Huffman K, Marcus CB, Tocco G, Malfroy E, Adinolfi CA, Kruk H, Baker K, Lazarowych N, Mascarenhas J, Malfroy B. Salen-manganese complexes as catalytic scavengers of hydrogen peroxide and cytoprotective agents: structure–activity relationship studies. *J. Med. Chem.* 45: 4549–4558 (2002).
26. Doctrow SR, Adinolfi C, Baudry M, Huffman K, Malfroy B, Marcus CB, Melov S, Pong K, Rong Y, Smart JL, Tocco G. Salen manganese complexes, combined superoxide dismutase/catalase mimetics, demonstrate potential for treating neurodegenerative and other age-associated diseases. In: Cutler RG, Rodriguez H (eds.) *Advances in Basic Science, Diagnostics, and Intervention*. World Scientific Publishing Company, Singapore, 2003.
27. Samlowski WE, Petersen R, Cuzzocrea S, Macarthur H, Burton D, McGreagor JR, Salvemini D. A nonpeptidyl mimic of superoxide dismutase, M40403, inhibits dose-limiting hypotension associated with interleukin-2 and increases its antitumor effects. *Nat. Med.* 9: 750–755 (2003).
28. Salvemini D, Mazzon E, Dugo L, Serraino I, De Sarro A, Caputi AP, Cuzzocrea S. Amelioration of joint disease in a rat model of collagen-induced arthritis by M 40403, a superoxide dismutase mimetic. *Arthritis Rheum.* 44: 2909–2921 (2001).
29. Masini E, Cuzzocrea S, Mazzon E, Marzocca C, Mannaioni PF, Salvemini D. Protective effects of M 40403, a selective superoxide dismutase mimetic, in myocardial ischemia and reperfusion injury *in vivo*. *Br. J. Pharmacol.* 136: 905–917 (2002).
30. Salvemini D, Cuzzocrea S. Superoxide, superoxide dismutase and ischemic injury. *Curr. Opin. Investig. Drugs* 3: 886–895 (2002).
31. Marzocca C, Vannacci A, Cuzzocrea S, Salvemini D, Mannaioni PF, Masini E. Effects of the SOD mimetic, M 40403, on prostaglandin production in an *in vivo* model of ischemia and reperfusion in rat heart. *Inflamm. Res.* 52 (Suppl. 1): S23–S24 (2003).

32. Wang ZQ, Porreca F, Cuzzocrea S, Galen K, Lightfoot R, Masini E, Muscoli C, Mollace V, Ndengele M, Ischiropoulos H, Salvemini D. A newly identified role for superoxide in inflammatory pain. *J. Pharmacol. Exp. Ther.* 309: 869–878 (2004).
33. Arbiser JL. Role of manganese superoxide dismutase in cancer. *Nat. Med.* 9: 1103 (2003).
34. Vujaskovic Z, Batinic-Haberle I, Rabbani ZN, Feng QF, Kang SK, Spasojevic I, Samulski TV, Fridovich I, Dewhirst MW, Anscher MS. A small molecular weight catalytic metalloporphyrin antioxidant with superoxide dismutase (SOD) mimetic properties protects lungs from radiation-induced injury. *Free Radic. Biol. Med.* 33: 857–863 (2002).

37 Nanoscale Antioxidant Therapeutics

Thomas Dziubla, Silvia Muro, Vladimir R. Muzykantov, and Michael Koval

1. Introduction

Drug efficacy is a function of both therapeutic activity and delivery to the proper location. Although highly active drugs with low toxicity can be delivered systemically, the ability to target delivery to specific tissues or intracellular compartments has the potential to increase drug efficacy and/or decrease toxicity. Targeted antioxidant nanoparticles are potentially applicable to contain oxidative stress and seem particularly well suited to be applied as intravenous agents to treat vascular oxidant stress.

Of recent interest are drug delivery vehicles in the nanoscale size range, typically 100–600 nm in diameter. In practice, particles less than 1 μm in diameter tend to have distinct properties compared to larger particles. For instance, small particles have been shown to migrate across biological barriers (e.g., blood–brain barrier, intestinal epithelium) and are internalized by cells much more readily than large particles. Efficacy is also influenced by the class of antioxidant scavenger or enzyme and the type of packaging agent. Other criteria that have significant effects on the recognition and processing of nanoparticles include particle geometry, valence, and binding affinity to target cells.

2. Antioxidants

Antioxidants can be divided into two main categories, oxidant scavengers and antioxidant enzymes (AOEs).[1] Organic antioxidant scavengers are small molecular compounds that readily reduce free radicals, peroxides, and oxidized molecules, thereby neutralizing their effect and protecting functionally sensitive proteins, lipids, and nucleic acids from oxidative damage. This scavenging capability is usually insensitive to the form of reactive oxygen species (ROS); hence, their use is not typically limited by variations in ROS forms.

Some of the common molecules in this group include tocopherol (vitamin E) and *N*-acetyl cysteine.[2–4] The advantage of free radical scavengers is that they are well tolerated, stable during long-term storage, and resistant to formulation processing. Also, hydrophobic molecules, such as tocopherol, readily partition into biological membranes and enhance protection of the membrane lipids and proteins from radical damage.[5] However, since scavengers reduce oxidants in stoichiometric fashion, large doses are often required for appreciable protective effects.[6] In theory, targeted application of antioxidants might help reduce the effective dose.

AOEs are an alternative to organic free radical scavengers that theoretically have the capacity to detoxify multiple copies of ROS molecules. Enzymatic defense against oxidative stress include "classic" AOE (Fig. 1), such as superoxide dismutases (SOD), catalase, glutathione peroxidase,

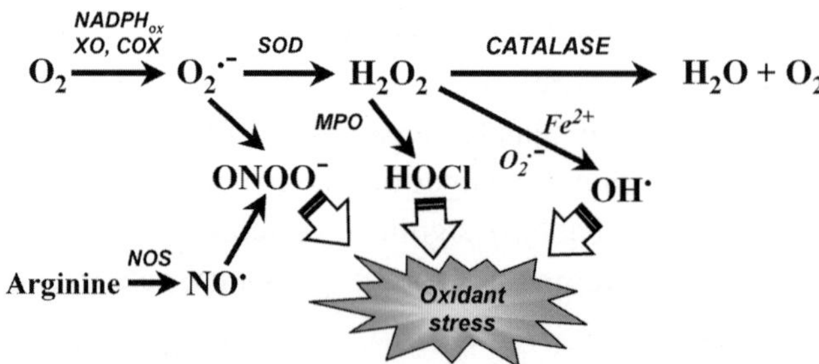

Fig. 1. Antioxidant enzyme reaction pathways. SOD prevents inactivation of NO• and generation of ONOO− by accelerating $O_2^{\bullet -}$ dismutation into H_2O_2. H_2O_2 can form strong oxidants in reactions with MPO and transient metals. Catalase reduces H_2O_2 into water. XO, xanthine oxidase; MPO, myeloperoxidase; NOS, nitric oxide synthase; COX, cyclooxygenase.

glutathione reductase, and other enzymes, such as heme oxygenase and peroxiredoxins.[7–13]

As catalysts, AOEs are effective against specific oxidant species, although AOEs can also generate oxidant by-products. For instance, SODs catalyze the conversion of superoxide into hydrogen peroxide (H_2O_2), which has a beneficial effect by reducing oxidant load. However, the reaction product, H_2O_2, is highly diffusible and in the presence of transition metals (iron or copper) forms hydroxyl radical, a strong oxidant. H_2O_2 is also catalyzed by myeloperoxidase into a toxic by-product, hypochlorous acid (HOCl).[14,15] Therefore, in the absence of clearance mechanism for H_2O_2, SOD may aggravate oxidative stress.[16,17]

One potential clearance mechanism for H_2O_2 is catalase, a heme-containing, 240-kD tetrameric AOE that safely degrades H_2O_2 to water and oxygen with extremely rapid kinetics ($2.5–5.0 \times 10^6$ H_2O_2 degraded per minute).[18] This suggests the possibility that multifunctional particles containing a combination of AOEs might be a useful approach to maximizing the antioxidant capacity of potential therapeutic agents.

Preventing loss of enzyme activity is another potential pitfall in the application of AOEs to treat oxidative stress. Also, it is neither cost effective nor practical to apply AOEs systemically to prevent oxidative stress in an intact animal or human. To date, high doses of AOEs have only produced significant protective effects in either cultured cells or perfused organ systems. Thus, the effective use of AOEs as a therapeutic agent requires a strategy to promote delivery to specific target organs and to protect their activity. Nanocarriers provide a particularly attractive method for pharmacologic application of AOEs.

3. Classes of Nanocarriers

The small size of nanocarriers offers several inherent advantages. One of these is a targeting strategy known as passive targeting. By limiting particle size to the nanoscale range, non-specific organ distribution is impeded and hepatic uptake is enhanced without requiring an active targeting strategy. This allows for the passive targeting of diseases such as acute and chronic liver disease,[19,20] where ROS generation is believed to be a primary causative factor. Hepatic clearance is extremely rapid, where typically 90% of circulating material is cleared after 5 min in mice.[21–24]

However, the lifetime of particles can be greatly extended with the use of "stealth" technology, by coating nanoparticles with an inert substance, such as poly(ethylene) glycol (PEG). PEG polymers form a hydrophilic shell, or brush, that repels plasma opsonins, complement, and phagocytes.[25,26] PEGylation has been successfully applied to proteins, liposomes, and polylactic acid (PLA) nanoparticles to enhance circulation time.[26–28] This enhanced circulation time can vary from a few hours to days for nanosphere structures.

Another form of passive targeting used by nanoparticles, which is especially useful for long-circulating stealth nanoparticles, is through the enhanced permeation and retention effect (EPR).[29,30] At sites where tumor cells or leukocytes are migrating across the vasculature (diapedesis), vessel barrier function is disrupted, creating small leaks that can be permeated by nanoscale particles. Sites of cell diapedesis also have the potential to disrupt blood flow. Turbulent flow patterns can cause "dead zones" where nanocarriers can accumulate to enhance drug delivery.

The first pass phenomenon is another passive targeting strategy related to patterns of vessel flow, since infusion into an afferent blood vessel permits preferential uptake in the downstream microvascular bed. For example, intravenously injected agents first encounter the pulmonary vasculature, which represents about 30% of the total vascular surface in the body and receives 100% of the cardiac first pass venous blood output. The first pass phenomenon combined with immunotargeting (see below) provides a particularly powerful approach to targeting the pulmonary endothelium. However, if needed, this effect can be circumvented by injecting agents locally via catheters inserted in a conduit artery, facilitating delivery toward downstream vascular areas.[31,32]

Nanoparticle size also helps control internalization by target cells, where smaller particles are more readily internalized than particles greater than 1–2 μm.[33] This provides the opportunity to control residence time at the cell surface by controlling particle size. For instance, small, internalized, antioxidant nanoparticles are better suited to treat oxidative stress derived from intracellular sources, such as mitochondrial ROS induced by ischemia/reperfusion or hypoxia.

Small particles might also be best suited for uptake and transcytosis to permeate vascular barriers (see Sec. 4). In contrast, large antioxidant nanoparticles retained on the cell surface are better suited to treat oxidative stress derived from extracellular sources, such as ROS generated by leukocytes during inflammation, or superoxide anion produced by plasma membrane NADPH-oxidase due to pathological shear stress. It is plausible that a combination of small and large particles could be used to target both the cell surface and intracellular compartments.

3.1. *Liposomes*

One of the first classes of nanocarriers pursued for drug delivery are liposomes, which are chemically produced membrane vesicles composed of either naturally occurring lipids or synthetic amphiphiles.[34–37] Liposome membranes are organized into spheriod shells, which can be either uni- or multilamellar and can vary in diameter from 50 nm up to 10 or more micrometers.

The two most commonly used methods to produce drug encapsulated liposomes are extrusion and sonication.[38] Extrusion through permeable polycarbonate filters is particularly useful for lab-scale liposome formation, since liposome size is controlled by filter pore size. Extrusion also avoids the pitfalls related to membrane or cargo damage that can be induced by the energy input required to produce liposomes using sonication.

Liposome loading is determined by the equilibrium partitioning of solute inside and outside the liposome. Since partitioning decreases with increasing solute molecular weight (MW), liposomes are useful for packaging small antioxidants. In this case, the entrapped volume for liposomes is well suited to encapsulation of aqueous molecules, as opposed to the relatively low hydrophobic capacity of liposomes (∼10–20% for 100 nm lipsomes). On the other hand, large enzymes are often difficult to encapsulate into liposomes. Freeze-drying, freeze/thaw, and pH gradients have been used to improve the loading of AOEs such as SOD and catalase into liposomes.[39,40]

While liposomes have been successfully used as a commercial pharmacologic agent,[41,42] their use for the delivery of antioxidants has several drawbacks. First, liposomal formulations have a relatively short circulation half-life. The most stable liposome preparations have a 12 h half-life, which may not be significant enough for applications to chronic diseases. Also, unblocked liposome preparations are preferentially cleared by the hepatic system through passive targeting and thus need to be blocked in order to be targeted to other organ systems.

3.2. *Solid lipid nanoparticles*

Solid lipid nanoparticles (SLNs)[43,44] are emulsion-derived nanocarriers related to liposomes, except that they are composed of lipids, such as trigylcerides and waxes, that are solid at room and physiological temperatures, yet are emulsified at elevated temperatures and/or in the presence of surfactants. Since these carriers can be composed of naturally occurring lipids, they are likely to be well tolerated.

SLNs have a significantly larger hydrophobic component than liposomes and are thus capable of carrying high loads of small hydrophobic compounds (e.g., doxorubicin, pacitaxol).[45,46] Consistent with the therapeutic use of SLNs, antioxidants such as tocopherol and TEMPO were loaded with fair success.[47,48] However, SLN-loaded antioxidants have not yet been tested using *in vitro* or *in vivo* models of oxidative stress. Furthermore, SLNs are not expected to be an effective means for delivery of AOEs, since the high temperatures used during SLN formation will denature and inactivate AOEs.

3.3. *Protein immunoconjugates*

The biotin–streptavidin crosslinking pair can be used to synthesize nanocarriers exclusively from protein components.[18,49] These conjugates are typically characterized by (a) their high drug incorporation efficiency, (b) high drug to carrier weight ratio, (c) a wide tunable range of particle sizes with the comparable composition, and (d) a relatively rigid and biodegradable structure.

Biotin/avidin complexes are extremely specific and widely used in biology and medicine. The binding between biotin and avidin (or avidin-related proteins, such as streptavidin and neutravidin) is arguably the strongest known biochemical noncovalent interaction. Conjugate size can be controlled by a number of parameters, including controlling the level of protein biotinylation, the ratio of biotinylated protein to avidin and incubation time and temperature. However, due to the relative speed of the binding reaction and heterogeneity of protein biotinylation, batch to batch variations can be rather significant. Thus, stringent quality control is critical when using protein conjugates. Dynamic light scattering can be used to insure that protein conjugate nanocarrier preparations are in the correct size range prior to use, although this method has some limitations.[50]

Avidin and streptavidin form tetramers to theoretically bind four biotins per complex, although the binding capacity of biotinylated proteins will be limited by steric interference. Small oligomeric conjugates are typically formed by proteins containing less than two biotin residues per protein, which minimizes the possibility of forming large crosslinked aggregates. However, when the average biotinylation level of the proteins exceeds two per protein, polymeric structures are usually formed, resulting in multimeric structures that are into the micrometer range of particle diameter. Binding valence is also controlled by the binding capacity of different classes of avidin substrates. Crosslinked monomeric avidin or anti-biotin antibodies offer alternatives when a sub-tetrameric biotin binding capacity is desired.

Since protein nanoconjugates can be produced from pure proteins under fairly mild conditions, they are ideal for the formation of nanoscale AOE therapeutic agents. They can also include antibodies to help promote active targeting (see below). Immunoconjugates represent the current state of the art in antioxidant therapeutics and have been used to successfully deliver therapeutic levels of AOEs to the pulmonary endothelium.[33,51–55]

3.4. *Biodegradable polymeric nanocarriers*

Encapsulation of drugs into biodegradable polymer nanocarriers (PNCs) may help to protect AOEs from inactivation and proteolysis, while enabling controlled release in the appropriate environment (e.g., optimum pH). Poly(lactic acid) (PLA) and the related copolymer poly(lactic acid-*co*-glycolic acid) (PLGA) have been used to prepare injectable microspheres and nanoparticles as controlled release agents.[56,57] These are quite stable. Micelles prepared from short-chain mPEG–PLA polymer were stable for

6 weeks in PBS at 37°C,[58] which is considerably more stable than liposomes.[59]

Nanoparticle synthesis of higher molecular weight mPEG–PLA can be done using either emulsification followed by solvent extraction/evaporation, or polymer micellization.[60–63] As a result of partitioning effects, these techniques are effective for loading hydrophobic, but not hydrophilic drugs. However, with multiple emulsification steps, hydrophilic agents, including proteins, can be incorporated within aqueous domains contained within the nanoparticle core.[64–66]

For instance, catalase has been encapsulated using diblock copolymers to form PNCs. These particles can be formulated in the size range of 200–500 nm with at least 25% of loaded catalase was fully protected from external proteases by loading into these PNCs.[67] Diblock copolymer also offers native stealth characteristics gained by PEG as well as providing derivatizable sites for tethering targeting moieties (such as antibodies) to the PNC surface.

A type of hybrid carrier that is an alternative to PNCs is polymersomes, which are polymer-derived analogs of liposomes.[68,69] Like liposomes, these structures have a large internal aqueous domain, which is theoretically ideal for AOE loading. The membrane bilayer of polymersomes is much thicker than liposomes (~8 nm compared to ~3 nm), resulting in a more durable carrier with a greatly enhanced circulation half-life.

Preparation and loading of polymersomes are equivalent to liposomes, except that polymers called "super-amphiphiles" are used in place of lipids or small surfactants. They are called super-amphiphiles due to the presence of exaggerated hydrophilic/hydrophobic domains, which are significantly larger than comparable domains found in common surfactants and phospholipids.[69] Some of the polymers used for synthesis of stable polymersomes include the block copolymers, PEG–poly(butadiene), PEG–poly(ethylethylene), and PEG–poly(propylene sulfide)–PEG (PEG–PPS–PEG).[70] PEG–PPS–PEG is of unique interest in that the sulfide group of the polymer is sensitive to oxidative stress. This hydrophobic block can be converted into the more hydrophilic poly(propylene sulfoxide), resulting in the destabilization of the polymer vesicle. Such a mechanism has the potential to allow triggered release of cargo in the presence of an oxidative environment.

Small solutes such as impermeant osmolytes, sucrose and glucose are encapsulated into polymersomes at concentrations comparable to their bulk concentrations. Also, small hydrophobic drugs can be encapsulated in 100 nm vesicles at 1 mole per mole copolymer. From a MW series of dextrans, hydrophilic drugs with sizes up to 500 kD (~20 nm) can be encapsulated, although the efficiency of encapsulation generally decreases with increasing MW.[71] Yet, due to the more rigorous encapsulation conditions required in overcoming the more durable nature of these materials (e.g., high temperature, pressure), protein stability and activity remains a concern. Also, the efficacy of antioxidant therapeutic agents formulated with super amphiphiles requires further study, since the biocompatibility and clearance mechanisms for polymersomes remain poorly understood at present.

4. Nanocarrier Immunotargeting and Internalization

In contrast to passive targeting based on nanoparticle size alone, active targeting takes advantage of a specific interaction to direct a therapeutic agent to the proper cell type. Immunotargeting has been a particularly effective approach, using antibodies directed against cell surface antigens. When considering a targeting strategy, the ultimate fate of the engaged nanoparticle needs to be considered to insure maximum efficacy (Fig. 2). For instance, nanocarriers targeted to the extracellular surface are susceptible to shedding from the cell surface, as well as phagocyte clearance and dissociation. Nanoparticle uptake can help prevent this by sequestering particles in endocytic vesicles. This strategy is well suited to internalized catalase nanoparticles, since H_2O_2 can readily permeate endosome membranes and be neutralized. However, internalized SOD might not have optimum antioxidant effect, since superoxide is believed to be too charged and too unstable to permeate into endosomes. However, restricting SOD to the cell surface, either through nanocarrier size or ligand type, might be an ideal approach to treat extracellular superoxide generated by activated leukocytes or by the NADPH complex as a result of ischemia/reperfusion injury.

Cells employ multiple mechanisms for vesicle-mediated membrane transport, which is dictated by the plasma membrane proteins used by a given extracellular ligand. As an illustration of immunotargeting strategies,

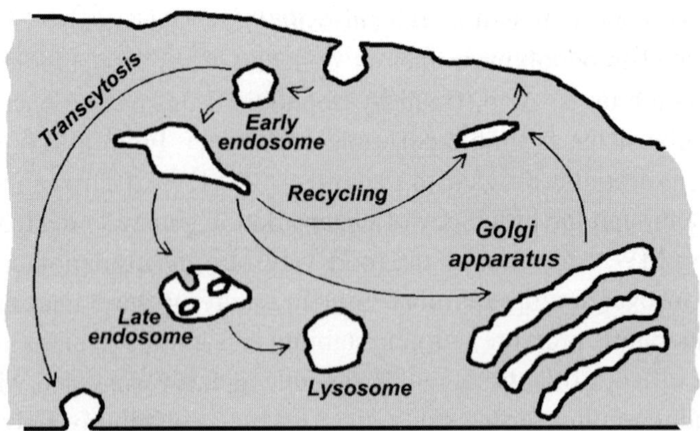

Fig. 2. Intracellular membrane trafficking pathways. Endocytic vesicles, containing membrane receptors and their respective ligands, are targeted to different sub-cellular compartments. These include trafficking to lysosomes for degradation or to other intracellular compartments, such as the Golgi apparatus or endoplasmic reticulum (not shown). Intracellular compartments, such as early endosomes are significantly less degradative than lysosomes, and thus provide an environment that can stabilize internalized nanocarriers. Alternatively, vesicles can be retargeted to the plasma membrane (recycling) or transported through the cell body to the abluminal space (transcytosis). Transcytosis can be used to circumvent barriers, such as the blood–brain barrier.

we emphasize vascular immunotargeting, i.e., coupling drugs with carrier antibodies to endothelial cell determinants.[1,18,72,73]

4.1. *Angiotensin-converting enzyme*

Angiotensin-converting enzyme (ACE) is a transmembrane glycoprotein expressed on the endothelial luminal surface, which regulates vasoconstriction. Nearly all of the alveolar capillary endothelium expresses ACE as opposed to less than 15% of the extra-pulmonary capillary endothelium.[31] Anti-ACE-conjugated antioxidant enzymes, such as catalase, accumulate in rat lungs *in vivo*[74] and protect perfused rat lungs against H_2O_2.[51]

In some instances, ROS and cytokines suppress anti-ACE targeting.[75] Also, ACE sheds from the endothelial surface, which can affect the targeting efficiency. This depends on the anti-ACE antibody used, since some ACE antibodies block its active site and/or facilitate ACE shedding from the endothelium.[76,77] However, other ACE antibodies enable ACE to retain its function. Therefore, using ACE antibodies directed to different epitopes enables targeting strategies to be developed that either retain or inhibit ACE activity. Inhibiting ACE activity might also be a useful strategy to inhibit hypertension and inflammation accompanying vascular oxidative stress.

4.2. *Selectins/clathrin-mediated endocytosis*

Endothelial cells exposed to inflammatory mediators and abnormal shear stress show cell surface expression of P-selectin, normally stored intracellularly and mobilized rapidly to the surface, and E-selectin, which is newly synthesized by activated endothelial cells.[78] Therefore, selectins are transiently exposed on the surface of stressed endothelial cells and may permit, in theory, targeting inflammation.[79–81] However, endothelial cells expose selectins transiently and at relatively low density. Also, selectins and their ligands rapidly traffic to lysosomes for degradation.[82,83] This is the case for anti-E-selectin immunoliposomes or conjugates of anti-E-selectin and dexamethasone, which are delivered intracellularly to activated endothelial cells.[84,85]

Endothelial cells internalize E- and P-selectins as well as nanocarriers targeted to these molecules via clathrin-mediated endocytosis.[82,86] This is the predominant form of receptor-mediated endocytosis in most cell types, although it is less prominent in endothelial cells than caveolar-mediated endocytosis. As mentioned above, most internalized E- and P-selectin is routed to the endo-lysosomal pathway. Degradation of P-selectin occurs in lysosomes as a consequence of frequent passage through endocytic vesicles; also, internalized E-selectin-targeted conjugates are delivered to degradative compartments.[83,86] However, in epithelial cells, IgA is internalized by clathrin-mediated endocytosis and subsequently transcytosed from the basolateral to the apical plasma membrane.[87] Whether a comparable pathway also operates in endothelial cells remains to be determined.

4.3. *Caveolar proteins*

There are many caveolar-associated surface antigens, such as gp60.[88–90] Caveolar-mediated endocytosis is preferentially inhibited by cholesterol chelators (e.g., filipin or cyclodextrin) and is mediated by interactions of the coat protein caveolin with cell signaling and cytoskeletal molecules. Ligands internalized by caveolar-mediated endocytosis can be sorted to intracellular compartments other than lysosomes. For instance, cholera toxin traffics through early and late endosomes,[91] SV40 is sorted from early endosomes to Golgi and finally ER,[92] and folate is directly transported across the plasma membrane and delivered to the cytoplasm by potocytosis.[93] Other caveolar localized proteins, such as alkaline phosphatase, bradykinin, acetylcholine, and endothelin, are returned to the cell surface after their internalization.[94,95]

Caveolar-mediated uptake has been used as a drug delivery strategy.[96] Importantly, caveolar-mediated endocytosis serves as an entry point for transcytosis of many compounds through the endothelial monolayer, from the bloodstream to sub-endothelial tissues. Consistent with this, some ligands of caveolar-localized surface molecules accumulate in the pulmonary vasculature after intravenous injection in rats, enter endothelial cells, and traverse the endothelial barrier.[89] Thus, caveolar-localized determinants might provide an opportunity for targeted trans-endothelial drug delivery or for permeating the blood–brain barrier.

4.4. *Phagocytosis*

Clathrin- and caveolar-mediated endocytosis account for internalization of nanocarriers in the 100–300 nm diameter size range, given restrictions on the natural size of the endocytic vesicles produced by these pathways. However, phagocytosis and macropinocytosis can be used for intracellular delivery of much larger particles. Phagocytosis, typically displayed by macrophages and antigen presenting cells, accounts for the internalization of large particulate ligands ($>1\ \mu m$), which are rapidly delivered to lysosomes.[97] This requires initial binding of the particle to particular receptors (e.g., scavenger receptor, C3 receptor, or Fc receptor), resulting in activation of specific signaling cascades (e.g., phosphatidyl inositol 3 kinase, Rho family GTPases[98]), and redistribution of the actin cytoskeleton. Although the extent of phagocytosis varies with cell type, most cells have some phagocytic capacity. For instance, vascular endothelial cells phagocytose and degrade aged red blood cells and apoptotic cells via phosphatidylserine receptors (LOX-1).[99]

4.5. *Ig-family cell adhesion molecules*

Platelet-endothelial cell adhesion molecule-1 (PECAM, CD31) is a pan-endothelial transmembrane Ig superfamily glycoprotein, predominantly localized in the sites of cellular contacts in the endothelial monolayer.[100] PECAM is also expressed by platelets and leukocytes, although to a lesser extent than endothelium.[74] PECAM is involved in the cellular recognition, adhesion, signaling, and trans-endothelial migration of leukocytes.[100] In addition, PECAM is a stable endothelial cell antigen where the expression and surface density is not changed by cytokines or ROS. This promises robust PECAM-targeted drug delivery to either normal or pathologically altered endothelial cells for either prophylaxis or therapies. Anti-PECAM targeting may also provide secondary benefits for management of inflammation, since PECAM plays a role in regulating leukocyte transmigration. Consistent with this, anti-PECAM suppresses inflammation and protects organs against leukocyte-mediated oxidative stress.[101]

Intercellular adhesion molecule-1 (ICAM-1, CD54) is another Ig superfamily surface glycoprotein.[102,103] It is normally expressed by endothelial cells at relatively high surface density (2×10^4–2×10^5 surface copies per cell) and is further upregulated by inflammation. Like PECAM, ICAM-1 also contributes to leukocyte binding to endothelial cells and thus contributes to inflammation.[104] Antibodies (including humanized murine mAbs) directed against ICAM-1 suppress leukocyte adhesion, thus preventing inflammation associated with vascular injury.[105–107]

Interestingly, ICAM-1 and PECAM-1 are internalized by endothelial cells using a novel pathway called CAM-mediated endocytosis, which is distinct from classical clathrin- or caveolar-mediated uptake as well as phagocytosis.[108] In particular, internalization of anti-ICAM-1 or anti-PECAM-1 conjugates was dependent on antigen clustering, and required Rho kinase- and protein kinase C-mediated rearrangements of the actin cytoskeleton.[108]

CAM-mediated endocytosis is uniquely suited to nanoparticles, since it requires PECAM or ICAM-1 clustering via a multivalent particle. Neither cell adhesion molecules nor monovalent ligands (such as monomeric antibodies) show significant uptake in the absence of clustering. This suggests both that monovalent anti-CAM nanoparticles can be surface targeted and that CAM-mediated endocytosis is a stimulated process.[33,52,53,108]

5. Efficacy of CAM-Targeted Nanoparticles

The efficacy of CAM-mediated endocytosis for treating oxidant stress has been demonstrated using anti-CAM/catalase. Catalase nanoparticles bind to and enter cultured endothelial cells and protect them from H_2O_2-induced cell death.[52,55] In lung transplantation, where ROS generated by the ischemia reperfusion has been implicated as one of the primary injurious mechanisms limiting transplantation success, injection of anti-PECAM/catalase conjugates into a donor animal prior to lung transplantation greatly extended the functional window between organ harvest and implantation.[54] Also, in artificial oxidative stress models such as pulmonary targeted glucose oxidase, anti-PECAM/catalase conjugates allowed for complete protection, even with low injection levels.[33]

There are several features of CAM-targeted nanoparticles that promote their efficacy. CAM-mediated endocytosis delivers materials to lysosomal compartments with unusually slow kinetics (around 3 h) and is therefore ideal for preserving AOEs in the relatively mild endosomal environment as a safe haven.[108,109] This has been demonstrated using catalase conjugated to either anti-ICAM-1 or anti-PECAM-1 antibodies.[108,109] The protective effect of anti-CAM delivered catalase can be further prolonged either in the presence of drugs acting on the microtubule network (i.e., nocodazole),[109] which is required for vesicle traffic to lysosomes.[110] Alternatively, application of weak bases such as chloroquine, which increase lysosome pH, reduce their degradative capacity and increase the active lifetime of AOEs.

Also, ICAM-1, which rapidly disappears from to the plasma membrane following nanocarrier internalization, does not traffic to lysosomes.[111] Instead, internalized ICAM-1 recycles back to the cell surface, providing a source for recurrent delivery of AOEs via anti-ICAM nanocarriers. Moreover, saturation of cell lysosomes with a first dose of anti-ICAM nanocarriers delays lyososomal traffic and degradation of a subsequent dose of anti-ICAM nanocarriers. This saturation effect further promotes sustained AOE activity by inhibiting nanocarrier degradation.[111]

An alternative approach in extending the activity of delivered catalase is to load catalase inside polymeric nanocarriers. By providing a physical barrier between proteolytic lysosomal enzymes and catalase, the therapeutic duration of targeted catalase can be increased. Indeed, by loading catalase into 200–300 nm PEG–PLGA nanoparticles, 25% of enzyme activity remained stable for at least 18 h *in vitro*. By comparison, free catalase lost 90% activity under identical conditions after 1 h incubation.[67] One additional advantage of this strategy is that the therapeutic duration of delivered catalase can be directly controlled by the degradation rate of the encapsulating biodegradable polymer. Also, polymers or lipsosomes that are pH sensitive are another strategy that can be used protect nanocarrier cargo by enabling unloading in the appropriate endocytic compartment.[39,79]

6. Conclusion and Perspectives

A successful drug delivery strategy takes into account properties of both the vehicle and target system. Until recently, development of new nanocarriers has primarily focused on size and evading hepatic clearance. Modulating parameters such as nanocarrier charge, binding affinity, valence, and crosslinking capacity are parameters that can be adjusted to further control the uptake and fate of targeted drugs.

Crosslinkers sensitive to minute changes in pH or specific cellular proteases (e.g., lysosomal cathepsin G) are just beginning to be employed. This approach will be best suited for release of active drugs at selected stages of their intracellular traffic. Conjugation of drugs or drug vehicles with membrane fusion and chaperone peptides also has the potential to help achieve even more precise subcellular localization to the cytosol or to organelles that are critical for regulation of cell redox capacity, such as mitochondria and peroxysomes. Nuclear targeting could conceivably be used to either protect the genome from oxidant damage or to deliver DNA-based gene therapies.

Designing nanocarrier antioxidants that take advantage of different binding sites, entry mechanisms, and trafficking pathways will help serve diverse therapeutic goals. In the case of antioxidants targeted to the vascular endothelium, there are many options for specifically recognizing the endothelium and intracellular compartments. Targeting strategies are likely to be fine tuned by taking advantage of surface molecules specific for different classes of endothelial cells, such as microcirculation versus large vessels. Also, the availability of different endothelial target molecules with different fates helps provide further parameters to help control delivery and turnover of internalized nanocarriers.

Besides being a clinically relevant treatment strategy, AOE nanocarriers provide a proving ground for determining the potential success of targeting, delivery, and turnover of other enzyme-based therapies, such as enzyme replacement therapy, which would otherwise be cost prohibitive to pursue in exploratory studies. As such, future progress in understanding the foundations of nanoparticle–endothelial interactions will help set the stage for future novel targeted treatments in addition to treatment of oxidant stress.

References

1. Muzykantov VR. *J. Control Release* 71: 1–21 (2001).
2. Dekhuijzen PN. *Eur. Respir. J.* 23: 629–636 (2004).
3. Antoniades C, Tousoulis D, Tentolouris C, Toutouzas P, Stefanadis C. *Herz* 28: 628–638 (2003).
4. Berger TM, Polidori MC, Dabbagh A, Evans PJ, Halliwell B, Morrow JD, Roberts LJ, II, Frei B. *J. Biol. Chem.* 272: 15656–15660 (1997).
5. Wang X, Quinn PJ. *Chem. Phys. Lipids* 114: 1–9 (2002).
6. Stephens NG, Parsons A, Schofield PM, Kelly F, Cheeseman K, Mitchinson MJ. *Lancet* 347: 781–786 (1996).
7. Wei Z, Costa K, Al-Mehdi AB, Dodia C, Muzykantov V, Fisher AB. *Circ. Res.* 85: 682–689 (1999).
8. Manevich Y, Al-Mehdi A, Muzykantov V, Fisher AB. *Am. J. Physiol. Heart. Circ. Physiol.* 280: H2126–H2135 (2001).
9. Christou H, Morita T, Hsieh CM, Koike H, Arkonac B, Perrella MA, Kourembanas S. *Circ. Res.* 86: 1224–1249 (2000).
10. Otterbein LE, Kolls JK, Mantell LL, Cook JL, Alam J, Choi AM. *J. Clin. Invest.* 103: 1047–1054 (1999).
11. Fridovich I. *Annu. Rev. Biochem.* 64: 97–112 (1995).
12. Connolly ES, Jr., Winfree CJ, Springer TA, Naka Y, Liao H, Yan SD, Stern DM, Solomon RA, Gutierrez-Ramos JC, Pinsky DJ. *J. Clin. Invest.* 97: 209–216 (1996).
13. Jin LH, Bahn JH, Eum WS, Kwon HY, Jang SH, Han KH, Kang TC, Won MH, Kang JH, Cho SW, Park J, Choi SY. *Free. Radic. Biol. Med.* 31: 1509–1519 (2001).

14. Britigan BE, Roeder TL, Shasby DM. *Blood* 79: 699–707 (1992).
15. Louie S, Halliwell B, Cross CE. *Adv. Pharmacol.* 38: 457–490 (1997).
16. Nguyen TT, Cox CS, Jr., Herndon DN, Biondo NA, Traber LD, Bush PE, Zophel A, Traber DL. *J. Appl. Physiol.* 78: 2161–2168 (1995).
17. McCord JM. *J. Free. Radic. Biol. Med.* 2: 307–310 (1986).
18. Muzykantov VR. *Antioxid. Redox Signal.* 3: 39–62 (2001).
19. Loguercio C, Federico A. *Free Radic. Biol. Med.* 34: 1–10 (2003).
20. Feher J, Lengyel G, Blazovics A. *Scand. J. Gastroenterol. Suppl.* 228: 38–46 (1998).
21. Seki J, Sonoke S, Saheki A, Fukui H, Sasaki H, Mayumi T. *Int. J. Pharm.* 273: 75–83 (2004).
22. Panagi Z, Beletsi A, Evangelatos G, Livaniou E, Ithakissios DS, Avgoustakis K. *Int. J. Pharm.* 221: 143–152 (2001).
23. Fernandez-Urrusuno R, Fattal E, Feger J, Couvreur P, Therond P. *Biomaterials* 18: 511–517 (1997).
24. Fernandez-Urrusuno R, Fattal E, Rodrigues JM, Jr., Feger J, Bedossa P, Couvreur P. *J. Biomed. Mater. Res.* 31: 401–408 (1996).
25. Photos PJ, Bacakova L, Discher B, Bates FS, Discher DE. *J. Control Release* 90: 323–334 (2003).
26. Abuchowski A, McCoy JR, Palczuk NC, van Es T, Davis FF. *J. Biol. Chem.* 252: 3582–3586 (1977).
27. Moghimi SM, Szebeni J. *Prog. Lipid. Res.* 42: 463–478 (2003).
28. Avgoustakis K, Beletsi A, Panagi Z, Klepetsanis P, Livaniou E, Evangelatos G, Ithakissios DS. *Int. J. Pharm.* 259: 115–127 (2003).
29. Gao X, Cui Y, Levenson RM, Chung LW, Nie S. *Nat. Biotechnol.* 22: 969–976 (2004).
30. Brannon-Peppas L, Blanchette JO. *Adv. Drug. Deliv. Rev.* 56: 1649–1659 (2004).
31. Danilov SM, Gavrilyuk VD, Franke FE, Pauls K, Harshaw DW, McDonald TD, Miletich DJ, Muzykantov VR. *Am. J. Physiol. Lung. Cell. Mol. Physiol.* 280: L1335–L13347 (2001).
32. Scherpereel A, Rome JJ, Wiewrodt R, Watkins SC, Harshaw DW, Alder S, Christofidou-Solomidou M, Haut E, Murciano JC, Nakada M, Albelda SM, Muzykantov VR. *J. Pharmacol. Exp. Ther.* 300: 777–786 (2002).
33. Wiewrodt R, Thomas AP, Cipelletti L, Christofidou-Solomidou M, Weitz DA, Feinstein SI, Schaffer D, Albelda SM, Koval M, Muzykantov VR. *Blood* 99: 912–922 (2002).
34. Szoka F, Jr., Papahadjopoulos D. *Proc. Natl. Acad. Sci. USA* 75: 4194–4198 (1978).

35. Kosloski MJ, Rosen F, Milholland RJ, Papahadjopoulos D. *Cancer. Res.* 38: 2848–2853 (1978).
36. Lasic DD. *Trends. Biotechnol.* 16: 307–321 (1998).
37. Lasic DD, Papahadjopoulos D. *Science* 267: 1275–1276 (1995).
38. Winterhalter M, Lasic DD. *Chem. Phys. Lipids.* 64: 35–43 (1993).
39. Zhou F, Rouse BT, Huang L. *J. Immunol. Methods* 145: 143–152 (1991).
40. Vemuri S, Rhodes CT. *J. Pharm. Pharmacol.* 46: 778–783 (1994).
41. Ceh B, Winterhalter M, Frederik PM, Vallner JJ, Lasic DD. *Adv. Drug. Deliv. Rev.* 24: 165–177 (1997).
42. Johnston SR, Gore ME. *Eur. J. Cancer* 37 (Suppl 9): S8–S14 (2001).
43. Muller RH, Radtke M, Wissing SA. *Adv. Drug. Deliv. Rev.* 54 (Suppl 1): S131–S155 (2002).
44. Rao GC, Kumar MS, Mathivanan N, Rao ME. *Pharmazie* 59: 5–9 (2004).
45. Wong HL, Bendayan R, Rauth AM, Wu XY. *J. Pharm. Sci.* 93: 1993–2008 (2004).
46. Miglietta A, Cavalli R, Bocca C, Gabriel L, Gasco MR. *Int. J. Pharm.* 210: 61–67 (2000).
47. Pegi A, Julijana K, Slavko P, Janez S, Marjeta S. *J. Pharm. Sci.* 92: 58–66 (2003).
48. Dingler A, Blum RP, Niehus H, Muller RH, Gohla S. *J. Microencapsul.* 16: 751–767 (1999).
49. Muzykantov VR. *Biotechnol. Appl. Biochem.* 26: 103–109 (1997).
50. Shuvaev VV, Dziubla T, Wiewrodt R, Muzykantov VR. *Methods Mol. Biol.* 283: 3–19 (2004).
51. Atochina EN, Balyasnikova IV, Danilov SM, Granger DN, Fisher AB, Muzykantov VR. *Am. J. Physiol.* 275: L806–L817 (1998).
52. Muzykantov VR, Christofidou-Solomidou M, Balyasnikova I, Harshaw DW, Schultz L, Fisher AB, Albelda SM. *Proc. Natl. Acad. Sci. USA* 96: 2379–2384 (1999).
53. Murciano JC, Muro S, Koniaris L, Christofidou-Solomidou M, Harshaw DW, Albelda SM, Granger DN, Cines DB, Muzykantov VR. *Blood* 101: 3977–3984 (2003).
54. Kozower BD, Christofidou-Solomidou M, Sweitzer TD, Muro S, Buerk DG, Solomides CC, Albelda SM, Patterson GA, Muzykantov VR. *Nat. Biotechnol.* 21: 392–398 (2003).
55. Sweitzer TD, Thomas AP, Wiewrodt R, Nakada MT, Branco F, Muzykantov VR. *Free Radic. Biol. Med.* 34: 1035–1046 (2003).
56. Dunne M, Corrigan I, Ramtoola Z. *Biomaterials* 21: 1659–1668 (2000).
57. Cao X, Schoichet MS. *Biomaterials* 20: 329–339 (1999).

58. Piskin E, Kaitian X, Denkbas EB, Kucukyavuz Z. *J. Biomater. Sci. Polym. Ed.* 7: 359–373 (1995).
59. Shive MS, Anderson JM. *Adv. Drug. Deliv. Rev.* 28: 5–24 (1997).
60. Matsumoto J. *Int. J. Pharm.* 185: 93–101 (1999).
61. Perez C, Sanchez A, Putnam D, Ting D, Langer R, Alonso MJ. *J. Control. Release* 75: 211–224 (2001).
62. Avgoustakis K. *J. Control. Release* 79: 123–135 (2002).
63. Zambaux MF, Bonneaux F, Gref R, Dellacherie E, Vigneron C. *J. Biomed. Mater. Res.* 44: 109–115 (1999).
64. Hans ML, Lowman AM. *Curr. Opin. Solid State Mater. Sci.* 6: 319–327 (2002).
65. Li Y-P, Pei Y-Y, Zhang X-Y, Gu Z-H, Zhou Z-H, Yuan W-F, Zhou J-J, Zhu J-H, Gao X-J. *J. Control Release* 71: 203–211 (2001).
66. Zambaux MF, Faivra-Fiorina B, Bonneaux F, Marchal S, Merlin J-L, Dellacherie E, Labrude P, Vigneron C. *Biomaterials* 21: 975–980 (2000).
67. Dziubla TD, Lowman AM. *J. Biomed. Mater. Res.* 68A: 603–614 (2004).
68. Lee J-M, Bermudez H, Discher BM, Sheehan MA, Won Y-Y, Bates FS, Discher DE. *Biotechnol. Bioeng.* 73: 135–145 (2001).
69. Discher DE, Eisenberg A. *Science* 297: 967–973 (2002).
70. Napoli A, Valentini M, Tirelli N, Muller M, Hubbell JA. *Nat. Mater.* 3: 183–189 (2004).
71. Ahmed F, Discher DE. *J. Control Release* 96: 37–53 (2004).
72. Schnitzer JE. *N. Engl. J. Med.* 339: 472–474 (1998).
73. Muro S, Koval M, Muzykantov V. *Curr. Vasc. Pharmacol.* 2: 281–299 (2004).
74. Muzykantov VR, Atochina EN, Ischiropoulos H, Danilov SM, Fisher AB. *Proc. Natl. Acad. Sci. USA* 93: 5213–5218 (1996).
75. Atochina EN, Muzykantov VR, Al-Mehdi AB, Danilov SM, Fisher AB. *Am. J. Respir. Crit. Care Med.* 156: 1114–1119 (1997).
76. Sadhukhan R, Santhamma KR, Reddy P, Peschon JJ, Black RA, Sen I. *J. Biol. Chem.* 274: 10511–10516 (1999).
77. Balyasnikova IV, Karran EH, Albrecht RF, II, Danilov SM. *Biochem. J.* 362: 585–595 (2002).
78. Bevilacqua MP, Nelson RM, Mannori G, Cecconi O. *Annu. Rev. Med.* 45: 361–378 (1994).
79. Spragg DD, Alford DR, Greferath R, Larsen CE, Lee KD, Gurtner GC, Cybulsky MI, Tosi PF, Nicolau C, Gimbrone MA, Jr. *Proc. Natl. Acad. Sci. USA* 94: 8795–8800 (1997).
80. Harari OA, Wickham TJ, Stocker CJ, Kovesdi I, Segal DM, Huehns TY, Sarraf C, Haskard DO. *Gene. Ther.* 6: 801–807 (1999).

81. Lindner JR, Song J, Christiansen J, Klibanov AL, Xu F, Ley K. *Circulation* 104: 2107–2112 (2001).
82. von Asmuth EJ, Smeets EF, Ginsel LA, Onderwater JJ, Leeuwenberg JF, Buurman WA. *Eur. J. Immunol.* 22: 2519–2526 (1992).
83. Kuijpers TW, Raleigh M, Kavanagh T, Janssen H, Calafat J, Roos D, Harlan JM. *J. Immunol.* 152: 5060–5069 (1994).
84. Kessner S, Krause A, Rothe U, Bendas G. *Biochim. Biophys. Acta* 1514: 177–190 (2001).
85. Everts M, Kok RJ, Asgeirsdottir SA, Melgert BN, Moolenaar TJ, Koning GA, van Luyn MJ, Meijer DK, Molema G. *J. Immunol.* 168: 883–889 (2002).
86. Straley KS, Green SA. *J. Cell. Biol.* 151: 107–116 (2000).
87. Sheff DR, Daro EA, Hull M, Mellman I. *J. Cell. Biol.* 145: 123–139 (1999).
88. Jacobson BS, Schnitzer JE, McCaffery M, Palade GE. *Eur. J. Cell. Biol.* 58: 296–306 (1992).
89. McIntosh DP, Tan XY, Oh P, Schnitzer JE. *Proc. Natl. Acad. Sci. USA* 99: 1996–2001 (2002).
90. Ghitescu LD, Crine P, Jacobson BS. *Exp. Cell. Res.* 232: 47–55 (1997).
91. Tran D, Carpentier JL, Sawano F, Gorden P, Orci L. *Proc. Natl. Acad. Sci. USA* 84: 7957–7961 (1987).
92. Parton RG, Lindsay M. *Immunol. Rev.* 168: 23–31 (1999).
93. Kamen BA, Smith AK, Anderson RG. *J. Clin. Invest.* 87: 1442–1449 (1991).
94. Chun M, Liyanage UK, Lisanti MP, Lodish HF. *Proc. Natl. Acad. Sci. USA* 91: 11728–11732 (1994).
95. Parton RG, Joggerst B, Simons K. *J. Cell. Biol.* 127: 1199–1215 (1994).
96. Schnitzer JE. *Adv. Drug Deliv. Rev.* 49: 265–280 (2001).
97. Koval M, Preiter K, Adles C, Stahl PD, Steinberg TH. *Exp. Cell. Res.* 242: 265–273 (1998).
98. Etienne-Manneville S, Hall A. *Nature* 420: 629–635 (2002).
99. Oka K, Sawamura T, Kikuta K, Itokawa S, Kume N, Kita T, Masaki T. *Proc. Natl. Acad. Sci. USA* 95: 9535–9540 (1998).
100. Newman PJ. *J. Clin. Invest.* 100: S25–S29 (1997).
101. Mulligan MS, Miyasaka M, Tamatani T, Jones ML, Ward PA. *J. Immunol.* 152: 832–840 (1994).
102. Springer TA. *Nature* 346: 425–434 (1990).
103. Albelda SM. *Am. J. Respir. Cell Mol. Biol.* 4: 195–203 (1991).
104. Steeber DA, Tedder TF. *Immunol. Res.* 22: 299–317 (2000).
105. Rothlein R, Mainolfi EA, Kishimoto TK. *Res. Immunol.* 144: 735–739; discussion 754–762 (1993).

106. Murohara T, Delyani JA, Albelda SM, Lefer AM. *J. Immunol.* 156: 3550–3557 (1996).
107. Kumasaka T, Quinlan WM, Doyle NA, Condon TP, Sligh J, Takei F, Beaudet A, Bennett CF, Doerschuk CM. *J. Clin. Invest.* 97: 2362–2369 (1996).
108. Muro S, Wiewrodt R, Thomas AP, Koniaris L, Albelda SM, Muzykantov VR, Koval M. *J. Cell Sci.* 116: 1599–1609 (2003).
109. Muro S, Cui X, Gajewski C, Murciano JC, Muzykantov VR, Koval M. *Am. J. Physiol. Cell Physiol.* 285: C1339–C1347 (2003).
110. Bomsel M, Parton R, Kuznetsov SA, Schroer TA, Gruenberg J. *Cell* 62: 719–731 (1990).
111. Muro S, Gajewski C, Koval M, Muzykantov VR. *Blood* 105: 650–658 (2005).

38 Use of Biomarkers of Oxidative Stress in Human Studies

Chung-Yen Chen and Jeffrey B. Blumberg

1. Introduction

In human studies, biomarkers can be employed to reflect environmental pro-oxidant exposures and dietary antioxidant intake or to serve as a surrogate measure of a disease process like carcinogenesis.[1–3] To be truly useful, the biomarker must have some degree of predictive validity, but full substantiation of this relationship is still lacking for the antioxidant hypothesis. While a number of challenges must be overcome in using biomarkers to obtain a better understanding of the contributions of reactive species to carcinogenesis and other diseases, a rational application of biomarkers of oxidative stress to observational studies and clinical trials examining antioxidants and disease can still be employed if the constraints associated with them are fully appreciated.[4–6] Without measuring parameters relevant to the status of antioxidant defenses and oxidative stress in clinical trials, it is not possible to determine whether the selection, dose, and duration of an antioxidant intervention achieves its intended biochemical or physiological endpoint or whether the enrolled subjects even present with oxidative stress. Identification and application of suitable biomarkers should shorten the time it takes to demonstrate that an agent has a beneficial, untoward, or null effect on health promotion and disease prevention or a therapeutic value in disease treatment. However, some proposed biomarkers of oxidative stress might simply prove to be general markers of oxidative damage and relate poorly to disease process and outcome.

Considerations about the application of biomarkers of oxidative stress and the interpretation of study results must account for their adequacy in measuring relevant physiologic functions or relating to established pathological signs, particularly with regard to their accuracy, precision, and reliability.[7] Such efforts must consider the potential for artifacts produced during sample collection, processing, storage, and instrumental analyses, as well as confounding by the presence of related factors such as the status of facets of the antioxidant defense network that are not under direct study. The validation of biomarkers must include an assessment of the degree of bias in their measurement, especially the characterization of their prevalence and variability within large-scale population studies. An important issue for continued study is the determination of whether specific biomarkers reflect short- or long-term exposure to an antioxidant status or oxidative stress.

When establishing the Dietary Reference Intakes, the Institute of Medicine[8] defined dietary antioxidants by using biomarkers of oxidative stress. The IOM definition of dietary antioxidants includes their ability to significantly decrease the adverse effects of reactive species, such as reactive oxygen and nitrogen species, on normal physiologic function in humans. However, it is not clear whether a sufficient scientific agreement yet exists about the validity of these biomarkers to reflect the action and efficacy of dietary antioxidants. This issue is confused by an apparent difficulty in many studies to demonstrate an antioxidant effect without oxidative stress first being significantly elevated, e.g., as found in smokers or patients with active inflammatory conditions.

One common working definition of oxidative stress is the disturbance in the pro-oxidant/antioxidant balance in favor of the former, which leads to potential cellular damage. However, measuring oxidative stress can be difficult due to the presence of complex endogenous systems for correction and repair, e.g., as may occur when a brief elevation in oxidative stress rapidly induces various antioxidant defenses, particularly antioxidant enzymes such as superoxide dismutase, catalase, and glutathione peroxidase, that quickly reduce the stress and limit our ability to detect a change.[9] Oxidative stress can result from diminished antioxidant protection as well as increased free radical production. Therefore, investigating antioxidant depletion as a biomarker of oxidative stress may involve determining decreases in antioxidant concentrations or increases in their metabolites. However, such changes may not reflect a clinically significant or pathogenic event but merely may be an indication that the antioxidant defense system is functioning.

Three general approaches are commonly employed in assessing oxidative stress: induction of antioxidant enzymes, reduction of endogenous antioxidants, and production of oxidatively modified lipids, protein, and/or DNA (Fig. 1). The latter approach, measuring biomarkers of lipid peroxidation like malondialdehyde (MDA) and $F_{2\alpha}$-isoprostanes ($iPF_{2\alpha}$), protein oxidation products like carbonyls (PC) and oxidized amino acids, and oxidized DNA (oxDNA) including modified bases and strand breaks, is discussed first with regard to their biochemical reactions and the methods used to measure them and later concerning their application in human studies. While many other biomarkers could well be considered here, they are either less practical in their application to observational studies and clinical trials, e.g., L-band electron spin resonance with nitroxyl probes and magnetic resonance imaging spin trapping,[10] or less well characterized, e.g., isoketal adducts.[11] However, this chapter is focused on the practical application of

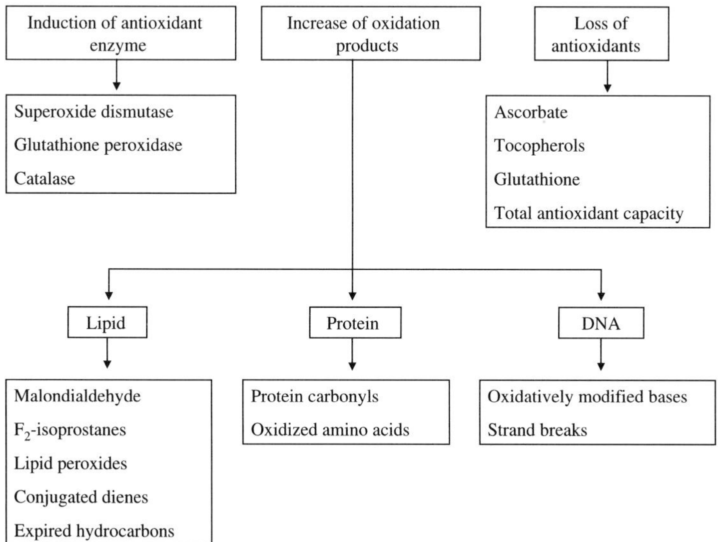

Fig. 1. Oxidative stress sorted as functionality of antioxidants and products of oxidation.

biomarkers of oxidative stress currently available and often employed in human studies.

2. Methods to Determine Biomarkers of Oxidative Damage

2.1. *Biomarkers for lipid peroxidation*

Products of lipid peroxidation reactions have been widely employed as biomarkers. While the biochemical pathways of these reactions have been well reviewed,[12] their intermediate and end-products generated are briefly summarized in Fig. 2.

2.1.1. *TBARS and MDA measurement*

MDA is most commonly measured by a thiobarbituric acid-reactive substances (TBARS) assay with a simple spectrophotometric method. The

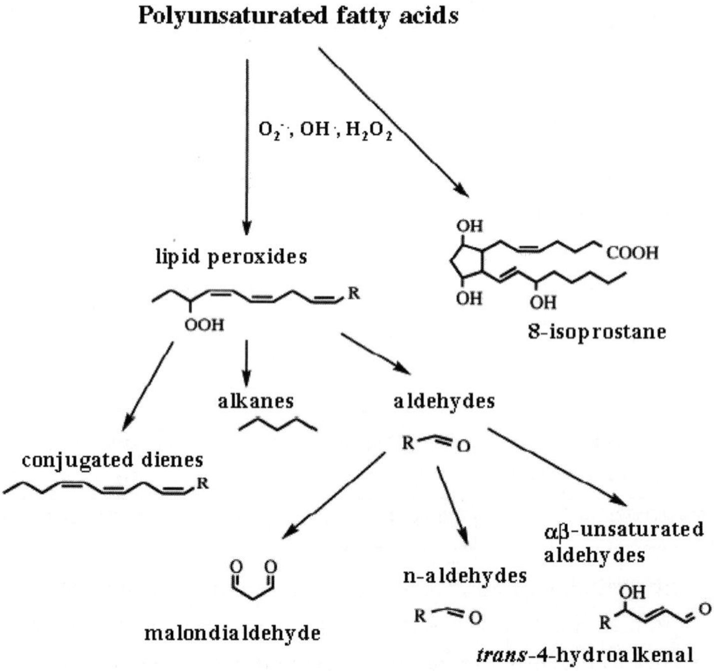

Fig. 2. Intermediate and end-products derived from lipid peroxidation.

amount of MDA corresponds to the chromogen formed from MDA and thiobarbituric acid (TBA) with a maximum absorption at 532–535 nm.[13] The acidity and Fe^{2+} in the reaction mixture can markedly influence the final concentration of the MDA–TBA. Total MDA is measured after protein-bound MDA is released by alkaline hydrolysis. However, the low sensitivity and specificity attributed to a cross-reaction of TBA with other substrates (including other alkanals, protein, sucrose, amino acids, sialic acid, urea, biliverdin, acetaldehyde–sucrose, and reducing sugars) make this method obsolete for human studies.[14,15] Employing high-performance liquid chromatography (HPLC) with fluorescence detection significantly improves the inadequacy of the TBARS method,[16,17] but may still overestimate the actual magnitude of lipid peroxidation through an artifact of inducing lipid peroxidation from the high temperature necessary for the TBA reaction.

In part due to various modifications of the assay, the range of plasma and urine MDA measured by HPLC varies between laboratories, but is generally about 1 μmol/l and 1 nmol/mg creatinine, respectively.[16] The limit of detection is typically about 0.1 μmol/l for plasma with an intra-assay coefficient of variation (CV) of 4–10% and inter-assay CV of 4–12%.[17]

2.1.2. $F_{2\alpha}$-*isoprostanes*

$iPF_{2\alpha}$ were first demonstrated in humans *in vivo* by Morrow *et al.*[18] with the potential for 64 different isomers to be generated through a cyclo-oxygenase independent peroxidation of arachidonic acid (AA) via endoperoxide and dioxethane/endoperoxide pathways.[19] As 8-isoprostane $F_{2\alpha}$ (8-$iPF_{2\alpha}$) is the mostly widely measured isomer in human studies, its formation is illustrated in Fig. 3.

$iPF_{2\alpha}$ are generally accepted as the best validated biomarker of lipid peroxidation *in vivo*.[20] However, it is important to appreciate the $iPF_{2\alpha}$ possess a biological half-life of only 18 min in plasma and are rapidly excreted in the urine. $iPF_{2\alpha}$ are formed systemically and constantly to maintain a steady-state plasma concentration.[21] It has been suggested that $iPF_{2\alpha}$ in urine could prove a more reliable biomarker of lipid peroxidation than in plasma, as a more integrated whole-body measure and less susceptible to artifact formation *ex vivo*.[20] Collection of plasma for the determination of $iPF_{2\alpha}$ requires rapid addition of butylated hydroxytoluene or tetraphenylporphine and

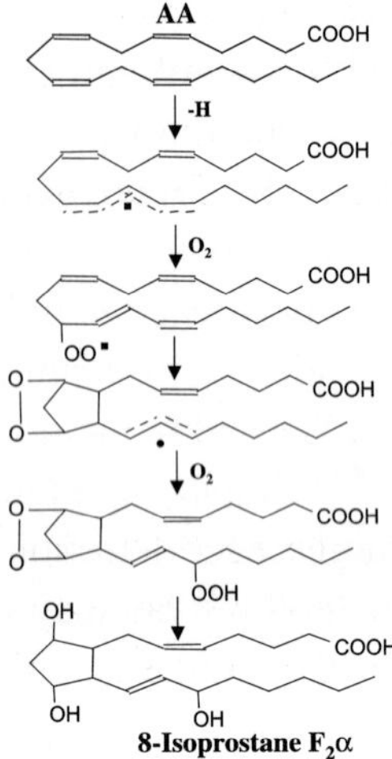

Fig. 3. Formation of 8-isoprostane $F_{2\alpha}$ from the peroxidation of arachidonic acid.

freezing (−70°C) of the sample to ensure stability.[20,22] Optimal determination of $iPF_{2\alpha}$ in urine requires collection of 24 h samples, though adjustment with urinary creatinine appears to improve the accuracy of those specimens collected for less than one day.

Several methods have been developed to determine $iPF_{2\alpha}$, including gas chromatography (GC)–mass spectrometry (MS),[20,23,24] enzyme immunoassay (EIA),[25] and HPLC–MS^2.[26] As most plasma $iPF_{2\alpha}$ are bound to phospholipids, total $iPF_{2\alpha}$ are obtained after alkaline hydrolysis with subsequent extraction via solid phase or HPLC methods and derivatization and silyation using pentafluorobenzyl bromide and N,O-bis(trimethysilyl)-trifluoroacetamide and internal standards such as $[^2H_4]$-9α,11β-$iPF_{2\alpha}$.[20] LC–MS^2 can require less labor-intensive derivatization procedures.[26,27] Both GC–MS or LC–MS methods possess a high degree of sensitivity and specificity, but their cost and technology limit their routine use, especially in large-scale human studies.[20] Commercially available EIA kits present a simple and cost-effective technique, but typically determine only 8-$iPF_{2\alpha}$ with a low specificity due to cross-reactivity with other $iPF_{2\alpha}$ isomers and related prostaglandin compounds. Correlations between MS and EIA methods are not strong.

$iPF_{2\alpha}$ concentrations in the plasma and urine of healthy individuals typically range between 5–40 pg/ml and 500–4000 pg/mg creatinine, respectively.[19] GC–MS methods provide a precision about 6% and an accuracy of 96%.[20] Intra- and inter-assay CV are generally <8%[28] and <6%,[29] respectively.

2.2. *Biomarkers for protein oxidation*

Proteins can be damaged directly by free radical attacks or indirectly via reactions with secondary by-products of lipid peroxidation[30] leading to formation of PC and oxidatively modified amino acid.

2.2.1. *Protein carbonyls*

PC can be generated through several different mechanisms, including Michael addition reactions of α,β-unsaturated aldehydes, glycation and glycoxidation, direct oxidation of amino acid side chains, and oxidative cleavage of proteins,[31] as illustrated in Fig. 4.

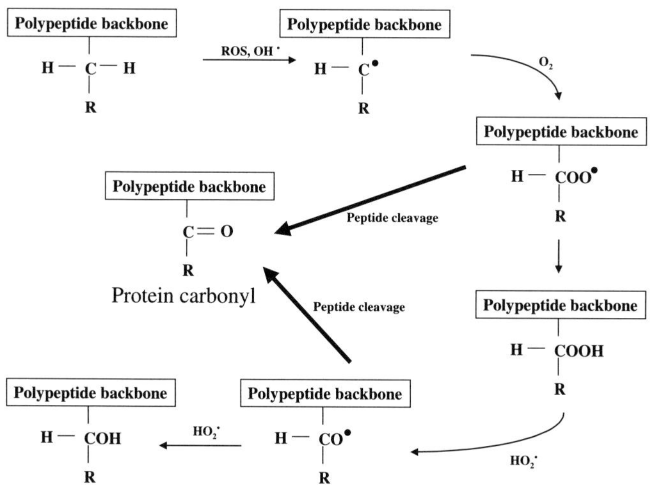

Fig. 4. Protein carbonyl formation after reactive oxygen species (ROS) attack and peptide cleavage.

PC are the most commonly employed biomarker for protein oxidation in human studies.[31,32] Although PC in tissues and body fluids can be measured by simple spectrometric,[33,34] enzyme-linked immunosorbent assay (ELISA),[35,36] and HPLC methods,[37] all these methods are based on formation of a hydrazone chromophore resulting from the reaction between PC and dinitrophenyl hydrazine (DNPH). The conventional spectrometric assay has a relatively low degree of reproducibility because of varied loss of PC during washing procedures.[34,38,39] Commercially available ELISA kits appear sensitive and capable of high throughput; however, its results are dependent upon the response of HOCl-generated PC standards to DNPH. Results from ELISA and spectrometric assays of plasma PC are relatively well correlated, but their absolute values may differ markedly.[35] HPLC works to separate DNPH–PC adducts from interfering compounds and improves overall sensitivity and reproducibility compared to other methods.[40]

Plasma PC from healthy individuals generally ranges between 0.1 and 1 nmol/mg protein.[41] The limit of PC detection in plasma with ELISA is 0.01 nmol/mg with intra- and inter-assay CV of 1–3% and 5–9%, respectively.[35,36]

2.2.2. *Oxidized amino acid products*

As PC are rather generic biomarkers of protein oxidation, specific oxidized amino acid products have been suggested as better reflecting specific radical reactions with protein.[42] With the capacity to delocalize charges, some amino acids are especially susceptible to oxidative attack with the generation of oxidized products, such as 3-chlorotyrosine (Cl-tyr), 3-nitrotyrosine (N-tyr), and dityrosine (di-tyr),[32,43] as illustrated in Fig. 5.

In contrast to PC, tyrosine products can reflect the specific radical species involved in protein oxidation.[44–47] However, the concentration of oxidized amino acids are orders of magnitude lower than PC.[43] Oxidized amino acids can be determined by HPLC with electrochemical detection (ECD)[48,49] and GC–MS,[50,51] often allowing for the concurrent measurement of all the compounds of interest.

Unlike lipid oxidation products, which can be readily generated during sample preparation, storage, and analysis, oxidized tyrosine is formed exclusively *in vivo* and not subject to artifacts.[31]

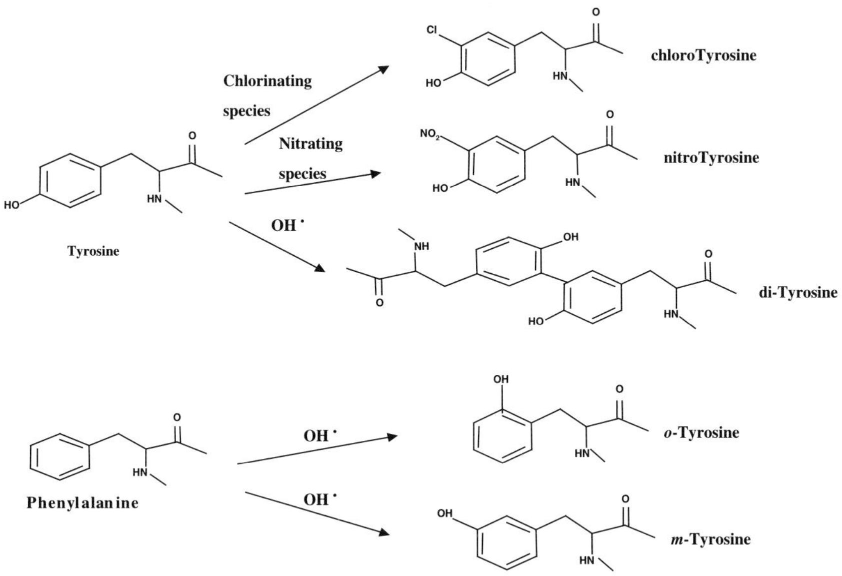

Fig. 5. Formation of oxidation products from tyrosine and phenylalanine.

Plasma N-tyr, Cl-tyr, and di-tyr determined by HPLC have been reported to be 0.1, 0.08, and 0.002 nmol/mol tyrosine, respectively.[21] Elevated concentrations of Cl-tyr have been found in low-density lipoproteins (LDL) from human atherosclerotic intima ($300/10^6$ tyrosyl residues), 30-fold higher than found in peripheral blood LDL.[52] Inter-assay variability in the measurement of oxidized tyrosine is about 9% with the limit of detection at 2 pmol.[21]

2.3. *Biomarkers of DNA damage*

A low steady-state level of DNA damaged by reactive species is present in healthy cells with increased concentrations associated with cancer cells.[53–55] Oxidized DNA bases have been assessed in urine, serum, and tissues by HPLC–ECD, GC–MS, and LC–MS, and ELISA and radical-induced DNA strand breaks have been investigated in single cells by gel electrophoresis.[53] Lymphocyte oxDNA is most commonly measured as a biomarker of DNA damage; however, the relationship between lymphocyte oxDNA and oxDNA present in other cells has not been established, so caution is warranted in extrapolating results from readily available blood cells to other tissues.[21,56] Similarly, the status of urinary oxDNA must be attributed not only to systemic DNA damage but also to DNA repair, so interpretation to other tissues is limited.[53] While there continues to be some discussion on the quantification of basal oxDNA levels and units employed to express oxDNA, The European Standards Committee on Oxidative DNA Damage (ESCODD) has proposed that oxDNA should be expressed in terms of altered bases (or nucleosides) per 10^6 unaltered bases (nucleosides).[21]

2.3.1. *Detection of DNA base oxidation*

Reactive oxygen species, particularly hydroxyl radicals, attack all four DNA bases, leading to the generation of a multiplicity of products, including thymine glycol, 8-hydroxy-guanine (8-oxo-Gua), 8-hydroxy-adenine (8-OH-A), 5-hydroxy-cytosine (5-OH-C), and 5-hydroxy-uracil (5-OH-U).[53] As 8-hydroxyguanosine (8-oxo-dG) is among the most commonly measured oxDNA products, its formation is illustrated in Fig. 6.

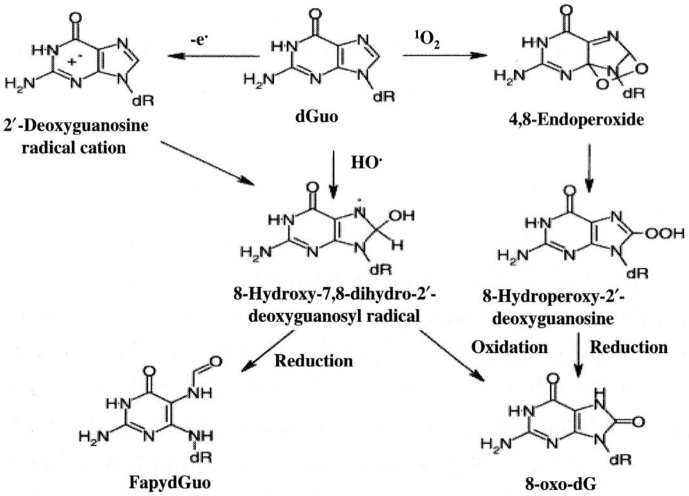

Fig. 6. The formation of 8-hydroxy-2′-deoxyguanosine (8-oxo-dG) by reactive oxygen species.

2.3.1.1. HPLC–ECD detection of oxDNA

HPLC–ECD has been widely used to measure oxDNA in biological samples with good sensitivity.[57,58] Before oxDNA bases are determined, the DNA must be isolated and purified through cell lysis, DNA release, RNA and protein digestion, chloroform/isoamyl alcohol extraction, and DNA hydrolysis. As each of these steps can be associated with the oxidative induction of artifacts, preventive steps including sodium iodide for DNA precipitation, endonucleases (nuclease P1 and alkaline phosphatase) for releasing DNA bases, addition of antioxidants, and elimination of ambient oxygen are required.[21,59] Similar caution is not required with DNA from serum and urine as oxDNA bases are determined after pre-purification by HPLC, solid-phase extraction, or immunoaffinity chromatography without other isolation and hydrolysis procedures.[21,53,60]

oxDNA bases with electroactive properties, such as 8-oxo-Gua, 8-OH-A, 5-OH-C, and 5-OH-U, can be measured by HPLC–ECD. Typically, their corresponding nucleosides are determined due to the greater resolution of these compounds with HPLC columns.[53] The amounts of oxDNA bases are determined according to calibrated curve of authenticated standards. HPLC–ECD sensitivity is within the picomole range for a DNA sample $\geq 20\,\mu g$.[53] An internal standard, 2,6-diamino-8-oxopurine, has been incorporated in HPLC–ECD to increase sensitivity.[61] Lymphocytes have been reported to contain between two and 40 8-oxo-Gua/10^6 cells.[62,63] Urinary 8-oxo-dG in humans is about 280 pmol/kg body weight (bw)/day with intra- and inter-assay CV about 2 and 4%, respectively.[64]

2.3.1.2. GC–MS and LC–MS–MS detection of oxDNA

GC–MS and LC–MS analysis of oxDNA provide positive identification and high sensitivity.[59,65,66] The caveats concerning the care necessary to avoid artifacts during extraction and hydrolysis are the same as those described for HPLC–ECD. In contrast to HPLC–ECD, DNA bases rather than nucleotides are determined with greater sensitivity.[53] Quantification is achieved with appropriate internal standards, such as stable isotope-labeled analogs of modified bases.[65] LC–MS^2 with electrospray ionization (ESI) or atmospheric pressure ionization chemical ionization (API-CI) provides several advantages in oxDNA analysis, particularly the reduction of derivatization steps required in GC–MS.[67–69]

The sensitivity of GC–MS in determining 8-oxo-dG at 2 fmol is at least an order of magnitude greater than that of LC–MS[70] and requires about 2 μg DNA, 20-fold less material than necessary for LC injection.[53] Typically, white blood cells contain about 300 8-oxo-Gua/10^6 guanine measured by GC–MS.[71–73] Intra- and inter-assay CV for GC–MS are 9–21 and 10%, respectively.[21,53] Urine specimens (24 h collections) tested with LC–MS contain 136 (1943 pmol/kg bw/day) 8-oxo-Gua and 28 nmol (400 pmol/kg bw/day) 8-oxo-dG.[74] Intra- and inter-assay CV for measuring 8-oxo-dG by LC–MS is about 2–5 and 3–7%, respectively.[74]

2.3.1.3. ELISA detection of oxDNA

Commercial ELISA kits provide a simple and high-throughput method for the determination of 8-oxo-dG in urine and, to a lesser extent, in some other specimens.[53] Reproducibility with the ELISA method is good and sensitivity comparable to HPLC–ECD though the actual concentration of 8-oxo-dG may be overestimated due to cross-reactivity of the antibody with 8-oxoguanosine from oxidized RNA and 8-oxo-dG in DNA oligomers.[75,76] The sensitivity of the assay for isolated DNA is about one adduct/10^8 nucleotides[53] with intra- and inter-assay CV both estimated at $<10\%$.[77]

2.3.2. *Single cell gel electrophoresis (Comet assay) detection of oxDNA*

The single cell gel electrophoresis or "Comet" assay was originally developed to monitor DNA strand breaks in individual cells.[78] With hydrolysis of endonucleases III (endo III) or formamidopyrimidine DNA glycosylase (FPG), this assay has been employed to detect oxidized pyrimidines and altered purines including 8-oxo-Gua.[79] Further, the resistance of cellular DNA against *in vitro* oxidant challenges, usually H_2O_2, in this assay reflect endogenous cellular antioxidant defenses and the adequacy of DNA repair systems.[80]

In the assay, cells are embedded in agarose, lysed with detergent plus high salt, and then subjected to alkaline electrophoresis to produce the image of a "comet" under the fluorescence microscopy.[81–83] Quantification of the comet image can be achieved by a visual scoring system or, preferably, with computer image analysis.

In contrast to HPLC or MS methods, the Comet assay is not particularly subject to artifact.[21] However, quantitation of the Comet results is indirect and relative, expressed as percent DNA in the tail or in arbitrary units. Further, the extent of oxDNA damage may be underestimated when lesions occur in clusters. As FPG recognizes all altered purines, the assay is not truly specific to individual bases, e.g., 8-oxo-Gua.[21] Interpretation of Comet assay results also requires caution because differences in cell cycle and lifespan among different cells in a heterogeneous mixture, such as leukocytes, can be confounding.[83,84]

Typically, analysis of white blood cells by the Comet assay indicates 0.5 8-oxo-dG/10^6 base[71,72] and CV of $<0.1\%$.[85]

3. Application of Biomarkers of Oxidative Stress in Human Studies

3.1. $F_{2\alpha}$-isoprostanes as biomarkers of pathogenesis

While oxidative stress is clearly associated with the risk of many chronic diseases, its role in the etiology and/or progression of critical pathogenic stages versus the potential of it merely being an outcome or epiphenomenon continues to be debated.[86,87] $iPF_{2\alpha}$ has been employed in many studies as a validated biomarker of lipid peroxidation useful to address this issue as well as to examine its practical application in diagnosis and prognosis.

Acute T lymphocyte and macrophage activation during the development of type 1 or insulin-dependent diabetes mellitus (IDDM) may lead to increased generation of reactive species and oxidative stress.[88,89] In a cross-sectional study, urinary 8-$iPF_{2\alpha}$ (determined by ELISA) was measured in 23 newly diagnosed IDDM patients <18 years and 23 age- and gender-matched patients with established disease.[90] All IDDM patients had urinary 8-$iPF_{2\alpha}$ concentrations greater than two standard deviations above the mean of matched healthy children. The newly diagnosed patients had significantly higher urinary 8-$iPF_{2\alpha}$ (500 pg/mg creatinine) than those living with the disease for >1 year. A reduction in urinary 8-$iPF_{2\alpha}$ was observed in 65% of the newly diagnosed group when they were re-examined 1 year later, a change highly correlated with a reduction in inflammation as assessed by interleukin-6 and tumor necrosis factor-α. Similarly, Handelman *et al.*[91] found a sixfold greater concentration of total plasma esterified $iPF_{2\alpha}$ (using

GC–MS) in patients with end-stage renal disease compared to healthy controls with this biomarker directly related to inflammatory status assessed by C-reactive protein.

Oxidative stress can serve as a potent stimulus for apoptosis in cardiomyocytes and may contribute to the progression of heart failure.[92,93] Mallat *et al.*[94] monitored 8-iPF$_{2\alpha}$ (measured by ELISA) in pericardial fluid collected immediately after incision from 51 patients, 39–78 years, with ischemic or valvular heart disease. 8-iPF$_{2\alpha}$ in symptomatic patients was significantly higher than in asymptomatic patients at 27.0 versus 11.1 pg/ml, respectively. The increase in 8-iPF$_{2\alpha}$ was directly associated with the functional severity of the heart failure, indicating a role of lipid peroxidation in the progression of the disease and its potential value in prognosis.

Infection with hepatitis C virus (HCV) is associated with the development of liver damage and necrosis. Although the pathogenic mechanism(s) in this relationship have not been elucidated, oxidative stress and inflammation may play an important role here. Jain *et al.*[95] observed that compared to 49 healthy volunteers, 42 HCV patients had significantly elevated 8-iPF$_{2\alpha}$ in their urine (1.08 versus 0.26 pg/mg creatinine) and plasma (96.0 versus 8.8 pg/ml), measured by ELISA, as well as a compromised antioxidant status. Urinary 8-iPF$_{2\alpha}$ in the cirrhotic group was threefold greater or equal than in the non-cirrhotic group, but there was no difference in plasma 8-iPF$_{2\alpha}$ between these two sets of patients. In contrast, the fibrosis score was positively correlated with both urinary and plasma 8-iPF$_{2\alpha}$ at $r = 0.639$ ($P < 0.001$) and $r = 0.416$ ($P = 0.017$), respectively. Interestingly, while 8-iPF$_{2\alpha}$ appears to predict the progression of liver damage in HCV patients, this relationship was not apparent with MDA.

Oxidative stress has been associated with human immunodeficiency virus (HIV-1) infection in several studies. Hulgan *et al.*[96] monitored the association between 8-iPF$_{2\alpha}$, infection, and anti-retroviral therapy in HIV-1 patients. Plasma 8-iPF$_{2\alpha}$ was determined by GC-MS in 120 non-fasting subjects with a mean age of 41 years and $\geq$1 year of HIV-1 infection. The median concentration of this biomarker was not significantly different from that in healthy volunteers at 31 versus 35 ± 6 pg/ml, respectively; however, the range of 8-iPF$_{2\alpha}$ among the patients was very large at 12–149 pg/ml. Patients treated with anti-retroviral therapy and having lower HIV-1 RNA levels had significantly higher plasma 8-iPF$_{2\alpha}$ than untreated patients, suggesting an untoward effect of long-term pharmacotherapy.

The oxidative modification of LDLs and other molecules has been proposed as a key event in the initiation and progression of atherogenesis, though whether $iPF_{2\alpha}$ in plasma or urine can adequately reflect changes in arterial lesions such as plaque is not clear. Due to their much greater abundance, hydroxyoctadecaenoic (HODE) and hydroxyeicosatetraenoic (HETE) acid have been proposed as biomarkers of the progression and rupture of atherosclerotic plaques.[97,98] Nonetheless, Gniwotta *et al.*[99] observed higher concentrations of $iPF_{2\alpha}$ (measured by GC–MS) in atherosclerotic lesions in anterior, aortic, femoralis, poplitea, tibialis, and vertebralis arteries from 10 patients than in human umbilical cord (75.9 versus 11.7 pg/mg dry weight). However, Waddington *et al.*[100] found that neither $iPF_{2\alpha}$ (measured by GC–MS), HODE, or HETE in the internal carotid arteries of 50 endarterectomy patients (mean age = 70 years) were different between those who were symptomatic (transient ischemic episode or stroke) and asymptomatic patients (with $\geq$70% carotid artery occlusion), suggesting that lipid peroxidation is not predictive of plaque instability.

Oxidative stress has been linked with the initiation and progression of Alzheimer's disease (AD) in cell culture and animal models, but data from human studies are limited.[101,102] Montine *et al.*[103] determined $iPF_{2\alpha}$ in urine as well as a urinary metabolite of 8-$iPF_{2\alpha}$ by GC–MS in 56 AD patients and 34 matched healthy subjects but detected no significant differences between these groups. Nevertheless, it is worth noting that in cerebrospinal fluid, $iPF_{2\alpha}$ in a subset of 32 patients (36.8 pg/ml) was significantly greater than that in six control subjects (24.2 pg/ml). These results suggest that $iPF_{2\alpha}$ in readily accessible tissue like plasma and urine may not adequately reflect oxidative stress status in certain localized lesions.

3.2. *Oxidized amino acids as biomarkers of atherosclerosis*

The recruitment of inflammatory cells during the early stages of atherogenesis is associated with the generation of reactive nitrogen species and myeloperoxidase (MPO)-derived reactive halogen species.[104] These free radicals lead to formation of Cl-tyr and N-tyr, a reaction that is not inhibited by the lipid-soluble, chain-breaking antioxidant vitamin E.[105–107] This is an interesting observation in light of the null outcome of some clinical trials of vitamin E in patients with heart disease.[107–109] Oxidized amino acids have been found to be abundant in human atheroma and LDL recovered from atherosclerotic laden versus normal aorta.[43,110] Consistent with the hypothesis that protein oxidation may play a role in atherogenesis is the observation of a reduced risk of heart disease in people with MPO deficiency people.[111]

Statin drugs are commonly employed in the treatment of hypercholesterolemia and their efficacy in reducing the risk of coronary heart disease mortality is well established. However, in addition to their ability to antagonize cholesterol synthesis, statins also possess the capacity to inhibit protein oxidation. Shishehbor *et al.*[112] administered 10 mg atorvastatin daily to 35 hypercholesterolemic subjects without frank coronary artery disease for 12 weeks and found significantly reduced plasma levels of protein-bound Cl-tyr and di-tyr (determined by GC–MS) and N-tyr (determined by LC–MS^2). These reductions in oxidized amino acids were largely independent of the statin-induced reduction in blood lipids.

Endothelial dysfunction, which can be triggered by oxidative stress, is part of the atherogenic process and a strong clinical correlate of functional decline preceding cardiac events.[108,113] Frustaci *et al.*[114] have proposed a causative link between N-tyr production and endothelial dysfunction. Ceriello *et al.*[115] conducted a placebo-controlled, cross-over study with 40 mg/day simvastatin in type II non-insulin dependent diabetic patients for 12 weeks and found both significant reductions in plasma N-tyr (determined by ELISA) and endothelial dysfunction assessed by flow-mediated vasodilation of the brachial artery. These outcomes, most marked during postprandial hyperglycemia and hypertriglyceridemia, were independent of the hypocholesterolemic effect of the drug and, thus, potentially linked to its antioxidant actions. In contrast, Kinlay *et al.*[116] provided 800 IU RRR-α-tocopherol and 1 g ascorbic acid daily to 25 cardiovascular patients for 6 months but were unable to improve endothelium-dependent vasomotor function in coronary and brachial arteries; it is worth noting that this intervention did not significantly reduce in plasma $iPF_{2\alpha}$ (determined by GC–MS). These results suggest not only that oxidized amino acids may be a useful marker of oxidative stress in cardiovascular disease but that testing antioxidant interventions effective in modifying protein oxidation are warranted.

3.3. *Oxidized DNA as a biomarker of oxidative stress induced by physical activity*

In part because oxidized bases are mutagenic, oxidative DNA damage has been proposed to contribute significantly to the development of cancer.[21,117,118] Further evidence linking oxDNA to carcinogenesis are observations associating elevated oxDNA in human carcinoma cells relative to adjacent tissue free of cancer.[54,55] Interestingly, strenuous physical activity is associated with inflammatory reactions and a marked increase in oxidative stress due to $\geq$10-fold increases in oxygen consumption but a decreased risk of several forms of cancer.[119–122] As physical activity presents a useful model for human studies of oxidative stress, it is worth reviewing the results of some studies examining the relationship between exercise and oxDNA damage.

Some investigators have found that habitual, moderate levels of exercise are not associated with increases in leukocyte 8-oxo-dG, although, for reasons noted above, the range in values can be broad, e.g., between 5 and 15 8-oxo-dG/10^6 dG as determined by HPLC–ECD.[62,123] Similarly, others have found no difference in urinary 8-oxo-dG (determined by ELSA) between trained athletes and sedentary healthy young men.[124] Indeed, lower leukocyte oxDNA appears more typical in physically active individuals than in sedentary people, suggesting an upregulation of antioxidant defenses and/or DNA repair mechanisms induced by regular exercise.[125,126] In contrast, exercise in healthy but untrained individuals may be associated with increases in oxDNA, although differences in the type, intensity, and duration of exercise make comparisons between studies difficult.

Sato *et al.*[125] tested seven active and eight sedentary non-smoking, young men, 19–29 years, in a mild 30 min exercise protocol (50% VO_{2max} on a bicycle ergometer) and found a decrease leukocyte oxDNA from 2.75 versus 2.0 8-oxo-Gua/10^6Gua (determined by HPLC–ECD) in the sedentary subjects at 48 h post-exercise accompanied by an increase in the mRNA expression of the DNA repair enzyme human MutT homolog, hMTH1. However, with their higher basal 8-oxo-Gua and mRNA hMTH1, the active men showed no change in these parameters. Similarly, Asami *et al.*[125] found that an increase in DNA repair enzyme activity was linked to reduction in leukocyte 8-oxo-dG (determined by HPLC–ECD) in 23 non-smoking men (including 10 moderately trained athletes), 19–50 years, immediately following a bicycle ergometer test. In contrast, Sumida *et al.*[127] challenged 14 non-smoking untrained young men with a single bout of high-intensity concentric exercise (bicycle ergometer) until exhaustion but found no change in urinary 8-oxo-dG excretion from baseline values of 1.8 nmol/mmol creatinine (determined by HPLC–ECD) for 3 days. Similarly, employing a strenuous 45 min bout of eccentric exercise (75% VO_{2max} with downhill running) in 32 moderately active but untrained men, Sacheck *et al.*[128] found no change in leukocyte 8-oxo-dG (determined by HPLC–ECD) from baseline levels of 4.5 8-oxo-dG/dG after 24 h.

Understanding regulatory mechanisms of DNA injury and repair induced by exercise may be improved by comparing oxDNA in leukocytes and urine. For example, Okamura *et al.*[129] examined lymphocyte 8-oxo-dG in 10 young trained marathon runners and found basal levels of 2.0 8-oxo-dG/10^6dG (determined by HPLC–ECD) were not altered after running 30 km/day for 8 days. However, amount of urinary 8-oxo-dG excretion was significantly greater after the training period than during a 3 day control period, 336 versus 266 pmol/kg bw/day. These results suggest urinary oxDNA excretion may serve as a systemic biomarker of oxDNA damage, essentially integrating rates of increased oxDNA formation and repair by removal of oxDNA bases. Consistent with this observation, Radák *et al.*[130] monitored five ultra-marathon runner training at 93, 120, 56, and 59 km in four successive days and found urinary 8-oxo-dG (determined by ELISA) increased from a baseline of 53.0 to 66.2 8-oxo-dG nmol/l on the first day, remained elevated during the training period, and decreased thereafter. However, caution is warranted in interpreting these results as the urinary 8-oxo-dG was not adjusted for creatinine or body weight. No adaptation effect to oxidative stress was observed by Almar *et al.*[131] in eight professional cyclists participating in two races. Their urinary 8-oxo-dG concentrations (determined by HPLC–ECD) before the races (175 pmol/kg bw/day) increased significantly by 121% during the first week of a 3-week race and by 47% after the first day of a 4-day race, and were not increased further in the race indicating oxDNA is sustained as long as very high intensity exercise is continued. In contrast, Hartmann *et al.*[132] found in six non-smoking young athletes that the less strenuous exercise of a short-distance of 2.5 h triathlon was not associated with a change in urinary 8-oxo-dG (determined by HPLC–ECD) from a baseline of 2.42 nmol/mmol creatinine up to 4 days following the competition.

Using ELISA, Radák *et al.*[133] determined oxDNA in biopsies of quadriceps femoris muscle taken from 12 young female athletes after isometric plus eccentric contraction exercises and after isometric exercise only and found higher 8-oxo-dG in the former group at 0.044 versus 0.035 nmol/mmol DNA. Radák *et al.*[134] also examined DNA repair enzyme activity by measuring endonuclease III and 8-oxoG DNA glycosylase (hOOG1) in quadriceps femoris muscle from six young athletes 16–18 h after completion of a 42 km marathon. They found significantly enhanced hOOG1 activity (though no change in endo III) suggesting an adaptive response to increases in the formation of 8-oxo-dG; however, oxDNA was not determined in this study. A clearer understanding of the relationship between oxDNA injury and DNA repair would be apparent if studies were to employ direct measures of both.

3.4. *Oxidized DNA as a biomarker in dietary antioxidant interventions*

Increased consumption of foods rich in dietary antioxidants is strongly associated with a reduced risk of cancer, although the extent to which the antioxidant ingredients contribute to this relationship is not clear.[135,136] One approach to examine this problem is to assess oxDNA following dietary interventions, and several studies have employed the Comet assay in this regard. For example, using the Comet assay, Collins *et al.*[137] demonstrated a reduction in lymphocyte pyrimidine and purine base damage in 14 healthy, non-smoking volunteers after consuming 1–3 kiwi/day for 3 weeks. In contrast, in a parallel design study, Moller *et al.*[138] gave 43 healthy volunteers 600 g fruits and vegetables, the equivalent dose of antioxidant vitamins in a supplement or a produce-free diet for 24 days but found no change in mononuclear cell oxDNA assessed with the Comet assay. Interestingly, Riso *et al.*[139] fed 60 g tomato puree (containing 16.5 mg lycopene) to 10 healthy women for 21 days and increased by 37.5% the resistance of their lymphocyte DNA to H_2O_2 challenge in the Comet assay, while Astley *et al.*[140] found no lymphocyte changes with the Comet assay after administering 15 mg/day of supplemental lycopene or lutein for 4 weeks to 28 healthy men and a significant increase in oxDNA in those given the same dose of β-carotene.

Arab *et al.*[141] employed a randomized clinical trial with 23 healthy non-smoking subjects exposed for 2 h to 0.4 ppm ozone before and 2 weeks after consumption of a carotenoid-rich vegetable juice, 250 mg vitamin C plus 50 IU α-tocopherol or placebo and found pulmonary epithelial cell oxDNA (measured with the Comet assay) reduced only in the first group and no change in leukocyte oxDNA in any group. While the many differences between the cohorts, antioxidant ingredients and matrices, and duration of studies make direct comparisons between these studies difficult, they do suggest that oxDNA assessed by the Comet assay is dependent on each of these factors as well as the choice of cell selected for the assessment. Importantly, similar limitations are found using proxy cells with other oxDNA biomarkers; e.g., in randomly assigning 26 men with prostate cancer to receive 30 mg lycopene from a tomato oleoresin extract or placebo for 3 weeks before radical prostatectomy, Kucuk *et al.*[142] found the treatment effective in reducing tumor size and prostate-specific antigen but without effect on lymphocyte 5-hydroxymethyl-deoxyuridine (determined by GC–MS).

4. Conclusions

DNA, lipid, and protein oxidation products provide an extensive, often practical, and growing array of potential biomarkers of oxidative stress. However, our understanding of the relationship between their status in the most readily accessible human matrices, i.e., blood cells, plasma, and urine, and the site of disease lesions remains to be elucidated. Current investigations are targeted to developing a broader panel of biomarkers that examine both pro- and antioxidant reactions including: the capacity of a biological sample to resist oxidation *in vitro* or *ex vivo*, modulation of redox-sensitive transcription factors or related alterations in signal transduction pathways, assessment of genomic factors relevant to antioxidant defenses and oxidative stress, and clinical assessments employing non-invasive technology such as magnetic resonance imaging. A balanced approach examining both the generation of reactive species (including their "footprint" biomarkers) and antioxidant defenses (including both enzymatic and non-enzymatic protection) may best describe the panel of assays necessary to examine the role of free radicals and antioxidants in biology and medicine. In practice, single elements from these facets of pro- and antioxidant reactions are often employed with the change in a single analyte incorrectly interpreted to characterize oxidative stress status. While much remains to be learned about the most effective ways to assess oxidative stress, human studies should no longer employ a "black box" approach, assessing antioxidant intake in a cohort or administering an antioxidant-rich food or supplement in a randomized clinical trial and then measuring clinical outcomes without determining any of the biological actions that were postulated to underlie the efficacy of the antioxidant.

References

1. Milbury P, Blumberg JB. Dietary antioxidants — human studies overview. In: Rodriguez H, Cutler RG (eds.) *Critical Reviews of Oxidative Stress and Aging: Advances in Basic Science, Diagnostics, and Intervention*. World Scientific Publishing Co., New Jersey, 2003, pp. 487–502.
2. Ohshima H, Pignatelli B, Li CQ, Baflast S, Gilibert I, Boffetta P. Analysis of oxidized and nitrated proteins in plasma and tissues as biomarkers for exposure to reactive oxygen and nitrogen species. *IARC Sci. Publ.* 156: 393–394 (2002).
3. Bartsch H. Studies on biomarkers in cancer etiology and prevention: a summary and challenge of 20 years of interdisciplinary research. *Mutat. Res.* 462: 255–279 (2000).
4. Taniyama Y, Griendling KK. Reactive oxygen species in the vasculature: molecular and cellular mechanisms. *Hypertension* 42: 1075–1081 (2003).
5. Inoue M, Sato EF, Nishikawa M, Park AM, Kira Y, Imada I, Utsumi K. Mitochondrial generation of reactive oxygen species and its role in aerobic life. *Curr. Med. Chem.* 10: 2495–2505 (2003).
6. Okada F. Inflammation and free radicals in tumor development and progression. *Redox Rep.* 7: 357–368 (2002).
7. Schisterman EF, Faraggi D, Browne R, Freudenheim J, Dorn J, Muti P, Armstrong D, Reiser B, Trevisan M. Minimal and best linear combination of oxidative stress and antioxidant biomarkers to discriminate cardiovascular disease. *Nutr. Metab. Cardiovasc. Dis.* 12: 259–266 (2002).

8. Institute of Medicine of the National Academies. *Dietary Reference Intakes for Vitamin C, Vitamin E, Selenium, and Carotenoids*. National Academies Press, Washington, DC, 2000.
9. Halliwell B. Antioxidant defense mechanisms: from the beginning to the end (of the beginning). *Free Radic. Res.* 31: 261–272 (1999).
10. Halliwell B, Whiteman M. Measuring reactive species and oxidative damage *in vivo* and in cell culture: how should you do it and what do the results mean? *Br. J. Pharmacol.* 142: 231–255 (2004).
11. Davies SS, Talati M, Wang X, Mernaugh RL, Amarnath V, Fessel J, Meyrick BO, Sheller J, Roberts LJ. Localization of isoketal adducts *in vivo* using a single-chain antibody. *Free Radic. Biol. Med.* 36: 1163–1174 (2004).
12. Abuja PM, Albertini R. Methods for monitoring oxidative stress, lipid peroxidation and oxidation resistance of lipoproteins. *Clin Chim Acta* 306: 1–17 (2001).
13. Yu TC, Sinnhuber RO. An improved 2-thiobarbituric acid (TBA) procedure for the measurement of autoxidation in fish oils. *J. Am. Oil. Chem. Soc.* 44: 256–258 (1967).
14. Gutteridge JM. Thiobarbituric acid-reactivity following iron-dependent free-radical damage to amino acids and carbohydrates. *FEBS Lett.* 128: 343–346 (1981).
15. Halliwell B, Gutteridge JM. Formation of thiobarbituric acid-reactive substance from deoxyribose in the presence of iron salts: the role of superoxide and hydroxyl radicals. *FEBS Lett.* 128: 347–352 (1981).
16. Agarwal R, Chase SD. Rapid fluorimetric-liquid chromatographic determination of malondialdehyde in biological samples. *J. Chromatogr. B* 775: 121–126 (2002).
17. Behrens WA, Madere R. Malondialdehyde determination in tissue and biological fluids by ion-paring high-performance liquid chromatography. *Lipids* 26: 232–236 (1991).
18. Morrow JD, Hill KE, Burk RF, Nammour TM, Badr KF, Roberts LJ II. A series of prostaglandin F2-like compounds are produced *in vivo* in humans by a non-cyclooxygenase, free radical-catalyzed mechanism. *Proc. Natl. Acad. Sci. USA* 87: 9383–9387 (1990).
19. Roberts LJ II, Morrow JD. The generation and actions of isoprostanes. *Biochim. Biophys. Acta.* 1345: 121–135 (1997).
20. Morrow JD, Roberts LJ II. Mass spectrometric quantification of F_2-isoprostanes in biological fluids and tissues as measure of oxidant stress. *Methods Enzymol.* 300: 3–12 (1999).

21. Griffiths HR, Moller L, Bartosz G, Bast A, Bertoni-Freddari C, Collins A, Cooke M, Coolen S, Haenen G, Hoberg AM, Loft S, Lunec J, Olinski R, Parry J, Pompella A, Poulsen H, Verhagen H, Astley SB. Biomarkers. *Mol. Aspects Med.* 23: 101–208 (2002).
22. Fam SS, Morrow JD. The isoprostanes: unique products of arachidonic acid oxidation — a review. *Curr. Med. Chem.* 10: 1723–1740 (2003).
23. Walter MF, Blumberg JB, Dolnikowski GG, Handelman GJ. Streamlined F2-isoprostane analysis in plasma and urine with high-performance liquid chromatography and gas chromatography/mass spectroscopy. *Anal. Biochem.* 280: 73–79 (2000).
24. Bachi A, Zuccato E, Baraldi M, Fanelli R, Chiabrando C. Measurement of urinary 8-Epi-prostaglandin F_{2alpha}, a novel index of lipid peroxidation *in vivo*, by immunoaffinity extraction/gas chromatography-mass spectrometry. Basal levels in smokers and non-smokers. *Free Radic. Biol. Med.* 20: 619–624 (1996).
25. Proudfoot J, Barden A, Mori TA, Burke V, Croft KD, Beilin LJ, Puddey IB. Measurement of urinary F(2)-isoprostanes as markers of *in vivo* lipid peroxidation-A comparison of enzyme immunoassay with gas chromatography/mass spectrometry. *Anal. Biochem.* 272: 209–215 (1999).
26. Liang Y, Wei P, Duke RW, Reaven PD, Harman SM, Cutler RG, Heward CB. Quantification of 8-iso-prostaglandin-F(2alpha) and 2,3-dinor-8-iso-prostaglandin-F(2alpha) in human urine using liquid chromatography-tandem mass spectrometry. *Free Radic. Biol. Med.* 34: 409–418 (2003).
27. Li H, Lawson JA, Reilly M, Adiyaman M, Hwang SW, Rokach J, FitzGerald GA. Quantitative high performance liquid chromatography/tandem mass spectrometric analysis of the four classes of F(2)-isoprostanes in human urine. *Proc. Natl. Acad. Sci. USA* 96: 13381–13386 (1999).
28. Hodgson JM, Watts GF, Playford DA, Burke V, Croft KD. Coenzyme Q10 improves blood pressure and glycemic control: a controlled trial in subjects with type 2 diabetes. *Eur. J. Clin. Nutr.* 56: 1137–1142 (2002).
29. Dietrich M, Block G, Hudes M, Morrow JD, Norkus EP, Traber MG, Cross CE, Packer L. Antioxidant supplementation decreases lipid peroxidation biomarker F(2)-isoprostanes in plasma of smokers. *Cancer Epidemiol. Biomarkers Prev.* 11: 7–13 (2002).
30. Berlett BS, Stadtman ER. Protein oxidation in aging, disease, and oxidative stress. *J. Biol. Chem.* 272: 20313–20316 (1997).
31. Dalle-Donne I, Giustarini D, Colombo R, Rossi R, Milzani A. Protein carbonylation in human diseases. *Trends Mol. Med.* 9: 169–176 (2003).

32. Beal MF. Oxidatively modified proteins in aging and disease. *Free Radic. Biol. Med.* 32: 797–803 (2002).
33. Levine RL, Garland D, Oliver CN, Amici A, Climent I, Lenz AG, Ahn BW, Shaltiel S, Stadtman ER. Determination of carbonyl content in oxidatively modified proteins. *Methods Enzymol.* 186: 464–478 (1990).
34. Reznick AZ, Packer L. Oxidative damage to proteins: spectrophotometric method for carbonyl assay. *Methods Enzymol.* 233: 357–363 (1994).
35. Buss H, Chan TP, Sluis KB, Domigan NM, Winterbourn CC. Protein carbonyl measurement by a sensitive ELISA method. *Free Radic. Biol. Med.* 23: 361–366 (1997).
36. Carty JL, Bevan R, Waller H, Mistry N, Cooke M, Lunec J, Griffiths HR. The effects of vitamin C supplementation on protein oxidation in healthy volunteers. *Biochem. Biophys. Res. Commun.* 273: 729–735 (2000).
37. Levine RL, Williams JA, Stadtman ER, Shacter E. Carbonyl assays for determination of oxidatively modified proteins. *Methods Enzymol.* 233: 346–357 (1994).
38. Cao G, Cutler RG. Protein oxidation and aging. I. Difficulties in measuring reactive protein carbonyls in tissues using 2,4-dinitrophenylhydrazine. *Arch. Biochem. Biophys.* 320: 106–114 (1995).
39. Lyras L, Evans PJ, Shaw PJ, Ince PG, Halliwell B. Oxidative damage and motor neurone disease difficulties in the measurement of protein carbonyls in human brain tissue. *Free Radic. Res.* 24: 397–406 (1996).
40. Levine RL, Wehr N, Williams JA, Stadtman ER, Shacter E. Determination of carbonyl groups in oxidized proteins. *Methods Mol. Biol.* 99: 15–24 (2000).
41. Levine R. Carbonyl modified proteins in cellular regulation, aging, and disease. *Free Radic. Biol. Med.* 32: 790–796 (2002).
42. Dean RT, Gieseg S, Davies MJ. Reactive species and their accumulation on radical-damaged proteins. *Trends Biochem. Sci.* 18: 437–441 (1993).
43. Davies MJ, Fu S, Wang H, Dean RT. Stable markers of oxidant damage to proteins and their application in the study of human disease. *Free Radic. Biol. Med.* 27: 1151–1163 (1999).
44. Winterbourn CC, Kettle AJ. Biomarkers of myeloperoxidase-derived hypochlorous acid. *Free Radic. Biol. Med.* 29: 403–409 (2000).
45. Crow JP, Ischiropoulos H. Detection and quantitation of nitrotyrosine residues in proteins: *in vivo* marker of peroxynitrite. *Methods Enzymol.* 269: 185–194 (1996).
46. Daneshvar B, Frandsen H, Dragsted LO, Knudsen LE, Autrup H. Analysis of native human plasma proteins and haemoglobin for the presence of bityrosine

by high-performance liquid chromatography. *Pharmacol. Toxicol.* 81: 205–208 (1997).

47. Leeuwenburgh C, Hansen PA, Holloszy JO, Heinecke JW. Hydroxyl radical generation during exercise increases mitochondrial protein oxidation and levels of urinary dityrosine. *Free Radic. Biol. Med.* 27: 186–192 (1999).
48. Ishida N, Hasegawa T, Mukai K, Watanabe M, Nishino H. Determination of nitrotyrosine by HPLC-ECD and its application. *J. Vet. Med. Sci.* 64: 401–404 (2002).
49. Crow JP. Measurement and significance of free and protein-bound 3-nitrotyrosine, 3-chlorotyrosine, and free 3-nitro-4-hydroxyphenylacetic acid in biologic samples: a high-performance liquid chromatography method using electrochemical detection. *Methods Enzymol.* 301: 151–160 (1999).
50. Heinecke JW, Hsu FF, Crowley JR, Hazen SL, Leeuwenburgh C, Mueller DM, Rasmussen JE, Turk J. Detecting oxidative modification of biomolecules with isotope dilution mass spectrometry: sensitive and quantitative assays for oxidized amino acids in proteins and tissues. *Methods Enzymol.* 300: 124–144 (1998).
51. Gaut JP, Byun J, Tran HD, Heinecke JW. Artifact-free quantification of free 3-chlorotyrosine, 3-bromotyrosine, and 3-nitrotyrosine in human plasma by electron capture-negative chemical ionization gas chromatography mass spectrometry and liquid chromatography–electrospray ionization tandem mass spectrometry. *Anal. Biochem.* 300: 252–259 (2002).
52. Hazen SL, Heinecke JW. 3-Chlorotyrosine, a specific marker of myeloperoxidase-catalyzed oxidation, is markedly elevated in low density lipoprotein isolated from human atherosclerotic intima. *J. Clin. Invest.* 99: 2075–2081 (1997).
53. Guetens G, Boeck GD, Highley M, van Oosterom AT, de Bruijn EA. Oxidative DNA damage: biological significance and methods of analysis. *Crit. Rev. Clin. Lab. Sci.* 39: 331–457 (2002).
54. Toyokuni S, Okamoto K, Yodoi J, Hiai H. Persistent oxidative stress in cancer. *FEBS Lett.* 358: 1–3 (1995).
55. Olinski R, Gackowski D, Rozalski R, Foksinski M, Bialkowski K. Oxidative DNA damage in cancer patients: a cause or a consequence of the disease development? *Mutat. Res.* 531: 177–190 (2003).
56. Foksinski M, Kotzbach R, Szymanski W, Olinski R. The level of typical biomarker of oxidative stress 8-hydroxy-2′-deoxyguanosine is higher in uterine myomas than in control tissues and correlates with the size of the tumor. *Free Radic. Biol. Med.* 29: 597–601 (2000).

57. Berger M, Anselmino C, Mouret JF. High performance liquid chromatography-electrochemical assay for monitoring the formation. *J. Liq. Chromatogr.* 13: 929–940 (1990).
58. Loft S, Poulsen HE. Markers of oxidative damage to DNA: antioxidants and molecular damage. *Methods Enzymol.* 300: 166–184 (1998).
59. Jaruga P, Speina E, Gackowski D, Tudek B, Olinski R. Endogenous oxidative DNA base modifications analyzed with repair enzymes and GC/MS technique. *Nucleic Acids Res.* 28: E16 (2000).
60. Hakim IA, Harris RB, Brown S, Chow HH, Wiseman S, Agarwal S, Talbot W. Effect of increased tea consumption on oxidative DNA damage among smokers: a randomized controlled study. *J. Nutr.* 133: 3303S–3309S (2003).
61. Cadet J, D'Ham C, Douki T, Pouget JP, Ravanat JL, Sauvaigo S. Facts and artifacts in the measurement of oxidative base damage to DNA. *Free Radic. Res.* 29: 541–550 (1998).
62. Nakajima M, Takeuchi T, Takeshita T, Morimoto K. 8-Hydroxydeoxyguanosine in human leukocyte DNA and daily health practice factors: effects of individual alcohol sensitivity. *Environ. Health Perspect.* 104: 1336–1338 (1996).
63. Degan P, Bonassi S, De Caterina M, Korkina LG, Pinto L, Scopacasa F, Zatterale A, Calzone R, Pagano G. *In vivo* accumulation of 8-hydroxy-2′-deoxyguanosine in DNA correlates with release of reactive oxygen species in Fanconi's anaemia families. *Carcinogenesis* 16: 735–741 (1995).
64. Lengger C, Schoch G, Topp H. A high-performance liquid chromatographic method for the determination of 8-oxo-7,8-dihydro-2′-deoxyguanosine in urine from man and rat. *Anal. Biochem.* 287: 65–72 (2000).
65. Dizdaroglu M. Chemical determination of oxidative DNA damage by GC–MS. *Methods Enzymol.* 234: 3–16 (1994).
66. Ravanat JL, Duretz B, Guiller A. Isotope dilution high performance liquid chromatography-electrospray tandem mass spectrometry assay. *J. Chromatogr. B* 715: 349–356 (1998).
67. Smith RD, Loo JA, Edmonds CG. New development in biochemical mass spectrometry: electrospray ionization. *Anal. Chem.* 62: 882–899 (1990).
68. Reddy DM, Iden CR. Analysis of modified deoxynucleosides by electrospray ionization mass spectrometry. *Nucleosides Nucleotides* 12: 815–826 (1993).
69. Dizdaroglu M, Jaruga P, Rodriguez H. Measurement of 8-hydroxy-2′-deoxyguanosine in DNA by high-performance liquid chromatography–mass spectrometry: comparison with measurement by gas chromatography-mass spectrometry. *Nucleic Acids Res.* 29: E12 (2001).

70. Dizdaroglu M, Jaruga P, Birincioglu M, Rodriguez H. Free radical-induced damage to DNA. *Free Radic. Biol. Med.* 32: 1102–1115 (2002).
71. Collins AR, Dusinska M, Gedik CM, Stetina R. Oxidative damage to DNA: do we have a reliable biomarker? *Environ. Health. Perspect.* 104(Suppl 3): 465–469 (1996).
72. Pflaum M, Will O, Epe B. Determination of steady-state levels of oxidative DNA base modifications in mammalian cells by means of repair endonucleases. *Carcinogenesis* 18: 2225–2231 (1997).
73. Podmore ID, Griffiths HR, Herbert KE, Mistry N, Mistry P, Lunec J. Vitamin C exhibits pro-oxidant properties. *Nature* 392: 559 (1998)
74. Weimann A, Belling D, Poulsen HE. Quantification of 8-oxo-guanine. *Nucleic Acids Res.* 30: E7 (2002).
75. Toyokuni S, Tanaka T, Hattori Y, Nishiyama Y, Yoshida A, Uchida K, Hiai H, Ochi H, Osawa T. Quantitative immunohistochemical determination of 8-hydroxy-2′-deoxyguanosine by a monoclonal antibody N45.1: its application to ferric nitrilotriacetate-induced renal carcinogenesis model. *Lab. Invest.* 76: 365–374 (1997).
76. Ahmad J, Cooke MS, Hussieni A, Evans MD, Patel K, Burd RM, Bleiker TO, Hutchinson PE, Lunec J. Urinary thymine dimers and 8-oxo-2′-deoxyguanosine in psoriasis. *FEBS Lett.* 460: 549–553 (1999).
77. Cooke MS, Evans MD, Podmore ID, Herbert KE, Mistry N, Mistry P, Hickenbotham PT, Hussieni A, Griffiths HR, Lunec J. Novel repair action of vitamin C upon *in vivo* oxidative DNA damage. *FEBS Lett.* 439: 363–367 (1998).
78. Lovell DP, Thomas G, Dubow R. Issues related to the experimental design and subsequent statistical analysis of *in vivo* and *in vitro* comet studies. *Teratog. Carcinog. Mutagen* 19: 109–119 (1999).
79. Collins AR. Measurement of oxidative DNA damage using the comet assay. In: Griffiths HR, Lunec J. (eds.). *Measuring In Vivo Oxidative Damage: A Practical Approach*. Wiley, New York, 2000, pp. 83–94.
80. Collins AR, Ma AG, Duthie SJ. The kinetics of repair of oxidative DNA damage (strand breaks and oxidized pyrimidines) in human cells. *Mutat. Res.* 336: 69–77 (1995).
81. Singh NP, McCoy MT, Tice RR, Schneider EL. A simple technique for quantitation of low levels of DNA damage in individual cells. *Exp. Cell Res.* 175: 184–191 (1988).
82. Olive PL, Banath JP, Durand RE. Heterogeneity in radiation-induced DNA damage and repair in tumor and normal cells measured using the "comet" assay. *Radiat. Res.* 122: 86–94 (1990).

83. Rojas E, Lopez MC, Valverde M. Single cell gel electrophoresis assay: methodology and applications. *J. Chromatogr. B* 722: 225–254 (1999).
84. Fairbairn DW, Olive PL, O'Neill KL. The comet assay: a comprehensive review. *Mutat. Res.* 339: 37–59 (1995).
85. Sampson MJ, Astley S, Richardson T, Willis G, Davies IR, Hughes DA, Southon S. Increased DNA oxidative susceptibility without increased plasma LDL oxidizability in type II diabetes: effects of alpha-tocopherol supplementation. *Clin. Sci.* 101: 235–241 (2001).
86. Meagher E, Rader DJ. Antioxidant therapy and atherosclerosis: animal and human studies. *Trends Cardiovasc. Med.* 11: 162–165 (2001).
87. Willcox JK, Ash SL, Catignani GL. Antioxidants and prevention of chronic disease. *Crit. Rev. Food Sci. Nutr.* 44: 275–295 (2004).
88. Hanninen A, Jalkanen S, Salmi M, Toikkanen S, Nikolakaros G, Simell O. Macrophages, T cell receptor usage, and endothelial cell activation in the pancreas at the onset of insulin-dependent diabetes mellitus. *J. Clin. Invest.* 90: 1901–1910 (1992).
89. Freiesleben De Blasio B, Bak P, Pociot F, Karlsen AE, Nerup J. Onset of type 1 diabetes: a dynamical instability. *Diabetes* 48: 1677–1685 (1999).
90. Davi G, Chiarelli F, Santilli F, Pomilio M, Vigneri S, Falco A, Basili S, Ciabattoni G, Patrono C. Enhanced lipid peroxidation and platelet activation in the early phase of type 1 diabetes mellitus: role of interleukin-6 and disease duration. *Circulation* 107: 3199–3203 (2003).
91. Handelman GJ, Walter MF, Adhikarla R, Gross J, Levin NW, Blumberg JB. Elevated plasma F_2 isoprostanes in patients on long-term hemodialysis. *Kidney Int.* 59: 1960–1966 (2001).
92. Diaz-Velez CR, Garcia-Castineiras S, Mendoza-Ramos E, Hernandez-Lopez E. Increased malondialdehyde in peripheral blood of patients with congestive heart failure. *Am. Heart J.* 131: 146–152 (1996).
93. Kumar D, Jugdutt BI. Apoptosis and oxidants in the heart. *J. Lab. Clin. Med.* 142: 288–297 (2003).
94. Mallat Z, Philip I, Lebret M, Chatel D, Maclouf J, Tedgui A. Elevated levels of 8-iso-prostaglandin F_{2alpha} in pericardial fluid of patients with heart failure: a potential role for *in vivo* oxidant stress in ventricular dilatation and progression to heart failure. *Circulation* 97: 1536–1539 (1998).
95. Jain SK, Pemberton PW, Smith A, McMahon RF, Burrows PC, Aboutwerat A, Warnes TW. Oxidative stress in chronic hepatitis C: not just a feature of late stage disease. *J. Hepatol.* 36: 805–811 (2002).

96. Hulgan T, Morrow J, D'Aquila RT, Raffanti S, Morgan M, Rebeiro P, Haas DW. Oxidant stress is increased during treatment of human immunodeficiency virus infection. *Clin. Infect. Dis.* 37: 1711–1717 (2003).
97. Carpenter KL, Taylor SE, van-der-Veen C, Williamson BK, Ballantine JA, Mitchinson MJ. Lipids and oxidized lipids in human atherosclerotic lesions at different stages of development. *Biochim. Biophys. Acta.* 1256: 141–150 (1995).
98. Mallat Z, Nakamura T, Chan J, Leséche G, Tedgui A, Maclouf J, Murphy RC. The relationship of hydroxyeicosatetraenoic acids and F_2-isoprostanes to plaque instability in human carotid atherosclerosis. *J. Clin. Invest.* 103: 421–427 (1999).
99. Gniwotta C, Morrow JD, Roberts LJ II, Kuhn H. Prostaglandin F_2-like compounds, F_2-isoprostanes, are present in increased amounts in human atherosclerotic lesions. *Arterioscler. Thromb. Vasc. Biol.* 17: 3236–3241 (1997).
100. Waddington EI, Croft KD, Sienuarine K, Latham B, Puddey IB. Fatty acid oxidation products in human atherosclerotic plaque: an analysis of clinical and histopathological correlates. *Atherosclerosis* 167: 111–120 (2003).
101. Montine TJ, Beal MF, Cudkowicz ME, O'Donnell H, Margolin RA, McFarland L, Bachrach AF, Zackert WE, Roberts LJ, Morrow JD. Increased CSF F_2-isoprostane concentration in probable AD. *Neurology* 52: 562–565 (1999).
102. Montine TJ, Kaye JA, Montine KS, McFarland L, Morrow JD, Quinn JF. Cerebrospinal fluid abeta42, tau, and f_2-isoprostane concentrations in patients with Alzheimer disease, other dementias, and in age-matched controls. *Arch. Pathol. Lab. Med.* 125: 510–512 (2001).
103. Montine TJ, Quinn JF, Milatovic D, Silbert LC, Dang T, Sanchez S, Terry E, Roberts LJ II, Kaye JA, Morrow JD. Peripheral F_2-isoprostanes and F_4-neuroprostanes are not increased in Alzheimer's disease. *Ann Neurol.* 52: 175–179 (2002).
104. Upston JM, Niu X, Brown AJ, Mashima R, Wang H, Senthilmohan R, Kettle AJ, Dean RT, Stocker R. Disease stage-dependent accumulation of lipid and protein oxidation products in human atherosclerosis. *Am. J. Pathol.* 160: 701–710 (2002).
105. Podrez EA, Schmitt D, Hoff HF, Hazen SL. Myeloperoxidase-generated reactive nitrogen species convert LDL into an atherogenic form *in vitro*. *J. Clin. Invest.* 103: 1547–1560 (1999).

106. Rubbo H, Radi R, Anselmi D, Kirk M, Barnes S, Butler J, Eiserich JP, Freeman BA. Nitric oxide reaction with lipid peroxyl radicals spares alpha-tocopherol during lipid peroxidation. Greater oxidant protection from the pair nitric oxide/alpha-tocopherol than alpha-tocopherol/ascorbate. *J. Biol. Chem.* 275: 10812–10818 (2000).
107. Heinecke JW. Is the emperor wearing clothes? Clinical trials of vitamin E and the LDL oxidation hypothesis. *Arterioscler. Thromb. Vasc. Biol.* 21: 1261–1264 (2001).
108. Diaz MN, Frei B, Vita JA, Keaney JF Jr. Antioxidants and atherosclerotic heart disease. *N. Engl. J. Med.* 337: 408–416 (1997).
109. Witztum JL, Steinberg D. The oxidative modification hypothesis of atherosclerosis: does it hold for humans? *Trends Cardiovasc. Med.* 11: 93–102 (2001).
110. Podrez EA, Abu-Soud HM, Hazen SL. Myeloperoxidase-generated oxidants and atherosclerosis. *Free Radic. Biol. Med.* 28: 1717–1725 (2000).
111. Kutter D, Devaquet P, Vanderstocken G, Paulus JM, Marchal V, Gothot A. Consequences of total and subtotal myeloperoxidase deficiency: risk or benefit ? *Acta Haematol.* 104: 10–15 (2000).
112. Shishehbor MH, Aviles RJ, Brennan ML, Fu X, Goormastic M, Pearce GL, Gokce N, Shishehbor MH, Brennan ML, Aviles RJ, Fu X, Penn MS, Sprecher DL, Hazen SL. Statins promote potent systemic antioxidant effects through specific inflammatory pathways. *Circulation* 108: 426–431 (2003).
113. Gryglewski RJ, Palmer RMJ, Moncada S. Superoxide anion is involved in the breakdown of endothelium-derived vascular relaxing factor. *Nature* 320: 454–456 (1986).
114. Frustaci A, Kajstura J, Chimenti C, Jakoniuk I, Leri A, Maseri A, Nadal-Ginard B, Anversa P. Myocardial cell death in human diabetes. *Circ. Res.* 87: 1123–1132 (2000).
115. Ceriello A, Taboga C, Tonutti L, Quagliaro L, Piconi L, Bais B, Da Ros R, Motz E. Evidence for an independent and cumulative effect of postprandial hypertriglyceridemia and hyperglycemia on endothelial dysfunction and oxidative stress generation: effects of short- and long-term simvastatin treatment. *Circulation* 106: 1211–1218 (2002).
116. Kinlay S, Behrendt D, Fang JC, Delagrange D, Morrow J, Witztum JL, Rifai N, Selwyn AP, Creager MA, Ganz P. Long-term effect of combined vitamins E and C on coronary and peripheral endothelial function. *J. Am. Coll. Cardiol.* 43: 629–634 (2004).

117. Cheng KC, Cahill DS, Kasai H, Nishimura S, Loeb LA. 8-Hydroxyguanine, an abundant form of oxidative DNA damage, causes G–T and A–C substitutions. *J. Biol. Chem.* 267: 166–172 (1992).
118. Halliwell B. Effect of diet on cancer development: is oxidative DNA damage a biomarker? *Free Radic. Biol. Med.* 32: 968–974 (2002).
119. Sacheck JM, Blumberg JB. The role of vitamin E and oxidative stress in exercise. *Nutrition* 17: 809–814 (2001).
120. Friedenreich CM, Orenstein MR. Physical activity and cancer prevention: etiologic evidence and biological mechanisms. *J. Nutr.* 132: 3456S–3464S (2002).
121. Loft S, Astrup A, Buemann B, Poulsen HE. Oxidative DNA damage correlates with oxygen consumption in humans. *FASEB J.* 8: 534–537 (1994).
122. Camus G, Deby-Dupont G, Duchateau J, Deby C, Pincemail J, Lamy M. Are similar inflammatory factors involved in strenuous exercise and sepsis? *Intensive Care Med.* 20: 602–610 (1994).
123. Lodovici M, Casalini C, Cariaggi R, Michelucci L, Dolara P. Levels of 8-hydroxydeoxyguanosine as a marker of DNA damage in human leukocytes. *Free Radic. Biol. Med.* 28: 13–17 (2000).
124. Tsai K, Hsu TG, Hsu KM, Cheng H, Liu TY, Hsu CF, Kong CW. Oxidative DNA damage in human peripheral leukocytes induced by massive aerobic exercise. *Free Radic. Biol. Med.* 31: 1465–1472 (2001).
125. Sato Y, Nanri H, Ohta M, Kasai H, Ikeda M. Increase of human MTH1 and decrease of 8-hydroxydeoxyguanosine in leukocyte DNA by acute and chronic exercise in healthy male subjects. *Biochem. Biophys. Res. Commun.* 305: 333–338 (2003).
126. Asami S, Hirano T, Yamaguchi R, Itoh H, Kasai H. Reduction of 8-hydroxyguanine in human leukocyte DNA by physical exercise. *Free Radic. Res.* 29: 581–584 (1998).
127. Sumida S, Okamura K, Doi T, Sakurai M, Yoshioka Y, Sugawa-Katayama Y. No influence of a single bout of exercise on urinary excretion of 8-hydroxy-deoxyguanosine in humans. *Biochem. Mol. Biol. Int.* 42: 601–609 (1997).
128. Sacheck JM, Milbury PE, Cannon JG, Roubenoff R, Blumberg JB. Effect of vitamin E and eccentric exercise on selected biomarkers of oxidative stress in young and elderly men. *Free Radic. Biol. Med.* 34: 1575–1588 (2003).
129. Okamura K, Doi T, Hamada K, Sakurai M, Yoshioka Y, Mitsuzono R, Migita T, Sumida S, Sugawa-Katayama Y. Effect of repeated exercise on urinary 8-hydroxy-deoxyguanosine excretion in humans. *Free Radic. Res.* 26: 507–514 (1997).

130. Radák Z, Pucsuk J, Boros S, Josfai L, Taylor AW. Changes in urine 8-hydroxydeoxyguanosine levels of super-marathon runners during a four-day race period. *Life Sci.* 66: 1763–1767 (2000).
131. Almar M, Villa JG, Cuevas MJ, Rodriguez-Marroyo JA, Avila C, Gonzalez-Gallego J. Urinary levels of 8-hydroxydeoxyguanosine as a marker of oxidative damage in road cycling. *Free Radic. Res.* 36: 247–253 (2002).
132. Hartmann A, Pfuhler S, Dennog C, Germadnik D, Pilger A, Speit G. Exercise-induced DNA effects in human leukocytes are not accompanied by increased formation of 8-hydroxy-2′-deoxyguanosine or induction of micronuclei. *Free Radic. Biol. Med.* 24: 245–251 (1998).
133. Radák Z, Pucsok J, Mecseki S, Csont T, Ferdinandy P. Muscle soreness-induced reduction in force generation is accompanied by increased nitric oxide content and DNA damage in human skeletal muscle. *Free Radic. Biol. Med.* 26: 1059–1063 (1999).
134. Radák Z, Apor P, Pucsok J, Berkes I, Ogonovszky H, Pavlik G, Nakamoto H, Goto S. Marathon running alters the DNA base excision repair in human skeletal muscle. *Life Sci.* 72: 1627–1633 (2003).
135. WCRF/AICR. *Food, Nutrition and the Prevention of Cancer: A Global Perspective.* WCRF/AICR, Washington, DC, 1997.
136. Joshipura KJ, Hu FB, Manson JE, Stampfer MJ, Rimm EB, Speizer FE, Colditz G, Ascherio A, Rosner B, Spiegelman D, Willett WC. The effect of fruit and vegetable intake on risk for coronary heart disease. *Ann. Intern. Med.* 134: 1106–1114 (2001).
137. Collins AR, Harrington V, Drew J, Melvin R. Nutritional modulation of DNA repair in a human intervention study. *Carcinogenesis* 24: 511–515 (2003).
138. Moller P, Vogel U, Pedersen A, Dragsted LO, Sandstrom B, Loft S. No effect of 600 grams fruit and vegetables per day on oxidative DNA damage and repair in healthy non-smokers. *Cancer Epidemiol. Biomarkers Prev.* 12: 1016–1022 (2003).
139. Riso P, Pinder A, Santangelo A, Porrini M. Does tomato consumption effectively increase the resistance of lymphocyte DNA to oxidative damage? *Am. J. Clin. Nutr.* 69: 712–718 (1999).
140. Astley SB, Hughes DA, Wright AJ, Elliott RM, Southn S. DNA damage and susceptibility to oxidative damage in lymphocytes: effects of carotenoids *in vitro* and *in vivo*. *Br. J. Nutr.* 91: 53–61 (2004).
141. Arab L, Steck-Scott S, Fleishauer AT. Lycopene and the lung. *Exp. Biol. Med.* 227: 894–899 (2002).
142. Kucuk O, Sarkar FH, Djuric Z, Sakr W, Pollak MN, Khachik F, Banerjee M, Bertram JS, Wood DP Jr. Effects of lycopene supplementation in patients with localized prostate cancer. *Exp. Biol. Med.* 227: 881–885 (2002).

Index